Litt's

DRUG
ERUPTION
REFERENCE MANUAL
INCLUDING DRUG INTERACTIONS
with CD-ROM

10th EDITION

Litt's DRUG ERUPTION REFERENCE MANUAL

INCLUDING DRUG INTERACTIONS

with CD-ROM

10th EDITION

Jerome Z. Litt, MD

Assistant Clinical Professor of Dermatology
Case Western Reserve University School of Medicine
Cleveland, Ohio, USA

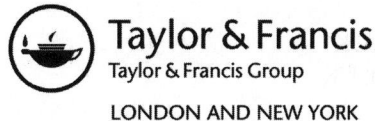

Taylor & Francis
Taylor & Francis Group

LONDON AND NEW YORK

A PARTHENON BOOK

©2004 Taylor & Francis an imprint of the Taylor & Francis Group

First published in the United Kingdom in 2004
by Taylor & Francis,
an imprint of the Taylor & Francis Group,
11 New Fetter Lane,
London EC4P 4EE

Tel.:   +44 (0) 20 7583 9855
Fax.:   +44 (0) 20 7842 2298
Website: www.tandf.co.uk

Although every effort has been made to ensure that all owners of copyright material have been acknowledged in this publication, we would be glad to acknowledge in subsequent reprints or editions any omissions brought to our attention.

Library of Congress Cataloging-in-Publication Data

British Library Cataloguing in Publication Data

Data available on application

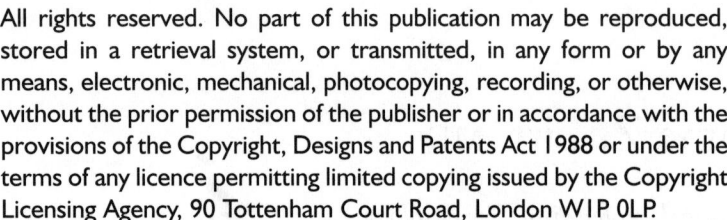

ISBN: 1-84214-250-X

Typeset by AMA DataSet Limited, Preston, UK
Printed and bound by The Bath Press, Bath, UK

CONTENTS

To Vel – my Muse

Introduction

Any drug can cause any rash.

According to the World Health Organization, an adverse reaction (ADR) – or and adverse event (ADE) – to a drug has been defined as any noxious or unintended reaction to a drug that has been administered in standard doses by the proper route for the purposes of prophylaxis, diagnosis, or treatment. This definition does not include abuse, overdose, withdrawal, or error of administration. It appears that most ADRs are related to the dose. Death is the ultimate adverse drug event, and has now been incorporated into the manual.

ADRs are underreported and thus are an underestimated cause of morbidity and mortality. The incidence and severity of ADRs can be influenced by age, sex, disease, genetic factors, type of drug, route of administration, duration of therapy, dosage, and bioavailability, as well as interactions with other drugs. It has been estimated that fatal ADRs are the third or fourth leading cause of death in the US.

Adverse drug reactions have been arbitrarily classified into six types:

1. Dose-related (e.g. Digoxin toxicity)
2. Non-dose-related (e.g. Immunological reactions)
3. Dose-related and Time-related (e.g. Corticosteroids)
4. Time-related (e.g. Tardive dyskinesia)
5. Withdrawal (e.g. Opiate or beta-blocker withdrawal)
6. Unexpected failure of therapy (e.g. Inadequate dosage of an oral contraceptive)

Cutaneous drug eruptions can mimic almost any inflammatory dermatosis. While most eruptions are mild and self-limited, severe and life-threatening eruptions do occur, as seen in Stevens–Johnson syndrome and Toxic epidermal necrolysis.

More and more people – primarily the older population – are taking more and more prescription and over-the-counter medications. New drugs are appearing in the medical marketplace on an almost daily basis. More and more drug reaction – in the form of cutaneous eruptions – are developing from all drugs. It has been reported that more than 100,000 hospitalized people in the United States alone died in 1999 as a result of medications.

Dermatologists and general physicians are often perplexed by the nature of some of these problems. The few sources that are available to identify the causes of many of these side effects cannot be accessed by proprietary (trade, brand) names.

This Manual is a Drug Eruption Reference guide that describes and catalogues the adverse cutaneous side effects of more than **950** commonly prescribed and over-the-counter generic drugs. The drugs have been listed and indexed by both their **Generic** and **Trade** (**Brand**) names for easy accessibility.

Some of the additional, newer generic drugs in the past year that have been catalogued for this latest edition include (the **Trade/Brand** name drugs are in bold):

Adefovir (**Hepsera**), Alefacept (**Amevive**), Anakinra (**Kineret**), Aprepitant (**Emend**), Bortezomid (**Velcade**), Drotrecogin alfa (**Xigris**), Dutasteride (**Avodart**), Enfuvirtide (**Fuzeon**), Eplerenone (**Inspra**), Escitalopram (**Lexapro**), Ezetimbe (**Zetia**), Fomepizole (**Antizol**), Gemifloxacin (**Factive**), Gefitinib (**Iressa**), Glatiramer (**Copaxone**), Interferon beta-1B (**Betaseron**), Mecamylamine (**Inversine**), Nitazoxanide (**Alinia**), Nitisinone (**Orfadin**), Paricalcitol (**Zemplar**), Pegvisomant (**Somavert**), Rasburicase (**Elitek**), Sermorelin (**Geref**), Tegaserod (**Zelnorm**), Teriparatide (**Forteo**), Urofollitropin, and Valrubicin (**Valstar**). The number of herbals and supplements has also increased, and vaccines have been added.

In addition to adverse cutaneous reactions, there are many severe, hazardous interactions between two or more drugs. Unlike the voluminous interaction details in previous editions of the Manual, some of which were either moderate or mild, I have incorporated only the highly, clinically significant drug interactions that can trigger potential harm, and could be life-threatening. These interactions are predictable and well documented in controlled studies; they should be avoided. This section denoting hazardous interactions has been omitted from those drugs where no such interactions have been reported.

Since the last edition, many generic drugs have been withdrawn from the marketplace and, therefore, have been deleted from this edition.

For each drug, I have listed all the known adverse side effects – in the form of drug reactions – that can develop from the use of the corresponding drug. These side effects include those that primarily involve the skin, the hair, the nails and the mucous membranes. The section entitled 'other' has been expanded to include such reactions as rhabdomyolysis, depression, and dysgeusia.

Appropriate references (author, journal or book, volume, date and page) for each side effect for every drug have been cited. Where there is more than one reference to a particular side effect, I have employed the most illustrative and most recent citation(s) in the literature.

In this new, 2004 state-of-the-art tenth edition, I have cited more than **25,000** references and sources from journals articles, books and observations from dermatologists all over the world via the Internet and from personal communications.

The first part of the Manual lists, in alphabetical order, all the listed **950+ Generic** and **Trade** drugs with their corresponding names for easy access to the **A-Z** section – main body of the Manual.

Next comes a listing of the various **Classes** of drugs, and those **Generic** drugs that belong to each class.

The major portion of the Manual – the body of the work – lists the **950+ Generic** drugs, herbals and supplements in alphabetical order and the adverse reactions that can arise from their use along with the appropriate references.

The last parts of the Manual include a description of the **31** most common **Reaction Patterns**; a listing of those drugs that can occasion more than **100** different reaction patterns, including, among others, **Acne, Acute generalized exanthematous pustulosis, Alopecia, Aphthous stomatitis, Bullous eruptions, Bullous pemphigoid, Erythema multiforme, Erythema nodosum, Exanthems, Exfoliative dermatitis, Fixed eruptions, Lichenoid eruptions, Lupus erythematosus, Onycholysis, Pemphigus, Photosensitivity, Pityriasis rosea, Pruritus, Psoriasis, Purpura, Pustular eruptions, Stevens-Johnson syndrome, Toxic epidermal necrolysis, Urticaria,** and **Vasculitis.** This is followed by color photographs of some of these reactions.

USAGE, STYLE & CONVENTIONS EMPLOYED IN THIS MANUAL

The **Generic Drug** name is at the top of each page.

The **Trade (Brand) Name(s)** are then listed alphabetically. When there are many **Trade Names**, the ten (or so) most commonly recognized ones are listed. This compilation lists and cross-references both the **Trade** *and* **Generic** names of all the cataloged drugs. Following the more common **Trade Name** drugs are recorded – in parentheses – the latest name of the pharmaceutical company that is marketing the drug. As a result of acquisitions, mergers, and other factors in the pharmaceutical industry, many of the names of the companies have changed from earlier editions of this Manual.

Beneath the **Trade Name** listing is a list of **Other Common Trade Names**, those drugs from other countries. Then appears the **Indication(s),** the **Category** in which the drug belongs, and the **Half-Life** of each drug, when known. On occasion, an important or pertinent **Note** will follow.

Reactions: These are the **Adverse Reactions** to the particular **Generic** drug. They are classified in four **Categories: Skin, Hair, Nails,** and **Other. (Other** refers to **Mucous Membrane, Teeth, Muscle** and various other forms of **Reactions.) Reactions** are listed alphabetically in each **Category.**

Under each **Reaction Pattern** are listed the **References** (the sources of the information). These are arranged in reverse chronological order – the most recent reference appearing first on the list.

References in the English language predominate. For the few foreign references, we have resorted to the summary or abstract. The majority of the citations come from the *J Am Acad Dermatol, Arch Dermatol, Cutis, Int J Dermatol, Contact Dermatitis, Br J Dermatol, JAMA, Lancet, BMJ, Aust J Dermatol, N Engl J Med, Ann Intern Med,* and other prominent and easily accessible journals.

Many reference works have been consulted in the course of compiling this manual. These include:

(2002): Stockley IH, *STOCKLEY'S DRUG INTERACTIONS,* Pharmaceutical Press, London and Chicago

(1998): Kauppinen K et al, *SKIN REACTIONS TO DRUGS,* CRC Press, Boca Raton

(1996): Bruinsma W, *A GUIDE TO DRUG ERUPTIONS,* The File of Medicines, PO Box 21, 1474 HJ Oosthuizen, Netherlands.

(1994): Goldstein S & Wintroub BU, *ADVERSE CUTANEOUS REACTIONS TO MEDICATION,* CoMedica, New York.

(1992): Zürcher K & Krebs A, *CUTANEOUS DRUG REACTIONS,* Karger, Basel.

(1992): Breathnach SM & Hintner H, *ADVERSE DRUG REACTIONS and the SKIN,* Blackwell, Oxford.

(1988): Bork K, *CUTANEOUS SIDE EFFECTS OF DRUGS,* WB Saunders, Philadelphia.

Other references, based on package inserts, have been obtained from:

(2003): *LEXI-COMP'S CLINICAL REFERENCE LIBRARY,* Hudson, Ohio

(2003): *DRUG FACTS & COMPARISONS,* St. Louis, Missouri.

(2003): *PDR GENERICS,* Montvale, New Jersey.

There are occasions when there are very few adverse reactions to a specific drug. These drugs are still included in the Manual since there is often a **positive significance in negative findings.**

As a departure from the official, conventional and established style guide, and as a function of space constraints, the order of each **Reference** will appear as follows:

• The year in parentheses. The most recent citation appearing first.

• Last name and initial(s) of the principal author.

• A plus sign (+) after the author's name denotes one or more co-authors.

• Journal name (standard abbreviation where possible), in *italics.*

- Volume Number (often followed by a parenthetical Part or Supplemental Number).

- First page of the article

- Books when cited are italicised, followed by the publisher and page number.

  Other notes:

- (sic) means **just so.** This is how the authors designated the **REACTION.**

- For example, **Rash** (sic); **Dermatitis** (sic); **Skin Rash** (sic)*

- I have used the term **passim** to mean ;**in passing.**' Forgive me.

There are occasional allusions to the incidence of many of the listed **Reactions**. Percentages – which for the most part are essentially vague and meaningless – are obtained from articles, from Zürcher & Krebs, and from Bork.

I have simplified the references to the many **Reaction Patterns** by eliminating, for the most part, tags such as '-like' as in **Psoriasis-Like**, '-reactivation,' '-syndrome,' '-dissemination,' '-iform,' etc.

'**Observation**' means just that. **Observations** (read: **Anecdotes**) are derived from information obtained from reliable dermatologists from the Internet and from personal correspondence. And if you send me your observations, they will be cataloged and you will be given appropriate attribution and recognition in the next Edition.

Enjoy!

Jerome Z. Litt, M.D.
January, 2004

* The term **Skin Rash** is a deplorable and reprehensible idiotism adored by non-dermatologists and the writers of the PDR (read Package Inserts). Can you have a **Rash** on any other organ?

INDEX OF GENERIC AND TRADE NAMES

Generic drug names are in **bold**

MabCampath	**alemtuzumab**	mesna	Mesnex
Macrobid	**nitrofurantoin**	Mesnex	**mesna**
Macrodantin	**nitrofurantoin**	mesoridazine	Serentil
mafenide	Sulfamylon	Metadate CD	**methylphenidate**
Maigret-50	**phenylpropanolamine**	Metaglip	**glipizide, metformin**
Malarone	**atovaquone**	Metahydrin	**trichlormethiazide**
Mandelamine	**methenamine**	Metandren	**methyltestosterone**
Mandol	**cefamandole**	metaxalone	Skelaxin
Mapap	**acetaminophen**	metformin	Avandamet, Glucophage, Glucovance, Metaglip
maprotiline	Ludiomil	methadone	Dolophine
Marax	**ephedrine, hydroxyzine**	methamphetamine	Desoxyn
Marazide	**benzthiazide**	methantheline	Banthine
Marcillin	**ampicillin**	Methazolamide	**methazolamide**
Marihuana	**marihuana**	methenamine	Hiprex, Mandelamine, Prosed, Urised, Uroqid
Marinol	**dronabinol**	methicillin	Staphcillin
Marmine	**dimenhydrinate**	methimazole	Tapazole
Marplan	**isocarboxazid**	methocarbamol	Robaxin
Matulane	**procarbazine**	methohexital	Brevital
Mavik	**trandolapril**	methotrexate	Rheumatrex
Maxair	**pirbuterol**	methoxsalen	8-MOP, Oxsoralen
Maxalt	**rizatriptan**	methoxyflurane	Penthrane
Maxaquin	**lomefloxacin**	methsuximide	Celontin
Maxidex	**corticosteroids**	methyclothiazide	Aquatensen, Enduronyl
Maxidone	**hydrocodone**	methyldopa	Aldoclor, Aldomet, Aldoril
Maxipime	**cefepime**	Methylin	**methylphenidate**
Maxitrol	**corticosteroids, neomycin**	methylphenidate	Concerta, Metadate CD, Methylin, Ritalin
Maxzide	**hydrochlorothiazide, triamterene**	methyltestosterone	Android, Estratest, Metandren, Oreton, Testred, Virilon
Mazanor	**mazindol**		
mazindol	Mazanor, Sanorex	methysergide	Sansert
MDMA	Ecstacy	Meticorten	**corticosteroids**
Measurin	**aspirin**	metoclopramide	Reglan
Mebaral	**mephobarbital**	metolazone	Mykrox, Zaroxolyn
mebendazole	Vermox	metoprolol	Lopressor, Toprol XL
mecamylamine	Inversine	Metrocream	**metronidazole**
mechlorethamine	Mustargen	Metrodin	**urofollitropin**
meclizine	Antivert	Metrogel	**metronidazole**
Meclofenamate	**meclofenamate**	Metrolotion	**metronidazole**
Medihaler-ISO	**isoproterenol**	**metronidazole**	Flagyl, Helidac, Metrocream, Metrogel, Metrolotion, Noritate, Protostat, Satric
MedihalerEpi	**epinephrine**		
Medilax	**phenolphthalein**	Mevacor	**lovastatin**
Medipren	**ibuprofen**	mexiletine	Mexitil
Medispaz	**hyoscyamine**	Mexitil	**mexiletine**
Medrol	**corticosteroids**	Mezlin	**mezlocillin, penicillins**
medroxyprogesterone	Amen, Cycrin, Depo-Provera, Lunelle, Premphase, Prempro, Provera	**mezlocillin**	Mezlin
		Miacalcin	**calcitonin**
mefenamic acid	Ponstel	Micardis	**hydrochlorothiazide, telmisartan**
mefloquine	Lariam	miconazole	Lotrimin, Monistat
Mefoxin	**cefoxitin**	Micronase	**glyburide**
Megace	**progestins**	Micronor	**progestins**
Megacillin	**penicillins**	Microsulfon	**sulfadiazine**
Mellaril	**thioridazine**	Microzide	**hydrochlorothiazide**
meloxicam	Mobic	Midamor	**amiloride**
melphalan	Alkeran	**midazolam**	Versed
Menest	**estrogens**	midodrine	Proamatine
Mepergan	**meperidine**	Midol 220	**ibuprofen**
meperidine	Demerol, Mepergan	Mifeprex	**mifepristone**
mephenytoin	Mesantoin	**mifepristone**	Mifeprex
mephobarbital	Mebaral	miglitol	Glyset
Mephyton	**phytonadione**	Migranal	**dihydroergotamine**
meprobamate	Equagesic, Miltown	Milontin	**phensuximide**
Mepron	**atovaquone**	Miltown	**meprobamate**
mercaptopurine	Purinethol	Minipress	**prazosin**
Meridia	**sibutramine**	Minitran	**nitroglycerin**
Mersol	**thimerosal**	Minizide	**polythiazide, prazosin**
Merthiolate	**thimerosal**	Minocin	**minocycline**
mesalamine	Asacol, Canasa, Pentasa, Rowasa	**minocycline**	Arestin, Dynacin, Minocin
Mesantoin	**mephenytoin**	Minoxidil	**minoxidil**

INDEX OF HERBALS

Herbal drug names are in **bold**

CLASSES OF DRUGS

ACE inhibitors
benazepril
candesartan*
captopril
enalapril
eprosartan*
fosinopril
irbesartan*
lisinopril
losartan*
moexipril
olmesartan
perindopril
quinapril
ramipril
spirapril
telmisartan*
trandolapril
valsartan*
*Angiotenin II receptor antagonist

Alpha adrenergic receptor inhibitors
brimonidine
doxazosin
phenoxybenzamine
phentolamine
prazosin
tamsulosin
terazosin

Alpha adrenoreceptor agonists
apraclonide
clonidine
guanabenz
guanethidine
guanfacine
tizanidine

Aminoglycoside antibiotics
amikacin
gentamicin
kanamycin
neomycin
paromomycin
streptomycin
tobramycin

Amphetamines
amphetamine sulfate
dextroamphetamine
diethylpropion
mazindol
methamphetamine
methylphenidate
phendimetrazine
phentermine

Antiarrhythmic agents and class
acebutolol
adenosine
amiodarone III
atropine
belladonna
beta-blockers II
bretylium III
chlorothiazide
digoxin
diltiazem IV
disopyramide IV
dofetilide III
edrophonium
esmolol II
flecainide IC
ibutilide III
indecainide IC
isoproterenol
lidocaine IB
magnesium sulfate
metoprolol
mexiletine IB
minoxidil
moricizine IA
phenytoin IB
procainamide IA
propafenone IC
propranolol II
quinidine IA
sotalol III
tocainide IB
verapamil IV

Anticholinergic agents
albuterol
amantadine
atropine
belladonna
benztropine
biperiden
bromocriptine
buclizine
carbidopa
clidinium
dicyclomine
diphenhydramine
glycopyrrolate
homatropine
hyoscyamine
ipratropium
levodopa
methantheline
orphenadrine
pergolide
physostigmine

procyclidine
propantheline
scopolamine
selegiline
tacrine
tolterodine
trihexiphenidyl

Anticoagulants [1]
Antiplatelets [2]
Thrombolytics [3]
abciximab [2]
alteplase [3]
anagrelide [2]
anisindione [1]
anistreplase [3]
ardeparin [1]
argatroban [1]
aspirin [2]
bivalirudin [1]
cilostazol [2]
clopidogrel [2]
dalteparin [1]
danaparoid [1]
dicumarol [1]
dipyridamole [2]
enoxaparin [1]
heparin [1]
reteplase [3]
streptokinase [3]
tenecteplase [3]
ticlopidine [2]
tinzaparin [1]
torsemide [1]
urokinase [3]
warfarin [1]

Anticonvulsants
acetazolamide
amobarbital
carbamazepine
chlorpromazine
clonazepam
clorazepate
diazepam
divalproex
ethosuximide
ethotoin
felbamate
fosphenytoin
gabapentin
hydroxyzine
lamotrigine
levetiracetam
lorazepam
mephenytoin

mephobarbital
methsuximide
oxazepam
oxcarbazepine
paraldehyde
paramethadione
pentobarbital
phenobarbital
phensuximide
phenytoin
primidone
thiopental
tiagabine
topiramate
trimethadione
valproic acid
vigabatrin
zonisamide

Antidepressants

Tricyclics I = 1st generation
Tricyclics II = 2nd generation
Tricyclics III = 3rd generation

amitriptyline I
amoxapine II
benactyzine
bupropion II
citalopram III
clomipramine I
desipramine I
divalproex
doxepin I
escitalopram
fluoxetine III
fluvoxamine III
imipramine I
isocarboxazid
lithium
loxapine
maprotiline II
methylphenidate
mirtazapine III
nefazodone III
nortriptyline I
paroxetine III
perphenazine
phenelzine
protriptyline I
sertraline III
thioridazine
tranylcypromine
trazodone II
trimipramine I
venlafaxine III

Antidiabetic agents

acarbose
acetohexamide
chlorpropamide
glimepiride
glipizide
glucagon

glyburide
insulin
metformin
miglitol
nateglinide
pioglitazone
repaglinide
rosiglitazone
tolazamide
tolbutamide
troglitazone

Antifungals

amphotericin B
caspofungin
clotrimazole
fluconazole
flucytosine
griseofulvin
itraconazole
ketoconazole
metronidazole
miconazole
nystatin
terbinafine
vorinconazole

Antihypertensives

acebutolol
amiloride
amlodipine
atenolol
benazepril
bendroflumethiazide
benzthiazide
betaxolol
bisoprolol
bumetanide
candesartan
captopril
carteolol
carvedilol
chlorothiazide
chlorthalidone
clonidine
cyclothiazide
diazoxide
diltiazem
doxazosin
enalapril
eplerenone
eprosartan
esmolol
ethacrynic acid
felodipine
fosinopril
furosemide
guanabenz
guanethidine
guanfacine
hydralazine
hydrochlorothiazide

hydroflumethiazide
indapamide
isradipine
labetalol
lisinopril
losartan
mecamylamine
meclofenamate
methyclothiazide
methyldopa
methylphenidate
metolazone
metoprolol
minoxidil
moexipril
nadolol
nicardipine
nifedipine
nimodipine
nisoldipine
nitroglycerin
penbutolol
phentolamine
pindolol
polythiazide
prazosin
propantheline
propranolol
quinapril
quinethazone
ramipril
reserpine
spironolactone
terazosin
timolol
torsemide
triamterene
trichlormethiazide
valsartan
verapamil
yohimbine

Antimalarial agents

chloroquine
hydroxychloroquine
mefloquine
primaquine
pyrimethamine
quinacrine
quinine

Antimigraine drugs

5-HT, receptor agonists
almotriptan
frovatriptan
naritriptan
rizatriptan
sumatritan
zolmitriptan

Antimycobacterial agents

aminosalicylic acid

capreomycin
clofazimine
cycloserine
dapsone
ethambutol
ethionamide
isoniazid
kanamycin
pyrazinamide
rifampin
rifapentine
streptomycin

Antineoplastics
aldesleukin
alemtuzumab
altretamine
anastrazole
azathioprine
asparaginase
bleomycin
bortezomib
busulfan
caraway
carboplatin
carmustine
chlorambucil
chlorotrianisene
cisplatin
clomiphene
cyclophosphamide
cyclosporine
cytarabine
dacarbazine
dactinomycin
danazol
daunorubicin
diethylstilbestrol
docetaxel
doxorubicin
estradiol
estramustine
etoposide
exemestane
floxuridine
fluorouracil
fluoxymesterone
flutamide
fluvestrant
gemcitabine
hydroxyprogesterone
hydroxyurea
ibritumomab
idarubicin
ifosfamide
imatinib
interferon
leucovorin
leuprolide
levamisole
lomustine
masoprocol

mechlorethamine
medroxyprogesterone
megestrol
melphalan
mercaptopurine
mesna
methotrexate
methyltestosterone
mitomycin
mitotane
mitoxantrone
nafarelin
octreotide
oxaliplatin
paclitaxel
pentostatin
plicamycin
procarbazine
progesterone
somastatin
streptozocin
tamoxifen
taxol
testosterone
thioguanine
thiotepa
topotecan
trimetrexate
triptorelin
valrubicin
vinblastine
vincristine
vinorelbine

Antiparkinsonian agents
amantadine
benztropine
biperiden
bromocriptine
cabergoline
carbidopa
entacapone
levodopa/carbidopa
pergolide
pramipexole
procyclidine
ropinirole
selegiline
tolcapone
trihexyphenidyl

Antipsychotic agents
acetophenazine
aripiprazole
chlorpromazine
chlorprothixene
clozapine
droperidol
fluphenazine
haloperidol
lithium
loxapine

mesoridazine
molindone
olanzapine
perphenazine
prochlorperazine
pimozide
promazine
quetiapine
riluzole
risperidone
sertindole
thioridazine
thiothixene
trifluoperazine
ziprasidone

Antiretroviral agents
Nucleoside analog reverse transcriptase inhibitors (NRTIs)
abacavir
didanosine
lamivudine
stavudine
tenofovir
zalcitabine
zidovudine
Non-nucleoside reverse transcriptase inhibitors (NNRTIs)
delavirdine
efavirenz
nevirapine
Protease inhibitors
amprenavir
indinavir
lopinavir
nelfinavir
ritonavir
saquinavir
valacyclovir

Anxiolytics, sedatives and hypnotics
alprazolam
amobarbital
aprobarbital
buspirone
butabarbital
chloral hydrate
chlordiazepoxide
chlormezanone
chlorzoxazone
clonazepam
clorazepate
diazepam
droperidol
estazolam
ethchlorvynol
fentanyl
flurazepam
glutethimide
hydroxyzine
ketamine
lorazepam

mephobarbital
meprobamate
methohexital
midazolam
opium alkaloids
oxazepam
paraldehyde
paroxetine
pentobarbital
phenobarbital
prazepam
prochlorperazine
promethazine
propofol
quazepam
secobarbital
sertraline
temazepam
thiopental
triazolam
trifluoperazine
zaleplon
zolpidem

Benzodiazepines
alprazolam
amitriptyline
chlordiazepoxide
clonazepam
clorazepate
diazepam
estazolam
flurazepam
halazepam
lorazepam
midazolam
olanzapine
oxazepam
prazepam
quazepam
temazepam
triazolam

Beta-blockers
acebutolol
atenolol
betaxolol
bisoprolol
carteolol
carvedilol
esmolol
labetalol
levobetaxolol
levobunolol
metipranolol
metoprolol
nadolol
penbutolol
pindolol
propranolol
sotalol
timolol

Beta-lactam antibiotics
aztreonam
cefixime
cefoxitin
imipenen/cilastin
loracarbef
meropenem
moxalactam
tazobactam

Bronchodilators
albuterol
aminophylline
atropine
bitolterol
ephedrine
epinephrine
ipratropium
isoetharine
isoproterenol
levalbuterol
metaproterenol
montelukast
pirbuterol
salmeterol
terbutaline
theophylline
zafirlukast
zileuton

Calcium channel blockers
amlodipine
bepridil
diltiazem
enalapril
felodipine
isradipine
nicardipine
nifedipine
nimodipine
nisoldipine
trandolapril
verapamil

Cephalosporin antibiotics
By generation
First generation
cefadroxil
cefazolin
cephalexin
cephalothin
cephapirin
cephradine
Second generation
cefaclor
cefamandole
cefmetazole
cefonicid
ceforanide
cefotetan
cefoxitin
cefprozil

cefuroxime
loracarbef
Third generation
cefdinir
cefditoren
cefixime
cefoperazone
cefotaxime
cefpodoxime
ceftazidime
ceftibuten
ceftizoxime
ceftriaxone
Fourth generation
cefepime

Diuretics
acetazolamide
amiloride
bendroflumethiazide
benzthiazide
bumetanide
chlorthalidone
chorothiazide
cyclothiazide
ethacrynic acid
furosemide
hydrochlorothiazide
hydroflumethiazide
indapamide
isosorbide
mannitol
methyclothiazide
metolazone
polythiazide
potassium chloride
quinethazone
spironolactone
torsemide
triamterene
trichlormethiazide
urea

Diuretics, loop
bumetanide
ethacrynic acid
furosemide
torsemide

Fluoroquinolones + Quinolones
alatrofloxacin
cinoxacin
ciprofloxacin
enoxacin
gatifloxacin
gemifloxacin
grepafloxacin
levofloxacin
lomefloxacin
moxifloxacin
norfloxacin

ofloxacin
sparfloxacin
trovafloxacin

H₂ antagonists

cimetidine
famotidne
nizatidine
ranitidine
roxatidine

Hypnotics

aprobarbital
ethchlorvynol
flurazepam
glutethimide
L-tryptophan
methohexital
opium alkaloids
pentobarbital
phenobarbital
propofol
quazepam
secobarbital
temazepam
thiopental
triazolam
zolpidem

Hypolipidemic agents HMG-CoA reductase inhibitors (statins)

atorvastatin
cerivastatin
cholestyramine
clofibrate
colesevelam
colestipol
dextrothyroxine
fenofibrate
fluvastatin
gemfibrozil
lovastatin
niacin
pravastatin
probucol
simvastatin

Macrolide antibiotics

azithromycin
clarithromycin
dirithromycin
erythromycin
lincomycin
troleandomycin

Monamine oxidase inhibitors

isocarboxazid
pargyline
phenelzine
tranylcypromine

Narcotic agonists

alfentanil
buprenorphine
butorphanol
codeine
fentanyl
hydrocodone
hydromorphone
levorphanol
meperidine
methadone
morphine
nalbuphine
oxycodone
pentazocine
propoxyphene
remifentanil
sufentanil

Neuroleptics

amitriptyline
chlorpromazine
fluphenazine
haloperidol
lithium
loxapine
molindone
pimozide
prochlorperazine
thioridazine
thiothixene
tranylcypromine
trifluoperazine

Neuromuscular blocking agents

atracurium
cisatracurium
doxacurium
gallimine
metocurine
mivacurium
pancuronium
pipecuronium
rapacuronium
rocuronium
succinylcholine
tubocurarine
vecuronium

NSAIDs

aspirin
bromfenac
celecoxib
choline salicylate
diclofenac
diflunisal
etodolac
fenoprofen
flurbiprofen
ibuprofen
indomethacin
ketoprofen
ketorolac
magnesium salicylate
meclofenamate
mefenamic acid
meloxicam
mesalamine
methotrexate
nabumetone
naproxen
olsalazine
oxaprozin
oxyphenbutazone
phenylbutazone
piroxicam
rofecoxib
salsalate
sodium salicylate
sulindac
tolmetin
valdecoxib

Penicillin antibiotics

amoxicillin
ampicillin
carbenicillin
cloxacillin
dicloxacillin
methicillin
mezlocillin
nafcillin
oxacillin
penicillin
piperacillin
ticarcillin

Selective serotonin reuptake inhibitors (SSRIs)

almotriptan
citalopram
eletriptan
escitalopram
fluoxetine
fluvoxamine
nefazodone
paroxetine
sertraline
trazodone
venlafaxine

Sulfonamide derivatives

Antimicrobial agents
mafenide acetate
silver sulfadiazine
sodium sulfacetamide
sulfadiazine
sulfamethiazole
sulfamethoxazole
sulfisoxazole
Diuretic, carbonic anhydrase inhibitor
acetazolamide
dichlorphenamide

methazolamide
Diuretics, loop
  bumetanide
  furosemide
  torsemide
Diuretics, thiazide
  bendroflumethiazide
  benzthiazide
  chlorothiazide
  chlorthalidone
  cyclothiazide
  hydrochlorothiazide
  hydroflumethiazide
  indapamide
  methyclothiazide
  metolazone
  polythiazide
  quinethazone
  trichlormethiazide
Hypoglycemic agents, oral
  acetohexamide
  chlorpropamide
  glipizide
  glyburide
  tolazamide
  tolbutamide
Other agents

cyclamate
dorzolamide
saccharin
sulfasalazine

Tranquilizers
amitriptyline
buspirone
chlordiazepoxide
chlormezanone
chlorpromazine
clorazepate
diazepam
doxepin
droperidol
fluphenazine
haloperidol
hydroxyzine
lorazepam
loxapine
meprobamate
mesoridazine
molindone
oxazepam
perphenazine
pimozide
prochlorperazine

promazine
promethazine
reserpine
risperidone
thioridazine
thiothixene
trifluoperazine

Tetracycline antibiotics
demeclocycline
doxycycline
minocycline
oxytetracycline
tetracycline

Vasodilators
hydralazine
isoxusprine
minoxidil
nesiritide
nitroglycerin
nitroprusside
papaverine
tolazoline
treprostinil

ABACAVIR

Trade names: Trizivir (GSK); Ziagen (GSK)
Indications: HIV infections in combination with other antiretrovirals
Category: Antiretroviral; Nucleoside reverse transcriptase inhibitor (NRTI)
Half-life: 1.5 hours
Clinically important, potentially hazardous interactions with: arbutamine, argatroban, arsenic

Reactions

Skin

Chills
　(1999): Escaut L+, *AIDS* 13, 1419
Edema
　(1999): Spruance SL, *Skin and Allergy News* October, 37
Erythroderma
　(2001): Shapiro M+, *The AIDS Reader* 11, 222
Exanthems
　(1999): Nathanson N (from Internet) (observation) (generalized)
　(1999): Spruance SL, *Skin and Allergy News* October, 37
　(1998): Saag M+, *AIDS* 12, F203
Kawasaki syndrome
　(2002): Toerner JG+, *Clin Infect Dis* 34(1), 131
Pruritus
　(1998): Saag M+, *AIDS* 12, F203
Rash (sic) (10%)
　(2002): Kessler HA+, *Clin Infect Dis* 34(4), 535
　(2001): Hetherington S+, *Clin Ther* 23(10), 1603
　(2000): Hervey PS+, *Drugs* 60, 447 (5%)
　(1999): Hughes W+, *Antimicrob Agents Chemother* 43, 609 (9%)
　(1999): Spruance SL, *Skin and Allergy News* October, 37 (69%)
　(1998): Foster RH+, *Drugs* 55, 729
　(1998): Kessler H+, *36th Meeting of the Infectious Disease Society of America, Denver* Abstract 453 (10–15%)
　(1998): Saag M+, *AIDS* 12, F203 (10–15%)
　(1998): Staszewski S+, *AIDS* 12, F197 (10–15%)
Stevens–Johnson syndrome
　(2002): Bossi P+, *Clin Infect Dis* 35(7), 902

Other

Anaphylactoid reactions
　(2001): Frissen PH+, *AIDS* 15, 289
　(1999): Spruance SL, *Skin and Allergy News* October, 37 (3–4%)
　(1999): Walensky RP+, *AIDS* 13, 999
Cough
　(2002): Peyriere H+, *Allerg Immunol* (Paris) 34(10), 359
　(2001): Hetherington S+, *Clin Ther* 23(10), 1603 (10%)
Death
Headache
Hypersensitivity (5%)
　(2002): Dargere S+, *AIDS* 16(12), 1696
　(2002): Flexner C, *Hopkins HIV Rep* 14(3), 5
　(2002): Hetherington S+, *Lancet* 359(9312), 1121
　(2002): Hewitt RG+, *Clin Infect Dis* 34(8), 1137 (3.7%)
　(2002): *AIDS Patient Care STDS* 16(5), 242
　(2002): Kessler HA+, *Clin Infect Dis* 34(4), 535
　(2002): Mallal S+, *Lancet* 359, 727 (5%)
　(2002): Symonds W+, *Clin Ther* 24(4), 565
　(2002): Toerner JG+, *Clin Infect Dis* 34(1), 131
　(2001): Cutrell A+, *International AIDS Society Conference on HIV Buenos Aires* Abstract 527
　(2001): Frissen PH+, *AIDS* 15, 289
　(2001): Hetherington S, *AIDS Read* 11(12), 620
　(2001): Hetherington S+, *Clin Ther* 23(10), 1603 (4.3%)

　(2001): Keiser P+, *8th Conferences on Retroviruses* (Chicago) Abstract 622
　(2001): Loeliger AE+, *AIDS* 15(10), 1325
　(2001): Peyrieere H+, *Ann Pharmacother* 35(10), 1291
　(2001): Shapiro M+, *The AIDS Reader* 11, 222
　(2001): Wit FW+, *AIDS* 15(18), 2423
　(2000): Clay PG+, *Ann Pharmacother* 34, 247
　(2000): GlaxoWellcome, *Important Drug Warning* July (severe or fatal)
　(2000): Hervey PS+, *Drugs* 60, 447 (3–5%)
　(2000): *AIDS Read* 10, 525
　(2000): *AIDS Treat News* 337, 7
　(2000): *Prescrire Int* 9, 67
　(2000): Keiser P+, *Conference on Retroviruses & Opportunistic Infections* (Chicago) Abstract 622
　(1999): Escaut L+, *AIDS* 13, 1419
　(1999): Miller JL, *Am J Health Syst Pharm* 56, 304
　(1998): Foster RH+, *Drugs* 55, 729 (2–3%)
　(1998): *AIDS Patient Care SDS* 12, 405
　(1998): *Newsline People AIDS Coalit N Y* Feb, 35
　(1998): Saag M+, *AIDS* 12, F203 (2–5%)
　(1998): Staszewski S+, *AIDS* 12, F197
　(1997): James JS, *AIDS Treat News* 285, 1, 5
Lipodystrophy
　(2002): Bernasconi E+, *J Acquir Immune Defic Syndr* 31(1), 50
Mouth vesiculation
　(2002): Fantry LE+, *AIDS Patient Care STDS* 16(1), 5
Myalgia
　(1999): Escaut L+, *AIDS* 13, 1419
　(1999): Spruance SL, *Skin and Allergy News* October, 37
Oral ulceration
　(1999): Spruance SL, *Skin and Allergy News* October, 37
Paresthesias
Perioral paresthesias
　(2001): McMahon D+, *Antivir Ther* 6(2), 105

ABCIXIMAB

Synonym: C7E3
Trade name: Reopro (Lilly)
Indications: Thrombotic arterial disease
Category: Antiplatelet; Glycoprotein IIb/IIIa inhibitor
Half-life: 10–30 minutes – given intravenously
Clinically important, potentially hazardous interactions with: fondaparinux, reteplase

Reactions

Skin

Cellulitis (0.3%)
Edema
　(2002): Pharand C+, *Pharmacotherapy* 22(3), 380
Peripheral edema (1.6%)
Petechiae (0.3%)
Pruritus (0.3%)
　(2002): Pharand C+, *Pharmacotherapy* 22(3), 380

Other

Anaphylactoid reactions
　(2002): Pharand C+, *Pharmacotherapy* 22(3), 380
　(2001): Iakovou Y+, *Cardiology* 95(4), 215
　(1999): Guzzo JA+, *Catheter Cardiovasc Interv* 48, 71
Headache
Hyperesthesia (1%)
Injection-site reactions (3.6%)
Myalgia (0.3%)
Myopathy (0.3%)

ACARBOSE

Trade name: Precose (Bayer)
Other common trade names: *Glucobay; Glumida; Prandase*
Indications: Non-insulin dependent diabetes type II
Category: Oral antidiabetic (alpha-glucosidase inhibitor)
Half-life: 2.7–9 hours

Reactions

Skin
Erythema (<1%)
  (2000): Schmutz JL+, *Ann Dermatol Venereol* 127, 869
    (polymorphous)
Erythema multiforme
  (1999): Kono T+, *Lancet* 354, 396 (generalized)
Rash (sic)
Urticaria (<1%)

Other
Ageusia
  (1996): Martin Bun N+, *Med Clin (Barc)* (Spanish) 28, 399

ACEBUTOLOL

Trade name: Sectral (ESP Pharma)
Other common trade names: *Acecor; Acetanol; Alol; Apo-Acebutolol; Monitan; Neptal; Novo-Acebutolol; Nu-Acebutolol; Prent; Rhodiasectral; Rhotral*
Indications: Hypertension, angina, ventricular arrhythmias
Category: Antiarrhythmic; Antihypertensive; Beta-adrenoceptor blocker
Half-life: 3–7 hours
Clinically important, potentially hazardous interactions with: clonidine, verapamil

Note: Cutaneous side effects of beta-receptor blockaders are clinically polymorphous. They apparently appear after several months of continuous therapy. Atypical psoriasiform, lichen planus-like, and eczematous chronic rashes are mainly observed. (1983): Hödl St, *Z Hautkr* (German) 1:58, 17

Reactions

Skin
Dermatitis (sic)
Diaphoresis
  (1995): Schmutz JL+, *Dermatology* 190, 86
Edema (1–10%)
Erythema multiforme (<1%)
Exanthems (4%)
  (1985): Singh BN+, *Drugs* 29, 531
Exfoliative dermatitis
Facial edema (<1%)
Hyperkeratosis (palms and soles)
Lichenoid eruption
  (1982): Taylor AEM+, *Clin Exp Dermatol* 7, 219
  (1978): Savage RL+, *BMJ* 1, 987
Lupus erythematosus (<1%)
  (1997): Burlingame RW, *Clin Lab Med* 17, 367
  (1992): Rubin RL+, *J Clin Invest* 90, 165
  (1992): Stevens MB, *Hosp Pract* 27, 27
  (1987): Doktor D, *Rev Fr Allergol Immunol* (French) 27, 77
  (1985): Hourdebaight-Larrusse P+, *Ann Cardiol Angeiol* (Paris) (French) 34, 421

  (1985): Singh BN+, *Drugs* 29, 531
  (1984): Bigot MC+, *Therapie* (French) 39, 571
  (1984): Meyer O+, *Rev Rhum Mal Osteoartic* (French) 51, 303
  (1983): Homberg JC+, *J Pharmacol* (French) 14, 61
  (1982): Taylor AE+, *Clin Exp Dermatol* 7, 219
  (1981): Record NB, *Ann Intern Med* 95, 326
  (1981): Simon P+, *Nouv Presse Med* (French) 10, 105
Pigmentation
Pityriasis rubra pilaris
  (1978): Finlay AY+, *BMJ* 1, 987
Pruritus (<2%)
Psoriasis
  (1986): Czernielewski J+, *Lancet* 1, 808
  (1984): Arntzen N+, *Acta Derm Venereol* (Stockh) 64, 346
Rash (sic) (1–10%)
Raynaud's phenomenon
  (1984): Eliasson K+, *Acta Med Scand* 215, 333
  (1976): Marshall AJ+, *BMJ* 1, 1498
Toxic epidermal necrolysis
Urticaria
  (1977): Ashford R+, *Lancet* 2, 462
Vasculitis
  (1988): Bonnefoy M+, *Ann Dermatol Venereol* (French) 115, 27
  (1977): Ashford R+, *Lancet* 2, 462
Xerosis

Hair
Hair – alopecia

Nails
Nails – bluish
Nails – dystrophy
Nails – onycholysis
Nails – pincer (reverse transverse curvature of the nails)
  (1998): Greiner D+, *J Am Acad Dermatol* 39, 486

Other
Dysgeusia
Hyperesthesia (<2%)
Myalgia (1–10%)
Oculo-mucocutaneous syndrome
  (1982): Cocco G+, *Curr Ther Res* 31, 362
Oral lichenoid eruption
Peyronie's disease
  (1979): Pryor JP+, *Lancet* 1, 331
Xerostomia (<1%)

ACETAMINOPHEN

Synonyms: APAP; paracetamol

Trade names: Anacin-3 (Wyeth); Bromo-Seltzer; Darvocet-N (Lilly); Datril; Excedrin (Bristol-Myers Squibb); Liquiprin; Lorcet (Forest); Mapap; Neopap; Panadol (GSK); Percogesic; Percoset (Endo); Phenaphen; Sinutab; Tylenol (Ortho-McNeil); Valadol; Vicodin (Abbott)

Other common trade names: *Abenol; Anaflon; Ben-U-Ron; Doliprane; Geluprane; Panadol*

Indications: Pain, fever

Category: Non-narcotic antipyretic analgesic

Half-life: 1–3 hours

Clinically important, potentially hazardous interactions with: alcohol, cholestyramine, didanosine, **dong quai, melatonin**

Note: Acetaminophen is the active metabolite of phenacetin

Reactions

Skin

Acute generalized exanthematous pustulosis (AGEP)
  (2001): Cohen AD+, *Int J Dermatol* 40(7), 458
  (1998): Leger F+, *Acta Derm Venereol* 78, 222
  (1996): DeConinck AL+, *Dermatology* 193, 338
  (1995): Moreau A+, *Int J Dermatol* 34, 263 (passim)
  (1991): Roujeau J-C+, *Arch Dermatol* 127, 1333
Angioedema (<1%)
  (2002): Litt JZ, Beachwood, OH (personal case) (observation)
    (patient inadvertently re-challenged herself)
  (1997): de Almeida MA+, *Allergy Asthma Proc* 18, 313
  (1990): Van Diem L+, *Eur J Clin Pharmacol* 38, 389
  (1986): Idoko JA+, *Trans R Soc Trop Med Hyg* 80, 175
  (1985): Stricker BH+, *BMJ* 291, 938
  (1970): Henriques CC, *JAMA* 214, 2336
Dermatitis (sic)
  (1997): Mathelier-Fusada P+, *Contact Dermatitis* 36, 267
  (1996): Szczurko C+, *Contact Dermatitis* 35, 299
  (1995): Barbaud A+, *Lancet* 346(8979), 902
Diaphoresis
Erythema (sic)
  (1985): Stricker BH+, *BMJ* 291, 938
Erythema multiforme
  (1995): Dubey NK+, *Indian Pediatr* 32, 1117
  (1984): Hurvitz H+, *Isr J Med Sci* 20, 145
Erythema nodosum (<1%)
Exanthems
  (1997): Foong H, Malaysia (from Internet) (observation)
  (1985): Matheson I+, *Pediatrics* 76, 651
  (1985): Stricker BH+, *BMJ* 291, 938
  (1975): Michelson PA, *Ann Intern Med* 83, 374
  (1970): Henriques CC, *JAMA* 214, 2336
Exfoliative dermatitis
  (1984): Guerin C+, *Therapie* (French) 39, 47
Fixed eruption (<1%)
  (2001): Silva A+, *Pediatr Dermatol* 18(2), 163
  (2000): Bernand S+, *Dermatology* 201, 184 (similar to ondansetron)
  (2000): Galindo PA+, *J Investig Allergol Clin Immunol* 9, 399
  (2000): Ko R+, *Clin Exp Dermatol* 25, 96
  (2000): Ozkaya-Bayazit E+, *Eur J Dermatol* 10, 288
  (1999): Sehgal VN, *Pediatr Dermatology* 16, 165 (multiple)
  (1998): Hern S+, *Br J Dermatol* 139, 1129,
  (1998): Litt JZ, Beachwood, OH (personal case) (observation)
  (1998): Mahboob A+, *Int J Dermatol* 37, 833

(1996): Gomez-Martinez M+, *J Investig Allergol Clin Immunol* 6, 131
(1996): Kawada A+, *Int J Dermatol* 35, 148
(1996): Laude TA, *Cosmetic Dermatology* 9, 7
(1995): Harris A+, *Br J Dermatol* 133, 790
(1994): Rademaker M+, *N Z Med J* 107, 295
(1992): Cohen HA+, *Ann Pharmacother* 26, 1596
(1992): Zemtsov A+, *Cutis* 50, 281
(1991): Thankappen TP+, *Int J Dermatol* 30, 867
(1990): Duhra P+, *Clin Exp Dermatol* 15, 293
(1990): Gaffoor PMA+, *Cutis* 45, 242 (passim)
(1989): Valsecchi R, *Dermatologica* 179, 51
(1988): Guin J+, *Cutis* 41, 107
(1987): Bharija SC+, *Australas J Dermatol* 28, 85
(1987): Guin J+, *J Am Acad Dermatol* 17, 399
(1986): Meyrick-Thomas RH+, *Br J Dermatol* 115, 357
(1985): Verbov J, *Dermatologica* 171, 60 (with chlormezanone)
(1975): Wilson HTH, *Br J Dermatol* 92, 213
(1970): Henriques CC, *JAMA* 214, 2336
(1965): Fitzpatrick TB, *Arch Dermatol* 92(4), 484 (phenacetin)
Flushing
  (1985): Stricker BH+, *BMJ* 291, 938
Linear IgA bullous dermatosis
  (2003): Avci O+, *J Am Acad Dermatol* 48(2), 299
Neutrophilic eccrine hidradenitis
  (1988): Kuttner BJ+, *Cutis* 41, 403
Pemphigus
  (1990): Brenner S+, *Acta Derm Venereol* 70, 357
Penile edema
  (1997): Cabanes Higuero N+, *Med Clin (Barc)* (Spanish) 109, 685
Photosensitivity
  (1999): Popescu C, Bucharest, Romania (from Internet) (observation)
Pityriasis rosea
  (1993): Yosipovitch G+, *Harefuah* (Israel) 124, 198; 247
Progressive pigmentary purpura (Schamberg's disease)
  (1992): Abeck D+, *J Am Acad Dermatol* 27, 123
Pruritus
  (2001): Grant JA+, *Ann Allergy Asthma Immunol* 87(3), 227 (rare)
  (1985): Stricker BH+, *BMJ* 291, 938
Purpura
  (1998): Kwon SJ+, *J Dermatol* 25, 756
  (1993): Guccione JL+, *Arch Dermatol* 129, 1267
  (1992): Abeck D+, *J Am Acad Dermatol* 27, 123
  (1980): Miescher PA+, *Clin Haematol* 9, 505
  (1977): Ameer B+, *Ann Intern Med* 87, 202
  (1973): Skokan JD+, *Cleve Clin Quart* 40, 89
Purpura fulminans
  (1993): Guccione JL+, *Arch Dermatol* 129, 1267
Rash (sic) (<1%)
Sensitivity (sic)
  (1998): Mendizabal SL+, *Allergy* 53, 457
Stevens–Johnson syndrome
  (1995): Kuper K+, *Ophthalmologue* (German) 92, 823
  (1985): Ting HC+, *Int J Dermatol* 24, 587
Toxic epidermal necrolysis
  (2002): Cordova M, (Lima) (Peru) March AAD Poster
  (2002): Thakker J+, *World Congress Dermatol* Poster, 0129 (with nimesulide)
  (2000): Halevi A+, *Ann Pharmacother* 34, 32
  (1991): Sakellariou G+, *Int J Artif Organs* 14, 634
  (1986): Roupe G+, *Int Arch Allergy Appl Immunol* 80, 145
Urticaria
  (2002): Litt JZ, Beachwood, OH (personal case) (observation) (patient inadvertently re-challenged herself)
  (2001): Grant JA+, *Ann Allergy Asthma Immunol* 87(3), 227 (rare)
  (2000): Samanta BB, *J Assoc Physicians India* 47, 464
  (1997): de Almeida MA+, *Allergy Asthma Proc* 18, 313

(1997): Ownby DR, *J Allergy Clin Immunol* 99, 151
(1985): Cole TO, *Clin Exp Dermatol* 10, 404
(1985): Stricker BH+, *BMJ* 291, 938
(1975): Michelson PA, *Ann Intern Med* 83, 374
(1970): Henriques CC, *JAMA* 214, 2336
Vasculitis
(1995): Harris A+, *Br J Dermatol* 133, 790
(1988): Dussarat GV+, *Presse Med* (French) 17, 1587

Hair

Hair – alopecia
(1998): Litt JZ, Beachwood, OH (personal case) (observation)

Nails

Nails – changes (sic)
(1975): Michelson PA, *Ann Intern Med* 83, 374

Other

Anaphylactoid reactions
(2002): Bachmeyer C+, *South Med J* 95(7), 759
(2002): Liao CM+, *Acta Paediatr Taiwan* 43(3), 147
(2001): Verma S, Baroda, India (from Internet)(observation)
(with ibuprofen)
(2000): Ayonrinde OT+, *Postgrad Med J.* 76, 501
(2000): de Paramo BJ+, *Ann Allergy Asthma Immunol* 85, 508 (4
patients)
(2000): Stephenson I+, *Postgrad Med* 76, 503
(1999): Kumar RK+, *Hosp Med* 60, 66
(1999): Spitz E, *Ann Allergy Asthma Immunol* 82, 591
(1998): Galindo PA+, *Allergol Immunopathol (Madr)* (Spanish)
26, 199
(1998): Huitema AD+, *Hum Exp Toxicol* 17, 406
(1990): Van Diem L+, *Eur J Clin Pharmacol* 38, 389
(1988): *Allergy Observer* (Janssen Pharmaceutica) 5(7), 1
(1985): Stricker BH+, *BMJ* 291, 938
Death
(2001): Stevenson R+, *Scott Med J* 46(3), 84 (overdose)
Dysgeusia
(1976): Rollin H, *Laryngol Rhinol Otol* (Stuttgart) (German)
55, 873
Headache
Hypersensitivity (<1%)
(2001): Grant JA+, *Ann Allergy Asthma Immunol* 87(3), 227 (rare)
(1999): Kivity S+, *Allergy* 54, 187
(1997): Vidal C+, *Ann Allergy Asthma Immunol* 79, 320
(1996): Ibanez MD+, *Allergy* 51, 121
(1993): Martin JA+, *Med Clin (Barc)* (Spanish) 100, 158
Rhabdomyolysis
(2001): Yang CC+, *Vet Hum Toxicol* 43(6), 344 (overdose)
(1999): Moneret-Vautrin DA+, *Allergy* 54(10), 1115
(1996): Riggs JE+, *Mil Med* 161(11), 708 (with alcohol)

ACETAZOLAMIDE

Trade name: Diamox (Wyeth)
Other common trade names: *Acetazolam; Ak-Zol; Dazamide; Defiltran; Diuramid; Novo-Zolamide*
Indications: Epilepsy, glaucoma
Category: Anticonvulsant; Carbonic anhydrase inhibitor; Sulfonamide diuretic
Half-life: 2–6 hours
Clinically important, potentially hazardous interactions with: ephedra, lithium

Reactions

Skin

Acute generalized exanthematous pustulosis (AGEP)
(1995): Moreau A+, *Int J Dermatol* 34, 263 (passim)
(1992): Ogoshi M+, *Dermatology* 184, 142
Bullous eruption (<1%)
(1957): Ellis FA, *Arch Dermatol* 75, 836
Erythema multiforme
(1961): Baer RL+, *Year Book of Dermatology* 9 Year Book Medical
Publishers
(1956): Spring M, *Ann Allergy* Jan/Feb, 41
Exanthems
(1967): Lockey SD, *Med Sci* 18, 43
(1956): Spring M, *Ann Allergy* Jan/Feb, 41
Frostbite
(2001): Laemmle T, *Wilderness Environ Med* 12(4), 290
Lupus erythematosus
(1966): Cohen P+, *JAMA* 197, 817
Photosensitivity
Pruritus
Purpura
(1976): Underwood LC, *JAMA* 161, 1477
Pustular psoriasis
(1995): Kuroda K+, *J Dermatol* 22, 784
Pustules
(1992): Ogoshi M+, *Dermatology* 184, 142
Rash (sic) (<1%)
Rosacea
(1993): Shah P+, *Br J Dermatol* 129, 647
Stevens–Johnson syndrome
Toxic epidermal necrolysis (<1%)
(1957): Ellis FA, *Arch Dermatol* 75, 836
Urticaria

Hair

Hair – hirsutism
(1974): Weiss IS, *Am J Ophthalmol* 78, 327

Other

Ageusia
Anaphylactoid reactions
(2002): Gallerani M+, *Am J Emerg Med* 20(4), 371
(2000): Gerhards LJ+, *Ned Tijdschr Geneeskd* (Dutch) 144, 1228
(1998): Tzanakis N+, *Br J Ophthalmol* 82, 588
Anosmia
Dysgeusia (>10%) (metallic taste)
(1997): Martinez-Mir I+, *Ann Pharmacother* 31, 373
(1990): Miller LG+, *J Fam Pract* 31, 199
(1981): Lichter PR, *Ophthalmol* 88, 266
Extravasation
(1994): Callear A+, *Br J Ophthalmol* 78, 731
Headache

Paresthesias (<1%)
   (1981): Lichter PR, *Ophthalmol* 88, 266
Tinnitus
Xerostomia (<1%)

*Note: Acetazolamide is a sulfonamide and can be absorbed systemically. Sulfonamides can produce severe, possibly fatal, reactions such as toxic epidermal necrolysis and Stevens–Johnson syndrome

ACETOHEXAMIDE

Trade name: Dymelor (Lilly)
Other common trade names: *Dimelin; Dimelor*
Indications: non-insulin dependent diabetes type II
Category: Oral hypoglycemic; Sulfonylurea antidiabetic
Half-life: 1–6 hours
Clinically important, potentially hazardous interactions with: phenylbutazones

Reactions

Skin
Diaphoresis
Eczema (sic)
Erythema (<1%)
Exanthems (<1%)
Lichenoid eruption
Photosensitivity (1–10%)
Pruritus (<1%)
Rash (sic) (1–10%)
Urticaria (1–10%)

Hair
Hair – alopecia
   (1962): Boshell BR+, *Clin Pharmacol Ther* 3, 750

Other
Headache
Paresthesias
Porphyria cutanea tarda

*Note: Acetohexamide is a sulfonamide and can be absorbed systemically. Sulfonamides can produce severe, possibly fatal, reactions such as toxic epidermal necrolysis and Stevens–Johnson syndrome

ACETYLCYSTEINE

Synonyms: N-acetylcysteine; L-Cysteine; NAC
Trade names: Mucomyst (Apothecon); Mucomyst-10 (Geneva); Mucosil-10 (DEY); Parvolex
Other common trade names: *Agisolvan; Alveolex; Ecomucyl; Encore; Exomuc; Fabrol; Fluimicil; Mucofillin; Mucolit; Mucolitico; Mucoloid; Mucomiste; Siran*
Indications: Emphysema, bronchitis, tuberculosis, bronchiectasis, tracheostomy care, antidote for acetaminophen toxicity
Category: Diagnostic aid; mucolytic
Half-life: N/A
Clinically important, potentially hazardous interactions with: carbamazepine, nitroglycerin

Reactions

Skin
Angioedema
   (2001): Tas S+, *Br J Dermatol* 145(5), 856
   (1999): Schmidt LE+, *Ugeskr Laeger* 161(18), 2669
   (1997): Mroz LS+, *Ann Emerg Med* 30(2), 240
   (1984): Mant TG+, *Br Med J* 289(6439), 217
   (1984): Tenenbein M, *Vet Hum Toxicol* 26(Suppl 2), 3
Chills
Clammy skin
Dermatitis
   (2002): Davison SC+, *Contact Dermatitis* 47(4), 238
Flushing
   (1999): Schmidt LE+, *Ugeskr Laeger* 161(18), 2669
   (1992): Bonfiglio MF+, *Ann Pharmacother* 26(1), 22
Pruritus
   (1999): Schmidt LE+, *Ugeskr Laeger* 161(18), 2669
   (1984): Tenenbein M, *Vet Hum Toxicol* 26(Suppl 2), 3
Rash (sic)
   (1999): Schmidt LE+, *Ugeskr Laeger* 161(18), 2669
   (1994): Chan TY+, *Hum Exp Toxicol* 13(8), 542
   (1984): Mant TG+, *Br Med J* 289(6439), 217
Urticaria
   (1984): Tenenbein M, *Vet Hum Toxicol* 26(Suppl 2), 3

Other
Anaphylactoid reactions
   (2002): Appelboam AV+, *Emerg Med J* 19(6), 594 (fatal)
   (2001): Recasens M+, *Med Clin* (Barc) 117(14), 558
   (1999): Schmidt LE+, *Ugeskr Laeger* 161(18), 2669
   (1998): Bailey B+, *Ann Emerg Med* 31(6), 710
   (1997): Stavem K, *Tidsskr Nor Laegeforen* 117(4), 2038
   (1992): Bonfiglio MF+, *Ann Pharmacother* 26(1), 22
   (1992): Sunman W+, *Lancet* 339(8803), 1231
   (1984): Gervais S+, *Clin Pharm* 3(6), 586
   (1982): Vale JA+, *Lancet* 2(8305), 988
   (1979): Walton NG+, *Lancet* 2(8155), 1298
Death
   (1997): Ardissino D+, *J Am Coll Cardiol* 29(5), 941
Fever
   (1994): Chan TY+, *Hum Exp Toxicol* 13(8), 542
Hypersensitivity
   (1984): Tenenbein M, *Vet Hum Toxicol* 26, 3
Injection-site pain
   (1984): Casola G+, *Radiology* 152(1), 233
Status epilepticus
   (1996): Hershkovitz E+, *Isr J Med Sci* 32(11), 1102
Stomatitis

ACITRETIN

Trade name: Soriatane (Roche)
Other common trade name: *Neotigason*
Indications: Psoriasis
Category: Antipsoriatic retinoid
Half-life: 49 hours
**Clinically important, potentially hazardous interactions
with: alcohol,** bexarotene, chloroquine, cholestyramine,
corticosteroids, danazol, ethanolamine, isotretinoin, lithium,
medroxyprogesterone, methotrexate, minocycline, progestins,
tetracycline, vitamin A

Reactions

Skin

Atrophy (10–25%)
Bullous eruption (1–10%)
Cheilitis (>75%)
   (2001): Berbis P, *Ann Dermatol Venereol* 128(6), 737
   (1999): Katz HI+, *J Am Acad Dermatol* 41, S7 (>75%)
   (1997): Buccheri L+, *Arch Dermatol* 133, 711 (100%)
   (1996): Lacour M+, *Br J Dermatol* 134, 1023
   (1991): Murray HE+, *J Am Acad Dermatol* 24, 598 (49%)
   (1990): Ruzicka T+, *Arch Dermatol* 126, 482 (80%)
   (1989): Gupta AK+, *J Am Acad Dermatol* 21, 1088 (100%)
   (1988): Geiger J-M+, *Dermatologica* 176, 182 (82%)
Chills
   (2001): Liss WA, Pleasanton, CA (from Internet) (observation)
Cold, clammy skin (1–10%)
Dermatitis (sic) (1–10%)
Diaphoresis (1–10%)
   (1997): Buccheri L+, *Arch Dermatol* 133, 711 (18.2%)
   (1988): Geiger J-M+, *Dermatologica* 176, 182 (9%)
Edema
   (2001): Liss WA, Pleasanton, CA (from Internet) (observation)
Erythema (sic)
   (1997): Buccheri L+, *Arch Dermatol* 133, 711 (18.2%)
Erythroderma
   (2001): Liss WA, Pleasanton, CA (from Internet) (observation)
Exanthems (10–25%)
   (1999): Katz HI+, *J Am Acad Dermatol* 41, S7
   (1990): Ruzicka T+, *Arch Dermatol* 126, 482 (2%)
Exfoliation
   (1999): Katz HI+, *J Am Acad Dermatol* 41, S7 (25–50%)
   (1997): Buccheri L+, *Arch Dermatol* 133, 711 (36.4%)
Exfoliative dermatitis
   (2001): Blumenthal HL, Beachwood, OH (observation)
Fissures (1–10%)
Milia
   (1993): Chang A+, *Acta Derm Venereol* 73, 235
Palmar–plantar desquamation
   (1991): Murray HE+, *J Am Acad Dermatol* 24, 598 (29%)
   (1990): Ruzicka T+, *Arch Dermatol* 126, 482 (20–25%)
   (1989): Gupta AK+, *J Am Acad Dermatol* 21, 1088 (50–80%)
   (1988): Geiger J-M+, *Dermatologica* 176, 182 (26%)
Palmar–plantar peeling
   (2001): Berbis P, *Ann Dermatol Venereol* 128(6), 737
   (2001): *Ami* (from Internet) (observation) (severe)
Phototoxicity
   (1999): Katz HI+, *J Am Acad Dermatol* 41, S7
Pruritus (25–50%)
   (1999): Katz HI+, *J Am Acad Dermatol* 41, S7
   (1997): Buccheri L+, *Arch Dermatol* 133, 711 (54.5%)
   (1996): Lacour M+, *Br J Dermatol* 134, 1023
   (1991): Murray HE+, *J Am Acad Dermatol* 24, 598 (32%)

   (1990): Ruzicka T+, *Arch Dermatol* 126, 482 (37%)
   (1989): Gupta AK+, *J Am Acad Dermatol* 21, 1088 (10–20%)
   (1988): Geiger J-M+, *Dermatologica* 176, 182 (16%)
Psoriasis (1–10%)
Purpura (1–10%)
Pyogenic granuloma (1–10%)
   (2002): Diederen PVMM+, *World Congress Dermatol*
     Poster, 0099
Rash (sic) (>10%)
Seborrhea (1–10%)
Shaking (sic)
Stickiness (10–25%)
   (1999): Katz HI+, *J Am Acad Dermatol* 41, S7
   (1997): Buccheri L+, *Arch Dermatol* 133, 711 (18%)
   (1991): Murray HE+, *J Am Acad Dermatol* 24, 598 (8%)
   (1989): Schröder K+, *Acta Derm Venereol* (Stockh) 69, 111 (3%)
   (1988): Geiger J-M+, *Dermatologica* 176, 182 (2.5%)
Sunburn (1–10%)
Ulcerations (1–10%)
Urticaria
Xerosis (25–50%)
   (2001): Berbis P, *Ann Dermatol Venereol* 128(6), 737
   (1999): Katz HI+, *J Am Acad Dermatol* 41, S7 (15–25%)
   (1997): Buccheri L+, *Arch Dermatol* 133, 711 (45.5%)
   (1991): Murray HE+, *J Am Acad Dermatol* 24, 598 (24%)
   (1990): Ruzicka T+, *Arch Dermatol* 126, 482 (48%)
   (1989): Gupta AK+, *J Am Acad Dermatol* 21, 1088 (10–20%)
   (1989): Schröder K+, *Acta Derm Venereol* (Stockh) 69, 111 (65%)
   (1988): Geiger J-M+, *Dermatologica* 176, 182 (30%)

Hair

Hair – alopecia (50–75%)
   (2001): Berbis P, *Ann Dermatol Venereol* 128(6), 737
   (2001): Popescu C, Bucharest, Romania (from Internet)
     (observation)
   (2001): Thaler D, Monona, WI (from Internet) (observation)
     (diffuse)
   (2001): Vedamurthy V, Chennai, India (from Internet)
     (observation) (scalp, mustache, eyebrows & beard)
   (1999): Katz HI+, *J Am Acad Dermatol* 41, S7 (10–25%)
   (1997): Buccheri L+, *Arch Dermatol* 133, 711 (45.5%)
   (1991): Murray HE+, *J Am Acad Dermatol* 24, 598 (33%)
   (1990): Ruzicka T+, *Arch Dermatol* 126, 482 (12%)
   (1989): Gupta AK+, *J Am Acad Dermatol* 21, 1088 (30–70%)
   (1989): Schröder K+, *Acta Derm Venereol* (Stockh) 69, 111
     (13%)
   (1988): Geiger J-M+, *Dermatologica* 176, 182 (20%)
Hair – alopecia (totalis)
   (2002): Chave TA+, *World Congress Dermatol* Poster 0092
     (regrowth in 6 months)
Hair – alopecia universalis
   (1998): Haycox CL, Seattle, WA (from Internet) (observation)
   (1998): Nadel RS, Springfield, MA (from Internet) (observation)
Hair – pili torti
   (2001): Davidson DM, Groton, CT (from Internet) (observation)

Nails

Nails – brittle (sic)
   (1991): Murray HE+, *J Am Acad Dermatol* 24, 598 (27%)
   (1990): Ruzicka T+, *Arch Dermatol* 126, 482
   (1988): Geiger J-M+, *Dermatologica* 176, 182 (10%)
Nails – changes (sic) (25–50%)
Nails – paronychia (10–25%)
   (2002): Hirsch R, Brooklyn, NY (from Internet) (observation)
   (1999): Katz HI+, *J Am Acad Dermatol* 41, S7
   (1997): Buccheri L+, *Arch Dermatol* 133, 711 (18.2%)
   (1991): Murray HE+, *J Am Acad Dermatol* 24, 598 (7%)
Nails – periungual granuloma
   (1997): Buccheri L+, *Arch Dermatol* 133, 711 (9.1%)

Nails – pyogenic granulomas
(1999): Guzick N, Houston, TX (from Internet) (observation)

Other

Bromhidrosis (1–10%)
(2001): Liss WA, Pleasanton, CA (from Internet) (observation)
(2000): Liss WA, Pleasanton, CA (from Internet) (observation)
Dry mucous membranes
(2001): Berbis P, *Ann Dermatol Venereol* 128(6), 737
Gingivitis (1–10%)
Gouty tophi
(1998): Vanhooteghem O+, *Clin Exp Dermatol* 23, 274
Hyperesthesia (10–25%)
(1999): Katz HI+, *J Am Acad Dermatol* 41, S7
Myopathy
(1996): Lister RK+, *Br J Dermatol* 134, 989
Oral mucosal lesions
(1988): Geiger J-M+, *Dermatologica* 176, 182 (6%)
Paresthesias (10–25%)
(1999): Katz HI+, *J Am Acad Dermatol* 41, S7
Pseudotumor cerebri
(1999): Katz HI+, *J Am Acad Dermatol* 41, S7
Sialorrhea (1–10%)
Stomatitis (1–10%)
Ulcerative stomatitis (1–10%)
Vulvovaginal candidiasis
(1995): Sturkenboom MC+, *J Clin Epidemiol* 48, 991
Xerostomia (10–25%)
(1999): Katz HI+, *J Am Acad Dermatol* 41, S7
(1997): Buccheri L+, *Arch Dermatol* 133, 711 (63.6%)
(1989): Schröder K+, *Acta Derm Venereol* (Stockh) 69, 111 (60%)
(1988): Geiger J-M+, *Dermatologica* 176, 182 (30%)

ACTINOMYCIN-D

(See DACTINOMYCIN)

ACYCLOVIR

Synonyms: aciclovir; ACV; acycloguanosine
Trade name: Zovirax (GSK)
Other common trade names: *Acifur; Acyclo-V; Acyvir; Avirax; Herpefug; Zyclir*
Indications: Herpes simplex, herpes zoster
Category: Antiherpes; Antiviral
Half-life: 3 hours (adults)
Clinically important, potentially hazardous interactions with: meperidine, tenofovir

Reactions

Skin

Acne (<3%)
Dermatitis (sic)
(2001): Lammintausta K+, *Contact Dermatitis* 45(3), 181
(2000): Serpentier-Daude A+, *Ann Dermatol Venereol* 127, 191
(1996): Bourezane Y+, *Allergy* 51, 755
(1995): Koch P, *Contact Dermatitis* 33, 255
(1991): Goday J+, *Contact Dermatitis* 24, 381
(1990): Baes H+, *Contact Dermatitis* 23, 200
(1990): Valsecchi R+, *Contact Dermatitis* 23, 372
(1989): Gola M+, *Contact Dermatitis* 20, 394
(1989): O'Brien JJ+, *Drugs* 37, 233 (vesicular)

(1988): Camarasa JG+, *Contact Dermatitis* 19, 235
(1985): Robinson GE+, *Genitourin Med* 61, 62 (palms and soles)
Diaphoresis
Edema
(1991): Medina S+, *Int J Dermatol* 30, 305
Erythema
(2002): Carrasco L+, *Clin Exp Dermatol* 27(2), 132
Erythema nodosum
(1983): Richards DM+, *Drugs* 26, 378
Exanthems (1–5%)
(1991): Whitley R+, *N Engl J Med* 324, 444
(1985): Robinson GE+, *Genitourin Med* 61, 62
(1984): Strauss SE+, *N Engl J Med* 301, 1545
(1983): Balfour HH+, *N Engl J Med* 308, 1448
(1983): Richards DM+, *Drugs* 26, 378
Facial edema (3–5%)
(2000): Colin J+, *Ophthalmology* 107, 1507
Fixed eruption
(1997): Montoro J+, *Contact Dermatitis* 36, 225
Herpes zoster (recurrent)
(1993): Murphy F, *The Schoch Letter* 43, 28, #104 (observation)
Lichenoid eruption
(1985): Robinson GE+, *Genitourin Med* 61, 62
Periorbital edema (3–5%)
(2000): Colin J+, *Ophthalmology* 107, 1507
Peripheral edema
(1991): Medina S+, *Int J Dermatol* 30, 305
(1988): Hisler BM+, *J Am Acad Dermatol* 18, 1142
Photosensitivity
(2001): Schmutz JL+, *Ann Dermatol Venereol* 128, 184
Pruritus (1–10%)
(1993): Goldberg LH+, *Arch Dermatol* 129, 582 (passim)
Radiation recall
(2002): Carrasco L+, *Clin Exp Dermatol* 27(2), 132
(2001): *Ann Dermatol Venereol* 128(2), 184
Rash (sic) (<3%)
(1985): Lundgren G+, *Scand J Infect Dis* Suppl 47, 137
(1983): Balfour HH+, *N Engl J Med* 308, 1448
(1983): Masaoka T+, *Gan To Kagaku Ryoho* (Japanese) 10, 944
Stevens–Johnson syndrome
(1995): Fazal BA+, *Clin Infect Dis* 21, 1038
Urticaria (1–5%)
(1985): Robinson GE+, *Genitourin Med* 61, 62
(1983): Richards DM+, *Drugs* 26, 378
(1982): Smith CI+, *Am J Med* 73, 267
(1981): Balfour HH+, *Minn Med* 64, 739
Vasculitis
(1983): Richards DM+, *Drugs* 26, 378
Vesicular eruptions
(1993): Buck ML+, *Ann Pharmacother* 27, 1458

Hair

Hair – alopecia (<3%)

Other

Anaphylactoid reactions (<1%)
Dysgeusia (0.3%)
Headache
Hypersensitivity
(2001): Kawsar M+, *Sex Transm Infect* 77(3), 204
Injection-site inflammation (>10%)
(1989): O'Brien JJ+, *Drugs* 37, 233
Injection-site necrosis
(1987): Fayol J+, *Therapie* (French) 42(2), 249
Injection-site thrombophlebitis (9%)
(1988): Arndt KA, *J Am Acad Dermatol* 18, 188
Injection-site vesicular eruption
(1986): Sylvester RK+, *JAMA* 255, 385

Paresthesias (<1%)
  (1993): Goldberg LH+, *Arch Dermatol* 129, 582 (passim)
Tremor
Vaginitis (candidal)
  (1993): Goldberg LH+, *Arch Dermatol* 129, 582 (passim)

ADALIMUMAB

Synonym: D2E7
Trade name: Humira (Abbott)
Indications: Rheumatoid arthritis
Category: Anti-TNF-alpha monoclonal antibody
Half-life: 10–20 days

Reactions

Skin
Allergic reactions (sic) (1%)
Carcinoma
Cellulitis
Erysipelas
Flu-like syndrome (7%)
Fungal infections
Herpes zoster
Infections (5%)
Lupus erythematosus (<0.1%)
Lymphoma
  (1998): Baecklund E+, *BMJ* 317(7152), 180
Melanoma
Peripheral edema
Rash (sic) (12%)
Upper respiratory infection (17%)

Other
Back pain (6%)
Death
Headache
Injection-site edema (15.2%)
Injection-site erythema (15.2%)
Injection-site pain (12%)
Myasthenia
Paresthesias
Tendon disorder (sic)
Tremor

Note: TNF blocking agents may lead to serious infections, lymphoma, or fatalities, particularly in patients receiving concomitant immunosuppressive therapy. Patients should be evaluated for latent tuberculosis prior to treatment with adalimumab.

ADAPALENE

Trade names: Adaferin; Differin (Galderma)
Indications: Acne vulgaris
Category: Retinoid (topical)
Half-life: N/A
Clinically important, potentially hazardous interactions with: resorcinol, salicylates

Reactions

Skin
Acne (<1%)

Burning (<1%)
  (2001): Nyirady J+, *J Dermatolog Treat* 12(3), 149
  (2001): Tu P+, *J Eur Acad Dermatol Venereol* 15 (Suppl 3), 31
  (1998): Ellis CN+, *Br J Dermatol* 139, Suppl 52:41
Dermatitis (sic) (<1%)
Eczema (<1%)
Erythema (<1%)
  (2001): Leyden J+, *Cutis* 67(6 Suppl), 17
  (2001): Nyirady J+, *J Dermatolog Treat* 12(3), 149
  (2001): Tu P+, *J Eur Acad Dermatol Venereol* 15, (Suppl 3) 31
  (1998): Ellis CN+, *Br J Dermatol* 139, Suppl 52:41
Eyelid edema (<1%)
Irritation (sic) (<1%)
  (2001): Queille-Roussel C+, *Clin Ther* 23(2), 205
  (1998): Bonardeaux C+, *Rev Med Liege* 53(2), 109 (mild)
Pruritus (<1%)
  (2001): Nyirady J+, *J Dermatolog Treat* 12(3), 149
  (2001): Tu P+, *J Eur Acad Dermatol Venereol* 15 (Suppl 3), 31
  (1998): Ellis CN+, *Br J Dermatol* 139, Suppl 52:41
Rash (sic) (<1%)
Scaling (<1%)
  (2001): Tu P+, *J Eur Acad Dermatol Venereol* 15 (Suppl 3), 31
  (1998): Ellis CN+, *Br J Dermatol* 139, Suppl 52:41
Xerosis (<1%)
  (2001): Leyden J+, *Cutis* 67(6 Suppl), 17
  (2001): Tu P+, *J Eur Acad Dermatol Venereol* 15 (Suppl 3), 31
  (1998): Dunlap FE+, *Br J Dermatol* 139 (Suppl 52), 17 (3 cases)
  (1998): Ellis CN+, *Br J Dermatol* 139, Suppl 52:41

Other
Conjunctivitis

ADEFOVIR

Synonym: GS840
Trade name: Hepsera (Gilead)
Other common trade name: *Preveon*
Indications: HIV infection, Hepatitis B infection
Category: Nucleotide reverse transcriptase inhibitor (NRTI)
Half-life: 16–18 hours
Clinically important, potentially hazardous interactions with: amikacin, amphotericin B, delavirdine, drugs causing kidney toxicity, foscarnet, gentamicin, hydroxyurea, pentamidine, tobramycin

Reactions

Skin
Hot flashes

Other
Headache

ADENOSINE

Trade names: Adenocard (Fujisawa); Adenoscan (Fujisawa)
Other common trade names: *Adenic; Adeno-Jec; Adenocur; Adenoject; Adrecar; Atp; Krenosin; Krenosine*
Indications: Paroxysmal supraventricular tachycardia, varicose vein complications with stasis dermatitis
Category: Antiarrhythmic
Half-life: seconds
Clinically important, potentially hazardous interactions with: carbamazepine, dipyridamole, theophylline

Reactions

Skin
Burning (<1%)
Diaphoresis (<1%)
Flushing (18%)
Rash (sic)

Other
Dizziness (1%)
Dysgeusia (<1%)
Headache
Numbness (1%)
Paresthesias (1%)
Tendinitis

ALBENDAZOLE

Trade name: Albenza (GSK)
Other common trade names: *ABZ; Albezole; Alzol; Bendex; Eskazole; Vermin; Zentel*
Indications: Nematode infections, hydatid cyst disease
Category: Antihelmintic
Half-life: 8–12 hours

Reactions

Skin
Adverse effects (sic)
   (2002): Supali T+, *Trop Med Int Health* 7(10), 894 (with diethylcarbamazine)
Allergic reactions (sic) (<1%)
Dermatitis
   (1991): Macedo NA+, *Contact Dermatitis* 25, 73
Fixed eruption
   (1998): Mahboob A+, *Int J Dermatol* 37, 833
   (1998): Mahboob A+, *JPMA J Pak Med Assoc* 48, 316
Pruritus (<1%)
   (2002): Supali T+, *Trop Med Int Health* 7(10), 894 (with diethylcarbamazine)
Rash (sic) (<1%)
Stevens–Johnson syndrome
   (1997): Dewardt S+, *Acta Derm Venereol* 77, 411
Urticaria (<1%)
   (1991): Macedo NA+, *Contact Dermatitis* 25, 73

Hair
Hair – alopecia (<1%)
   (1993): Tomas S+, *Enferm Infecc Microbiol Clin* (Spanish) 11, 113
   (1990): Pilar-Garcia-Muret M+, *Int J Dermatol* 29, 669

Other
Myalgia
   (2002): Supali T+, *Trop Med Int Health* 7(10), 894 (with diethylcarbamazine)
Xerostomia (<1%)

ALBUTEROL

Synonym: salbutamol
Trade names: AccuNeb (DEY); Airet (Medeva); Combivent (Boehringer Ingelheim); Duoneb (DEY); Proventil (Schering); Ventolin (GSK); Volmax (Muro)
Other common trade names: *Asmaven; Broncho-Spray; Cobutolin; Salbulin; Ventoline*
Indications: Bronchospasm associated with asthma
Category: Beta-2-adrenergic agonist; Bronchodilator (sympathomimetic)
Half-life: 3–6 hours
Clinically important, potentially hazardous interactions with: atomoxetine, epinephrine

Combivent is albuterol and ipratropium

Reactions

Skin
Angioedema
Chills
Dermatitis
   (1994): Smeenk G+, *Contact Dermatitis* 31, 123
Diaphoresis (1–10%)
   (1989): Price AH+, *Drugs* 38, 77
Erythema (palmar) (with infusion)
   (1992): Lebre C+, *Ann Dermatol Venereol* (French) 119, 293
   (1990): Morin Leport LRM+, *Br J Dermatol* 122, 116
Exanthems
Flushing (1–10%)
Lupus erythematosus (pseudo-lupus)
   (1987): Lacour JP+, *Presse Med* (French) 16, 1599
Pallor
Pruritus
   (1991): Hatton MQ+, *Lancet* 337, 1169
Shaking (sic)
Urticaria
   (1991): Hatton MQ+, *Lancet* 337, 1169

Other
Dysgeusia (1–10%)
Headache
Tinnitus
Tremor
Xerostomia (1–10%)

ALDESLEUKIN

Synonyms: IL-2; interleukin-2
Trade name: Proleukin (Chiron)
Other common trade names: *Aerovent; Atem; Atronase; Narilet*
Indications: Metastatic renal cell carcinoma
Category: Antineoplastic; Biologic response modulator
Half-life: 6–85 minutes
**Clinically important, potentially hazardous interactions
with:** altretamine, amikacin, aminoglycosides, antineoplastics,
bleomycin, busulfan, carboplatin, carmustine, chlorambucil,
cisplatin, corticosteroids, cyclophosphamide, cytarabine,
dacarbazine, dactinomycin, daunorubicin, docetaxel, doxorubicin,
estramustine, etoposide, fludarabine, fluorouracil, gemcitabine,
gentamicin, hydroxyurea, idarubicin, ifosfamide, indomethacin,
kanamycin, levamisole, lomustine, mechlorethamine, melphalan,
mercaptopurine, methotrexate, mitomycin, mitotane,
mitoxantrone, neomycin, pentostatin, plicamycin, procarbazine,
streptomycin, streptozocin, thioguanine, thiotepa, tobramycin,
tretinoin, uracil, vinblastine, vincristine, vinorelbine

Reactions

Skin

Allergic reactions (sic) (<1%)
Angioedema
  (1992): Baars JW+, *Ann Oncol* 3, 243
Bullous eruption
  (1991): Staunton MR, *J Natl Cancer Inst* 83, 56
Bullous pemphigoid
  (1993): Fellner MJ, *Clin Dermatol* 11, 515
Dermatitis (sic)
  (1989): Kerker BJ+, *Semin Dermatol* 8, 173
  (1987): Gaspari AA+, *JAMA* 258, 1624 (1–5%)
Desquamation
  (2001): Chi KH+, *Oncology* 60, 110
Eczema reactivation
  (1997): Cork MJ+, *Br J Dermatol* 136, 644
Edema (47%)
  (1994): Rosenberg SA+, *JAMA* 271, 907
  (1990): Chien CH+, *Pediatrics* 86, 937
Erythema (sic) (41%)
  (1993): Wolkenstein P+, *J Am Acad Dermatol* 28, 66
  (1992): Blessing K+, *J Pathol* 167, 313
  (1988): Lee RE+, *Arch Dermatol* 124, 1811
  (1987): Gaspari AA+, *JAMA* 258, 1624
Erythema nodosum
  (1989): Kerker BJ+, *Semin Dermatol* 8, 173
  (1987): Weinstein A+, *JAMA* 258, 3120
Erythroderma
  (1992): Blessing K+, *J Pathol* 167, 313
  (1991): Siegel JP+, *J Clin Oncol* 9, 694 (>5%)
  (1989): Kerker BJ+, *Semin Dermatol* 8, 173
  (1987): Gaspari AA+, *JAMA* 258, 1624
Exanthems
  (1991): Dummer R+, *Dermatologica* 183, 95
  (1991): Siegel JP+, *J Clin Oncol* 9, 694 (>5%)
  (1989): Jost LM+, *Schweiz Med Wochenschr* (German) 119, 137
  (1987): Gaspari AA+, *JAMA* 258, 1624
Exfoliative dermatitis (14%)
  (1993): Larbre B+, *Ann Dermatol Venereol* (French) 120, 528
Graft-versus-host reaction
  (1995): Costello R+, *Bone Marrow Transplant* 16, 199
Granulomatous dermatitis (Churg–Strauss syndrome)
  (1997): Shiota Y+, *Inren Med* 36, 709
Intertriginous cutaneous eruption (sic)

  (1996): Prussick R+, *J Am Acad Dermatol* 35, 705
Kaposi's sarcoma
  (1989): Krigel RL+, *J Biol Response Mod* 8, 359
Linear IgA bullous dermatosis
  (2002): Cohen LM+, *J Am Acad Dermatol* 46, S32 (passim)
  (1996): Tranvan A+, *J Am Acad Dermatol* 35, 865
  (1993): Oeda E+, *Am J Hematol* 44, 213
  (1990): Guillaume JC+, *Ann Dermatol Venereol* (French) 117, 899
Necrosis
  (1993): Wolkenstein P+, *J Am Acad Dermatol* 28, 66
  (1988): Rosenberg SA+, *Ann Intern Med* 108, 853 (3%)
Pemphigus
  (1995): Wolkenstein P+, *Arch Dermatol* 130, 890
  (1994): Prussick R+, *Arch Dermatol* 130, 890
  (1989): Ramseur WL+, *Cancer* 63, 2005 (fatal)
Peripheral edema (1–10%)
Petechiae (4%)
Photosensitivity
  (1992): Blessing K+, *J Pathol* 167, 313
Pruritus (48%)
  (2001): Chi KH+, *Oncology* 60(2), 110
  (1995): Wahlgren CF+, *Arch Dermatol Res* 287, 572
  (1994): Rosenberg SA+, *JAMA* 271, 907
  (1993): Wolkenstein P+, *J Am Acad Dermatol* 28, 66
  (1988): Lee RE+, *Arch Dermatol* 124, 1811
  (1987): Gaspari AA+, *JAMA* 258, 1624
Psoriasis
  (1991): Siegel JP+, *J Clin Oncol* 9, 694 (>5%)
  (1989): Kerker BJ+, *Semin Dermatol* 8, 173
  (1988): Lee RE+, *Arch Dermatol* 124, 1811 (exacerbation)
  (1987): Gaspari AA+, *JAMA* 258, 1624
Purpura (4%)
  (1989): Kerker BJ+, *Semin Dermatol* 8, 173
Rash (sic) (26%)
Sarcoidosis
  (2000): Blanche P+, *Clin Infect Dis* 31, 1493
Scleroderma
  (1994): Boni R, *Dermatology* 189, 330
  (1994): Puett DW+, *J Rheumatol* 21, 752
Toxic epidermal necrolysis
  (1992): Wiener JS+, *South Med J* 85, 656
Urticaria (2%)
  (1993): Wolkenstein P+, *J Am Acad Dermatol* 28, 66
  (1992): Baars JW+, *Ann Oncol* 3, 243
Vitiligo
  (1996): Rosenberg SA+, *J Immunother Emphasis Tumor Immunol*
    19, 81
  (1995): Wolkenstein P+, *Arch Dermatol* 130, 890
  (1994): Scheibenbogen C+, *Eur J Cancer* (30A) 8, 1209
Xerosis (15%)

Hair
Hair – alopecia (<1%)
  (1989): Jost LM+, *Schweiz Med Wochenschr* (German) 119, 137
  (1987): Gaspari AA+, *JAMA* 258, 1624 (10%)

Other
Aphthous stomatitis
  (1987): Gaspari AA+, *JAMA* 258, 1624 (5%)
Death
Depression
  (2001): Maes M+, *Mol Psychiatry* 6(4), 475
Dysgeusia (7%)
Glossitis
  (1987): Gaspari AA+, *JAMA* 258, 1624 (30%)
Headache
Injection-site inflammation
  (1999): Asadullah K+, *Arch Dermatol* 135, 187

Injection-site nodules (sic)
  (1993): Klapholtz L+, *Bone Marrow Transplant* 11, 443
Injection-site panniculitis
  (1992): Baars JW+, *Br J Cancer* 66, 698
Injection-site reactions (sic) (3%)
  (2002): Assmann K+, *Hautarzt* 53(8), 554
Myalgia (6%)
Oral mucosal eruption
  (1989): Kerker BJ+, *Semin Dermatol* 8, 173
  (1987): Gaspari AA+, *JAMA* 258, 1624
Oral ulceration
  (1990): Chien CH+, *Pediatrics* 86, 937
Rhabdomyolysis
  (1995): Anderlini P+, *Cancer* 76(4), 678
Stomatitis (32%)
Xerostomia
  (2001): Chi KH+, *Oncology* 60, 110

ALEFACEPT

Trade name: Amevive (Biogen)
Indications: Chronic plaque psoriasis (in adults)
Category: Immunomodulator; recombinant human LFA-3/imunoglobulin G-1 fusion protein; T-cell blocker
Half-life: 270 hours

Reactions

Skin
Adverse effects (sic) (2.5%)
  (2002): Krueger GG+, *J Am Acad Dermatol* 47(6), 821
  (2001): Ellis CN+, *N Engl J Med* 345(4), 248
Angioedema
  (2002): Cather J+, *Am J Clin Dermatol* 3(3), 159
Chills (transient) (<2%)
  (2003): Kimball AB+, *Poster, American Academy of Dermatology Meeting* San Francisco, CA
  (2002): Krueger GG+, *J Am Acad Dermatol* 47(6), 821
  (2001): Ellis CN+, *N Engl J Med* 345(4), 248
Eruptions
Flu-like syndrome
  (2002): Cather J+, *Am J Clin Dermatol* 3(3), 159
Herpes simplex
  (2002): Cather J+, *Am J Clin Dermatol* 3(3), 159
Infections (0.7–1.5%)
  (2002): Krueger GG+, *J Am Acad Dermatol* 47(6), 821
  (2001): Ellis CN+, *N Engl J Med* 345(4), 248
Itching
Lymphoma (3 cases)
Malignancies (1.3%)
Necrotizing cellulitis
Pruritus (2–5%)
Urticaria (<1%)

Other
Cough (<2%)
  (2001): Ellis CN+, *N Engl J Med* 345(4), 248
Dizziness (<2%)
  (2001): Ellis CN+, *N Engl J Med* 345(4), 248
Headache
Hypersensitivity
Injection-site bleeding (4%)
Injection-site edema (2%)
Injection-site hypersensitivity
Injection-site inflammation (4%)

Injection-site pain (7%)
Myalgia (2–5%)
Pharyngitis (<2%)
  (2002): Krueger GG+, *J Am Acad Dermatol* 47(6), 821
  (2001): Ellis CN+, *N Engl J Med* 345(4), 248

ALEMTUZUMAB

Synonyms: Campath-1H; DNA-derived Humanized Monoclonal Antibody; Humanized IgG1 Anti-CD52 Monoclonal Antibody
Trade names: Campath (Berlex); MabCampath (Schering)
Indications: B-cell chronic lymphocytic leukemia, non-Hodgkin's lymphoma
Category: Antineoplastic; Recombinant DNA-derived humanized monoclonal antibody
Half-life: 12 days

Note: Prophylactic therapy against PCP pneumonia and herpes viral infections is recommended upon initiation of therapy and for at least 2 months following last dose

Reactions

Skin
Allergic reactions (sic) (<1%)
Angioedema (<1%)
Bullous eruption (<1%)
Cellulitis (<1%)
Chills
  (2000): Flynn JM+, *Curr Opin Oncol* 12(6), 574
Facial edema (<1%)
Flushing
  (2000): Tang SC+, *Leuk Lymphoma* 24(1-2), 93
Hematomas (<1%)
Infections (sic)
  (2002): Keating MJ+, *J Clin Oncol* 20(1), 205
  (2002): Lundin J+, *Blood* 100(3), 768
  (2002): Rai KR+, *J Clin Oncol* 20(18), 3891
  (2001): Khorana A+, *Leuk Lymphoma* 41(1), 77
  (2000): Tang SC+, *Leuk Lymphoma* 24(1-2), 93
  (1998): Lundin J+, *J Clin Oncol* 16(10), 3257
Peripheral edema (13%)
Purpura (8%)
Squamous cell carcinoma (<1%)
Urticaria
  (2000): Tang SC+, *Leuk Lymphoma* 24(1-2), 93

Other
Anaphylactoid reactions (<1%)
Death
  (2002): Keating MJ+, *J Clin Oncol* 20(1), 205 (2 cases)
  (1998): Lundin J+, *J Clin Oncol* 16(10), 3257
Depression (7%)
Dysesthesia (15%)
Dysgeusia (<1%)
Gingivitis (<1%)
Headache
Injection-site pruritus (30–40%)
Injection-site rash (14–24%)
Injection-site reactions (sic)
  (2002): Keating MJ+, *Blood* 99(10), 3554
  (2002): Keating MJ+, *J Clin Oncol* 20(1), 205
  (2002): Lundin J+, *Blood* 100(3), 768 (90%)
  (2001): Khorana A+, *Leuk Lymphoma* 41(1), 77
Lymphoproliferative disease (64% to 70%)

Malignant lymphoma (<1%)
Myalgia (11%)
Myositis (<1%)
Phlebitis (<1%)
Polymyositis (<1%)
Stomatitis (14%)
Stomatodynia
Thrombophlebitis (<1%)

ALENDRONATE

Trade name: Fosamax (Merck)
Other common trade name: *Fosalan*
Indications: Osteoporosis in postmenopausal women, Paget's disease
Category: Biphosphonate; Inhibitor of bone resorption
Half-life: >10 years

Reactions

Skin
Erythema (<1%)
  (1996): Keen RW+, *Br J Clin Pract* 50, 211
Erythema multiforme
  (2000): Madnani N, Mumbai, India (from Internet) (observation)
Exanthems
  (2000): Madnani N, Mumbai, India (from Internet) (observation)
Fixed eruption
  (1998): McCarthy J, Ft. Worth, TX (from Internet) (observation)
Peripheral edema
Petechiae
  (1997): Berger R, St. George, UT (from Internet) (observation)
Pruritus (0.6%)
  (2000): Madnani N, Mumbai, India (from Internet) (observation)
  (1997): Kyriakidou-Himonas M+, *Advances in Therapy* 14, 281
Rash (sic) (<1%)
  (1997): Berger R, St. George, UT (from Internet) (observation)
  (1996): Freedholm D+, *Osteoporosis Int* 6, 261
  (1996): Keen RW+, *Br J Clin Pract* 50, 211
  (1996): Selby PL, *Osteoporosis Int* 6, S21
  (1995): Chestnut CH+, *Am J Med* 99, 144

Other
Conjunctivitis
  (2003): Frauenfelder FW+, *N Engl J Med* 348, 1187
Dysgeusia (0.6%)
  (1997): Kyriakidou-Himonas M+, *Advances in Therapy* 14, 281
Headache
Hypersensitivity
  (1996): Kirk JK+, *Am Fam Physician* 54, 2053
Ocular inflammation
  (1999): Mbekeani JN+, *Arch Ophthalmol* 117, 837
Ocular irritation
  (2003): Frauenfelder FW+, *N Engl J Med* 348, 1187
Oral ulceration
  (1999): Demerjian N+, *Clin Rheumatol* 18, 349
Seizures
  (2002): MacIsaac RJ+, *J R Soc Med* 95(12), 615

ALFENTANIL

Trade name: Alfenta (Taylor)
Other common trade name: *Rapifen*
Indications: General anesthesia, post-operative pain
Category: Narcotic agonist analgesic
Half-life: 83–97 minutes (adults)
Clinically important, potentially hazardous interactions with: erythromycin, ranitidine, ritonavir

Reactions

Skin
Clammy skin (<1%)
Pruritus (<1%)
  (1999): Kyriakides K+, *Br J Anaesth* 82, 439
Rash (sic) (<1%)
Shivering (sic) (3–9%)
Urticaria (<1%)

Other
Dysesthesia

ALITRETINOIN

Trade name: Panretin (Ligand)
Indications: Kaposi's sarcoma cutaneous lesions
Category: Antineoplastic retinoic acid derivative
Half-life: N/A

Reactions

Skin
Abrasion
Adverse effects (sic)
  (2000): Duvic M+, *Arch Dermatol* 136, 1461 (17%)
Bullous eruption
Burning
  (2002): Morganroth GS, *Arch Dermatol* 138, 542
Edema (3–8%)
  (2000): Duvic M+, *Arch Dermatol* 136, 1461 (3%)
Exfoliative dermatitis (3–9%)
Flushing
Photosensitivity
Pigmentation (3%)
  (2000): Duvic M+, *Arch Dermatol* 136, 1461 (3%)
Pruritus (8–11%)
Rash (sic) (25–77%)
  (2000): Duvic M+, *Arch Dermatol* 136, 1461 (69%)
Toxicity (sic)
  (2002): Miles SA+, *AIDS* 16(3), 421
Ulcerations (2%)
  (2000): Duvic M+, *Arch Dermatol* 136, 1461
Xerosis (10%)
  (2000): Duvic M+, *Arch Dermatol* 136, 1461 (10%)

Hair
Hair – alopecia

Other
Application-site dermatitis
  (2002): Morganroth GS, *Arch Dermatol* 138, 542
Application-site reactions
  (1999): Walmsley S+, *J Acquir Immune Defic Syndr* 22, 325

Myalgia
Pain
   (2000): Duvic M+, *Arch Dermatol* 136, 1461 (18%)
Paresthesias (3–22%)

ALLOPURINOL

Trade name: Zyloprim (Promtheus)
Other common trade names: *Allo 300; Allo-Puren; Alloprin; Atisuril; Bleminol; Caplenal; Hamarin; Novo-Purol; Purinol; Unizuric; Zyloric*
Indications: Gouty arthritis
Category: Antigout; Uricosuric
Half-life: 1–3 hours
Clinically important, potentially hazardous interactions with: amoxicillin, ampicillin, azathioprine, dicumarol, mercaptopurine

Reactions

Skin

Acute generalized exanthematous pustulosis (AGEP)
   (1995): Moreau A+, *Int J Dermatol* 34, 263 (passim)
Allergic reactions (sic) (severe)
   (1999): Tanna SB+, *Ann Pharmacother* 33 1180
Angiitis (<1%)
Angioedema
   (1996): Yale SH+, *Hosp Pract Off Ed* 31, 92
Chills (1–10%)
Diaphoresis (<1%)
Ecchymoses (<1%)
Edema (periorbital)
   (1981): McInnes GT+, *Ann Rheum Dis* 40, 245
Erythema multiforme (<1%)
   (2001): Perez A+, *Contact Dermatitis* 44, 113 (with amoxicillin)
   (1999): Fonseka MM+, *Ceylon Med J* 44, 190
   (1996): Kumar A+, *BMJ* 312, 173
   (1984): Pennell DJ+, *Lancet* 1, 463
   (1979): Lupton GP+, *J Am Acad Dermatol* 1, 365
Exanthems (1–5%)
   (2003): Masaki T+, *Acta Derm Venereol* 83(2), 128
   (2001): Fam AG+, *Arthritis Rheum* 44, 231
   (1998): Dintiman B, Fairfax, VA (from Internet) (observation)
   (1992): Fam AG+, *Am J Med* 93, 299
   (1989): Chan SH+, *Dermatologica* 179, 32
   (1987): Hoigné R+, *N Engl J Med* 316, 1217
   (1984): Hande KR+, *Am J Med* 76, 47
   (1981): Jick H+, *J Clin Pharmacol* 21, 456 (with ampicillin 14%)
   (1981): McInnes GT+, *Ann Rheum Dis* 40, 245
   (1979): Lang GP+, *South Med J* 72, 1361
   (1979): Lupton GP+, *J Am Acad Dermatol* 1, 365
   (1976): Lockard O+, *Ann Intern Med* 85, 333
   (1976): Utsinger PD+, *Am J Med* 61, 287
   (1971): Mills RM, *JAMA* 216, 799
Exanthems (generalized)
   (2003): Masaki T+, *Acta Derm Venereol* 83(2), 128
Exfoliative dermatitis (>10%)
   (2001): Dominguez Ortega J+, *An Med Intern* 18(1), 27
   (1996): Emmerson BT, *N Engl J Med* 334, 445
   (1996): Sigurdsson V+, *J Am Acad Dermatol* 35, 53
   (1989): Chan SH+, *Dermatologica* 179, 32
   (1984): Vinciullo C, *Aust J Dermatol* 25, 59
   (1979): Lang GP+, *South Med J* 72, 1361
   (1979): Lupton GP+, *J Am Acad Dermatol* 1, 365
   (1977): Boyer TD+, *West J Med* 126, 143
   (1976): McMenamin RA+, *Aust N Z J Med* 6, 583

   (1975): Sisca TS, *J Clin Pharmacol* 15, 566
   (1973): Feuerman EJ+, *Br J Dermatol* 89, 83
   (1966): Rundles RW+, *Ann Intern Med* 64, 229
Fixed eruption (<1%)
   (2001): Dominguez Ortega J+, *An Med Intern* 18(1), 27
   (1999): Sehgal VN+, *J Dermatol* 26, 198 (transitory giant)
   (1998): Mahboob A+, *Int J Dermatol* 37, 833
   (1998): Umpierrez A+, *J Allergy Clin Immunol* 101, 286
   (1996): Gimbel Moral LF+, *Med Clin (Barc)* (Spanish) 106, 119
   (1996): Kelso JM+, *J Allergy Clin Immunol* 97, 1171
   (1990): Audicana M+, *Clin Exp Allergy* 20(Supp 1), 121
Graft-versus-host reaction
   (1998): Jappe U+, *Hautarzt* (German) 49, 126
Granuloma annulare (disseminated)
   (1995): Becker D+, *Hautarzt* (German) 46, 343
Ichthyosis
   (1968): Auerbach R+, *Arch Dermatol* 98, 104
Lichen planus (<1%)
Lupus erythematosus
   (1980): Condemi JJ, *Geriatrics* 35(3), 81
   (1978): Pereyo-Torrellas N, *Arch Dermatol* 114, 1097
   (1975): Lee SL+, *Semin Arthritis Rheum* 5, 83
Lymphocytoma cutis
   (1988): Raymond JZ+, *Cutis* 41, 323
Necrotizing angiitis
Perforating foot ulceration
   (1997): Bouloc A+, *Clin Exp Dermatol* 21, 351
Petechiae
   (1977): Chan HL+, *Aust N Z J Med* 7, 518
Photosensitivity
   (1986): Lerman S, *Ophthalmology* 93, 304
Pruritus (<1%)
   (2001): Dominguez Ortega J+, *An Med Intern* 18(1), 27
   (2001): Fam AG+, *Arthritis Rheum* 44, 231
   (1998): Dintiman B, Fairfax, VA (from Internet) (observation)
   (1979): Lang GP+, *South Med J* 72, 1361
   (1979): Lupton GP+, *J Am Acad Dermatol* 1, 365
   (1965): Klinenberg JR+, *Ann Intern Med* 62, 639
Purpura (>10%)
   (1979): Lang GP+, *South Med J* 72, 1361
   (1977): Boyer TD+, *West J Med* 126, 143
Pustules
   (2002): Lun K+, *Australas J Dermatol* 43(2), 140
Pustuloderma
   (1994): Fitzgerald DA+, *Clin Exp Dermatol* 19, 243
Rash (sic) (>10%)
   (2001): Dominguez Ortega J+, *An Med Intern* 18(1), 27
   (1996): Yale SH+, *Hosp Pract Off Ed* 31, 92
Sensitivity (sic)
   (1979): Haughey DB+, *Am J Hosp Pharm* 36, 1377
Stevens–Johnson syndrome (>10%)
   (1995): Roujeau JC+, *N Engl J Med* 333, 1600
   (1993): Leenutaphong V+, *Int J Dermatol* 32, 428
   (1992): Goodglick TA+, *Ophthalmic Surg* 23, 557
   (1989): Chan SH+, *Dermatologica* 179, 32
   (1985): Edwards R+, *Dimens Crit Care Nurs* 4, 335
   (1985): Renwick IG, *BMJ* 291, 485
   (1985): Ting HC+, *Int J Dermatol* 24, 587
   (1984): Pennell DJ+, *Lancet* 1, 463 (fatal)
   (1979): Lupton GP+, *J Am Acad Dermatol* 1, 365
   (1978): Assaad D+, *Can Med Assoc* 118, 154
   (1977): Chan HL+, *Aust N Z J Med* 7, 518
Toxic epidermal necrolysis
   (2002): Correia O+, *Arch Dermatol* 138, 29 (2 cases)
   (2001): Hammer B+, *Dtsch Med Wochenschr* 126(47), 1331
   (1999): Sorkin MJ, Denver, CO (from Internet) (observation)
   (1995): Roujeau JC+, *N Engl J Med* 333, 1600
   (1995): Wolkenstein P+, *Arch Dermatol* 131, 544

(1994): Alfandari S+, *Infection* 22, 365
(1993): Correia O+, *Dermatology* 186, 32
(1993): Leenutaphong V+, *Int J Dermatol* 32, 428
(1991): Sakellariou G+, *Int J Artif Organs* 14, 634
(1987): Guillaume JC+, *Arch Dermatol* 123, 1166
(1986): Kumar L, *Indian J Dermatol* 31, 53
(1985): Auboeck J+, *BMJ* 290, 1969
(1985): Renwick IG, *BMJ* 291, 485
(1985): Zakraoui L+, *Tunis Med* (French) 63, 167
(1984): Chan HL, *J Am Acad Dermatol* 10, 973
(1984): Dan M+, *Int J Dermatol* 23, 142
(1979): Lang GP+, *South Med J* 72, 1361
(1979): Lupton GP+, *J Am Acad Dermatol* 1, 365
(1978): Assaad D+, *Can Med Assoc* 118, 154
(1977): Bennett TO+, *Arch Ophthalmol* 95, 1362 (ocular)
(1977): Chan HL+, *Aust N Z J Med* 7, 518
(1976): Fellner MJ, *Arch Dermatol* 112, 1327
(1975): Ellman MH+, *Arch Dermatol* 111, 986
(1975): Sisca TS, *J Clin Pharmacol* 15, 566
(1975): Trentham DE+, *N Engl J Med* 292, 870
(1972): Stratigos JD+, *Br J Dermatol* 86, 564
(1970): Kantor GL, *JAMA* 212, 478 (fatal)
Toxic erythema
    (1995): Rademaker M, *N Z Med J* 108, 165
Toxic pustuloderma
    (1994): Boffa MJ+, *Br J Dermatol* 131, 447
    (1994): Fitzgerald DA+, *Clin Exp Dermatol* 19, 243
    (1993): Yu RC+, *Br J Dermatol* 128, 95
Urticaria (>10%)
    (2001): Dominguez Ortega J+, *An Med Interna* 18(1), 27
    (1999): Litt JZ, Beachwood, OH (personal case) (observation)
    (1992): Breathnach SM+, *Adverse Drug Reactions and the Skin* Blackwell, Oxford, 193 (passim)
    (1991): Anderson MH+, *Ann Allergy* 66, 207
Vasculitis (<1%)
    (2001): Dominguez Ortega J+, *An Med Intern* 18(1), 27
    (1998): Choi HK+, *Clin Exp Rheumatol* 16, 743
    (1996): Emmerson BT, *N Engl J Med* 334, 445
    (1977): Boyer TD+, *West J Med* 126, 143
    (1976): Bailey RR+, *Lancet* 2, 907
    (1971): Mills RM, *JAMA* 216, 799

Hair
Hair – alopecia (1–10%)
    (1974): Lovatt GE, *Br J Dermatol* 91, 115
    (1968): Auerbach R+, *Arch Dermatol* 98, 104

Nails
Nails – onycholysis (<1%)

Other
Death
    (2002): Correia O+, *Arch Dermatol* 138, 29 (one case)
    (2001): Hammer B+, *Dtsch Med Wochenschr* 126(47), 1331
DRESS syndrome
    (2001): Descamps V+, *Arch Dermatol* 137, 301 (passim)
Dysgeusia
Headache
Hypersensitivity*
    (2003): Masaki T+, *Acta Derm Venereol* 83(2), 128
    (2002): Perez Pimiento AJ+, *Rev Clin Esp* 202(6), 339
    (2002): Sommers LM+, *Arch Intern Med* 162(10), 1190
    (2001): Arakawa M+, *Intern Med* 40(4), 331
    (2001): Benito-Leon J+, *Eur Neurol* 45, 186
    (2001): Dominguez Ortega J+, *An Med Interna* 18(1), 27
    (2001): Hammer B+, *Dtsch Med Wochenschr* 126(47), 1331
    (2001): Rivas Gonzalez P+, *Rev Clin Esp* 201(8), 493
    (1999): Gillott TJ+, *Rheumatology* (Oxford) 38, 85
    (1999): Melsom RD, *Rheumatology* 38, 1301 (familial)
    (1999): Morel D+, *Nephrol Dial Transplant* 14, 780
    (1998): Kluger E, *Ugeskr Laeger* (Danish) 160, 1179

(1998): Pluim HJ+, *Neth J Med* 52, 107
(1997): Carpenter C, *Tenn Med* 90, 151
(1996): Kumar A+, *BMJ* 312, 173
(1995): Elasy T+, *West J Med* 162, 360
(1994): Lee SS+, *Chung Hua Min Kuo Wei Sheng Wu Chi Mien I Hsueh Tsa Chih* 27, 140
(1994): Salinas Martin A+, *Aten Primaria* (Spanish) 14, 694
(1989): Puig JG+, *J Rheumatol* 16, 842
(1988): McDonald J+, *J Rheumatol* 15, 865
(1985): Stein CM, *S Afr Med J* 67, 935
(1984): Vinciullo C, *Aust J Dermatol* 25, 59
(1984): Vinciullo C, *Med J Aust* 141, 449
(1979): Lupton GP+, *J Am Acad Dermatol* 1, 365
(1976): Utsinger PD+, *Am J Med* 61, 287
Mucocutaneous eruption
Myalgia
    (2002): Terawaki H+, *Nippon Jinzo Gakkai Shi* 44, 50
    (1996): Ghanem BM+, *J Egypt Soc Parasitol* 26, 619
Myopathy (<1%)
Oral ulceration
    (1984): Chau NY+, *Oral Surg Oral Med Oral Pathol* 58, 397 (lichenoid)
    (1979): Lang GP+, *South Med J* 72, 1361
Paresthesias (<1%)
Polyarteritis nodosa
    (1976): Bailey RR+, *Lancet* 2, 907
    (1974): Young JL+, *Arch Intern Med* 134, 553
    (1970): Jarzobski J+, *Am Heart J* 79, 116
Pseudolymphoma
    (1993): Kerl H+, *Dermatology in General Medicine* McGraw-Hill New York
Stomatitis
    (1981): McInnes GT+, *Ann Rheum Dis* 40, 245
    (1977): Chan HL+, *Aust N Z J Med* 7, 518 (ulcerative)
Thrombophlebitis (<1%)
Tinnitus
Tongue edema (<1%)

*Note: The antiepileptic drug hypersensitivity syndrome is a severe, occasionally fatal, disorder characterized by any or all of the following: pruritic exanthem, toxic epidermal necrolysis, Stevens–Johnson syndrome, exfoliative dermatitis, fever, hepatic abnormalities, eosinophilia, and renal failure

ALMOTRIPTAN

Trade name: Axert (Pharmacia)
Indications: Migraine headaches
Category: Serotonin 5-Ht1d receptor agonist
Half-life: 3–4 hours
Clinically important, potentially hazardous interactions with: dihydroergotamine, ergotamine, ketoconazole, methysergide

Reactions

Skin
Chills (<1%)
Dermatitis (sic)
Diaphoresis (<1%)
Erythema (<1%)
Flu-like syndrome (12%)
    (2001): Cabarrocas X+, *Headache* 41, 57 (5.62%)
Photosensitivity (<1%)
Pruritus (<1%)
Rash (sic) (<1%)
Upper respiratory infection (20%)

Other

Arthralgia (<1%)
Bone or joint pain
  (2002): Keam SJ+, *Drugs* 62(2), 387
Depression (<1%)
Dizziness
  (2002): Balbisi EA, *Am J Health Syst Pharm* 59(22), 2184
Dysgeusia (<1%)
Fatigue
  (2002): Balbisi EA, *Am J Health Syst Pharm* 59(22), 2184
Headache
Hyperesthesia (<1%)
Injection-site irritation
  (2001): Cabarrocas X, *Clin Ther* 23(11), 1867
Myalgia (<1%)
Myopathy (<1%)
Paresthesias (1%)
  (2002): Balbisi EA, *Am J Health Syst Pharm* 59(22), 2184
  (2002): Keam SJ+, *Drugs* 62(2), 387
  (2001): Dodick DW, *Headache* 41(5), 449
Parosmia (<1%)
Sialorrhea (<1%)
Tinnitus (<1%)
Xerostomia (1%)
  (2002): Balbisi EA, *Am J Health Syst Pharm* 59(22), 2184

ALOE VERA (GEL, JUICE, LEAF)

Scientific names: *Aloë africana; Aloë barbadensis; Aloë ferox; Aloë spicata*
Family: Liliaceae
Trade and other common names: Barbados aloe; Curacau aloe; Kumari; Lu Hui; SaliCept Patch (Carrington Labs)
Category: Anti-inflammatory; Antiseptic
Purported indications and other uses: Oral: anesthetic, antiseptic, antipyretic, antipruritic, vasodilator, anti-inflammatory, vermifuge, antifungal. antiulcer, diabetes, asthma. Topical: promote healing, cold sores, ulceration, radiations injuries, psoriasis, frostbite. Also used in cosmetics and for its moisturizing and emollient properties
Half-life: N/A

Reactions

Skin

Allergic reactions (sic)
  (1999): Reynolds T+, *J Ethnopharmacol* 68(1–3), 3
  (1974): Diba SA, *Zh Ushn Nos Gorl Bolezn* Mar-Apr 0(2), 108
    (from juice)
Dermatitis

Other

Anaphylactoid reactions
  (1970): Trakhtenberg SB, *Klin Med* (Mosk) (following injection)
Hypersensitivity
  (1980): Morrow DM+, *Arch Dermatol* 116, 1064
Side effects (sic)
  (2000): Ernst E, *Br J Dermatol* 143(5), 923

Note: *"I have perfumed my bed with myrrh, aloes and cinnamon" (Proverbs 7:17)
* Cleopatra regarded the gel as a fountain of youth and used it to preserve her skin against the ravages of the Egyptian sun.
* One blade of aloe can be used for weeks. The severed end of the blade is self healing.

ALOSETRON

Trade name: Lotronex (GSK)
Indications: Irritable bowel syndrome
Category: 5-HT3 receptor antagonist
Half-life: 1.5 hours

Reactions

Skin

Acne (<1%)
Allergic reactions (sic) (<1%)
Bacterial infections
Folliculitis (<1%)
Hematomas (<1%)

Other

Dysgeusia (<1%)
Parosmia (<1%)

ALPRAZOLAM

Trade name: Xanax (Pharmacia)
Other common trade names: *Alprox; APO-Alpraz; Cassadan; Kalma; Nu-Alprax; Ralozam; Tafil*
Indications: Anxiety, depression, panic attacks
Category: Benzodiazepine anxiolytic
Half-life: 11–16 hours
Clinically important, potentially hazardous interactions with: alcohol, aprepitant, clarithromycin, CNS depressants, delavirdine, digoxin, efavirenz, fluconazole, fluoxetine, fluvoxamine, **grapefruit juice**, indinavir, itraconazole, ivermectin, **kava**, ketoconazole, propoxyphene, ritonavir, saquinavir

Reactions

Skin

Acne
  (1985): Levy MH+, *Semin Oncol* 12, 411
Allergic reactions (sic)
  (1996): Bhatia MS, *Indian J Med Sci* 50, 285 (to the tartrazine
    dye)
Dermatitis (sic) (3.8%)
  (1984): Elie R+, *J Clin Psychopharmacol* 4, 125
  (1982): Fawcett JA+, *Pharmacotherapy* 2, 243
  (1981): Evans RL, *Drug Intell Clin Pharm* 15, 633
  (1981): Kolin IS+, *J Clin Psychiatry* 42, 169
  (1976): Fabre LF, *Curr Ther Res* 19, 661
Diaphoresis (15.8%)
Edema (4.9%)
Exanthems
  (1988): Warnock JK+, *Am J Psychiatry* 145, 425
Photosensitivity
  (1999): Watanabe Y+, *J Am Acad Dermatol* 40, 832
  (1998): Pazzagli L+, *Pharm World Sci* 20, 136 (with fluoxetine)
  (1994): Shelley WB+, *Cutis* 54, 70 (observation)
  (1990): Kanwar AJ+, *Dermatologica* 181, 75
Phototoxicity
  (1993): Litt JZ, Beachwood, OH (personal case) (observation)
  (1991): Shelley WB+, *Cutis* 48, 187 (observation)
Pruritus
  (1988): Islas JA+, *Curr Ther Res* 43, 384
  (1982): Chouinard G+, *Psychopharmacol* 77, 229

Purpura
Rash (sic) (10.8%)
  (1987): Fyer AJ+, *Am J Psychiatry* 144, 303
  (1985): Jerram TC, *Side Eff Drugs Annu* 9, 39
  (1985): Rush AJ+, *Arch Gen Psychiatry* 42, 1154
  (1983): Davison K+, *Psychopharmacol* 80, 308
Urticaria
Xerosis
  (1982): Chouinard G+, *Psychopharmacol* 77, 229

Other
Dysgeusia (<1%)
  (1982): Chouinard G+, *Psychopharmacol* 77, 229
Galactorrhea
Gynecomastia
Headache
Oral ulceration
Paresthesias (2.4%)
Pseudolymphoma
  (1995): Magro CM+, *J Am Acad Dermatol* 32, 419
Sialopenia (32.8%)
Sialorrhea (4.2%)
Tinnitus
Xerostomia (14.7%)
  (1988): Islas JA+, *Curr Ther Res* 43, 384
  (1984): Elie R+, *J Clin Psychopharmacol* 4, 125
  (1982): Chouinard G+, *Psychopharmacol* 77, 229
  (1982): Fawcett JA+, *Pharmacotherapy* 2, 243
  (1981): Evans RL, *Drug Intell Clin Pharm* 15, 633

ALPROSTADIL

Synonyms: PGE; prostaglandin E₁
Trade names: Caverject (Pharmacia); Edex (Schwartz); Muse (Vivus); Prostin VR (Pharmacia)
Other common trade names: *Lyple; Minprog; Palux; Prostine VR; Prostivas*
Indications: Impotence, to maintain patent ductus arteriosus
Category: Erectile dysfunction agent; Prostaglandin
Half-life: 5–10 minutes

Reactions

Skin
Balanitis (<1%)
Diaphoresis (<1%)
Ecchymoses
  (1996): Linet OI+, *N Engl J Med* 334, 873 (8%)
Edema (1%)
Flushing (>10%)
Lichen sclerosus (penile shaft hypopigmentation)
  (1998): English JC+, *J Am Acad Dermatol* 39, 801
Penile edema (1%)
Penile pruritus (<1%)
Penile rash (1–10%)
Rash (sic) (<1%)
Toxic epidermal necrolysis
  (1996): Lecorvaisier-Pieto C+, *J Am Acad Dermatol* 35, 112
Urticaria
  (2000): Carter EL+, *Pediatr Dermatol* 17, 58

Other
Hyperesthesia (<1%)
Injection-site ecchymoses (1–10%)
  (1996): Linet OI+, *N Engl J Med* 334, 873 (8%)

Injection-site hematoma (3%)
Injection-site inflammation (<1%)
Injection-site pain (2%)
  (1996): Hellstrom WJG, *Urology* 48, 851
Injection-site pruritus (<1%)
Penile pain (37%)
  (1997): Padma-Nathan H+, *N Engl J Med* 336, 1 (32.7%)
  (1996): Linet OI+, *N Engl J Med* 334, 873 (50%)
Priapism (4%)
  (1999): Lue TF, *J Urol* 161, 725
  (1998): Bettocchi C+, *Br J Urol* 81, 926
  (1997): *Med Lett Drugs Ther* 39, 32
  (1996): Hellstrom WJG, *Urology* 48, 851
  (1996): Linet OI+, *N Engl J Med* 334, 873 (1%)
Thrombophlebitis
  (2002): Barthelmes L+, *Int J Impot Res* 14(3), 199
Xerostomia (<1%)

ALTEPLASE

Trade name: Activase (Genentech)
Other common trade names: *Actilyse; Activacin; Lysatec-rt-PA*
Indications: Acute myocardial infarction, acute pulmonary embolism
Category: Thrombolytic (tissue plasminogen activator)
Half-life: 30–45 minutes
Clinically important, potentially hazardous interactions with: nitroglycerin, ticlopidine

Reactions

Skin
Angioedema
  (2002): Molinaro G+, *Stroke* 33(6), 1712
  (2001): Pechlaner C+, *Blood Coagul Fibrinolysis* 12(6), 491
  (2000): Hill MD+, *CMAJ* 162, 1281
  (2000): Rudolf J+, *Neurology* 55, 599
Ecchymoses (1–10%)
Purpura (<1%)
  (1990): De Trana+, *Arch Dermatol* 126, 690 (painful) (<1%)
Rash (sic) (<0.02%)
Urticaria (<1%)
  (1989): Collen D+, *Drugs* 38, 346

Other
Anaphylactoid reactions (<0.02%)
  (2001): Pechlaner C+, *Blood Coagul Fibrinolysis* 12(6), 491
  (2000): Hill MD+, *CMAJ* 162, 1281 (fatal)
  (1999): Rudolf J+, *Stroke* 30, 1142
Death
Gingivitis (<1%)
Headache
Hypersensitivity
  (2001): Pechlaner C+, *Blood Coagul Fibrinolysis* 12(6), 491

ALTRETAMINE

Synonym: hexamethylmelamine
Trade name: Hexalen (MGI)
Other common trade names: *Hexamethylmelamin; Hexastat; Hexinawas*
Indications: Palliative treatment of recurrent ovarian cancer
Category: Antineoplastic
Half-life: 13 hours
Clinically important, potentially hazardous interactions with: aldesleukin

Reactions

Skin
Dermatitis (sic)
Exanthems
Pruritus (<1%)
Rash (sic) (<1%)

Hair
Hair – alopecia (<1%)

Other
Mucocutaneous reactions (sic)
  (1978): Levine LR, *Cancer Treat Rev* 5, 67
Paresthesias
  (2001): Rothenberg ML+, *Gynecol Oncol* 82(2), 317
Tremor (<1%)

AMANTADINE

Trade name: Symmetrel (Endo)
Other common trade names: *Amixx; Endantadine; Grippin-Merz; Mantadix; PK-Merz; Protexin; Tregor*
Indications: Parkinsonism, influenza A viral infection
Category: Antidyskinetic; Antiparkinsonian; Antiviral
Half-life: 10–28 hours

Note: Fifty to 90% of patients receiving amantadine for Parkinsonism develop 'a more or less livedo reticularis'

Reactions

Skin
Ankle edema
  (1972): Calne DB+, *Drugs* 4, 49
  (1972): Schwab RS+, *JAMA* 222, 792
  (1971): Parkes JD+, *Lancet* 1, 1085
  (1971): Vollum DI+, *BMJ* 2, 628
Dermatitis (sic) (0.1%)
  (1997): Jauregui I+, *J Invest Allergol Clin Immunol* 7, 260
  (1990): Patruno C+, *Contact Dermatitis* 22, 187
  (1988): van Ketel WG, *Derm Beruf Umwelt* (German) 36, 23
  (1987): Angelini G+, *Contact Dermatitis* 15, 114
  (1987): Miranda A+, *Contact Dermatitis* 17, 55
  (1987): van Joost T+, *Ned Tijdschr Geneeskd* (Dutch) 131, 21
  (1987): van Ketel WG, *Ned Tijdschr Geneeskd* (Dutch) 131, 461
  (1985): Tosti A+, *Contact Dermatitis* 13, 339
  (1985): Valsecchi R+, *Contact Dermatitis* 13, 341
  (1984): Agathos M+, *Derm Beruf Umwelt* (German) 32, 157
  (1984): Lembo G+, *Contact Dermatitis* 10, 317
  (1984): Santucci B+, *Contact Dermatitis* 10, 317
  (1983): Przybilla B, *J Am Acad Dermatol* 9, 165
  (1982): Brandao FM+, *Contact Dermatitis* 8, 140
  (1982): van der Walle HB+, *Ned Tijdschr Geneeskd* (Dutch) 126, 1033
  (1982): van Ketel WG, *Contact Dermatitis* 8, 71
  (1980): Przybilla B+, *MMW Munch Med Wochenschr* (German) 122, 1195
  (1978): Miescher P+, *Hautarzt* (German) 29, 337
  (1976): Fanta D+, *Contact Dermatitis* 2, 282
  (1972): Schwab RS+, *JAMA* 222, 792
Discoloration (sic)
  (1971): Parkes JD+, *Lancet* 1, 1083
Eczema (sic)
  (1983): Hellgren L+, *Dermatologica* 167, 267
Edema
  (1975): Butzer JF+, *Neurology* 25, 603
Edema of leg
  (2002): Litt JZ, Beachwood, OH (observation)
Erythema multiforme
  (2000): Mitchell D, Thomasville, GA (from Internet) (observation)
Exanthems
  (1971): Vollum DI+, *BMJ* 2, 627
Eyelid edema
Livedo reticularis (50–90%)
  (2002): Litt JZ, Beachwood, OH (observation)
  (2001): Vaughn K, (from Internet) (observation)
  (2000): Litt JZ, Beachwood, OH (personal case) (observation)
  (1998): Loffler H+, *Hautarzt* (German) 49, 224
  (1996): Eisner J, Mount Vernon, WA (from Internet) (observation)
  (1995): Paulson GW+, *Clin Neuropharmacol* 18, 466
  (1975): Butzer JF+, *Neurology* 25, 603 (25%)
  (1974): Kalsbeek GL+, *Ned Tijdschr Geneeskd* (Dutch) 118, 66
  (1972): Schwab RS+, *JAMA* 222, 792
  (1972): Silver DE+, *Neurology* 22, 665
  (1971): Marchoul JC+, *Bull Soc Fr Dermatol Syphiligr* (French) 78, 236
  (1971): Parkes JD+, *Lancet* 1, 1083 (90%)
  (1971): Vollum DI+, *BMJ* 2, 627
  (1970): Shealy CN+, *JAMA* 212, 1522 (55%)
Peripheral edema (1–10%)
Photosensitivity
  (1983): van den Berg WH+, *Contact Dermatitis* 9, 165
  (1974): van Ketel WG+, *Dermatologica* 148, 124
Pruritus (<1%)
  (2002): Litt JZ, Beachwood, OH (observation)
  (1972): Schwab RS+, *JAMA* 222, 792
Rash (sic) (<1%)
Urticaria

Hair
Hair – alopecia
  (1975): Butzer JF+, *Neurology* 25, 603 (8%)
Hair – hypertrichosis
  (1975): Butzer JF+, *Neurology* 25, 603

Nails
Nails – growth
  (1975): Butzer JF+, *Neurology* 25, 603

Other
Headache
Xerostomia (1–10%)
  (1972): Schwab RS+, *JAMA* 222, 792
  (1971): Parkes JD+, *Lancet* 1, 1085

AMIFOSTINE

Synonyms: ethiofos; gammaphos
Trade name: Ethyol (Medimmune)
Other common trade name: *Ethyol 500*
Indications: Nephrotoxicity prophylaxis
Category: Antidote (cisplatin); Cytoprotective
Half-life: 9 minutes

Reactions

Skin
Allergic reactions (sic)
Chills (sic) (>10%)
  (2000): Sriswasdi C+, *J Med Assoc Thai* 83, 374
Flushing (>10%)
  (2001): Awasthy BS+, *J Assoc Physicians India* 49, 236 (19%)
  (2001): Genvresse I+, *Anticancer Drugs* 12(4), 345
  (2000): Sriswasdi C+, *J Med Assoc Thai* 83, 374
Rash (sic) (<1%)
  (1998): Buresh CM+, *J Pediatr Hematol Oncol* 20, 361
Toxic epidermal necrolysis
  (2002): Demiral AN+, *Jpn J Clin Oncol* 32(11), 477

Other
Dysgeusia
  (2001): Genvresse I+, *Anticancer Drugs* 12(4), 345
  (2000): Sriswasdi C+, *J Med Assoc Thai* 83, 374
Xerostomia
  (2002): Anne PR+, *Semin Radiat Oncol* 12(1), 18
  (2001): Genvresse I+, *Anticancer Drugs* 12(4), 345

AMIKACIN

Trade name: Amikacin Sulfate (Elkins-Sinn)
Other common trade names: *Amicacina; Amicasil; Amikan; Biclin; Biklin; Gamikal; Kanbine; Lukadin; Miacin; Yectamid*
Indications: Short-term treatment of serious infections due to gram-negative bacteria
Category: Aminoglycoside
Half-life: 1.5–2.5 hours (adults)
Clinically important, potentially hazardous interactions with: adefovir, aldesleukin, aminoglycosides, atracurium, bumetanide, cephalexin, doxacurium, ethacrynic acid, furosemide, succinylcholine, torsemide

Reactions

Skin
Dermatitis (sic)
  (1989): Rudzki E+, *Contact Dermatitis* 20, 391
  (1985): Holdiness MR, *Int J Dermatol* 24, 280
Exanthems
  (1977): Pollack AA+, *JAMA* 237, 562 (3.7%)
  (1977): Yu VL+, *JAMA* 238, 943 (3.7%)
Pruritus
  (1985): Holdiness MR, *Int J Dermatol* 24, 280
Rash (sic) (<1%)
  (1995): Rodriguez-Noriega E+, *J Chemother* 7, 155
Urticaria

Other
Injection-site induration
Injection-site necrosis

  (1993): Plantin P+, *Presse Med* (French) 22, 1366
Injection-site pain
Paresthesias (<1%)
Tremor (<1%)

AMILORIDE

Trade names: Midamor (Merck); Moduretic (Merck)
Other common trade names: *Amikal; Kaluril; Medamor; Midoride; Modamide; Nirulid; Ride*
Indications: Prevention of hypokalemia associated with kaliuretic diuretics, management of edema in hypertension
Category: Potassium-sparing antihypertensive diuretic
Half-life: 6–9 hours
Clinically important, potentially hazardous interactions with: ACE inhibitors, benazepril, captopril, cyclosporine, enalapril, fosinopril, lisinopril, moexipril, potassium salts, quinapril, quinidine, ramipril, spironolactone, trandolapril

Moduretic is amiloride and hydrochlorothiazide

Reactions

Skin
Diaphoresis
Exanthems
  (1972): *Drug Ther Bull*
Flushing (>1%)
Photosensitivity
  (1981): *Aust Prescriber* 5, 23
Pruritus (<1%)
Purpura
Rash (sic) (<1%)
Urticaria
Vasculitis
Xerosis (<1%)

Hair
Hair – alopecia (<1%)

Other
Anaphylactoid reactions
Dysgeusia (<1%)
Gynecomastia (1–10%)
Headache
Paresthesias (<1%)
Tinnitus
Tremor
Xerostomia (<1%)

AMINOCAPROIC ACID

Trade name: Amicar (Immunex)
Other common trade names: *Capramol; Caproamin; Caprolisin; Ipron; Ipsilon; Resplamin*
Indications: To provide hemostasis in the treatment of fibrinolysis
Category: Antifibrinolytic; Hemostatic
Half-life: 1–2 hours

Reactions

Skin
Bullous eruption
  (1992): Brooke CP+, *J Am Acad Dermatol* 27, 880
Dermatitis (sic)
  (2000): Miyamoto H+, *Contact Dermatitis* 42, 50
  (1999): Villarreal O, *Contact Dermatitis* 40, 114 (systemic)
  (1989): Shono M, *Contact Dermatitis* 21, 106
Eczema (sic)
Edema
Exanthems
  (1995): Gonzalez-Gutierrez ML+, *Allergy* 50, 745
Kaposi's sarcoma
Pruritus
Purpura
  (1985): Verstraete M, *Drugs* 29, 236
  (1980): Chakrabarti A+, *BMJ* 281, 197
Rash (sic) (1–10%)
Urticaria

Other
Anaphylactoid reactions
Death
  (2001): Fanashawe MP+, *Anesthesiology* 95(6), 1525 (2 cases)
Headache
Injection-site erythema
Injection-site phlebitis
Injection-site reactions (sic)
Muscle necrosis
Myalgia
Myopathy (1–10%)
  (1988): Kane MJ+, *Am J Med* 85, 861
Rhabdomyolysis
  (1997): Seymour BD+, *Ann Pharmacother* 31(1), 56
  (1983): Luliri P+, *Haematologica* 68(5), 664 (2 cases)
  (1983): Morris CD+, *S Afr Med J* 64(10), 363
  (1982): Brown JA+, *J Neurosurg* 57(1), 130
  (1982): Vanneste JA+, *Eur Neurol* 21(4), 242
  (1980): Britt CW+, *Arch Neurol* 37(3), 187
  (1980): Le Porrier M+, *Nouv Presse Med* 9(33), 2347
  (1978): Griffin JD+, *Semin Thromb Hemost* 5(1), 27
  (1969): Korsan-Bengtsen K+, *Acta Med Scand* 185(4), 341
Thrombophlebitis
Tinnitus

AMINOGLUTETHIMIDE

Trade name: Cytadren (Novartis)
Other common trade names: *Orimeten; Orimetene; Rodazol*
Indications: Suppression of adrenal function, metastatic carcinoma
Category: Antineoplastic
Half-life: 7–15 hours

Reactions

Skin
Angioedema
  (1967): Horky K+, *Schweiz Med Wochenschr* (German) 98, 1843
Erythema
  (1987): Williams DS+, *Br J Radiology* 60, 1226
Exanthems
  (1990): Vanek N+, *Med Pediatr Oncol* 18, 162
  (1987): Williams DS+, *Br J Radiology* 60, 1226
  (1986): Leloire O+, *Presse Med* (French) 15, 34
  (1984): Coltart RS, *Br J Radiol* 57, 531
  (1982): Naysmith A+, *N Engl J Med* 306, 45 (26%)
  (1982): Santen RJ+, *Ann Intern Med* 96, 94 (29%)
  (1980): Savaraj N+, *Med Pediatr Oncol* 8, 251
  (1967): Horky K+, *Schweiz Med Wochenschr* (German) 98, 1843
    (4–30%)
Exfoliative dermatitis
  (1967): Horky K+, *Schweiz Med Wochenschr* (German) 98, 1843
Lupus erythematosus (>10%)
  (1980): McCraken M+, *BMJ* 281, 1254
Pruritus (5%)
Purpura
  (1994): Stratakis CA+, *Am J Hosp Pharm* 51, 2589
Pustular psoriasis
  (1984): Coltart RS, *Br J Radiol* 57, 531
Rash (sic) (>10%)
Urticaria

Hair
Hair – hirsutism (1–10%)

Other
Anaphylactoid reactions
  (1986): Leloire O+, *Presse Med* (French) 15, 34
Headache
Myalgia (3%)
Oral mucosal eruption
  (1984): Coltart RS, *Br J Radiol* 57, 531
  (1967): Horky K+, *Schweiz Med Wochenschr* (German) 98, 1843
Oral ulceration
  (1984): Coltart RS, *Br J Radiol* 57, 531

AMINOLEVULINIC ACID

Trade name: Levulan Kerastick* (Dusa)
Indications: Non-hyperkeratotic actinic keratoses of face & scalp
Category: Photosensitizer; Porphyrin
Half-life: 30 ± 10 hours

Reactions

Skin
Burning (>50%)
  (1997): Jeffes EW+, *Arch Dermatol* 133, 727
  (1996): Stender IM+, *Br J Dermatol* 135, 454

Crusting (64–71%)
   (2000): Hongcharu W+, *J Invest Dermatol* 115, 183
   (1995): Lang S+, *Laryngorhinootologie* (German) 74, 85
Dermatitis
   (1998): Gnaizdowska B+, *Contact Dermatitis* 38, 348
Edema (35%)
   (1997): Jeffes EW+, *Arch Dermatol* 133, 727
   (1995): Lang S+, *Laryngorhinootologie* (German) 74, 85
Erosions (14%)
Erythema (99%)
   (1997): Jeffes EW+, *Arch Dermatol* 133, 727
   (1995): Lang S+, *Laryngorhinootologie* 74, 85
Exfoliation (when treated for acne)
   (2000): Hongcharu W+, *J Invest Dermatol* 115, 183
   (1996): Stender IM+, *Br J Dermatol* 135(3), 454
Hypopigmentation (22%)
Koebner phenomenon (psoriasis)
   (1996): Stender IM+, *Acta Derm Venereol* 76, 392
Melanoma
   (1997): Wolf P+, *Dermatology* 194, 53 (on scalp)
Photosensitivity
Pigmentation (when treated for acne) (22%)
   (2000): Hongcharu W+, *J Invest Dermatol* 115, 183
Pruritus (25%)
Pustules (<4%)
Scaling (64–71%)
Stinging (>50%)
   (1997): Jeffes EW+, *Arch Dermatol* 133, 727
Ulcerations (4%)
Vesiculation (4%)

Other
Dysesthesia (2%)

*Note: To be used in conjunction with the Blue Light Photodynamic Therapy Illuminator

AMINOPHYLLINE

Synonym: theophylline ethylenediamine
Trade names: Aerolate; Aminophyllin; Bronkodyl; Choledyl; Elixophyllin (Forest); Norphyl; Phyllocontin (Napp); Quibron (Monarch); Slo-Bid; Somophyllin; Theo-Dur; Truphylline
Other common trade names: *Corophyllin; Euphyllin; Palaron; Phyllotemp; Planphylline; Tefamin*
Indications: Prevention or treatment of reversible bronchospasm
Category: Xanthine bronchodilator
Half-life: 3–15 hours (in adult nonsmokers)
Clinically important, potentially hazardous interactions with: cimetidine, erythromycin, halothane

Reactions

Skin
Allergic reactions (sic) (<1%)
   (1986): Cusano F+, *G Ital Dermatol Venereol* (Italian) 121, 443
   (1985): Editorial, *Lancet* 1, 289
   (1983): Gibb W+, *Br Med J (Clin Res Ed)* 13, 501
   (1983): Hardy C+, *Br Med J (Clin Res Ed)* 286, 2051
Baboon syndrome
   (1999): Guin JD+, *Contact Dermatitis* 40, 170
Dermatitis
   (1994): Corazza M+, *Contact Dermatitis* 31, 328
   (1984): Editorial, *Lancet* 2, 1192
   (1983): Berman BA+, *Cutis* 31, 594

   (1983): van den Berg WH+, *Ned Tijdschr Geneeskd* (Dutch) 127, 1801
   (1980): Vazquez Botet M, *Bol Asoc Med P R* (Spanish) 72, 14
   (1978): Tsyrkunova LP+, *Gig Tr Prof Zabol* (Russian) October, 52
   (1959): Baer RL+, *Arch Dermatol* 79, 647
Diaphoresis
Exanthems
   (1985): Editorial, *Lancet* 2, 1192
   (1984): Thompson PJ+, *Thorax* 39, 600
   (1983): Hardy C+, *BMJ* 286, 2051
   (1981): de Shazo RD+, *Ann Allergy* 46, 152
   (1980): Lawyer CH+, *J Allergy Clin Immunol* 65, 353
Exfoliative dermatitis
   (1984): Thompson PJ+, *Thorax* 39, 600
   (1982): Nierenberg DW+, *West J Med* 137, 328
   (1981): Elias JA+, *Am Rev Respir Dis* 123, 550
   (1979): Bernstein JE+, *Arch Dermatol* 115, 360
   (1976): Petrozzi JW+, *Arch Dermatol* 112, 525
   (1958): Tas J+, *Acta Allergologica* 12, 39
Flushing
Pruritus
   (1980): Lawyer CH+, *J Allergy Clin Immunol* 65, 353
   (1971): Davidson MB, *N Engl J Med* 285, 689
   (1971): Wong D+, *J Allergy* 48, 165
Rash (sic) (<1%)
   (1983): Hardy C+, *BMJ* 286, 2051
Shaking (sic)
Side effects (sic)
   (1995): Simon PA+, *JAMA* 273, 1737
Stevens–Johnson syndrome
   (1989): Hidalgo HA, *Pediatr Pulmonol* 6, 209 (theophylline)
Urticaria
   (1994): Urbani CE, *Contact Dermatitis* 31, 198
   (1985): Editorial, *Lancet* 2, 1192
   (1984): Thompson PJ+, *Thorax* 39, 600
   (1982): Neumann H, *Dtsch Med Wochenschr* (German) 107, 116
   (1979): Booth BH+, *Ann Allergy* 43, 289
   (1971): Wong D+, *J Allergy* 48, 165

Hair
Hair – alopecia

Other
Headache
Hypersensitivity
   (1999): Yoshizawa A+, *Arerugi* (Japanese) 48, 1206 (from ethylenediamine)
   (1985): Gibb WR, *Lancet* 1, 49
   (1981): Elias JA+, *Am Rev Respir Dis* 123, 550
   (1970): Foussereau J+, *Bull Soc Fr Dermatol Syphiligr* (French) 77, 415
   (1967): Sonnischen N, *Allerg Asthma Leipz* (German) 13, 215
   (1967): Sonnischen N, *Allerg Asthma Leipz* (German) 13, 259
Parosmia
Rhabdomyolysis
   (2001): Teweleit S+, *Med Klin* 96(1), 40
   (2000): Iwano J+, *J Med Invest* 47(1), 9
   (1999): Shimada N+, *Nippon Jinzo Gakkai Shi* 41(4), 460 (with clarithromycin)
   (1991): Aoshima M+, *Nihon Kyobu Shikkan Gakki Zasshi* 29(8), 1064

AMINOSALICYLATE SODIUM

Synonyms: para-aminosalicylate sodium; PAS
Trade names: Paser Granules (Jacobus); Sodium P.A.S. (Lannett) (Palisades); Tubasal
Other common trade names: Aminox; Eupasal; Nemasol
Indications: Tuberculosis
Category: anti-inflammatory; Antimycobacterial
Half-life: 45–60 minutes

Reactions

Skin
Allergic reactions (sic)
  (1988): Fardy JM+, J Clin Gastroenterol 10, 635
Angioedema
  (1964): Lajouanine P+, Ann Pédiatr (Paris) (French) 40, 620
  (1959): Bereston ES, J Invest Dermatol 33, 427
Bullous eruption
  (1964): Lajouanine P+, Ann Pédiatr (Paris) (French) 40, 620
  (1959): Bereston ES, J Invest Dermatol 33, 427
Eczema (sic) (<1%)
Erythema multiforme
  (1963): Van Ketel WG, Ned Tijdschr Geneeskd (Dutch) 107, 952
Exanthems
  (1988): Gron I+, Ugeskr Laeger (Danish) 150, 32
  (1982): Nagaratnam N, Postgrad Med J 58, 729
  (1968): Sarkany I, Proc R Soc Med 61, 891
  (1964): Duncan JT, Am Rev Respir Dis 89, 103
  (1964): Lajouanine P+, Ann Pédiatr (Paris) (French) 40, 620
  (1963): Filoz-Diaz JA+, Archos Méd Panama (Spanish) 12, 68
  (1960): Simpson DG+, Am J Med 29, 297 (1–5%)
  (1959): Bereston ES, J Invest Dermatol 33, 427 (1–5%)
  (1950): Cuthbert J, Lancet 2, 209
Exfoliative dermatitis
  (1972): Kauppinen K, Acta Derm Venereol (Stockh) 52 (suppl), 68
  (1967): Coleman WP, Med Clin North Am 51, 1073
  (1965): Griffiths HED+, J Bone Joint Surg (Edinburgh) 47, 86
  (1964): Bower G, Am Rev Respir Dis 89, 440
  (1964): Lajouanine P+, Ann Pédiatr (Paris) (French) 40, 620
  (1961): Gupta SK, Indian J Dermatol 6, 115
Fixed eruption
  (1972): Levantine A+, Br J Dermatol 86, 604
  (1965): Laszczka C, Gruzlica (Polish) 33, 935
  (1965): Snelling MRJ+, Tubercle 46, 284
  (1961): Welch AL+, Arch Dermatol 84, 1004
  (1952): Warring FC+, Am Rev Tuberc Pulm Dis 65, 235
  (1949): Kierland RR+, Proc Staff Meet Mayo Clin 24, 539
Lichenoid eruption
  (1971): Almeyda J+, Br J Dermatol 95, 604
  (1964): Baker H+, Br J Dermatol 76, 186
  (1953): Shatin H+, J Invest Dermatol 21, 135
Lupus erythematosus
  (1985): Holdiness MR, Int J Dermatol 24, 280
  (1980): Agarwal MB+, J Postgrad Med 26(4), 263
  (1961): Bickers JN+, N Engl J Med 265, 131
Lymphoma (benign)
  (1982): Nagaratnam N, Postgrad Med J 58, 729
Photosensitivity
  (1972): Kuokkanen K, Acta Allergol 27, 407
  (1971): Girard JP, Helv Med Acta 36, 3
  (1964): Lajouanine P+, Ann Pédiatr (Paris) (French) 40, 620
Pruritus
  (1968): No Author, BMJ 3, 664
  (1964): Berté SJ+, Am Rev Respir Dis 90, 598
  (1960): Simpson DG+, Am J Med 29, 297
Purpura

  (1980): Miescher PA+, Clin Haematol 9, 505
  (1963): Filoz-Diaz JA+, Archos Méd Panama (Spanish) 12, 68
  (1959): Bereston ES, J Invest Dermatol 33, 427
  (1952): Warring FC+, Am Rev Tuberc Pulm Dis 65, 235
Toxic epidermal necrolysis
  (1963): Filoz-Diaz JA+, Archos Méd Panama (Spanish) 12, 68
Urticaria
  (1964): Lajouanine P+, Ann Pédiatr (Paris) (French) 40, 620
  (1961): Gupta SK, Indian J Dermatol 6, 115
  (1960): Simpson DG+, Am J Med 29, 297
  (1959): Bereston ES, J Invest Dermatol 33, 427
  (1952): Warring FC+, Am Rev Tuberc Pulm Dis 65, 235
Vasculitis (<1%)
  (1972): Levantine A+, Br J Dermatol 87, 646

Hair
Hair – alopecia
  (1982): Kutty PK+, Ann Intern Med 97, 785
  (1965): Griffiths HED+, J Bone Joint Surg (Edinburgh) 47, 86
  (1960): Simpson DG+, Am J Med 29, 297
  (1951): Grandjean LC, Acta Derm Venereol (Stockh) 31, 615

Other
Hypersensitivity
Oral lichenoid eruption
Oral mucosal eruption
  (1964): Lajouanine P+, Ann Pédiatr (Paris) (French) 40, 620
  (1960): Simpson DG+, Am J Med 29, 297

AMIODARONE

Trade names: Cordarone (Wyeth); Pacerone (Upsher-Smith)
Other common trade names: Aratac; Corbionax; Cordarex; Cordarone X; Tachydaron
Indications: Ventricular fibrillation, ventricular tachycardia
Category: Class III antiarrhythmic
Half-life: 26–107 days
Clinically important, potentially hazardous interactions with: amprenavir, anisindione, anticoagulants, arsenic, ciprofloxacin, dicumarol, digoxin, diltiazem, enoxacin, fentanyl, gatifloxacin, lomefloxacin, methotrexate, moxifloxacin, norfloxacin, ofloxacin, quinidine, quinolones, rifabutin, rifampin, rifapentine, ritonavir, sparfloxacin, verapamil, warfarin

Reactions

Skin
Allergic reactions (sic)
  (1989): Reingardene DI, Klin Med Mosk (Russian) 67, 128
Angioedema
  (2000): Burches E+, Allergy 55, 1199
Basal cell carcinoma
  (1995): Monk BE, Br J Dermatol 133, 148
Diaphoresis
  (1985): Raeder EA+, Am Heart J 109, 979 (0.5%)
  (1983): McGovern B+, BMJ 287, 175 (2.5%)
Ecchymoses (<1%)
Edema (1–10%)
Erythema multiforme
  (2002): Yung A+, Australas J Dermatol 43(1), 35
Erythema nodosum (<1%)
  (1983): Fogoros RN+, Circulation 68, 88 (1%)
  (1976): Rosenbaum MB+, Am J Cardiol 38, 934
Exanthems
  (1985): Raeder EA+, Am Heart J 109, 975 (0.9%)
  (1984): Rotmensch HH+, Ann Intern Med 101, 462 (0.7%)

(1983): Fogoros RN+, *Circulation* 68, 88 (2%)
(1983): Harris L+, *Circulation* 67, 45
(1969): Kappart A, *Z Ther* (German) #8, 474

Exfoliative dermatitis
(1988): Moots RJ+, *BMJ* 296, 1332

Facial erythema (3.1%)
(1984): Rotmensch HH+, *Ann Intern Med* 101, 462
(1983): Harris L+, *Circulation* 67, 45

Flushing (1–10%)

Iododerma
(1997): Ricci C+, *Ann Dermatol Venereol* (French) 124, 260
(1975): Porters JE+, *Arch Dermatol* 111, 1656
(1975): Zantkuyl CF+, *Dermatologica* 151, 311

Keratosis pilaris
(1999): Capper N, Mobile, AL (from Internet) (observation)

Linear IgA bullous dermatosis
(2002): Cohen LM+, *J Am Acad Dermatol* 46, S32 (passim)
(1996): Primka EJ+, *J Cutan Pathol* 23, 58
(1996): Tranvan A+, *J Am Acad Dermatol* 35, 865
(1994): Primka EJ+, *J Am Acad Dermatol* 31, 809
(1990): Espagne E+, *Ann Dermatol Venereol* (French) 117, 898

Lupus erythematosus
(2003): Kundu AK, *J Assoc Physicians India* 51, 216
(2002): Sheikhzadeh A+, *Arch Intern Med* 162(7), 834
(1999): Susano R+, *Ann Rheum Dis* 58, 655
(1985): Raeder EA+, *Am Heart J* 109, 979 (4.6%)

Photosensitivity (10–30%)
(2000): Burns KE+, *Can Respir* 7, 193 (passim)
(1997): O'Reilly FM+, American Academy of Dermatology Meeting, Poster #14
(1995): Collins P+, *Br J Dermatol* 132, 956
(1995): Tisdale JE+, *J Clin Pharmacol* 35, 351
(1995): Zehender M, *Circulation* 92, 1665
(1993): Allen JE, *Clin Pharm* 12, 580
(1993): Ettler K+, *Sb Ved Pr Lek Fak Karlovy Univerzity Hradci Kralove* (Czech) 36, 305 (9.4%)
(1992): Editorial, *JAMA* 267, 3322
(1992): Gosselink AT+, *JAMA* 267, 3289
(1990): Monk B, *Clin Exp Dermatol* 15, 319
(1989): Rappersberger K+, *J Invest Dermatol* 93, 201
(1988): Hyatt RH+, *Age Aging* 17, 116 (10%)
(1988): Parodi A, *Photodermatol* 5, 146
(1987): Roupe G+, *Acta Derm Venereol* (Stockh) 67, 76
(1987): Waitzer S+, *J Am Acad Dermatol* 16, 779
(1986): Boyle J, *Br J Dermatol* 115, 253
(1986): Ferguson J, *Br J Clin Pract Symp Suppl* 44, 63
(1986): Ljunggren B+, *Photodermatol* 3, 26
(1986): Toback AC+, *Dermatol Clin* 4, 223
(1986): Török L+, *Hautarzt* (German) 37, 507 (24%)
(1985): Ferguson J+, *Br J Dermatol* 113, 537
(1985): Mulrow JP+, *Ann Int Med* 103, 68
(1985): Raeder EA+, *Am Heart J* 109, 979 (4.6%)
(1985): Stäubli M, *Postgrad Med J* 61, 245
(1985): Vila Serra MD+, *Med Clin (Barc)* (Spanish) 84, 379
(1984): Diffey BL+, *Clin Exp Dermatol* 9, 248
(1984): Ferguson J+, *Lancet* 2, 414
(1984): Guerciolini R+, *Lancet* 1, 962
(1984): Kaufmann G, *Lancet* 1, 51
(1984): Walter JF+, *Arch Dermatol* 120, 1591
(1984): Zachary CB+, *Br J Dermatol* 110, 451
(1983): Fogoros RN+, *Circulation* 68, 88 (11%)
(1983): Harris L+, *Circulation* 67, 45 (57%)
(1983): McGovern B+, *BMJ* 287, 175 (8.75%)
(1983): Nadamanee K+, *Ann Intern Med* 98, 577 (5.3%)
(1982): Chalmers RJ+, *Br Med J Clin Res Ed* 285, 341

Pigmentation
(2002): Marko P+, *Acta Dermatoven* 11(3), 110 (3 cases)
(2001): Dereure O, *Am J Clin Dermatol* 2(4), 253
(2001): Haas N+, *Arch Dermatol* 137, 313 (blue-gray)
(2001): High WA+, *N Engl J Med* 345, 1464

(2001): Rubegni P+, *Am Fam Physician* 63, 1409
(2000): Burns KE+, *Can Respir* 7, 193 (passim)
(2000): Gutknecht DR, *Cutis* 66, 294 (blue-gray)
(1999): Karrer S+, *Arch Dermatol* 135, 251
(1997): Sivaram CA+, *N Engl J Med* 337, 1813
(1996): Ammann R+, *Hautarzt* (German) 47, 930
(1996): Kounis NG+, *Clin Cardiol* 19, 592
(1995): Tisdale JE+, *J Clin Pharmacol* 35, 351 (blue-gray)
(1993): Balslev E+, *Ugeskr Laeger* (Danish) 155, 4014 (blue-gray)
(1993): Colquhoun JP, *Aust Fam Physician* 22, 2168
(1993): Ettler K+, *Sb Ved Pr Lek Fak Karlovy Univerzity Hradci Kralove* (Czech) 36, 305 (9.4%)
(1992): Editorial, *JAMA* 267, 3322
(1992): Fitzpatrick JE, *Derm Clinics* 10, 19
(1992): Son En Ai+, *Klin Med Mosk* (Russian) 70, 46
(1991): Blackshear JL+, *Mayo Clin Proc* 66, 721
(1991): Fazekas T+, *Szent Gyorgyi Albert Orvostudomanyi Egyetem* (Hungarian) 132, 2157
(1990): Brazzelli V+, *G Ital Dermatol Venereol* (Italian) 125, 521
(1989): Klein AD+, *Arch Dermatol* 125, 417
(1989): Rappersberger K+, *J Invest Dermatol* 93, 201
(1989): Reingardene DI, *Kardiologiia* (Russian) 29, 112
(1988): Beukema WP+, *Am J Cardiol* 62, 1146
(1988): Zadionchenko VS+, *Klin Med Mosk* (Russian) 66, 126
(1987): Goldstein GD+, *Chest* 91, 772
(1987): Waitzer S+, *J Am Acad Dermatol* 16, 779
(1986): Dowson JH+, *Arch Dermatol* 122, 244
(1986): Rappersberger K+, *Br J Dermatol* 114, 189
(1986): Török L+, *Hautarzt* (German) 37, 507
(1985): Alinovi A+, *J Am Acad Dermatol* 12, 563
(1985): Lakatos A, *Orv Hetil* (Hungarian) 126, 1343
(1985): Varotti C+, *G Ital Dermatol Venereol* (Italian) 120, 183
(1984): Miller RAW+, *Arch Dermatol* 120, 646
(1984): Onofrey BE+, *J Am Optom Assoc* 55, 337
(1984): Rotmensch HH+, *Ann Intern Med* 101, 462 (4.6%)
(1984): Weiss SR+, *J Am Acad Dermatol* 11, 898
(1984): Zachary CB+, *Br J Dermatol* 110, 451
(1983): Harris L+, *Circulation* 67, 45 (1.4%)
(1983): McGovern B+, *BMJ* 287, 175
(1983): Trimble JW+, *Arch Dermatol* 119, 914
(1982): Ferrer I+, *Med Clin (Barc)* (Spanish) 79, 355
(1982): Quintanilla E+, *Med Cutan Ibero Lat Am* (Spanish) 10, 177
(1981): Granstein RD+, *J Am Acad Dermatol* 5, 1 (blue-gray)
(1981): Korting HC+, *Hautarzt* (German) 32, 301
(1979): Nageli U+, *Schweiz Med Wochenschr* (German) 109, 1708
(1978): Cassilas-Ruiz JA+, *Rev Esp Cardiol* (Spanish) 31, 617
(1975): Delage C+, *Can Med Assoc J* 112(10), 1205
(1975): Lambert D+, *Ann Dermatol Syphiligr Paris* (French) 102, 277
(1974): Olmos L+, *Med Cutan Ibero Lat Am* (Spanish) 2, 447
(1972): Balouet G+, *Arch Anat Pathol* (Paris) (French) 20, 265
(1971): Labouche F+, *Bull Soc Fr Dermatol Syphiligr* (French) 78, 27
(1971): Thiers H+, *Bull Soc Fr Dermatol Syphiligr* (French) 78, 548

Pruritus (1–5%)
(1969): Kappart A, *Z Ther* (German) #8, 474 (4.1%)
(1968): Leutenegger A+, *Schweiz Med Wochenschr* (German) 98, 2020 (4.1%)

Psoriasis
(1986): Abel EA+, *J Am Acad Dermatol* 15, 1007
(1982): Muir AD, *N Z Med J* 95, 711

Purpura (2%)
(1983): Fogoros RN+, *Circulation* 68, 88

Pustular psoriasis
(1982): Muir AD, *N Z Med J* 95, 711

Rash (sic) (<1%)

Rosacea

(1987): Reifler DM+, *Am J Ophthalmol* 103, 594
Side effects (sic)
   (1994): Shukla R+, *Postgrad Med J* 70, 492
Stevens–Johnson syndrome (<1%)
Toxic epidermal necrolysis
   (2002): Yung A+, *Australas J Dermatol* 43(1), 35 (fatal)
   (2000): Danby WF, Manchester, NH (from Internet)
      (observation)
   (1985): Bencini PL+, *Arch Dermatol* 121, 838
Urticaria
   (1983): McGovern B+, *BMJ* 287, 175 (1.25%)
Vasculitis (<1%)
   (2001): Scharf C+, *Lancet* 358, 2045
   (1994): Dootson G+, *Clin Exp Dermatol* 19, 422
   (1994): Gutierrez R+, *Ann Pharmacother* 28, 537
   (1985): Starke ID+, *BMJ* 291, 940
   (1985): Stäubli M, *Postgrad Med J* 61, 245

Hair

Hair – alopecia (<1%)
   (2000): Litt JZ, Beachwood, OH (personal case) (observation)
      (after 2 weeks of therapy)
   (1995): Ahmad S, *Arch Intern Med* 155, 1106
   (1992): Samuel LM+, *Postgrad Med J* 68, 771
   (1985): Raeder EA+, *Am Heart J* 109, 979 (4.1%)
   (1984): Rotmensch HH+, *Ann Intern Med* 101, 462 (0.7%)
   (1983): McGovern B+, *BMJ* 287, 175 (2.5%)
Hair – hypertrichosis
   (1985): Ferguson J+, *Br J Dermatol* 113, 537

Other

Death
   (2002): Kharabsheh S+, *Am J Cardiol* 89(7), 896
   (2002): Yung A+, *Australas J Dermatol* 43(1), 35
Dyschromatopsia
   (2002): Ikaheimo K+, *Acta Ophthalmol Scand* 80(1), 59
Dysgeusia (1–10%)
   (1983): McGovern B+, *BMJ* 287, 175
Headache
Paresthesias (4–9%)
Parosmia (1–10%)
Pseudoporphyria
   (1988): Parodi A, *Photodermatology* 5, 146
Pseudotumor cerebri (<1%)
Sialorrhea (1–3%)
Torsades de pointes
   (2003): Atar S+, *Pacing Clin Electrophysiol* 26(3), 785 (with
      loratadine)
   (2003): Makai A+, *Orv Hetil* 144(5), 241
   (2003): Voigt L+, *Angiology* 54(2), 229
Tremor

AMITRIPTYLINE

Trade names: Elavil (AstraZeneca); Limbitrol (ICN)
Other common trade names: *Amineurin; Domical; Laroxyl; Lentizol; Levate; Novotriptyn; Saroten; Tryptanol; Tryptizol*
Indications: Depression
Category: Antimigraine; Tricyclic antidepressant
Half-life: 10–25 hours
Clinically important, potentially hazardous interactions with: amprenavir, clonidine, **ephedra**, epinephrine, guanethidine, isocarboxazid, linezolid, MAO inhibitors, phenelzine, quinolones, sparfloxacin, **St John's wort**, tranylcypromine

Limbitrol is amitriptyline and chlordiazepoxide

Reactions

Skin

Acne
Allergic reactions (sic) (<1%)
Angioedema
   (1999): Garcia-Doval I+, *Cutis* 63, 35 (passim)
Bullous eruption (<1%)
   (1979): Herschthal D+, *Arch Dermatol* 115, 499
Dermatitis (sic)
   (1966): Hollister LE+, *J Nerv Ment Dis* 142, 460
Dermatitis herpetiformis
   (1969): Rhyner K, *Diss Zürich* (German)
Diaphoresis (1–10%)
   (1995): Feder R, *J Clin Psychiatry* 56, 35
Edema
   (2002): *Prescrire Int* 11(60), 111
Erythema
Erythema annulare centrifugum
   (1999): Garcia-Doval I+, *Cutis* 63, 35
Erythroderma
   (1999): Garcia-Doval I+, *Cutis* 63, 35 (passim)
Exanthems
Exfoliative dermatitis
Facial edema
Fixed eruption
   (1998): McCarthy J, Ft. Worth, TX (from Internet) (observation)
Flushing
Lichen planus
   (1999): Garcia-Doval I+, *Cutis* 63, 35 (passim)
Lupus erythematosus
   (1993): Dove FB, *Hosp Pract Off Ed* 28, 14
Necrosis
   (1999): Fogarty BJ+, *Burns* 25, 768
Petechiae
Photosensitivity (<1%)
   (1999): Garcia-Doval I+, *Cutis* 63, 35 (passim)
   (1996): Taniguchi S+, *Am J Hematol* 53, 49
   (1966): Hollister LE+, *J Nerv Ment Dis* 142, 460
Pigmentation
   (1999): Garcia-Doval I+, *Cutis* 63, 35 (passim)
   (1988): Warnock JK+, *Am J Psychiatry* 145, 425
   (1985): Basler RS+, *J Am Acad Dermatol* 12, 577
Pruritus
   (1999): Garcia-Doval I+, *Cutis* 63, 35 (passim)
   (1988): Larrey D+, *Gastroenterology* 94, 200
   (1966): Hollister LE+, *J Nerv Ment Dis* 142, 460
Purpura
   (1999): Garcia-Doval I+, *Cutis* 63, 35 (passim)
   (1971): Kozakova M, *Cesk Dermatol* (Czech) 46, 158

Rash (sic)
Urticaria
Vasculitis
  (1969): Gisslén H+, *Dermatol Monatsschr* (German) 155, 783

Hair

Hair – alopecia (<1%)
  (1992): Breathnach SM+, *Adverse Drug Reactions and the Skin*
    Blackwell, Oxford, 196 (passim)

Other

Ageusia
Anaphylactoid reactions
Black tongue
Bromhidrosis
Dysgeusia (>10%)
Galactorrhea (<1%)
Glossitis
Gynecomastia (<1%)
Headache
Hypersensitivity
  (2000): Milionis HJ, *Postgrad Med J* 76, 361
Lymphoid hyperplasia
  (1995): Crowson AN+, *Arch Dermatol* 131, 925
Oral mucosal eruption
  (1964): Pollack B+, *Am J Psychiatry* 121, 384
Paresthesias
Parkinsonism
Pseudolymphoma
  (1995): Crowson AN+, *Arch Dermatol* 131, 925
  (1995): Magro CM+, *J Am Acad Dermatol* 32, 419
Rhabdomyolysis
  (1983): Caruana RJ+, *N C Med* 44(1), 18 (with lorazepam and
    perphenazine)
Sialopenia
  (1995): Loesche WJ+, *J Am Geriatr Soc* 43, 401
Sialorrhea
Stomatitis
  (1988): Larrey D+, *Gastroenterology* 94, 200
Stomatopyrosis
Tardive dyskinesia
  (1990): Miller LG+, *South Med J* 83(5), 525 (with perphenazine)
    (30%)
Tinnitus
Tongue edema
Tremor
Vaginitis
Xerostomia (>10%)
  (2002): Krymchantowski AV+, *Headache* 42(6), 510 (with
    fluoxetine)
  (1996): Rani PU+, *Anesth Analg* 83, 371
  (1995): Loesche WJ+, *J Am Geriatr Soc* 43, 401
  (1966): Hollister LE+, *J Nerv Ment Dis* 142, 467

AMLODIPINE

Trade names: Lotrel (Novartis); Norvasc (Pfizer)
Other common trade names: *Amdepin; Amlodin; Amlogard;
Amlopin; Amlor; Istin; Norvas*
Indications: Hypertension, angina
Category: Antianginal; Antihypertensive; Calcium channel
blocker
Half-life: 30–50 hours
**Clinically important, potentially hazardous interactions
with:** epirubicin, imatinib

Lotrel is amlodipine and benazepril

Reactions

Skin

Ankle edema
  (2001): Zanchetti A+, *J Cardiovasc Pharmacol* 38(4), 642
Dermatitis (sic) (1–10%)
Diaphoresis (<1%)
Discoloration (sic) (<1%)
Edema (5–14%)
  (2001): Chugh SK+, *J Cardiovasc Pharmacol* 38(3), 356
  (1996): Corea L+, *Clin Pharmacol Ther* 60, 341
  (1992): DiBianco R+, *Clin Cardiol* 15, 519
  (1992): Johnson BF+, *Am J Hypertens* 5, 727
  (1991): Elliott HL+, *Postgrad Med J* 67, S20
  (1991): Murdoch D+, *Drugs* 41, 478
  (1989): Chahine RA+, *Am Heart J* 118, 1128
  (1989): Doyle GD+, *Eur J Clin Pharmacol* 36, 205 (ankle)
  (1989): Estrada JN+, *Am Heart J* 118, 1130
  (1989): Osterloh I, *Am Heart J* 118, 1114
  (1988): Glasser SP+, *Am J Cardiol* 62, 518
Erythema multiforme
  (1993): Bewley AP+, *BMJ* 307, 241
Exanthems (2–4%)
  (1989): Doyle GD+, *Eur J Clin Pharmacol* 36, 205
Flushing (1–10%)
  (1992): *Med Lett Drugs Ther* 34, 99
  (1992): Johnson BF+, *Am J Hypertens* 5, 727
  (1991): Murdoch D+, *Drugs* 41, 478
  (1989): Osterloh I, *Am Heart J* 118, 1114
Granuloma annulare
  (2002): Lim AC+, *Australas J Dermatol* 43(1), 24
Lichen planus
  (2001): Swale VJ+, *Br J Dermatol* 144, 920
Lichenoid eruption
  (1998): Silver B, Deerfield, IL (from Internet) (observation)
Lupus erythematosus
  (2002): Boye T+, *World Congress Dermatol* Poster 0088
Peripheral edema (>10%)
  (2002): Litt JZ, Beachwood, OH (personal case) (observation)
  (2001): Lenz TL+, *Pharmacotherapy* 21(8), 898 (4 cases) (with
    nisoldipine)
  (1994): Clavijo GA+, *Am J Hosp Pharm* 51, 59
  (1993): Ellis JS+, *Lancet* 341, 1102
Petechiae (<1%)
Pruritus (2–4%)
  (1998): Litt JZ, Beachwood, OH (personal case) (observation)
  (1997): Orme S+, *BMJ* 315, 463
  (1994): Baker BA+, *Ann Pharmacother* 28, 118
  (1993): Ellis JS+, *Lancet* 341 1102
Purpura (<1%)
  (1994): Dacosta A+, *Therapie* (French) 49, 515
Rash (sic) (1–10%)
Telangiectasia (facial)

(2000): Grabczynska SA+, *Br J Dermatol* 142, 1255
(1999): van der Vleuten CJ+, *Acta Derm Venereol* 79, 323
(1997): Basarab T+, *Br J Dermatol* 136, 974 (photo-induced)
Urticaria (<1%)
Vasculitis
(1995): del Rio Fermandez MC+, *Rev Clin Esp* (Spanish) 195, 738
Xerosis (<0.1%)

Hair
Hair – alopecia (<1%)

Other
Acute intermittent porphyria
(1997): Kepple A+, *Ann Pharmacother* 31, 253
Dysgeusia (<1%)
Gingival hyperplasia
(2001): Morisaki I+, *Spec Care Dentist* 21(2), 60
(2000): James JA+, *J Clin Periodontol* 27, 109 (with cyclosporine)
(1999): Ellis JS+, *J Periodontol* 70, 63 (3.3%)
(1999): van der Vleuten CJ+, *Acta Derm Venereol* 79, 323
(1997): Infante-Cossio P+, *An Med Interna* (Spanish) 14, 83
(1997): Jorgensen MG, *J Periodontol* 68, 676
(1995): Salerno L+, *Clin Ter* (Italian) 146, 275
(1995): Wynn RL, *Gen Dent* 43, 218
(1994): Juncadella Garcia E+, *Med Clin (Barc)* (Spanish) 103, 358
(1994): Seymour RA+, *J Clin Periodontol* 21, 281
(1993): Ellis JS+, *Lancet* 341, 1102
(1993): Smith RG, *Br Dent J* 175, 279
(1991): Wynn RL, *Gen Dent* 39, 240
Gynecomastia
(1994): Zochling J+, *Med J Aust* 160, 807
Headache
Hyperesthesia (<1%)
Paresthesias (<1%)
Parkinsonism
(2003): *Prescrire Int* 12(64), 62
(2002): Teive HA+, *Mov Disord* 17(4), 833
Parosmia (<0.1%)
Tendinitis
(1999): Zambanini A+, *J Hum Hypertens* 13, 565 (Achilles)
Tinnitus
Tremor
Xerostomia (<1%)

AMOBARBITAL

Trade name: Amytal (Lilly)
Other common trade names: *Amytal Sodium; Isoamitil Sedante; Neur-Amyl; Novambarb; Sodium Amytal*
Indications: Insomnia, sedation
Category: Anticonvulsant; Barbiturate sedative-hypnotic
Half-life: initial: 40 minutes; terminal: 20 hours
Clinically important, potentially hazardous interactions with: alcohol, dicumarol, ethanolamine, warfarin

Reactions

Skin
Acne
Angioedema
Bullous eruption
Erythema
(1979): Rudzki E, *Przegl Dermatol* (Polish) 66, 415
Exanthems
Exfoliative dermatitis (<1%)
Photosensitivity

Purpura
Rash (sic) (<1%)
Stevens–Johnson syndrome (<1%)
Toxic epidermal necrolysis
(1969): Strom J, *Scand J Infect Dis* 1, 209
Urticaria (<1%)

Other
Headache
Hypersensitivity
Injection-site pain (>10%)
Rhabdomyolysis
(1990): Larpin R+, *Presse Med* 19(30), 1403
Serum sickness
Thrombophlebitis (<1%)

AMOXAPINE

Trade name: Amoxapine (Watson)
Other common trade names: *Amoxan; Asendis; Defanyl; Demolox*
Indications: Depression
Category: Tricyclic antidepressant
Half-life: 11–30 hours
Clinically important, potentially hazardous interactions with: amprenavir, clonidine, epinephrine, guanethidine, isocarboxazid, linezolid, MAO inhibitors, phenelzine, quinolones, sparfloxacin, tranylcypromine

Reactions

Skin
Acne
Acute generalized exanthematous pustulosis (AGEP)
(1998): Loche F+, *Acta Derm Venereol* 78, 224
(1994): Larbre B+, *Ann Dermatol Venereol* (French) 121, 40
Allergic reactions (sic) (<1%)
Dermatitis (sic)
Diaphoresis (1–10%)
Edema (>1%)
Erythema multiforme (observation)
(1982): Bishop L, *ADRRS* oral communication
Exanthems
(1996): Nagayama H+, *J Dermatol* 23, 899
(1982): Jue SG+, *Drugs* 24, 1
Flushing
Petechiae
Photosensitivity (<1%)
Pruritus (<1%)
(1988): Warnock JK+, *Am J Psychiatry* 145, 425
Pseudoparkinsonism (sic)
Purpura
Rash (sic) (>1%)
Side effects (sic) (5.1%)
(1982): Jue SG+, *Drugs* 24, 1
Toxic epidermal necrolysis
(1988): Warnock JK+, *Am J Psychiatry* 145, 425
(1983): Camisa C+, *Arch Dermatol* 119, 709
Urticaria (<1%)
Vasculitis (<1%)
(1988): Warnock JK+, *Am J Psychiatry* 145, 425
Xerosis

Hair
Hair – alopecia (<1%)

Other

Black tongue
Bromhidrosis
Dysgeusia (>10%)
Galactorrhea (<1%)
  (1979): Gelenberg AJ+, JAMA 242, 1900
  (1978): Jaffe K, J Clin Psychiatry 39, 821
Glossitis
Gynecomastia (<1%)
Headache
Paresthesias (<1%)
Sialorrhea
Stomatitis
Tinnitus
Tremor
Vaginitis
Xerostomia (14%)
  (1982): Jue SG+, Drugs 24, 1

AMOXICILLIN

Synonym: amoxycillin
Trade names: Amoxil (GSK); Augmentin (GSK); Prevpac (TAP);
Trimox (Geneva)
Other common trade names: A-Gram; Acimox; Almodan;
Amodex; Apo-Amoxi; Clamoxyl; Eupen; Fisamox; Lin-Amnox;
Novamoxin; Nu-Amoxi; Pro-Amox
Indications: Infections of the respiratory tract, skin and urinary
tract
Category: Broad-spectrum penicillin
Half-life: 0.7–1.4 hours
**Clinically important, potentially hazardous interactions
with:** allopurinol, chloramphenicol, demeclocycline, doxycycline,
erythromycin, methotrexate, minocycline, oxytetracycline,
sulfonamides, tetracycline

Augmentin is amoxicillin and clavulanate

Reactions

Skin

Acute generalized exanthematous pustulosis (AGEP)
  (2002): Pattee SF+, Arch Dermatol 138(8), 1091
  (2001): de Thier F+, Contact Dermatitis 44, 114
  (2000): Meadows KP+, Pediatric Dermatology 17, 399
  (1997): Gibert-Agullo A+, An Esp Pediatr (Spanish) 46, 285
  (1997): Zabawski, E, Dallas, TX (from Internet) (observation)
  (1996): Wolkenstein P+, Contact Dermatitis 35, 234
  (1995): Moreau A+, Int J Dermatol 34, 263 (passim)
  (1991): Roujeau J-C+, Arch Dermatol 127, 1333
  (1989): Epelbaum S+, Pediatrie (French) 44, 387
Angioedema (1–10%)
  (1998): Minguez MA+, Allergol Immunopathol (Madr) (Spanish)
    26, 43
  (1994): Galindo-Bonilla PA+, Contact Dermatitis 31, 319
  (1994): Vega JM+, Allergy 49, 317
  (1989): Chopra R+, Can Med Assoc J 140, 921 (in children)
Baboon syndrome
  (2002): Strub C+, Schweiz Rundsch Med Prax 91(6), 232
  (2000): Kick G+, Contact Dermatitis 43, 366
  (1996): Kohler LD+, Int J Dermatol 35, 502
  (1994): Duve S+, Acta Derm Venereol 74, 480
  (1993): Herfs H+, Hautarzt (German) 44, 466
Bullous pemphigoid
  (1997): Miralles J+, Int J Dermatol 36, 42

  (1988): Alcalay J+, J Am Acad Dermatol 18, 345
Dermatitis
  (2001): Petavy-Catala C+, Contact Dermatitis 44, 251 (consort)
  (1996): Garcia R+, Contact Dermatitis 35, 116
  (1995): Gamboa P+, Contact Dermatitis 32, 48 (occupational)
Diaper rash
  (1988): Honig PJ+, J Am Acad Dermatol 19, 275
Ecchymoses
Edema
  (1993): Echeverria-Arellano A+, An Esp Pediatr (Spanish) 39, 448
Erythema multiforme
  (2001): Perez A+, Contact Dermatitis 44, 113 (with allopurinol)
  (1999): Benjamin S+, Ann Pharmacother 33, 109
  (1999): Wakelin SH+, Clin Exp Dermatol 24, 71
  (1996): Webster GF, Philadelphia, PA (from Internet)
    (observation)
  (1995): Wolkenstein P+, Arch Dermatol 131, 544
  (1992): Gross AS+, J Am Acad Dermatol 27, 781
  (1990): Chan HL+, Arch Dermatol 126, 43
  (1990): Escallier F+, Rev Med Interne (French) 11, 73
  (1989): Chopra R+, Can Med Assoc J 140, 921 (in children)
  (1988): Massullo RE+, J Am Acad Dermatol 19, 358
  (1988): Platt R, J Infect Dis 158, 474
  (1986): Davidson NJ+, BMJ 292, 380
  (1986): Dikland WJ+, Pediatr Dermatol 3, 135
  (1982): Freeman T, Can Med Assoc J 127, 818
Exanthems (>5%)
  (2002): Renn CN+, Br J Dermatol 147(6), 1166 (4 cases, all with
    infectious mononucleosis)
  (1999): Wakelin SH+, Clin Exp Dermatol 24, 71 (flexural)
  (1997): Barbaud AM+, Arch Dermatol 133, 481
  (1997): Blumenthal HL, Beachwood, OH (personal case)
    (observation)
  (1995): Romano A+, Allergy 50, 113
  (1995): Wolkenstein P+, Arch Dermatol 131, 544
  (1994): Litt JZ, Beachwood, OH (personal case) (observation)
  (1993): Fellner MJ, Int J Dermatol 32, 308
  (1993): Romano A+, J Invest Allergol Clin Immunol 3, 53
  (1990): Pauszek ME, Indiana Med 83, 330
  (1989): Battegay M+, Lancet 2, 1100
  (1989): Chopra R+, Can Med Assoc J 140, 921 (in children)
  (1989): Kennedy C+, Contact Dermatitis 20, 313
  (1986): Bigby M+, JAMA 256, 3358 (5.14%)
  (1986): de Haan P+, Allergy 41, 75
  (1986): Sonntag MR+, Schweiz Med Wochenschr (German)
    116, 142 (7%)
  (1985): Levine LR, Pediatr Infect Dis 4, 358
  (1981): Odegaard OR, Tidsskr Nor Laegeforen (Norwegian)
    101, 1973
  (1977): Taylor B+, BMJ 2, 552 (3.7%)
  (1975): Brogden RN+, Drugs 9, 88 (1–22%)
  (1974): Wise PJ+, J Infect Dis 129 (Suppl), s266
  (1973): Dubb S, S A Med J 47, 1218
Exfoliative dermatitis
Fixed eruption
  (2001): Agnew KL+, Australas J Dermatol 42(3), 200
    (reproducible)
  (2000): Brabek E+, Dtsch Med Wochenschr 125(42), 1260
  (1998): Mahboob A+, Int J Dermatol 37, 833
  (1997): Jimenez I+, Allergol Immunopathol (Madr) 25, 247 (glans
    penis)
  (1997): Zabawski E, Dallas, TX (from Internet) (observation)
  (1995): Arias J+, Clin Exp Dermatol 20, 339
  (1995): Dhar S+, Pediatr Dermatol 12, 51 (tongue)
  (1994): Gil-Garcia JF+, Med Clin (Barc) (Spanish) 102, 438
  (1989): Shuttleworth D, Clin Exp Dermatol 14, 367 (pustular)
  (1982): Chowdhury FH, Practitioner 226, 1450 (penile)
Fixed eruption (neutrophilic)
  (2001): Agnew KI+, Aust J Dermatol 42, 200

Hematomas

Intertrigo
(1992): Wolf B+, *Acta Derm Venereol (Stockh)* 72, 441

Jarisch–Herxheimer reaction
(1998): Maloy AL+, *J Emerg Med* 16, 437

Keratosis pilaris
(1997): Kay M, North Hollywood, CA (from Internet) (observation)

Pemphigus
(1997): Brenner S+, *J Am Acad Dermatol* 36, 919
(1997): Landau M+, *Am J Dermatopathol* 19, 411
(1991): Escallier F+, *Ann Dermatol Venereol* (French) 118, 381
(1983): Toan ND+, *Ann Dermatol Venereol* (French) 110, 917

Perleche
(1982): Arata J+, *Jpn J Antibiot* (Japanese) 35, 394

Petechiae (Rumpel–Leede sign)
(1992): Gross AS+, *J Am Acad Dermatol* 27, 781

Pruritus
(2000): Blumenthal HL, Beachwood, OH (personal case) (observation)
(1996): Drouet M+, *Allerg Immunol Paris* (French) 28, 311
(1995): Shelley WB+, *Cutis* 55, 202 (observation)
(1993): Fellner MJ, *Int J Dermatol* 32, 308
(1989): Battegay M+, *Lancet* 2, 1100

Psoriasis
(1993): Litt JZ, Beachwood, OH (personal case) (observation)

Purpura

Pustular psoriasis
(1987): Katz M, *J Am Acad Dermatol* 17, 918

Pustules
(2000): Whittam LR+, *Clin Exp Dermatol* 25, 122
(1995): Wolkenstein P+, *Arch Dermatol* 131, 544
(1992): Trueb R+, *Hautarzt* (German) 43, 595
(1991): Armster H+, *Hautarzt* (German) 42, 713
(1991): Roujeau J-C+, *Arch Dermatol* 127, 1333
(1990): Guy C+, *Nouv Dermatol* (French) 9, 540
(1989): Epelbaum S+, *Pédiatrie* (French) 44, 387
(1989): Shuttleworth D, *Clin Exp Dermatol* 14, 367

Rash (sic) (1–10%)
(1997): Van Buchem FL+, *Lancet* 349, 683
(1989): Battegay M+, *Lancet* 2, 1100
(1982): Arata J+, *Jpn J Antibiot* (Japanese) 35, 394
(1982): Millard G, *Scott Med J* 27, S35
(1980): Porter J+, *Lancet* 1, 1037

Side effects (sic)
(1994): Paparello SF+, *AIDS* 8, 276

Stevens–Johnson syndrome
(1999): Limauro DL+, *Ann Pharmacother* 33, 560
(1996): Cullimore KC, Westminster, CO (from Internet) (observation)
(1992): Martin Mateos MA+, *J Investig Allergol Clin Immunol* 2, 278
(1988): Platt R, *J Infect Dis* 158, 474

Toxic epidermal necrolysis
(2001): Spies M+, *Pediatrics* 108, 1162
(1996): Blum L+, *J Am Acad Dermatol* 34, 1088
(1996): Surbled M+, *Ann Fr Anesth Reanim* (French) 15, 1095
(1993): Correia O+, *Dermatology* 186, 32
(1993): Romano A+, *J Invest Allergol Clin Immunol* 3, 53
(1988): Massullo RE+, *J Am Acad Dermatol* 19, 358
(1984): Herman TE+, *Pediatr Radiol* 14, 439

Toxic pustuloderma
(1992): Trueb R+, *Hautarzt* (German) 43, 595
(1991): Armster H+, *Hautarzt* (German) 42, 713

Urticaria (1–5%)
(2001): Torres MJ+, *Allergy* 56(9), 850
(2000): Blumenthal HL, Beachwood, OH (personal case) (observation)

(1998): Minguez MA+, *Allergol Immunopathol (Madr)* (Spanish) 26, 43
(1997): Delpre G+, *Dig Dis Sci* 42, 728
(1997): Thaler D, Monona, WI (from internet) (observation)
(1995): Litt JZ, Beachwood, OH (personal case) (observation)
(1994): Vega JM+, *Allergy* 49, 317
(1990): Fraj J+, *Clin Exp Allergy* 20, 121
(1989): Battegay M+, *Lancet* 2, 1100
(1989): Chopra R+, *Can Med Assoc J* 140, 921 (in children)
(1985): Goolamali SK, *Postgrad Med J* 61, 925

Vasculitis
(1999): Garcia-Porrua C+, *J Rheumatol* 26, 1942

Vesicular eruptions

Other

Anaphylactoid reactions
(2001): Torres MJ+, *Allergy* 56(9), 850
(1999): Salgado Fernandez J+, *Rev Esp Cardiol* (Spanish) 52, 622
(1998): Rich MW, *Tex Heart Inst J* 25, 194
(1994): Vega JM+, *Allergy* 49, 317
(1993): van der Klauw MM+, *Br J Clin Pharmacol* 35, 400
(1990): Fraj J+, *Clin Exp Allergy* 20, 121
(1988): Blanca M+, *Allergy* 43, 508

Black tongue

Dysgeusia

Glossitis

Glossodynia

Headache

Hypersensitivity
(2000): da Fonseca MA, *Pediatr Dent* 22(5), 401
(1995): Mokry C, *N Engl J Med* 333, 1151
(1993): Romano A+, *Contact Dermatitis* 28, 190
(1989): Kennedy C+, *Contact Dermatitis* 20, 313

Injection-site pain

Oral candidiasis

Serum sickness (1–10%)
(1995): Martin J+, *N Z Med J* 108, 123
(1992): Stricker BH+, *J Clin Epidemiol* 45, 1177
(1990): Heckbert SR+, *Am J Epidemiol* 132, 336
(1989): Chopra R+, *Can Med Assoc J* 140, 921 (in children)
(1988): Platt R+, *J Infect Dis* 158, 474

Stomatitis
(1996): Drouet M+, *Allerg Immunol Paris* (French) 28, 311

Stomatodynia

Tooth discoloration
(2001): Garcia-Lopez M+, *Pediatrics* 108(3), 819

Vaginitis (1%)
(1996): Drouet M+, *Allerg Immunol Paris* (French) 28, 311
(1978): Fang LST+, *N Engl J Med* 298, 413

Xerostomia

AMPHOTERICIN B

Trade names: Abelcet (Elan); AmBisome (Fujisawa); Amphocin (Pharmacia); Fungizone (Geneva)
Other common trade names: *Ampho-Moronal; Fungilin*
Indications: Potentially life-threatening fungal infections
Category: Antifungal; Antiprotozoal
Half-life: initial: 15–48 hours; terminal: 15 days
Clinically important, potentially hazardous interactions with: adefovir, aminoglycosides, cephalothin, cidofovir, cyclosporine, digoxin, fluconazole, ganciclovir, itraconazole, ketoconazole, probenecid

Reactions

Skin
Angioedema
Burning (sic) (from topical)
Chills
  (2002): Bowden R+, *Clin Infect Dis* 35(4), 359
Dermatitis
Diaphoresis
Erythema
Erythema multiforme
Exanthems (<1%)
  (1999): Cesaro S+, *Support Care Cancer* 7, 284
  (1976): Lorber B+, *Ann Intern Med* 84, 54
  (1966): Beaty HN+, *Ann Intern Med* 65, 641
Exfoliative dermatitis
  (1961): Sternberg TH+, *Med Clin North Am* 45, 781
Fixed eruption
  (1969): Kandil E, *Dermatologica* 139, 37
Flushing (1–10%)
  (1964): Martin WJ, *Med Clin North Am* 48, 255
  (1961): Sternberg TH+, *Med Clin North Am* 45, 781
Pigmentation
Pruritus
  (1999): Cesaro S+, *Support Care Cancer* 7, 284
  (1966): Beaty HN+, *Ann Intern Med* 65, 641
Purpura
  (1971): Costello MJ, *Arch Dermatol* 79, 184
  (1966): Beaty HN+, *Ann Intern Med* 65, 641
  (1961): Sternberg TH+, *Med Clin North Am* 45, 781
Rash (sic)
  (1995): Oppenheim BA+, *Clin Infect Dis* 21, 1145
Raynaud's phenomenon (cyanotic)
  (1997): Zernikow B+, *Mycoses* 40, 359
Red man syndrome
  (1990): Ellis ME+, *BMJ* 300, 1468
Toxicity (sic)
  (2002): Bowden R+, *Clin Infect Dis* 35(4), 359
Ulcerations
Urticaria
Vesicular eruptions
Xerosis

Hair
Hair – alopecia

Other
Anaphylactoid reactions
  (2001): Bishara J+, *Ann Pharmacother* 35, 308
  (1999): Cronin JE+, *Clin Infect Dis* 28, 1342
  (1998): Schneider P+, *Br J Haematol* 102, 1108
Death
  (2002): Johnson PC+, *Ann Intern Med* 137(2), 105

  (2001): Collazos J+, *Clin Infect Dis* 33(7), E75
Headache
Injection-site pain
Injection-site reactions (sic)
  (2003): Imhof A+, *Clin Infect Dis* 36(8), 943
  (2002): Johnson PC+, *Ann Intern Med* 137(2), 105
Injection-site thrombophlebitis
  (1995): Goodwin SD+, *Clin Infect Dis* 20, 755
Injection-site toxicity
  (2000): Karthaus M+., *Chemotherapy* 46, 293
Myalgia
Paresthesias (1–10%)
Rhabdomyolysis
  (1970): Drutz DJ+, *JAMA* 211(5), 824
Stomatitis
Thrombophlebitis (1–10%)
  (1993): Dietze R+, *Clin Infect Dis* 17, 981
Tinnitus
Xerostomia

AMPICILLIN

Trade names: D-Amp; Marcillin; Omnipen (Wyeth); Polycillin (Bristol-Myers Squibb); Principen (Geneva); Totacillin (GSK); Unasyn (Roerig)
Other common trade names: *Amfipen; Ampicin; Binotal; Penbritin; Penstabil; Pro-Ampi; Sinaplin; Taro-Ampicillin Trihydrate; Totapen; Vidopen*
Indications: Susceptible strains of gram-negative and gram-positive bacterial infections
Category: Broad-spectrum penicillin
Half-life: 1–1.5 hours
Clinically important, potentially hazardous interactions with: allopurinol, anticoagulants, chloramphenicol, cyclosporine, demeclocycline, doxycycline, erythromycin, methotrexate, minocycline, oxytetracycline, sulfonamides, tetracycline

Note: Five to 10% of people taking ampicillin develop eruptions between the 5th and 14th day following initiation of therapy. Also, there is a 95% incidence of exanthematous eruptions in patients who are treated for infectious mononucleosis with ampicillin. The allergenicity of ampicillin appears to be enhanced by allopurinol or by hyperuricemia. Ampicillin is clearly the more allergenic of the two drugs when given alone

Reactions

Skin
Acute generalized exanthematous pustulosis (AGEP)
  (1995): Moreau A+, *Int J Dermatol* 34, 263 (passim)
  (1994): Manders SM+, *Cutis* 54, 194
  (1991): Roujeau J-C+, *Arch Dermatol* 127, 1333
Allergic reactions (sic) (1–10%)
  (2003): Medrala W+, *Pol Merkuriusz Lek* 14(79), 39
  (1993): Grover JK+, *Indian J Physiol Pharmacol* 37, 247 (2.9%)
  (1974): Revuz J+, *Nouv Presse Med* (French) 3, 1169
Angioedema (<1%)
  (1982): Valsecchi R+, *Contact Dermatitis* 8, 278
  (1980): Kraemer MJ+, *Pediatrics in Review* 1, 197
Baboon syndrome
  (1993): Herfs H+, *Hautarzt* (German) 44, 466
  (1985): Rasmussen LP+, *Ugeskr Laeger* (Danish) 147, 1341
  (1984): Andersen KE+, *Contact Dermatitis* 10, 97
Bullous eruption (<1%)
  (1982): Stepien B+, *Przegl Dermatol* (Polish) 69, 65

Bullous pemphigoid
   (1990): Hodak E+, *Clin Exp Dermatol* 15, 50
Candidiasis
   (1973): Bass JW+, *J Pediatrics* 83, 106
Dermatitis
   (1997): Romano A+, *Clin Exp Allergy* 27, 1425
   (1995): Gamboa P+, *Contact Dermatitis* 32, 48
   (1988): Andersen KE, *Acta Derm Venereol* Suppl (Stockh) 135, 62
      (systemic)
   (1986): Pigatto PD+, *Contact Dermatitis* 14, 196
   (1978): Bruevich TS+, *Vest Dermatol Venerol* (Russian) March, 74
   (1970): Schulz KH+, *Berufsdermatosen* (German) 18, 132
   (1969): Braun W+, *Ther Ggw* (German) 108, 250
Diaper rash
   (1973): Bass JW+, *J Pediatrics* 83, 106 (4.5–13%)
Erythema annulare centrifugum
   (1975): Gupta HL+, *J Indian Med Assoc* 65, 307
Erythema multiforme (<1%)
   (1995): Dhar S+, *Dermatology* 191, 76
   (1994): Garty BZ+, *Ann Pharmacother* 28, 730
   (1990): Chan HL+, *Arch Dermatol* 126, 43
   (1985): Konstantinidis AB+, *J Oral Med* 40, 168
   (1984): Gebel K+, *Dermatologica* 168, 35
   (1979): Gupta HL+, *J Indian Med Assoc* 72, 188
   (1975): Böttiger LE+, *Acta Med Scand* 198, 229
   (1972): Kauppinen K, *Acta Derm Venereol* (Stockh) 52, 68
   (1970): Crow KD, *Trans A Rep St John's Hosp Dermatol Soc* 56, 35
Exanthems (>10%)
   (1997): Romano A+, *Clin Exp Allergy* 27, 1425
   (1996): Adcock BB+, *Arch Fam Med* 5, 301
   (1996): Marra CA+, *Ann Pharmacother* 30, 401
   (1995): Romano A+, *Allergy* 50, 113
   (1994): Grayson ML+, *Clin Infect Dis* 18, 683
   (1994): Shelley WB+, *Cutis* 53, 40 (observation)
   (1993): Romano A+, *J Invest Allergol Clin Immunol* 3, 53
   (1993): Warrington RJ+, *J Allergy Clin Immunol* 92, 626
   (1988): Hou SR, *Chung Hua Nei Ko Tsa Chih* (Chinese) 27, 36
   (1987): Pavithran K, *Indian J Lepr* 59, 309
   (1986): Cabo HA+, *Med Cutan Ibero Lat Am* (Spanish) 14, 177
   (1986): de Haan P+, *Allergy* 41, 75
   (1986): Sonntag MR+, *Schweiz Med Wochenschr* (German)
      116, 142 (8%)
   (1985): Bruynzeel DP+, *Dermatologica* 171, 429
   (1985): Hefelfinger DC, *Ala Med* 55, 16
   (1983): Bianchi C+, *Med Cutan Ibero Lat Am* (Spanish) 11, 113
   (1983): Scioli C+, *Boll Ist Sieroter Milan* (Italian) 62, 287
   (1982): Dourmischev AL+, *Dermatol Monatsschr* (German)
      168, 469
   (1982): Gatter KC+, *Clin Allergy* 12, 279
   (1981): Jick H+, *J Clin Pharmacol* 21, 456 (5.9%)
   (1981): Lin CS+, *Arch Dermatol* 117, 282
   (1980): Kraemer MJ+, *Pediatrics in Review* 1, 197
   (1980): Porter D+, *Lancet* 1, 1037
   (1980): Scherzer W+, *Derm Beruf Umwelt* (German) 28, 175
   (1979): Murphy TF, *Ann Intern Med* 91, 324
   (1978): Geyman JP+, *J Fam Pract* 7, 493
   (1978): Kouba K+, *Cesk Pediatr* (Czech) 33, 487
   (1978): Pollowitz JA, *Am J Dis Child* 132, 819
   (1977): Campbell AB+, *Pediatrics* 59, 638
   (1977): Gupta HL+, *J Indian Med Assoc* 68, 33
   (1977): Sokoloff B, *Pediatrics* 59, 637
   (1976): Arndt KA+, *JAMA* 235, 918 (5.2%)
   (1976): Fellner MJ+, *N Y State J Med* 76, 101
   (1976): Morris J, *Lancet* 1, 423
   (1976): Wuthrich B, *Dtsch Med Wochenschr* (German) 101, 470
   (1975): Editorial, *BMJ* 2, 708
   (1975): Esten H+, *Med Welt* (German) 26, 296
   (1975): Gleckman RA, *JAMA* 233, 427 (2.5%)
   (1975): Krsic B+, *Lijec Vjesn* (Serbo-Croatian-Roman) 97, 339
   (1975): Lehnhoff B, *Monatsschr Kinderheilkd* (German) 123, 548

   (1974): Spitzy KH, *Acta Med Austriaca* (German) 2, 46
   (1974): Webster AW+, *Clin Exp Immunol* 18, 553
   (1973): Bass JW+, *J Pediatrics* 83, 106 (4.75%)
   (1973): Boston Collaborative Drug Surveillance Program, *Arch
      Dermatol* 107, 74 (9.7%)
   (1973): Gregg I, *BMJ* 1, 295
   (1973): *BMJ* 1, 7
   (1973): *N Z Med J* 77, 105
   (1973): Kerns DL+, *Am J Dis Child* 125, 187
   (1973): Wemmer U, *Fortschr Med* (German) 91, 1232
   (1973): Zürcher K+, *Dermatologica* (German) 147, 1
   (1972): Almeyda J+, *Br J Dermatol* 87, 293
   (1972): Balfour HH+, *Clin Pediatr Phila* 11, 417
   (1972): Bierman CW+, *JAMA* 220, 1098
   (1972): Harris JR+, *BMJ* 1, 687
   (1972): *BMJ* 1, 195
   (1972): *BMJ* 1, 505
   (1972): *N Engl J Med* 286, 1217
   (1972): Kuokkanen K, *Acta Allergol* 27, 407
   (1972): Potter JPL, *BMJ* 1, 749
   (1972): Schulz KH, *Arch Dermatol Forsch* (German) 244, 309
   (1972): Steiniger U, *Dtsch Gesundheitsw* (German) 27, 1164
   (1972): Weuta H, *Arzneimittelforschung* (German) 22, 1300
   (1971): Beckmann H, *Munch Med Wochenschr* (German)
      113, 1423
   (1971): Bronsert U, *Med Klin* (German) 66, 352
   (1971): Kroidon EaP, *Antibiotiki* (Russian) 16, 549
   (1971): Pullen H, *BMJ* 2, 653
   (1971): Speck WT, *Clin Pediatr Phila* 10, 59
   (1970): Corless JD+, *South Med J* 63, 1341
   (1970): Crow KD, *Trans St Johns Hosp Dermatol Soc* 56, 35
   (1970): Fournier A+, *J Sci Med Lille* (French) 88, 529
   (1970): Jaffe IA, *Lancet* 1, 245
   (1970): Kerrebijn KF, *Lancet* 1, 245
   (1970): Knudsen ET+, *BMJ* 1, 469
   (1970): Kronig B+, *Arzneimittelforschung* (German) 20, 1930
   (1970): Shapiro S+, *Lancet* 1, 194 (9.5%)
   (1970): Weary PE+, *Arch Dermatol* 101, 86
   (1969): Hurwitz N+, *BMJ* 1, 531 (7.8%)
   (1969): No Author, *Lancet* 2, 993
   (1969): Sanders DY, *Clin Pediatr Phila* 8, 47
   (1969): Shapiro S+, *Lancet* 2, 969 (7.7%)
   (1968): Gabbert WR+, *J Ky Med Assoc* 66, 967
   (1968): Levene G+, *Br J Dermatol* 80, 417
   (1968): Loffler H+, *Med Welt* (German) 32, 1736
   (1966): Stevenson J+, *BMJ* 1, 1359
Exfoliative dermatitis
   (1985): Fong PH+, *Ann Acad Med Singapore* 14, 693
   (1974): Tay C, *Asian J Med* 10, 223
Fixed eruption
   (2000): Brabek E+, *Dtsch Med Wochenschr* 125(42), 1260
   (1998): Mahboob A+, *Int J Dermatol* 37, 833
   (1990): Bharija SC+, *Dermatologica* 181, 237
   (1990): Gaffoor PMA+, *Cutis* 45, 242
   (1987): Sharma SN, *J Assoc Physicians India* 35, 608
   (1986): Kanwar AJ+, *Dermatologica* 172, 315
   (1986): Panagariya A, *J Ass Physicians India* 34, 458
   (1984): Chan H-L, *Arch Dermatol* 120, 542
   (1983): Chan H-L, *Int J Dermatol* 23, 607
   (1970): Savin JA, *Br J Dermatol* 83, 546
Linear IgA bullous dermatosis
   (2002): Cohen LM+, *J Am Acad Dermatol* 46, S32 (passim)
   (1996): Tranvan A+, *J Am Acad Dermatol* 35, 865
   (1981): Boffety B+, *Journées Dermatologiques de Paris*
      (French), 53–53a
Pemphigus
   (1997): Brenner S+, *J Am Acad Dermatol* 36, 919
   (1996): Takizawa H+, *Am J Gastroenterol* 91, 1654
   (1993): Brenner S+, *Isr J Med Sci* 29, 44
   (1986): Brenner S+, *J Am Acad Dermatol* 14, 453

(1986): Wilson JP+, *Drug Intell Clin Pharm* 20, 219
(1980): Fellner MJ+, *Int J Dermatol* 19, 392
Pityriasis rosea
(1987): Olumide Y, *Int J Dermatol* 26, 234
Pruritus (1–5%)
(1996): Adcock BB+, *Arch Fam Med* 5, 301
(1982): Bernhard JD+, *Cutis* 29, 158
(1980): Kraemer MJ+, *Pediatrics in Review* 1, 197
(1973): Bass JW+, *J Pediatrics* 83, 106 (0.75%)
Psoriasis
(1993): Litt JZ, Beachwood, OH (personal case) (observation)
(1992): Breathnach SM+, *Adverse Drug Reactions and the Skin*
    Blackwell, Oxford, 141 (passim)
(1990): Saito S+, *J Dermatol* 17, 677
(1988): Tsankov N+, *J Am Acad Dermatol* 19, 629
Purpura
(1993): Pang BK+, *Ann Acad Med Singapore* 22, 870
(1990): Hannedouche T+, *J Antimicrob Chemother* 20, 3
(1982): Beeching NL+, *J Antimicrob Chemother* 10, 479
(1981): Valman HB, *Br Med J Clin Res Ed* 283, 970
(1973): Croydon EAP+, *BMJ* 1, 7
(1971): Parker JC+, *Arch Intern Med* 127, 474
Pustular psoriasis
(1987): Katz M+, *J Am Acad Dermatol* 17, 918
(1986): Verner E+, *Harefuah* (Hebrew) 110, 132
Pustules
(1995): Lim JT+, *Cutis* 56, 163
(1994): Jay S+, *Arch Dermatol* 130, 787 (localized)
(1991): Roujeau J-C+, *Arch Dermatol* 127, 1333
(1990): Guy C+, *Nouv Dermatol* (French) 9, 540
Rash (sic) (1–10%)
Stevens–Johnson syndrome
(1990): Cavanzo FJ+, *Gastroenterology* 99, 854
(1990): Chan HL+, *Arch Dermatol* 126, 43
(1987): Howell CG+, *J Pediatr Surg* 22, 994
(1985): Ting HC+, *Int J Dermatol* 24, 587
(1985): Turck M, *Hosp Pract Off Ed* 20, 49
(1979): Gupta HL+, *J Indian Med Assoc* 72, 188
(1978): Assaad D+, *Can Med Assoc* 118, 154
(1975): McArthur JE+, *N Z Med J* 81, 390
(1972): Kauppinen K, *Acta Derm Venereol* (Stockh) 52, 68
Toxic epidermal necrolysis (<1%)
(2002): Zelenkova H+, *World Congress Dermatol* Poster, 0136
(1997): Rodrigues-Ares MT+, *Int Ophthalmol* 21, 39
(1993): Romano A+, *J Invest Allergol Clin Immunol* 3, 53
(1991): Heng MC+, *J Am Acad Dermatol* 25, 778
(1985): Robbens EJ+, *Acta Clin Belg* 40, 115
(1983): Tagami H+, *Arch Dermatol* 119, 910
(1981): Berkel AI+, *Turk J Pediatr* 23, 37
(1980): Giuffre L+, *Minerva Pediatr* (Italian) 32, 633
(1979): Rosenthal AL+, *Cutis* 24, 437
(1978): Assaad D+, *Can Med Assoc* 118, 154
(1975): Böttiger LE+, *Acta Med Scand* 198, 229
(1975): McArthur JE+, *N Z Med J* 81, 390
(1975): Schopf E+, *Z Haut* (German) 50, 865
(1972): Carli-Basset C+, *Sem Hop* (French) 48, 497
Urticaria
(1997): Romano A+, *Clin Exp Allergy* 27, 1425
(1996): Adcock BB+, *Arch Fam Med* 5, 301
(1985): Goolamali SK, *Postgrad Med J* 61, 925
(1982): Valsecchi R+, *Contact Dermatitis* 8, 278
(1980): Kraemer MJ+, *Pediatrics in Review* 1, 197
(1977): Gupta HL+, *J Indian Med Assoc* 68, 33
(1975): Gleckman RA, *JAMA* 233, 427 (0.8%)
(1973): Croydon EAP+, *BMJ* 1, 7
(1972): Bierman CW+, *JAMA* 220, 1098
(1969): Coskey RJ+, *Arch Dermatol* 100, 717
(1969): Knudsen ET, *BMJ* 1, 846
(1969): Pullen H, *BMJ* 2, 247

(1963): Kennedy WPU+, *BMJ* 2, 962 (10%)
Vasculitis
(1991): Estrada-Rodriguez JL+, *J Investig Allergol Clin Immunol*
    1, 69
(1990): Hannedouche T+, *J Antimicrob Chemother* 20, 3
(1975): Pevny I+, *MMW Munch Med Wochenschr* (German)
    117, 9
(1974): Tay C, *Asian J Med* 10, 223

Other
Anaphylactoid reactions
(1998): Rich MW, *Tex Heart Inst J* 25, 194
(1997): Romano A+, *Clin Exp Allergy* 27, 1425
(1996): Adcock BB+, *Arch Fam Med* 5, 301
(1976): Fellner MJ, *Int J Dermatol* 15, 497
(1975): Pietzcker F+, *Z Hautkr* (German) 50, 437
(1973): Weck AL de, *Munch Med Wochenschr* (German)
    115, 1650
(1972): Ohela K+, *Duodecim* (Finnish) 88, 1177
Black tongue
(1966): Meyler L (ed), *Side Effects of Drugs* 5th ed. Amsterdam,
    Excerpta Medica
Glossitis
Hypersensitivity
(1996): Torricelli R+, *Hautarzt* (German) 47, 392
(1993): Romano A+, *Contact Dermatitis* 28, 190
(1987): Ackerman Z+, *Postgrad Med J* 63, 55
(1970): Klemola E, *Scand J Infect Dis* 2, 29
Injection-site pain (>10%)
Oral candidiasis
Oral mucosal eruption
(1984): Gebel K+, *Dermatologica* 168, 35
Phlebitis
Serum sickness
(1974): Caldwell JR+, *JAMA* 230, 77
Stomatitis
Thrombophlebitis
Vaginal candidiasis

AMPRENAVIR

Trade name: Agenerase (GSK)
Indications: HIV infection
Category: Protease inhibitor; Sulfonamide
Half-life: N/A
**Clinically important, potentially hazardous interactions
with:** amiodarone, amitriptyline, amoxapine, benzodiazepines,
bepridil, clomipramine, clonazepam, clorazepate, delavirdine,
desipramine, diazepam, dihydroergotamine, doxepin, ergotamine,
fentanyl, flurazepam, imipramine, lidocaine, lorazepam,
methysergide, midazolam, nortriptyline, oxazepam, phenytoin,
protriptyline, quazepam, quinidine, rifampin, sildenafil, **St John's
wort**, temazepam, tricyclic antidepressants, trimipramine,
vitamin E

Reactions

Skin
Exanthems
Pruritus
Rash (sic) (25%)
(2003): Justesen US+, *Br J Clin Pharmacol* 55(1), 100 (with
    delavirdine)
(2001): Scott T+, *Clin Ther* 23(2), 252 (8%)
(2000): Noble S+, *Drugs* 60(6), 1383
(2000): Pedneault L+, *Clin Ther* 22(12), 1378 (3%)

Stevens–Johnson syndrome (4%)

Other
Buffalo hump
Dysgeusia (10%)
Gynecomastia
Hyperesthesia
   (1999): Sadler BM+, *Antimicrob Agents Chemother* 14, 1686
Paresthesias (perioral) (26%)
   (2001): *Prescrire Int* 10(53), 70
   (2001): McMahon D+, *Antivir Ther* 6(2), 105
   (2000): Pedneault L+, *Clin Ther* 22(12), 1378

*Note: Protease inhibitors cause dyslipidemia which includes elevated triglycerides and cholesterol and redistribution of body fat centrally to produce the so-called 'protease paunch,' breast enlargement, facial atrophy, and 'buffalo hump'

**Note: Amprenavir is a sulfonamide and can be absorbed systemically. Sulfonamides can produce severe, possibly fatal, reactions such as toxic epidermal necrolysis and Stevens–Johnson syndrome

AMYL NITRITE

Synonym: isoamyl nitrite
Trade name: Amyl Nitrite (Lilly)
Other common trade name: *Nitrit*
Indications: Angina pectoris
Category: Antianginal; Coronary vasodilator
Half-life: N/A
Clinically important, potentially hazardous interactions with: furosemide, sildenafil

Reactions

Skin
Allergic reactions (sic)
   (1989): Dax EM+, *Am J Med* 86, 732
Dermatitis (sic)
   (1985): Bos JD+, *Contact Dermatitis* 12, 109
   (1984): Fisher AA, *Cutis* 34(2), 118
   (1982): Romaguera C+, *Contact Dermatitis* 8, 266
Diaphoresis
Edema
Flushing (1–10%)
Pallor
Rash (sic) (<1%)

Other
Headache

ANAGRELIDE

Trade name: Agrylin (Shire)
Indications: Essential thrombocytopenia. To reduce elevated platelet count and the risk of thrombosis
Category: Phospholipase A 2 inhibitor; Platelet aggregation inhibitor
Half-life: ~3 days
Clinically important, potentially hazardous interactions with: fondaparinux

Reactions

Skin
Adverse effects (sic) (<5%)
Chills (<5%)
Ecchymoses (<5%)
Edema (19.8%)
   (2002): Kornblihtt LI+, *Medicina (B Aires)* 62(3), 231
   (1998): Oertel MD, *Am J Health Syst Pharm* 55(19), 1979
Flu-like syndrome (<5%)
Peripheral edema (7.1%)
   (1992): Mazzucconi MG+, *Haematologica* 77(4), 315
Photosensitivity (<5%)
Pruritus (<5%)
Rash (sic) (7.8%)
Urticaria (7.8%)

Hair
Hair – alopecia (<5%)

Other
Aphthous stomatitis (<5%)
Arthralgia (<5%)
Back pain (6.4%)
Depression (<5%)
Headache
Leg cramps (<5%)
Myalgia (<5%)
Paresthesias (7.3%)
Tinnitus (<5%)

ANAKINRA

Synonym: IL-1RA
Trade name: Kineret (Amgen)
Indications: Rheumatoid arthritis
Category: Disease modifying antirheumatic (DMARD); Interleukin-1 receptor antagonist
Half-life: 4–6 hours
Clinically important, potentially hazardous interactions with: etanercept

Reactions

Skin
Flu-like syndrome (6%)
Infections (40%)
   (2003): Fleischmann RM+, *Arthritis Rheum* 48(4), 927 (2.1%)
   (2003): Kary S+, *Int J Clin Pract* 57(3), 231
Upper respiratory infection (4%)

Other
Headache

Hypersensitivity
Injection-site ecchymoses
Injection-site erythema
Injection-site inflammation
Injection-site pain
Injection-site reactions (sic) (71%)
  (2003): Fleischmann RM, *Rheumatology* (Oxford) 42(Suppl
    2), ii29
  (2003): Kary S+, *Int J Clin Pract* 57(3), 231
  (2002): Calabrese LH, *Ann Pharmacother* 36(7), 1204
  (2002): Cohen S+, *Arthritis Rheum* 46(3), 614
  (2001): Bresnihan B, *Semin Arthritis Rheum* 30(5 Suppl 2), 17
  (2001): Garces K, *Issues Emerg Health Technol* May(16), 1
  (1998): Bresnihan B+, *Arthritis Rheum* 41(12), 2196
Sinusitis (7%)

ANASTROZOLE

Trade name: Arimidex (AstraZeneca)
Indications: Breast carcinoma (localized-advanced or metastatic)
Category: Antineoplastic; Aromatase inhibitor
Half-life: 50 hours

Reactions

Skin
Chills
Diaphoresis
  (1997): Jonat W, *Oncology* 54 (Suppl 2), 15
Flu-like syndrome (6.9%)
Flushing (>5%)
Hot flashes (26.5%)
  (2002): Buzdar AU, *Expert Rev Anticancer Ther* 2(6), 623
  (1998): Higa GM+, *Am J Health* 55(5), 445
Infections (sic) (2–5%)
Peripheral edema (10.1%)
Pruritus (2–5%)
Rash (sic) (7.5%)
Shivering

Hair
Hair – alopecia (2–5%)

Other
Arthralgia (2–5%)
Bone or joint pain (10.7%)
Cough (10.9%)
Depression (4.5%)
Headache
Mastodynia (2–5%)
Myalgia (2–5%)
Pain (13.8%)
  (1998): Higa GM+, *Am J Health* 55(5), 445
Paresthesias
Thrombophlebitis (2–5%)
Tumor pain (>5%)
Vaginal dryness (1.7%)
Xerostomia

ANDROSTENEDIONE

Scientific names: *4-androstene-3,17-dione; Androst-4-ene-3,17-dione*
Family: N/A
Trade and other common names: Andro; Androstene
Category: Dietary supplement
Purported indications and other uses: Enhanced athletic performance, increased energy, to keep red blood cells healthy
Half-life: N/A

Reactions

Skin
Acne
  (1999): Pheatt N, *Sports Supplements. Pharmacist's Letter* 99, 1
  (1998): *Med Lett Drugs Ther* 40, 105
Coarsening of skin (sic)
  (1998): *Med Lett Drugs Ther* 40, 105

Hair
Hair – alopecia
  (1998): *Med Lett Drugs Ther* 40, 105
Hair – hirsutism (in women)
  (1999): Pheatt N, *Sports Supplements. Pharmacist's Letter* 99, 1

Other
Gynecomastia
Priapism
  (2000): Kachhi PN+, *Ann Emerg Med* 35, 391
Side effects (sic)
  (2002): Lawrence ME+, *J Clin Gastroenterol* 35(4), 299

Note: Androstenedione gained popularity as the supplement used by homerun-hitter, Mark McGuire. Recent evidence suggests that its use can cause abnormal elevations in serum estrogen, increase risk of developing prostate or pancreatic cancers, and reduce high-density lipoproteins thus increasing cardiovascular disease risk

ANISINDIONE

Trade name: Miradon (Schering)
Indications: Adjunct in treatment of coronary occlusion, Atrial fibrillation
Category: Indanedione oral anticoagulant
Half-life: 3–5 days
Clinically important, potentially hazardous interactions with: amiodarone, anabolic steroids, antithyroid agents, barbiturates, bivalirudin, cimetidine, clofibrate, clopidogrel, cyclosporine, delavirdine, dextrothyroxine, disulfiram, fluconazole, glutethimide, imatinib, itraconazole, ketoconazole, metronidazole, miconazole, penicillins, phenylbutazones, piperacillin, quinidine, quinine, rifabutin, rifampin, rifapentine, rofecoxib, salicylates, sulfinpyrazone, sulfonamides, testosterone, thyroid, zileuton

Reactions

Skin
Chills
Dermatitis (sic)
Ecchymoses
Erythema
Erythema multiforme

Exanthems
Exfoliative dermatitis
Necrosis
Petechiae
Purple toe syndrome
Urticaria

Hair

Hair – alopecia

Other

Death
Hypersensitivity
Oral ulceration
Priapism
Stomatitis
Stomatodynia

ANISTREPLASE

Synonym: APSAC
Trade name: Eminase (Shire)
Other common trade name: *Iminase*
Indications: Acute myocardial infarction
Category: Thrombolytic enzyme
Half-life: 70–120 minutes

Reactions

Skin

Allergic reactions (sic)
Angioedema
Chills (<1%)
Diaphoresis (<1%)
Ecchymoses
Exanthems
  (1995): Dykewicz MS+, *J Allergy Clin Immunol* 95, 1020
Flushing
Livedo reticularis
  (1994): Gianni R+, *Ann Ital Med Int* (Italian) 9, 105
Purpura
Rash (sic)
Ulcerations
  (1994): Gianni R+, *Ann Ital Med Int* (Italian) 9, 105
Urticaria
  (1995): Dykewicz MS+, *J Allergy Clin Immunol* 95, 1020
Vasculitis
  (1994): Gianni R+, *Ann Ital Med Int* (Italian) 9, 105
  (1992): Burrows N+, *J Am Acad Dermatol* 26, 508
  (1990): Burrows N+, *Br Heart J* 64, 289
  (1988): Bucknall C+, *Br Heart J* 59, 9
  (1988): Gemmill JD+, *Br Heart J* 60, 361

Other

Anaphylactoid reactions (1–10%)
  (1997): Cannas S+, *G Ital Cardiol* (Italian) 27, 278
Gingival hemorrhage
Hypersensitivity
  (1993): Lee HS+, *Eur Heart J* 14, 1640
Myalgia
  (1994): Gianni R+, *Ann Ital Med Int* (Italian) 9, 105
Serum sickness
  (1993): Lee HS+, *Eur Heart J* 14, 1640

ANTHRAX VACCINE

Trade names: Anthrax Vaccine Adsorbed [AVA] (BioPort);
Carbosap
Indications: Anthrax prophylaxis
Category: Vaccine
Half-life: Requires 1 month to achieve immunity (92.5%
efficient)

Reactions

Skin

Allergic reactions (sic)
  (2000): Captain James Bishop, *Citizen Airman* (0,002%)
  (1999): Ellenberg SS, *Center for Biologics Evaluation & Research,
    FDA Statement* (widespread)
Angioedema
  (2000): *MMWR* 49(RR15), 1
Cellulitis
  (2000): *MMWR* 49(RR15), 1
Chills (<0.06%)
  (2000): *MMWR* 49(RR15), 1
Diaphoresis
  (2001): Swanson-Biearman B+, *J Toxicol Clin Toxicol* 39(1), 81
  (1999): Dr. Sue Bailey, *Asst Sec Defense Health Affairs – Service
    Member #16* 21
Edema (3%)
  (2000): *MMWR* 49(RR15), 1
Erythema
  (2000): *MMWR* 49(RR15), 1
Eyelid edema
  (1999): Dr. Sue Bailey, *Asst Sec Defense Health Affairs – Service
    Member #16* 21
Flu-like syndrome (<0.2%)
  (2001): Swanson-Biearman B+, *J Toxicol Clin Toxicol* 39(1), 81
  (2000): Captain James Bishop, *Citizen Airman* (0.0006%)
  (1999): Dr. Sue Bailey, *Asst Sec Defense Health Affairs – Service
    Member #1*
Hot flashes
  (1999): Dr. Sue Bailey, *Asst Sec Defense Health Affairs – Service
    Member #31* 34, 37
Lupus erythematosus
  (2000): *MMWR* 49(RR15), 1
  (1999): Ellenberg SS, *Center for Biologics Evaluation & Research,
    FDA Statement*
Photosensitivity
  (1999): Dr. Sue Bailey, *Asst Sec Defense Health Affairs – Service
    Member #1*
Pruritus
  (2000): *MMWR* 49(RR15), 1
  (1999): Dr. Sue Bailey, *Asst Sec Defense Health Affairs – Service
    Member #5*
Rash (sic)
  (1999): Dr. Sue Bailey, *Asst Sec Defense Health Affairs – Service
    Members #5, 9,14, 25, 44*
  (1999): Ellenberg SS, *Center for Biologics Evaluation & Research,
    FDA Statement*
Scrotal edema
  (1999): Dr. Sue Bailey, *Asst Sec Defense Health Affairs – Service
    Members #9*
Urticaria
  (2001): Swanson-Biearman B+, *J Toxicol Clin Toxicol* 39(1), 81

Hair

Hair – alopecia

Other

Anaphylactoid reactions
(2000): *MMWR* 49(RR15), I
(1999): Dr. Sue Bailey, *Asst Sec Defense Health Affairs – Service Member #29*

Arthralgia
(2000): *MMWR* 49(RR15), I
(1999): Dr. Sue Bailey, *Asst Sec Defense Health Affairs – Service Member #46*

Asthenia
(2000): *MMWR* 49(RR15), I

Chronic fatigue syndrome
(1999): Dr. Sue Bailey, *Asst Sec Defense Health Affairs – Service Member #39*

Depression
(1999): Dr. Sue Bailey, *Asst Sec Defense Health Affairs – Service Member #23*

Fever (<1%)
(2000): *MMWR* 49(RR15), I

Gingivitis
(1999): Dr. Sue Bailey, *Asst Sec Defense Health Affairs – Service Member #32*

Guillain–Barré syndrome
(2000): *MMWR* 49(RR15), I
(1999): Ellenberg SS, *Center for Biologics Evaluation & Research, FDA Statement* (2 cases)

Hypersensitivity
(2001): Swanson-Biearman B+, *J Toxicol Clin Toxicol* 39(1), 81
(1999): Ellenberg SS, *Center for Biologics Evaluation & Research, FDA Statement* (2 cases)
(1996): Shlyakhov E+, *Med Trop (Mars)* 56(2), 148
(1996): Uhr JW, *Physiol Rev.* 46:359
(1994): Shlyakhov E+, *Med Trop (Mars)* 54(1):33

Injection-site burning
(1999): Dr. Sue Bailey, *Asst Sec Defense Health Affairs – Service Member #12,27*

Injection-site edema
(2000): *MMWR* 49(RR15), I
(1999): Dr. Sue Bailey, *Asst Sec Defense Health Affairs – Service Member #4, 12, 32*
(1999): Ellenberg SS, *Center for Biologics Evaluation & Research, FDA Statement*
(1962): Brachman PS+, *Am J Pub Health* 52, 632 (up to 48 hours)
(1954): Wright GG+, *J Immunol* 73, 387 (2.4%)

Injection-site erythema
(1999): Dr. Sue Bailey, *Asst Sec Defense Health Affairs – Service Member #21, 27, 47*
(1962): Brachman PS+, *Am J Pub Health* 52, 632

Injection-site hematoma
(1999): Dr. Sue Bailey, *Asst Sec Defense Health Affairs – Service Member #12*

Injection-site hypersensitivity
(2000): *MMWR* 49(RR15), I

Injection-site induration
(1962): Brachman PS+, *Am J Pub Health* 52, 632

Injection-site inflammation

Injection-site nodules (sic)
(1999): Dr. Sue Bailey, *Asst Sec Defense Health Affairs – Service Members #2, 24, 28, 37, 40, 47*
(1962): Brachman PS+, *Am J Pub Health* 52, 632 lasting up to several weeks

Injection-site numbness
(1999): Dr. Sue Bailey, *Asst Sec Defense Health Affairs – Service Members #6, 13, 15, 22, 26, 31, 39, 43*

Injection-site pain
(2001): Swanson-Biearman B+, *J Toxicol Clin Toxicol* 39(1), 81
(2000): *MMWR* 49(RR15), I

(1999): Bailey S MD, *Asst Sec Defense Health Affairs – Service Members #1, 4, 8, 13, 18, 19, 20, 42, 45, 47, 49*
(1962): Brachman PS+, *Am J Pub Health* 52, 632 (24–48 hours)

Injection-site pruritus
(1962): Brachman PS+, *Am J Pub Health* 52, 632
(1954): Wright GG+, *J Immunol* 73, 387 (2.4%)

Injection-site reaction (sic)
(2001): Swanson-Biearman B+, *J Toxicol Clin Toxicol* 39(1), 81 (30%)
(2000): Hayes SC+, *J R Army Med Corps* 146(3), 191 (47%)
(2000): *MMWR* 49(RR15), I
(1999): Ellenberg SS, *Center for Biologics Evaluation & Research, FDA Statement* (severe)
(1963): Puziss M+, *J. Bacteriol* 85, 230
(1956): Darlow HM+, *Lancet* 2, 476

Joint pains
(1999): Dr. Sue Bailey, *Asst Sec Defense Health Affairs – Service Members #6, 13, 15, 22, 26, 31, 39, 43*

Myalgia
(2000): *MMWR* 49(RR15), I
(1999): Dr. Sue Bailey, *Asst Sec Defense Health Affairs – Service Members #1, 6, 12, 22, 40, 41*
(1954): Wright GG+, *J Immunol* 73, 387 (0.7%)

Paresthesias
(1999): Dr. Sue Bailey, *Asst Sec Defense Health Affairs – Service Members #3, 4, 11, 17, 28, 31, 34, 36, 37, 49*

Systemic reactions (sic)
(2000): Hayes SC+, *J R Army Med Corps* 146(3), 191 (47%)

Tinnitus
(1999): Dr. Sue Bailey, *Asst Sec Defense Health Affairs – Service Members #1, 6, 7, 10, 11, 13, 14, 23, 24, 28, 29, 48, 49*

Tremor
(1999): Dr. Sue Bailey, *Asst Sec Defense Health Affairs – Service Members #1*

Note: Dr. Sue Bailey, Assistant Secretary for Health Affairs, released a statement on June 29, 1999 that 'almost one million shots given, the anthrax immunization is proving to be one of the safest vaccination programs on record.' The above reports occurred for '50 service members at one installation alone.' Note that no number of military personnel was mentioned at this installation, nor did it give any percentages of the above reaction patterns

ANTIRETROVIRAL AGENTS

(Please refer to individual generic drugs for reaction patterns)

PROTEASE INHIBITORS*
Generic names:
Amprenavir
Trade name: Agenerase (GSK)
Indinavir
Trade name: Crixivan (Merck)
Iopinavir (ABT-378/r)
Trade name: Kaletra (Abbott)
Nelfinavir
Trade name: Viracept (Agouron)
Ritonavir
Trade name: Norvir (Abbott)
Saquinavir
Trade names: Invirase (Roche); Fortovase (Roche)

***Note:** Protease inhibitors cause dyslipidemia which includes elevated triglycerides and cholesterol and redistribution of body fat centrally to produce the so-called 'protease paunch,' breast enlargement, facial atrophy, and 'buffalo hump.'

NUCLEOSIDE ANALOG REVERSE TRANSCRIPTASE INHIBITORS (NRTIs)
  Generic names:
    Abacavir (ABC)
      Trade name: Ziagen (GSK)
    Didanosine (ddl)
      Trade name: Videx (Bristol-Myers Squibb)
    Lamivudine (3TC)
      Trade names: Epivir (GSK), Combivir (GSK)
    Stavudine (d4T)
      Trade name: Zerit (Bristol-Myers Squibb)
    Zalcitabine (ddc)
      Trade names: ddC; Hivid (Roche)
    Zidovudine (AZT)
      Trade names: AZT; Retrovir (GSK)

NON-NUCLEOSIDE REVERSE TRANSCRIPTASE INHIBITORS (NNRTIs)
  Generic names:
    Delavirdine
      Trade name: Rescriptor (Agouron)
    Efavirenz
      Trade name: Sustiva (Bristol-Myers Squibb)
    Nevirapine
      Trade name: Viramune (Boehringer Ingelheim)

NUCLEOSIDE REVERSE TRANSCRIPTASE INHIBITORS (NRTIs)
    Tenofovir
      Trade name: Viread (Gilead)

*Note: Combivir is a combination of lamivudine and zidovudine

APRACLONIDINE

Trade name: Iopidine (Alcon)
Indications: Post-surgical intraocular pressure elevation
Category: Alpha-2-adrenoceptor stimulant; Sympathomimetic ophthalmic solution; Vasoconstrictor
Half-life: 8 hours

Reactions

Skin
  Allergic reactions (sic) (<1%)
    (2000): Geyer O+, *Graefes Arch Clin Exp Ophthalmol* 238, 149
    (1999): Britt MT+, *Br J Ophthalmol* 83, 992 (progressing to ectropion)
    (1998): Gordon RN+, *Eye* 12, 697
    (1995): Butler P+, *Arch Ophthalmol* 113, 293
    (1995): Feibel RM, *Arch Ophthalmol* 113, 1579
  Burning
    (1996): Stewart WC, *Klin Monatsbl Augenheilkd* (German) 209, A7
  Dermatitis (sic) (<1%)
    (2001): Holdiness MR, *Am J Contact Dermat* 12(4), 217
    (2001): Silvestre JF+, *Contact Dermatitis* 45(4), 251
    (1998): Armisen M+, *Contact Dermatitis* 39, 193
  Edema (eyelids) (<3%)
  Facial edema (<1%)
  Periocular dermatitis
    (2000): Williams GC+, *Glaucoma* 9, 235
  Pruritus (10%)
    (1996): Stewart WC, *Klin Monatsbl Augenheilkd* (German) 209, A7
  Xerosis

Other
  Dysgeusia (3%)
  Headache
  Myalgia (0.2%)
  Ocular inflammation
    (1999): Shin DH+, *Am J Ophthalmol* 127, 511
  Paresthesias (<1%)
  Parosmia (0.2%)
  Xerostomia (1–10%)
    (1987): Abrams DA+, *Arch Ophthalmol* 105, 1205 (52%)

APREPITANT

Synonyms: mk-869; l-754-030
Trade name: Emend (Merck)
Indications: Prevention of nausea and vomiting associated with cancer (cisplatin) chemotherapy*
Category: Antiemetic; P/neurokinin 1 (NK1) receptor antagonist
Half-life: 9-13 hours
Clinically important, potentially hazardous interactions with: alprazolam, astemizole, carbamazepine, cisapride, clarithromycin, dexamethasone, diltiazem, docetaxel, ifosfamide, imatinib, irinotecan, itraconazole, ketoconazole, methylprednisolone, midazolam, nefazodone, oral contraceptives, paroxetine, phenytoin, pimozide, rifampin, ritonavir, terfenadine, tolbutamide, troleandomycin, vinblastine, vincristine, warfarin

Reactions

Skin
  Angioedema
  Diaphoresis (>0.5%)
  Edema (>0.5%)
  Flushing (>0.5%)
  Infections
    (2003): Chawla SP+, *Cancer* 97(9), 2290 (13%)
  Rash (sic) (>0.5%)
  Stevens–Johnson syndrome
  Upper respiratory infection (>0.5%)
  Urticaria

Hair
  Hair – alopecia (>0.5%)

Other
  Abdominal pain (>0.5%)
  Asthenia (18%)
  Cough (>0.5%)
  Depression (>0.5%)
  Dizziness (6.6%)
  Dysgeusia (>0.5%)
  Fatigue (18%)
  Fever
  Headache
  Hiccups (11%)
  Mucous membrane disorder (sic)
  Myalgia (>0.5%)
  Sialorrhea (>0.5%)
  Tinnitus (3.7%)

*Note: Aprepitant treatment is given along with a 5-HT3-receptor antagonist and dexamethasone

APROBARBITAL

Trade name: Alurate (Roche)
Indications: Short-term sedation, sleep induction
Category: Barbiturate
Half-life: 14–34 hours
Clinically important, potentially hazardous interactions with: alcohol, brompheniramine, buclizine, dicumarol, ethanolamine, warfarin

Reactions

Skin

Angioedema
Exanthems
Exfoliative dermatitis
Purpura
Rash (sic)
Stevens–Johnson syndrome
Urticaria

Other

Rhabdomyolysis
    (1990): Larpin R+, *Presse Med* 19(30), 1403
Serum sickness

APROTININ

Trade name: Trasylol (Bayer)
Indications: For prophylactic use to reduce blood loss in patients undergoing coronary artery bypass surgery
Category: Hemostatic (natural protease inhibitor)
Half-life: 150 minutes

Reactions

Skin

Allergic reactions (sic) (0.5%)
    (1994): Bayo M+, *Rev Esp Anestesiol Reanim* (Spanish) 41, 123
    (1983): Freeman JG+, *Curr Med Res Opin* 8, 559 (2 cases)
Angioedema
Erythema
Exanthems
    (2000): Beierlein W+, *Transfusion* 40, 302 (generalized)
Pruritus
Rash (sic)
Urticaria

Other

Anaphylactoid reactions (0.5%)
    (2001): Dietrich W+, *Anesthesiology* 95(1), 64
    (2000): Beierlein W, *Ann Thorac Surg* 69, 1298
    (2000): Laxenaire MC+, *Ann Fr Anesth Reanim* (French) 19, 96
    (2000): Pecquet C+, *Ann Fr Anesth* 19(10), 755
    (1999): Cohen DM+, *Ann Thorac Surg* 67, 837
    (1999): Laxenaire MC, *Ann Fr Anesth Reanim* (French) 18, 796 (4 cases)
    (1999): Ong BC+, *Anaesth Intensive Care* 27, 538
    (1999): Ryckwaert Y+, *Ann Fr Anesth Reanim* (French) 18, 904
    (1998): Scheule AM+, *Gastrointest Endosc* 48, 83
    (1997): Dietrich W+, *J Thorac Cardiovasc Surg* 113, 194
    (1997): Orsel I+, *Ann Fr Anesth Reanim* (French) 16, 292
    (1997): Scheule AM+, *Ann Thorac Surg* 63, 242
    (1996): Martinelli L+, *Ann Thorac Surg* 61, 1288
    (1995): Ceriana P+, *J Cardiothorac Vasc Anesth* 9, 477

    (1995): Diefenbach C+, *Anesth Analg* 80, 830
    (1994): Kon NF+, *Masui* (Japanese) 43, 1606
    (1993): Cottineau C+, *Ann Fr Anesth Reanim* (French) 12, 590
    (1993): Schulze K+, *Eur J Cardiothorac Surg* 7, 495 (2 patients)
    (1984): *BMJ* 289, 1696
    (1984): LaFerla GA+, *BMJ* 289, 1176
    (1976): Proud G+, *Lancet* 2, 48
    (1971): Bauer J+, *Am J Gastroenterol* 56, 542
Hypersensitivity
    (2002): Jaquiss RD+, *Circulation* 106(12 Suppl 1), 190
    (2000): Beierlein W+, *Transfusion* 40, 302
    (1998): Dietrich W, *Ann Thoracic Surg* 65, S60 (1.8%)
    (1975): Ariani G+, *Minerva Anestesiol* (Italian) 41, 138
Lipohypertrophy
    (1985): Boag F+, *N Engl J Med* 312, 245 (in a diabetic)
    (1985): Dandona P+, *Diabetes Res* 2, 213 (in a diabetic)
Phlebitis (1–10%)
Shock (sic)
    (1971): Vashchuk VV, *Klin Med (Mosk)* (Russian) 49, 128

ARBUTAMINE

Trade name: GenESA (Gensia)
Indications: Diagnostic aid for coronary artery disease
Category: Adrenergic agonist; Nonradioactive diagnostic synthetic catecholamine
Half-life: 1.8 hours
Clinically important, potentially hazardous interactions with: abacavir, clidinium, clomipramine, desipramine, dicyclomine, digoxin, doxepin, flavoxate, glycopyrrolate, hyoscyamine, imipramine, methantheline, nortriptyline, oxybutynin, procyclidine, propantheline, protriptyline, scopolamine, trihexyphenidyl, trimipramine

Reactions

Skin

Diaphoresis (1.5%)
Flushing (3%)
    (2001): Wright DJ+, *Nucl Med Commun* 22(12), 1305 (35%)
Hot flashes (3%)
Rash (sic)

Other

Application-site reactions (0.1%)
Back pain (0.1%)
Cough (0.2%)
Dysgeusia (1.3%)
    (2001): Wright DJ+, *Nucl Med Commun* 22(12), 1305 (23%)
Hyperesthesia (1.0%)
Pain (1.8%)
Paresthesias (2%)
Tremor (15%)
    (1997): Cohen A+, *Am J Cardiol* 79(6), 713 (5.6%)
Twitching (0.3%)
Xerostomia (1.1%)

ARGATROBAN

Trade name: Acova (GSK)
Indications: Heparin-induced thrombocytopenia
Category: Anticoagulant; Thrombin inhibitor
Half-life: 40–50 minutes
Clinically important, potentially hazardous interactions with: abacavir, butabarbital

Reactions

Skin
Allergic reactions (sic)
Bullous eruption (<1%)
Infections (sic) (4%)
Rash (sic) (<1%)

Other
Headache
Injection-site bleeding (2–5%)

ARIPIPRAZOLE

Trade name: Abilify (Bristol-Myers Squibb)
Other common trade name: *Abilitat*
Indications: Schizophrenia
Category: Antipsychotic
Half-life: 75–94 hours
Clinically important, potentially hazardous interactions with: carbamazepine, ketoconazole, quinidine

Reactions

Skin
Acne
Blepharitis
Candidiasis
Cheilitis
Chills
Diaphoresis
Eczema
Exanthems
Exfoliative dermatitis
Flu-like syndrome
Neuroleptic malignant syndrome
Peripheral edema
Pruritus
Psoriasis
Rash (sic) (6%)
Seborrhea
Ulcerations
Upper respiratory infection
Urticaria
Vesiculobullous eruption
Xerosis

Hair
Hair – alopecia

Other
Akathisia (10%)
(2003): Bowles TM+, *Ann Pharmacother* 37(5), 687

Anxiety (15%)
Arthralgia
Arthritis
Bone or joint pain
Cough (3%)
Depression
Dry eyes
Dysgeusia
Fever (2%)
Gingival hemorrhage
Gingivitis
Glossitis
Gynecomastia
Headache
Hiccups
Hyperesthesia
Lacrimation
Mastodynia
Mouth vesiculation
Myalgia
Myasthenia
Oral candidiasis
Oral ulceration
Phlebitis
Priapism
Rhabdomyolysis
Seizures
Sialorrhea
Stomatitis
Tendinitis
Thrombophlebitis
Tinnitus
Tongue edema
Tremor (3%)
Twitching
Vaginal candidiasis
Xerostomia

ARISTOLOCHIA*

Scientific names: *Aristolochia clematitis; Aristolochia serpentaria*
Family: Aristolochiaceae
Trade and other common names: Birthwort; Long Birthwort; Pelican Flower; Red River Snakeroot; Sangree Root; Sangrel; Serpentaria; Snakeweed; Virginia Serpentary
Category: Immune stimulant
Purported indications and other uses: Aphrodisiac, anti-allergy, anticonvulsant, promotes menstruation
Half-life: N/A

Reactions

Skin
None

Other
Death

*__*Note:__ Aristolochia has been reported to cause severe kidney damage or 'Chinese herb nephropathy'. Eighteen patients developed carcinomas of the bladder, ureter and/or renal pelvis

__Note:__ Aristolochia is banned in the European Union and Japan

ARNICA

Scientific names: *Arnica fulgens; Arnica montana; Arnica sororia*
Family: Asteraceae; Compositae
Trade and other common names: Leopard's Bane; Mountain snuff; Mountain tobacco; Wolf's Bane
Category: Anti-inflammatory; Immune stimulant
Purported indications and other uses: Bruising, aches and sprains, insect bites, superficial phlebitis, diuretic, flavoring agent, found in hair tonic and shampoo
Half-life: N/A
Clinically important, potentially hazardous interactions with: warfarin

Reactions

Skin
Acute febrile neutrophilic dermatosis (Sweet's syndrome)
Adverse effects (sic)
   (2002): Haller CA+, *Adverse Drug React Toxicol Rev* 21(3), 143
Allergic reactions (sic)
   (2002): Knuesel O+, *Adv Ther* 19(5), 209 (1 case)
Dermatitis
   (2002): Schempp CM+, *Hautarzt* 53(2), 93
   (2001): *Int J Toxicol* 20, 1
   (2001): Reider N+, *Contact Dermatitis* 45(5), 269
Irritation (sic)
Sensitization
   (2002): Paulsen E, *Contact Dermatitis* 47(4), 189

Other
Death
   (2001): *Int J Toxicol* 20, 1
Mucous membrane irritation (sic)

ARSENIC

Trade names: Trisonex (Cell Therapeutics); Fowler's Solution (rarely employed); found in pesticides and herbal medicines
Indications: Acute promyelocytic leukemia, psoriasis (in the early 1900s), devitalization of pulp in dental procedures
Category: Trace metal
Half-life: N/A
Clinically important, potentially hazardous interactions with: abacavir, amiodarone, bretylium, chlorpromazine, ciprofloxacin, disopyramide, enoxacin, fluphenazine, gatifloxacin, lomefloxacin, mesoridazine, moxifloxacin, norfloxacin, ofloxacin, phenothiazines, procainamide, prochlorperazine, promethazine, quinidine, quinolones, sotalol, sparfloxacin, thioridazine, trifluoperazine

Reactions

Skin
Acrocyanosis
   (2002): Hall AH, *Toxicol Lett* 128(1), 69
Basal cell carcinoma
   (2002): Centeno JA+, *Environ Health Perspect* 110, 883 (chronic exposure)
   (2002): Dorfner B+, *Hautarzt* 53(8), 542
   (2001): Guo HR+, *Cancer Causes Control* 12(10), 909
Bowen's disease
   (2002): Centeno JA+, *Environ Health Perspect* 110, 883
   (2002): Park JY+, *J Dermatol* 29(7), 446

Bullous eruption
   (1993): Alain G+, *Int J Dermatol* 32, 899 (passim)
   (1992): Breathnach SM+, *Adverse Drug Reactions and the Skin* Blackwell, Oxford, 236 (passim)
   (1988): Bork K, *Cutaneous Side Effects of Drugs* WB Saunders, 114
   (1968): Privat Y+, *Bull Soc Med Afr Noire Lang Fr* (French) 13, 195
   (1955): Alexander HL, *Reactions with Drug Therapy* Philadelphia, WB Saunders
Carcinoma (sic)
   (2002): Hall AH, *Toxicol Lett* 128(1), 69
   (2002): Liu J+, *Environ Health Perspect* 110(2), 119
   (2001): Guo HR+, *Cancer Causes Control* 12(10), 909
   (2001): Rahman MM+, *J Toxicol Clin Toxicol* 39(7), 683
   (2001): Yu HS+, *J Dermatol* 28(11), 628
   (1997): Schwartz RA, *Int J Dermatol* 36, 241
   (1995): Fawell J, *Hum Exp Toxicol* 14, 464
   (1995): Hsueh YM+, *Br J Cancer* 71, 109
   (1993): Urbach F, *Recent Results Cancer Res* 128, 243
   (1992): Wong O+, *Int Arch Occup Environ Health* 64, 235
   (1989): Bickley LK+, *N J Med* 86, 377
   (1988): Chen CJ+, *Lancet* 1, 414
   (1988): Durocher LP+, *Union Med Can* (French) 117, 345
   (1976): Spoor HJ, *Cutis* 18, 631
   (1970): Thivolet J+, *Lyon Med* (French) 223, 457
   (1969): Thivolet J+, *Bull Soc Fr Dermatol Syphiligr* (French) 76, 892
Dermatitis (sic)
   (2001): Guo X+, *Mol Cell Biochem* 222(1), 137
   (1995): Barbaud A+, *Contact Dermatitis* 33, 272
   (1986): Wahlberg JE+, *Derm Beruf Umwelt* (German) 34, 10
   (1964): Gaffi A, *Gazz Int Med Chir* (Italian) 69, 3363
   (1955): Alexander HL, *Reactions with Drug Therapy* Philadelphia, WB Saunders
Dermatofibrosarcoma protuberans
   (1986): Shneidman D+, *Cancer* 58, 1585
Edema (non-pitting)
   (2002): Alam MG+, *Int J Environ Health Res* 12(3), 235 (chronic exposure)
Erythema multiforme
   (1990): Vassileva S+, *Int J Dermatol* 29, 381
   (1988): Bork K, *Cutaneous Side Effects of Drugs* WB Saunders, 145
   (1967): Coleman WP, *Med Clin North Am* 51, 1073
   (1955): Alexander HL, *Reactions with Drug Therapy* Philadelphia, WB Saunders
   (1945): Fletcher MWC+, *J Pediatr* 27, 465
Erythema nodosum
   (1988): Bork K, *Cutaneous Side Effects of Drugs* WB Saunders, 148
Exanthems
   (1993): Alain G+, *Int J Dermatol* 32, 899 (passim)
   (1974): *Med Lett* 16, 11
   (1974): Tay CH, *Aust J Dermatol* 15, 121 (16%)
   (1955): Alexander HL, *Reactions with Drug Therapy* Philadelphia, WB Saunders
   (1952): Sulzberger MB+, *Postgrad Med* 11, 549
Exfoliative dermatitis
   (1993): Alain G+, *Int J Dermatol* 32, 899 (passim)
   (1992): Breathnach SM+, *Adverse Drug Reactions and the Skin* Blackwell, Oxford, 236 (passim)
   (1973): Nicolis GD+, *Arch Dermatol* 108, 788
   (1967): Coleman WP, *Med Clin North Am* 51, 1073
   (1967): Lockey SD, *Med Sci* 18, 43
   (1965): Fellner MJ+, *Med Clin North Am* 49, 709
   (1963): Abrahams I+, *Arch Dermatol* 87, 96
   (1955): Alexander HL, *Reactions with Drug Therapy* Philadelphia, WB Saunders

Fixed eruption
(1988): Bork K, *Cutaneous Side Effects of Drugs* WB Saunders, 108
(1964): Browne SG, *BMJ* 2, 1041
(1961): Welsh AL, *The Fixed Drug Eruption* Thomas, Springfield
(1955): Alexander HL, *Reactions with Drug Therapy* Philadelphia, WB Saunders
Follicular keratosis (sic)
(1952): Sulzberger MB+, *Postgrad Med* 11, 549
Freckles
(1995): Gritiyarangsan P+, *Photodermatol Photoimmunol Photomed* 11, 174
Hyperhidrosis
(1993): Alain G+, *Int J Dermatol* 32, 899 (passim)
Hyperkeratosis (palms and soles) (40%)
(2002): Alam MG+, *Int J Environ Health Res* 12(3), 235 (chronic exposure)
(2002): Centeno JA+, *Environ Health Perspect* 110 Suppl 5, 883 (chronic exposure)
(2001): Kurokawa M+, *Arch Dermatol* 137, 102
(1996): Maloney ME, *Dermatol Surg* 22, 301 (passim)
(1965): Fierz U, *Dermatologica* 131, 41
Hypopigmentation
(2002): Kadono T+, *Int J Dermatol* 41(12), 841 (chronic exposure)
Keratoses
(2002): Alam MG+, *Int J Environ Health Res* 12(3), 235 (chronic exposure)
(2002): Centeno JA+, *Environ Health Perspect* 110 Suppl 5, 883 (chronic exposure)
(2002): Kadono T+, *Int J Dermatol* 41(12), 841 (chronic exposure)
(2002): Liu J+, *Environ Health Perspect* 110(2), 119
(2002): Park JY+, *J Dermatol* 29(7), 446
(2001): Rahman MM+, *J Toxicol Clin Toxicol* 39(7), 683
(2001): Yu HS+, *J Dermatol* 28(11), 628
(1999): Tondel M+, *Environmental Health Perspectives* 107, 727
(1998): Guha Mazumder DN+, *Int J Epidemiol* 27, 871
(1993): Alain G+, *Int J Dermatol* 32, 899 (passim)
(1992): Breathnach SM+, *Adverse Drug Reactions and the Skin* Blackwell, Oxford, 236 (passim)
(1988): Bork K, *Cutaneous Side Effects of Drugs* WB Saunders, 232
(1978): Reymann F+, *Arch Dermatol* 114, 378
(1969): Bartruff JK, *Arch Dermatol* 100, 382
(1965): Dobson RL+, *Arch Dermatol* 92, 553
Leukomelanosis (sic)
(2002): Alam MG+, *Int J Environ Health Res* 12(3), 235 (chronic exposure)
(2001): Kurokawa M+, *Arch Dermatol* 137, 102
(2001): Rahman MM+, *J Toxicol Clin Toxicol* 39(7), 683
(1999): Tondel M+, *Environmental Health Perspectives* 107, 727
(1993): Sass U+, *Dermatology* 186, 303
(1974): Tay CH, *Aust J Dermatol* 15, 121 (31%)
(1952): Sulzberger MB+, *Postgrad Med* 11, 549
Lichen planus (bullous)
(1970): Aguilera-Diaz LF, *Ann Dermatol Syphiligr Paris* (French) 97, 39
Livedo reticularis
(1974): Nagy G+, *Z Hautkr* (German) 25, 534
Melanoderma
(1992): Breathnach SM+, *Adverse Drug Reactions and the Skin* Blackwell, Oxford, 236 (passim)
Melanoma
(1984): Philipp R+, *Br Med J Clin Res Ed* 288, 237
(1980): Clough P, *BMJ* 280, 112
(1980): Evans S, *BMJ* 280, 403
(1976): Grobe JW, *Berufsdermatosen* (German) 24, 167
Melanosis

(2002): Alam MG+, *Int J Environ Health Res* 12(3), 235 (chronic exposure)
(2002): Kadono T+, *Int J Dermatol* 41(12), 841 (chronic exposure)
(2001): Rahman MM+, *J Toxicol Clin Toxicol* 39(7), 683
Merkel cell carcinoma
(1999): Huang-Chun L+, *J Am Acad Dermatol* 41, 641
(1998): Tsuruta D+, *Br J Dermatol* 139, 291
(1997): Ohnishi Y+, *J Dermatol* 24, 310
(1991): Huang HP+, *J Formos Med Assoc* 90, 900
Morphea
(1952): Sulzberger MB+, *Postgrad Med* 11, 549
Palmar–plantar erythema
(1952): Sulzberger MB+, *Postgrad Med* 11, 549
Palmar–plantar hyperhidrosis
(2000): Gerdssn R+, *Acta Derm Venereol* 80, 292
(1974): Tay CH, *Aust J Dermatol* 15, 121 (31%)
Palmar–plantar hyperkeratosis
(2002): Hall AH, *Toxicol Lett* 128(1), 69
(2000): Gerdsen R+, *Acta Derm Venereol* 80, 292
(1998): Tsuruta D+, *Br J Dermatol* 139, 291
(1997): Ohnishi Y+, *J Dermatol* 24, 310
(1996): Maloney ME, *Dermatol Surg* 22, 301 (passim)
(1996): Person JR, *Cutis* 58, 65
(1994): Hsieh LL+, *Cancer Lett* 86, 59
(1993): Alain G+, *Int J Dermatol* 32, 899 (passim)
(1992): Breathnach SM+, *Adverse Drug Reactions and the Skin* Blackwell, Oxford, 236 (passim)
(1989): Koh E+, *Eur Urol* 16, 398
(1989): Shannon RL+, *Hum Toxicol* 8, 99
(1988): Ismail R+, *J Dermatol* 15, 65
(1983): Heddle R+, *Chest* 84, 776
(1982): Ohyama K, *Dermatologica* 164, 161
(1982): Rosen T+, *J Am Acad Dermatol* 7, 364
(1979): Allen RB+, *Cutis* 23, 805
(1974): Tay CH, *Aust J Dermatol* 15, 121
(1973): Yeh S, *Human Path* 4, 469
Palmar–plantar keratoderma
(1996): Maloney ME, *Dermatol Surg* 22, 301 (passim)
(1996): Matsumura Y+, *Int J Cancer* 65, 778
(1994): McNutt NS+, *Arch Dermatol* 130, 225
(1993): Alain G+, *Int J Dermatol* 32, 899 (passim)
(1993): Sass U+, *Dermatology* 186, 303
(1993): Ziegler A+, *Proc Natl Acad*
(1992): Breathnach SM+, *Adverse Drug Reactions and the Skin* Blackwell, Oxford, 236 (passim)
(1987): Chakraborty AK+, *Indian J Med Res* 85, 326
(1986): Munzberger H+, *Z Arztl Fortbild Jena* (German) 80, 985
(1985): Kastl J+, *Dermatol Monatsschr* (German) 171, 158
(1984): Schroeder P+, *Fortschr Med* (German) 102, 1128
(1980): Weiss J+, *Hautarzt* (German) 31, 654
(1974): Tay CH, *Aust J Dermatol* 15, 121 (6%)
(1973): Yeh S, *Human Path* 4, 469
(1972): Hadida E+, *Bull Soc Fr Dermatol Syphiligr* (French) 79, 287
(1967): Schulz EJ, *S Afr Med J* 41, 819
(1965): Fierz U, *Dermatologica* 131, 41
Palmar–plantar punctate keratoses
(1996): Maloney ME, *Dermatol Surg* 22, 301 (passim)
(1992): Breathnach SM+, *Adverse Drug Reactions and the Skin* Blackwell, Oxford, 236 (passim)
Parapsoriasis
(1952): Sulzberger MB+, *Postgrad Med* 11, 549
Photosensitivity
(1992): Breathnach SM+, *Adverse Drug Reactions and the Skin* Blackwell, Oxford, 236 (passim)
Pigmentation
(2002): Hall AH, *Toxicol Lett* 128(1), 69
(2002): Liu J+, *Environ Health Perspect* 110(2), 119

(2002): Park JY+, *J Dermatol* 29(7), 446
(2001): Kurokawa M+, *Arch Dermatol* 137, 102
(2001): Yu HS+, *J Dermatol* 28(11), 628
(1999): Tondel M+, *Environmental Health Perspectives* 107, 727
(1998): Guha Mazumder DN+, *Int J Epidemiol* 27, 871
(1996): Maloney ME, *Dermatol Surg* 22, 301 (passim)
(1993): Alain G+, *Int J Dermatol* 32, 899 (passim)
(1992): Breathnach SM+, *Adverse Drug Reactions and the Skin*
        Blackwell, Oxford, 236 (passim)
(1989): Shannon RL+, *Hum Toxicol* 8, 99
(1981): Granstein RD+, *J Am Acad Dermatol* 5, 1 (bronze)
(1974): Tay CH, *Aust J Dermatol* 15, 121 (85%)
(1973): Levantine A+, *Br J Dermatol* 89, 105
Pityriasis rosea (from organic arsenic)
(1988): Bork K, *Cutaneous Side Effects of Drugs* WB Saunders,
        169
(1952): Sulzberger MB+, *Postgrad Med* 11, 549
Pruritus
(1967): Young AW, *J Am Geriatr Soc* 15, 750
Psoriasis
(1952): Sulzberger MB+, *Postgrad Med* 11, 549
Purpura
(1988): Bork K, *Cutaneous Side Effects of Drugs* WB Saunders,
        191
(1955): Alexander HL, *Reactions with Drug Therapy* Philadelphia,
        WB Saunders
Raynaud's phenomenon
(2002): Hall AH, *Toxicol Lett* 128(1), 69
Squamous cell carcinoma
(2002): Centeno JA+, *Environ Health Perspect* 110 Suppl 5, 883
        (chronic exposure)
(2001): Guo HR+, *Cancer Causes Control* 12(10), 909
(1996): Maloney ME, *Dermatol Surg* 22, 301 (passim)
(1993): Alain G+, *Int J Dermatol* 32, 899 (passim)
(1992): Breathnach SM+, *Adverse Drug Reactions and the Skin*
        Blackwell, Oxford, 236 (passim)
(1989): Shannon RL+, *Hum Toxicol* 8, 99
(1988): Ismail R+, *J Dermatol* 15, 65
(1988): Scholz S+, *Z Arztl Fortbild Jena* (German) 82, 1201
(1979): Brownstein MH+, *Int J Dermatol* 18, 1
(1979): Southwick GJ+, *J Surg Oncol* 12, 115
(1974): Tay CH, *Aust J Dermatol* 15, 121
(1973): Yeh S, *Human Path* 4, 469
Stevens–Johnson syndrome
(1990): Vassileva S+, *Int J Dermatol* 29, 381
(1967): Coleman WP, *Med Clin North Am* 51, 1073
(1945): Fletcher MWC+, *J Pediatr* 27, 465
Ulcerations
(2002): Liu J+, *Environ Health Perspect* 110(2), 119
Urticaria
(1955): Alexander HL, *Reactions with Drug Therapy* Philadelphia,
        WB Saunders
Vitiligo
(1989): Bickley LK+, *N J Med* 86, 377

Hair

Hair – alopecia
(1993): Alain G+, *Int J Dermatol* 32, 899 (passim)
(1992): Breathnach SM+, *Adverse Drug Reactions and the Skin*
        Blackwell, Oxford, 236 (passim)
(1988): Bork K, *Cutaneous Side Effects of Drugs* WB Saunders,
        249
(1974): Tay CH, *Aust J Dermatol* 15, 121 (5%)

Nails

Nails – leukonychia
(1988): Bork K, *Cutaneous Side Effects of Drugs* WB Saunders,
        262
Nails – pigmentation

(1988): Bork K, *Cutaneous Side Effects of Drugs* WB Saunders,
        261
(1978): Shah PC+, *Br J Dermatol* 98, 675 (passim)
Nails – transverse white bands
(1993): Alain G+, *Int J Dermatol* 32, 899 (passim)
(1993): Sass U+, *Dermatology* 186, 303

Other

Dysgeusia
(2002): Hall AH, *Toxicol Lett* 128(1), 69
Foetor ex ore (halitosis)
(1988): Bork K, *Cutaneous Side Effects of Drugs* WB Saunders,
        310
Gangrene
(2002): Alam MG+, *Int J Environ Health Res* 12(3), 235 (chronic
        exposure)
(1952): Sulzberger MB+, *Postgrad Med* 11, 549
Gynecomastia
(1992): Breathnach SM+, *Adverse Drug Reactions and the Skin*
        Blackwell, Oxford, 237 (passim)
Headache
Oral mucosal eruption (8%)
(1974): Tay CH, *Aust J Dermatol* 15, 121
(1966): Dummett CO, *J Oral Ther Pharmacol* 1, 106
(1952): Sulzberger MB+, *Postgrad Med* 11, 549
Oral mucosal pigmentation
(1988): Bork K, *Cutaneous Side Effects of Drugs* WB Saunders,
        288
Stomatitis
(1966): Dummett CO, *J Oral Ther Pharmacol* 1, 106
Tumors (malignant)
(2001): Kurokawa M+, *Arch Dermatol* 137, 102

ASCORBIC ACID

Synonym: vitamin C
Trade names: Ascorbicap; Cebid; Cecon; Cemill; Cetane;
Cevalin (Lilly); Cevi-Bid; Dull-C; Sunkist; Vita-C
Other common trade names: *Apo-C; Ce-Vi-Sol; Cebion; Cetebe;
Laroscorbine; Potent C; Pro-C; Redoxon*
Indications: Prevention of scurvy
Category: Water-soluble nutritional supplement
Half-life: N/A
**Clinically important, potentially hazardous interactions
with:** deferoxamine, penicillamine

Reactions

Skin

Angioedema
(1980): Bilyk MA+, *Vrach Delo* (Russian) May, 81
Eczema (sic)
(1980): Metz J+, *Contact Dermatitis* 6, 172
Erythema
Flushing (<1%)
Side effects (sic)
(1992): Breathnach SM+, *Adverse Drug Reactions and the Skin*
        Blackwell, Oxford, 265 (passim)
(1980): Bilyk MA+, *Vrach Delo* (Russian) May, 81

Other

Injection-site irritation

ASPARAGINASE

Synonym: L-asparaginase
Trade name: Elspar (Merck)
Other common trade names: *Crasnitin; Erwinase; Kidrolase; Laspar; Leunase*
Indications: Acute lymphocytic leukemia, lymphoma
Category: Antineoplastic; Protein synthesis inhibitor
Half-life: 8–30 hours (IV); 39–49 hours (IM)

Reactions

Skin

Angioedema
  (1983): Bronner AK+, *J Am Acad Dermatol* 9, 645 (15%)
  (1981): Weiss RB+, *Ann Intern Med* 94, 66
  (1971): Jacquillat C+, *Med Welt* (German) 22, 503 (<1.0%)
Chills
Diaphoresis
Edema
Exanthems
Flushing
  (1983): Bronner AK+, *J Am Acad Dermatol* 9, 645 (15%)
Pruritus (<1%)
  (1981): Weiss RB+, *Ann Intern Med* 94, 66
Rash (sic) (<1%)
Toxic epidermal necrolysis
  (1989): Stern RS+, *J Am Acad Dermatol* 21, 317
  (1980): Rodriguez AR, *J Med Assoc Ga* 69, 355
Urticaria (<1%)
  (1983): Bronner AK+, *J Am Acad Dermatol* 9, 645 (15%)
  (1981): Weiss RB+, *Ann Intern Med* 94, 66
  (1979): Ertel IJ+, *Cancer Res* 39, 3893
  (1971): Jacquillat C+, *Med Welt* (German) 22, 503 (<0.5%)

Hair

Hair – alopecia

Other

Anaphylactoid reactions (10–40%)
  (1983): Bronner AK+, *J Am Acad Dermatol* 9, 645 (15%)
  (1982): Dunagin WG, *Semin Oncol* 9, 14 (3%)
  (1979): Ertel IJ+, *Cancer Res* 39, 3893
Aphthous stomatitis (1–10%)
Headache
Hypersensitivity (10–40%)
  (2001): Bryant R, *J Intraven Nurs* 24(3), 169
  (1998): Bonno M+, *J Allergy Clin Immunol* 101, 571
  (1998): Larson RA+, *Leukemia* 12, 660
  (1992): Weiss RB, *Semin Oncol* 19, 458
  (1982): Dunagin WG, *Semin Oncol* 9, 14 (33%)
  (1981): Weiss RB+, *Ann Intern Med* 94, 66 (6–43%)
  (1978): Levine N+, *Cancer Treat Res* 5, 67 (5–20%)
  (1974): Levantine A+, *Br J Dermatol* 90, 239
Injection-site erythema
Oral mucosal lesions (26%)
Serum sickness
  (1983): Bronner AK+, *J Am Acad Dermatol* 9, 645 (15%)

ASPARTAME

Trade names: Equal; Nutrasweet*
Indications: No data
Category: Low-calorie artificial sweetener
Half-life: N/A

Reactions

Skin

Allergic reactions (sic)
  (1998): Garriga MM+, *Ann Allergy* 61, 63
  (1996): Roberts HJ, *Arch Intern Med* 156, 1027
Angioedema
  (1992): Downham TF, *Clin Cases in Dermatol* 4, 12 (observation)
  (1988): Metcalfe DD, *Skin and Allergy News* 19, 52 (observation)
Dermatitis (sic)
  (1992): Downham TF, *Clin Cases in Dermatol* 4, 12 (observation)
Exanthems
  (1986): *Arzneimittelinformation ATI Berlin GmbH* (German) 12, 121
Pruritus
  (1994): Shelley WB+, *Cutis* 53, 77 (observation)
  (1988): Metcalfe DD, *Skin and Allergy News* 19, 52 (observation)
Pruritus ani
  (1994): Shelley WB+, *Cutis* 53, 237 (observation)
Purpura
  (1999): Leal G, Fortaleza, Brazil (from Internet) (observation)
  (1992): Downham TF, *Clin Cases in Dermatol* 4, 12 (observation)
Rash (sic)
  (1988): Metcalfe DD, *Skin and Allergy News* 19, 52 (observation)
Urticaria
  (1995): Kulczycki A, *J Allergy Clin Immunol* 95, 639
  (1992): Downham TF, *Clin Cases in Dermatol* 4, 12 (observation)
  (1988): Metcalfe DD, *Skin and Allergy News* 19, 52 (observation)
  (1986): Kulczycki A, *Ann Intern Med* 104, 207
Vasculitis
  (1992): Downham TF, *Clin Cases in Dermatol* 4, 12 (observation)

Other

Anaphylactoid reactions
  (1996): Roberts HJ, *Arch Intern Med* 156, 1027
Panniculitis
  (1992): Geha RS, *J Am Acad Dermatol* 26, 277 (lobular)
  (1991): McCauliffe DP+, *J Am Acad Dermatol* 24, 298 (lobular)
  (1985): Novick NL, *Ann Intern Med* 102, 206 (granulomatous)

*Note: Aspartame can be found in instant breakfasts, breath mints, cereals, sugar-free chewing gum, cocoa mixes, coffee beverages, frozen desserts, gelatin desserts, juice beverages, laxatives, multivitamins, milk drinks, pharmaceuticals and supplements, shake mixes, soft drinks, tabletop sweeteners, tea beverages, instant teas and coffees, topping mixes, wine coolers, yogurt

ASPIRIN

Synonyms: acetylsalicylic acid; ASA
Trade names: Aggrenox (Boehringer Ingelheim); Alka-Seltzer; Anacin (Wyeth); Ascriptin (Novartis) (Wallace); Aspergum; Bufferin (Bristol-Myers Squibb); Coricidin D; Darvon Compound (Lilly); Ecotrin (GSK); Empirin; Equagesic (Women First); Excedrin (Bristol-Myers Squibb); Fiorinal (Watson); Gelprin; Halfprin; Measurin; Norgesic (3M); Percodan (Endo); Robaxisal; Soma Compound (Wallace); Talwin Compound (Sanofi-Synthelabo); Vanquish
Other common trade names: *ASA; Aspro; ASS; Bex; Caprin; Claragine; Disprin; Ecotrin; Novasen; Rhonal*
Indications: Pain, fever, inflammation
Category: Nonsteroidal anti-inflammatory (NSAID) analgesic; Salicylate
Half-life: 15–20 minutes
Clinically important, potentially hazardous interactions with: anticoagulants, bismuth, **capsicum**, cholestyramine, **devil's claw**, dicumarol, etodolac, **ginkgo biloba**, **ginseng**, heparin, ibuprofen, indomethacin, ketoprofen, ketorolac, methotrexate, NSAIDs, **phellodendron**, reteplase, sermorelin, tirofiban, urokinase, valdecoxib, valproic acid, verapamil, warfarin

Aggrenox is aspirin and dipyridamole

Reactions

Skin

Acute generalized exanthematous pustulosis (AGEP)
 (1993): Ballmer-Weber BK+, *Schweiz Med Wochenschr (German)* 123, 542
Allergic reactions (sic) (<1%) (with dipyridamole)
 (1991): VanArsdel PP Jr, *JAMA* 266, 3343
Angioedema (1–5%)
 (2003): Sanchez-Borges M+, *Clin Rev Allergy Immunol* 24(2), 125
 (2002): Higashi N+, *J Allergy Clin Immunol* 110(4), 666
 (2000): Ghislain PD+, *Ann Med Interne* (Paris) 151, 227 (Nuchal scalp)
 (2000): Pradalier A+, *Rev Med Interne* (French) 21, 75
 (2000): Wong JT+, *J Allergy Clin Immunol* 105, 997
 (1998): Grzelewska-Rzymowska I, *Pol Merkuriusz Lek* (Polish) 4, 233
 (1998): Quiralte J, *Ann Allergy Asthma Immunol* 81, 459 (periorbital)
 (1997): Tomaz EM+, *Allergy Asthma Proc* 18, 319
 (1996): Chan TY, *Br J Clin Pract* 50, 412
 (1993): Grzelewska-Rzymowska I+, *Pneumonol Alergol Pol* (Polish) 61, 29
 (1988): Botey J+, *Allergol Immunopathol Madr* (Spanish) 16, 43
 (1984): Botey J+, *Ann Allergy* 53, 265
 (1981): Juhlin L, *Br J Dermatol* 104, 369
 (1977): Abrishami MA+, *Ann Allergy* 39, 28
 (1977): Szczeklik A+, *J Allergy Clin Immunol* 60, 276
 (1974): Schlumberger HD+, *Acta Med Scand* 196, 451
 (1972): Kauppinen K, *Acta Derm Venereol* (Stockh) 52 (Suppl), 68
 (1970): Baker H+, *Br J Dermatol* 82, 319
 (1969): Girard JP+, *Helv Med Acta* 35, 86
 (1967): Moore-Robinson M+, *BMJ* 4, 263
Bullous eruption (<1%)
 (1989): Sfar Z +, *Tunis Med* 67, 805
 (1979): Odinokova VA+, *Arkh Patol* (Russian) 41, 37
 (1972): Kauppinen K, *Acta Derm Venereol* (Stockh) 52 (Suppl), 68
 (1960): Hejier A+, *Acta Derm Venereol* (Stockh) 40, 35
Dermatitis herpetiformis
 (1966): Brannen M+, *Tex State J Med* 62, 58
Dermatomyositis

 (1964): Shelley WB, *JAMA* 189, 986
Diaphoresis
Erythema multiforme (<1%)
 (1998): Lee SG+, *Eur J Dermatol* 8, 280
 (1985): Laurberg G+, *Ugeskr Laeger* 147, 1853
 (1985): Ting HC+, *Int J Dermatol* 24, 587
 (1982): Bailin PL+, *Clin Rheum Dis* 8, 493 (passim)
 (1977): Davis JD+, *Clin Pharm Ther* 21, 52
 (1975): Bottiger LE+, *Acta Med Scand* 198, 229
 (1968): Bianchine JR+, *Am Med J* 44, 390
 (1966): Brannen M+, *Tex State J Med* 62, 58
 (1960): Hejier A+, *Acta Derm Venereol* (Stockh) 40, 35
Erythema nodosum (<1%)
 (1996): Buckshee K+, *Int J Gynaecol Obstet* 55, 293
 (1996): Durden FM+, *Int J Dermatol* 35, 39
 (1994): Fernandes NC+, *Rev Inst Med Trop Sao Paulo* (Portuguese) 36, 507
 (1987): Blasetti P, *Clin Ter* 123(4), 303
 (1982): Bailin PL+, *Clin Rheum Dis* 8, 493 (passim)
 (1982): Ubogy Z+, *Acta Derm Venereol* 62, 265
 (1970): Baker H+, *Br J Dermatol* 82, 319
 (1966): Brannen M+, *Tex State J Med* 62, 58
 (1964): Shelley WB, *JAMA* 189, 985
Erythroderma
 (1974): Tay C, *Asian J Med* 10, 223
Exanthems
 (1993): Ballmer-Weber BK+, *Schweiz Med Wochenschr* 123, 542
 (1989): Hass WK+, *N Engl J Med* 321, 501 (5.2%)
 (1987): Castles JJ+, *Arch Intern Med* 138, 362 (2.8%)
 (1982): Morley PA+, *Drugs* 23, 250 (5%)
 (1980): Goerz G+, *Fortschr Med* 98, 726
 (1977): Chalem F+, *Curr Ther Res* 22, 769
 (1977): Davis JD+, *Clin Pharm Ther* 21, 52 (1–5%)
 (1975): Blechman WJ+, *JAMA* 233, 336 (2.5%)
 (1975): Bowers DE+, *Ann Intern Med* 83, 470 (18%)
 (1972): Kauppinen K, *Acta Derm Venereol* (Stockh) 52 (Suppl), 68
 (1960): Hejier A+, *Acta Derm Venereol* (Stockh) 40, 35
Exfoliative dermatitis
 (1969): Girard JP+, *Helv Med Acta* 35, 86
Fixed eruption (<1%)
 (1999): Galindo PA+, *J Investig Allergol Clin Immunol* 9, 399
 (1998): Mahboob A+, *Int J Dermatol* 37, 833
 (1997): Bhargava P+, *Int J Dermatol* 36, 236
 (1992): Hatzis J+, *Cutis* 50, 50
 (1991): Thankappen TP+, *Int J Dermatol* 30, 867 (1.7%)
 (1990): Bharija SC+, *Dermatologica* 181, 237
 (1990): Gaffoor PMA+, *Cutis* 45, 242
 (1989): Shiohara T+, *Arch Dermatol* 125, 1371
 (1986): Kanwar AJ, *Dermatologica* 172, 315
 (1986): Kanwar AJ+, *J Dermatol* 11, 383
 (1985): Gomez B+, *Allergol Immunopathol Madr* (Spanish) 13, 87
 (1985): Kauppinen K+, *Br J Dermatol* 112, 575
 (1984): Boyle J+, *Br Med J Clin Res Ed* 289, 802
 (1984): Chan HL, *Int J Dermatol* 23, 607
 (1984): Pandhi RK+, *Sex Transm Dis* 11, 164
 (1982): Bailin PL+, *Clin Rheum Dis* 8, 493 (passim)
 (1981): Shukla SR, *Dermatologica* 163, 160
 (1975): Gimenez-Camarasa JM+, *N Engl J Med* 292, 819
 (1974): Kuokkanen K, *Int J Dermatol* 13, 4
 (1972): Kauppinen K, *Acta Derm Venereol* (Stockh) 52 (Suppl), 68
 (1970): Savin JA, *Br J Dermatol* 83, 546
Flushing
 (1964): Shelley WB, *JAMA* 189, 986
Genital herpes
 (1964): Shelley WB, *JAMA* 189, 986
Graft-versus-host reaction
 (1998): Jappe U+, *Hautarzt* (German) 49, 126 (passim)
Granulomas
 (1982): Cozzutto C+, *Virchows Arch A Pathol Anat Histol* 397, 61

Herpes simplex
(1984): Boyle J, Moul B, *Br Med J (Clin Res Ed)* 289, 802

Jitters (sic)

Lichenoid eruption
(1988): Bharija SC+, *Dermatologica* 177, 19
(1966): Brannen M+, *Tex State J Med* 62, 58

Parapsoriasis
(1966): Brannen M+, *Tex State J Med* 62, 58

Pemphigus
(1986): Pisani M+, *G Ital Dermatol Venereol* (Italian) 121, 39

Periorbital edema
(1997): Price KS+, *Ann Allergy Asthma Immunol* 79, 420
(1993): Katz Y+, *Allergy* 48, 366

Petechiae
(1997): Blumenthal HL, Beachwood, OH (personal case) (observation)

Photo-recall phenomenon
(1998): Lee SG+, *Eur J Dermatol* 8, 280

Pigmented purpuric eruption
(1999): Lipsker D+, *Ann Dermatol Venereol* (French) 126, 321

Pityriasis rosea
(1993): Yosipovitch G+, *Harefuah* (Hebrew) 124, 198; 247
(1966): Brannen M+, *Tex State J Med* 62, 58

Pruritus
(1981): Settipane GA, *Arch Intern Med* 141, 328
(1977): Chalem F+, *Curr Ther Res* 22, 769 (1–5%)
(1977): Davis JD+, *Clin Pharm Ther* 21, 52 (>5%)
(1975): Blechman WJ+, *JAMA* 233, 336 (2%)
(1969): Girard JP+, *Helv Med Acta* 35, 86
(1967): Moore-Robinson M+, *BMJ* 4, 263

Psoriasis
(1966): Brannen M+, *Tex State J Med* 62, 58
(1964): Shelley WB, *JAMA* 189, 986

Purpura
(2001): Tsuda T+, *J Int Med Res* 29(4), 374
(1997): Sola-Alberich R+, *Ann Intern Med* 126, 665
(1989): Hass WK+, *N Engl J Med* 321, 501 (2%)
(1980): Miescher PA+, *Clin Haematol* 9, 505
(1976): Karchmer AW+, *N Engl J Med* 295, 451
(1972): Kauppinen K, *Acta Derm Venereol* (Stockh) 52 (Suppl), 68
(1971): Davis SL+, *Nebraska St Med J* 56, 432

Pustular psoriasis
(1976): Lindgren S+, *Acta Derm Venereol* (Stockh) 56, 139
(1964): Shelley WB, *JAMA* 189, 985

Rash (sic) (1–10%)

Stevens–Johnson syndrome
(1993): Leenutaphong V+, *Int J Dermatol* 32, 428
(1972): Monnat A, *Schweiz Med Wochenschr* (French) 102, 1876
(1968): Bianchine JR+, *Am Med J* 44, 390
(1966): Brannen M+, *Tex State J Med* 62, 58

Toxic epidermal necrolysis (<1%)
(2002): Correia O+, *Arch Dermatol* 138, 29
(1993): Leenutaphong V+, *Int J Dermatol* 32, 428
(1988): Dahle MG, *Tidsskr Nor Laegeforen* (Norwegian) 108, 1917
(1987): Guillaume JC+, *Arch Dermatol* 123, 1166
(1979): Hunziker N, *Schweiz Rundsch Med Prax* (French) 68, 283
(1972): Spahr A+, *Rev Med Suisse Romande* (French) 92, 935
(1970): Ocheret'ko MP, *Pediatriia* (Russian) 49, 86
(1967): Lowney ED+, *Arch Dermatol* 95, 359
(1967): Lyell A, *Br J Dermatol* 79, 662

Ulcerations (<1%) (with dipyridamole)

Urticaria (1–10%)
(2003): Grattan CE, *Clin Exp Dermatol* 28(2), 123
(2003): Sanchez-Börges M+, *Clin Rev Allergy Immunol* 24(2), 125
(2002): Higashi N+, *J Allergy Clin Immunol* 110(4), 666
(2001): Cousin F+, *Ann Dermatol Venereol* 128(10), 1166
(2001): Harada S+, *Br J Dermatol* 145(2), 336
(2000): Pradalier A+, *Rev Med Interne* (French) 21, 75

(2000): Wong JT+, *J Allergy Clin Immunol* 105, 997
(1999): Eseverri JL+, *Allergol Immunopathol (Madr)* (Spanish) 27, 104
(1998): Grzelewska-Rzymowska I, *Pol Merkuriusz Lek* (Polish) 4, 233
(1998): Ohnishi-Inoue Y+, *Br J Dermatol* 138, 483
(1997): Tomaz EM+, *Allergy Asthma Proc* 18, 319
(1995): Gebhardt M+, *Z Rheumatol* (German) 54, 405
(1995): Grzelewska-Rzymowska I+, *J Invest Allergol Clin Immunol* 5, 272
(1994): Paul E+, *Hautarzt* (German) 45, 12
(1994): Smith RJ+, *Br J Dermatol* 131, 583
(1993): Grzelewska-Rzymowska I+, *Pneumonol Alergol Pol* (Polish) 61, 29
(1992): Grzelewska-Rzymowska I+, *J Invest Alergol Clin Immunol* 2, 39
(1989): Alanko K+, *Acta Derm Venereol* (Stockh) 69, 223 (1–5%)
(1989): Grzelewska-Rzymowska I, *Allergol Immunopathol Madr* (Spanish) 16, 231
(1989): Hass WK+, *N Engl J Med* 321, 501 (0.3%)
(1988): Botey J+, *Allergol Immunopathol Madr* (Spanish) 16, 43
(1987): Asad SI+, *Ann Allergy* 59, 219
(1986): Dupont C, *Int J Dermatol* 25, 334
(1986): Finzi AF+, *Minerva Med* (Italian) 77, 1401
(1986): Nagy G+, *Dermatol Monatsschr* 72, 594
(1986): Wojnerowicz-Grajewska M+, *Przegl Dermatol* (Polish) 73, 115
(1984): Botey J+, *Ann Allergy* 53, 265
(1984): Kauppinen K+, *Allergy* 39, 469
(1983): Kaplan AP, *Postgrad Med* 74, 209
(1982): Kirchhof B+, *Dermatol Monatsschr* (German) 168, 513
(1981): Juhlin L, *Br J Dermatol* 104, 369
(1981): Settipane GA, *Arch Intern Med* 141, 328
(1980): Settipane RA+, *Allergy* 35, 149
(1980): Wuthrich B+, *Z Hautkr* (German) 55, 102
(1978): Hofmann C+, *Munch Med Wochenschr* (German) 120, 65
(1978): Oshima K+, *Nippon Hifuka Gakkai Zasshi* (Japanese) 88, 459
(1977): Abrishami MA+, *Ann Allergy* 39, 28
(1977): Chalem F+, *Curr Ther Res* 22, 769
(1977): Doeglas HM, *Dermatologica* 154, 308
(1977): Rudzki E, *Przegl Dermatol* (Polish) 64, 163
(1977): Szczeklik A+, *J Allergy Clin Immunol* 60, 276
(1976): Erlings M+, *Ned Tijdschr Geneeskd* (Dutch) 120, 1565
(1976): Ros AM+, *Br J Dermatol* 95, 19
(1976): Stubb S, *Acta Derm Venereol* (Stockh) 56 (Suppl 76), 16
(1975): Blechman WJ+, *JAMA* 233, 336 (0.5%)
(1975): Doeglas HM, *Br J Dermatol* 93, 135
(1974): Schlumberger HD+, *Acta Med Scand* 196, 451
(1973): Samter M, *Hosp Pract* 8, 85
(1972): Kauppinen K, *Acta Derm Venereol* (Stockh) 52 (Suppl), 68
(1972): Sheffer AL, *N Y State J Med* 72, 922
(1971): Davis SL+, *Nebraska St Med J* 56, 432
(1970): Baker H+, *Br J Dermatol* 82, 319
(1970): James J+, *Br J Dermatol* 82, 204
(1970): Naess K, *Tidsskr Nor Laegeforen* (Norwegian) 90, 112
(1969): Champion RH+, *Br J Dermatol* 81, 588
(1969): Girard JP+, *Helv Med Acta* 35, 86
(1967): Moore-Robinson M+, *BMJ* 4, 262
(1966): Brannen M+, *Tex State J Med* 62, 58
(1960): Hejier A+, *Acta Derm Venereol* (Stockh) 40, 35
(1960): Warin RP, *Br J Dermatol* 72, 350

Vasculitis
(1999): Crutchfield CE+, *Skin and Aging* May, 84 (leukocytoclastic)
(1984): Ekenstam E+, *Arch Dermatol* 120, 484
(1971): Meszaros C, *Börgyogy Vener Sz* (Hungarian) 47, 20

Hair

Hair – alopecia
(1968): Rawnsley HM+, *Lancet* 1, 561

Other
Ageusia (<1%) (with dipyridamole)
Anaphylactoid reactions (1–10%)
  (2003): Berkes EA, *Clin Rev Allergy Immunol* 24(2), 137
  (2001): Harada S+, *Br J Dermatol* 145(2), 336
  (1999): Kubota Y+, *Eur J Dermatol* 9, 559
  (1984): Stevenson DD, *J Allergy Clin Immunol* 74, 617
  (1972): Ohela K+, *Duodecim* (Finnish) 88, 1177
Aphthous stomatitis
  (2001): Vincent L+, *Ann Dermatol Venereol* 128, 57
  (1982): Bailin PL+, *Clin Rheum Dis* 8, 493 (passim)
  (1966): Brannen M+, *Tex State J Med* 62, 58
Dysgeusia
Gingivitis (<1%) (with dipyridamole)
Headache
Hypersensitivity
  (2001): Hinrichs R+, *Allergy* 56(8), 789
  (2001): Rueff F+, *Allergy* 56, 258
Myalgia (1.2%) (with dipyridamole)
Oral burn (sic)
  (1998): Dellinger TM+, *Ann Pharmacother* 32, 1107
Oral lichen planus
  (1989): Espana-Alonso A+, *An Med Interna* (Spanish) 6, 219
Oral mucosal eruption
  (1988): Bork K, *Cutaneous Side Effects of Drugs* WB Saunders, 283
  (1966): Brannen M+, *Tex State J Med* 62, 58
  (1964): Shelley WB, *JAMA* 189, 986
Oral ulceration
  (1975): Kawashima Z+, *JAMA* 91, 130
  (1974): Glick GL+, *N Y St Dent J* 40, 475
  (1970): Baker H+, *Br J Dermatol* 82, 319
  (1967): Claman HN, *JAMA* 202, 651
Paresthesias (<1%) (with dipyridamole)
Pseudolymphoma
  (1980): Olmos L+, *Rev Clin Esp* 157, 67
Pseudoporphyria
  (1994): Hazen PG, *J Am Acad Dermatol* 31, 500
Tinnitus

Infections (sic) (~50%)
Pallor
Peripheral edema
Photosensitivity
Pruritus
Purpura
Rash (sic) (20%)
Seborrhea
Urticaria
Vesiculobullous eruption
Xerosis

Hair
Hair – alopecia

Nails
Nails – changes (sic)

Other
Abdominal pain
Anxiety
Back pain (2%)
Buffalo hump
Cough
Dizziness (3%)
Dysgeusia
Fatigue (2%)
Fever
Gynecomastia
Headache (14%)
Hiccups
Hypesthesia
Lipoatrophy
Myasthenia
Myopathy
Pain (3%)
Tinnitus
Twitching

ATAZANAVIR

Trade name: Reyataz (Bristol-Myers Squibb)
Indications: HIV infection
Category: HIV-1 protease inhibitor
Half-life: 7 hours
Clinically important, potentially hazardous interactions with: bepridil, cisapride, dofetilide, ergot derivatives, fentanyl, **garlic**, indinavir, irinotecan, lovastatin, marihuana, midazolam, pimozide, proton-pump inhibitors, rifampin, sildenafil, simvastatin, **St John's Wort**, triazolam

Reactions

Skin
Allergic reactions (sic)
Aphthous stomatitis
Burning
Cellulitis
Diaphoresis
Ecchymoses
Eczema
Edema
Fungal infections

ATENOLOL

Trade names: Tenoretic (AstraZeneca); Tenormin (AstraZeneca)
Other common trade names: *Antipressan; Apo-Atenol; AteHexal; Atendol; Evitocor; Noten; Novo-Atenol; Nu-Atenol; Taro-Atenol; Tenolin; Tenormine*
Indications: Angina, hypertension, acute myocardial infarction
Category: Antianginal; Antihypertensive; Beta-adrenoceptor blocker
Half-life: 6–7 hours (adults)
Clinically important, potentially hazardous interactions with: clonidine, epinephrine, verapamil

Tenoretic is atenolol and chlorthalidone

Reactions

Skin
Acrocyanosis
  (1987): Naeyaert JM+, *Br J Dermatol* 117, 371
Dermatitis (sic)
  (1979): Harrison PV+, *Clin Exp Dermatol* 4, 547
Diaphoresis
Edema
Erythema multiforme

Exanthems
Facial edema
Fixed eruption
   (1999): Palungwachira P+, *J Med Assoc Thai* 82, 1158
Grinspan's syndrome*
   (1990): Lamey PJ+, *Oral Surg Oral Med Oral Pathol* 70, 184
Hyperkeratosis (palms and soles)
Lichenoid eruption
   (1978): Savage RL+, *BMJ* 1, 987
Lupus erythematosus
   (1997): McGuiness M+, *J Am Acad Dermatol* 37, 298
   (1986): Gouet D+, *J Rheumatol* 13, 446
Necrosis
   (1979): Gokal R+, *BMJ* 1, 721
   (1979): Rees PJ, *BMJ* 1, 955
   (1977): Simpson WT, *Postgrad Med J* 53, 162
Papulo-nodular lesions
   (1992): Shelley WB+, *Cutis* 50, 87 (observation)
Photosensitivity
Pityriasis rubra pilaris
   (1978): Finlay AY+, *BMJ* 1, 987
Pruritus (1–5%)
Psoriasis
   (2002): Yilmaz MB+, *Angiology* 53(6), 737
   (1990): Wakefield PL+, *Arch Dermatol* 126, 968 (exacerbation)
   (1990): Wolf R, *Dermatologica* 181, 51
   (1988): Gold MH+, *J Am Acad Dermatol* 19, 837
   (1988): Heng MCY+, *Int J Dermatol* 27, 619
   (1986): Abel EA+, *J Am Acad Dermatol* 15, 1007
   (1984): Gawkrodger DJ+, *Clin Exp Dermatol* 9, 92
Purpura
Pustular psoriasis
   (1990): Wakefield PE+, *Arch Dermatol* 126, 968
Rash (sic)
   (1987): Bolzano K+, *J Cardiovasc Pharmacol* 9 (Suppl 3), S43
Raynaud's phenomenon
   (1976): Marshall AJ+, *BMJ* 1, 1498 (35%)
Toxic epidermal necrolysis
Urticaria
   (1989): Wolf R+, *Cutis* 43, 231
   (1988): Howard PJ+, *Scott Med J* 33, 344
Vasculitis
   (1989): Wolf R+, *Cutis* 43, 231
Vitiligo
Xerosis

Hair
Hair – alopecia
   (1991): Shelley WB+, *Cutis* 48, 368 (observation)

Nails
Nails – bluish
Nails – dystrophy
Nails – onycholysis
Nails – splinter hemorrhages
   (1987): Naeyaert JM+, *Br J Dermatol* 117, 371

Other
Anaphylactoid reactions
   (1988): Howard PJ+, *Scott Med J* 33, 344
Death
   (2001): Briggs GG+, *Ann Pharmacother* 35(7), 859
Oculo-mucocutaneous syndrome
   (1982): Cocco G+, *Curr Ther Res* 31, 362
Oral lichenoid eruption
   (1990): Lamey PJ+, *Oral Surg Oral Med Oral Pathol* 70, 184
Peyronie's disease
Pseudolymphoma

   (1990): Henderson CA+, *Clin Exp Dermatol* 15, 119

***Note:** Grinspan's syndrome: the triad of oral lichen planus, diabetes mellitus, and hypertension

ATOMOXETINE

Trade name: Strattera (Lilly)
Indications: Attention deficit hyperactivity disorder (ADHD)
Category: Selective norepinephrine reuptake inhibitor
Half-life: 5 hours
Clinically important, potentially hazardous interactions with: albuterol, MAO inhibitors

Reactions

Skin
Allergic reactions (sic)
Angioedema
Pruritus (>2%)
Rash (sic)
Urticaria

Other
Depression (>2%)
Dizziness (>5%)
Headache
Tremor (>2%)
Xerostomia (>5%)

ATORVASTATIN

Trade name: Lipitor (Parke-Davis) (Pfizer)
Indications: Hypercholesterolemia
Category: Antihyperlipidemic; HMG-CoA reductase inhibitor
Half-life: 14 hours
Clinically important, potentially hazardous interactions with: azithromycin, bosentan, clarithromycin, cyclosporine, erythromycin, gemfibrozil, imatinib, itraconazole, niacin, verapamil

Reactions

Skin
Acne (<2%)
Allergic reactions (sic) (<2%)
Cheilitis (<2%)
Dermatitis (<2%)
Dermatomyositis
   (2001): Noel B+, *Am J Med* 110, 670
Dermographism
   (2001): Adcock BB+, *J Am Board Fam Prac* 14, 148
Diaphoresis (<2%)
Ecchymoses (<2%)
Eczema (sic) (<2%)
Edema (<2%)
Exanthems
Facial edema (<2%)
Flu-like syndrome (sic)
Lichenoid eruption
   (1998): Silver B, Deerfield, IL (from Internet) (observation)
Linear IgA bullous dermatosis
   (2001): König C+, *J Am Acad Dermatol* 44, 689

Lymphocytic infiltration
   (2001): Faivre M+, *Ann Dermatol Venereol* 128, 67
Petechiae (<2%)
Photosensitivity (<2%)
Pruritus (<2%)
Rash (sic) (>3%)
   (2001): Coverman M, *The Schoch Letter* 51, 23 (with simvastatin)
Seborrhea (<2%)
Toxic epidermal necrolysis
   (1998): Pfeiffer CM+, *JAMA* 279, 1613
Ulcerations (<2%)
Urticaria (<2%)
   (2002): Anliker MD+, *Allergy* 57(4), 366
Xerosis (<2%)

Hair

Hair – alopecia (<2%)
   (2002): Burrow W, Jackson MS (from Internet) (observation on himself)
   (2002): Litt JZ, Beachwood, OH (personal case)
   (2002): Segal AS, *Am J Med* 113(2), 171
   (2001): Altman E, West Orange, NJ (from Internet) (observation)
   (1999): Oakley A, Hamilton, New Zealand (from Internet) (observation)
   (1997): Litt JZ, Beachwood, OH (personal case) (observation)

Other

Ageusia (<2%)
Dysgeusia (<2%)
Glossitis (<2%)
Gynecomastia (<2%)
Headache
Limb pain
   (2001): Wright WL, Castro Valley, CA (from Internet) (observation)
Myalgia (>3%)
   (2003): Guis S+, *Arthritis Rheum* 49(2), 237
   (2003): Litt JZ, Beachwood, OH (personal case) (observation)
   (2003): Olsson AG+, *Clin Ther* 25(1), 119 (2.2%)
   (2002): Litt JZ, Beachwood, OH (personal observation)
   (2002): Patel DN+, *J Heart Lung Transplant* 21(2), 204
   (2002): Sinzinger H, *Wien Klin Wochenschr* 114(21), 943
   (2001): Litt JZ, Beachwood, OH (2 personal cases)
   (2001): Rehbein H, Jacksonville, FL (from Internet) (observation)
   (2001): Sorkin M, Denver, CO (from Internet) (observation)
   (2001): Wright W, Castro Valley, CA (from Internet) (2 observations)
   (1998): Malinowski JM, *Am J Health Syst Pharm* 55, 2253
Myopathy
   (2002): Leon Vazquez F+, *Aten Primaria* 30(3), 188
   (2002): Phillips PS+, *Ann Intern Med* 137(7), 581
Myositis
   (2002): Patel DN+, *J Heart Lung Transplant* 21(2), 204
Oral ulceration (<2%)
Paresthesias (<2%)
Parosmia (<2%)
Rhabdomyolysis
   (2003): Guis S+, *Arthritis Rheum* 49(2), 237
   (2003): Mah Ming JB+, *AIDS Patient Care STDS* 17(5), 207 (with clarithromycin, and lopinavir/ritonavir)
   (2003): Sipe BE+, *Ann Pharmacother* 37(6), 808 (with clarithromycin and esomeprazole)
   (2002): Castro JG+, *Am J Med* 112(6), 505 (with delavirdine)
   (2002): Patel DN+, *J Heart Lung Transplant* 21(2), 204
   (2000): Davidson MH, *Curr Atheroscler Rep* 2(1), 14
   (1999): Bottorff M, *Atherosclerosis* 147(Suppl 1), S23
   (1999): Maltz HC+, *Ann Pharmacother* 33(11), 1176 (with cyclosporine)
Stomatitis (<2%)

Tendinopathy
   (2001): Chazerain P+, *Joint Bone Spine* 68(5), 430

ATOVAQUONE

Trade names: Malarone (GSK); Mepron (GSK)
Other common trade name: *Wellvone*
Indications: *Pneumocystis carinii* infection
Category: Antiprotozoal
Half-life: 2.2–2.9 days
Clinically important, potentially hazardous interactions with: rifampin

Reactions

Skin

Diaphoresis (10%)
Erythema multiforme
Exanthems
   (1993): Haile LG+, *Ann Pharmacother* 27, 1488
Pruritus (11%)
   (1996): Radloff PD+, *Lancet* 347, 1511
Rash (sic) (23%)
   (1993): Artymowicz RJ+, *Clin Pharm* 12, 563

Other

Dysgeusia (3%)
Headache
Oral candidiasis (1–10%)

ATRACURIUM

Trade name: Tracrium (GSK)
Indications: Neuromuscular blockade, endotracheal intubation
Category: Neuromuscular blocker; Skeletal muscle relaxant
Half-life: initial: 2 minutes; terminal: 20 minutes
Clinically important, potentially hazardous interactions with: amikacin, aminoglycosides, anesthetics, antibiotics, gentamicin, halothane, kanamycin, neomycin, piperacillin, streptomycin, tobramycin

Reactions

Skin

Allergic reactions (sic)
   (1985): Aldrete JA, *Br J Anaesth* 57, 929
   (1983): Mirakhur RK+, *Anaesthesia* 38, 818
Edema
Erythema (<1%)
Flushing (1–10%)
Pruritus (<1%)
Urticaria (<1%)

Other

Injection-site reactions (sic)

ATROPINE SULFATE

Trade names: Belladenal*; Bellergal-S; Butibel; Donnagel; Donnatal; Donnazyme; Isopto Atropine (Alcon); Lofene; Logen; Lomanate; Lomotil (Pharmacia); Urised (PolyMedica)
Other common trade names: *Atropine Martinet; Atropt; Chibro-Atropine; Isopto; Tropyn Z; Vitatropine*
Indications: Salivation, sinus bradycardia, uveitis, peptic ulcer
Category: Anticholinesterase
Half-life: 2–3 hours
Clinically important, potentially hazardous interactions with: anticholinergics

Reactions

Skin
  Adverse effects
    (2002): Robenshtok E+, *Isr Med Assoc J* 4(7), 535
  Allergic reactions (sic)
    (2001): Decraene T+, *Contact Dermatitis* 45(5), 309
    (1997): Moyano P+, *Rev Esp Anestesiol Reanim* (Spanish) 44, 290
  Bullous eruption
    (1967): Coleman WP, *Med Clin North Am* 51, 1073
  Dermatitis
    (2003): de Misa RF+, *Clin Exp Dermatol* 28(1), 97
    (1988): Gutierrez-Ortega MC+, *Med Cutan Ibero Lat Am* (Spanish) 16, 430
    (1987): van der Willigen AH+, *Contact Dermatitis* 17, 56 (periocular)
    (1985): Yoshikama K+, *Contact Dermatitis* 12, 56
    (1982): Gallasch G+, *Klin Monatsbl Augenheilkd* (German) 181, 96 (periocular)
  Eccrine hidrocystomas
    (1992): Masri-Fridling GD+, *J Am Acad Dermatol* 26, 780
  Erythema multiforme (<1%)
    (1979): Guill MA, *Arch Dermatol* 115, 742
    (1967): Coleman WP, *Med Clin North Am* 51, 1073
  Exanthems
  Exfoliative dermatitis
    (1955): Alexander HL, *Reactions with Drug Therapy* Saunders, Philadelphia
  Eyelid edema
  Fixed eruption
    (1961): Welsh AL, *The Fixed Eruption* Thomas, Springfield
  Flushing
    (1992): Amitai Y+, *JAMA* 268, 630
  Hypohidrosis (>10%)
    (2001): Sanz-Sanchez T+, *Arch Dermatol* 137, 670 (local)
  Periocular dermatitis
    (2003): de Misa RF+, *Clin Exp Dermatol* 28(1), 97
  Photosensitivity (1–10%)
  Pruritus
  Rash (sic) (<1%)
  Sheet-like erythema
  Stevens–Johnson syndrome
    (1967): Coleman WP, *Med Clin North Am* 51, 1073
  Urticaria
    (1986): Bigby M+, *JAMA* 256, 3358
  Xerosis

Other
  Anaphylactoid reactions
    (2002): Robenshtok E+, *Isr Med Assoc J* 4(7), 535 (from eyedrops)
  Dry mucous membranes (sic)
    (1992): Amitai Y+, *JAMA* 268, 630

Dysgeusia
Headache
Injection-site irritation (>10%)
Tremor
Xerostomia (>10%)

*****Note:** Many of the above trade name drugs contain phenobarbital, scopolamine, hyoscyamine, hydrocodone, methenamine, etc

AURANOFIN

(See GOLD and GOLD COMPOUNDS)

AUROTHIOGLUCOSE

(See GOLD and GOLD COMPOUNDS)

AZATADINE

Trade name: Trinalin (Schering)
Other common trade names: *Idulamine; Idulian; Lergocil; Nalomet; Verben; Zadine*
Indications: Allergic rhinitis, urticaria
Category: Antihistamine H$_1$-blocker
Half-life: 9 hours
Clinically important, potentially hazardous interactions with: barbiturates, chloral hydrate, paraldehyde, phenylthiazines, zolpidem

Reactions

Skin
  Angioedema (<1%)
  Diaphoresis
  Edema (<1%)
  Exanthems
  Flushing
  Photosensitivity (<1%)
  Purpura
  Rash (sic) (<1%)
  Urticaria

Other
  Myalgia (<1%)
  Paresthesias (<1%)
  Tinnitus
  Xerostomia (1–10%)
    (1990): Small P+, *Ann Allergy* 64, 129

AZATHIOPRINE

Trade name: Imuran (Prometheus)
Other common trade names: *Azamedac; Azamune; Azatrilem; Imuprin; Imurek; Imurel; Thioprine*
Indications: Lupus nephritis, psoriatic arthritis, rheumatoid arthritis, autoimmune diseases, kidney transplant patients
Category: Immunosuppressant
Half-life: 12 minutes
Clinically important, potentially hazardous interactions with: allopurinol, chlorambucil, cyclophosphamide, mycophenolate, olsalazine, **vaccines**

Reactions

Skin

Acanthosis nigricans
(1980): L'Eplattenier JL+, *Schweiz Med Wochenschr* (German) 110, 1307 (0.5%)
(1974): Koranda FC+, *JAMA* 229, 419 (10%)
Acne
(1983): Schmoeckel C+, *Hautarzt* (German) 34, 413
Allergic reactions (sic)
(1996): Parnham AP+, *Lancet* 348, 542
Angioedema
(1988): Saway PA+, *Am J Med* 84, 960 (passim)
Basal cell carcinoma
(2001): Otley CC+, *Arch Dermatol* 137, 459
Carcinoma (sic)
(1992): Taylor AE+, *Acta Derm Venereol* 72, 115
Chills (>10%)
Dermatitis
(2001): Lauerma AI+, *Contact Dermatitis* 44, 129
(1996): Soni BP+, *Am J Contact Dermat* 7, 116
(1992): Burden AD+, *Contact Dermatitis* 27, 329
Edema of foot
(1996): Oakley A, Hamilton, New Zealand (from Internet) (observation)
Erythema gyratum repens
(2002): Gunther R+, *Med Klin* 97(7), 414
(2002): von Rainer Gunther ZB+, *Med Klin* 97(12), 759
Erythema multiforme
(1995): Knowles SR+, *Clin Exp Dermatol* 20, 353 (passim)
(1988): Saway PA+, *Am J Med* 84, 960 (passim)
Erythema nodosum
(1995): Knowles SR+, *Clin Exp Dermatol* 20, 353 (passim)
(1988): Saway PA+, *Am J Med* 84, 960 (passim)
Exanthems (<1%)
(1995): Knowles SR+, *Clin Exp Dermatol* 20, 353 (passim)
(1990): Jeurissen ME+, *Ann Rheum Dis* 49, 25 (4%)
(1988): Bergman SM+, *Ann Intern Med* 109, 83
(1988): Saway PA+, *Am J Med* 84, 960
(1978): Franchmont P+, *J Rheumatol* 5 (Suppl 4), 85 (5.4%)
(1972): Decker JL, *Ann Intern Med* 76, 619
(1972): King JO+, *Med J Aust* 2, 939
(1971): Harris J+, *BMJ* 4, 463 (1–5%)
(1969): Mason M+, *BMJ* 1, 420 (1–5%)
(1967): Adams DA+, *JAMA* 199, 459
Exfoliation (sic)
(1997): Hermanns-Le T+, *Dermatology* 194, 175
Fixed eruption
(1990): Black AK+, *Br J Dermatol* 123, 277 (observation)
Formication
(1992): Shelley WB+, *Advanced Dermatologic Diagnosis* WB Saunders, 1042 (passim)
Fungal infections

(1980): L'Eplattenier JL+, *Schweiz Med Wochenschr* (German) 110, 1307 (42%)
Herpes simplex
(1980): L'Eplattenier JL+, *Schweiz Med Wochenschr* (German) 110, 1307 (27%)
(1979): Spencer ES+, *BMJ* 2, 829
(1974): Koranda FC+, *JAMA* 229, 419 (35%)
Herpes zoster
(2001): Vergara M+, *Gastroenterol Hepatol* 24, 47
(1991): Callen JP+, *Arch Dermatol* 127, 515
(1982): Speerstra F+, *Ann Rheum Dis* 41, Suppl 37
(1980): L'Eplattenier JL+, *Schweiz Med Wochenschr* (German) 110, 1307 (27%)
(1974): Koranda FC+, *JAMA* 229, 419 (13%)
(1966): Rifkind D, *J Lab Clin Med* 68, 463 (8%)
Infections (sic)
(2003): Bernal I+, *Gastroenterol Hepatol* 26(1), 19
(1978): Bergfeld WF+, *Cutis* 22, 169 (62%)
(1974): Koranda FC+, *JAMA* 229, 419 (>5%)
(1973): Haim S+, *Br J Dermatol* 89, 169 (100%)
Intraepidermal carcinoma
(2001): Austin AS+, *Eur J Gastroenterol Hepatol* 13, 193
Kaposi's sarcoma
(1997): Aebischer MC+, *Dermatology* 195, 91
(1997): Halpern SM+, *Br J Dermatol* 137, 140
(1997): Lesnoni-La-Parola I+, *Dermatology* 194, 229
(1997): Vandercam B+, *Dermatology* 194, 180
(1996): Ozen S+, *Nephrol Dial Transplant* 11, 1162
(1991): Almog Y+, *Clin Exp Dermatol* 9, 285
(1984): Luderschmidt C+, *Klin Wochenschr* (German) 62, 803
(1982): Weiss VC+, *Arch Dermatol* 118, 183
(1980): Iversen OH+, *Scand J Urol Nephrol* 14, 125
(1974): Faye I+, *Bull Soc Fr Dermatol Syphiligr* (French) 81, 379
(1973): Haim S+, *Br J Dermatol* 89, 169
Keratoacanthoma
(1971): Walder BK+, *Lancet* 2, 1282
Lichenoid eruption
(1979): Beaaff D+, *Arch Dermatol* 115, 498
Neoplasms
(2003): Li AC+, *Eur J Gastroenterol Hepatol* 15(2), 185
Photosensitivity
Pigmentation (sun-exposed skin)
(1974): Koranda FC+, *JAMA* 229, 419 (37%)
Porokeratosis
(1997): Matsushita S+, *J Dermatol* 24, 110 (disseminated superficial actinic)
(1988): Neumann RA+, *Br J Dermatol* 119, 375 (disseminated superficial actinic)
(1987): Tatnall FM+, *J R Soc Med* 80, 180 (Mibelli)
(1974): Macmillan AL+, *Br J Dermatol* 90, 45
Purpura
Pyoderma gangrenosum
(1976): Haim S+, *Dermatologica* 153, 44
Rash (sic) (1–10%)
(1997): Lavaud F+, *Dig Dis Sci* 42, 823
(1990): Jeurissen ME+, *Ann Rheum Dis* 49, 25
(1975): Goldenberg DL+, *J Rheumatol* 2, 346
(1972): King JO+, *Med J Aust* 2, 939
Raynaud's phenomenon
Sarcoma
(1996): Csuka ME+, *Arch Intern Med* 156, 1573
Scabies
(1980): L'Eplattenier JL+, *Schweiz Med Wochenschr* (German) 110, 1307 (1%)
(1978): Bricklin AS+, *Cutis* 22, 81
(1976): Anolik MA+, *Arch Dermatol* 112, 73
(1973): Paterson WD+, *BMJ* 4, 211
Scleroderma
(1993): Choy E+, *Br J Rheumatol* 32, 160

Squamous cell carcinoma
  (2001): Otley CC+, *Arch Dermatol* 137, 459
  (2001): Werth V, *Dermatology Times* 15
  (1995): Bottomley WW+, *Br J Dermatol* 133, 460
  (1993): Nachbar F+, *Acta Derm Venereol* 73, 217
  (1992): McCain J, *Nurs Pract* 17, 13
  (1988): Krickeberg H, *Z Hautkr* (German) 63, 773
  (1973): Westburg SP+, *Arch Dermatol* 107, 893
  (1971): Walder BK+, *Lancet* 2, 1282
Tinea corporis
  (1980): L'Eplattenier JL+, *Schweiz Med Wochenschr* (German)
    110, 1307 (3%)
  (1974): Koranda FC+, *JAMA* 229, 419 (2%)
Tinea versicolor
  (1981): Burkhart CG+, *Cutis* 27, 56
  (1974): Koranda FC+, *JAMA* 229, 419 (18%)
Toxic epidermal necrolysis
  (1990): Black AK+, *Br J Dermatol* 123, 277
Urticaria
  (1995): Knowles SR+, *Clin Exp Dermatol* 20, 353 (passim)
  (1990): Wijnands MJ+, *Scand J Rheumatol* 19, 167
  (1988): Saway PA+, *Am J Med* 84, 960 (passim)
  (1972): Decker JL, *Ann Intern Med* 76, 619
  (1970): Drinkard JP+, *Medicine* (Baltimore) 49, 411
Vasculitis
  (1995): Blanco R+, *Arthritis Rheum* 39, 1016
  (1995): Knowles SR+, *Clin Exp Dermatol* 20, 353 (passim)
  (1988): Bergman SM+, *Ann Intern Med* 109, 83
Viral infections
  (1980): L'Eplattenier JL+, *Schweiz Med Wochenschr* (German)
    110, 1307 (45%)
  (1974): Koranda FC+, *JAMA* 229, 419 (43%)
Warts
  (1991): Callen JP+, *Arch Dermatol* 127, 515
  (1980): L'Eplattenier JL+, *Schweiz Med Wochenschr* (German)
    110, 1307 (21%)

Hair

Hair – alopecia (<1%)
  (1982): Bailin PL+, *Clin Rheum Dis* 8, 493 (passim)
  (1980): L'Eplattenier JL+, *Schweiz Med Wochenschr* (German)
    110, 1307 (27%)
  (1974): Koranda FC+, *JAMA* 229, 419 (54%)
Hair – curly
  (1996): van der Pijl JW+, *Lancet* 348, 622 (with isotretinoin)

Nails

Nails – discoloration (red lunulae)
  (1974): Koranda FC+, *JAMA* 229, 419 (2%)
Nails – onychomycosis
  (1980): L'Eplattenier JL+, *Schweiz Med Wochenschr* (German)
    110, 1307 (1%)
  (1974): Koranda FC+, *JAMA* 229, 419 (5%)

Other

Anaphylactoid reactions
  (1993): Jones JJ+, *J Am Acad Dermatol* 29, 795
Aphthous stomatitis (<1%)
Cicatricial pemphigoid
  (2000): Burgess MJA+, *Arch Dermatol* 136, 1274
Hypersensitivity (<1%)*
  (2001): Corbett M+, *Intern Med J* 31(6), 366
  (2001): Sofat N+, *Ann Rheum Dis* 60(7), 719
  (2001): Werth V, *Dermatology Times* 15
  (1999): Korelitz BI+, *J Clin Gastroenterol* 28, 341
  (1998): Fields CL+, *South Med J* 91, 471
  (1998): Garey KW+, *Ann Pharmacother* 32, 425
  (1998): Schlienger RG+, *Epilepsia* 39, S3 (passim)
  (1997): Caramaschi P+, *Lupus* 6, 616
  (1997): Knowles S+, *Muscle Nerve* 20, 1467

  (1996): Compton MR+, *Arch Dermatol* 132, 1254 (with
    rhabdomyolysis)
  (1995): Knowles SR+, *Clin Exp Dermatol* 20, 353
  (1982): Mosbech H+, *Ugeskr Laeger* (Danish) 144, 2424
  (1975): Goldenberg DL+, *J Rheumatol* 2, 346
  (1972): King JO+, *Med J Aust* 2, 939
Lymphoproliferative disease
  (1987): Phillips T+, *Clin Exp Dermatol* 12, 444
  (1987): Pitt PI+, *J R Soc Med* 80, 428
  (1982): Ulreich A+, *Z Rheumatol* (German) 41, 73
Myalgia (<1%)
Non-Hodgkin's lymphoma
  (2000): Lewis JD+, *Gastroenterology* 118, 1018
Oral ulceration
  (2000): Madinier I+, *Ann Med Interne (Paris)* (French) 151, 248
Rhabdomyolysis
  (1996): Compton MR+, *Arch Dermatol* 132, 1254
Rheumatoid nodules (sic)
  (1991): Langevitz P+, *Arthritis Rheum* 34, 123
Serum sickness
Stomatitis
  (1982): Bailin PL+, *Clin Rheum Dis* 8, 493 (passim)
Tumors (sic)
  (1986): Gupta AK+, *Arch Dermatol* 122, 1288 (5.3%) (malignant)
  (1982): Bailin PL+, *Clin Rheum Dis* 8, 493 (passim)
  (1980): L'Eplattenier JL+, *Schweiz Med Wochenschr* (German)
    110, 1307 (2.9%) (benign); (4.3%) (malignant)
  (1978): Bergfeld WF+, *Cutis* 22, 169 (4.6%) (malignant)
  (1974): Koranda FC+, *JAMA* 229, 419 (3.5%) (malignant)
  (1973): Westburg SP+, *Arch Dermatol* 107, 893
  (1973): Wishart J, *Arch Dermatol* 108, 563 (reticulosarcoma)
  (1971): Walder BK+, *Lancet* 2, 1282 (>5%) (malignant)
Xerostomia

*Note: The antiepileptic drug hypersensitivity syndrome is a severe,
occasionally fatal, disorder characterized by any or all of the
following: pruritic exanthems, toxic epidermal necrolysis, Stevens–
Johnson syndrome, exfoliative dermatitis, fever, hepatic
abnormalities, eosinophilia, and renal failure

AZELASTINE

Trade names: Astelin (Wallace); Optivar (Muro)
Other common trade names: *Allergodil; Azeptin*
Indications: Allergic rhinitis
Category: Antihistamine; anti-inflammatory
Half-life: 22 hours
**Clinically important, potentially hazardous interactions
with:** barbiturates, chloral hydrate, paraldehyde, phenothiazines,
zolpidem

Reactions

Skin

Allergic reactions (sic) (<2%)
Dermatitis (<2%)
Eczema (sic) (<2%)
Exanthems
  (1989): McTavish D+, *Drugs* 38, 19
Flushing (<2%)
Folliculitis (<2%)
Furunculosis (<2%)
Herpes simplex (<2%)

Other

Ageusia (<2%)

Aphthous stomatitis (<2%)
Dysgeusia (bitter taste) (19.7%)
  (1993): Davies RJ+, *Rhinology* 31, 159
  (1990): Tinkelman DG+, *Am Rev Respir Dis* 141, 569 (30–52%)
  (1988): Weiler JM+, *J Allergy Clin Immunology* 82, 801 (19.7%)
Glossitis (<2%)
Headache
Hyperesthesia (<2%)
Mastodynia (<2%)
Myalgia (1.5%)
Oral dryness
  (1989): McTavish D+, *Drugs* 38, 19
Oral mucosal eruption
  (1989): McTavish D+, *Drugs* 38, 19
Stomatitis (ulcerative) (<2%)
Xerostomia (2.8%)
  (1990): Tinkelman DG+, *Am Rev Respir Dis* 141, 569 (4–6%)

AZITHROMYCIN

Trade name: Zithromax (Pfizer)
Other common trade names: *Azenil; Azitrocin; Azitromax; Zeto; Zitromax*
Indications: Infections of the upper and lower respiratory tract, skin infections, sexually-transmitted diseases
Category: Macrolide antibiotic
Half-life: 68 hours
Clinically important, potentially hazardous interactions with: atorvastatin, cyclosporine, fluvastatin, lovastatin, pimozide, pravastatin, simvastatin, warfarin

Reactions

Skin

Allergic reactions (sic) (<1%)
  (1998): Salit IE+, *Infect Med* 15, 773 (0.4%)
Angioedema (<1%)
Dermatitis
  (2001): Milkovic-Kraus S+, *Contact Dermatitis* 45(3), 184
Diaper rash
  (1997): Arguedas A+, *Infections in Medicine* October, 807
Edema
Erythema
  (1991): Felstead SJ+, *J Int Med Res* 19, 363
Exanthems
  (2000): Schissel DJ+, *Cutis* 65, 123 (in a patient with infectious mononucleosis)
Facial edema
Fixed eruption
  (1999): Smith KC, Niagara Falls, Ontario (from Internet) (observation)
Granulomatous dermatitis (Churg–Strauss syndrome)
  (1998): Dietz A+, *Laryngorhinootologie* (German) 77, 111
  (1997): Kranke B+, *Lancet* 350, 1551
Photosensitivity (1%)
Pruritus
  (2000): Schissel DJ+, *Cutis* 65, 123 (in a patient with infectious mononucleosis)
Pustules
  (1994): Trevis P+, *Clin Exp Dermatol* 19, 280
Rash (sic) (<1%)
  (1991): Felstead SJ+, *J Int Med Res* 19, 363
  (1991): Hopkins S, *Am J Med* 91, 36s
Side effects (sic)

  (1993): Hopkins S, *J Antimicrob Chemother* 31 (Suppl E), 111
Stevens–Johnson syndrome
  (2001): Brett AS+, *South Med J* 94, 342
  (1998): Smith KC, Niagara Falls, Ontario (from Internet) (observation)
Toxic pustuloderma
  (1994): Trevisi P+, *Clin Exp Dermatol* 19, 280
Urticaria
  (2001): Thaler D, Monana, WI (from Internet) (observation) (2–year-old child 3 hours after initiation of drug)
  (1991): Hopkins S, *Am J Med* 91, 36s

Other

Anaphylactoid reactions
Headache
Hypersensitivity (0.6%)
  (2001): Cascaval RI+, *Am J Med* 110, 330
  (1998): Salit IE+, *Infect Med* 15, 773
Injection-site erythema
  (1997): Luke DR+, *Ann Pharmacother* 31, 965
Injection-site pain
  (2001): Zimmerman T+, *Clin Drug Invest* 21, 527 (67%)
  (1997): Luke DR+, *Ann Pharmacother* 31, 965
Torsades de pointes
  (2002): Shaffer D+, *Clin Infect Dis* 35(2), 197
Vaginitis (2%)
  (1991): Hopkins S, *Am J Med* 91, 36s

AZTREONAM

Synonym: azthreonam
Trade name: Azactam (Elan)
Other common trade names: *Primbactam; Urobactam*
Indications: Aerobic gram-negative bacillary infections
Category: Narrow-spectrum antibiotic (monobactam)
Half-life: 1.4–2.2 hours

Reactions

Skin

Angioedema
  (1990): Soto Alvarez J+, *Lancet* 335, 1094
Diaphoresis
Erythema multiforme
  (1997): Epstein ME+, *J Am Acad Dermatol* 37, 149 (passim)
Exanthems
  (1990): Adkinson NF, *Am J Med* 88 (Suppl 3C), 12S (1.6%)
  (1990): Fekete T+, *Drug Intell Clin Pharm* 24, 438 (1–5%)
  (1988): Pazmiño P, *Am J Nephrol* 8, 68
  (1986): Brogden RN+, *Drugs* 18, 241 (1.8%)
Exfoliative dermatitis
  (1997): Epstein ME+, *J Am Acad Dermatol* 37, 149 (passim)
Petechiae
  (1997): Epstein ME+, *J Am Acad Dermatol* 37, 149 (passim)
Pruritus
  (1997): Epstein ME+, *J Am Acad Dermatol* 37, 149 (passim)
  (1990): Adkinson NF, *Am J Med* 88 (Suppl 3C), 12S
  (1986): Brogden RN+, *Drugs* 18, 241 (1.8%)
Purpura
  (1997): Epstein ME+, *J Am Acad Dermatol* 37, 149 (passim)
  (1990): Adkinson NF, *Am J Med* 88 (Suppl 3C), 12S (0.1%)
Rash (sic) (1–10%)
  (1985): Newman TJ+, *Rev Infect Dis* 7, S648
Toxic epidermal necrolysis
  (1997): Epstein ME+, *J Am Acad Dermatol* 37, 149 (passim)
  (1992): McDonald BJ+, *Ann Pharmacother* 26, 34

Urticaria
  (1997): Epstein ME+, *J Am Acad Dermatol* 37, 149 (passim)
  (1993): de la Fuente-Prieto R+, *Allergy* 48, 634
  (1991): Hantson P+, *BMJ* 302, 294
  (1990): Adkinson NF, *Am J Med* 88 (Suppl 3C), 12S (0.2%)
  (1990): Soto Alvarez J+, *Lancet* 335, 1094

Other
  Anaphylactoid reactions (<1%)
  Aphthous stomatitis (<1%)
  Dysgeusia (<1%)
  Foetor ex ore (halitosis) (<1%)
  Hypersensitivity
  Injection-site pain (1–10%)

Injection-site phlebitis (1–10%)
Injection-site reactions (sic)
  (1985): Newman TJ+, *Rev Infect Dis* 7, S648
Mastodynia (<1%)
Myalgia (<1%)
Oral ulceration (<1%)
Paresthesias
Thrombophlebitis (1–10%)
Tinnitus
Tongue numb (sic) (<1%)
Vaginal candidiasis
Vaginitis (<1%)

BACAMPICILLIN

Synonym: carampicillin
Trade name: Spectrobid (Pfizer)
Other common trade names: *Albaxin; Ambacamp; Ambaxin; Bacacil; Bacampicine; Penglobe*
Indications: Respiratory tract infections, urinary tract infections, gonorrhea
Category: Beta-lactamase-sensitive aminopenicillin
Half-life: 65 minutes
Clinically important, potentially hazardous interactions with: anticoagulants, cyclosporine, demeclocycline, doxycycline, methotrexate, minocycline, oxytetracycline, tetracycline

Reactions

Skin
Acute generalized exanthematous pustulosis (AGEP)
  (1990): Guy C+, *Nouv Dermatol* (French) 9, 540
Angioedema
Dermatitis
  (1986): Stejskal VD+, *J Allergy Clin Immunol* 77, 411
Ecchymoses
Edema
  (2002): Liccardi G+, *Lancet* 359, 1700 (lips) ("deep kissing" husband who had taken bacampicillin)
Erythema multiforme
Exanthems
  (1989): Alanko K+, *Acta Derm Venereol* (Stockh) 69, 223
  (1988): Kohl PK+, *Aktuel Dermatol* 14, 104
  (1986): Pauwels R+, *J Int Med Res* 14, 110
Exfoliative dermatitis
Fixed eruption
  (1984): Chan HL, *Arch Dermatol* 120, 542
Hematomas
Jarisch–Herxheimer reaction
Pruritus
  (2002): Liccardi G+, *Lancet* 359, 1700 (lips) ("deep kissing" husband who had taken bacampicillin)
Pustules
  (1998): Isogai Z+, *J Dermatol* 25, 612
Rash (sic) (<1%)
Stevens–Johnson syndrome
Urticaria

Other
Anaphylactoid reactions
Black tongue
Dysgeusia
Glossitis
Glossodynia
Hypersensitivity (<1%)
Injection-site pain
Oral candidiasis
Serum sickness
Stomatitis
Stomatodynia
Vaginitis
Xerostomia

BACLOFEN

Trade names: Baclofen (Watson); Lioresal (Novartis)
Other common trade names: *Alpha-Baclofen; Baclon; Baclosal; Baklofen; Clofen; Dom-Baclofen; Gen-Baclofen; Lebic; Nu-Baclo; Pacifen; PMS-Baclofen; Spinax*
Indications: Spasticity resulting from multiple sclerosis
Category: Antispastic; Skeletal muscle relaxant
Half-life: 2.5–4 hours

Reactions

Skin
Ankle edema
  (1993): Albright AL+, *JAMA* 270, 2475
Dermatitis (sic)
Diaphoresis
Exanthems
  (1983): Lynde CW+, *Ann Neurol* 13, 216
Facial edema
Flushing
Pruritus
Rash (sic) (1–10%)
Side effects (sic) (1–2%)
  (1972): Birkmayer W, *Aspeckte der Muskelspastik Int Symp Wien* (German) Bern, Huber
Urticaria
  (1972): Birkmayer W, *Aspeckte der Muskelspastik Int Symp Wien* (German) Bern, Huber (2%)

Other
Dysgeusia (<1%)
  (1976): Rollin H, *Laryngol Rhinol Otol* (Stuttgart) (German) 55, 873
Headache
Paresthesias (<1%)
Tinnitus
Xerostomia (<1%)

BALSALAZIDE

Trade name: Colazal (Salix)
Indications: Mild to moderately active ulcerative colitis
Category: Aminosalicylate anti-inflammatory
Half-life: N/A

Reactions

Skin
Flu-like syndrome (1%)
Pruritus
Rash (sic)

Hair
Hair – alopecia

Other
Arthralgia (4%)
Headache
Hypersensitivity
  (2000): Adhiyaman V+, *BMJ* 320, 613
Myalgia (1%)
Xerostomia (1%)

BASILIXIMAB

Trade name: Simulect (Novartis)
Indications: Prophylaxis of organ rejection in renal transplantation
Category: Chimeric monoclonal antibody; Immunosuppressant
Half-life: 7.2 days
Clinically important, potentially hazardous interactions with: cyclosporine, mycophenolate

Reactions

Skin
Acne (>10%)
Candidiasis (>10%)
Cyst (3–10%)
Edema (generalized) (3–10%)
Edema of leg
Facial edema (3–10%)
Genital edema (sic) (3–10%)
Hematomas (3–10%)
Herpes simplex (3–10%)
Herpes zoster
Infections (sic) (3–10%)
Peripheral edema (>10%)
Pruritus (3–10%)
Rash (sic) (3–10%)
Ulcerations (3–10%)
Vascular disorder (sic)
Viral infections (>10%)

Hair
Hair – hypertrichosis (3–10%)

Other
Anaphylactoid reactions
Arthralgia (3–10%)
Depression (3–10%)
Gingival hyperplasia (3–10%)
Headache
Hyperesthesia (3–10%)
Hypersensitivity (17 cases)
Myalgia (3–10%)
Pain
Paresthesias (3–10%)
Sneezing
Stomatitis (3–10%)
Tremor (>10%)
Ulcerative stomatitis
Wound complications (sic) (>10%)

BENACTYZINE

Trade name: Deprol (Wallace)
Indications: Depression, anxiety
Category: Antidepressant
Half-life: N/A

Deprol is benactyzine and meprobamate

Note: Most of the adverse reactions are due to meprobamate (which see)

Reactions

Skin
Angioedema
Bullous eruption
Ecchymoses
Edema
Erythema multiforme
Exanthems
  (1964): Welsh AL, *Med Clin North Am* 48, 459
Exfoliative dermatitis
Fixed eruption
Petechiae
Pruritus
Urticaria

Other
Anaphylactoid reactions
Paresthesias
Stomatitis
Xerostomia

BENAZEPRIL

Trade names: Lotensin (Novartis); Lotensin-HCT (Novartis); Lotrel (Novartis)
Other common trade names: *Cibace; Cibacen; Cibacene*
Indications: Hypertension
Category: Angiotensin-converting enzyme (ACE) inhibitor; Antihypertensive
Half-life: 11–12 hours
Clinically important, potentially hazardous interactions with: amiloride, spironolactone, triamterene

Lotrel is benazepril and amlodipine; Lotensin-HCT is benazepril and hydrochlorothiazide

Reactions

Skin
Angioedema (<1%)
  (2001): Cohen EG+, *Ann Otol Rhinol Laryngol* 110(8), 701 (64 cases)
  (1996): O'Mara NB+, *Pharmacotherapy* 16, 675
  (1992): Kuhn M, *Clin Issues Crit Care Nurs* 3, 461
  (1991): Anon, *Med Lett Drugs Ther* 33, 83
  (1991): Balfour JA+, *Drugs* 42, 511
  (1991): MacNab M+, *Clin Cardiol* 14, IV33
Ankle edema
  (1990): Mirvis DM+, *Am J Med Sci* 300, 354
Dermatitis (sic)
Diaphoresis (<1%)

(1991): Morant J+ (eds), *Arzneimittel-Kompendium der Schweiz* Basel (German), Documed, 1990

Exanthems
(1991): Morant J+ (eds), *Arzneimittel-Kompendium der Schweiz* Basel (German), Documed, 1990

Flushing
(1991): Morant J+ (eds), *Arzneimittel-Kompendium der Schweiz* Basel (German), Documed, 1990

Linear IgA dermatosis
(2003): Femiano F+, *Oral Surg Oral Med Oral Pathol Oral Radiol Endod* 95(2), 169

Lupus erythematosus
(2002): Boye T+, *World Congress Dermatol* Poster 0088

Pemphigus foliaceus
(2000): Ong CS+, *Australas J Dermatol* 41(4), 242

Peripheral edema
Photosensitivity (<1%)
Pruritus
(1991): Morant J+ (eds), *Arzneimittel-Kompendium der Schweiz* Basel (German), Documed, 1990

Rash (sic) (<1%)
(1991): MacNab M+, *Clin Cardiol* 14, IV33

Urticaria
(1991): Moser M+, *Clin Pharmacol Ther* 49, 322

Other

Ageusia
Cough
(2001): Adigun AQ+, *West Afr J Med* 20(1), 46–7
(2001): Lee SC+, *Hypertension* 38(2), 166

Dysgeusia
(1991): MacNab M+, *Clin Cardiol* 14, IV33

Headache
Hypersensitivity
Myalgia (<1%)
Paresthesias (<1%)
Tinnitus

BENDROFLUMETHIAZIDE

Trade name: Corzide (Monarch)
Other common trade names: *Aprinox; Berkozide; Centyl; Naturine; Neo-Naclex; Pluryle*
Indications: Edema, diabetes insipidus, hypertension
Category: Antihypertensive; Thiazide diuretic
Half-life: 8.5 hours
Clinically important, potentially hazardous interactions with: digoxin, lithium

Corzide is bendroflumethiazide and nadolol

Reactions

Skin

Allergic reactions (sic)
Dermatitis
(1997): Pereira F+, *Contact Dermatitis* 35, 303

Diaphoresis
Exanthems
(1991): Morant J+ (eds), *Arzneimittel-Kompendium der Schweiz* Basel (German), Documed, 1990

Exfoliative dermatitis
Facial edema
Grinspan's syndrome**
(1990): Lamey PG+, *Oral Surg Oral Med Oral Pathol* 70, 184

Pemphigus (sic)
Photosensitivity
(1989): Diffey BL+, *Arch Dermatol* 125, 1355

Phototoxicity
(1997): Selvaag E, *Arzneimittelforschung* (German) 47, 97
(1997): Selvaag E+, *In Vivo* 11, 103

Pruritus
(1991): Morant J+ (eds), *Arzneimittel-Kompendium der Schweiz* Basel (German), Documed, 1990

Purpura
Rash (sic)
Urticaria
Vasculitis

Hair

Hair – alopecia

Other

Anaphylactoid reactions
Gynecomastia
Paresthesias
Tinnitus
Xanthopsia
Xerostomia

*Note: Bendroflumethiazide is a sulfonamide and can be absorbed systemically. Sulfonamides can produce severe, possibly fatal, reactions such as toxic epidermal necrolysis and Stevens–Johnson syndrome

**Note: Grinspan's syndrome: the triad of oral lichen planus, diabetes mellitus, and hypertension

BENZONATATE

Trade name: Tessalon (Forest)
Other common trade names: *Beknol; Benzonal; Pebegal; Tesalon; Tusehli*
Indications: Symptomatic relief of cough
Category: Non-narcotic antitussive
Half-life: Duration: 3–8 hours

Reactions

Skin

Chills
Eruptions (sic)
Ocular burning (1–10%)
Pruritus
Rash (sic) (1–10%)

Other

Death
(1998): Crouch BI+, *J Toxicol Clin Toxicol* 36(7), 713 (2 cases)
(1986): Cohan JA+, *Vet Hum Toxicol* 28(6), 543

Headache
Hypersensitivity
Numbness in chest (sic) (1–10%)
Seizures
(1998): Crouch BI+, *J Toxicol Clin* 36(7), 713

Tremor (overdose)

Note: Benzonatate is related to tetracaine and other anesthetics of the para-aminobenzoic acid class

BENZPHETAMINE

Trade name: Didrex (Pharmacia)
Other common trade name: *Inapetyl*
Indications: Adjunct to diet plan to reduce weight
Category: Anorexiant; CNS Stimulant; Sympathomimetic amine
Half-life: N/A
Clinically important, potentially hazardous interactions with: furazolidone, guanethidine, MAO inhibitors, SSRIs

Reactions

Skin
Allergic reactions (sic)
Diaphoresis
Erythema
Flushing
Rash (sic)
Urticaria

Hair
Hair – alopecia

Other
Anxiety
Depression (following withdrawal)
Dizziness
Gynecomastia
Headache
Hypersensitivity
Myalgia
Tremor
Xerostomia

BENZTHIAZIDE

Trade names: Aquatag; Exna (Wyeth); Hydrex; Marazide; Proaqua
Other common trade names: *Diurin; Fovane; Regulon*
Indications: Hypertension
Category: Antihypertensive; Thiazide diuretic
Half-life: N/A
Clinically important, potentially hazardous interactions with: digoxin, lithium

Reactions

Skin
Allergic reactions (sic) (<1%)
Photosensitivity
Purpura
Rash (sic)
Urticaria
Vasculitis

Other
Dysgeusia
Paresthesias (<1%)
Xanthopsia

*****Note:** Benzthiazide is a sulfonamide and can be absorbed systemically. Sulfonamides can produce severe, possibly fatal, reactions such as toxic epidermal necrolysis and Stevens–Johnson syndrome

BENZTROPINE

Trade name: Cogentin (Merck)
Other common trade names: *Akitan; Apo-Benzthioprine; Cogentine; Cogentinol; Phatropine; PMS-Benztropine*
Indications: Parkinsonism
Category: Antidyskinetic; Antiparkinsonian
Half-life: 6–48 hours
Clinically important, potentially hazardous interactions with: anticholinergics

Reactions

Skin
Exanthems
Hypohidrosis (>10%)
Photosensitivity (1–10%)
Pruritus
Rash (sic) (<1%)
Urticaria
Xerosis (>10%)

Other
Black tongue
  (2000): Heymann WR, *Cutis* 66, 25
Death
  (2001): Lynch MJ+, *Med Sci Law* 41(2), 155
Dysgeusia
  (2000): Heymann WR, *Cutis* 66, 25
Glossodynia
Paresthesias
Stomatodynia
Tinnitus
Xerostomia (>10%)
  (2000): Heymann WR, *Cutis* 66, 25
  (1989): Gelenberg AJ+, *J Clin Psychopharmacol* 9, 180

BEPRIDIL

Trade name: Vascor (Ortho-McNeil)
Other common trade names: *Bapadin; Bepricol; Cordium; Cruor*
Indications: Angina pectoris
Category: Antianginal; Calcium channel blocker
Half-life: 24 hours
Clinically important, potentially hazardous interactions with: amprenavir, atazanavir, ciprofloxacin, enoxacin, epirubicin, gatifloxacin, lomefloxacin, **mistletoe**, moxifloxacin, norfloxacin, ofloxacin, quinolones, ritonavir, sparfloxacin

Reactions

Skin
Diaphoresis (<2%)
Edema (1–10%)
Irritation (sic)
Peripheral edema (<1%)
Rash (sic) (<2%)
  (1988): Sharma MK+, *Am J Cardiol* 61, 1210

Other
Dysgeusia (<1%)
Myalgia (<1%)
Paresthesias (2.5%)

Tinnitus
Tremor (<9%)
Xerostomia (1–10%)
    (1988): Hasegawa GR, *Clin Pharm* 7, 97
    (1988): Krusell LR+, *Eur J Clin Pharmacol* 34, 221

BERGAMOT*

Scientific name: *Citrus aurantium* ssp *bergamia*
Family: Rutaceae
Trade and other common names: Bergamottin; Earl Grey tea; Florida Water; Kananga Water; Neroli oil; Oil of bergamot
Category: Mild stimulant
Purported indications and other uses: Headache, bronchitis, vitiligo, mycosis fungoides, psoriasis (in conjunction with UVA), insecticide, essential oil in perfumery, cosmetics, flavoring
Half-life: N/A

***Note:** two distinct species are known by the common name of bergamot. This profile does not refer to *Monarda didyma*

Reactions

Skin
Adverse effects (sic)
    (2001): Kaddu S+, *J Am Acad Dermatol* 45(3), 458
Berloque dermatitis
    (2002): Gruson LM+, *Arch Pediatr Adolesc Med* 156(11), 1091
    (2002): Wang L+, *Cutis* 70(1), 29
Blistering
    (2002): Gruson LM+, *Arch Pediatr Adolesc Med* 156(11), 1091
Bullous eruption
    (2001): Kaddu S+, *J Am Acad Dermatol* 45(3), 458
Burning
    (1998): Cocks H+, *Burns* 24(1), 82
Dermatitis
    (1984): Zacher KD+, *Derm Beruf Umwelt* 32(3), 95
    (1976): Urbach F+, *J Invest Dermatol* 67(1), 209
Erythema
    (2002): Gruson LM+, *Arch Pediatr Adolesc Med* 156(11), 1091
Photosensitivity
    (2001): Kaddu S+, *J Am Acad Dermatol* 45(3), 458
    (1993): Moysan A+, *Skin Pharmacol* 6(4), 282
    (1990): Morliere P+, *J Photochem Photobiol B* 7(2), 199
Phototoxicity
    (2001): Kaddu S+, *J Am Acad Dermatol* 45(3), 458
    (1993): Moysan A+, *Skin Pharmacol* 6(4), 282
    (1990): Dubertret L+, *J Photochem Photobiol B* 7(2), 251
    (1986): Maibach HI+, *Dermatol Clin* 4(2), 217
    (1979): Girard J+, *Dermatologica* 158(4), 229
    (1977): Zaynoun ST+, *Br J Dermatol* 96(5), 475
    (1977): Zaynoun ST+, *Contact Dermatitis* 3(5), 225
Pigmentation
    (2002): Gruson LM+, *Arch Pediatr Adolesc Med* 156(11), 1091
Tumors
    (1990): Young AR+, *J Photochem Photobiol B* 7(2), 231

Note: Oil of bergamot possesses photosensitive and melanogenic properties because of the presence of furocoumarins, primarily bergapten (5-methoxypsoralen [5-MOP]). Its use is restricted or banned in many countries

BETA-CAROTENE

Trade name: Solatene (Merck)
Other common trade names: *B-Tene; Betavin; Carotaben; Solvin*
Indications: Photosensitivity reactions
Category: Fat-soluble vitamin; Photosensitivity reaction suppressant
Half-life: N/A
Clinically important, potentially hazardous interactions with: bexarotene

Reactions

Skin
Carotenemia (>10%)
    (2000): Frieling UM+, *Arch Dermatol* 136, 179 (15.9%)
Dermatitis (sic)
    (1992): Zürcher K and Krebs A, *Cutaneous Drug Reactions*
        Karger, 280
Ecchymoses (<1%)
Purpura (<1%)

BETAXOLOL

Trade names: Betoptic [Ophthalmic] (Alcon); Kerlone (Pharmacia)
Other common trade names: *Betoptic S; Betoptima; Kerlon; Optipres*
Indications: Open-angle glaucoma, hypertension
Category: Antihypertensive; Beta-adrenoceptor blocker
Half-life: 14–22 hours
Clinically important, potentially hazardous interactions with: clonidine, verapamil

Note: Cutaneous side effects of beta-receptor blockaders are clinically polymorphic. They apparently appear after several months of continuous therapy. Atypical psoriasiform, lichen planus-like, and eczematous chronic rashes are mainly observed. (1983): Hödl St, *Z Hautkr* 1:58, 17

Reactions

Skin
Acne
Allergic reactions (sic) (<2%)
Angioedema
Cold extremities (sic)
Dermatitis
    (2001): Holdiness MR, *Am J Contact Dermat* 12(4), 217
    (1993): O'Donnell BF+, *Contact Dermatitis* 28, 121
Diaphoresis (<2%)
Edema (1.3%)
Erythema (1–10%)
Exanthems
Exfoliative dermatitis
Facial edema
Flushing (<2%)
Lupus erythematosus
    (1997): Hardee JT+, *West J Med* 167, 106
Photosensitivity
Pigmentation (palms)
    (1997): Adams DR+, *Am J Contact Dermat* 8, 183

Pruritus (1–10%)
Psoriasis
Purpura
Rash (sic) (1.2%)
  (1989): Burris JF+, *Arch Intern Med* 149, 2437
Raynaud's phenomenon
Toxic epidermal necrolysis
Urticaria
Xerosis

Hair

Hair – alopecia (following topical use) (<2%)
  (1990): Buckley MMT+, *Drugs* 40, 75
Hair – hypertrichosis (<2%)

Nails

Nails – pigmentation (bluish)

Other

Ageusia (<2%)
Anaphylactoid reactions
Depression
  (2001): Schweitzer I+, *Aust NZ J Psychiatry* 35(5), 569
Dysgeusia (<2%)
Glossitis (following topical use)
Headache
Mastodynia (<2%)
Myalgia (3.2%)
Myasthenia gravis
  (1997): Khella SL+, *Muscle Nerve* 20, 631
Oral ulceration (<2%)
Paresthesias (1.9%)
Peyronie's disease (<2%)
Sialorrhea (<2%)
Tinnitus
Xerostomia (<2%)

BETHANECHOL

Trade name: Urecholine (Odessey)
Other common trade names: *Muscaran; Myocholine-Glenwood; Myotonine Chloride; Urocarb*
Indications: Nonobstructive urinary retention
Category: Urinary tract cholinergic stimulant
Half-life: up to 6 hours
Clinically important, potentially hazardous interactions with: galantamine, physostigmine

Reactions

Skin

Diaphoresis (1–10%)
Flushing (<1%)
Miliaria
  (1967): Rochmis PG+, *Arch Dermatol* 95, 499

Other

Headache
Sialorrhea (<1%)

BEXAROTENE

Trade name: Targretin (Ligand)
Indications: Cutaneous T-cell lymphoma (CTCL), (mycosis fungoides)
Category: Retinoid (rexinoid)
Half-life: 7 hours
Clinically important, potentially hazardous interactions with: acitretin, beta-carotene, gemfibrozil, isotretinoin, tretinoin, vitamin A

Reactions

Skin

Acne (<10%)
Adverse effects (sic)
  (2001): Duvic M+, *Arch Dermatol* 137, 581 (13%)
Bacterial infections (1.2–13.2%)
Cellulitis
Cheilitis (<10%)
Chills (9.5%)
  (2001): Duvic M+, *Arch Dermatol* 137, 581
Cold extremities
  (2000): Bedikian AY+, *Oncol Rep* 7, 883
Erythema
  (2002): Breneman D+, *Arch Dermatol* 138, 352
  (2002): Liu HL+, *Arch Dermatol* 138, 398
Exanthems (<10%)
Exfoliative dermatitis (10–28%)
  (2001): Duvic M+, *Arch Dermatol* 137, 581 (7%)
Facial edema
  (2002): Breneman D+, *Arch Dermatol* 138, 325
Flu-like syndrome (sic) (3.6–13.2%)
Necrosis
  (2002): Breneman D+, *Arch Dermatol* 138, 325
Nodules (sic) (<10%)
Peripheral edema (13.1%)
Photosensitivity
Pruritus (20–30%)
  (2002): Breneman D+, *Arch Dermatol* 138, 325
  (2001): Duvic M+, *Arch Dermatol* 137, 581 (20%)
  (2000): Duvic M, *Dermatology Times*, August, 3 (25%)
Pustules
Rash (sic) (16.7%)
  (2001): Duvic M+, *Arch Dermatol* 137, 581
Ulcerations (<10%)
  (2002): Breneman D+, *Arch Dermatol* 138, 325
Vasculitis
  (2002): Breneman D+, *Arch Dermatol* 138, 325
Vesiculobullous eruption (<10%)
  (2002): Breneman D+, *Arch Dermatol* 138, 325
Xerosis (10.7%)
  (2003): Esteva FJ+, *J Clin Oncol* 21(6), 999 (34%)

Hair

Hair – alopecia (4–11%)

Other

Asthenia
  (2003): Esteva FJ+, *J Clin Oncol* 21(6), 999 (30%)
Gingivitis (<10%)
Headache
Hyperesthesia (<10%)
Mastodynia (<10%)
Myalgia (<10%)
  (2000): Bedikian AY+, *Oncol Rep* 7, 883

Pain
  (2002): Breneman D+, *Arch Dermatol* 138, 325
Xerostomia (<10%)

BICALUTAMIDE

Trade name: Casodex (AstraZeneca)
Indications: Metastatic prostatic carcinoma
Category: Antiandrogen
Half-life: up to 10 days

Reactions

Skin
  Diaphoresis (6%)
  Edema (2–5%)
  Exanthems (<1%)
  Hot flashes (49%)
    (2002): Chuang CK+, *Chang Gung Med J* 25(9), 577 (5.4%)
    (2002): Gommersall LM+, *Expert Opin Pharmacother* 3(12), 1685
    (2001): Kucuk O+, *Urology* 58(1), 53 (23%)
    (1996): Bales GT+, *Urology* 47, 38
    (1995): Lunglmayr G, *Anticancer Drugs* 6, 508
    (1994): Eri LM+, *Eur Urol* 26, 219
    (1990): Mahler C+, *J Steroid Biochem Mol Biol* 37, 921
  Peripheral edema (8%)
  Pruritus (2–5%)
  Rash (sic) (6%)
  Xerosis (2–5%)

Hair
  Hair – alopecia (2–5%)

Other
  Gynecomastia (38%)
    (2002): Iversen P, *Urology* 60(3 Suppl 1), 64
    (2002): Mcleod DG, *Urology* 60(3 Suppl 1), 13
    (2002): See WA+, *J Urol* 168(2), 429
    (2001): Wirth M+, *Urology* 58(2), 146 (17.4%)
    (1998): Goa KL+, *Drugs Aging* 12, 401
    (1996): Bales GT+, *Urology* 47, 38
    (1996): Kotake T+, *Hinyokika Kiyo* (Japanese) 42, 157
    (1995): Lunglmayr G, *Anticancer Drugs* 6, 508
    (1994): Eri LM+, *Eur Urol* 26, 219
    (1990): Mahler C+, *J Steroid Biochem Mol Biol* 37, 921
  Injection-site reactions (sic) (2–5%)
  Mastodynia (39%)
    (2002): Gommersall LM+, *Expert Opin Pharmacother* 3(12), 1685
    (2002): Iversen P, *Urology* 60(3 Suppl 1), 64
    (2002): Mcleod DG, *Urology* 60(3 Suppl 1), 13
    (2002): See WA+, *J Urol* 168(2), 429
    (2001): Wirth M+, *Urology* 58(2), 146 (17.6%)
    (1998): Goa KL+, *Drugs Aging* 12, 401
    (1996): Bales GT+, *Urology* 47, 38
    (1996): Kotake T+, *Hinyokika Kiyo* (Japanese) 42, 157
    (1995): Lunglmayr G, *Anticancer Drugs* 6, 508
    (1994): Eri LM+, *Eur Urol* 26, 219
    (1990): Mahler C+, *J Steroid Biochem Mol Biol* 37, 921
  Myalgia (2–5%)
  Paresthesias (6%)
  Xerostomia (2–5%)

BIMATOPROST

Trade name: Lumigan (Allergan)
Indications: Open-angle glaucoma, ocular hypertension
Category: Ophthalmic; Prostamide
Half-life: 45 minutes

Reactions

Skin
  Blepharitis (3–10%)
  Eyelid erythema (3–10%)
  Eyelid pigmentation (3–10%)
    (2003): Herndon LW+, *Am J Ophthalmol* 135(5), 713
  Ocular pruritus (>10%)
  Upper respiratory infection (10%)

Hair
  Eyelashes – change in color
  Eyelashes – growth (>10%)
    (2003): Noecker RS+, *Am J Ophthalmol* 135(1), 55
    (2002): Eisenberg DL+, *Surv Ophthalmol* 47(Suppl 1), S105
  Hair – eyelash lengthening
    (2003): Herndon LW+, *Am J Ophthalmol* 135(5), 713
  Hirsutism (1–5%)

Other
  Conjunctival hyperemia (>10%)
    (2001): DuBiner H+, *Surv Ophthalmol* 45(Suppl 4), S353–60
    (2001): Gandolfi S+, *Adv Ther* 18(3), 110
    (2001): Laibovitz RA+, *Arch Ophthalmol* 119(7), 994
    (2001): Sherwood M+, *Surv Ophthalmol* 45(Suppl 4), S361–8
  Eyelid irritation (3–10%)
  Eyelid pain (3–10%)
  Eyelid xerosis (3–10%)
  Headache
  Ocular pigmentation (1–3%)
    (2002): Novack GD+, *J Am Geriatr Soc* 50(5), 956
    (2002): Stjernschantz JW+, *Surv Ophthalmol* 47(Suppl 1), S162
    (2001): Sherwood M+, *Surv Ophthalmol* 45(Suppl 4), S361–8
    (1.1%)
  Pigmentation – eye color

BIPERIDEN

Trade name: Akineton (Abbott)
Other common trade names: *Biperen; Bipiden; Dekinet; Desiperiden; Dyskinon*
Indications: Parkinsonism
Category: Anticholinergic; Antiparkinsonian
Half-life: 18–24 hours
Clinically important, potentially hazardous interactions with: anticholinergics

Reactions

Skin
  Dermatitis
    (1995): Torinuki W, *Tohoku J Exp Med* 176, 249
  Diaphoresis
    (2001): Richardson C+, *Am J Psychiatry* 158(8), 1329
  Exanthems
  Flushing
  Rash (sic)
  Urticaria

Other
Glossodynia
Paresthesias
Stomatodynia
Xerostomia

BISACODYL

Trade names: Biscolax; Carter's Little Pills; Dacodyl; Dulcagen; Dulcolax (Novartis); Fleet Laxative (Fleet)
Other common trade names: Apo-Bisacodyl; Dulcolan; Laxit
Indications: Constipation
Category: Irritant/stimulant laxative
Onset of action: 6–10 hours

Reactions

Skin
Diaphoresis
Exanthems
Fixed eruption
 (1997): Burrow WH, Jackson, MS (from Internet) (observation)
 (1961): Welsh AL+, Arch Dermatol 84, 1004
Urticaria

BISMUTH

Trade names: Bismuth subcitrate; Bismuth subgallate (colostomy deodorant); Bismuth subnitrate and Bismuth idoform paraffin paste (BIPP); Bismuth sucralfate; Helidac (Prometheus); Pepto-Bismol (Procter & Gamble)
Other common trade names: Bismatrol; Caved-S; Colo-Fresh; De-Nol; Devrom; Diotame; Pepto-Bismol (Procter & Gamble); Pink Bismuth
Indications: As part of 'triple therapy' (antibiotics + bismuth) for eradication of H. pylori. Bismuth subgallate initiates clotting via activation of factor XII, and is used for bleeding during tonsillectomy and adenoidectomy. BIPP impregnated ribbon gauze is used for packing following ear surgery. Bismuth subsalicylate is in OTC products for gastrointestinal complaints and peptic ulcer disease.
Category: Antidiarrheal
Half-life: 21–72 days
Clinically important, potentially hazardous interactions with: aspirin, ciprofloxacin, doxycycline, hypoglycemics, lomefloxacin, methotrexate, minocycline, tetracycline, warfarin

Reactions

Skin
Adverse effects (sic) (triple therapy)
 (2001): Danese S+, Hepatogastroenterology 48(38), 465
 (2001): Sotudehmanesh R+, J Gastroenterol Hepatol 16(3), 264
 (2000): de Boer WA+, Am J Gastroenterol 95(3), 641
 (2000): Malekzadeh R+, Aliment Pharmacol Ther 14(3), 299
 (2000): Spinzi GC+, Aliment Pharmacol Ther 14(3), 325
 (1999): Monkemuller KE+, Aliment Pharmacol Ther 13(5), 661
 (1999): Olafsson S+, Aliment Pharmacol Ther 13(5), 651
 (1999): Xiao SD+, Aliment Pharmacol Ther 13(3), 311
 (1998): Cammarota G+, Aliment Pharmacol Ther 12(6), 539
 (1998): Cestari R, Aliment Pharmacol Ther 12(10), 991

 (1998): Dobrucali A+, Wien Med Wochenschr (German) 148(20), 464
 (1998): Lerang F+, Am J Gastroenterol 93(2), 212
 (1998): Ricciardiello L+, Aliment Pharmacol Ther 12(6), 533
 (1998): Spadaccini A+, Aliment Pharmacol Ther 12(10), 997
 (1998): van der Wouden EJ+, Am J Gastroenterol 93(8), 1228
 (1997): Henriksen M+, Am J Gastroenterol 92, 653
 (1997): Huang JQ+, J Gastroenterol Hepatol 12(8), 590
 (1997): Kolkman JJ+, Aliment Pharmacol Ther 11(6), 1123
 (1997): Kung NN+, Am J Gastroenterol 92(3), 438
 (1997): Laine L+, Am J Gastroenterol 92(12), 2213
 (1996): Thijs JC+, Am J Gastroenterol 91(1), 93
 (1996): van der Hulst RW+, Helicobacter 1(1), 6
 (1996): Weldon MJ+, Aliment Pharmacol Ther 10(3), 279
 (1995): al-Assi MT+, Am J Gastroenterol 90(3), 403
 (1995): Hoffenberg P+, Rev Med Chil 123(2), 185
 (1995): Rauws EA+, Drugs 50(6), 984
 (1995): Webb DD+, Am J Gastroenterol 90(8), 1273
 (1994): Borody TJ+, Am J Gastroenterol 89(1), 33
 (1994): Hentschel E, Wien Klin Wochenschr (German) 106(17), 543
 (1994): Park KN+, Eur J Gastroenterol Hepatol 6 (Suppl 1), S103
 (1994): Reijers MH+, Aliment Pharmacol Ther 8(3), 351 (sucralfate)
 (1994): Wilhelmsen I+, Hepatogastroenterol 41(1), 43
 (1993): Malfertheiner P, Scand J Gastroenterol Suppl 196, 34
 (1992): Berstad K+, Scand J Gastroenterol 27(12), 1006
 (1992): Burgess E+, Drug Saf 7(4), 282
 (1992): Wilhelmsen I+, Tidsskr Nor Laegeforen (Norwegian) 112(25), 3197
 (1990): Steffen R, Rev Infect Dis 12(Suppl1), S80 (subsalicylate)
 (1989): Bradley B+, J Clin Pharm Ther 14(6), 423 (subsalicylate and subcitrate)
 (1988): Borsch G, Med Klin (German) 83(18), 605
 (1988): Dipalma JR, Am Fam Physician 38(5), 244
 (1988): Eskens GT, Postgrad Med J 64(755), 724
 (1980): Fournier PE, Therapie (French) 35(3), 319
 (1980): Henderson IW, Can Med Assoc J 123(9), 848
 (1977): Glozman VN+, Vestn Dermatol Venerol (Russian) 4, 88
 (1976): Martin-Bouyer G, Therapie (French) 31(6), 683
 (1976): Rebattu JP+, JFORL J Fr Otorhinolaryngol Audidphonol Chir Maxillofac 25(9), 627 (suppositories)
 (1974): Lowe DJ, Med J Aust 2(18), 664
Allergic reactions (sic)
 (1985): Jones PH, J Laryngol Otol 99(4), 389
 (1981): Anchupane IS+, Vestn Dermatol Venerol (Russian) 11, 63
Angioedema (subcitrate)
 (1994): Ottervanger JP+, Ned Tijdschr Geneeskd (Dutch) 138(3), 152
Black granules on skin (subsalicylate)
 (1997): Ruiz-Maldonado R+, J Am Acad Dermatol 37(3), 489
Dermatitis
 (2001): Wictorin A+, Contact Dermatitis 45(5), 318 (ointment)
 (1987): Goh CL+, Contact Dermatitis 16(2), 109 (subnitrate)
Erythema (subcitrate)
 (1994): Ottervanger JP+, Ned Tijdschr Geneeskd (Dutch) 138(3), 152
Exanthems (subcitrate)
 (1994): Ottervanger JP+, Ned Tijdschr Geneeskd (Dutch) 138(3), 152
Exfoliative dermatitis
 (1969): Singh R, Indian J Dermatol 15(1), 13
Fixed eruption
 (1981): Granstein RD+, J Am Acad Dermatol 5, 1
Pigmentation
 (1993): Zala L+, Dermatology 187(4), 288
 (1981): Granstein RD+, J Am Acad Dermatol 5(1), 1
 (1973): Levantine A+, Br J Dermatol 89(1), 105
 (1970): Plisek V+, Vnitr Lek (Czech) 16(11), 1085

Prurigo pigmentosa
  (1987): Dijkstra JW+, *Int J Dermatol* 26(6), 379
Pruritus (triple therapy)
  (1998): Pozzato P+, *Aliment Pharmacol Ther* 12(5), 447
Rash (sic)
  (1990): Burnett JW, *Cutis* 45(4), 220
Vasculitis

Hair

Hair – alopecia
  (1990): Gollnick H+, *Z Haut* (German) 65, 1128

Other

Arthopathy
  (1993): Kendel K+, *Dtsch Med Wochenschr* (German)
    118(7), 221 (subgallate)
  (1981): Emile J+, *Clin Toxicol* 18(11), 1285
  (1980): Gaucher A+, *Rev Rhum Mal* 47(1), 31
  (1979): Emile J+, *Ann Med Interne* 130(2), 75
  (1979): Gaucher A+, *Med J Aust* 1(4), 129
  (1979): Murray JR, *Med J Aust* 1(11), 522
  (1979): Netter P+, *Pathol Biol* (Paris) (French) 27(5), 300
  (1978): Sany J+, *Rev Rhum Mal Osteosrtic* 45(12), 729
  (1976): Monseu G+, *Acta Neurol Belg* 76(5), 301
  (1975): Buge A+, *Rev Rhum Mal Osteoartic* 42(12), 721
Death
  (1991): Sainsbury SJ, *West J Med* 155(6), 637 (subsalicylate)
  (1990): Jones JA, *Oral Surg Oral Med Oral Pathol* 69(6), 668 (BIPP)
  (1989): Hudson M+, *BMJ* 299(6692), 159 (subcitrate)
  (1985): Sanz Gallen P+, *Med Clin* (Barc) (Spanish) 84(13), 538
  (1980): Allain P+, *Therapie* (French) 35(3), 303
  (1978): Lhermitte F+, *Nouv Presse Med* (French) 7(24), 2170
  (1978): Martin-Bouyer G, *Gastroenterol Clin Biol* 2(4), 349
  (1978): Rouzaud P+, *Toxicol Eur Res* 1(4), 273
  (1977): Robert JF, *Infirm Fr* 780(188), 24
  (1976): Loiseau P+, *J Neurol Sci* 27(2), 133
Depression
Dysgeusia (46%) (triple therapy)
  (2001): Gisbert JP+, *Helicobacter* 6(2), 157
  (2001): Kaviani MJ+, *Eur J Gastroenterol Hepatol* 13(8), 915
  (1998): Scott BB, *Aliment Pharmacol Ther* 12(3), 277 (10%)
  (1997): Chey WD+, *Am J Gastroenterol* 92(9), 1483 (39%)
  (1993): Ateshkadi A+, *Clin Pharm* 12(1), 34
  (1993): Friedland RP+, *Clin Neuropharmacol* 16(2), 173
    (subgallate)
Gingivitis
  (1989): Slikkerveer A+, *Med Toxicol Adverse Drug Exp* 4(5), 303
    (subnitrate, subcarbonate and subgallate)
Headache
Hypersensitivity
  (1998): Lim PV+, *J Laryngol Otol* 112(4), 335 (impregnated tape)
  (1981): Anchupane IS+, *Vestn Dermatol Venerol* (Russian) Nov
    11, 63
Injection-site lymphoma
  (1984): Krivitzky A+, *Ann Med Interne* (Paris) (French)
    135(3), 205
Oral mucosal pigmentation
  (1984): Sutak J+, *Prakt Zuban Lek* (Czech) 32(6), 166
  (1983): Dayan D+, *Clin Prev Dent* 5(3), 25 (after root canal filling
    with AH-26)
  (1971): Dummett CO, *Postgrad Med* 49(1), 78
Pain (10%) (triple therapy)
  (1998): Scott BB, *Aliment Pharmacol Ther* 12(3), 277 (10%)
Porphyria cutanea tarda
  (1966): Bielicky T, *Dermatol Wochenschr* (German) 152(30), 761
Stomatitis
  (1990): Burnett JW, *Cutis* 45(4), 220
  (1989): Slikkerveer A+, *Med Toxicol Adverse rug Exp* 4(5), 303
    (subnitrate, subcarbonate and subgallate)

  (1966): Jackson JA, *Oral Surg Oral Med Oral Pathol* 21(2), 154
  (1955): Nagel V, *Hautarzt* (German) 6, 232
Tinnitus
  (1987): DuPont HL+, *JAMA* 257(10), 1347 (subsalicylate)
Tongue discoloration (>10%)
  (2001): Ioffreda MD+, *Arch Dermatol* 137(7), 968 (black)
  (1987): DuPont HL+, *JAMA* 257(10), 1347 (black)
Tooth discoloration
  (1990): Burnett JW, *Cutis* 45(4), 220
Tremor
  (1993): Kendel K+, *Dtsch Med Wochenschr* (German)
    118(7), 221 (subgallate)
  (1975): Aimard G+, *Nouv Presse Med* (French) 4(39), 2816
Xerostomia (41%) (triple therapy)
  (2001): Kaviani MJ+, *Eur J Gastroenterol Hepatol* 13(8), 915

BISOPROLOL

Trade names: Zebeta (Wyeth); Ziac (Wyeth)
Other common trade names: *Concor; Cordalin; Detensiel;
Emcor; Fondril; Monocor; Soprol*
Indications: Hypertension
Category: Beta-adrenoceptor blocker
Half-life: 9–12 hours

Ziac is bisoprolol and hydrochlorothiazide

Reactions

Skin

Acne
Angioedema
Ankle edema (1–10%)
Diaphoresis (1%)
Eczema (sic)
Edema (3%)
Exanthems
Exfoliative dermatitis
Facial edema
Flushing
Lupus erythematosus
Photosensitivity
Pigmentation
Pruritus
Psoriasis
Purpura
Rash (sic) (1–10%)
Raynaud's phenomenon (1–10%)
Urticaria
Xerosis

Hair

Hair – alopecia

Nails

Nails – bluish

Other

Anaphylactoid reactions
Dysgeusia
Headache
Hyperesthesia (1.5%)
Myalgia (1–10%)
Paresthesias
Peyronie's disease
Tinnitus
Xerostomia (1.3%)

BIVALIRUDIN

Synonym: Hirulog
Trade name: Angiomax (The Medicines Company)
Indications: Angioplasty adjunct
Category: Anticoagulant; Thrombin inhibitor
Half-life: 25 minutes
Clinically important, potentially hazardous interactions with: anisindione, dicumarol, heparin, reteplase, streptokinase, tenecteplase, urokinase, warfarin

Reactions

Skin
Infections (sic)

Other
Back pain (42%)
Headache
Injection-site pain (8%)
Pain (15%)

BLACK COHOSH

Scientific names: *Actaea macrotys; Actaea racemosa; Cimicifuga racemosa*
Family: Ranunculaceae
Trade and other common names: Baneberry; Black Snake root; Bugbane; Bugwort; Macrotys; Rattletop; Rattleweed; Remifemin (PhytoPharmica/Enzymatic Therapy; Schaper & Brummer); Shengma; Squawroot
Category: Phytoestrogen
Purported indications and other uses: Anxiety, arthritis, asthma, cardiovascular and circulatory problems, climacteric, menstrual and premenstrual disorders, colds, cough, constipation, depression, kidney disorders, malaria, sore throat, tinnitus
Half-life: N/A
Clinically important, potentially hazardous interactions with: estrogens, salicylates, tamoxifen

Reactions

Skin
Diaphoresis
(1996): Newell CA+, *Herbal Medicine: A Guide for Healthcare Professionals*. London: The Pharmaceutical Press
(1985): Duke JA, *Handbook of Medicinal Herbs*, CRC Press, Boca Raton, FL (overdose)
Jaundice
(2002): Whiting PW+, *Med J Aust* 177(8), 440
Petechiae (forearms)
Pruritus
(2002): Whiting PW+, *Med J Aust* 177(8), 440
Rash (sic)
(2003): Huntley A+, *Menopause* 10(1), 58

Other
Arthralgia (overdose)
Dizziness
(2002): Mahady GB+, *Nutr Clin Care* 5(6), 283
Mastodynia
(2002): Mahady GB+, *Nutr Clin Care* 5(6), 283
Seizures
(1999): McFarlin BL+, *J Nurse Midwifery* 44, 295

(1996): Shuster EA, *Mayo Clin Proc* 71(10), 991 (with *Vitex agnus-castusl* and evening primrose) (reversible)
(1996): Shuster J, *Hosp Pharm* 31, 1553
Tremor (overdose)

Note: In 2001, the American College of Obstetricians and Gynecologists stated that black cohosh might be helpful in the short term (6 months or less) for women with vasomotor symptoms of menopause

BLEOMYCIN

Synonyms: bleo; BLM
Trade name: Blenoxane (Bristol-Myers Squibb)
Other common trade names: *Bleo; Bleocin; Bleomycine; Bleomycinum; BLM*
Indications: Melanomas, sarcomas, lymphomas, testicular carcinoma
Category: Antineoplastic antibiotic
Half-life: 1.3–9 hours
Clinically important, potentially hazardous interactions with: aldesleukin

Reactions

Skin
Acral erythema
(1982): Burgdorf WHC+, *Ann Intern Med* 97, 61
Acral gangrene
(1998): Reiser M+, *Eur J Clin Microbiol Infect Dis* 17, 58
(1997): Hladunewich M+, *J Rheumatol* 24, 2371
Acral sclerosis
(1984): Snauwaert J+, *Dermatologica* 169, 172
Acrocyanosis
(1983): Bork K+, *Hautarzt* (German) 34, 10
Allergic reactions (sic)
(1998): Mullai N+, *J Clin Oncol* 16, 1625
(1998): Yeo W+, *J Clin Oncol* 16, 1626
Angioedema
(1984): Khansur T+, *Arch Intern Med* 144, 2267
Bullous eruption (1–5%)
Chills (>10%)
Dermatitis (sic)
Erythema
(2003): Nayak N+, *Clin Exp Dermatol* 28(1), 105
(2001): Robinson JB+, *Gynecol Oncol* 82(3), 550
Erythema multiforme
(1990): Cortina P+, *Dermatologica* 180(2), 106
(1985): Fernandez-Obregon AC+, *J Am Acad Dermatol* 13(3), 464
Exanthems
(1993): Haerslev T+, *Cutis* 52, 45 (linear and symmetrical)
(1980): Lincke-Plewig H, *Hautarzt* (German) 31, 616
(1976): Werner Y+, *Acta Derm Venereol* (Stockh) 56, 155
Fixed eruption
(1987): Lindae ML+, *Arch Dermatol* 123(3), 395
Flagellate erythema
(1999): Rubeiz NG+, *Int J Dermatol* 38, 140 (urticarial)
(1998): Yamamoto T+, *Dermatology* 197, 399
(1997): Polsky D+, New York, American Academy of Dermatology Meeting (SF), (gross and microscopic)
(1995): Watanabe T+, *Dermatology* 190, 230
(1994): Mowad CM+, *Br J Dermatol* 131, 700
(1994): Zaki I+, *Clin Exp Dermatol* 19, 366
(1992): Barduagni O+, *Dermatol Clin* (Italian) 3, 169
(1992): Jolin-Garijo L+, *An Med Interna* (Spanish) 9, 520

(1991): Duhra P+, *Clin Exp Dermatol* 16, 216
(1990): Cortina P+, *Dermatologica* 180, 106
(1990): Miori L+, *Am J Dermatopathol* 12, 598
(1990): Miori L+, *Dermatologica* 181, 238
(1987): Lindae ML+, *Arch Dermatol* 123, 395

Flagellate pigmentation
(2003): Nayak N+, *Clin Exp Dermatol* 28(1), 105
(2001): Nigro MG+, *Cutis* 68, 285
(1998): Wenzel FG+, *J Am Acad Dermatol* 38(1), 1
(1994): Templeton SF+, *Arch Dermatol* 130(5), 577
(1993): Lincke-Plewig H, *Hautarzt* (German) 44, 331
(1993): Tsuji T+, *J Am Acad Dermatol* 28, 503
(1992): Albig J+, *Hautarzt* (German) 43, 376
(1990): Vicente MA+, *Med Cutan Ibero Lat Am* (Spanish) 18, 148
(1988): Lazar AP+, *Cutis* 42(5), 397
(1986): Polla BS+, *J Am Acad Dermatol* 14, 690
(1985): Fernandez-Obregon AC+, *J Am Acad Dermatol* 13, 464
(1972): Yagoda A+, *Ann Intern Med* 77, 861
(1970): Moulin G+, *Bull Soc Fr Dermatol Syphiligr* 77, 293

Flushing
(2001): Robinson JB+, *Gynecol Oncol* 82(3), 550

Hyperkeratosis (palms and soles)
(1976): Werner Y+, *Acta Derm Venereol* (Stockh) 56, 155
(1971): de Bast C+, *Arch Dermatol* 104, 509

Ichthyosis
(1971): de Bast C+, *Arch Dermatol* 104, 509

Intertrigo
(1971): de Bast C+, *Arch Dermatol* 104, 509

Linear streaking (sic)
(1989): Vignini M+, *Clin Exp Dermatol* 14, 261
(1988): Lazar A+, *Cutis* 42, 397
(1987): Rademaker M+, *Clin Exp Dermatol* 12, 457
(1975): Lowitz BB, *N Engl J Med* 292, 1300

Lymphangitis
(1998): Allen AL+, *J Am Acad Dermatol* 39, 295

Neutrophilic eccrine hidradenitis
(1998): Wenzel FG+, *J Am Acad Dermatol* 38(1), 1
(1988): Scallan PJ+, *Cancer* 62, 2532

Painful erythema (elbows, knees, palms)
(1980): Lincke-Plewig H, *Hautarzt* (German) 31, 616
(1976): Werner Y+, *Acta Derm Venereol* (Stockh) 56, 155

Palmar nodules (sic)
(1993): Haerslev T+, *Cutis* 52, 45

Palmar–plantar erythema
(1990): Pagliuca A+, *Postgrad Med J* 66, 242

Papulo-nodular lesions
(1997): Polsky D+, New York, American Academy of Dermatology Meeting (SF), (gross and microscopic)

Pigmentation (~50%)
(2001): Mutafoglu-Uysal K+, *Turk J Pediatr* 43(2), 172
(1999): Susser WS+, *J Am Acad Dermatol* 40(3), 367
(1998): Behrens S+, *Hautarzt* (German) 49, 725
(1993): Tsuji T+, *J Am Acad Dermatol* 28, 503 (in striae distensae)
(1992): Gallais V+, *Ann Dermatol Venereol* (French) 119, 471
(1990): Wright AL+, *Dermatologica* 181, 255 (reticulate)
(1988): Massone L+, *G Ital Dermatol Venereol* (Italian) 123, 225 (striae)
(1986): Guillet G+, *Arch Dermatol* 122, 381 (in stripes)
(1985): Polla L+, *Ann Dermatol Venereol* (French) 112, 821
(1984): Schuler G+, *Hautarzt* (German) 35, 383 (linear)
(1983): Bork K+, *Hautarzt* (German) 34, 10
(1982): Kukla LJ+, *Cancer* 50, 2283
(1981): Granstein RD+, *J Am Acad Dermatol* 5, 1 (brown-black)
(1981): Nixon DW+, *Cutis* 27, 181
(1978): Perrot H+, *Arch Dermatol Res* 261, 245
(1973): Cohen IS+, *Arch Dermatol* 107, 553
(1973): Kiefer O, *Dermatologica* 146, 229

Pruritus (>5%)
(2001): Robinson JB+, *Gynecol Oncol* 82(3), 550

(1995): Watanabe T+, *Dermatology* 190(3), 230
(1994): Templeton SF+, *Arch Dermatol* 130(5), 577 (generalized)
(1990): Caumes E+, *Lancet* 336, 1593
(1990): Cortina P+, *Dermatologica* 180(2), 106
(1985): Fernandez-Obregon AC+, *J Am Acad Dermatol* 13(3), 464

Radiation recall
(1993): Stelzer KJ+, *Cancer* 71, 1322

Raynaud's phenomenon (>10%)
(2001): Vanhooteghem O+, *Pediatr Dermatol* 18(3), 249
(1998): Reiser M+, *Eur J Clin Microbiol Infect Dis* 17, 58
(1997): Emmerich J, *Presse Med* (French) 26, 1580
(1997): Hladunewich M+, *J Rheumatol* 24, 2371
(1997): Sibilia J+, *Presse Med* (French) 26, 1564 (12.6%)
(1996): Epstein E, *The Schoch Letter* 46, 34 (observation)
(1996): Munn SE+, *Br J Dermatol* 135, 969
(1993): von Gunten CF+, *Cancer* 72, 2004
(1992): de Pablo P+, *Acta Derm Venereol* (Stockh) 72, 465
(1992): Doll DC+, *Semin Oncol* 19(5), 580
(1992): Gregg LJ, *J Am Acad Dermatol* 26, 279
(1991): Epstein E, *J Am Acad Dermatol* 24, 785
(1990): Cortina P+, *Dermatologica* 180(2), 106
(1985): Adoue D+, *Ann Dermatol Venereol* (French) 112, 151
(1985): Bovenmyer DA, *J Am Acad Dermatol* 13, 470
(1985): Epstein E, *J Am Acad Dermatol* 13, 468
(1984): Adoue D+, *Ann Intern Med* 100, 770
(1984): Snauwaert J+, *Dermatologica* 169, 172
(1981): Kukla LJ+, *Arch Dermatol* 117, 604

Scleroderma
(2000): D'Cruz D, *Toxicol Lett* 112 and 421
(1999): Passiu G+, *Clin Rheumatol* 18, 422
(1998): Behrens S+, *Hautarzt* (German) 49, 725 (pseudoscleroderma)
(1997): Komosinska K+, *Postepy Hig Med Dosw* (Polish) 51, 285
(1994): Marck Y+, *Ann Dermatol Venereol* (French) 121, 712,
(1992): Kerr LD+, *J Rheumatol* 19, 294
(1991): Bourgeois P+, *Baillieres Clin Rheumatol* 5, 13
(1991): Guseva NG, *Revmatologiia Mosk* (Russian) 1, 33
(1985): Haustein UF+, *Int J Dermatol* 24, 147
(1984): Rush PJ+, *J Rheumatol* 11, 262
(1983): Bork K+, *Hautarzt* (German) 34, 10
(1980): Finch WR+, *J Rheumatol* 7, 651
(1973): Cohen IS+, *Arch Dermatol* 107, 533
(1971): de Bast C+, *Arch Dermatol* 104, 509

Stevens–Johnson syndrome
(1989): Brodsky A+, *J Clin Pharmacol* 29, 821
(1986): Giaccone G+, *Tumori* 72, 331

Thickening (sic)

Urticaria

Xerosis
(1973): Cohen IS+, *Arch Dermatol* 107, 555

Hair

Hair – alopecia (~50%)
(1999): Susser WS+, *J Am Acad Dermatol* 40(3), 367
(1992): Breathnach SM+, *Adverse Drug Reactions and the Skin* Blackwell, Oxford, 292 (passim)
(1990): Siegel RD+, *Chest* 98, 507
(1982): Kukla LJ+, *Cancer* 50, 2283
(1973): Cohen IS+, *Arch Dermatol* 107, 553
(1973): Kiefer O, *Dermatologica* 146, 229
(1971): de Bast C+, *Arch Dermatol* 104, 509

Hair – gray

Nails

Nails – Beau's lines (transverse nail bands)
(1994): Ben-Dyan D+, *Acta Haematol* 91, 89

Nails – dystrophy
(1984): Miller RAW, *Arch Dermatol* 120, 963

Nails – growth reduced

(1999): Susser WS+, *J Am Acad Dermatol* 40(3), 367
(1971): de Bast C+, *Arch Dermatol* 104, 509
Nails – loss
(1999): Susser WS+, *J Am Acad Dermatol* 40(3), 367
(1986): Gonzalez FU+, *Arch Dermatol* 122, 974
(1973): Cohen IS+, *Arch Dermatol* 107, 553
Nails – onychodystrophy
(1999): Susser WS+, *J Am Acad Dermatol* 40(3), 367
(1985): Baran R, *Ann Dermatol Venereol* (French) 112, 463
Nails – onycholysis
(1999): Susser WS+, *J Am Acad Dermatol* 40(3), 367
(1998): Roussou P+, *Acta Derm Venereol* 78, 303
(1984): Snauwaert J+, *Dermatologica* 169, 172
Nails – pigmentation (banding)
(1977): Shetty MR, *Cancer Treatment Reports* 61, 501

Other
Anaphylactoid reactions (<1%)
Calcinosis
(1983): Bork K+, *Hautarzt* (German) 34, 10
(1975): Ihde DC+, *Cancer Chemother* 59, 1039 (penis)
Digital necrosis
(1997): Emmerich J, *Presse Med* (French) 26, 1580
(1997): Sibilia J+, *Presse Med* (French) 26, 1564
Gangrene (digital)
(1998): Reiser M+, *Eur J Clin Microbiol Infect Dis* 17, 58
(1998): Surville-Barland J+, *Eur J Dermatol* 8, 221
(1993): Vayssairat M+, *J Rheumatol* 20, 921
Glossitis
(1992): Breathnach SM+, *Adverse Drug Reactions and the Skin* Blackwell, Oxford, 292 (passim)
Hyperesthesia
Hypersensitivity (1–10%)
(2001): Mutafoglu-Uysal K+, *Turk J Pediatr* 43(2), 172
(2001): Robinson JB+, *Gynecol Oncol* 82(3), 550
(1992): Weiss RB, *Semin Oncol* 19, 458
Injection-site phlebitis (1–10%)
Oral papillomatosis
(1978): Hagedorn M+, *Hautarzt* (German) 29, 425
Oral ulceration
(1992): Breathnach SM+, *Adverse Drug Reactions and the Skin* Blackwell, Oxford, 292 (passim)
(1971): de Bast C+, *Arch Dermatol* 104, 509
Paresthesias
Stomatitis (>10%)
(1999): Susser WS+, *J Am Acad Dermatol* 40(3), 367
(1993): Haerslev T+, *Cutis* 52, 45
(1990): Siegel RD+, *Chest* 98, 507
(1983): Bronner AK+, *J Am Acad Dermatol* 9, 645
(1976): Werner Y+, *Acta Derm Venereol* (Stockh) 56, 176
(1975): Khlebnov AV+, *Klin Med Mosk* (Russian) 52, 78
(1973): Cohen IS+, *Arch Dermatol* 107, 553
(1973): Kiefer O, *Dermatologica* 146, 229
Tongue erosions
(1973): Cohen IS+, *Arch Dermatol* 107, 553

BLOODROOT

Scientific name: *Sanguinaria canadensis*
Family: Papaveraceae
Trade and other common names: Coon Root; Indian Plant; Indian Red Paint; Red Puccoon; Red Root; Snakebite; Sweet Slumber; Tetterwort; Viadent
Category: Anti-inflammatory; Antispasmodic
Purported indications and other uses: Oral: emetic, cathartic, expectorant. Topical: debriding agent, bronchitis, asthma, croup, laryngitis, pharyngitis, scabies, eczema, athlete's foot, nasal polyps, rheumatism, fever, anemia
Half-life: N/A

Reactions

Skin
Dermatitis
(1998): Brinker F, *Contraindications and Drug Interactions* Eclectic Medical Publications
Irritation (sic)

Other
Keratosis
(2000): Eversole LR+, *Oral Surg Oral Med Oral Pathol Oral Radiol Endod* 89(4), 455
Leukoplakia
(2001): Allen CL+, *Gen Dent* 49(6), 608
(2000): Eversole LR+, *Oral Surg Oral Med Oral Pathol Oral Radiol Endod* 89(4), 455

BLUE COHOSH

Scientific name: *Caulophyllum thalictroides*
Family: Berberidaceae
Trade and other common names: Beechdrops; Blue ginseng; Blueberry root; Papoose root; Squawroot; Yellow ginseng
Category: Anthelmintic; Antispasmodic diuretic; Diaphoretic; Expectorant; Oxytocic
Purported indications and other uses: Rheumatism, dropsy, epilepsy, hysteria, uterine inflammation, thrush, menopause, headache, sexual debility, aphthous stomatitis, laxative, colic, sore throat, hiccups
Half-life: N/A
Clinically important, potentially hazardous interactions with: cardioactive drugs

Reactions

Skin
Allergic reactions (sic)
Diaphoresis
(2002): Rao RB+, *Vet Hum Toxicol* 44(4), 221

Other
Mucous membrane irritation (sic)
Myalgia
(2002): Rao RB+, *Vet Hum Toxicol* 44(4), 221
Shock
(1998): Jones TK+, *J Pediatr* 132(3 Pt 1), 550

Note: Cohosh is from the Algonquin word 'rough', referring to the appearance of the roots. It is a toxic herb and should not be confused with the safer, unrelated herb, Black Cohosh

BORTEZOMIB

Synonyms: PS-341; LDP-341
Trade name: Velcade (Millennium)
Indications: Multiple myeloma
Category: Antineoplastic; Proteasome inhibitor
Half-life: 9–15 hours

Reactions

Skin
Edema (25%)
Herpes zoster (11%)
Pruritus (11%)
  (2002): Aghajanian C+, *Clin Cancer Res* 8(8), 2505
Rash (sic) (21%)
  (2002): Aghajanian C+, *Clin Cancer Res* 8(8), 2505
Upper respiratory infection (18%)

Other
Anaphylactoid reactions
Arthralgia (26%)
Asthenia (65%)
Back pain (14%)
Bone or joint pain (14%)
Cough (17%)
Death
Dizziness (21%)
Dysesthesia (23%)
Dysgeusia (13%)
Dysphagia
Fatigue (65%)
  (2003): Richardson PG+, *N Engl J Med* 348(26), 2609 (12%)
  (2002): Aghajanian C+, *Clin Cancer Res* 8(8), 2505
Fever (36%)
  (2002): Aghajanian C+, *Clin Cancer Res* 8(8), 2505
Headache
Hypersensitivity
Injection-site irritation (5%)
Limb pain (26%)
Myalgia (14%)
Paresthesias (26%)
Pneumonia (10%)
Rigors (12%)
Seizures
Stomatitis
Thrombocytopenia
  (2003): Richardson PG+, *N Engl J Med* 348(26), 2609 (28%)

BOSENTAN

Trade name: Tracleer (Actelion)
Indications: Pulmonary arterial hypertension
Category: Endothelial receptor antagonist
Half-life: ~5 hours
**Clinically important, potentially hazardous interactions
with:** atorvastatin, cyclosporine, fluvastatin, glyburide,
itraconazole, ketoconazole, lovastatin, simvastatin, **St John's
wort**, warfarin

Reactions

Skin
Edema (8%)
Flushing (9%)
Peripheral edema (8%)
Pruritus (4%)

Other
Headache

BOTULINUM TOXIN (A & B)

Trade names: Botox (Allergan); Dysport (Speywood); Myobloc
(Elan)
Indications: Blepharospasm, hemifacial spasm, spasmodic
torticollis, sialorrhea, hyperhidrosis, strabismus, oromandibular
dystonia, cervical dystonia, spasmodic dysphonia. Cosmetic
application for wrinkles
Category: Neuromuscular blocker; Toxin
Half-life: 3–6 months

Reactions

Skin
Acne
Allergic reactions (sic)
Depigmentation
  (1999): Roehm PC+, *J Neuroophthalmol* 19(1), 7
Erythema multiforme
Eyelid edema
  (1990): NIH Consensus Statement 8(8), 1
Flu-like syndrome (2–10%)
  (2002): Madalinski MH+, *Eur J Gastroenterol Hepatol* 14(8), 853
    (3 cases)
  (2002): Molloy F, *eMedicine Journal* 3(2)
  (1990): NIH Consensus Statement 8(8), 1
Hematomas
  (1997): Heinen F+, *Neuropediatrics* 28(6), 307 (local)
  (1997): Nussgens Z+, *Graefes Arch Clin Exp Opthalmol*
    235(4), 197
Hypohidrosis
  (2003): Dressler D+, *Eur Neurol* 49(1), 34
Infections (sic) (13–19%)
Intertrigo
  (2002): Madalinski MH+, *Eur J Gastroenterol Hepatol* 14(8), 853
    (1 case)
Peripheral edema (1–10%)
Pruritus (1–10%)
Psoriasis
Purpura (1–10%)
Rash (sic)
Urticaria

Other

Anaphylactoid reactions
  (1997): LeWitt PA+, *Mov Disord* 12(6), 1064 (localized)
Arthralgia (<7%)
Death
Depression
  (1999): Brenner R+, *South Med J* 92(7), 738
Dry eyes (6.3%)
Dysgeusia (1–10%)
  (2003): Murray C+, *Dermatol Surg* 29(5), 562
Ectropion
  (1990): *NIH Consensus Statement* 8(8), 1
Entropion
Headache
Hyperesthesia (1–10%)
Injection-site bruising
  (2002): Molloy F, *eMedicine Journal* 3(2)
  (1998): Goodman G, *Australas J Dermatol* 39(3), 158
Injection-site burning
  (2000): Karamfilov T+, *Arch Dermatol* 136(4), 487
Injection-site ecchymoses
  (1997): Guerrissi J+, *Ann Plast Surg* 39(5), 447
  (1990): NIH, *Consensus Statement* 8(8), 1
Injection-site edema
  (2000): Ahn KY+, *Plast Reconstr Surg* 105(2), 778
  (2000): Wissel J+, *J Pain Symptom Manage* 20(1), 44
  (1997): Guerrissi J+, *Ann Plast Surg* 39(5), 447
Injection-site pain (2–10%)
  (2002): Madalinski MH+, *Eur J Gastroenterol Hepatol* 14(8), 853
    (4 cases)
  (2002): Molloy F, *eMedicine Journal* 3(2)
  (2001): de Almeida+, *Dermatol Surg* 27(1), 34
  (2000): Karamfilov T+, *Arch Dermatol* 136(4), 487
  (2000): Wissel J+, *J Pain Symptom Manage* 20(1), 44
  (1990): *NIH Consensus Statement* 8(8), 1
Injection-site rash (sic)
  (1997): LeWitt PA+, *Mov Disord* 12(6), 1064
Limb pain
Oral candidiasis
  (2003): Dressler D+, *Eur Neurol* 49(1), 34
Pain (6–13%)
  (1997): Truong DD+, *Mov Disord* 12(5), 772
Ptosis (14–20%)
  (2002): Molloy F, *eMedicine Journal* 3(2) (10%)
  (1997): Nussgens Z+, *Graefes Arch Clin Exp Ophthalmol*
    235(4), 197
  (1990): *NIH Consensus Statement* 8(8), 1
Stomatitis (1–10%)
Tinnitus (1–10%)
Tremor (1–10%)
  (1997): Truong DD+, *Mov Disord* 12(5), 772
Vaginal candidiasis (1–10%)
Xerostomia (3–34%)
  (2003): Dressler D+, *Eur Neurol* 49(1), 34

Note: An antitoxin is available in the event of overdose or misinjection

BRETYLIUM

Trade name: Bretylol (Abbott)
Other common trade names: *Bretylate; Critifib*
Indications: Ventricular tachycardia and fibrillation
Category: Antiarrhythmic class III
Half-life: 4–17 hours
**Clinically important, potentially hazardous interactions
with:** arsenic, ciprofloxacin, enoxacin, gatifloxacin, lomefloxacin, moxifloxacin, norfloxacin, ofloxacin, quinolones, sparfloxacin

Reactions

Skin

Diaphoresis (<1%)
Flushing (<1%)
Rash (sic) (<1%)

Other

Injection-site atrophy (<1%)
Injection-site necrosis (<1%)

BRIMONIDINE

Trade name: Alphagan (Allergan)
Indications: Open-angle glaucoma, ocular hypertension
Category: Alpha-2-adrenoceptor stimulant
Half-life: 12 hours

Reactions

Skin

Allergic reactions (sic) (<1%)
  (1999): thoe Schwartzenberg GW+, *Ophthalmology* 106, 1616
  (1998): Gordon RN+, *Eye* 12, 697
Blepharitis (1–10%)
Eyelid crusting (1–10%)
Eyelid edema (1–10%)
Eyelid erythema (1–10%)
Ocular pruritus (<10%)
Upper respiratory infection (1–10%)

Other

Depression
Dysgeusia (1–10%)
Headache
Ocular allergy (sic) (4.2%)
  (2000): Melamed S+, *Clin Ther* 22, 103
  (1999): Shin DH+, *Am J Ophthalmol* 127, 511
  (1998): LeBlanc RP, *Ophthalmology* 105, 1960
  (1996): Schuman JS, *Surv Ophthalmol* 41, Suppl 1:S27
Ocular burning (<10%)
  (1998): LeBlanc RP, *Ophthalmology* 105, 1960
  (1997): Schuman JS+, *Arch Ophthalmol* 115, 847 (28.1%)
  (1996): Schuman JS, *Surv Ophthalmol* 41, Suppl 1:S27
Ocular erythema
  (2001): Stewart WC+, *Am J Ophthalmol* 131(5), 631
Ocular stinging (<10%)
  (1998): LeBlanc RP, *Ophthalmology* 105, 1960
  (1997): Schuman JS+, *Arch Ophthalmol* 115, 847 (28.1%)
  (1996): Schuman JS, *Surv Ophthalmol* 41, Suppl 1:S27
Periocular dermatitis
  (2000): Williams GC+, *Glaucoma* 9, 235
Teardrop sign*

(2000): Scruggs JT+, *Br J Ophthalmol* 84, 671
Xerostomia (<10%)
  (2000): Detry-Morel M+, *J Fr Ophthalmol* 23, 763
  (1998): LeBlanc RP, *Ophthalmology* 105, 1960
  (1997): Derick RJ+, *Ophthalmology* 104, 131
  (1997): Schuman JS+, *Arch Ophthalmol* 115, 847 (33%)
  (1996): Schuman JS, *Surv Ophthalmol* 41, Suppl 1:S27
  (1996): Walters TR, , *Surv Ophthalmol* 41, Suppl 1:S19

*Note: The Teardrop sign is a laceration or deformity of the limbus of the eye

BRINZOLAMIDE

Trade name: Azopt (Alcon)
Indications: Open-angle glaucoma, ocular hypertension
Category: Carbonic anhydrase inhibitor; Ophthalmic
Half-life: 111 days
Clinically important, potentially hazardous interactions with: salicylates

*Note: Brinzolamide is a sulfonamide and can be absorbed systemically. Sulfonamides can produce severe, possibly fatal, reactions such as toxic epidermal necrolysis and Stevens–Johnson syndrome.

Reactions

Skin
Allergic reactions (sic) (<1%)
Blepharitis (1–5%)
Dermatitis (sic) (1–5%)
Eyelid crusting (<1%)
Ocular burning
  (2000): Barnebey H+, *Clin Ther* 22(10), 1204
  (2000): Sall K, *Surv Ophthalmol* 44, S155
  (1998): Silver LH, *Am J Ophthalmol* 126(3), 400 (1–5%)
Ocular pruritus (1–5%)
Urticaria (<1%)

Hair
Hair – alopecia (<1%)

Other
Blurred vision (5–10%)
  (2001): Seong GJ+, *Ophthalmologica* 215(3), 188
  (2000): Sugrue MF, *Prog Retin Eye Res* 19(1), 87
Dry eyes (1–5%)
  (2002): Novack GD+, *J Am Geriatr Soc* 50, 956
Dysgeusia (5–10%)
  (2002): Novack GD+, *J Am Geriatr* 50(5), 956
  (2000): Sall K, *Surv Ophthalmol* 44, S155
Foreign body sensation (5–10%)
Ocular irritation (1–5%)
Ocular stinging
  (2000): Barnebey H+, *Clin Ther* 22(10), 1204
  (2000): Sall K, *Surv Ophthalmol* 44, S155
  (1998): Silver LH, *Am J Ophthalmol* 126(3), 400 (1–5%)
Xerostomia (<1%)
  (2002): Novack GD+, *J Am Geriatr* 50(5), 956

BROMOCRIPTINE

Trade name: Parlodel (Novartis)
Other common trade names: *Apo-Bromocriptine; Bromed; Cryocriptina; Kripton; Parilac; Pravidel; Serocryptin*
Indications: Amenorrhea, parkinsonism, infertility
Category: Antidyskinetic; Antihyperprolactinemic; Antiparkinsonian; Dopamine agonist; Growth hormone suppressant; Infertility therapy adjunct; Lactation inhibitor
Half-life: initial: 6–8 hours; terminal: 50 hours
Clinically important, potentially hazardous interactions with: erythromycin, pseudoephedrine, sympathomimetics

Reactions

Skin
Exanthems
Flushing
  (1992): Shelley WB+, *Advanced Dermatologic Diagnosis* WB Saunders, 582 (passim)
Livedo reticularis
  (1985): Hoehn MMM+, *Neurology* 35, 199
  (1978): Calne DB+, *Lancet* 1, 735
  (1978): Lees AJ+, *Arch Neurol* 35, 503 (2%)
Morphea
  (1989): Leshin B+, *Int J Dermatol* 28, 177
Nodules
Purpura
Rash (sic)
Raynaud's phenomenon (1–10%)
  (1987): Quagliarello J+, *Fertility and Sterility* 48, 877
  (1978): Lees AJ+, *Arch Neurol* 35, 503 (5%)
  (1978): Pearce I+, *BMJ* 1, 1402
  (1976): Duvoisin RC, *Lancet* 2, 204
  (1976): Wass JAH+, *Lancet* 1, 1135
Scleroderma
  (1989): Leshin B+, *Int J Dermatol* 28, 177
  (1983): Dupont E+, *Neurology* 33, 670
Urticaria
Vasculitis
  (1978): Lees AJ+, *Arch Neurol* 35, 503

Hair
Hair – alopecia
  (1993): Fabre N+, *Clin Neuropharmacol* 16, 266
  (1980): Blum I+, *N Engl J Med* 303, 1418

Other
Anaphylactoid reactions
  (1980): Parkes S, *N Engl J Med* 302, 750
Dysgeusia (metallic taste)
Erythromelalgia
  (1983): Dupont E+, *Neurology* 33, 670
  (1981): Eisler T+, *Neurology* 31, 1368
  (1979): Eisler T+, *Neurology* 29, 571
  (1978): Calne DB+, *Lancet* 1, 735 (11%)
Headache
Paresthesias
  (1985): Hoehn MMM+, *Neurology* 35, 199
Priapism (clitoral)
Seizures
  (2003): Burckard E+, *Ann Fr Anesth Reanim* 22(1), 46
Stomatopyrosis
  (1985): Hoehn MMM+, *Neurology* 35, 199
Xerostomia (4–10%)
  (1985): Hoehn MMM+, *Neurology* 35, 199
  (1982): Gauthier G+, *Eur Neurol* 21, 217

BROMPHENIRAMINE

Trade names: Bromfed (Muro); Dimethane (Wyeth); Rondec (Biovail)
Other common trade names: *Bromine; Brommine; Bromphen; Dimegan; Ilvin; Kinmedon; Nasahist; ND-Stat; Neo-Meton*
Indications: Allergic rhinitis, urticaria
Category: Antihistamine H₁-blocker
Half-life: 12–48 hours
Clinically important, potentially hazardous interactions with: aprobarbital, butabarbital, chloral hydrate, etchlorvynol, mephobarbital, pentobarbital, phenobarbital, phenothiazines, primidone, secobarbital, zolpidem

Reactions

Skin
Angioedema (<1%)
Exanthems (<1%)
Photosensitivity (<1%)
Rash (sic) (<1%)

Other
Headache
Myalgia (<1%)
Paresthesias (<1%)
Xerostomia (1–10%)

BUCLIZINE

Trade names: Bucladin-S (Stuart); Vibazine
Other common trade names: *Aphilan; Buclixin; Longifene; Odetin; Postafeno; Vibazina*
Indications: Motion sickness, nausea/vomiting
Category: Anticholinergic; Antiemetic; Antihistamine
Half-life: N/A
Clinically important, potentially hazardous interactions with: aprobarbital, butabarbital, chloral hydrate, etchlorvynol, mephobarbital, pentobarbital, phenobarbital, phenothiazines, primidone, secobarbital, zolpidem

Reactions

Other
Tremor
Xerostomia

BUMETANIDE

Trade name: Bumex (Roche)
Other common trade names: *Bumedyl; Burinex; Fondiuran; Fontego; Lunetoron; Miccil; Primex*
Indications: Edema associated with congestive heart failure
Category: Antihypertensive; Sulfonamide loop diuretic
Half-life: 1–1.5 hours
Clinically important, potentially hazardous interactions with: amikacin, aminoglycosides, digoxin, gentamicin, kanamycin, neomycin, streptomycin, tobramycin

Reactions

Skin
Allergic reactions (sic)
Bullous eruption
  (1990): Leitao EA+, *J Am Acad Dermatol* 23, 129
Bullous pemphigoid
  (1998): Boulinguez S+, *Br J Dermatol* 138, 549
Dermatitis
  (1989): Moller NE+, *Contact Dermatitis* 20, 393
Diaphoresis (0.1%)
Edema (periorbital)
  (1981): Handler B+, *J Clin Pharmacol* 21, 691
Erythema multiforme (<1%)
  (1975): Ring-Larsen H, *Acta Med Scand* 195, 411
Exanthems
Exfoliative dermatitis
  (1981): Handler B+, *J Clin Pharmacol* 21, 691
Photosensitivity
  (1990): Leitao EA+, *J Am Acad Dermatol* 23, 129
Pruritus (<1%)
  (1992): Shelley WB+, *Cutis* 50, 17 (observation)
  (1984): Ward A+, *Drugs* 28, 426 (1–5%)
Purpura
Rash (sic) (0.2%)
Side effects (sic) (1.1%)
  (1984): Ward A+, *Drugs* 28, 426 (1–5%)
Urticaria (0.2%)
  (1981): Handler B+, *J Clin Pharmacol* 21, 691
Vasculitis

Other
Headache
Nipple tenderness (0.1%)
Pseudoporphyria
  (1990): Leitao EA+, *J Am Acad Dermatol* 23, 129
Xerostomia (0.1%)

*Note: Bumetanide is a sulfonamide and can be absorbed systemically. Sulfonamides can produce severe, possibly fatal, reactions such as toxic epidermal necrolysis and Stevens–Johnson syndrome

BUPROPION

Trade names: Wellbutrin (GSK); Zyban (GSK)
Indications: Depression, aid to smoking cessation
Category: Aid to smoking cessation; Heterocyclic antidepressant
Half-life: 14 hours
Clinically important, potentially hazardous interactions with: isocarboxazid, phenelzine, ritonavir, tranylcypromine, trimipramine

Reactions

Skin

Acne (1–10%)
Angioedema
Aquagenic pruritus
  (2002): Moreno Caballero B+, *Aten Primaria* 30(10), 662
Diaphoresis (5%)
  (1983): Feighner JP, *J Clin Psychiatry* 44, 49
  (1981): Halaris AE+, *Psychopharmacol Bull* 17, 140
Ecchymoses (<0.1%)
Edema (>1%)
  (1999): Peloso PM+, *JAMA* 282, 1817
Erythema multiforme
  (2002): Drago F+, *Arch Intern Med* 162(7), 843
  (2001): Carrillo-Jimenez R+, *Arch Intern Med* 161(12), 1556
  (2001): Lineberry TW+, *Mayo Clin Proc* 76, 664
Exanthems (<0.1%)
  (1983): Fabre LF+, *J Clin Psychiatry* 44, 88
  (1981): Halaris AE+, *Psychopharmacol Bull* 17, 140
Exfoliative dermatitis
Flushing (4%)
Hot flashes
Lupus panniculitis
  (1986): Ottuso P, *The Schoch Letter*, 46, 37 (observation)
Peripheral edema
  (1999): Peloso PM+, *JAMA* 282, 1817
Photosensitivity (<0.1%)
Pruritus (4%)
  (2003): Litt JZ, Beachwood, OH (personal case) (observation)
  (1983): Cato AE+, *J Clin Psychiatry* 44, 187
Rash (sic) (4%)
  (2000): McCollom RA+, *Ann Pharmacother* 34, 471
  (1985): Golden RN+, *Am J Psychiatry* 142, 1459 (vascular)
Stevens–Johnson syndrome
Urticaria
  (2003): Chiaverini C+, *Ann Dermatol Venereol* 130(2), 208
  (2003): Fays S+, *Br J Dermatol* 148(1), 177 (8 cases)
  (2003): Litt JZ, Beachwood, OH (personal case) (observation)
    (generalized)
  (1999): Peloso PM+, *JAMA* 282, 1817
  (1983): Cato AE+, *J Clin Psychiatry* 44, 187
  (1983): Fabre LF+, *J Clin Psychiatry* 44, 88
  (1983): Feighner JP, *J Clin Psychiatry* 44, 49
  (1983): Mendels J+, *J Clin Psychiatry* 44, 118
  (1978): Fann WE+, *Curr Ther Res* 23, 222
Xerosis (1–10%)

Hair

Hair – alopecia (<1%)
  (2002): Klein AD, Statesboro, GA (from Internet) (observation)
Hair – color change (sic) (<1%)
Hair – hirsutism (1–10%)

Other

Anaphylactoid reactions
Bromhidrosis

Bruxism (<0.1%)
Death
  (2002): *Prescrire Int* 11(60), 117
  (2002): Wooltorton E, *CMAJ* 166(1), 68
DRESS syndrome
  (2003): Bagshaw SM+, *Ann Allergy Asthma Immunol* 90(5), 572
Dry mouth
  (2002): Zwar N+, *Aust Fam Physician* 31(5), 443
Dysgeusia (4%)
  (1999): Berigan TR, *JAMA* 281, 233 (letter)
Gingivitis
Glossitis
Gynecomastia (<1%)
Headache
Hyperesthesia (<0.1%)
Hypersensitivity
  (2003): Ferry L+, *Int J Clin Pract* 57(3), 224 (0.12%)
  (2002): *Prescrire Int* 11(58), 49
  (2002): Zwar N+, *Aust Fam Physician* 31(5), 443
  (2001): Benson E, *Med J Aust* 174(12), 650
Myalgia (6%)
  (1999): Peloso PM+, *JAMA* 282, 1817
Oral edema (<1%)
Painful erection
Paresthesias (2%)
Parkinsonism
  (2001): Jerome L, *Can J Psychiatry* 46(6), 560
Priapism
  (1995): Levenson JL, *Am J Psychiatry* 152, 813
Rhabdomyolysis
  (1999): David D+, *J Clin Psychopharmacol* 19(2), 185
Seizures
  (2003): Balit CR+, *Med J Aust* 178(2), 61
  (2003): Ferry L+, *Int J Clin Pract* 57(3), 224 (0.1%)
  (2003): Gamarra M+, *Aten Primaria* 31(3), 202
  (2003): Oncken CA+, *Nicotine Tob Res* 5(1), 131
  (2002): Bergmann F+, *J Clin Psychopharmacol* 22(6), 630
  (2002): Welsh CJ+, *N Engl J Med* 347(12), 951
  (2002): Wooltorton E, *CMAJ* 166(1), 68
  (2002): Zwar N+, *Aust Fam Physician* 31(5), 443
  (2001): Enns MW, *J Clin Psychiatry* 62(6), 476 (with trimipramine)
Serum sickness
  (2002): Wooltorton E, *CMAJ* 166(1), 68
  (2001): Davis JS+, *Med J Aust* 174, 479
  (2000): McCollom RA+, *Ann Pharmacother* 34, 471
  (1999): Peloso PM+, *JAMA* 282, 1817
  (1999): Tripathi A+, *Ann Allergy Asthma Immunol* 83, 165
  (1999): Yolles JC+, *Ann Pharmacother* 33, 931
Sialorrhea
Stomatitis (>1%)
Tinnitus
Tongue edema (0.1%)
  (2000): McCollom RA+, *Ann Pharmacother* 34, 471
Tremor (>10%)
Twitching (2%)
Vaginitis
Xerostomia (up to 64%)
  (2003): Litt JZ, Beachwood, OH (personal case) (observation)
  (2002): George TP+, *Biol Psychiatry* 52(1), 53
  (1999): Settle EC+, *Clin Ther* 21, 454
  (1997): Hurd RD+, *N Engl J Med* 337, 1195
  (1991): James WA+, *South Med J* 84, 222
  (1986): Feighner JP+, *J Clin Psychopharmacol* 6, 27
  (1983): Chouinard G, *J Clin Psychiatry* 44, 121
  (1983): Feighner JP, *J Clin Psychiatry* 44, 49
  (1981): Halaris AE+, *Psychopharmacol Bull* 17, 140

BUSPIRONE

Trade name: BuSpar (Bristol-Myers Squibb)
Other common trade names: *Ansail; Apo-Buspirone; Bespar; Biron; Busirone; Bustab; Kallmiren; Narol; Neurosine; Nu-Buspirone*
Indications: Anxiety
Category: Nonbenzodiazepine anxiolytic tranquilizer; Serotonin antagonist
Half-life: 2–3 hours
Clinically important, potentially hazardous interactions with: nefazodone, ritonavir

Reactions

Skin
Acne (<0.1%)
Bullous eruption (<1%)
Diaphoresis
  (1986): Newton RE+, *Am J Med* 3B:80, 17
Ecchymoses
Edema
Exanthems
Facial edema (1%)
Flushing
Hypopigmentation
  (2002): Chapman MS+, *Am J Contact Dermat* 13(1), 46
Pruritus (1%)
Purpura (1%)
Radiation recall
  (1989): Vassal G+, *Cancer Chemother Pharmacol* 23, 117
Rash (sic) (<1%)
Seborrheic dermatitis
  (1993): Litt JZ, Beachwood, OH (personal case) (observation)
Urticaria (<1%)
Xerosis (1%)

Hair
Hair – alopecia (1%)
  (2000): Mercke Y+, *Ann Clin Psychiatry* 12, 35
  (1995): Ljungman P+, *Bone Marrow Transplant* 15, 869

Nails
Nails – thinning (<0.1%)

Other
Dysgeusia (<1%)
Galactorrhea (<0.1%)
Glossodynia
Glossopyrosis
Headache
Myalgia
Paresthesias (1%)
  (1986): Newton RE+, *Am J Med* 3B:80, 17
Parkinsonism
  (2003): Clay PG+, *Ann Pharmacother* 37(2), 202 (with ritonavir)
Parosmia (1%)
Serotonin syndrome
  (2000): Manos GH, *Ann Pharmacother* 34(7–8), 871 (with fluoxetine)
Sialorrhea
Sicca syndrome
  (1977): Sidi Y+, *JAMA* 238, 1951
Tinnitus
Xerostomia (3%)

BUSULFAN

Trade name: Myleran (GSK)
Other common trade names: *Citosulfan; Leukosulfan; Mablin; Misulban*
Indications: Chronic myelogenous leukemia, bone marrow disorders
Category: Antineoplastic
Half-life: 3.4 hours (after first dose)
Clinically important, potentially hazardous interactions with: aldesleukin

Reactions

Skin
Bullous eruption
  (1970): Dosik H+, *Blood* 35, 543
Cheilitis
  (1980): Wintroub B+, *Clinical Cancer Medicine* GK Hall and Company, 206
  (1961): Haut A+, *Blood* 17, 1
Eccrine squamous syringometaplasia
  (1997): Valks R+, *Arch Dermatol* 133, 873
Erythema (macular) (>10%)
  (1985): Hymes SR+, *J Cutan Pathol* 12, 125
Erythema multiforme (<1%)
  (1981): Weiss RB+, *Ann Intern Med* 94, 66
  (1980): Adrian RM+, *CA* 30, 143
  (1978): Levine N+, *Cancer Treat Rev* 5, 67
  (1974): Levantine A+, *Br J Dermatol* 90, 239
  (1970): Dosik H+, *Blood* 35, 543
Erythema nodosum (<1%)
  (1978): Levine N+, *Cancer Treat Rev* 5, 67
  (1961): Kyle BA+, *Blood* 18, 497
  (1956): Marinko HM+, *Arq Brasil Med* (Portuguese) 46, 161
Exanthems
  (1992): Fitzpatrick JE, *Derm Clinics* 10, 19 (passim)
  (1978): Leyden MJ+, *Lancet* 2, 797
Granulomatous dermatitis
  (2002): Longo M+, *World Congress Dermatol* Poster, 0110
Kaposi's sarcoma
  (1998): Roszkiewicz A+, *Cutis* 61, 137
Pigmentation (1–10%) ("busulfan tan")
  (1999): Simonart T+, *Ann Dermatol Venereol* (French) 126, 439
  (1992): Fitzpatrick JE, *Derm Clinics* 10, 19 (passim)
  (1985): Hymes SR+, *J Cutan Pathol* 12, 125
  (1983): Bronner AK+, *J Am Acad Dermatol* 9, 645
  (1981): Granstein RD+, *J Am Acad Dermatol* 5, 1 (brown-black)
  (1980): Adam BA+, *J Dermatol* 7, 405
  (1971): Burns WA+, *Med Ann DC* 40, 567
  (1966): Harrold BP, *BMJ* 1, 463
  (1966): Sprunt JG+, *BMJ* 5489, 736
  (1965): Desai RG, *N Engl J Med* 272, 808
  (1963): Marchal G+, *Sem Ther* (French) 39, 565
  (1961): Haut A+, *Blood* 17, 1
  (1961): Kyle RA+, *Blood* 18, 497
Purpura
  (2001): Chuang C+, *Movement Disorders* 16, 990 (with cyclophosphamide)
Urticaria (>10%)
  (1981): Spiegel RJ, *Cancer Treat Rev* 8, 197
  (1981): Weiss RB+, *Ann Intern Med* 94, 66
  (1978): Levine N+, *Cancer Treat Rev* 5, 67
  (1961): Kyle BA+, *Blood* 18, 497
  (1960): Ducach C+, *Rev Med Chile* (Spanish) 88, 36
Vasculitis

(1992): Breathnach SM+, *Adverse Drug Reactions and the Skin*
   Blackwell, Oxford, 288 (passim)
(1982): Weiss RB, *Sem Oncology* 9, 5
(1967): Coleman WP, *Med Clin North Am* 51, 1073
Xerosis
   (1961): Haut A+, *Blood* 17, 1

Hair

Hair – alopecia (>10%)
   (2000): Tran D+, *Australas J Dermatology* 41, 106
   (1995): Ljungman P+, *Bone Marrow Transplant* 15, 869
   (1993): Vowels M+, *Bone Marrow Transplant* 12, 347
   (1977): Moschella S, *Cutis* 19, 603
   (1975): Dreizen S+, *Postgrad Med* 58, 150
   (1961): Haut A+, *Blood* 17, 1

Nails

Nails – pigmentation

Other

Anhidrosis
   (1961): Haut A+, *Blood* 17, 1
Dysgeusia
   (1961): Haut A+, *Blood* 17, 1
Gynecomastia (<1%)
   (1979): Harrington WJ, *Adv Intern Med* 24, 141
   (1979): White DR+, *N C Med J* 40, 73
   (1977): Moschella SL, *Cutis* 19, 603
Headache
Oral mucosal pigmentation
   (1965): Desai RG, *N Engl J Med* 272, 808
Oral mucositis
   (2000): Wardley AM+, *Br J Haematol* 110, 292
Parkinsonism
Porphyria cutanea tarda
   (1983): Bronner AK+, *J Am Acad Dermatol* 9, 645
   (1964): Kyle BA+, *Blood* 23, 776
Stomatitis

BUTABARBITAL

Trade names: Butalan; Buticaps; Butisol (Wallace)
Other common trade name: *Day-Barb*
Indications: Sedation
Category: Sedative-hypnotic barbiturate
Half-life: 40–140 hours
**Clinically important, potentially hazardous interactions
with: alcohol,** antihistamines, ardeparin, argatroban,
brompheniramine, buclizine, chlorpheniramine, dalteparin,
danaparoid, dicumarol, enoxaparin, ethanolamine, heparin,
imatinib, tinzaparin, warfarin

Reactions

Skin

Acne
Angioedema (<1%)
Bullous eruption
   (1970): Groeschel D+, *N Engl J Med* 283, 409
Erythema multiforme
   (1975): Böttiger LE, *Acta Med Scand* 198, 229
Exanthems
   (1943): Davison TC, *Curr Res Anesth Analg* 22, 52
Exfoliative dermatitis (<1%)
   (1944): Potter JK+, *Ann Intern Med* 21, 1041
Fixed eruption

   (1970): Savin JA, *Br J Dermatol* 83, 546
Herpes simplex
Lupus erythematosus
   (1967): Williams DI, *Proc R Soc Med* 60, 299
   (1951): Grant Peterkin GA, *Edinb Med J* 58, 41
Necrosis
   (1972): Almeyda J+, *Br J Dermatol* 86, 313
Photosensitivity
   (1939): Stryker GV, *J Mo Med Assn* 36, 484
Pruritus
Purpura
   (1946): Grant Peterkin GA, *BMJ* 2, 52
Rash (sic) (<1%)
Stevens–Johnson syndrome (<1%)
Toxic epidermal necrolysis
   (1973): Stüttgen G, *Br J Dermatol* 88, 291
Urticaria
Vasculitis

Other

Oral ulceration
Porphyria variegata
Rhabdomyolysis
   (1990): Larpin R+, *Presse Med* 19(30), 1403
Thrombophlebitis (<1%)

BUTALBITAL

Trade name: Esgic (Wyeth); Fioricet (Watson); Fiorinal
(Watson)
Other common trade names: *Amaphen; Anoquan; Axotal;
Butace; Fioricet; Marnal; Medigesic; Phrenilin; Tecnal*
Indications: Tension headaches
Category: Sedative-analgesic barbiturate
Half-life: 35 hours
**Clinically important, potentially hazardous interactions
with: alcohol,** dicumarol

Reactions

Skin

Bullous eruption
   (1970): Groeschel D+, *N Engl J Med* 283, 409
Erythema multiforme
   (1984): Gebel K+, *Dermatologica* 168, 35
   (1975): Böttiger LE, *Acta Med Scand* 198, 229
Exanthems
   (1943): Davison TC, *Curr Res Anesth Analg* 22, 52
Exfoliative dermatitis (<1%)
   (1944): Potter JK+, *Ann Intern Med* 21, 1041
Fixed eruption
   (1970): Savin JA, *Br J Dermatol* 83, 546
Herpes simplex
Lupus erythematosus
   (1967): Williams DI, *Proc R Soc Med* 60, 299
   (1951): Grant Peterkin GA, *Edinb Med J* 58, 41
Necrosis
   (1972): Almeyda J+, *Br J Dermatol* 86, 313
Photosensitivity
   (1939): Stryker GV, *J Mo Med Assn* 36, 484
Pruritus
Purpura
   (1946): Grant Peterkin GA, *BMJ* 2, 52
Rash (sic) (1–10%)
Stevens–Johnson syndrome (<1%)

Toxic epidermal necrolysis
 (1973): Stüttgen G, *Br J Dermatol* 88, 291
Urticaria
 (1993): Litt JZ, Beachwood, OH (personal case) (observation)
Vasculitis

Other

Anaphylactoid reactions (1–10%)
Headache
Oral erythema multiforme
 (1984): Gebel K+, *Dermatologica* 168, 35
Oral ulceration
Porphyria variegata
Rhabdomyolysis
 (1990): Larpin R+, *Presse Med* 19(30), 1403

BUTORPHANOL

Trade name: Stadol (Bristol-Myers Squibb) (Geneva)
Other common trade names: *Biforal; Busphen; Stadol NS*
Indications: Pain, migraine
Category: Analgesic; Narcotic
Half-life: 2.5–4 hours
**Clinically important, potentially hazardous interactions
with:** cimetidine

Reactions

Skin

Clammy skin (sic)
Diaphoresis (1–10%)
Edema (<1%)
Exanthems
Flushing (1–10%)
Gooseflesh (sic)
Pruritus (1–10%)
 (1989): Ackerman WE+, *Can J Anaesth* 36, 388
 (1981): Bernstein JE+, *J Am Acad Dermatol* 5, 227
Rash (sic) (<1%)
Urticaria (<1%)

Other

Dysgeusia (3–9%)
Headache
Injection-site reactions (sic)
Paresthesias
Tinnitus
Xerostomia (3–9%)

BUTTERBUR

Scientific names: *Petasites hybridus; Petasites officinalis*
Family: Asteraceae; Compositae
Trade and other common names: Blatterdock; bog rhubarb;
bogshorn; butterdock; butterfly dock; capdockin; flapperdock;
Petadolex* (Weber & Weber)
Category: Anodyne; Anti-inflammatory; Antispasmodic
Purported indications and other uses: Allergic rhinitis,
asthma, bronchitis, chills, cough, dysmenorrhea, hay fever,
headache, heart tonic, migraine, peptic ulcer, appetite stimulant,
irritable bladder, poultice for wounds or skin ulcers
Half-life: N/A

*****Note:** Petadolex formulation has had the potentially carcinogenic
pyrrolizidine alkaloids removed

Reactions

Skin

Edema (<0.1%)
 (2000): Grossmann WM+, *Int J Clin Pharmacol Ther* 38(9), 430
 (1996): Grossman W, *Der Freie Arzt* (German) 3, 44
Erythema (<0.1%)
 (2000): Grossmann WM+, *Int J Clin Pharmacol Ther* 38(9), 430
 (1996): Grossman W, *Der Freie Arzt* (German) 3, 44
Ocular pruritus (<1%)
 (2002): Schapowal A, *Br Med J* 324(733), 144
Pruritus (<1%)
 (2002): Schapowal A, *Br Med J* 324(7330), 144
Rash (sic)
 (2000): Grossmann WM+, *Int J Clin Pharmacol Ther* 38(9), 430
 (1996): Grossman W, *Der Freie Arzt* (German) 3, 44

Other

Hypersensitivity (<0.1%)
 (2000): Grossmann WM+, *Int J Clin Pharmacol Ther* 38(9), 430
 (1996): Grossman W, *Der Freie Arzt* (German) 3, 44

CABERGOLINE

Trade name: Dostinex (Pharmacia)
Indications: Hyperprolactinemia, parkinsonism
Category: Dopamine receptor agonist; Ergot alkaloid
Half-life: 63–69 hours

Reactions

Skin
Acne (1%)
  (1997): Rademaker M, New Zealand (from Internet) (observation)
Ankle edema (1%)
Facial edema (1%)
Fixed eruption
  (1997): Rademaker M, New Zealand (from Internet) (observation)
Flu-like syndrome (sic) (1%)
Hot flashes (3%)
Periorbital edema (1%)
Peripheral edema (1%)
Pruritus (1%)

Other
Mastodynia (2%)
Paresthesias (5%)
Toothache (1%)
Xerostomia (2%)

CAFFEINE

Scientific names: *Coffea arabica; Coffea canephora; Coffea robusta; Cola acuminata;* guarana *(Paullinia cupana); Thea sinensis; Theobroma cacao*
Family: Rubiales
Trade and other common names: 1, 3, 7 trimethylxanthine; Anacin; Aqua-Ban; Black tea; Cafergot; Cola; Coryban-D; Darvon Compound; Dexatrim; Dristan; Elsinore; Endolor; Esgic; Excedrin; Fioricet; Fiorinal; Guanara; Midol; Migralam; NoDoz; Norgesic; Norgesic Forte; Synalgos-DC; Synalgos-DC-A; Triaminicin; Vanquish; Vivarin (GSK). Ingredient in: Adipokinetix
Category: CNS stimulant; Somnolytic
Purported indications and other uses: with ergotamine for migraine, with NSAIDs in analgesics, headache, respiratory depression in neonates, postprandial hypotension, enhances seizure duration in electroconvulsive therapy. Ingredient in cough and cold remedies
Half-life: 2–7 hours
Clinically important, potentially hazardous interactions with: carbamazepine, cimetidine, clozapine, **ephedra**, ginseng, idrocilamide, methoxsalen, mexiletine, phenylpropanolamine, zonisamide

Note: Caffeine is an addictive psychoactive substance. Spontaneous abortion and low birthweight babies have occurred in pregnant women consuming 150 mg caffeine per day. Abuse can lead to cardiac damage or death
Physical Dependence & Withdrawal of Caffeine
Common symptoms of caffeine withdrawal are headache; drowsiness; yawning, impaired concentration; lassitude; irritability; decreased contentedness, well-being and self-confidence; decreased sociability; flu-like symptoms; muscle aches and stiffness; hot or cold spells; nausea or vomiting; and blurred vision

Reactions

Skin
Angioedema
Bullous eruption
Burning (feet)
  (1982): Young JJ+, *Drug Intell Clin Pharm* 16(10), 779
Chills
  (1988): Mattila M+, *Int Clin Psychopharmacol* 3(3), 215
Ecchymoses
Exfoliation
Facial edema
Pemphigus
  (1990): Brenner S+, *Acta Derm Venereol* 70(4), 357
    (+paracetamol, chlorpheniramine, phenylephrine)
Pruritus
Purpura
Rash (sic)
Rosacea
  (2001): Goldman D, *J Am Acad Dermatol* 44(6), 995
Urticaria
  (2002): Fernandez-Nieto M+, *Allergy* 57(10), 967 (cola drink)
  (1999): Kubota Y+, *Eur J Dermatol* 9(7), 559 (+aspirin)
  (1993): Caballero T+, *J Investig Allergol Clin Immunol* 3(3), 160
  (1991): Quirce Gancedo+, *J Allergy Clin Immunol* 88(4), 680
  (1988): Pola J+, *Ann Allergy* 60(3), 207
Xanthoderma

Other
Anaphylactoid reactions
  (1999): Kubota Y+, *Eur J Dermatol* 9(7), 559 (+aspirin)
  (1983): Przybilla B+, *Hautarzt* (German) 34(2), 73
Death (from abuse/overdose)
  (2003): Kanstrup MH+, *Ugeskr Laeger* 165(3), 239 (with ephedrine)
  (2001): Ahrendt DM, *Am Fam Physician* 63(5), 913
  (2000): Le Coz, *Presse Med* (French) 29(1), 33
  (2000): Tanskanen A+, *Eur J Epidemiol* 16(9), 789
  (2000): Zivkovic R, *Acta Med Croatica* 54(1), 33
  (1999): Zahn KA+, *J Emerg Med* 17(2), 289 (herbal ecstasy)
  (1998): Ferslew KE+, *J Forensic Sci* 43(5), 1082 (+clozapine, fluoxetine)
  (1997): Shum S+, *Vet Hum Toxicol* 39(4), 228
  (1990): Lake CR+, *Int J Obes* 14(7), 575
    (+phenylpropanolamine)
  (1989): Mrvos RM+, *Vet Hum Toxicol* 31(6), 571 (diet pills)
  (1986): Hanzlick R+, *J Anal Toxicol* 10(3), 126
  (1985): Garriott JC+, *J Anal Toxicol* 9(3), 141
  (1985): Winek CL+, *Forensic Sci Int* 29(3–4), 207
  (1985): Zimmerman PM+, *Ann Emerg Med* 14(12), 1227
  (1981): Bryant J, *Arch Pathol Lab Med* 105, 685
  (1980): McGee MB, *J Forensic Sci* 25(1), 29
  (1977): Turner JE+, *Clin Toxicol* 10(3), 341
  (1974): Dimaio VJ+, *Forensic Sci* 3(3), 275
  (1973): Alstott RL+, *J Forensic Sci* 18(2), 135
  (1959): Jokela S+, *Acta Pharmacologica et Toxilogica* 15, 331
Depression
  (2002): Patten SB, *Expert Opin Pharmacother* 3(10), 1405
  (1996): Rapoport A+, *Headache* 36(1), 14 (+migraine medication)
Hallucinations
  (2002): Gulbranson SH+, *Pharmacotherapy* 22(1), 126 (with ergotamine)
Headache
Hypersensitivity

(2002): Hinrichs R+, *Allergy* 57(9), 859
Paresthesias
  (2000): Yates KM+, *N Z Med* 113(1114), 315 (herbal ecstasy)
Rhabdomyolysis
  (1999): Kamijo Y+, *Vet Hum Toxicol* 41(6), 381 (oolong tea)
  (1998): Kasamatsu Y+, *Intern Med* 37(2), 169 (cold remedy)
  (1995): Dawson JK+, *J Accid Emerg Med* 12(1), 49 (+ephedrine, theophylline)
  (1991): Michaelis HC+, *J Toxicol Clin Toxicol* 29(4), 521 (overdose, +acetaminophen, phenazone)
  (1989): Wrenn KD+, *Ann Emerg Med* 18(1), 94 (overdose)
Tic disorder
  (1998): Davis RE+, *Pediatrics* 101(6), E4
Tremor
  (1992): Astrup A+, *Int J Obes Relat Metab Disord* 16(4), 269 (+ephedrine)
  (1991): Hughes JR+, *Arch Gen Psychiatry* 48(7), 611
  (1988): Mattila M+, *Int Clin Psychopharmacol* 3(3), 215 (+yohimbine)
  (1981): Malchow-Moller A+, *Int J Obes* 5(2), 183 (Elsinore[ephedrine])
Xerostomia
  (2002): Boozer CN+, *Int J Obes Relat Metab Disord* 26(5), 593 (with ephedra)

CALCITONIN

(See HUMAN and SALMON)
Trade names: Calcimar (Aventis); Miacalcin (Novartis)
Other common trade names: *Caltine; Cibacalcine; Clasynar; Miacalcic*
Indications: Paget's disease of bone
Category: Bone resorption inhibitor; Calcium regulator; Osteoporosis therapy adjunct
Half-life: 70–90 minutes

Reactions

Skin
Allergic reactions (sic)
  (2001): Rodriguez A+, *Allergy* 56(8), 801
Edema of feet
Exanthems
Flushing (>10%)
  (1995): Kobayashi T+, *J Endocrinol* 146, 431
  (1975): Goldsmith RS, *JAMA* 232, 1156
  (1975): *Med Lett* 17, 97
Granuloma annulare
  (1993): Goihman YM, *Int J Dermatol* 32, 150
Pruritus
Rash (sic) (<1%)
Tender palms and soles (sic)
Urticaria (<1%)
  (1975): *Med Lett* 17, 97

Other
Anaphylactoid reactions
Dysgeusia (metallic or salty)
Hypersensitivity
Injection-site edema (>10%)
Injection-site inflammation (>10%)
  (1975): Goldsmith RS, *JAMA* 232, 1156
  (1975): *Med Lett* 17, 97
Injection-site pain
  (1988): Warrell RP+, *Ann Intern Med* 108, 669 (62%)
Paresthesias (<1%)

CALFACTANT

Trade name: Infasurf (Forest)
Indications: Prevention of respiratory distress syndrome
Category: Lung surfactant (intratracheal)
Half-life: N/A

Reactions

Other
None

CANDESARTAN

Trade name: Atacand (AstraZeneca)
Other common trade name: *Amias*
Indications: Hypertension
Category: Angiotensin II receptor antagonist; Antihypertensive
Half-life: 9 hours

Reactions

Skin
Angioedema
  (2003): Hille K+, *Am J Ophthalmol* 135(2), 224
  (2002): Lo KS, *Pharmacotherapy* 22(9), 1176
Diaphoresis (>0.5%)
Edema
Exanthems (<1%)
Linear IgA bullous dermatosis
  (2003): Pena-Penabad C+, *Am J Med* 114(2), 163
Peripheral edema (>1%)
Rash (sic) (>0.5%)

Other
Cough
  (2002): Cuspidi C+, *J Hypertens* 20(11), 2293
Headache
Myalgia (>0.5%)
Paresthesias (>0.5%)

CAPECITABINE

Trade name: Xeloda (Roche)
Indications: Metastatic breast cancer
Category: Antimetabolite (prodrug of 5-FU); Antineoplastic
Half-life: 0.5–1 hour

Reactions

Skin
Acral erythema
Blistering
Dermatitis (sic) (37%)
  (2003): Wagstaff AJ+, *Drugs* 63(2), 217 (25%)
  (1999): Dooley M+, *Drugs* 58, 69
Diaphoresis (0.2%)
Edema (9%)
  (1996): Bajetta E+, *Tumori* 82, 450
Erythema
Exfoliative dermatitis (31–37%)
Hand-foot syndrome (57%)

(2003): Wagstaff AJ+, *Drugs* 63(2), 217 (25%)
(2002): Abushullaih S+, *Cancer Invest* 20(1), 3 (68.3%)
(2002): Liu X+, *Zhonghua Zhong Liu Za Zhi* 24(1), 71
(2002): Wenzel C+, *Am J Kidney Dis* 39(1), 48 (7.7%)
(2001): Elasmar SA+, *Jpn J Clin Oncol* 31(4), 172 (passim)
(2001): McGavin JK+, *Drugs* 61(15), 2309
(2001): O'Shaughnessy JA+, *Ann Oncol* 12(9), 1247
(2001): Seitz JF, *Semin Oncol* 28(1 Suppl 1), 41
(1999): Blum JL+, *J Clin Oncol* 17, 485 (10%)
(1999): Blum JL, *Oncology* 57, 16
(1999): Dooley M+, *Drugs* 58, 69
(1999): Mrozek-Orlowski ME+, *Oncol Nurs Forum* 26, 753
(1998): Budman DR+, *J Clin Oncol* 16, 1795
Infections (sic) (<1%)
Photosensitivity (<1%)
Pigmentation
    (2002): Liu X+, *Zhonghua Zhong Liu Za Zhi* 24(1), 71
Pruritus
Purpura (0.2%)
Pyogenic granuloma
    (2002): Piguet V+, *Br J Dermatol* 147(6), 1270
Radiation recall (<1%)
    (2002): Camidge R+, *J Clin Oncol* 20(19), 4130
    (2002): Ortmann E+, *J Clin Oncol* 20(13), 3029
Repigmentation (of vitiligo)
    (2001): Schmid-Wendtner M-H+, *Lancet* 358, 1575
Vitiligo
    (2001): Schmid-Wendtner MH+, *Lancet* 358(9293), 1575
Xerosis

Hair

Hair – alopecia (<1%)
    (2001): Hoff PM+, *J Clin Oncol* 19(8), 2282
    (2001): McGavin JK+, *Drugs* 61(15), 2309
    (2001): Oshaughnessy JA+, *Ann Oncol* 12(9), 1247

Nails

Nails – changes (sic) (7%)
Nails – hyponychial dermatitis
    (2003): Chen GY+, *Br J Dermatol* 148, 1071 (also taking
        docetaxel)
Nails – onycholysis
    (2003): Munoz A+, *J Natl Cancer Inst* 95(16), 1252 (with
        irinotecan)
    (2001): Chen G-Y+, *Br J Dermatol* 145(3), 521
Nails – onychomadesis
    (2001): Chen G-Y+, *Br J Dermatol* 145(3), 521

Other

Fatigue
    (2003): Wagstaff AJ+, *Drugs* 63(2), 217 (25%)
Headache
Hypersensitivity (<1%)
Mucositis
    (2001): Bell KA+, *J Am Acad Dermatol* 45(5), 790
Myalgia (9%)
Oral candidiasis (0.2%)
Oral ulceration
Paresthesias (21%)
Stomatitis (24%)
    (2002): Liu X+, *Zhonghua Zhong Liu Za Zhi* 24(1), 71
    (2001): Hoff PM+, *J Clin Oncol* 19(8), 2282
    (2001): McGavin JK+, *Drugs* 61(15), 2309
Thrombophlebitis (0.2%)

CAPSICUM

Scientific names: *Capsicum annuum; Capsicum baccatum; Capsicum chinense; Capsicum frutescens; Capsicum pubscens*
Family: Solanaceae
Trade and other common names: African chili; Bell pepper; Bird pepper; Capsaicin; Capsicool; Capsin; Capzasin-P; Cayenne; Cayenne Pepper; Chili; Dolorac; Goat's pod; Ici Fructus; Jalapeno; Louisiana long pepper; No Pain-HP; Oleoresin; Pain Doctor; Pain-X; Paprika; Pimento; R-Gel; Zanzibar pepper; Zostrix
Trade names: Capsin, Capzasin-P, Dolorac, No Pain-HP, Pain Doctor (with methyl-salicylate and menthol), Pain-X, R-Gel, Zostrix. Oral: Cajun Seasoning, Capsicool, Cayenne Extra Hot, Cayenne Pepper Capsules, Kidney Blend, Tabasco sauce
Category: Antiseptic; Spasmolytic; Stimulant; Stomachic
Purported indications and other uses: nausea, neuropathic pain, osteoarthritis, fibromyalgia, anticarcinogen, rheumatoid arthritis, diabetic neuropathy, postherpetic neuralgia (shingles), psoriasis, pruritus, vitiligo, dyspepsia, flatulence, ulcers, stomach cramps, hypertension, improved circulation, weight-loss.
Half-life: N/A
Clinically important, potentially hazardous interactions with: ACE inhibitors, antiplatelet drugs, aspirin, disulfiram, heparin, latex, salicylic acid, theophylline, warfarin

Note: Pepper spray or gas contains 5% oleoresin capsicum (OC). It is used by police and in personal defense sprays

Reactions

Skin

Acute febrile neutrophilic dermatosis (Sweet's syndrome)
    (1993): Greer JM+, *Cutis* 51(2), 112
Adverse effects (sic)
    (2001): Keitel W+, *Arzneimittelforschung* 51(11), 896 (mild)
    (2001): Stam C+, *Br Homeopath J* 90(1), 21 (11%)
    (1991): Govindarajan VS+, *Crit Rev Food Sci Nutr* 29(6), 435
Allergic reactions (sic)
    (2002): Groenewoud GC+, *Clin Exp Allergy* 32(3), 434
    (1996): Sastre J+, *Allergy* 51(2), 117
    (1979): Meneghini CL+, *Contact Dermatitis* 5(3), 197
Bullous eruption
    (1993): Greer JM+, *Cutis* 51(2), 112
Burning
    (1998): Busker RW+, *Am J Forensic Med Pathol* 19(4), 309 (spray)
    (1990): Chan OY+, *J Soc Occup Med* 40(3), 111
    (1987): Jones LA+, *J Toxicol Clin Toxicol* 25(6), 483
Dermatitis
    (1996): Kanerva L+, *Contact Dermatitis* 35(3), 157
    (1995): Williams SR+, *Ann Emerg Med* 25(5), 713
    (1989): Burnett JW, *Cutis* 43(6), 534
Diaphoresis
    (1985): Locock, *Can Pharm J* 118, 517
Erosions
    (2000): Zollman TM+, *Ophthalmology* 107(12), 2186 (21%)
        (spray)
Erythema
    (1996): Watson WA+, *Ann Pharmacother* 30(7), 733
    (1993): Greer JM+, *Cutis* 51(2), 112
    (1987): Jones LA+, *J Toxicol Clin Toxicol* 25(6), 483
Erythema multiforme
    (1995): Raccagni AA+, *Contact Dermatitis* 33(5), 353
Flushing
    (1985): Locock, *Can Pharm J* 118, 517
Inflammation

(1998): Busker RW+, *Am J Forensic Med Pathol* 19(4), 309 (spray)

Irritation
  (2001): Babakhanian RV+, *Sud Med Ekspert* 44(1), 9 (spray)

Pustules
  (1993): Greer JM+, *Cutis* 51(2), 112

Rhinoconjunctivitis
  (1998): Vega de la Osada F+, *Med Clin* (Barc) 111(7), 263

Sensitization
  (1997): Gallo R+, *Contact Dermatitis* 37(1), 36

Toxicoderma
  (1985): Rogov VD, *Vestn Dermatol Venerol* comp(5), 53

Urticaria
  (2003): Feldman H+, *Am J Emerg Med* 21(2), 159
  (1997): Foti C+, *Contact Dermatitis* 37(3), 135

Other

Application-site burning
  (1992): Tandan R+, *Diabetes Care* 15(1), 8

Conjunctivitis
  (2003): Holopainen JM+, *Toxicol Appl Pharmacol* 186(3), 155
    (spray)
  (1996): Lee RJ+, *J Am Optom Assoc* 67(9), 548 (spray)
  (1995): Steffee CH+, *Am J Forensic Med Pathol* 16(3), 185 (spray)

Cough
  (1991): Blanc P+, *Chest* 99(1), 27

Death
  (2001): Olajos EJ+, *J Appl Toxicol* 21(5), 355 (spray)
  (1998): Pollanen MS+, *CMAJ* 158(12), 1603 (spray)
  (1995): Steffee CH+, *Am J Forensic Med Pathol* 16(3), 185 (spray)
  (1989): Mack RB, *N C Med J* 50(11), 627 (spray)

Fibrosis
  (1988): Escobar CH, *Rev ADM* 45(6), 369

Gingivitis
  (1991): Serio FG+, *J Periodontol* 62(6), 390

Hypersensitivity
  (2002): Groenewoud GC+, *Clin Exp Allergy* 32(3), 434
  (1998): Busker RW+, *Am J Forensic Med Pathol* 19(4), 309 (spray)

Lacrimation
  (1996): Lee RJ+, *J Am Optom Assoc* 67(9), 548 (spray)

Mucosal bleeding
  (1987): Myers BM+, *Am J Gastroenterol* 82(3), 211

Ocular burning
  (1996): Watson WA+, *Ann Pharmacother* 30(7), 733 (spray)

Pain
  (2000): Zollman TM+, *Ophthalmology* 107(12), 2186 (spray)
  (1995): Steffee CH+, *Am J Forensic Med Pathol* 16(3), 185 (spray)
  (1992): Landau O+, *JAMA* 268(13), 1686
  (1991): Marabini S+, *Eur Arch Otorhinolaryngol* 248(4), 191
  (1987): Jones LA+, *J Toxicol Clin Toxicol* 25(6), 483

Tooth pigmentation
  (1987): Schuurs AH+, *Oral Surg Oral Med Oral Pathol* 64(4), 427
    (with wine)

CAPTOPRIL

Synonym: ACE
Trade names: Captopen (Par); Captozide (Par)
Other common trade names: *Acenorm; Acepril; Adocor; APO-Capto; Captolane; Captoril; Lopirin; Lopril; Nu-Capto; Precaptil*
Indications: Hypertension
Category: Angiotensin-converting enzyme (ACE) inhibitor;
Antihypertensive
Half-life: <3 hours
**Clinically important, potentially hazardous interactions
with:** amiloride, spironolactone, triamterene

Capozide is captopril and hydrochlorothiazide

Reactions

Skin

Allergic reactions (sic)
  (2001): Martinez JC+, *Allergol Immunopathol* (Madr) 29(6), 279
  (1998): Lluch-Bernal M+, *Contact Dermatitis* 39, 316

Angioedema (<1%)
  (2002): Arzi H+, *Harefuah* 141(10), 869, 931 (tongue and
    oropharynax)
  (2001): Cohen EG+, *Ann Otol Rhinol Laryngol* 110(8), 701 (64
    cases)
  (1998): Smoger SH+, *South Med J* 91, 1060
  (1997): Brown NJ+, *JAMA* 278, 232
  (1997): Tisch M+, *Anaesthesiol Intensivmed Notfallmed
    Schmerzther* (German) 32, 122
  (1996): Ekborn A+, *Lakartidningen* (Swedish) 93, 468
  (1996): Pillans PI+, *Eur J Clin Pharmacol* 51, 123
  (1995): Bauwens LJ+, *Ned Tijdschr Geneeskd* (Dutch) 139, 674
  (1995): Kozel MM+, *Clin Exp Dermatol* 20, 60
  (1993): Chu TJ+, *Ann Intern Med* 118, 314
  (1993): Thompson T+, *Laryngoscope* 103, 10
  (1992): Diehl KL+, *Dtsch Med Wochenschr* (German)117, 727
  (1992): Dobroschke B+, *Anasthesiol Intensivmed Notfallmed
    Schmerzther* (German) 27, 510
  (1992): Hedner T+, *BMJ* 304, 941
  (1992): Jason DR, *J Forensic Sci* 37, 1418 (fatal)
  (1992): Sanchez-Hernandez J+, *An Med Interna* (Spanish) 9, 572
  (1991): Pek F, *HNO D* (German) 39, 410
  (1991): Roberts JR+, *Ann Emerg Med* 20, 555
  (1990): Cameron DI, *Can J Cardiol* 6, 265
  (1990): DiNardo LJ+, *Trans Pa Acad Ophthalmol Otolaryngol*
    42, 998
  (1990): Gannon TH+, *Laryngoscope* 100, 1156
  (1990): McAreavey D+, *Drugs* 40, 326
  (1990): Motel PJ, *J Am Acad Dermatol* 23, 124
  (1990): Seidman MD+, *Otolaryngol Head Neck Surg* 102, 727
  (1990): Zech J+, *HNO* (German) 38, 143
  (1989): Barna JS+, *Va Med* 116, 147
  (1989): Werber JL+, *Otolaryngol Head Neck Surg* 101, 96
  (1988): Brogden RN+, *Drugs* 36, 540
  (1988): Slater EE+, *JAMA* 260, 967 (0.1%)
  (1988): Wernze H, *Z Kardiol* (German) 77, 61
  (1987): Edwards IR+, *Br J Clin Pharmacol* 23, 529
  (1987): Ferner RE+, *BMJ* 294, 1119
  (1987): No Author, *Am J Med* 82 576
  (1987): Wood SM+, *BMJ* 294, 91
  (1986): Suarez M+, *Am J Med* 81, 336
  (1984): Jett GK, *Ann Emerg Med* 13, 489
  (1984): Materson BJ+, *Ann Intern Med* 144, 1947 (2.1%)
  (1984): Smit AJ+, *Clin Allergy* 14, 413 (2%)
  (1982): Vidt DG+, *N Engl J Med* 306, 214 (passim)
  (1980): Wilkin JK+, *Arch Dermatol* 116, 903 (15%)

Bullous eruption

(1989): Klein LE+, *Cutis* 44, 393
Bullous pemphigoid
(2000): Popescu C, Bucharest, Romania (from Internet)
(observation)
(1993): Fitzgerald DA, *Clin Exp Dermatol* 18, 196
(1989): Mallet L+, *Drug Intell Clin Pharm* 23, 63
Dermatitis (sic)
(2001): Martinez JC+, *Allergol Immunopathol (Madr)* 29(6), 279
(positive patch test)
(1990): Cnudde F+, *Contact Dermatitis* 23, 375
Erythroderma
(1989): Allegue F+, *Rev Clin Esp (Spanish)* 184, 210
(1985): Goodfield MJ+, *BMJ* 290, 1111
Exanthems (4–7%)
(1993): Fitzgerald DA, *Clin Exp Dermatol* 18, 196 (passim)
(1990): Cnudde F+, *Contact Dermatitis* 23, 375
(1990): McAreavey D+, *Drugs* 40, 326 (0.5–4%)
(1990): Motel PJ, *J Am Acad Dermatol* 23, 124
(1989): Clemens G+, *Verh Dtsch Ges Inn Med (German)* 95, 721
(1989): Gomez-Martino-Arroyo JR+, *Rev Clin Esp (Spanish)*
184, 497
(1988): Bretin N+, *Dermatologica* 177, 11
(1988): Brogden RN+, *Drugs* 36, 540 (0.5–4%)
(1988): Warner NJ+, *Drugs* 35 (Suppl 5) 89 (4–7%)
(1985): Goodfield MJ+, *BMJ* 290, 1111
(1985): Todd PA+, *Drugs* 31, 198
(1984): Smit AJ+, *Clin Allergy* 14, 413 (7%)
(1983): Romankiewicz JA+, *Drugs* 25, 6 (4.6%)
(1983): Steinman TI+, *Am J Med* 75, 154
(1982): Luderer JR+, *J Clin Pharm* 22, 151
(1982): Vidt DG+, *N Engl J Med* 306, 214 (passim)
(1980): Heel RC+, *Drugs* 20, 409 (8–14%)
(1980): Wilkin JK+, *Arch Dermatol* 116, 903
(1978): Gavras H+, *N Engl J Med* 298, 991 (10%)
Exfoliative dermatitis (<2%)
(1990): Motel PJ, *J Am Acad Dermatol* 23, 124
(1989): O'Neill PG+, *Tex Med* 85, 40
(1988): Lai KN+, *Singapore Med J* 29, 526
(1982): Solinger AM, *Cutis* 29, 437
Flushing (<1%)
(1989): Healy LA+, *N Engl J Med* 321, 763
(1987): Ferner RE+, *Br Med J Clin Res Ed* 294, 1119
Graft-versus-host reaction
(1998): Jappe U+, *Hautarzt (German)* 49, 126 (passim)
Kaposi's sarcoma
(1991): Larbre JP, *J Rheumatol* 18, 476
(1990): Puppin D+, *Lancet* 336, 1251
Lichen planus (pemphigoides)
(1986): Flageul B+, *Dermatologica* 173, 248
Lichenoid eruption
(2002): Feijoo A+, *World Congress Dermatol* Poster, 0100
(generalized)
(1996): Revenga-Arranz F+, *Rev Clin Esp (Spanish)* 196, 412
(1994): Phillips WG+, *Clin Exp Dermatol* 19, 317
(1992): Perez-Roldan E+, *Rev Clin Esp (Spanish)* 191, 501
(1992): Wong SS+, *Acta Derm Venereol (Stockh)* 72, 358
(1990): Pascual J+, *Nephron* 56, 110
(1989): Cox NH+, *Br J Dermatol* 120, 319
(1989): Rotstein E+, *Australas J Dermatol* 30, 9
(1988): Bretin N+, *Dermatologica* 177, 11
(1984): Smit AJ+, *Clin Allergy* 14, 413 (1%)
(1983): Bravard P+, *Ann Dermatol Venereol (French)* 110, 433
(1983): Bravard P+, *Presse Med (French)* 12, 577
(1983): Reinhardt LA+, *Cutis* 31, 98
Linear IgA bullous dermatosis
(2002): Cohen LM+, *J Am Acad Dermatol* 138, 29 (two cases)
(1998): Friedman IS+, *Int J Dermatol* 37, 608
(1994): Kuechle MK+, *J Am Acad Dermatol* 30, 187
(1989): Klein LE+, *Cutis* 44, 393

Lupus
(2002): Ratliff NB 3rd, *J Rheumatol* 29(8), 1807
Lupus erythematosus
(1995): Fernandez-Diaz ML+, *Lancet* 345, 398
(1994): Yung RL+, *Rheum Dis Clin North Am* 20, 61
(1993): Bertin P+, *Clin Exp Rheumatol* 11, 695
(1993): Pelayo M+, *Ann Pharmacother* 27, 1541
(1990): Sieber C+, *BMJ* 301, 669
(1985): Patri P+, *Acta Derm Venereol (Stockh)* 65, 447
Mycosis fungoides
(1995): Carroll J+, *Cutis* 56, 276 (pustular)
(1986): Furness PN+, *J Clin Pathol* 39, 902
Palmar–plantar pustulosis
(1995): Eriksen JG+, *Ugeskr Laeger (Danish)* 157, 3335
Pemphigus (<2%)
(1995): Butt A+, *Br J Dermatol* 132, 315
(1994): Kuechle MK+, *Mayo Clin Proc* 69, 1166
(1994): Trinidad-Paz JM+, *Rev Clin Esp (Spanish)* 194, 999
(1992): Kaplan RP+, *J Am Acad Dermatol* 26, 364
(1992): Pinto GM+, *J Am Acad Dermatol* 27, 281 (vegetans)
(1992): Ruocco V+, *Int J Dermatol* 31, 33
(1991): Beaulieu P+, *Ann Dermatol Venereol (French)* 118, 547
(1991): Korman NJ+, *J Invest Dermatol* 96, 273
(1990): Black AK+, *Br J Dermatol* 123, 277
(1990): Motel PJ, *J Am Acad Dermatol* 23, 124
(1990): Ruocco V+, *Arch Dermatol* 126, 965
(1988): Blanken R+, *Acta Derm Venereol (Stockh)* 68, 456
(1988): Bretin N+, *Dermatologica* 177, 11
(1987): Arnoux D+, *Ann Dermatol Venereol (French)* 114, 1241
(1987): Katz RA+, *Arch Dermatol* 123, 20
(1986): Ricci G+, *Recenti Prog Med (Italian)* 77, 321
(1985): Bernard P+, *Ann Dermatol Venereol (French)* 112, 661
(1982): Christeler A+, *Schweiz Med Wochenschr (German)*
112, 1483
(1982): Ruocco V+, *Arch Dermatol Res* 274, 123
(1981): Clement MI, *Arch Dermatol* 117, 525
(1980): Parfrey PS+, *BMJ* 281, 194
Pemphigus foliaceus
(2000): Ong CS+, *Australas J Dermatol* 41(4), 242
Penile ulcers
(1983): Romankiewicz JA+, *Drugs* 25, 6 (4.6%)
(1981): Nicholls MG+, *Ann Intern Med* 94, 695
Photosensitivity
(1994): Shelley WB+, *Cutis* 54, 70 (observation)
(1990): Motel PJ, *J Am Acad Dermatol* 23, 124
(1988): Mauduit G+, *Ann Dermatol Venereol (French)* 115, 167
Phototoxicity (<2%)
Pigmentation
(1990): Black AK+, *Br J Dermatol* 123, 277
(1987): O'Neill MB+, *BMJ* 295, 33
Pityriasis rosea (<2%)
(1990): Ghersetich I+, *G Ital Dermatol Venereol (Italian)* 125, 457
(1990): Motel PJ, *J Am Acad Dermatol* 23, 124
(1990): Wolf R+, *Dermatologica* 181, 51
(1988): Bretin N+, *Dermatologica* 177, 11
(1983): Reinhardt LA+, *Cutis* 31, 98
(1982): Wilkin JK+, *Arch Dermatol* 118, 186
Pruritus (4–7%)
(1992): Shelley WB+, *Cutis* 49, 391 (observation)
(1990): Motel PJ, *J Am Acad Dermatol* 23, 124
(1984): Materson BJ+, *Ann Intern Med* 144, 1947 (0.2%)
(1983): Daniel F+, *Ann Dermatol Venereol (French)* 110, 441
(10%)
(1983): Romankiewicz JA+, *Drugs* 25, 6 (4%)
(1983): Steinman TI+, *Am J Med* 75, 154
(1982): Liebau G, *Klin Wochenschr (German)* 60, 107
(1982): Vidt DG+, *N Engl J Med* 306, 214 (passim)
(1980): Luderer JR+, *Clin Res* 28, 589A
Psoriasis

(1995): Ikai K, *J Am Acad Dermatol* 32, 819
(1993): Coulter DM+, *N Z Med J* 106, 392
(1992): Shelley WB+, *Cutis* 50, 87 (observation)
(1990): Sieber C+, *BMJ* 301, 669
(1990): Wolf R+, *Dermatologica* 181, 51
(1987): Hamlet DW+, *BMJ* 295, 1352
(1987): Wolf R+, *Cutis* 40, 162
(1986): Hauschild TT+, *Hautarzt* (German) 37, 274

Purpura
(1989): Grosbois B+, *BMJ* 298, 189

Rash (sic) (4–7%)
(1990): Kahan A+, *Clin Pharmacol Ther* 47, 483
(1985): Jenkins AC+, *J Cardiovasc Pharmacol* 7, S96
(1984): Kubo SH+, *Ann Intern Med* 100, 616
(1984): Martin MF+, *Lancet* 1, 1325
(1983): Romankiewicz JA+, *Drugs* 25, 6
(1983): Rotmensch HH+, *Pharmacotherapy* 3, 131
(1983): Steinman TI+, *Am J Med* 75, 154
(1982): Liebau G, *Klin Wochenschr* (German) 60, 107
(1982): Rosendorff C, *S Afr Med J* 62, 593
(1981): Luderer JR+, *Am J Med* 71, 493

Stevens–Johnson syndrome
(1984): Pennell DJ+, *Lancet* 1, 463 (fatal)

Toxic epidermal necrolysis
(2003): Alkurtass DA+, *Ann Pharmacother* 37(3), 380
(1999): Winfred RI+, *South Med J* 92, 918
(1983): Sala F+, *G Ital Dermatol Venereol* (Italian) 118, 89

Urticaria
(1996): Pillans PI+, *Eur J Clin Pharmacol* 51, 123
(1993): Fitzgerald DA, *Clin Exp Dermatol* 18, 196 (passim)
(1988): Bretin N+, *Dermatologica* 177, 11
(1988): Slater EE+, *JAMA* 260, 967
(1987): Wood SM+, *BMJ* 294, 91
(1985): Goodfield MJD+, *BMJ* 290, 1111
(1984): Materson BJ+, *Ann Intern Med* 144, 1947 (1.4%)
(1984): Smit AJ+, *Clin Allergy* 14, 413 (7%)
(1980): Wilkin JK+, *Arch Dermatol* 116, 902

Vasculitis
(1994): Dorman RL+, *AJR Am J Roentgenol* 163, 840
(1990): Black AK+, *Br J Dermatol* 123, 277 (fatal)
(1988): Lotti T+, *G Ital Dermatol Venereol* (Italian) 123, 657
(1988): Miralles R+, *Ann Intern Med* 109, 514
(1987): Laaban J+, *European Heart J* 8, 319
(1984): Goodfield MJD+, *Lancet* 2, 517
(1984): Smit AJ+, *Clin Allergy* 14, 413

Xerosis
(1983): Smit AJ+, *Nephron* 34, 196

Hair

Hair – alopecia (<2%)
(1994): Shelley WB+, *Cutis* 52, 264 (observation)
(1990): Motel PJ, *J Am Acad Dermatol* 23, 124
(1984): Leaker B+, *Aust N Z J Med* 14, 866
(1984): Smit AJ+, *Clin Allergy* 14, 413 (3%)
(1983): Smit AJ+, *Nephron* 34, 196

Nails

Nails – dystrophy
(1984): Brueggemeyer CD+, *Lancet* 1, 1352
(1983): Smit AJ+, *Nephron* 34, 196

Nails – onycholysis
(1986): Borders JV, *Ann Intern Med* 105, 305
(1984): Brueggemeyer CD+, *Lancet* 1, 1352

Other

Ageusia (2–4%)
(1997): Acanfora D+, *Am J Ther* 4, 181
(1993): Fitzgerald DA, *Clin Exp Dermatol* 18, 196 (passim)
(1988): Rumboldt Z+, *Int J Clin* 8(3), 181
(1987): Edwards IR+, *Br J Clin Pharmacol* 23, 529

(1987): O'Connor DT+, *J Clin Hypertens* 3(4), 405
(1984): Martin MF+, *Lancet* 1, 1325
(1983): Smit AJ+, *Nephron* 34, 196
(1982): Liebau G, *Klin Wochenschr* (German) 60, 107
(1982): Vidt DG+, *N Engl J Med* 306, 214 (passim)
(1979): McNeil JJ+, *BMJ* 6204, 1555
(1979): Vlasses PH+, *Lancet* 2, 526

Anaphylactoid reactions (during hemodialysis)
(2002): Peces R, *Nephrol Dial Transplant* 17(10), 1859

Aphthous stomatitis (<2%)
(1983): Daniel F+, *Ann Dermatol Venereol* (French) 110, 441
(1982): Vidt DG+, *N Engl J Med* 306, 214 (passim)
(1980): Heel RC+, *Drugs* 20, 409
(1979): Seedat YK, *Lancet* 2, 1297

Cough
(2001): Adigun AQ+, *West Afr J Med* 20(1), 46–7
(2001): Lee SC+, *Hypertension* 38(2), 166

Death

Dysgeusia (2–4%) (metallic or salty taste)
(2000): Zervakis J+, *Physiol Behav* 68, 405
(1993): Boyd I, *Lancet* 342, 304
(1993): Zazgornik J+, *Lancet* 341, 1542
(1990): Kahan A+, *Clin Pharmacol Ther* 47, 483
(1985): Jenkins AC+, *J Cardiovasc Pharmacol* 7, S96
(1985): Mauersberger H+, *Lancet* 1, 517
(1983): Kayanakis JG+, *Arch Mal Coeur Vaiss* (French) 76, 1065
(1983): Romankiewicz JA+, *Drugs* 25, 6
(1979): McNeil JJ+, *BMJ* 6204, 1555

Glossitis
(1989): Drucker CR+, *Arch Dermatol* 125, 1437 (atrophic)
(1983): Romankiewicz JA+, *Drugs* 25, 6
(1981): Nicholls MG+, *Ann Intern Med* 94, 659

Glossopyrosis
(1989): Drucker CR+, *Arch Dermatol* 125, 1437

Gynecomastia
(2000): Hugues FC+, *Ann Med Interne (Paris)* (French) 151, 10 (passim)
(1990): Nakamura Y+, *BMJ* 300, 541
(1988): Markusse HM+, *BMJ* 296, 1262

Headache

Lymphadenopathy
(1981): Aberg H+, *BMJ* 283, 1297

Myalgia

Oral mucosal eruption
(1989): Firth NA+, *Oral Surg Oral Med Oral Pathol* 67, 41 (lichenoid)
(1985): Todd PA+, *Drugs* 31, 198
(1980): Heel RC+, *Drugs* 20, 409

Oral ulceration
(2000): Madinier I+, *Ann Med Interne (Paris)* (French) 151, 248
(1993): Fitzgerald DA, *Clin Exp Dermatol* 18, 196 (passim)
(1982): Viraben R+, *Arch Dermatol* 118, 959

Paresthesias (<2%)

Pseudolymphoma
(1986): Furness PN+, *J Clin Pathol* 39, 902
(1980): Wilkin JK+, *Arch Dermatol* 116, 902

Scalded mouth (sic)
(1982): Vlasses PH+, *BMJ* 284, 1672

Tongue ulceration
(1982): Viraben R+, *Arch Dermatol* 118, 959
(1982): Vlasses PH+, *BMJ* 284, 1672 (passim)
(1981): Nicholls MG+, *Ann Intern Med* 94, 659

Xerostomia (<2%)

CARAWAY

Scientific names: *Apium carvi; Carum carvi*
Family: Apiaceae Umbelliferae
Trade and other common trade names: *Caraway seed; Carvene; Kummel*
Category: Analgesic; Anti-inflammatory; Antimicrobial; Antineoplastic; Antipyretic; Carminative; Stimulant
Purported indications: Hypotensive, dyspepsia, hysteria, tonic, stomachic. flatulent indigestion, flatulent colic of infants, fragrance, flavoring in foods, toothpaste, and cosmetics
Half-life: N/A

Reactions

Skin

Adverse effects (sic)
  (1999): Madisch A+, *Arzneimittelforschung* 49(11), 925
  (1996): May B+, *Arzneimittelforschung* 46(12), 1149
Allergic reactions (sic)
  (1981): Niinimaki A+, *Allergy* 36(7), 487
Dermatitis
  (2003): Ali BH+, *Phytother Res* 17(4), 299
Rhinoconjunctivitis
  (2002): Garcia-Gonzalez JJ+, *Ann Allergy Asthma Immunol* 88(5), 518
Urticaria
  (1985): Wuthrich B+, *Schweiz Med Wochenschr* 115(11), 258

Other

Anaphylactoid reactions
  (1985): Wuthrich B+, *Schweiz Med Wochenschr* 115(11), 258
Cough
  (1988): Zuskin E+, *Environ Res* 47(1), 95 (occupational)
Hypersensitivity
  (1984): Wuthrich B+, *Dtsch Med Wochenschr* 109(25), 981 (26%)
Sensitivity
  (2002): Moneret-Vautrin DA+, *Allerg Immunol (Paris* (Paris) 34(4), 135 (2%)

CARBAMAZEPINE

Trade names: Carbatrol (Shire); Tegretol (Novartis)
Other common trade names: *Apo-Carbamazepine; Atreol; Foxsalepsin; Kodapan; Lexin; Mazepine; Sirtal; Tegretol XR; Teril; Timonil*
Indications: Epilepsy, pain or trigeminal neuralgia
Category: Anticonvulsant; Antimanic; Antineuralgic; Antipsychotic
Half-life: 18–55 hours
Clinically important, potentially hazardous interactions with: acetylcysteine, adenosine, aprepitant, aripiprazole, **caffeine**, charcoal, clarithromycin, clorazepate, clozapine, diltiazem, doxacurium, erythromycin, felodipine, imatinib, midazolam, **St John's wort**, troleandomycin, verapamil, voriconazole

Reactions

Skin

Acne keloid
  (1990): Grunwald MH+, *Int J Dermatol* 29, 559
Acute generalized exanthematous pustulosis (AGEP)

  (1999): Lachgar T, *Allerg Immunol* (Paris) (French) 31, 151
  (1999): Poster Exhibit #163, AAD Meeting, March 1999 (Reported by ED and WB Shelley)
  (1996): Wolkenstein P+, *Contact Dermatitis* 35, 234
  (1995): Moreau A+, *Int J Dermatol* 34, 263 (passim)
  (1991): Roujeau J-C+, *Arch Dermatol* 127, 1333
Adverse effects (sic)
  (2003): Matthews R+, *Br Dent J* 194(3), 121
Allergic reactions (sic)
  (1999): Pasmans SG+, *Allergy* 54, 649
  (1995): Tijhuis GJ+, *Ned Tijdschr Geneeskd* (Dutch) 139, 2265 (42 cases)
  (1993): Beran RG, *Epilepsia* 34, 163
  (1992): Dzianott A+, *Wiad Lek* (Polish) 45, 465
  (1985): Moore NC+, *Am J Psychiatry* 142, 974
Angioedema (<1%)
  (2001): Grieco A+, *Eur J Gastroenterol Hepatol* 13(8), 973
  (1977): Houwerzijl J+, *Clin Exp Immunol* 29, 272
  (1971): Virolainen M, *Clin Exp Immunol* 9, 429
  (1967): Livingston S+, *JAMA* 200, 204
Ankle edema
Bullous eruption (<1%)
  (2001): Grieco A+, *Eur J Gastroenterol Hepatol* 13(8), 973
  (1990): Gebauer K+, *Australas J Dermatol* 31, 89 (passim)
  (1988): Warnock JK+, *Am J Psychiatry* 145, 425
  (1983): Godden DJ+, *Postgrad Med J* 59, 336
Collagen disease (sic)
  (1966): Simpson JR, *BMJ* 2, 1434
Dermatitis (sic)
  (1992): Duhra P+, *Contact Dermatitis* 27, 325
  (1991): Ljunggren B+, *Contact Dermatitis* 24, 259
  (1991): Rodriguez-Mosquera M+, *Contact Dermatitis* 25, 137
  (1989): Malanin G+, *Duodecim* (Finnish) 105, 784
  (1989): Terui T+, *Contact Dermatitis* 20, 260
  (1981): Roberts DL+, *Arch Dermatol* 117, 273
  (1967): Arieff AJ+, *Dis Nerv Syst* 28, 820
Diaphoresis (1–10%)
Eczema (sic)
  (1999): Ozkaya-Bayazit E+, *J Eur Acad Dermatol Venereol* 12, 182
  (1992): Duhra P+, *Contact Dermatitis* 27, 325
Edema
Edema of feet
  (2002): Valikhani M+, *World Congress Dermatol* Poster, 0131
  (1998): Heyer G+, *Hautarzt* (German) 49, 123
Eosinophilic pustular folliculitis (Ofuji's disease)
  (1998): Mizoguchi S+, *J Am Acad Dermatol* 38, 641
Epidermolysis bullosa
  (1992): Kong LN, *Chung Hua Hu Li Tsa Chih* (Chinese) 27, 495
Erythema
  (2001): Gaida-Hommernick B+, *Epilepsia* 42(6), 793
Erythema multiforme
  (2003): Emmet SD, Solan Beach, CA (from Internet) (observation)
  (1999): Frederickson K (from Internet) (observation)
  (1994): Friedmann PS+, *Arch Dermatol* 130, 598
  (1993): Alanko K, *Contact Dermatitis* 29, 254
  (1993): Bruynzeel I+, *Br J Dermatol* 129, 45
  (1992): Chevenet C+, *Ann Dermatol Venereol* (French) 119, 929
  (1989): Alanko K+, *Acta Derm Venereol* (Stockh) 69, 223
  (1989): Busch RL, *N Engl J Med* 321, 692
  (1988): McDanal CE, *J Clin Psychiatr* 49, 369
  (1988): Warnock JK+, *Am J Psychiatry* 145, 425
  (1987): Fawcett RG, *J Clin Psychiatry* 48, 416
  (1986): Green ST, *Clin Neuropharmacol* 9, 561
  (1985): Delafuente JC, *Drug Intell Clin Pharm* 19, 114
  (1985): Patterson JF, *J Clin Psychopharmacol* 5, 185
  (1984): Meisel S+, *Clin Pharm* 3, 15
  (1975): Böttiger LE+, *Acta Med Scand* 198, 229
Erythema nodosum (<1%)

Erythroderma
  (2002): Kansky A+, *Acta Dermatoven* 11(3), 105
  (2000): Bugatti L (Italy) (from Internet) (observation)
  (1998): Tayoro J+, *Therapie* 53, 513
  (1996): Okuyama R+, *J Dermatol* 23, 489
  (1995): Koga T+, *Contact Dermatitis* 33, 275
  (1993): Blasco-Sarramian A+, *An Med Interna* (Spanish) 10, 341
  (1990): Ruiz-Ezquerro JJ+, *An Med Interna* (Spanish) 31, 89
  (1989): Romaguera C+, *Contact Dermatitis* 20, 304
  (1987): Granier F+, *Rev Med Interne* (French) 8, 206
  (1986): Silva R+, *Contact Dermatitis* 15, 254
  (1982): Chennebault JM+, *Therapie* (French) 37, 106
  (1980): Gaulier A+, *Nouv Presse Med* (French) 9, 1388
Exanthems (>5%)
  (2002): Kansky A+, *Acta Dermatoven* 11(3), 105
  (2002): Maradeix S+, *World Congress Dermatol* Poster, 0112
  (2000): Thaler D, Monona, WI (from Internet) (observation)
  (1999): Lombardi SM+, *Ann Pharmacother* 33, 571
  (1998): Nathan D+, *J Am Acad Dermatol* 38, 806
  (1997): Hyson C+, *Can J Neurol Sci* 24, 245
  (1995): Wolkenstein P+, *Arch Dermatol* 131, 544
  (1993): Alanko K, *Contact Dermatitis* 29, 254
  (1993): Hermle L+, *Nervenarzt* (German) 64, 208 (generalized)
  (1993): Konishi T+, *Eur J Pediatr* 152, 605
  (1990): Garavelli PL+, *Minerva Med* (Italian) 81, 115
  (1990): Gebauer K+, *Australas J Dermatol* 31, 89 (passim)
  (1989): Eames P, *Lancet* 1, 509
  (1988): Shear NH+, *J Clin Invest* 82, 1826
  (1988): Warnock JK+, *Am J Psychiatry* 145, 425
  (1984): Chadwick D+, *J Neurol Neurosurg Psychiatry* 47, 642
     (17%)
  (1982): Breathnach SM+, *Clin Exp Dermatol* 7, 585 (4%)
  (1981): Sillanpää M, *Acta Neurol Scand* 64 (Suppl 88), 145
  (1981): Taylor MW+, *Practitioner* 225, 219
  (1977): Houwerzijl J+, *Clin Exp Immunol* 29, 272
  (1974): Livingston S+, *Dis Nerv Syst* 35, 103 (2.7%)
  (1972): Levantine A+, *Br J Dermatol* 87, 646 (3–4%)
  (1971): Virolainen M, *Clin Exp Immunol* 9, 429
Exfoliative dermatitis
  (2001): Dintiman B, Fairfax, VA (from Internet)
  (1999): Lombardi SM+, *Ann Pharmacother* 33, 571
  (1996): Sigurdsson V+, *J Am Acad Dermatol* 35, 53
  (1996): Troost RJ+, *Pediatr Dermatol* 13, 316
  (1995): Bahamdan KA+, *Int J Dermatol* 34, 661
  (1995): Corazza M+, *Contact Dermatitis* 33, 447
  (1995): Koga T+, *Contact Dermatitis* 32, 181
  (1993): Alanko K, *Contact Dermatitis* 29, 254
  (1991): Blin O+, *Therapie* (French) 46, 91
  (1990): Gebauer K+, *Australas J Dermatol* 31, 89 (passim)
  (1989): Alanko K+, *Acta Derm Venereol* (Stockh) 69, 223
  (1989): Romaguera C+, *Contact Dermatitis* 20, 304
  (1989): Vaillant L+, *Arch Dermatol* 125, 299
  (1988): Cox NH+, *Postgrad Med J* 64, 249
  (1987): Gimenez Garcia RM+, *Rev Clin Esp* (Spanish) 181, 542
  (1987): Granier F+, *Rev Med Interne* 8, 206
  (1985): Camarasa JG, *Contact Dermatitis* 12, 49
  (1984): Shuttleworth D+, *Clin Exp Dermatol* 9, 421
  (1982): Reed MD+, *Clin Pharm* 1, 78
  (1981): Roberts DL+, *Arch Dermatol* 117, 273
  (1977): Houwerzijl J+, *Clin Exp Immunol* 29, 272
  (1968): Ford GR+, *N Z Med J* 68, 386
Facial edema
  (2002): Kansky A+, *Acta Dermatoven* 11(3), 105
Fixed eruption (<1%)
  (1997): Chan HL+, *J Am Acad Dermatol* 36, 259
  (1997): de Argila D+, *Allergy* 52, 1039
  (1993): Alanko K, *Contact Dermatitis* 29, 254
  (1990): Gaffoor PMA+, *Cutis* 45, 242 (passim)
  (1989): Stubb S+, *Br J Dermatol* 120, 583
  (1988): Bhariga JC+, *Sex Transm Dis* 15, 177

  (1988): Warnock JK+, *Am J Psychiatry* 145, 425
  (1985): Kauppinen K+, *Br J Dermatol* 112, 575
  (1984): Shuttleworth D+, *Clin Exp Dermatol* 9, 424
Lichenoid eruption
  (1994): Thompson DF+, *Pharmacotherapy* 14, 561
  (1990): Atkin SL+, *Clin Exp Dermatol* 15, 382
  (1990): Gebauer K+, *Australas J Dermatol* 31, 89 (passim)
  (1989): Ohtsuyama M+, *Nishinihon J Dermatol* (Japanese)
     51, 958
  (1988): Yasuda S+, *Photodermatology* 5, 206 (photosensitive)
  (1981): Roberts DL+, *Arch Dermatol* 117, 273
Linear IgA bullous dermatosis
  (2002): Cohen LM+, *J Am Acad Dermatol* 46(2), S32
Lupus erythematosus
  (1998): Bachmeyer C+, *Presse Med* (French) 27, 966
  (1998): Toepfer M+, *Eur J Clin Pharmacol* 54, 193 (late onset)
  (1997): Milesi-Lecat AM+, *Mayo Clin Proc* 72, 1145
  (1997): Reiffers-Mettelock J+, *Dermatology* 195, 306
  (1996): Ghorayeb I+, *Rev Med Interne* (French) 17, 503
  (1993): Drory VE+, *Clin Neuropharmacol* 16, 19 (passim)
  (1993): Ohashi T+, *Rinsho Shinkeigaku* (Japanese) 33, 1094
  (1992): Boon DM+, *Ned Tijdschr Geneeskd* (Dutch) 136, 2085
     (disseminated)
  (1992): Kanno T+, *Intern Med* 31, 1303
  (1992): Schmidt S+, *Br J Psychiatry* 161, 560
  (1992): Yust I+, *Intern Med* 31, 1303
  (1991): De Giorgio CM+, *Epilepsia* 32, 128
  (1991): Jain KK, *Drug Saf* 6, 350
  (1990): Gebauer K+, *Australas J Dermatol* 31, 89 (passim)
  (1990): Oner A+, *Clin Neurol Neurosurg* 92, 261
  (1989): Drory VE+, *Clin Neuropharmacol* 12, 115
  (1987): Alballa S+, *J Rheumatol* 14, 599
  (1986): Leyh F+, *Z Haut* (German) 61, 611
  (1985): Bateman DE, *Br Med J Clin Res Ed* 291, 632
  (1985): *Br Med J Clin Res Ed* 291, 1125
  (1985): Lovisetto P+, *Recenti Prog Med* (Italian) 76, 84
  (1985): McNicholl B, *BMJ* 291, 1126
  (1983): Kolstee HJ, *Ned Tijdschr Geneeskd* (Dutch) 127, 1588
  (1976): Takigawa M+, *Arch Dermatol* 112, 845
  (1974): Livingston S+, *Dis Nerv Syst* 35, 103 (2.7%)
  (1969): Gayford JJ+, *Proc R Soc Med* 62, 615
  (1967): Livingston S+, *JAMA* 200, 204
  (1966): Simpson JR, *BMJ* 2, 1434
Lymphoma
  (2003): Cohen Y+, *Isr Med Assoc J* 5(6), 457
  (2001): Di Lernia V+, *Arch Dermatol* 137, 675
Mucocutaneous lymph node syndrome (Kawasaki syndrome)
  (1990): Gebauer K+, *Australas J Dermatol* 31, 89 (passim)
  (1987): Hicks RA+, *Pediatr Infect Dis J* 7, 525
Mycosis fungoides
  (1991): Rijlaarsdam U+, *J Am Acad Dermatol* 24(2 Pt 1), 219
     (with phenytoin)
  (1991): Rijlaarsdam U+, *J Am Acad Dermatol* 24, 216
  (1990): Welykyi S+, *J Cutan Pathol* 17, 111
Pemphigus
  (2003): Patterson CR+, *Clin Exp Dermatol* 28(1), 98
Periorbital edema
  (2001): Dintiman B, Fairfax, VA (from Internet) (observation)
Petechiae
  (1993): Konishi T+, *Eur J Pediatr* 152, 605
Photosensitivity
  (2001): Hebert AA+, *J Clin Psychiatry* 62(suppl 14), 22
  (1991): Ljunggren B+, *Contact Dermatitis* 24, 259
  (1990): Gebauer K+, *Australas J Dermatol* 31, 89 (passim)
  (1989): Terui T+, *Contact Dermatitis* 20, 260
  (1988): Warnock JK+, *Am J Psychiatry* 145, 425
  (1988): Yasuda S+, *Photodermatology* 5, 206
  (1986): Silva R+, *Contact Dermatitis* 15, 54
  (1981): Sillanpää M, *Acta Neurol Scand* 64 (Suppl 88), 145

(1972): Levantine A+, *Br J Dermatol* 87, 646

Pigmentation

Pruritus (<1%)
(2002): Kansky A+, *Acta Dermatoven* 11(3), 105
(2001): Gaida-Hommernick B+, *Epilepsia* 42(6), 793
(1969): Davis EH, *Headache* 9, 77
(1967): Livingston S+, *JAMA* 200, 204
(1964): Spillane D, *Practitioner* 192, 71

Psoriasis
(1994): Brenner S+, *Isr J Med Sci* 30, 283

Purpura
(2001): Hebert AA+, *J Clin Psychiatry* 62(suppl 14), 22
(1988): Warnock JK+, *Am J Psychiatry* 145, 425
(1984): Staughton RCD+, *J R Soc Med* 77 (Suppl 4), 6
(1972): Levantine A+, *Br J Dermatol* 87, 646
(1969): Peterkin GAG+, *Practitioner* 202, 117
(1967): Harman RRM, *Br J Dermatol* 79, 500
(1967): Livingston S+, *JAMA* 200, 204
(1964): Spillane D, *Practitioner* 192, 71

Pustules
(1991): Kleier RS+, *Arch Dermatol* 127, 1361
(1990): Gebauer K+, *Australas J Dermatol* 31, 89 (passim)
(1988): Commens CA+, *Arch Dermatol* 124, 178
(1984): Staughton RCD+, *J R Soc Med* 77 (Suppl 4), 6

Rash (sic) (>10%)
(1999): van Ginneken EE+, *Neth Med J* 54, 158
(1998): Cates M+, *Ann Pharmacother* 32, 884
(1996): Boyle N+, *Am J Psychiatry* 152, 1234
(1996): Puig L+, *Contact Dermatitis* 34, 435
(1994): Kramlinger KG+, *J Clin Psychopharmacol* 14, 408 (12%)
(1993): Hosoda N+, *Jpn J Psychiatry Neurol* 47, 300
(1993): Konishi T+, *Eur J Pediatr* 152, 605
(1991): Frederick TE, *Neurology* 41, 1328
(1991): Murphy JM+, *Neurology* 41, 144
(1990): Garavelli PL+, *Minerva Med* (Italian) 81, 115
(1983): Ponte CD, *Drug Intell Clin Pharm* 17, 642
(1983): Vick NA, *N Engl J Med* 309, 1193

Schamberg's disease

Sheet-like erythema

Side effects (sic)
(1994): Jones M+, *Dermatology* 188, 18 (4%)
(1967): Livingston S+, *JAMA* 200, 204 (4.5%)

Stevens–Johnson syndrome (1–10%)
(2002): Garcia M+, *Dig Dis Sci* 47(1), 177
(2001): Duggal HS+, *J Assoc Physicians India* 49, 591
(2001): Hebert AA+, *J Clin Psychiatry* 62(suppl14), 22
(2000): Straussberg R+, *Pediatr Neurol* 22, 231
(2000): Suarez Moro R+, *An Med Interna* (Spanish) 17, 105
(1999): Dhar S+, *Dermatology* 199, 194
(1999): Petter G+, *Hautarzt* (German) 50, 884
(1999): Ruble R+, *CNS Drugs* 12, 215
(1999): Rzany B+, *Lancet* 353, 2190
(1995): Huang SC+, *Gen Hosp Psychiatry* 17, 458
(1995): Hughes-Davies L, *N Engl J Med* 332, 959
(1995): Keating A+, *Ann Pharmacother* 29, 538
(1995): Wolkenstein P+, *Arch Dermatol* 131, 544
(1993): Konishi T+, *Eur J Pediatr* 152, 605
(1993): Leenutaphong V+, *Int J Dermatol* 32, 428
(1993): Pagliaro LA+, *Hosp Community Psychiatry* 44, 999
(1993): Server Climent M, *Aten Primaria* (Spanish) 11, 377
(1992): Chevenet C+, *Ann Dermatol Venereol* (French) 119, 929 (with brain irradiation)
(1990): Gebauer K+, *Australas J Dermatol* 31, 89 (passim)
(1990): Hoang-Xuan K+, *Neurology* 40, 1144 (with cranial irradiation)
(1990): Khe HX+, *Neurology* 40, 1144
(1990): Roustan G+, *Actas Dermosifiliogr* (Spanish) 81, 775
(1990): Wong KE, *Singapore Med J* 31, 432
(1989): Alanko K+, *Acta Derm Venereol* (Stockh) 69, 223

(1988): McDanal CE, *J Clin Psychiatr* 49, 369
(1988): Warnock JK+, *Am J Psychiatry* 145, 425
(1987): Fawcett RG, *J Clin Psychiatry* 48, 416
(1975): Böttiger LE+, *Acta Med Scand* 198, 229 (4 of 77 cases)
(1965): Coombs BW, *Med J Aust* 1, 895
(1965): Inglis W, *Med J Aust* 2, 94

Toxic epidermal necrolysis (1–10%)
(2002): Correia O+, *Arch Dermatol* 138, 29 (2 cases)
(2002): Jackel R+, *Anaesthesist* 51(10), 815
(2002): Kansky A+, *Acta Dermatoven* 11(3), 105
(2001): Udawat H+, *J Assoc Physicians India* 49, 918
(1999): Dhar S+, *Dermatology* 199, 194
(1999): Egan CA+, *J Am Acad Dermatol* 40, 458
(1999): Petter G+, *Hautarzt* (German) 50, 884
(1999): Ruble R+, *CNS Drugs* 12, 215
(1999): Rzany B+, *Lancet* 353, 2190
(1997): Belgodere X+, *Arch Pediatr* (French) 4, 1020
(1997): Jarrett P+, *Clin Exp Dermatol* 22, 146
(1996): Blum L+, *J Am Acad Dermatol* 34, 1088
(1995): Sterker M+, *Int J Clin Pharmacol Ther* 33, 595
(1995): Urbanowski S+, *Wiad Lek* (Polish) 48, 154
(1995): Wolkenstein P+, *Arch Dermatol* 131, 544
(1994): Friedmann PS+, *Arch Dermatol* 130, 598
(1993): Correia O+, *Dermatology* 186, 32
(1993): Leenutaphong V+, *Int J Dermatol* 32, 428
(1993): Pagliaro LA+, *Hospital and Community Psychiatry* 44, 999
(1992): Park BK+, *Br J Clin Pharmacol* 34. 377
(1992): Weller M+, *Am J Psychiatry* 149, 1114
(1992): Weller M+, *Nervenarzt* (German) 63, 308
(1991): Sakellariou G+, *Int J Artif Organs* 14, 634
(1990): Gebauer K+, *Australas J Dermatol* 31, 89 (passim)
(1990): Roujeau JC+, *Arch Dermatol* 126, 37
(1988): Shear NH+, *J Clin Invest* 82, 1826
(1987): Guillaume JC+, *Arch Dermatol* 123, 1166
(1986): Rusciani L+, *G Ital Dermatol Venereol* (Italian) 121, 149
(1984): Husegaard HC+, *Ugeskr Laeger* (Danish) 146, 2784
(1984): Staughton RCD+, *J R Soc Med* 77 (Suppl 4), 6
(1982): Breathnach SM+, *Clin Exp Dermatol* 7, 585
(1977): Houwerzijl J+, *Clin Exp Immunol* 29, 272
(1976): Mutina ES+, *Klin Med Mosk* (Russian) 54, 124
(1972): Carli-Basset C+, *Sem Hop* (French) 48, 497

Toxic pustuloderma (sic) (probably AGEP [ed])
(1990): Gebauer K+, *Australas J Dermatol* 31, 89
(1988): Commens CA+, *Arch Dermatol* 124, 178
(1984): Staughton RCD+, *J R Soc Med* 77 (Suppl 4), 6

Toxic-allergic shock (sic)
(1979): Rummel GL, *ZFA* (Stuttgart) 55, 627

Toxicoderma (sic)
(1983): Rozov VD+, *Vestn Dermatol Venerol* (Russian) September, 48

Urticaria
(2001): Hebert AA+, *J Clin Psychiatry* 62(suppl 14), 22
(1993): Alanko K, *Contact Dermatitis* 29, 254
(1993): Konishi T+, *Eur J Pediatr* 152, 605
(1990): Gebauer K+, *Australas J Dermatol* 31, 89 (passim)
(1988): Warnock JK+, *Am J Psychiatry* 145, 425
(1987): Johannessen AC+, *Ugeskr Laeger* (Danish) 149, 376
(1984): Staughton RCD+, *J R Soc Med* 77 (Suppl 4), 6
(1977): Houwerzijl J+, *Clin Exp Immunol* 29, 272
(1976): Al-Ubaidy SS+, *Br J Oral Surg* 13, 289 (4.2%)
(1969): Rull JA+, *Diabetologia* 5, 215 (6.6%)
(1967): Arieff AJ+, *Dis Nerv Syst* 28, 820
(1964): Spillane D, *Practitioner* 192, 71

Vasculitis
(1993): Drory VE+, *Clin Neuropharmacol* 16, 19 (passim)
(1990): Gebauer K+, *Australas J Dermatol* 31, 89 (passim)
(1987): Harats N+, *J Neurol Neurosurg Psychiatry* 50, 1241
(1978): Nieme KM+, *Acta Derm Venereol* (Stockh) 58, 337
(1967): Harman RRM, *Br J Dermatol* 79, 500

Hair

Hair – alopecia
(2000): Mercke Y+, *Ann Clin Psychiatry* 12, 35 (~6%)
(1997): Ikeda A+, *J Neurol Neurosurg Psychiatry* 63, 549
(1996): McKinney PA+, *Ann Clin Psychiatry* 8, 183
(1988): Warnock JK+, *Am J Psychiatry* 145, 425
(1985): Shuper A+, *Drug Intell Clin Pharm* 19, 924
(1982): Breathnach SM+, *Clin Exp Dermatol* 7, 585

Nails

Nails – discoloration (bluish-black)
(1989): Mishra D+, *Int J Dermatol* 28, 460
Nails – hypoplasia
(1985): Niesen M+, *Neuropediatrics* 16, 167
Nails – lichen planus
(1989): Ohtsuyama M+, *Nishinihon J Dermatol* (Japanese) 51, 958
Nails – loss (sic)
(1982): Breathnach SM+, *Clin Exp Dermatol* 7, 585
Nails – onychomadesis
(1989): Mishra D+, *Int J Dermatol* 28, 460

Other

Acute intermittent porphyria
(1984): Doss M+, *Lancet* 1, 1026
(1983): Liawah AC+, *Lancet* 1, 1442
(1983): Rideout JM+, *Lancet* 2, 464
(1983): Shanley BC, *Lancet* 1, 1229
(1983): Yeung Laiwah AACY+, *Lancet* 1, 790
Anticonvulsant hypersensitivity syndrome
(2003): Bin-Nakhi HA+, *Med Princ Pract* 12(3), 197
(2002): Metin A+, *World Congress Dermatol* Poster, 0116
(2002): Romero Maldonado N+, *Eur J Dermatol* 12(5), 503
(2000): Moore, SJ+, *J Med Genet* 37, 489
(2000): Popescu C, Bucharest, Romania (from Internet) (observation)
Death
(2002): Correia O+, *Arch Dermatol* 138, 29
DRESS syndrome
(2002): Maradeix S+, *World Congress Dermatol* Poster, 0112
(2001): Descamps V+, *Arch Dermatol* 137, 301 (5 patients)
(2001): Queyrel V+, *Rev Med Interne* 22(6), 582
Dyschromatopsia
(2000): Nousiainen I+, *Ophthalmology* 107, 884
Dysgeusia
(1976): Rollin H, *Laryngol Rhinol Otol* (Stuttgart) (German) 55, 873
Fetal anticonvulsant syndrome
(2000): Moore SJ+, *J Med Genet* 37, 489
Glossitis
Headache
Hypersensitivity*
(2002): Kaur S+, *Pediatr Dermatol* 19(2), 142
(2001): Bessmertny O+, *Ann Pharmacother* 35(5), 533
(2001): Nashed MH+, *Pharmacotherapy* 21(4), 502
(2001): Sekine N+, *JAMA* 285(9), 1153
(2000): Bugatti L, Italy (from Internet) (observation)
(2000): Elstner S+, *Fortschr Neurol Psychiatr* (German) 68, 188
(2000): Ivry S+, *Harefuah* (Hebrew) 138, 545
(2000): Straussberg R+, *Pediatr Neurol* 22, 231
(1999): Balasbrananian S+, *Indian Pediatr* 36, 98
(1999): Brown KL+, *Dev Med Child Neurol* 41, 267
(1999): Hamer HM+, *Seizure* 8, 190
(1999): Lombardi SM+, *Ann Pharmacother* 33, 571
(1999): Mesec A+, *J Neurol Neurosurg Psychiatry* 66, 249
(1999): Moss DM+, *J Emerg Med* 17, 503
(1998): Dertinger S+, *J Hepatol* 28, 356
(1998): Schlienger RG+, *Epilepsia* 39, S3 (passim)
(1997): Morkunas AR+, *Crit Care Clin* 13, 727

(1997): Pichler WJ+, *New Engl J Med* 336, 377
(1997): Stein J+, *Dtsch Med Wochenschr* (German) 122, 314
(1997): Tennis P+, *Neurology* 49, 542
(1997): Waagner DC, *New Engl J Med* 336, 376
(1996): Callot V+, *Arch Dermatol* 132, 1315
(1996): *New Engl J Med* 335, 577
(1996): Knowles SR+, *J Clin Psychopharmacol* 16, 263
(1996): Koopman R, Enschede, The Netherlands (from Internet) (observation)
(1996): Oakley A, Hamilton, New Zealand (from Internet) (observation)
(1995): Bellman B+, *J Am Acad Child Adolesc Psychiatry* 34, 1405
(1995): De Vriese AS+, *Medicine* Baltimore 74, 144
(1995): Periole B+, *Ann Dermatol Venereol* (French) 122, 121
(1994): Alldredge BK+, *Pediatr Neurol* 10, 169
(1994): Gall H+, *Hautarzt* (German) 45, 494
(1994): Naranjo CA+, *Clin Pharmacol Ther* 56, 564
(1993): Handfield-Jones SE+, *Br J Dermatol* 129, 175
(1993): Parha S+, *Eur J Pediatr* 152, 1040
(1993): Scerri L+, *Clin Exp Dermatol* 18, 540
(1991): Baguena F+, *Med Clin* (Barc) (Spanish) 96, 237
(1991): Hosoda N+, *Arch Dis Child* 66, 722
(1989): Malanin G+, *Duodecim* (Finnish) 105, 784
(1983): Bernstein DI+, *Clin Pediatr* (Phila) 22, 524
(1978): Stephan WC+, *Chest* 74, 463 (pneumonitis)
(1977): Houwerzijl J+, *Clin Exp Immunol* 29, 272
Lymphoproliferative disease
(1992): Schlaifer D+, *Eur J Dermatol* 48, 274
(1992): Sigal-Nahum M+, *Br J Dermatol* 127, 545
(1990): Katzin WE+, *Arch Pathol Lab Med* 114, 1244
(1987): Severson GS+, *Am J Med* 83, 597
(1984): Shuttleworth D+, *Clin Exp Dermatol* 9, 421
Mucocutaneous eruption
(1999): Edwards SG+, *Postgrad Med J* 75, 680
(1993): Konishi T+, *Eur J Pediatr* 152, 605
(1979): Pollack MA+, *Ann Neurol* 5, 262
(1975): Böttiger LE+, *Acta Med Scand* 198, 229
Oral lichenoid eruption
(1989): Ohtsuyama M+, *Nishinihon J Dermatol* (Japanese) 51, 958
Oral mucosal eruption
(1964): Spillane D, *Practitioner* 192, 71
Oral ulceration
(2001): Hebert AA+, *J Clin Psychiatry* 62(suppl 14), 22
Porphyria cutanea tarda
(1996): Leo RJ+, *Am J Psychiatry* 153, 443
Porphyria variegata
(2001): Grieco A+, *Eur J Gastroenterol Hepatol* 13(8), 973
Pseudolymphoma
(2001): Cogrel O+, *Br J Dermatol* 144, 1235
(1999): Saeki H+, *J Dermatol* 26, 329
(1998): d'Incan M+, *Ann Dermatol Venereol* 125, 52
(1998): Nathan D+, *J Am Acad Dermatol* 38, 806
(1997): Kim ST+, Korea, American Academy of Dermatology Meeting (SF), Poster #82
(1997): Paramesh H+, *Indian Pediatr* 34, 829
(1996): Callot V+, *Arch Dermatol* 132, 1315
(1995): Magro CM+, *J Am Acad Dermatol* 32, 419
(1993): Rondas AA+, *Ned Tijdschr Geneeskd* (Dutch) 137, 1258
(1993): Sigal M+, *Ann Dermatol Venereol* (French) 120, 175
(1991): Rijlaarsdam U+, *J Am Acad Dermatol* 24(2), 216
(1990): Sinnige HAM+, *J Intern Med* 227, 355
(1986): Yates P+, *J Clin Pathol* 39, 1224
(1984): Shuttleworth D+, *Clin Exp Dermatol* 9, 424
Rhabdomyolysis
(1992): Zele I+, *Minerva Med* 83(12), 847
Seizures
(2003): Yang MT+, *Brain Dev* 25(1), 51
(2002): Gansaeuer M+, *Clin Electroencephalogr* 33(4), 174

Serum sickness
  (1993): Igarashi M+, *Int Arch Allergy Immunol* 100, 378
Stomatitis
Thrombophlebitis
Tinnitus
Tongue ulceration
  (1998): Melgarejo Moreno PJ+, *An Otorrinolaringol Ibero Am*
    (Spanish) 25, 167
  (1964): Spillane D, *Practitioner* 192, 71
Xerostomia

*Note: The antiepileptic drug hypersensitivity syndrome is a severe, occasionally fatal, disorder characterized by any or all of the following: pruritic exanthems, toxic epidermal necrolysis, Stevens–Johnson syndrome, exfoliative dermatitis, fever, hepatic abnormalities, eosinophilia, and renal failure

CARBENICILLIN

Trade name: Geocillin (Pfizer)
Other common trade names: *Carbecin; Carbelin; Geopen; Pyopen*
Indications: Urinary tract infections
Category: Penicillinase-sensitive penicillin
Half-life: 1.0–1.5 hours
Clinically important, potentially hazardous interactions with: anticoagulants, cyclosporine, demeclocycline, doxycycline, gentamicin, methotrexate, minocycline, oxytetracycline, tetracycline

Reactions

Skin

Allergic reactions (sic)
  (1994): Pleasants RA+, *Chest* 106, 1124 (in patients with cystic
    fibrosis)
Angioedema
Bullous eruption
Ecchymoses
Edema
Erythema multiforme
Erythema nodosum
Exanthems
Exfoliative dermatitis
Hematomas
Jarisch–Herxheimer reaction
Pruritus
Purpura
  (1976): Karchmer AW+, *N Engl J Med* 295, 451
  (1970): McClure PD+, *Lancet* 2, 1307
Rash (sic) (<1%)
Stevens–Johnson syndrome
Toxic epidermal necrolysis
  (1984): Westly ED+, *Arch Dermatol* 120, 721
Urticaria (<1%)
Vasculitis
Vesicular eruptions

Other

Anaphylactoid reactions
Black tongue
Dysgeusia (1–10%)
Glossitis (1–10%)
Glossodynia
Hypersensitivity

Injection-site pain
Oral candidiasis
Serum sickness
Stomatitis
Stomatodynia
Thrombophlebitis (<1%)
Tongue furry
Vaginitis (<1%)
Xerostomia

CARBIDOPA

(See LEVODOPA)

CARBOPLATIN

Trade name: Paraplatin (Bristol-Myers Squibb)
Other common trade names: *Carboplat; Carbosin; Ercar; Oncocarbin; Paraplatine*
Indications: Various carcinomas and sarcomas
Category: Antineoplastic
Half-life: terminal: 22–40 hours
Clinically important, potentially hazardous interactions with: aldesleukin

Reactions

Skin

Allergic reactions (sic)
  (2001): Yu DY+, *J Pediatr Hematol Oncol* 23(6), 349 (11.1%)
Depigmentation
  (1990): Costello SA+, *Clin Oncol R Coll Radiol* 2, 182
Erosion of body folds (sic)
  (1996): Prussick R+, *J Am Acad Dermatol* 35, 705
Erythema (2%)
  (2001): Robinson JB+, *Gynecol Oncol* 82(3), 550
  (1995): Inbar M+, *Anticancer Drugs* 6, 775
Exanthems
  (1995): Inbar M+, *Anticancer Drugs* 6, 775
  (1992): Beyer J+, *Bone Marrow Transplant* 10, 491
  (1989): Wagstaff AJ+, *Drugs* 37, 162
Facial edema
  (1992): Beyer J+, *Bone Marrow Transplant* 10, 491
Flushing
  (2001): Robinson JB+, *Gynecol Oncol* 82(3), 550
Pigmentation
  (1992): Beyer J+, *Bone Marrow Transplant* 10, 491
  (1991): Singal R+, *Pediatr Dermatology* 8, 231
Pruritus (2%)
  (2001): Robinson JB+, *Gynecol Oncol* 82(3), 550
Rash (sic) (2%)
Urticaria (2%)
  (1996): Broome CB+, *Med Pediatr Oncol* 26, 105
  (1995): Sredni B+, *J Clin Oncol* 13, 2342

Hair

Hair – alopecia (3%)
  (2002): de Jonge ME+, *Bone Marrow Transplantation* 30, 593
    (permanent) (with cyclophosphamide and thiotepa)
  (2002): *Lancet* 360(9332), 505 (with paclitaxel)
  (2002): Rein DT+, *Gynecol Oncol* 87(1), 98 (with docetaxel)
  (2002): Sehouli J+, *Gynecol Oncol* 85(2), 321 (with paclitaxel)
  (1989): Wagstaff AJ+, *Drugs* 37, 162
Hair – alopecia areata

(2003): Motl SE+, *Pharmacotherapy* 23(1), 104 (recurrent) (with paclitaxel)
(2002): Rein DT+, *Gynecol Oncol* 87(1), 98

Other

Anaphylactoid reactions (<1%)
  (2003): Herzinger T+, *Dtsch Med Wochenschr* 128(30), 1595
  (2002): Ogle SK+, *J Pediatr Oncol Nurs* 19(4), 122
Hypersensitivity (2%)
  (2003): Jones R+, *Gynecol Oncol* 89(1), 112
  (2003): Rose PG+, *Gynecol Oncol* 89(3), 429 (4 cases, on rechallenge)
  (2002): Chasen MR+, *Cancer Chemother Pharmacol* 50(5), 429
  (2002): Markman M, *Gynecol Oncol* 84(2), 353
  (2001): Robinson JB+, *Gynecol Oncol* 82(3), 550 (with paclitaxel)
  (1999): Menczer J+, *Eur J Gynaecol Oncol* 20, 214 (4 patients)
  (1999): Schiavetti A+, *Med Pediatr Oncol* 32, 183 (9.2%)
  (1999): Shukunami K+, *Gynecol Oncol* 72, 431
  (1998): Kook H+, *Bone Marrow Transplant* 21, 727
  (1996): Broome CB+, *Med Pediatr Oncol* 26, 105
Injection-site pain (>10%)
Mucositis
  (2002): Rein DT+, *Gynecol Oncol* 87(1), 98 (with docetaxel)
Oral mucosal lesions
  (1989): Wagstaff AJ+, *Drugs* 37, 162
Parkinsonism
  (2001): Chuang C+, *Movement Disorders* 16, 990 (with paclitaxel)
Stomatitis (>10%)

CARISOPRODOL

Synonyms: carisoprodate; isobamate
Trade name: Soma (Wallace)
Other common trade names: *Artifar; Carisoma; Myolax; Sanoma; Sodol; Somadril; Soridol*
Indications: Painful musculoskeletal disorders
Category: Skeletal muscle relaxant
Half-life: 4–6 hours

Reactions

Skin

Angioedema (1–10%)
Diaphoresis
  (1983): Rollings HE+, *Curr Ther Res* 34, 926
Edema
  (1983): Rollings HE+, *Curr Ther Res* 34, 926
Erythema multiforme (<1%)
Exanthems
  (1962): Honeycutt WM+, *JAMA* 180, 691 (passim)
Fixed eruption (<1%)
  (1965): Gore HC, *Arch Dermatol* 91, 627
  (1962): Honeycutt WM+, *JAMA* 180, 691
Flushing (1–10%)
Photosensitivity
  (1994): Hazen PG, *J Am Acad Dermatol* 31, 498
Pruritus (<1%)
Rash (sic) (<1%)
Urticaria (<1%)
  (1962): Honeycutt WM+, *JAMA* 180, 691 (passim)

Other

Anaphylactoid reactions
Headache
Paresthesias

(1983): Rollings HE+, *Curr Ther Res* 34, 926
Pseudoporphyria
  (1994): Hazen PG, *J Am Acad Dermatol* 31, 498
Tinnitus
Trembling (sic) (1–10%)
Xerostomia
  (1983): Rollings HE+, *Curr Ther Res* 34, 926

CARMUSTINE

Synonym: BCNU
Trade names: BiCNU (Bristol-Myers Squibb); Gliadel Wafer (Aventis)
Other common trade names: *Becenun; Carmubris; Nitrumon*
Indications: Brain tumors, Hodgkin's disease, multiple myeloma
Category: Antineoplastic
Half-life: initial: 1.4 minutes; secondary: 20 minutes
Clinically important, potentially hazardous interactions with: aldesleukin, cimetidine, clorazepate

Reactions

Skin

Dermatitis (sic) (<1%)
  (1994): Zackheim HS, *Semin Dermatol* 13, 202
  (1990): Zackheim HS+, *J Am Acad Dermatol* 22, 802
Eccrine squamous syringometaplasia
  (1997): Valks R+, *Arch Dermatol* 133, 873
Erythema
  (1992): Breathnach SM+, *Adverse Drug Reactions and the Skin* Blackwell, Oxford, 292
Exanthems
  (1978): Levine N+, *Cancer Treat Rev* 5, 67
Flushing (1–10%)
  (1978): Levine N+, *Cancer Treat Rev* 5, 67
  (1971): Young RC+, *N Engl J Med* 285, 475
Pigmentation (on accidental contact)
  (1982): Dunagin WG, *Semin Oncol* 9, 14
  (1966): Frost P+, *Arch Dermatol* 94, 265
Telangiectasia
  (1994): Zackheim HS, *Semin Dermatol* 13, 202
  (1992): Breathnach SM+, *Adverse Drug Reactions and the Skin* Blackwell, Oxford, 292
Tenderness (sic)
  (1992): Breathnach SM+, *Adverse Drug Reactions and the Skin* Blackwell, Oxford, 292

Hair

Hair – alopecia (1–10%)

Other

Gynecomastia
Headache
Injection-site burning (>10%)
Injection-site necrosis
  (1987): Dufresne RG, *Cutis* 39, 197
Injection-site pain
Oral mucositis
  (2000): Wardley AM+, *Br J Haematol* 110, 292
Stomatitis (1–10%)

CARTEOLOL

Trade names: Cartrol (Abbott); Ocupress (ophthalmic) (Novartis)
Other common trade names: *Arteolol; Arteoptic; Calte; Carteol; Endak; Mikelan; Teoptic*
Indications: Glaucoma, hypertension
Category: Beta-adrenoceptor blocker
Half-life: 6 hours
Clinically important, potentially hazardous interactions with: clonidine, epinephrine, verapamil

Note: Cutaneous side effects of beta-receptor blockaders are clinically polymorphous. They apparently appear after several months of continuous therapy. Atypical psoriasiform, lichen planus-like, and eczematous chronic rashes are mainly observed. (1983): Hödl St, *Z Hautkr* (German) 1:58, 17

Reactions

Skin
Acne
Angioedema
Ankle edema (<1%)
Cold extremities (sic)
Dermatitis (sic) (eye-drops)
  (2001): Holdiness MR, *Am J Contact Dermat* 12(4), 217
  (2000): Quiralte J+, *Contact Dermatitis* 42, 245
Diaphoresis (<1%)
  (1997): Schmutz JL+, *Dermatology* 194, 197 (from topical)
Edema
Exanthems
Exfoliative dermatitis
Facial edema
Flushing
Lupus erythematosus
Peripheral edema (1.7%)
Photosensitivity
Pigmentation
Pruritus
Psoriasis
Purpura (<1%)
Rash (sic) (2.5%)
Raynaud's phenomenon (<1%)
Vesiculobullous eruption
Xerosis

Hair
Hair – alopecia

Nails
Nails – discoloration (bluish)

Other
Anaphylactoid reactions
Dysgeusia (from topical application)
Headache
Myalgia
Paresthesias (2%)
Peyronie's disease
Tinnitus
Xerostomia

CARVEDILOL

Trade name: Coreg (GSK)
Other common trade names: *Dibloc; Dilatrend; Dimitone; Kredex; Querto*
Indications: Hypertension
Category: Antihypertensive; Beta-adrenoceptor blocker
Half-life: 7–10 hours

Reactions

Skin
Allergic reactions (sic) (<1%)
  (1998): Simpson SH+, *Can J Cardiol* 14, 1277
Angioedema
  (1988): Ogihara G+, *Drugs* 36, 75 (<1%)
Diaphoresis (2.9%)
Edema (generalized) (5.1%)
Exanthems (<1%)
  (2000): Litt JZ, Beachwood, OH (personal case) (observation)
  (1988): Ogihara G+, *Drugs* 36, 75 (2%)
Exfoliative dermatitis (<1%)
Infections (sic) (2.2%)
Peripheral edema (1.4%)
Photosensitivity (<1%)
Pruritus (<1%)
  (2000): Litt JZ, Beachwood, OH (personal case) (observation)
Psoriasis (<1%)
Purpura (1–10%)
Rash (sic) (<1%)
Stevens–Johnson syndrome
  (1997): Kowalski BJ+, *Am J Cardiol* 80, 669

Hair
Hair – alopecia (<0.1%)

Other
Anaphylactoid reactions (<1%)
Headache
Hyperesthesia (<1%)
Myalgia (3.4%)
Pain (8.6%)
Paresthesias (2%)
Xerostomia (<1%)

CASCARA

Scientific names: *Frangula purshianus; Rhamnus purshiana*
Family: Rhamnaceae
Trade and other common names: Bitter bark; Buckthorn; Californian buckthorn; Cascara sagrada; Chittem bark; Pursh's buckthorn; Yellow bark
Category: Antiparasitic; Bitter digestive tonic; Cholagogue; Laxative; Mild purgative; Stomachic
Purported indications and other uses: Atonic constipation, dyspepsia, Colitis, Diverticulitis, Dyspepsia, Gallstones, Gout, Hemorrhoids, hypertension, Indigestion, Insomnia, Jaundice, Liver disease, Nervous disorders, Parasites, Stomach disorders
Half-life: N/A
Clinically important, potentially hazardous interactions with: antiarrhythmics, cardiac glycosides, corticosteroids, **licorice**, thiazide diuretics

Reactions

Skin
None

CASPOFUNGIN

Trade name: Cancidas (Merck)
Indications: Invasive Aspergillus infection
Category: Antifungal (parenteral) (Glucan synthesis inhibitor)
Half-life: Beta phase: 9–11 hours; terminal: 40–50 hours
Clinically important, potentially hazardous interactions with: cyclosporine

Reactions

Skin
Chills (~3%)
Diaphoresis (<1%)
Edema (~3%)
Erythema (1–2%)
Facial edema (3%)
Flu-like syndrome (3%)
Flushing (3%)
Pruritus (2–3%)
Rash (sic) (1–4%)
Vasculitis (2%)

Other
Anaphylactoid reactions (<2%)
Headache
Injection-site induration (~3%)
Injection-site reactions (2–12%)
  (2002): *Prescrire Int* 11(61), 142
  (2001): Keating GM+, *Drugs* 61(8), 1121
Myalgia (~3%)
Pain (1–5%)
Paresthesias (1–3%)
Phlebitis (~16%)
Tremor (<2%)

CEFACLOR

Trade name: Ceclor (Lilly)
Other common trade names: *Alfatil; Apo-Cefaclor; CEC 500; Cefabiocin; Distaclor; Kefolor; Panoral; Sigacefal*
Indications: Various infections caused by susceptible organisms
Category: Second generation cephalosporin
Half-life: 0.6–0.9 hours

Note: Penicillin and cephalosporins share a common beta-lactam structure. People who are allergic to penicillin are approximately 4 times more likely to develop an allergic reaction to a cephalosporin than those people who have no penicillin allergy. (From 5 to 16% of patients allergic to penicillin develop reactions to cephalosporins)

Reactions

Skin
Acute generalized exanthematous pustulosis (AGEP)
  (1995): Moreau A+, *Int J Dermatol* 34, 263 (passim)
  (1992): Ogoshi M+, *Dermatology* 184, 142
Angioedema (<1%)
  (1998): Litt JZ, Beachwood, OH (personal case) (observation)
Candidiasis (vaginal)
  (1992): Stotka JL+, *Postgrad Med J* 68, S73
Dermatitis (sic)
  (1986): Hirata M+, *Kokyu To Junkan* (Japanese) 34, 791
Edema
  (1995): Dark DS+, *Infections in Medicine* October, 551
Erythema multiforme
  (2000): Ibia EO+, *Arch Dermatol* 136, 849
  (1999): Joubert GI+, *Can J Clin Pharmacol* 6, 197 (17 cases)
  (1988): Platt R+, *J Infect Dis* 158, 474 (0.6%)
  (1985): Levine LR, *Ped Infect Dis* 4, 358 (0.6%)
  (1982): Lovell SJ+, *Can Med Assoc J* 126, 1032
  (1980): Murray DL+, *N Engl J Med* 303, 1003
Exanthems
  (2000): Ibia EO+, *Arch Dermatol* 136, 849
  (1996): Nagayama H+, *J Dermatol* 23, 899
  (1994): Litt JZ, Beachwood, OH (personal case) (observation)
  (1994): Shelley WB+, *Cutis* 53, 40 (observation)
  (1987): Norrby SR, *Drugs* 34 (Suppl 2), 105 (1–5%)
  (1986): Ascher H, *Lakartidningen* (Swedish) 83, 411
  (1985): Murray DL+, *Pediatr Infect Dis* 4, 706
  (1983): Johnson T, *J Ark Med Soc* 80, 110
  (1982): Lovell SJ+, *Can Med Assoc J* 126, 1032
  (1981): Ackley AM+, *Southern Med J* 74, 1550
  (1980): Murray DL+, *N Engl J Med* 303, 1003
Flushing
Pruritus (<1%)
  (1998): Litt JZ, Beachwood, OH (personal case) (observation)
  (1988): Platt R+, *J Infect Dis* 158, 474
  (1982): Lovell SJ+, *Can Med Assoc J* 126, 1032
  (1981): Ackley AM+, *Southern Med J* 74, 1550
  (1980): Murray DL+, *N Engl J Med* 303, 1003
Purpura
  (2002): Kurokawa I, *Int J Antimicrob Agents* 20(5), 393
  (1980): Murray DL+, *N Engl J Med* 303, 1003
Pustules
  (1992): Ogoshi M+, *Dermatology* 184, 142
Rash (sic) (1–1.5%)
  (2002): Siddiqui SJ+, *J Pak Med Assoc* 52(10), 451 (1 case)
Stevens–Johnson syndrome (<1%)
  (1988): Platt R+, *J Infect Dis* 158, 474
Toxic epidermal necrolysis
  (1987): Guillaume JC+, *Arch Dermatol* 123, 1166
Urticaria (<1%)

(2000): Ibia EO+, *Arch Dermatol* 136, 849
(1999): Joubert GI+, *Can J Clin Pharmacol* 6, 197 (26 cases)
(1998): Litt JZ, Beachwood, OH (personal case) (observation)
(1995): Blumenthal HL, Beachwood, OH (personal case)
   (observation)
(1994): Litt JZ, Beachwood, OH (personal case) (observation)
(1993): Litt JZ, Beachwood, OH (2 personal cases) (observation)
(1991): Hebert AA+, *J Am Acad Dermatol* 25, 805
(1985): Levine LR, *Pediatr Infect Dis* 4, 358 (1–5%)
(1982): Lovell SJ+, *Can Med Assoc J* 126, 1032

Other

Anaphylactoid reactions (<1%)
   (1999): Grouhi M+, *Pediatrics* 103, e50
   (1986): Nishioka K+, *J Dermatol* 13, 226
Dysgeusia
   (1995): Dark DS+, *Infections in Medicine* October, 551
Glossitis
Hypersensitivity
Oral candidiasis
Paresthesias
Serum sickness (<1%)
   (2002): Sanklecha MU, *Indian J Pediatr* 69(10), 921
   (2000): Ibia EO+, *Arch Dermatol* 136, 849
   (1999): Joubert GI+, *Can J Clin Pharmacol* 6, 197 (31 cases)
   (1999): Parshuram CS+, *J Paediatr Child Health* 35, 223
   (1999): Phillips R, *Aust Fam Physician* 28, 539
   (1998): Boyd IW, *Med J Aust* 169, 443
   (1998): Kearns GL+, *Clin Pharmacol Ther* 63, 686 (10 patients)
   (1997): Szalai Z+, *Orv Hetil* (Hungarian) 138, 855
   (1996): Grammer LC, *JAMA* 275, 1152
   (1996): *Can Med Assoc J* 155, 913
   (1996): Reynolds RD, *JAMA* 276, 950
   (1995): Kearns GL+, *J Pediatr* 125, 805
   (1995): Martin J+, *N Z Med J* 108, 123
   (1992): Parra FM+, *Allergy* 47, 439
   (1992): Stricker BH+, *J Clin Epidemiol* 45, 1177
   (1992): Vial T+, *Ann Pharmacother* 26, 910
   (1991): Hebert AA+, *J Am Acad Dermatol* 25, 805
   (1990): Heckbert SB+, *Am J Epidemiol* 132, 336
   (1988): Platt R+, *J Infect Dis* 158, 474
   (1987): Norrby SR, *Drugs* 34 (Suppl 2), 105 (1–5%)
   (1985): Callahan CW+, *J Am Osteopath Assoc* 85, 450
   (1985): Levine LR, *Ped Infect Dis* 4, 358 (0.5%)
   (1985): Murray DL+, *Pediatr Inf Dis* 4, 706
   (1983): Johnson T+, *J Ark Med Soc* 80, 110
   (1982): Lovell SJ+, *Can Med Assoc J* 126, 1032
   (1980): Murray DL+, *N Engl J Med* 303, 1003
Stomatitis
   (2002): Siddiqui SJ+, *J Pak Med Assoc* 52(10), 451 (1 case)
Vaginitis
   (1992): Stotka JL+, *Postgrad Med J* 68, S73 (candidiasis)

CEFADROXIL

Trade name: Duricef (Warner Chilcott)
Other common trade names: *Baxan; Bidocef; Cedrox; Cefamox; Duracef; Moxacef; Oracefal; Sumacef*
Indications: Various infections caused by susceptible organisms
Category: First generation cephalosporin
Half-life: 1.2–1.5 hours

Note: Penicillin and cephalosporins share a common beta-lactam structure. People who are allergic to penicillin are approximately 4 times more likely to develop an allergic reaction to a cephalosporin than those people who have no penicillin allergy. (From 5 to 16% of patients allergic to penicillin develop allergic reactions to cephalosporins)

Reactions

Skin

Angioedema (<1%)
Candidiasis
Erythema
   (1986): Tanrisever B+, *Drugs* 32(Suppl 3), 1
Erythema multiforme (<1%)
Exanthems (<1%)
   (1986): Tanrisever B+, *Drugs* 32(Suppl 3), 1 (0.3%)
Pemphigus
   (1986): Wilson JP+, *Drug Intell Clin Pharm* 20, 219
Pruritus (<1%)
   (1986): Tanrisever B+, *Drugs* 32(Suppl 3), 1 (0.3%)
Rash (sic) (<1%)
Stevens–Johnson syndrome (<1%)
Toxic epidermal necrolysis
Urticaria (<1%)
   (1993): Shelley WB+, *Cutis* 52, 262 (observation)
   (1986): Tanrisever B+, *Drugs* 32(Suppl 3), 1 (0.1%)

Other

Anaphylactoid reactions (<1%)
Glossitis
   (1986): Tanrisever B+, *Drugs* 32 (Suppl 3), 1, 21, 43
Hypersensitivity
Oral candidiasis
Oral mucosal eruption
   (1986): Tanrisever B+, *Drugs* 32(Suppl 3), 1 (0.1%)
Oral ulceration
   (1986): Wilson JP+, *Drug Intell Clin Pharm* 20, 219
Serum sickness (<1%)
Vaginitis (<1%)
   (1986): Tanrisever B+, *Drugs* 32(Suppl 3), 1

CEFAMANDOLE

Trade name: Mandol (Lilly)
Other common trade names: *Cedol; Cefadol; Kefadol; Kefdole; Mancef; Mandokef*
Indications: Various infections caused by susceptible organisms
Category: Second generation cephalosporin
Half-life: 0.5–1.0 hours

Note: Penicillin and cephalosporins share a common beta-lactam structure. People who are allergic to penicillin are approximately 4 times more likely to develop an allergic reaction to a cephalosporin than those people who have no penicillin allergy. (From 5 to 16% of patients allergic to penicillin develop allergic reactions to cephalosporins)

Reactions

Skin
Acne
Diaper rash
Diaphoresis
Edema
Erythema multiforme
　(1987): Argenyi ZB+, *Cleve Clin J Med* 54, 445
Exanthems
　(1985): Richards DM+, *Drugs* 29, 281 (1.7%)
　(1985): Sanders CV+, *Ann Intern Med* 103, 70 (2%)
Flushing
Linear IgA bullous dermatosis
　(1987): Argenyi ZB+, *Cleve Clin J Med* 54, 445
Pruritus (<1%)
Purpura
Rash (sic) (<1%)
Stevens–Johnson syndrome (<1%)
Toxic epidermal necrolysis
　(1985): Sanders CV+, *Ann Intern Med* 103, 70 (2%)
　(1982): Seifter EJ+, *Johns Hopkins Med J* 151, 326
Toxic erythema
　(1995): Rademaker M, *N Z Med J* 108, 165
Urticaria (<1%)

Other
Anaphylactoid reactions (<1%)
　(1992): Lin RY, *Arch Intern Med* 152, 930
Dysgeusia
Glossitis
Hypersensitivity
Injection-site burning
Injection-site cellulitis
Injection-site edema
Injection-site inflammation
Injection-site pain (<1%)
　(1985): Sanders CV+, *Ann Intern Med* 103, 70 (7%)
Injection-site thrombophlebitis (1–10%)
　(1985): Sanders CV+, *Ann Intern Med* 103, 70 (15%)
Oral candidiasis (<1%)
Paresthesias
Serum sickness (<1%)
Vaginal candidiasis
Vaginitis

CEFAZOLIN

Trade names: Ancef (GSK); Kefzol (Lilly)
Other common trade names: *Basocef; Cefacidal; Cefamezin; Elzogram; Gramaxin; Kefarin; Totacef; Zolin*
Indications: Various infections caused by susceptible organisms
Category: First generation cephalosporin
Half-life: 1.4–1.8 hours

Note: Penicillin and cephalosporins share a common beta-lactam structure. People who are allergic to penicillin are approximately 4 times more likely to develop an allergic reaction to a cephalosporin than those people who have no penicillin allergy. (From 5 to 16% of patients allergic to penicillin develop allergic reactions to cephalosporins)

Reactions

Skin
Acute generalized exanthematous pustulosis (AGEP)
　(1995): Moreau A+, *Int J Dermatol* 34, 263 (passim)
　(1994): Manders SM+, *Cutis* 54, 194 (with metronidazole)
Allergic reactions (sic)
　(1994): Pleasants RA+, *Chest* 106, 1124 (in patients with cystic fibrosis)
　(1993): Faulk D+, *Nurse Anesth* 4, 188 (3–5%)
Dermatitis
　(2000): Straube MD+, *Contact Dermatitis* 42, 44
Erythema multiforme
Exanthems
　(1990): Flax SH+, *Cutis* 46, 59
　(1988): Fayol J+, *J Am Acad Dermatol* 19, 571
　(1986): Szylit JA+, *Cutis* 37, 390
Fixed eruption (linear)
　(1988): Sigal-Nahum M+, *Br J Dermatol* 118, 849
Pemphigus
　(1997): Brenner S+, *J Am Acad Dermatol* 36, 919
Photo-recall phenomenon (sic)
　(1990): Flax SH+, *Cutis* 46, 59
Photosensitivity
　(1990): Flax SH+, *Cutis* 46, 59
Pruritus (<1%)
　(1987): Stough D+, *J Am Acad Dermatol* 16, 1051
Pruritus ani
Pustules
　(1990): Rustin MHA+, *Br J Dermatol* 123, 119
　(1988): Fayol J+, *J Am Acad Dermatol* 19, 571
　(1987): Stough D+, *J Am Acad Dermatol* 16, 1051
Rash (sic) (<1%)
Stevens–Johnson syndrome (<1%)
Toxic epidermal necrolysis
　(1999): Egan CA+, *J Am Acad Dermatol* 40, 458 (6 cases)
　(1994): Julsrud ME, *J Foot Ankle Surg* 33, 255
Urticaria (<1%)

Other
Anaphylactoid reactions (<1%)
　(2003): Gibbs MW+, *Acta Anaesthesiol Scand* 47(2), 230
　(1996): Warrington RJ+, *J Allergy Clin Immunol* 98, 460
　(1995): Konno R+, *J Obstet Gynaecol* 21, 577
　(1992): Lin RY, *Arch Intern Med* 152, 930
Hypersensitivity
　(2001): Romano AG+, *Allergy Clin Immunol* 107, 134 (delayed)
Injection-site induration
Injection-site pain (<1%)
Injection-site phlebitis (<1%)
Oral candidiasis (<1%)

Phlebitis
Serum sickness (<1%)
Vaginitis (<1%)

CEFDINIR

Synonym: CFDN
Trade name: Omnicef (Abbott)
Indications: Community-acquired pneumonia and various infections caused by susceptible organisms
Category: Third generation cephalosporin
Half-life: 1–2 hours

Note: Penicillin and cephalosporins share a common beta-lactam structure. People who are allergic to penicillin are approximately 4 times more likely to develop an allergic reaction to a cephalosporin than those people who have no penicillin allergy. (From 5 to 16% of patients allergic to penicillin develop allergic reactions to cephalosporins)

Reactions

Skin
Candidiasis (1%)
Erythema multiforme
Erythema nodosum
Exanthems (0.2%)
Exfoliative dermatitis
Facial edema
Pruritus (0.2%)
Purpura
Rash (sic) (3%)
Stevens–Johnson syndrome (<1%)
Toxic epidermal necrolysis
Urticaria (<1%)
Vasculitis

Other
Anaphylactoid reactions
Headache
Serum sickness (<1%)
Stomatitis
Vaginal candidiasis (5%)
Vaginitis (1%)

CEFDITOREN

Trade name: Spectracef (TAP)
Indications: Various infections caused by susceptible organisms
Category: Third generation cephalosporin
Half-life: ~1.6 hours
Clinically important, potentially hazardous interactions with: famotidine

Reactions

Skin
Allergic reactions (sic) (<1%)
Diaphoresis (<1%)
Erythema multiforme
Fungal infections (<1%)
Peripheral edema (<1%)
Pruritus (<1%)

Rash (sic) (<1%)
Stevens–Johnson syndrome
Toxic epidermal necrolysis
Urticaria (<1%)

Other
Anaphylactoid reactions
Dysgeusia (<1%)
Headache
Myalgia (<1%)
Oral candidiasis (<1%)
Oral ulceration (<1%)
Pain (<1%)
Serum sickness
Stomatitis (<1%)
Vaginal candidiasis (3–6%)
Vaginitis (<1%)
Xerostomia (<1%)

CEFEPIME

Trade name: Maxipime (Elan)
Other common trade name: *Maxcef*
Indications: Various infections caused by susceptible organisms
Category: Fourth generation cephalosporin
Half-life: 2–2.3 hours

Note: Penicillin and cephalosporins share a common beta-lactam structure. People who are allergic to penicillin are approximately 4 times more likely to develop an allergic reaction to a cephalosporin than those people who have no penicillin allergy. (From 5 to 16% of patients allergic to penicillin develop allergic reactions to cephalosporins)

Reactions

Skin
Angioedema
Candidiasis (<1%)
Erythema multiforme
Exanthems (1.8%)
Pruritus (1–10%)
Rash (sic) (51%)
  (2000): Sheng WH+, *J Microbiol Immunol Infect* 33, 109
  (1996): Holloway WJ+, *Am J Med* 100, 52S
  (1994): Okamoto MP+, *Am J Hosp Pharm* 51, 463
Stevens–Johnson syndrome
Toxic epidermal necrolysis
Urticaria (1.8%)

Other
Anaphylactoid reactions
Headache
Hypersensitivity
Injection-site inflammation (0.6%)
Injection-site pain (0.6%)
Injection-site phlebitis (1.3%)
Injection-site rash (1.1%)
Oral candidiasis
Status epilepticus
  (2001): Martinez-Rodriguez JE+, *Am J Med* 111, 115
Vaginitis (<1%)

CEFIXIME

Trade name: Suprax (Wyeth)
Other common trade names: *Cefspan; Cephoral; Fixime; Oroken; Supran; Uro-cephoral*
Indications: Various infections caused by susceptible organisms
Category: Third generation cephalosporin
Half-life: 3–4 hours

Note: Penicillin and cephalosporins share a common beta-lactam structure. People who are allergic to penicillin are approximately 4 times more likely to develop an allergic reaction to a cephalosporin than those people who have no penicillin allergy. (From 5 to 16% of patients allergic to penicillin develop allergic reactions to cephalosporins)

Reactions

Skin
Candidiasis
Erythema multiforme (<2%)
Pruritus (<2%)
  (1987): Tally FP+, *Pediatr Infect Dis J* 6, 976
Pruritus ani
Rash (sic) (<2%)
  (2001): Ho MW+, *J Microbiol Immunol Infect* 34(3), 185 (3.2%)
  (1987): Tally FP+, *Pediatr Infect Dis J* 6, 976
Stevens–Johnson syndrome (<2%)
Urticaria (<2%)
  (1987): Tally FP+, *Pediatr Infect Dis J* 6, 976

Other
Anaphylactoid reactions
  (1996): Vilas Martinez F+, *Med Clin (Barc)* (Spanish) 106, 439
Hypersensitivity
  (1999): Gaig P+, *Allergy* 54(8), 901
Pseudolymphoma
  (1998): Jabbar A+, *Br J Haematol* 101, 209
Serum sickness (<2%)
  (1987): Tally FP+, *Pediatr Infect Dis J* 6, 976
Vaginal candidiasis
Vaginitis (<2%)
Xerostomia
  (1987): Tally FP+, *Pediatr Infect Dis J* 6, 976

CEFMETAZOLE

Trade name: Zefazone (Pharmacia)
Other common trade names: *Cefmetazon; Cefotazol; Cemetol; Cetazone; Gomcefa; Metalin*
Indications: Various infections caused by susceptible organisms
Category: Second generation cephalosporin
Half-life: 72 minutes

Note: Penicillin and cephalosporins share a common beta-lactam structure. People who are allergic to penicillin are approximately 4 times more likely to develop an allergic reaction to a cephalosporin than those people who have no penicillin allergy. (From 5 to 16% of patients allergic to penicillin develop allergic reactions to cephalosporins)

Reactions

Skin
Allergic reactions (sic)

  (1989): Saito A, *J Antimicrob Chemother* 23, 131
Candidiasis (<1%)
Hot flashes (<1%)
Periorbital edema
Pruritus (<1%)
Purpura
Rash (sic) (1–10%)
Stevens–Johnson syndrome (<1%)
Toxic epidermal necrolysis
Urticaria (<1%)

Other
Anaphylactoid reactions
  (1989): Saito A, *J Antimicrob Chemother* 23, 131
Disulfiram-like reaction*
  (1989): Saito A, *J Antimicrob Chemother* 23, 131
Dysgeusia
Headache
Hypersensitivity
Injection-site edema
Injection-site induration
Injection-site pain
Injection-site thrombophlebitis (<1%)
Phlebitis (<1%)
Serum sickness (<1%)
Vaginitis (<1%)

*****Note:** The disulfiram-like reaction consists of facial flushing, diaphoresis, tachycardia, and pounding headache

CEFONICID

Trade name: Monocid (GSK)
Other common trade names: *Dinacid; Monocef; Monocidur*
Indications: Various infections caused by susceptible organisms
Category: Second generation cephalosporin
Half-life: 3–6 hours

Note: Penicillin and cephalosporins share a common beta-lactam structure. People who are allergic to penicillin are approximately 4 times more likely to develop an allergic reaction to a cephalosporin than those people who have no penicillin allergy. (From 5 to 16% of patients allergic to penicillin develop allergic reactions to cephalosporins)

Reactions

Skin
Allergic reactions (sic)
  (1994): Martin JA+, *Ann Allergy* 72, 341
Candidiasis (<1%)
Erythema (<1%)
Erythema multiforme
Pruritus (<1%)
Purpura
Rash (sic) (<1%)
Stevens–Johnson syndrome (<1%)
Toxic epidermal necrolysis
Urticaria (<1%)

Other
Anaphylactoid reactions (<1%)
Disulfiram-like reaction*
  (1990): Marcon G+, *Recenti Prog Med* (Italian) 81, 47
Hypersensitivity
Injection-site edema (>1%)

Injection-site induration (>1%)
Injection-site pain (5.7%)
Injection-site phlebitis (>1%)
Myalgia
Serum sickness (<1%)
  (1995): Ortega Calvo M+, *An Med Interna* (Spanish) 12, 289
Vaginitis

*Note: The disulfiram-like reaction consists of facial flushing, diaphoresis, tachycardia, and pounding headache

CEFOPERAZONE

Trade name: Cefobid (Roerig)
Other common trade names: *Cefobis; Cefogram; Cefozone; CPZ; Mediper; Tomabef; Zoncef*
Indications: Various infections caused by susceptible organisms
Category: Third generation cephalosporin
Half-life: 1.6–2.6 hours

Note: Penicillin and cephalosporins share a common beta-lactam structure. People who are allergic to penicillin are approximately 4 times more likely to develop an allergic reaction to a cephalosporin than those people who have no penicillin allergy. (From 5 to 16% of patients allergic to penicillin develop allergic reactions to cephalosporins)

Reactions

Skin
Candidiasis (<1%)
Erythema multiforme
Exanthems (<1%)
Pruritus (<1%)
Rash (sic) (2%)
  (1983): Lyon JA, *Drug Intell Clin Pharm* 17, 7
Stevens–Johnson syndrome (<1%)
Toxic epidermal necrolysis
Urticaria (<1%)
  (1983): Lyon JA, *Drug Intell Clin Pharm* 17, 7

Other
Disulfiram-like reaction*
  (1981): Vonhogen LH+, *Ned Tijdschr Geneeskd* (Dutch) 125, 1610
  (1980): Foster TS+, *Am J Hosp Pharm* 37, 858
Hypersensitivity (>2%)
Injection-site induration (<1%)
Injection-site pain (<1%)
  (1983): Lyon JA, *Drug Intell Clin Pharm* 17, 7
Phlebitis (<1%)
  (1983): Lyon JA, *Drug Intell Clin Pharm* 17, 7
Serum sickness (<1%)
Thrombophlebitis

*Note: The disulfiram-like reaction consists of facial flushing, diaphoresis, tachycardia, and pounding headache

CEFOTAXIME

Trade name: Claforan (Aventis)
Other common trade names: *Alfotax; Benaxima; Biosint; Cefaxim; Cefotax; Molelant; Oritaxim; Primafen; Spirosine; Zariviz*
Indications: Various infections caused by susceptible organisms
Category: Third generation, broad-spectrum cephalosporin
Half-life: adults: 60 minutes

Note: Penicillin and cephalosporins share a common beta-lactam structure. People who are allergic to penicillin are approximately 4 times more likely to develop an allergic reaction to a cephalosporin than those people who have no penicillin allergy. (From 5 to 16% of patients allergic to penicillin develop allergic reactions to cephalosporins)

Reactions

Skin
Candidiasis
Erythema multiforme
  (1990): Todd PA+, *Drugs* 40, 608
  (1986): Green ST+, *Postgrad Med J* 62, 415
Exanthems
  (1990): Todd PA+, *Drugs* 40, 608
  (1984): Smith CR+, *Ann Intern Med* 101, 469 (3.4%)
  (1983): Carmine AA+, *Drugs* 25, 223 (2%)
Pruritus (2.4%)
  (1990): Todd PA+, *Drugs* 40, 608
  (1983): Carmine AA+, *Drugs* 25, 223 (2%)
Rash (sic) (2.4%)
  (1982): LeFrock JL+, *Clin Ther* 5, 19
Stevens–Johnson syndrome
  (2003): *Ann Pharmacother* 37(6), 812
Toxic epidermal necrolysis
Urticaria (2.4%)

Other
Anaphylactoid reactions (2.4%)
Headache
Hypersensitivity
  (1993): Papakonstantinou G+, *Clin Investig* 71, 165
Injection-site inflammation (4.3%)
  (1983): Carmine AA+, *Drugs* 25, 223 (5%)
Injection-site pain (1–10%)
  (1983): Carmine AA+, *Drugs* 25, 223 (32%)
Injection-site thrombophlebitis
Paresthesias
Phlebitis (<1%)
Serum sickness
Vaginitis (<1%)

CEFOTETAN

Trade name: Cefotan (AstraZeneca)
Other common trade names: *Apacef; Apatef; Ceftenon; Cepan; Yamatetan*
Indications: Various infections caused by susceptible organisms
Category: Second generation cephalosporin
Half-life: 3–5 hours

Note: Penicillin and cephalosporins share a common beta-lactam structure. People who are allergic to penicillin are approximately 4 times more likely to develop an allergic reaction to a cephalosporin than those people who have no penicillin allergy. (From 5 to 16% of patients allergic to penicillin develop allergic reactions to cephalosporins)

Reactions

Skin
Candidiasis (<1%)
Erythema multiforme
Exanthems
Pruritus (<1%)
Rash (sic) (<1%)
Stevens–Johnson syndrome (<1%)
Toxic epidermal necrolysis
Urticaria (<1%)

Other
Anaphylactoid reactions (<1%)
　(1990): Faro S+, *Am J Obstet Gynecol* 162, 296
　(1988): Bloomberg RJ, *Am J Obstet Gynecol* 159, 125
Hypersensitivity (1.2%)
　(2001): Romano A+, *Allergy* 56, 260
Injection-site pain (<1%)
Phlebitis (<1%)
Serum sickness (<1%)
Thrombophlebitis

CEFOXITIN

Trade name: Mefoxin (Merck)
Other common trade names: *Cefmore; Cefoxin; Lephocin; Mefoxil; Mefoxitin*
Indications: Various infections caused by susceptible organisms
Category: Second generation, broad-spectrum cephalosporin
Half-life: 40–60 minutes

Note: Penicillin and cephalosporins share a common beta-lactam structure. People who are allergic to penicillin are approximately 4 times more likely to develop an allergic reaction to a cephalosporin than those people who have no penicillin allergy. (From 5 to 16% of patients allergic to penicillin develop allergic reactions to cephalosporins)

Reactions

Skin
Angioedema (<1%)
Candidiasis (<1%)
Exanthems
　(1979): Brogden RN+, *Drugs* 17, 1 (2.2%)
Exfoliative dermatitis (<1%)
　(1987): Norrby SR, *Drugs* 34 (Suppl 2) 105
　(1985): Sanders CV+, *Ann Intern Med* 103, 70 (2%)

　(1983): Tietze KJ+, *Clin Pharmacy* 2, 582
　(1982): Kannangara DW+, *Arch Intern Med* 142, 1031
Flushing
　(1985): Sanders CV+, *Ann Intern Med* 103, 70
Pruritus (<1%)
　(1983): Tietze KJ+, *Clin Pharmacy* 2, 582
　(1979): Brogden RN+, *Drugs* 17, 1
Purpura
　(1990): Burstein M+, *Drug Intell Clin Pharm* 24, 206
Pustules
　(1994): Spencer JM+, *Br J Dermatol* 130, 514
Rash (sic) (<1%)
Stevens–Johnson syndrome (<1%)
Toxic epidermal necrolysis (<1%)
Urticaria

Other
Anaphylactoid reactions (<1%)
　(1992): Lin RY, *Arch Intern Med* 152, 930 (11 cases)
Injection-site induration
Injection-site pain
　(1985): Sanders CV+, *Ann Intern Med* 103, 70 (10%)
　(1979): Brogden RN+, *Drugs* 17, 1 (>5%)
Serum sickness (<1%)
　(1986): Panwalker AP+, *Drug Intell Clin Pharm* 20, 953
Thrombophlebitis

CEFPODOXIME

Trade name: Vantin (Pharmacia)
Other common trade names: *Cefodox; Orelox; Podomexef*
Indications: Various infections caused by susceptible organisms
Category: Third generation cephalosporin
Half-life: 2.1–2.8 hours

Note: Penicillin and cephalosporins share a common beta-lactam structure. People who are allergic to penicillin are approximately 4 times more likely to develop an allergic reaction to a cephalosporin than those people who have no penicillin allergy. (From 5 to 16% of patients allergic to penicillin develop allergic reactions to cephalosporins)

Reactions

Skin
Acne
Candidiasis (<1%)
Diaper rash (12.1%)
Diaphoresis
Edema
Erythema multiforme
Exfoliation (sic) (<1%)
Flushing (<1%)
Pruritus (<1%)
Rash (sic) (1.4%)
　(2001): Fulton B+, *Paediatr Drugs* 3(2), 137
Stevens–Johnson syndrome (<1%)
Toxic epidermal necrolysis
Urticaria (<1%)

Other
Anaphylactoid reactions (<1%)
Dysgeusia (<1%)
Glossitis
Hypersensitivity
Injection-site burning

Injection-site cellulitis
Injection-site edema
Injection-site inflammation
Injection-site thrombophlebitis
Oral candidiasis
Paresthesias
Serum sickness (<1%)
Sialopenia (<1%)
Tinnitus
Vaginal candidiasis (<1%)
Vaginitis
  (1991): Tack KJ+, *Drugs* 42, 51

CEFPROZIL

Trade name: Cefzil (Bristol-Myers Squibb)
Indications: Various infections caused by susceptible organisms
Category: Second generation cephalosporin
Half-life: 1.3 hours

Note: Penicillin and cephalosporins share a common beta-lactam structure. People who are allergic to penicillin are approximately 4 times more likely to develop an allergic reaction to a cephalosporin than those people who have no penicillin allergy. (From 5 to 16% of patients allergic to penicillin develop allergic reactions to cephalosporins)

Reactions

Skin
Angioedema (<1%)
Candidiasis
Diaper rash (1.5%)
Erythema multiforme (<1%)
Exanthems
Genital pruritus (1.6%)
Pruritus
Rash (sic) (<1%)
Stevens–Johnson syndrome (<1%)
Toxic epidermal necrolysis
Urticaria (<1%)

Other
Anaphylactoid reactions (<1%)
Glossitis
Headache
Hypersensitivity
Oral candidiasis
Paresthesias
Serum sickness (<1%)
  (1994): Lowery N+, *J Pediatr* 125, 325
Vaginitis (1.6%)

CEFTAZIDIME

Trade names: Ceptaz (GSK); Fortaz (GSK); Tazicef (GSK); Tazidime (Lilly)
Other common trade names: *Ceftazim; Fortum; Tagal; Taloken; Waytrax*
Indications: Various infections caused by susceptible organisms
Category: Third generation cephalosporin
Half-life: 1–2 hours

Note: Penicillin and cephalosporins share a common beta-lactam structure. People who are allergic to penicillin are approximately 4 times more likely to develop an allergic reaction to a cephalosporin than those people who have no penicillin allergy. (From 5 to 16% of patients allergic to penicillin develop allergic reactions to cephalosporins)

Reactions

Skin
Acne
Acute generalized exanthematous pustulosis (AGEP)
  (2003): Mysore V+, *J Dermatolog Treat* 14(1), 54
Allergic reactions (sic)
  (1994): Pleasants RA+, *Chest* 106, 1124 (in patients with cystic fibrosis)
Angioedema (2%)
Candidiasis (<1%)
Diaper rash
Diaphoresis
Edema
Erythema multiforme (2%)
  (1983): Pierce TH+, *J Antimicrob Chemother* 12 (Suppl A), 21
Exanthems
  (1985): Richards DM+, *Drugs* 29, 105 (1.6%)
Flushing
Pemphigus erythematosus (sic)
  (1993): Iannantuono M+, *Int J Dermatol* 32, 675
  (1993): Pellicano R+, *Int J Dermatol* 32, 675
Photosensitivity
  (1993): Vinks SA+, *Lancet* 341, 1221
Pruritus (2%)
  (1996): Holloway WJ+, *Am J Med* 100, 52S
  (1985): Richards DM+, *Drugs* 29, 105
Rash (sic) (2%)
  (1996): Holloway WJ+, *Am J Med* 100, 52S
Stevens–Johnson syndrome (2%)
Toxic epidermal necrolysis (2%)
Toxic erythema
  (1995): Rademaker M, *N Z Med J* 108, 165
Toxic pustuloderma
  (1990): Rustin MHA+, *Br J Dermatol* 123, 119
Urticaria (<1%)

Other
Anaphylactoid reactions (2%)
  (1985): Richards DM+, *Drugs* 29, 105
Dysgeusia
Glossitis
Hypersensitivity (2%)
  (2001): Romano A+, *Allergy* 56, 84
Injection-site burning
Injection-site cellulitis
Injection-site edema
Injection-site inflammation (2%)
Injection-site pain (1.4%)

(1989): Gaut PL+, *Am J Med* 87 (Suppl 5A), 169S
Injection-site thrombophlebitis (2%)
Oral candidiasis
Paresthesias (<1%)
Phlebitis (<1%)
Serum sickness
Vaginal candidiasis
Vaginitis (1%)

CEFTIBUTEN

Trade name: Cedax (Biovail)
Other common trade names: *Ceten; Cilecef; Keimax; Seftem*
Indications: Various infections caused by susceptible organisms
Category: Third generation cephalosporin
Half-life: 2 hours

Note: Penicillin and cephalosporins share a common beta-lactam structure. People who are allergic to penicillin are approximately 4 times more likely to develop an allergic reaction to a cephalosporin than those people who have no penicillin allergy. (From 5 to 16% of patients allergic to penicillin develop allergic reactions to cephalosporins)

Reactions

Skin
Candidiasis (<1%)
Diaper rash (<1%)
Pruritus (0.3%)
Rash (sic) (0.3%)
Stevens–Johnson syndrome (<1%)
Toxic epidermal necrolysis
Urticaria (<1%)

Other
Dysgeusia (<1%)
Hypersensitivity
Oral candidiasis
Paresthesias (<1%)
Serum sickness (<1%)
Vaginitis (<1%)
Xerostomia (<1%)

CEFTIZOXIME

Trade name: Cefizox (Fujisawa)
Other common trade names: *Ceftix; Ceftrax; Epocelin; Lyceft; Tefidox; Ultracef*
Indications: Various infections caused by susceptible organisms
Category: Third generation cephalosporin
Half-life: 1.6 hours

Note: Penicillin and cephalosporins share a common beta-lactam structure. People who are allergic to penicillin are approximately 4 times more likely to develop an allergic reaction to a cephalosporin than those people who have no penicillin allergy. (From 5 to 16% of patients allergic to penicillin develop allergic reactions to cephalosporins)

Reactions

Skin
Candidiasis (<1%)
Pruritus (1–5%)

Rash (sic) (1–5%)
Stevens–Johnson syndrome (<1%)
Toxic epidermal necrolysis
Urticaria (<1%)

Other
Anaphylactoid reactions (<1%)
Injection-site edema
Injection-site induration
Injection-site pain (1–5%)
Injection-site phlebitis (1–5%)
Oral candidiasis
Paresthesias (1–5%)
Phlebitis (<1%)
Serum sickness (<1%)
Vaginitis (<1%)

CEFTRIAXONE

Trade name: Rocephin (Roche)
Other common trade names: *Benaxona; Cefaxona; Cefaxone; Rocefin; Rocephalin; Tacex; Triaken; Zefone*
Indications: Various infections caused by susceptible organisms
Category: Third generation cephalosporin
Half-life: 5–9 hours

Note: Penicillin and cephalosporins share a common beta-lactam structure. People who are allergic to penicillin are approximately 4 times more likely to develop an allergic reaction to a cephalosporin than those people who have no penicillin allergy. (From 5 to 16% of patients allergic to penicillin develop allergic reactions to cephalosporins)

Reactions

Skin
Angioedema
  (1984): Richards DM+, *Drugs* 27, 469
Candidiasis (sic) (5%)
  (2002): Lamb HM+, *Drugs* 62(7), 1041
  (1983): Bittner MJ+, *Antimicrob Agents Chemother* 23, 261
    (superficial) (sic)
  (1983): Harrison CJ+, *Am J Dis Child* 137, 1048 (superficial) (sic)
    (5%)
Chills (<1%)
Dermatitis (sic)
  (1989): Baba S+, *Jap J Antibiotics* 42, 212 (4%)
  (1984): Richards DM+, *Drugs* 27, 469 (0.4%)
Diaphoresis (0.2%)
  (1984): Moskowitz BL, *Am J Med* 77 (Suppl 4C) 84
Erythema multiforme
  (1984): Richards DM+, *Drugs* 27, 469
Exanthems
  (1990): Schaad UB+, *N Engl J Med* 322, 141 (4%)
  (1988): Richards DM+, *Drugs* 35, 604
  (1985): Judson FN+, *JAMA* 253, 1417 (1.2%)
  (1984): Moskowitz BL, *Am J Med* 77 (Suppl 4C), 84 (1.74%)
  (1984): Richards DM+, *Drugs* 27, 469 (1.4%)
  (1983): Eron LJ+, *J Antimicrob Chemother* 12, 65 (6%)
Flushing (<1%)
  (1984): Moskowitz BL, *Am J Med* 77 (Suppl 4C), 84 (0.15%)
  (1983): Harrison CJ+, *Am J Dis Child* 137, 1048
Jarisch–Herxheimer reaction
  (1994): Strominger MB+, *J Neuroophthalmol* 14, 77
Linear IgA bullous dermatosis
  (1999): Yawalker N+, *Dermatology* 199, 25
Pemphigus
  (1992): Ruocco V+, *Acta Derm Venereol* (Stockh) 72, 48

Pruritus (<1%)
  (1984): Moskowitz BL, *Am J Med* 77 (Suppl 4C) 84 (0.34%)
  (1984): Richards DM+, *Drugs* 27, 469 (0.3%)
Purpura
Rash (sic) (1.7%)
  (2002): Lamb HM+, *Drugs* 62(7), 1041
  (1992): Francioli P+, *JAMA* 267, 264
  (1983): Eron LJ+, *J Antimicrob Chemother* 12, 65
Side effects (sic) (3%)
  (1984): Richards DM+, *Drugs* 27, 469
Stevens–Johnson syndrome
Toxic epidermal necrolysis
Urticaria (0.1%)
  (2002): Litt JZ, Beachwood, OH (personal case) (observation)
  (1984): Richards DM+, *Drugs* 27, 469

Other

Anaphylactoid reactions
  (2002): Baumgartner-Bonnevay C+, *Arch Pediatr* 9(10), 1050
  (1999): Romano A+, *J Allergy Clin Immunol* 104, 1113
  (1992): Lin RY, *Arch Intern Med* 152, 930 (17 cases)
  (1984): Richards DM+, *Drugs* 27, 469
Dysgeusia (<1%)
  (1992): Francioli P+, *JAMA* 267, 264
Glossitis
  (1984): Moskowitz BL, *Am J Med* 77 (Suppl 4C), 84
  (1984): Richards DM+, *Drugs* 27, 469
Hypersensitivity
  (2002): Hausermann P+, *Contact Dermatitis* 47(5), 311
  (2000): Demoly P+, *Allergy* 55, 418 (immediate)
  (2000): Romano A+, *Allergy* 55, 415 (immediate)
Injection-site induration
Injection-site pain (1–10%)
  (1992): Francioli P+, *JAMA* 267, 264
  (1984): Moskowitz BL, *Am J Med* 77 (Suppl 4C), 84 (1%)
  (1984): Richards DM+, *Drugs* 27, 469 (1–15%)
Injection-site phlebitis (<1%)
  (1984): Moskowitz BL, *Am J Med* 77 (Suppl 4C), 84 (0.95%)
  (1984): Richards DM+, *Drugs* 27, 469
Oral mucosal eruption
  (1984): Richards DM+, *Drugs* 27, 469
Serum sickness
  (1984): Moskowitz BL, *Am J Med* 77 (Suppl 4C), 84 (0.04%)
Status epilepticus
  (2001): Martinez-Rodriguez JE+, *Am J Med* 111
Vaginitis (<1%)

CEFUROXIME

Trade names: Ceftin (GSK); Kefurox (Lilly); Zinacef (GSK)
Other common trade names: *Cefuril; Cepazine; Elobact; Froxal; Zinacet; Zinat; Zinnat; Zoref*
Indications: Various infections caused by susceptible organisms
Category: Second generation cephalosporin
Half-life: 1–2 hours

Note: Penicillin and cephalosporins share a common beta-lactam structure. People who are allergic to penicillin are approximately 4 times more likely to develop an allergic reaction to a cephalosporin than those people who have no penicillin allergy. (From 5 to 16% of patients allergic to penicillin develop allergic reactions to cephalosporins)

Reactions

Skin

Acute generalized exanthematous pustulosis (AGEP)

(2001): Cohen AD+, *Int J Dermatol* 40(7), 458
(1995): Moreau A+, *Int J Dermatol* 34, 263 (passim)
Angioedema (<1%)
Erythema multiforme (<1%)
Exanthems
  (1997): Litt JZ, Beachwood, OH (personal case) (observation)
  (1990): Schaad UB+, *N Engl J Med* 332, 141 (6%)
  (1979): Brogden RN+, *Drugs* 17, 233 (4.4–6.7% in penicillin-allergic patients)
Jarisch–Herxheimer reaction
  (1992): Nadelman RB+, *Ann Intern Med* 117, 273
Pemphigus
  (1997): Brenner S+, *J Am Acad Dermatol* 36, 919
Perianal thrush
  (1987): Carson JWK+, *J Antimicrob Chemother* 19, 109
Pruritus (<1%)
Purpura
Pustules
  (1990): Rustin MHA+, *Br J Dermatol* 123, 119
Rash (sic) (<1%)
  (1988): *Med Lett* 30, 57
Stevens–Johnson syndrome (<1%)
Toxic epidermal necrolysis (<1%)
  (1997): Yossepowitch O+, *Eur J Med Res* 2, 182
  (1993): Correia O+, *Dermatology* 186, 32
Urticaria (<1%)
  (2002): Namyslowski G+, *J Chemother* 14(5), 508
  (1995): Litt JZ, Beachwood, OH (personal case) (observation)
  (1987): Parish LC+, *Int J Dermatol* 26, 389

Other

Anaphylactoid reactions (<1%)
  (2002): Prosser DP+, *Paediatr Anaesth* 12(1), 73
Hypersensitivity
  (1998): Romano A+, *J Allergy Clin Immunol* 101, 564
  (1992): Romano A+, *Contact Dermatitis* 27, 270
  (1991): Powell DA+, *Drug Intell Clin Pharm* 25, 1236
Injection-site pain (<1%)
Oral candidiasis
  (1985): Cooper TJ+, *J Antimicrobial Chemother* 16, 373
Serum sickness (<1%)
Thrombophlebitis (1–10%)
Vaginitis (<1%)
  (1988): *Med Lett* 30, 57

CELECOXIB

Trade name: Celebrex (Pfizer)
Indications: Osteoarthritis, rheumatoid arthritis
Category: NSAID Cox-2 inhibitor
Half-life: 11 hours

Reactions

Skin

Acute febrile neutrophilic dermatosis (Sweet's syndrome)
  (2001): Fye KH+, *J Am Acad Dermatol* 45, 300
Allergic reactions (sic) (<2%)
Angioedema
  (2002): Schneider F+, *Lancet* 359, 852
  (2001): Kelkar PS+, *J Rheumatol* 28(11), 2553
Bacterial infections (sic) (<2%)
Candidiasis (<2%)
  (1999): McClain SA, Bronx, NY (from Internet) (observation)
Dermatitis (sic) (<2%)

Diaphoresis (<2%)
Ecchymoses (<2%)
Edema (<2%)
Erythema
(2002): Friedman B+, *South Med J* 95(10), 1213
Erythema multiforme
(1999): Puritz E, Smithtown, NY (from Internet) (observation)
Exanthems (<2%)
(2002): Schneider F+, *Lancet* 359, 852
(2002): Verbeiren S+, *Ann Dermatol Venereol* 129(2), 203
(2000): Valentine MC, Everett, WA (from internet) (observation)
(patient was allergic to sulfa)
(1999): Fisher BJ, Toronto, Ontario (from Internet) (observation)
(1999): Graedon J+, *People's Pharmacy* (anecdote from a reader)
(1999): Jaffe PG, Columbia, SC (from Internet) (observation)
patient had "trouble" with sulfa years back
(1999): Litt JZ, Beachwood, OH (personal case) (observation)
(1999): Rudolph RI, Wyomissing, PA (from Internet)
(observation)
Exfoliative dermatitis
(2002): Friedman B+, *South Med J* 95(10), 1213
Facial edema (<2%)
Herpes simplex (<2%)
Herpes zoster (<2%)
Hot flashes (<2%)
Infections (sic) (<2%)
Lupus
(2003): Poza-Guedes P+, *Rheumatology* (Oxford) 42(7), 916
Nodules (sic) (<2%)
Peripheral edema (2.1%)
(2002): Chan FK+, *N Engl J Med* 347(26), 2104
(2000): Fetterman MR, Miami, FL (from Internet) (observation)
(leg)
(2000): Panagotacos PJ, San Francisco, CA (from Internet)
(observation) (pedal)
(1999): Simon LS+, *JAMA* 282, 1921
Photosensitivity (<2%)
(1999): Zabawski E, Dallas, TX (from Internet) (observation)
Pruritus (<2%)
(1999): Rudolph RI, Wyomissing, PA (from Internet)
(observation)
Psoriasis (palmoplantar)
(2000): Catalano PM, Bradenton, FL (from Internet)
(observation)
Rash (sic) (2.2%)
Stevens–Johnson syndrome
(1999): Puritz E, Smithtown, NY (from Internet) (observation)
Toxic epidermal necrolysis
(2003): Giglio P, *South Med J* 96(3), 320
(2002): Berger P+, *Pharmacotherapy* 22(9), 1193
(2002): Friedman B+, *South Med J* 95(10), 1213
(2000): Mitchell D, Thomasville, GA (from Internet)
(observation)
Urticaria (<2%)
(2002): Schneider F+, *Lancet* 359, 852
(2001): Kelkar PS+, *J Rheumatol* 28(11), 2553
Vasculitis
(2002): Gscheidel D+, *Hautarzt* 53(7), 488
(2002): Jordan KM+, *Rheumatology* (Oxford) 41(12), 1453
(2002): Schneider F+, *Lancet* 359, 852
Viral infections (sic) (<2%)
Xerosis (<2%)

Hair
Hair – alopecia (<2%)

Nails
Nails – changes (sic) (<2%)

Other
Anaphylactoid reactions
(2003): Gagnon R+, *J Allergy Clin Immunol* 111(6), 1404
(2001): Habki R+, *Ann Med Interne* (Paris) 152(5), 355
(2001): Levy MB+, *Ann Allergy Asthma Immunol* 87, 72
Application-site cellulitis (<2%)
Application-site reactions (<2%)
Death
(2002): Schneider F+, *Lancet* 359, 852
(2001): Weaver J+, *Am J Gastroenterol* 96(12), 3449
Dysgeusia (<2%)
Hyperesthesia (<2%)
Mastodynia (<2%)
Myalgia (<2%)
Paresthesias (<2%)
Pseudoporphyria
(2000): Cummins R+, *J Rheumatol* 27, 2938
Stomatitis (<2%)
Tendinitis (<2%)
Thrombophlebitis (<0.1%)
Tooth disorder (sic) (<2%)
Torsades de pointes
(2002): Pathak A+, *Ann Pharmacother* 36(7), 1290
Vaginal candidiasis (<2%)
Vaginitis (<2%)
Xerostomia (<2%)

*Note: Celecoxib is a sulfonamide and can be absorbed systemically. Sulfonamides can produce severe, possibly fatal, reactions such as toxic epidermal necrolysis and Stevens–Johnson syndrome

CEPHALEXIN

Trade names: Keflex (Dista); Keftab (DJ Pharma)
Other common trade names: *Apo-Cephalex; Biocet; Ceforal; Ceporex; Ceporexine; Kefarol; Novo-Lexin; Ospexin*
Indications: Various infections caused by susceptible organisms
Category: First generation cephalosporin
Half-life: 0.9–1.2 hours
Clinically important, potentially hazardous interactions with: amikacin, gentamicin

Note: Penicillin and cephalosporins share a common beta-lactam structure. People who are allergic to penicillin are approximately 4 times more likely to develop an allergic reaction to a cephalosporin than those people who have no penicillin allergy. (From 5 to 16% of patients allergic to penicillin develop allergic reactions to cephalosporins)

Reactions

Skin
Acute generalized exanthematous pustulosis (AGEP)
(2002): Arroyo MP+, *J Drugs Dermatol* 1(1), 63
(1995): Moreau A+, *Int J Dermatol* 34, 263 (passim)
Angioedema (<1%)
(1971): Griffith RS+, *Lancet* 1, 452 (0.7%)
Bullous pemphigoid
(2001): Czechowicz RT, *Australas J Dermatol* 42(2), 132
Dermatitis
(1986): Milligan A+, *Contact Dermatitis* 15, 91
Erythema multiforme (<1%)
(1998): Blumenthal HL, Beachwood, OH (personal case)
(observation)
(1992): Murray KM+, *Ann Pharmacotherapy* 26, 1230
(1988): Platt R+, *J Infect Dis* 158, 474

(1987): Norrby SR, *Drugs* 34 (Suppl 2), 105
Exanthems
  (1999): Litt JZ, Beachwood, OH (personal case) (observation)
  (1997): McCloskey GL+, *Cutis* 59, 251
  (1995): Litt JZ, Beachwood, OH (personal case) (observation)
  (1972): Speight TM+, *Drugs* 3, 9
  (1970): 8, 18 (1–5%)
Fixed eruption
  (1991): Baran R+, *Br J Dermatol* 125, 592
Pemphigus
  (1992): Vaillant L+, *Int J Dermatol* 31, 67
  (1991): Wolf R+, *Int J Dermatol* 30, 213
Pruritus
  (1999): Litt JZ, Beachwood, OH (personal case) (observation)
  (1988): Kumar A+, *Antimicrob Agents Chemother* 32, 882
  (1977): Okita K+, *Jpn J Antibiot* (Japanese) 30, 911
  (1971): Griffith RS+, *Lancet* 1, 452 (0.7%)
Pruritus ani et vulvae
Purpura
Pustules
  (1994): Spencer JM+, *Br J Dermatol* 130, 514
  (1988): Jackson H+, *Dermatologica* 177, 292
Rash (sic) (<1%)
Side effects (sic) (2%)
  (1972): Speight TM+, *Drugs* 3, 9
  (1971): Griffith RS+, *Lancet* 1, 452 (0.9%)
Stevens–Johnson syndrome (<1%)
  (1992): Murray KM+, *Ann Pharmacother* 26, 1230
  (1988): Platt R+, *J Infect Dis* 158, 474
  (1975): McArthur JE+, *N Z Med J* 81, 390
Toxic epidermal necrolysis (<1%)
  (1995): Jick H+, *Pharmacotherapy* 15, 428
  (1991): Dave J+, *J Antimicrob Chemotherapy* 28, 477
  (1987): Harnar TJ+, *J Burn Care Rehabil* 8, 554
  (1987): Hogan DJ+, *J Am Acad Dermatol* 17, 852
Urticaria (<1%)
  (1993): Litt JZ, Beachwood, OH (personal case) (observation)
  (1971): Griffith RS+, *Lancet* 1, 452 (0.7%)

Nails

Nails – paronychia
  (1991): Baran R+, *Br J Dermatol* 125, 592

Other

Anaphylactoid reactions (<1%)
  (1999): Nordt SP+, *Am J Emerg Med* 17, 492
  (1992): Lin RY, *Arch Intern Med* 152, 930 (17 cases)
  (1989): Hoffman DR+, *Ann Allergy* 62, 91 (fatal)
Hypersensitivity
Oral candidiasis
Serum sickness (<1%)
  (1988): Platt R+, *J Infect Dis* 158, 474
Vaginitis

CEPHALOTHIN

Trade name: Keflin (Lilly)
Other common trade names: *Ceftina; Ceporacin; Cepovenin; Keflin Neutral; Keflin Neutro; Keflin-N; Practogen*
Indications: Various infections caused by susceptible organisms
Category: First generation, broad-spectrum cephalosporin
Half-life: 30–50 minutes
Clinically important, potentially hazardous interactions with: amphotericin B, gentamicin

Note: Penicillin and cephalosporins share a common beta-lactam structure. People who are allergic to penicillin are approximately 4 times more likely to develop an allergic reaction to a cephalosporin than those people who have no penicillin allergy. (From 5 to 16% of patients allergic to penicillin develop allergic reactions to cephalosporins)

Reactions

Skin

Allergic reactions (sic)
  (1975): Braun WP, *Contact Dermatitis* 1, 190
  (1966): Thoburn R+, *JAMA* 198, 345 (8%)
Candidiasis (<1%)
Erythema multiforme
  (1996): Munoz-D+, *Contact Dermatitis* 34, 227
Exanthems (<1%)
  (1974): Sanders WE+, *N Engl J Med* 290, 424 (>5%)
  (1966): Merrill SL+, *Ann Intern Med* 64, 1 (1–5%)
  (1966): Thoburn R+, *JAMA* 198, 345 (5.5%)
  (1964): Griffith RS+, *JAMA* 189, 823 (5%)
  (1964): Weinstein L+, *JAMA* 189, 829 (1–5%)
Pruritus (<1%)
  (1966): Beaty HN+, *Ann Intern Med* 65, 641
Purpura
  (1980): Miescher PA+, *Clin Haematol* 9, 505
  (1968): Sheiman L+, *JAMA* 203, 601
Rash (sic)
Stevens–Johnson syndrome (<1%)
Toxic epidermal necrolysis
  (1988): Dreyfuss DA+, *Ann Plast Surg* 20, 146
Urticaria
  (1979): Branch DR+, *JAMA* 241, 495
  (1966): Beaty HN+, *Ann Intern Med* 65, 641
  (1966): Perkins RL+, *Ann Intern Med* 64, 13 (>5%)
  (1966): Thoburn R+, *JAMA* 198, 345 (4%)

Other

Anaphylactoid reactions
  (1987): Norrby SR, *Drugs* 34 (Suppl 2) 105
  (1974): Spruill FG+, *JAMA* 229, 440 (2 patients; both fatal)
  (1971): Petz LD, *Postgrad Med J* 47 Suppl, 64 (2 cases)
  (1966): Rothschild PD+, *JAMA* 196, 372
Injection-site induration (<1%)
Injection-site pain (<1%)
Phlebitis
  (1980): Meguro S+, *Jpn J Antibiot* 33, 1163
  (1976): Sorrentino AP+, *Am J Hosp Pharm* 33, 642
  (1973): Carrizosa J+, *Antimicrob Agents Chemother* 3, 306
  (1973): Inagaki J+, *Curr Ther Res Clin Exp* 15, 37
  (1973): Lane AZ+, *Antimicrob Agents Chemother* 2, 234
Serum sickness (<1%)
  (1974): Sanders WE+, *N Engl J Med* 290, 424

CEPHAPIRIN

Trade name: Cefadyl (Bristol-Myers Squibb)
Other common trade names: *Brisfirina; Cefaloject; Cefatrex; Cefatrexyl; Lopitrex; Unipirin*
Indications: Various infections caused by susceptible organisms
Category: First generation cephalosporin
Half-life: 36–60 minutes

Note: Penicillin and cephalosporins share a common beta-lactam structure. People who are allergic to penicillin are approximately 4 times more likely to develop an allergic reaction to a cephalosporin than those people who have no penicillin allergy. (From 5 to 16% of patients allergic to penicillin develop allergic reactions to cephalosporins)

Reactions

Skin
Candidiasis (<1%)
Erythema multiforme
Pruritus (1–5%)
Rash (sic) (1–5%)
Stevens–Johnson syndrome (<1%)
Toxic epidermal necrolysis
Urticaria (<1%)

Other
Anaphylactoid reactions
  (1979): Barnett AS+, *Anesth Analg* 58, 337
Hypersensitivity
Injection-site pain (1–5%)
Injection-site phlebitis (1–5%)
Paresthesias (1–5%)
Phlebitis
  (1980): Meguro S+, *Jpn J Antibiot* 33, 1163
  (1976): Sorrentino AP+, *Am J Hosp Pharm* 33, 642
  (1973): Carrizosa J+, *Antimicrob Agents Chemother* 3, 306
  (1973): Inagaki J+, *Curr Ther Res Clin Exp* 15, 37
  (1973): Lane AZ+, *Antimicrob Agents Chemother* 2, 234
Serum sickness (<1%)
Vaginitis

CEPHRADINE

Trade name: Velosef (Bristol-Myers Squibb)
Other common trade names: *Anspor; Cefro; Celex; Doncef; Eskacef; Maxisporin; Opebrin; Sefril; Veracef*
Indications: Various infections caused by susceptible organisms
Category: First generation cephalosporin
Half-life: 1–2 hours

Note: Penicillin and cephalosporins share a common beta-lactam structure. People who are allergic to penicillin are approximately 4 times more likely to develop an allergic reaction to a cephalosporin than those people who have no penicillin allergy. (From 5 to 16% of patients allergic to penicillin develop allergic reactions to cephalosporins)

Reactions

Skin
Acute generalized exanthematous pustulosis (AGEP)
  (1995): Moreau A+, *Int J Dermatol* 34, 263 (passim)
Erythema multiforme
Exanthems
  (1976): Brillinberg Wurth GH+, *Curr Res Med Opin* 4, 139

Pruritus (<1%)
Purpura
Pustules
  (1986): Kalb RE+, *Cutis* 38, 58
Rash (sic) (<1%)
Stevens–Johnson syndrome (<1%)
Toxic epidermal necrolysis
  (1990): Balcar-Boron A+, *Wiad Lek* (Polish) 43, 988
Toxic pustuloderma
  (1990): Rustin MHA+, *Br J Dermatol* 123, 119
Urticaria (<1%)

Other
Anaphylactoid reactions
Hypersensitivity
Injection-site pain (<1%)
Injection-site phlebitis (<1%)
Serum sickness
Vaginitis

CETIRIZINE

Synonyms: P-071; UCB-P071
Trade name: Zyrtec (Pfizer)
Other common trade names: *Alercet; Alerid; Cetrine; Cezin; Reactine; Triz; Virlix; Zirtin*
Indications: Allergic rhinitis, urticaria
Category: Antihistamine
Half-life: 8–11 hours
Clinically important, potentially hazardous interactions with: alcohol, CNS depressants

Reactions

Skin
Acne (<2%)
Angioedema (<2%)
Bullous eruption (<2%)
Dermatitis (sic) (<2%)
Diaphoresis (<2%)
Edema (periorbital, facial, ankle, generalized, peripheral)
Exanthems (<2%)
  (1998): Rehbein H, Jacksonville, FL (generalized) (from Internet)
    (observation)
  (1997): Stingeni L+, *Contact Dermatitis* 37, 249
Facial edema
  (2002): Schroer S+, *Clin Exp Dermatol* 27, 185
Fixed eruption
  (2002): Assouere MN+, *Ann Dermatol Venereol* 129(11), 1295
  (2002): Inamadar AC+, *Br J Dermatol* 147(5), 1025
  (2000): Kranke B+, *J Allergy Clin Immunol* 106(5), 988
    (multilocalized and bullous)
Flushing (<2%)
Furunculosis (<2%)
Hyperkeratosis (<2%)
Photosensitivity (<2%)
Phototoxicity (<2%)
Pruritus (<2%)
  (2002): Schroer S+, *Clin Exp Dermatol* 27, 185
Purpura (<2%)
Rash (sic) (<2%)
Seborrhea (<2%)
Urticaria (<2%)
  (2002): Schroer S+, *Clin Exp Dermatol* 27, 185

(2001): Calista D+, *Br J Dermatol* 144, 196
(1999): Karamfilov T+, *Br J Dermatol* 140, 979
(1997): Stingeni L+, *Contact Dermatitis* 37, 249
Xerosis (<2%)

Hair

Hair – alopecia (<2%)
  (1998): Reed BR, Denver, CO (from Internet) (observation)
Hair – hypertrichosis (<2%)

Other

Ageusia (<2%)
Anaphylactoid reactions (<2%)
Dysgeusia (<2%)
Fixed eruption
  (2002): Assouere MN+, *Ann Dermatol Venereol* 129(11), 1295
  (2002): Inamadar AC+, *Br J Dermatol* 147(5), 1025
Headache
Hyperesthesia (<2%)
Mastodynia (<2%)
Myalgia (<2%)
Paresthesias (<2%)
Parosmia (<2%)
Sialorrhea (<2%)
Stomatitis (<2%)
Tongue discoloration (<2%)
Tongue edema (<2%)
Vaginitis (<2%)
Xerostomia (5.7%)
  (1995): Breneman D+, *J Am Acad Dermatol* 33, 192

CETRORELIX

Trade name: Cetrotide (Serono)
Indications: Inhibition of premature luteinizing hormone surges in women undergoing controlled ovarian stimulation
Category: Antigonadotropic
Half-life: 5 hours

Reactions

Skin

Peripheral edema

Other

Anaphylactoid reactions
Injection-site edema
Injection-site erythema
  (1994): Leroy I+, *Fertil Steril* 62, 461
Injection-site pruritus
  (1994): Leroy I+, *Fertil Steril* 62, 461
Injection-site purpura

CEVIMELINE

Trade name: Exovac (SnowBrand)
Indications: Sicca syndrome in patients with Sjøgren's syndrome
Category: Cholinergic; Muscarinic agonist
Half-life: 3–4 hours

Reactions

Skin

Allergic reactions (sic) (1–10%)
Bullous eruption (<1%)
Dermatitis (sic) (<1%)
Diaphoresis (20%)
Eczema (<1%)
Edema (1–10%)
Exanthems (1–10%)
Flu-like syndrome (sic) (1–10%)
Fungal infections (sic) (1–10%)
Genital pruritus (<1%)
Hot flashes (2%)
Peripheral edema (1–10%)
Photosensitivity (<1%)
Pruritus (1–10%)
Rash (sic) (4%)
Ulcerations (<1%)
Vasculitis (<1%)
Xerosis (<1%)

Hair

Hair – alopecia (<1%)

Other

Dysgeusia (<1%)
Gingival hyperplasia (<1%)
Headache
Hyperesthesia (1–10%)
Myalgia (1–10%)
Paresthesias (<1%)
Parosmia (<1%)
Sialorrhea (2%)
Stomatitis (<1%)
Tendinitis (<1%)
Thrombophlebitis (<1%)
Tongue discoloration (<1%)
Tongue ulceration (<1%)
Tooth disorder (sic) (1–10%)
Tremor (1–10%)
Ulcerative stomatitis (1–10%)
Vaginitis (1–10%)
Xerostomia (1–10%)

CHAMOMILE

Scientific names: *Chamomilla recutita; Matricaria chamomilla; Matricaria recutita*
Family: Asteraceae; Compositae
Trade and other common names: Camomille; German Chamomile; Manzanilla; Pin Heads
Category: Sedative; Stomachic
Purported indications and other uses: Flatulence, travel sickness, nervous diarrhea, restlessness, menstrual cramps, hemorrhoids, mastitis, leg ulcers, inflammation of the respiratory tract. Used in flavoring, cosmetics, soaps and mouthwashes
Half-life: N/A
Clinically important, potentially hazardous interactions with: warfarin

Reactions

Skin
Allergic reactions (sic) (to those allergic to ragweed, marigolds, daisies)
Dermatitis
   (2002): Schempp CM+, *Hautarzt* 53(2), 93
   (2000): Foti C+, *Contact Dermatitis* 42(6), 360
   (2000): Giordano-Labadie F+, *Contact Dermatitis* 42(4), 247
Irritation
Sensitization
   (2002): Paulsen E, *Contact Dermatitis* 47(4), 189

Other
Anaphylactoid reactions
   (2001): Thien FC, *Med J Aust* 175(1), 54 (from enema)
   (1989): Subiza J+, *J Allergy Clin Immunol* 84, 353
Hypersensitivity

CHASTEBERRY

Scientific name: *Vitex agnus-castus*
Family: Verbenaceae
Trade and other common names: Abraham's Balm; Agno Casto; Agnocasto; Agnolyt (Madaus); Bish Barmagh Aghaji; Chaste Lamb-Tree; Chaste tree*; Daribrahim; Gatilier; Hayit; Hemp Tree; Kaff Maryam; Keuschlamm; Lygos; Monks Pepper; Panjangusht; Ranukabija; Safe Tree; Sauzgatillo; Seiyo-Ninzin-Boku; Shajerat Ebrahim; Strotan; Vitex; Ze 440
Category: Hormonal modulator
Half-life: N/A
Clinically important, potentially hazardous interactions with: dopamine-receptor antagonists

Reactions

Skin
Abscess
   (2001): Schellenberg R, *BMJ* 322(7279), 134 (mild)
Acne
   (2001): Schellenberg R, *BMJ* 322(7279), 134 (mild)
Adverse effects (sic)
   (2001): Schellenberg R, *BMJ* 322(7279), 134 (mild)
   (2000): Loch EG+, *J Womens Health Gend Based Med* 9(3), 315
      (1.2%)
Formication
Itching

Rash (sic)
Urticaria
   (2001): Schellenberg R, *BMJ* 322(7279), 134 (mild)

Other
Fatigue
   (2000): Berger D+, *Arch Gynecol Obstet* 264(3), 150
Headache
   (2000): Berger D+, *Arch Gynecol Obstet* 264(3), 150

Note: Chasteberry is not a phytoestrogen, it appears to stimulate progesterone production

*Note: The Catholic church once placed it in the pockets of neophyte monks to help them to maintain their vow of chastity

CHICORY

Scientific name: *Cichorium intybus*
Family: Compositae
Trade and other common names: Barbe de Capucin; Belgian endive; Hendibeh; Succory; Wild Succory
Category: Diuretic; Laxative; Tonic
Purported indications and other uses: coffee substitute, jaundice, liver enlargement, gout, rheumatism, skin eruptions connected with gout, inflammation. Topical: leaves used for swelling and inflammation. Culinary spice, flavoring
Half-life: N/A

Reactions

Skin
Allergic reactions (sic)
   (2003): Cadot P+, *Int Arch Allergy Immunol* 131(1), 19
   (1997): Helbling A+, *J Allergy Clin Immunol* 99(6), 854
   (1996): Cadot P+, *Clin Exp Allergy* 26(8), 940
Dermatitis
   (1983): Malten KE, *Contact Dermatitis* 9(3), 232

CHLORAL HYDRATE

Synonyms: chloral; hydrated chloral
Trade names: Aquachloral (Alcon); Noctec (Bristol-Myers Squibb)
Other common trade names: *Chloraldurat; Medianox; Novochlorhydrate; Somnox; Welldorm*
Indications: Insomnia, sedation
Category: Sedative-hypnotic
Half-life: 8–11 hours
Clinically important, potentially hazardous interactions with: antihistamines, azatadine, azelastine, brompheniramine, buclizine, chlorpheniramine, clemastine, dexchlorpheniramine, diphenhydramine, meclizine, tripelennamine

Reactions

Skin
Acne
   (1967): Hitch JM, *JAMA* 200, 879
   (1956): Christianson HB+, *Arch Dermatol* 74, 232
Angioedema
   (1973): Almeyda J+, *Br J Dermatol* 86, 313
   (1956): Christianson HB+, *Arch Dermatol* 74, 232
Bullous eruption

(1967): Coleman WP, *Med Clin North Am* 51, 1073
Dermatitis (sic)
  (1987): de Groot AC+, *Contact Dermatitis* 16, 229
  (1956): Christianson HB+, *Arch Dermatol* 74, 232
Eczema (sic)
  (1956): Christianson HB+, *Arch Dermatol* 74, 232
Erythema
  (1956): Christianson HB+, *Arch Dermatol* 74, 232
Erythema multiforme
  (1991): Porteous DM+, *Arch Dermatol* 127, 740 (in AIDS)
  (1956): Christianson HB+, *Arch Dermatol* 74, 232
Exanthems
  (1990): Lindner K+, *Dermatol Monatsschr* (German) 176, 483
  (1976): Arndt KA+, *JAMA* 235, 918 (0.02%)
  (1956): Christianson HB+, *Arch Dermatol* 74, 232
Fixed eruption
  (1973): Almeyda J+, *Br J Dermatol* 86, 313
  (1972): Verbov J, *Br J Dermatol* 86, 438
  (1966): Miller LH+, *Arch Dermatol* 94, 60
  (1961): Welsh AL+, *Arch Dermatol* 84, 1004
  (1956): Christianson HB+, *Arch Dermatol* 74, 232
Flushing
  (1956): Christianson HB+, *Arch Dermatol* 74, 232
Lichenoid eruption
  (1956): Christianson HB+, *Arch Dermatol* 74, 232
Perioral dermatitis
  (2001): Caksen H+, *Pediatr Dermatol* 18(5), 454
Pruritus
  (1990): Lindner K+, *Dermatol Monatsschr* (German) 176, 483
  (1956): Christianson HB+, *Arch Dermatol* 74, 232
Purpura
  (1973): Almeyda J+, *Br J Dermatol* 86, 313
  (1956): Christianson HB+, *Arch Dermatol* 74, 232
Rash (sic) (1–10%)
Ulcerations
  (1956): Christianson HB+, *Arch Dermatol* 74, 232
Urticaria (1–10%)
  (1973): Almeyda J+, *Br J Dermatol* 86, 313
  (1956): Christianson HB+, *Arch Dermatol* 74, 232

Other

Acute intermittent porphyria
Death
  (2003): Thurau K+, *Arch Kriminol* 211(3), 90
  (2001): Gaulier JM+, *J Forensic Sci* 46(6), 1507 (2 cases)
Dysgeusia
Headache
Hypersensitivity
Oral mucosal lesions
  (2001): Caksen H+, *Pediatr Dermatol* 18(5), 454
  (1956): Christianson HB+, *Arch Dermatol* 74, 232
Oral ulceration
  (1956): Christianson HB+, *Arch Dermatol* 74, 232
Stomatitis
  (1956): Christianson HB+, *Arch Dermatol* 74, 232

CHLORAMBUCIL

Trade name: Leukeran (GSK)
Other common trade names: *Chloraminophene; Linfolysin*
Indications: Chronic lymphocytic leukemia, lymphomas, carcinomas
Category: Antineoplastic
Half-life: 1.5 hours
Clinically important, potentially hazardous interactions with: aldesleukin, antineoplastics, azathioprine, bone marrow suppressants, **vaccines**

Reactions

Skin

Angioedema
  (1977): Millard LG+, *Arch Dermatol* 113, 1298
Edema
Edema of foot
  (1987): Schmutz JL+, *Ann Dermatol Venereol* (French) 114, 569
Erythema multiforme
  (1987): Hitchens RN+, *Aust N Z J Med* 17, 600
Exanthems
  (1992): Breathnach SM+, *Adverse Drug Reactions and the Skin* Blackwell, Oxford, 289 (passim)
  (1987): Hitchens RN+, *Aust N Z J Med* 17, 600
  (1986): Peterman A+, *Arch Dermatol* 122, 1358
  (1978): Franchimont P+J, *Rheumatol* 5, 85 (1.3%)
  (1977): Millard LG+, *Arch Dermatol* 113, 1298
  (1971): Knisely RE+, *Arch Dermatol* 104, 77
  (1968): Vissian L+, *Bull Soc Fr Dermatol Syphiligr* (French) 75, 570
Exfoliative dermatitis
  (1987): Hitchens RN+, *Aust N Z J Med* 17, 600
Facial erythema
  (1986): Peterman A+, *Arch Dermatol* 122, 1358
Herpes simplex
  (1984): Sahgal SM+, *J R Soc Med* 77, 144
  (1971): Degos R+, *Bull Soc Fr Dermatol Syphiligr* (French) 78, 631
Herpes zoster
  (2002): Goldstein DA+, *Ophthalmology* 109(2), 370
  (1972): Decker JL, *Ann Intern Med* 76, 619 (>5%)
Kaposi's sarcoma
  (1974): Faye I+, *Bull Soc Fr Dermatol Syphiligr* (French) 81, 379
Lupus erythematosus
  (1986): Peterman A+, *Arch Dermatol* 122, 1358
Necrosis
  (1972): Decker JL, *Ann Intern Med* 76, 619
Periorbital edema
  (1992): Breathnach SM+, *Adverse Drug Reactions and the Skin* Blackwell, Oxford, 289 (passim)
  (1986): Peterman A+, *Arch Dermatol* 122, 1358
  (1977): Millard LG+, *Arch Dermatol* 113, 1298
Photosensitivity
  (1987): Schmutz JL+, *Ann Dermatol Venereol* (French) 114, 569
Pruritus
  (1971): Knisely RE+, *Arch Dermatol* 104, 77
  (1968): Vissian L+, *Bull Soc Fr Dermatol Syphiligr* (French) 75, 570
Psoriasis (exacerbation)
  (1968): Vissian L+, *Bull Soc Fr Dermatol Syphiligr* (French) 75, 570
Purpura
  (1990): Pietrantonio F+, *Cancer Lett* 54, 109
Rash (sic) (1–10%)
Sezary syndrome
  (1981): Ferme F+, *Leuk Res* 5, 169
Side effects (sic)
  (1968): Moore GE+, *Cancer Chemother Abstr* 52, 661 (20%)

Stevens–Johnson syndrome
Toxic epidermal necrolysis
  (1997): Aydogdu I+, *Anticancer Drugs* 8, 468
  (1990): Barone C+, *Eur J Cancer* 26, 1262
  (1990): Pietrantonio F+, *Cancer Lett* 54, 109
  (1968): Vissian L+, *Bull Soc Fr Dermatol Syphiligr* (French) 75, 570
Urticaria
  (1992): Breathnach SM+, *Adverse Drug Reactions and the Skin*
    Blackwell, Oxford, 289 (passim)
  (1977): Millard LG+, *Arch Dermatol* 113, 1298
  (1971): Knisely RE+, *Arch Dermatol* 104, 77
  (1968): Vissian L+, *Bull Soc Fr Dermatol Syphiligr* (French) 75, 570

Hair

Hair – alopecia
  (1992): Breathnach SM+, *Adverse Drug Reactions and the Skin*
    Blackwell, Oxford, 289 (passim)
  (1978): Franchimont P+, *J Rheumatol* 5, 85 (1.3%)
  (1978): Levine N+, *Cancer Treat Rev* 5, 67
  (1973): Snaith ML+, *BMJ* 2, 197

Other

Acute intermittent porphyria
Hypersensitivity (<1%)
  (1971): Knisley RE+, *Arch Dermatol* 104, 77
Oral mucosal lesions
  (1968): Moore GE+, *Cancer Chemother Abstr* 52, 661 (2%)
Oral ulceration (<1%)
  (1987): Hitchens RN+, *Aust N Z J Med* 17, 600
Stomatitis

CHLORAMPHENICOL

Trade names: AK-Chlor (Akorn); Chloromycetin (Parke-Davis);
Chloroptic (Allergan); Ophthochlor (Parke-Davis)
Other common trade names: *Aquamycetin; Cebenicol;
Diochloram; Kloramfenicol; Oleomycetin; Pentamycetin;
Sopamycetin; Tifomycine*
Indications: Various infections caused by susceptible organisms
Category: Broad-spectrum antibiotic
Half-life: 1.5–3.5 hours
**Clinically important, potentially hazardous interactions
with:** amoxicillin, ampicillin, ethotoin, fosphenytoin,
mephenytoin, phenytoin

Reactions

Skin

Acute generalized exanthematous pustulosis (AGEP)
  (2000): Lee AY+, *Acta Derm Venereol* 79, 412
  (1995): Moreau A+, *Int J Dermatol* 34, 263 (passim)
Angioedema (<1%)
  (1985): Schewach-Millet M+, *Arch Dermatol* 121, 587
Bullous eruption
  (1963): Ory EM+, *JAMA* 185, 273
Dermatitis (sic)
  (2001): Sachs B+, *Allergy* 56(1), 69
  (1998): Le Coz CJ+, *Contact Dermatitis* 38, 108 (face)
  (1996): Moyano JC+, *Allergy* 51, 67
  (1992): Urrutia I+, *Contact Dermatitis* 26, 66
  (1991): Vincenzi C+, *Contact Dermatitis* 25, 64
  (1987): Kubo Y+, *Contact Dermatitis* 17, 245
  (1987): Raulin C+, *Derm Beruf Umwelt* 35, 64
  (1986): Rebandel P+, *Contact Dermatitis* 15, 92
  (1986): van Joost T+, *Contact Dermatitis* 14, 176
  (1985): Linss G+, *Dermatol Monatsschr* (German) 171, 250

  (1978): Blondeel A+, *Contact Dermatitis* 4, 270
  (1976): Rudzki E+, *Contact Dermatitis* 2, 181
  (1975): Braun WP, *Contact Dermatitis* 1, 241
  (1975): Wereide K, *Contact Dermatitis* 1, 271
  (1973): Ebner H, *Wien Klin Wochenschr* (German) 85, 203
  (1967): Schubert H, *Allerg Asthma Leipz* (German) 13, 25
  (1966): Eberhartinger C+, *Arch Klin Exp Dermatol* (German)
    224, 463
  (1966): Korossy S+, *Z Haut Geschlechtskr* (German) 41, 375
Eczema (sic)
Edema of foot
Erythema multiforme (<1%)
  (1996): Lazarov A+, *Cutis* 58, 263 (from eyedrops)
  (1986): Fisher AA, *Cutis* 37, 158 (topical application)
  (1969): Ting HC+, *Int J Dermatol* 24, 587
  (1967): Coleman WP, *Med Clin North Am* 51, 1073
  (1965): Mathé P+, *J Med Bordeaux* (French) 42, 1367
  (1965): Pieris EV, *Ceylon Med J* 10, 67
Exanthems (1–5%)
  (1992): Breathnach SM+, *Adverse Drug Reactions and the Skin*
    Blackwell, Oxford, 157 (passim)
  (1972): Kauppinen K, *Acta Derm Venereol* (Stockh) 52, (Suppl) 68
  (1969): Török H, *Dermatol Int* 8, 57
  (1951): Altemeier WA+, *JAMA* 145, 489 (1.7%)
  (1951): Usndek HE+, *Arch Dermatol* 64, 217
Fixed eruption
  (1985): Pandhi RK+, *Australasian J Dermatol* 26, 88
Gray syndrome*
Leucoderma
  (1980): Chalfin J+, *Ophthalmic Surg* 11, 194 (eyelid)
Pruritus (<1%)
  (1992): Breathnach SM+, *Adverse Drug Reactions and the Skin*
    Blackwell, Oxford, 157 (passim)
Purpura
  (1967): Singh S+, *Indian J Pediatr* 4, 451
  (1965): Horowitz HI+, *Semin Hematol* 2, 287
Pustules
  (1973): Macmillan AL, *Dermatologica* 146, 285
  (1971): Stevanovic DN, *Br J Dermatol* 85, 134
Rash (sic) (<1%)
Sensitization (sic)
  (1992): Urrutia I+, *Contact Dermatitis* 26, 66
  (1986): van Joost T+, *Contact Dermatitis* 14, 176
Sheet-like erythema
Stevens–Johnson syndrome
  (1965): Pieris EV, *Ceylon Med J* 10, 67
Systemic eczematous contact dermatitis
Toxic epidermal necrolysis (<1%)
  (1975): Munstermann M+, *Dtsch Med Wochenschr* (German)
    100, 2337
  (1965): Mathé P+, *J Med Bord* (French) 142, 1367
Urticaria
  (1992): Breathnach SM+, *Adverse Drug Reactions and the Skin*
    Blackwell, Oxford, 157 (passim)
  (1987): Perkins JB+, *Drug Intell Clin Pharm* 21, 343
  (1985): Schewach-Millet M+, *Arch Dermatol* 121, 587
Vasculitis
  (1965): McCombs RP, *JAMA* 194, 1059

Hair

Hair – alopecia
  (1977): Kapp JP+, *Clinical Pediatrics* 16, 64

Nails

Nails – photo-onycholysis
  (1985): Kechijian P, *J Am Acad Dermatol* 12, 552
  (1984): Daniel CR+, *J Am Acad Dermatol* 10, 250

Other
Acute intermittent porphyria
Anaphylactoid reactions
  (1976): Kozakova M, Cesk Dermatol (Slovak) 51, 82
Black tongue
  (1954): Annotations, Lancet 2, 179
Glossitis
  (1951): Altemeier WA+, JAMA 145, 489
Headache
Hypersensitivity
  (1978): Simon N, Z Hautkr (German) 53, 341
  (1974): Hegyi E+, Cesk Dermatol (Slovak) 49, 96
Oral mucosal eruption
  (1951): Altemeier WA+, JAMA 145, 489
Oral ulceration
Paresthesias
  (1988): Ramilo O+, Pediatr Infect Dis 7, 358
Porphyria
  (1976): Panica D+, Folia Med Plovdiv 18, 161
Stomatitis (<1%)
Xerostomia

*Note: Gray syndrome: toxic reactions in premature infants and newborns. Signs and symptoms include: abdominal distension, blue-gray skin color, low body temperature, and uneven breathing

CHLORDIAZEPOXIDE

Trade names: Libritabs (ICN); Librium (ICN); Limbitrol (ICN)
Other common trade names: Corax; Huberplex; Medilium; Mitran; Multum; Novopoxide; Psicofar; Reposans-10; Solium; Tropium
Indications: Anxiety
Category: Antianxiety; Antipanic; Antitremor; Benzodiazepine sedative-hypnotic
Half-life: 6–25 hours
Clinically important, potentially hazardous interactions with: chlorpheniramine, clarithromycin, efavirenz, esomeprazole, imatinib, indinavir, ketoconazole, nelfinavir, ritonavir

Limbitrol is amitriptyline and chlordiazepoxide

Reactions

Skin
Angioedema (<1%)
  (1971): Almeyda J, Br J Dermatol 84, 299
  (1964): Welsh AL, Med Clin North Am 48, 459
Dermatitis (sic) (1–10%)
Diaphoresis (>10%)
Edema (1–10%)
Erythema multiforme (<1%)
  (1992): Breathnach SM+, Adverse Drug Reactions and the Skin Blackwell, Oxford, 200 (passim)
  (1985): Kauppinen K+, Br J Dermatol 112, 575
  (1981): Edwards JG, Drugs 22, 495 (passim)
  (1974): Tay C, Asian J Med 10, 223
  (1971): Almeyda J, Br J Dermatol 84, 299
Erythema nodosum (<1%)
  (1981): Edwards JG, Drugs 22, 495 (passim)
  (1971): Almeyda J, Br J Dermatol 84, 299
Exanthems
  (1976): Arndt KA+, JAMA 235, 918 (0.42%)
  (1971): Almeyda J, Br J Dermatol 84, 299
Fixed eruption (<1%)
  (1990): Gaffoor PMA+, Cutis 45, 242 (passim)

  (1981): Edwards JG, Drugs 22, 495 (passim)
  (1974): Blair HM, Arch Dermatol 109, 914
  (1970): Savin JA, Br J Dermatol 83, 546
  (1964): Welsh AL, Med Clin North Am 48, 459
  (1961): Gaul LE, Arch Dermatol 83, 1010
Lupus erythematosus
  (1973): Hicks JH, Cutis 11, 33
  (1973): McCarthy J, Arch Dermatol 108, 733 (discussion)
  (1965): Grupper CH+, Bull Soc Franc Derm Syphiligr (French) 72, 714
Photosensitivity
  (1986): Morliere P, Biochemie 68, 849
  (1981): Edwards JG, Drugs 22, 495 (passim)
  (1980): Bjellerup M+, J Invest Dermatol 75, 228
  (1973): Torre D, Arch Dermatol 108, 733 (discussion)
  (1971): Almeyda J, Br J Dermatol 84, 299
  (1965): Luton EF+, Arch Dermatol 91, 362
Pigmented purpuric eruption
  (1989): Nishioka K+, J Dermatol (Tokio) 16, 220
Pruritus
  (1977): Ghosh JS, BMJ 1, 902
Purpura
  (2001): Alexopoulou A+, Arch Intern Med 161(14), 1778 (with clidinium)
  (1981): Edwards JG, Drugs 22, 495 (passim)
  (1977): Celada A+, BMJ 1, 268
  (1971): Almeyda J, Br J Dermatol 84, 299
  (1967): Copperman IJ, BMJ 4, 485
Rash (sic) (>10%)
  (1960): Tobin JM, JAMA 174, 1242
Urticaria
  (1981): Edwards JG, Drugs 22, 495 (passim)
  (1974): Tay C, Asian J Med 10, 223
  (1971): Almeyda J, Br J Dermatol 84, 299
  (1964): Welsh AL, Med Clin North Am 48, 459
Vasculitis
  (1989): Nishioka K+, J Dermatol 16, 220
  (1971): Almeyda J, Br J Dermatol 84, 299

Hair
Hair – alopecia
  (1977): Celada A+, BMJ 1, 268
  (1973): Hicks JH, Cutis 11, 33
  (1965): Luton EF+, Arch Dermatol 91, 362

Other
Acute intermittent porphyria
  (1967): de Matteis F, Pharmacol Rev 19, 523
Galactorrhea
  (1971): Almeyda J, Br J Dermatol 84, 299
  (1961): Hooper JH+, JAMA 178, 506
  (1956): Marshall WK+, Lancet 1, 152
Gynecomastia
  (1965): Vavala V+, Endocr Metabol 36, 43
Headache
Injection-site phlebitis
Paresthesias
Porphyria
  (1983): Eubanks SW+, Int J Dermatol 22, 337
Sialopenia (>10%)
Sialorrhea (1–10%)
Xerostomia (>10%)

CHLORHEXIDINE

Trade names: BactoShield; Betasept (Purdue Frederick); Dyna-Hex; Exidine Scrub; Hibiclens (Regent); Hibistat; Peridex; PerioChip; Periogard
Other common trade names: Alcloxidine; Bactoscrub; Chlorhexamed; Corsodyl; Hexol; Hibident; Hibidil; Hibiscrub; Hibitane; Savlon; Spectro Gram
Indications: Skin antisepsis, gingivitis
Category: Topical anti-infective
Half-life: N/A

Reactions

Skin

Allergic reactions (sic)
  (2003): Jayathillake A+, *Urology* 61(4), 837
  (2001): Garvey LH+, *Acta Anaesthesiol Scand* 45(10), 1290
    (4 cases)
  (1995): Yong D+, *Med J Aust* 162, 257
  (1992): Ramselaar CG+, *Br J Urol* 70, 451
  (1985): Cheung J+, *Anaesth Intensive Care* 13, 429
  (1982): Staab W+, *Stomatol DDR* (German) 32, 700
Dermatitis (sic)
  (2001): Barnett L+, *Ostomy Wound Manage* 47(9), 47
  (2001): Barrazza V, *Contact Dermatitis* 45(1), 42
  (1998): Ebo DG+, *J Allergy Clin Immunol* 101, 128
  (1998): Thune P, *Tidsskr Nor Laegeforen* (Norwegian) 18, 3295
  (1995): Stingeni L+, *Contact Dermatitis* 33, 172
  (1990): Reynolds NJ+, *Contact Dermatitis* 22, 103
  (1988): Bergqvist-Karlsson A, *Contact Dermatitis* 18, 84
  (1987): Osmundsen PE+, *Ugeskr Laeger* (Danish) 149, 3048
  (1985): Lasthein Andersen B+, *Contact Dermatitis* 13, 307
    (5.4%)
  (1983): Shoji A, *Contact Dermatitis* 9, 156
  (1982): Osmundsen PE, *Contact Dermatitis* 8, 81
  (1981): Roberts DL+, *Contact Dermatitis* 7, 326
  (1972): Ljunggren B+, *Acta Derm Venereol* (Stockh) 52, 308
  (1972): Neering H+, *Ned Tijdschr Geneeskd* (Dutch) 116, 1742
Facial edema (<1%)
Fixed eruption
  (1991): Moghadam BK+, *Oral Surg Oral Med Oral Pathol* 71, 431
Photosensitivity
  (1971): Wahlberg JE+, *Dermatologica* 143, 376
Rash (sic)
  (2001): Garvey LH+, *Acta Anaesthesiol Scand* 45(10), 1290
    (4 cases)
Urticaria
  (1998): Stables GI+, *Br J Urol* 82, 756
  (1990): Wong WK+, *Contact Dermatitis* 22, 52 (contact)
  (1989): Fisher AA, *Cutis* 43, 17
  (1988): Bergqvist-Karlsson A, *Contact Dermatitis* 18, 84

Other

Anaphylactoid reactions
  (2001): Garvey LH+, *Acta Anaesthesiol Scand* 45(10), 1204
    (4 cases)
  (2001): Knight BA+, *Intern Med J* 31(7), 436
  (2001): Lockhart AS+, *Br J Anaesth* 87(6), 940
  (2001): Stephens R+, *Br J Anaesth* 87(2), 306 (with sulfadiazine)
  (2000): Pham NH+, *Clin Exp Allergy* 30, 1001
  (1999): Autegarden JE+, *Contact Dermatitis* 40, 215
  (1999): Snellman E+, *J Am Acad Dermatol* 40, 771
  (1998): Ebo DG+, *J Allergy Clin Immunol* 101, 128
  (1998): Nikaido S+, *Masui* (Japanese) 47, 330
  (1998): Olivieri J+, *Schweiz Med Wochenschr* 128, 1508
  (1998): Terazawa E+, *Anesthesiology* 89, 1296
  (1998): Thune P, *Tidsskr Nor Laegeforen* (Norwegian) 118, 3295

  (1997): Chisholm DG+, *BMJ* 315, 785
  (1997): Fujita S+, *Masui* (Japanese) 46, 1118 (2 cases)
  (1996): Torricelli R, *Clin Exp Allergy* 26, 112
  (1995): Parker F+, *Anaesth Intensive Care* 23, 126
  (1994): de Groot AC+, *Ned Tijdschr Geneeskd* (Dutch) 138, 1342
  (1994): Okuda T+, *Masui* (Japanese) 43, 1352
  (1994): Russ BR+, *Anaesth Intensive Care* 22, 611
  (1994): Visser LE+, *Ned Tijdschr Geneeskd* (Dutch) 138, 778
  (1992): Evans RJ, *BMJ* 304, 686
  (1992): Harukuni I+, *Masui* (Japanese) 41, 455
  (1992): Peutrell JM, *Anaesthesia* 47, 1013
  (1990): Wong WK+, *Contact Dermatitis* 22, 52
Dysgeusia (>10%)
  (1978): Schaupp H+, *HNO* (German) 26, 335
Gingivitis
  (1984): Asikainen S+, *J Clin Periodontol* 11, 87
  (1982): Ainamo J+, *J Clin Periodontol* 9, 337
Glossitis (1–10%)
Hypersensitivity
  (2001): Lauerma AL, *Contact Dermatitis* 44(1), 59
  (1998): Burlington B, *Ostomy Wound Manage* 44, 84
  (1994): Aalto-Korte K+, *Duodecim* (Finnish) 110, 2013
  (1989): Okano M+, *Arch Dermatol* 125, 50 (6 cases)
  (1988): Bergqvist-Karlsson A, *Contact Dermatitis* 18, 84
  (1986): Ohtoshi T+, *Clin Allergy* 16, 155
  (1986): Yaacob H+, *J Oral Med* 41, 145
  (1971): Wahlberg JE+, *Dermatologica* 143, 376
Oral mucosal reaction
  (1982): Skoglund LA+, *Int J Oral Surg* 11, 380 (3 cases)
Stomatitis (1–10%)
Tongue irritation (1–10%)
Tongue pigmentation (>10%)
Tooth pigmentation
  (2002): Moshrefi A, *J West Soc Periodontol Periodontal Abstr* 50(1), 5

CHLORMEZANONE

Trade name: Trancopal (Sanofi-Synthelabo)
Indications: Anxiety
Category: Antianxiety
Half-life: 24 hours

Reactions

Skin

Ankle edema
Edema
Erythema multiforme
Exanthems
  (1989): Alanko K+, *Acta Derm Venereol* (Stockh) 69, 223
  (1964): Welsh AL, *Med Clin North Am* 48, 459
Fixed eruption
  (1998): Leal G, Fortaleza, Brazil (from Internet) (observation)
  (1998): Lee AY, *Contact Dermatitis* 38(5), 258
  (1998): Mahboob A+, *Int J Dermatol* 37, 833
  (1995): Rademacher D+, *Contact Dermatitis* 32, 117
  (1992): el-Sayed F+, *Ann Dermatol Venereol* (French) 119, 671
  (1991): Lee AY+, *Drug Intell Clin Pharm* 25, 604
  (1989): Alanko K+, *Acta Derm Venereol* (Stockh) 69, 223
  (1988): McFadden N, *Dermatologica* 176, 106
  (1985): Kauppinen K+, *Br J Dermatol* 112, 575
  (1985): Verbov J, *Dermatologica* 171, 60 (with acetaminophen)
  (1983): Mohamed KN+, *Int J Dermatol* 22, 548
  (1974): Kuokkanen K, *Int J Dermatol* 13, 4

(1964): Welsh AL, *Med Clin North Am* 48, 459
Flushing
Pruritus
  (1964): Welsh AL, *Med Clin North Am* 48, 459
Rash (sic)
  (1991): Lee AY+, *Drug Intell Clin Pharm* 25, 604 (passim)
Stevens–Johnson syndrome
  (1995): Roujeau JC+, *N Engl J Med* 333, 1600
  (1995): Wolkenstein P+, *Drug Saf* 13, 56
Toxic epidermal necrolysis
  (1998): von Boxberg C+, *Dtsch Med Wochenschr* (German)
    123, 866 (fatal)
  (1996): Blum L+, *J Am Acad Dermatol* 34, 1088
  (1995): Roujeau JC+, *N Engl J Med* 333, 1600
  (1993): Correia O+, *Dermatology* 186, 32
  (1992): Saiag P+, *J Am Acad Dermatol* 26, 567
  (1991): Rosenthal E+, *Presse Med* (French) 20, 1459
  (1987): Guillaume JC+, *Arch Dermatol* 123, 1166
  (1983): Tagami H+, *Arch Dermatol* 119, 910
Urticaria

Other

Acute intermittent porphyria
Death
Dysgeusia
  (1976): Rollin H, *Laryngol Rhinol Otol* (Stuttgart) (German)
    55, 873
Xerostomia
  (1964): Welsh AL, *Med Clin North Am* 48, 459

CHLOROQUINE

Trade name: Aralen (Sanofi-Synthelabo)
Other common trade names: *Avloclor; Chlorquin; Emquin;
Heliopar; Lagaquin; Malarivon*
Indications: Malaria, rheumatoid arthritis, lupus erythematosus
Category: Antimalarial; Antiprotozoal; Antirheumatic; Lupus
erythematosus suppressant
Half-life: 3–5 days
**Clinically important, potentially hazardous interactions
with:** acitretin, antacids, cholestyramine, dapsone, furazolidone,
hydroxychloroquine, methotrexate, methoxsalen, penicillamine,
sulfonamides

Reactions

Skin

Acute generalized exanthematous pustulosis (AGEP)
  (1998): Janier M+, *Dermatology* 196, 271
Angioedema (<1%)
  (1993): *Lakartidningen* (Swedish) 90, 54
Bullous pemphigoid
  (1999): Millard TP+, *Clin Exp Dermatol* 24, 263
Dermatitis
  (1984): Kellett JK+, *Contact Dermatitis* 11, 47
  (1975): Skog E, *Contact Dermatitis* 1, 187
Desquamation
  (2002): Pages F+, *Trop Med Int Health* 7(11), 919 (with
    proguanil)
Ephelides
  (1985): Dupre A+, *Arch Dermatol* 121, 1164
Erythema annulare centrifugum
  (1982): Koralewski F, *Dermatosen* (German) 30, 125
  (1967): Ashurst PJ, *Arch Dermatol* 95, 37
Erythema multiforme (<1%)

Erythroderma
  (1990): Simoneaux PW, *Curr Concept Skin Dis* Winter, 15
  (1986): Langtry JA+, *Br Med J Clin Res Ed* 292, 1107
  (1985): Slagel GA+, *J Am Acad Dermatol* 12, 857
Exanthems (1–5%)
  (1991): Ochsendorf FR+, *Hautarzt* (German) 42, 140
  (1990): Simoneaux PW, *Curr Concept Skin Dis* Winter, 15
  (1973): Rees RB+, *Arch Dermatol* 88, 280 (passim)
Exfoliative dermatitis
  (1986): Lavrijsen APM+, *Acta Derm Venereol* (Stockh) 66, 536
  (1985): Slagel GA+, *J Am Acad Dermatol* 12, 857
  (1980): Koranda FC, *J Am Acad Dermatol* 4, 650 (passim)
  (1973): Rees RB+, *Arch Dermatol* 88, 280 (passim)
Fixed eruption (<1%)
Lichenoid eruption
  (1990): Simoneaux PW, *Curr Concept Skin Dis* Winter, 15
  (1981): Koranda FC, *J Am Acad Dermatol* 4, 650 (passim)
  (1979): Krebs A, *Hautarzt* (German) 30, 281
  (1973): Rees RB+, *Arch Dermatol* 88, 280 (passim)
  (1958): Savage J, *Br J Dermatol* 70, 181
  (1948): Alving AS+, *J Clin Invest* 27, 56
Photosensitivity
  (2002): Pages F+, *Trop Med Int Health* 7(11), 919 (with
    proguanil)
  (1993): *Lakartidningen* (Swedish) 90, 54
  (1992): Seideman P+, *Scand J Rheumatol* 21, 101
  (1991): Ochsendorf FR+, *Hautarzt* (German) 42, 140
  (1989): Ortel B+, *Dermatologica* 178, 39
  (1982): van Weelden H, *Arch Dermatol* 118, 290
  (1973): Rees RB+, *Arch Dermatol* 88, 280 (passim)
Pigmentation
  (1998): Guedira N+, *Rev Rhum Engl Ed* 65, 58
  (1991): Ochsendorf FR+, *Hautarzt* (German) 42, 140
  (1987): Krebs A, *Schweiz Rundsch Med Prax* (German) 76, 1069
  (1982): Levy H, *S Afr Med J* 62, 735
  (1981): Koranda FC, *J Am Acad Dermatol* 4, 650 (passim)
  (1980): Bentsi-Enchill KO, *Trop Geogr Med* 32, 216
  (1975): Marriott P+, *Proc R Soc Med* 68, 535
  (1968): Stewart TW+, *Acta Derm Venereol* 48, 47
  (1963): Tuffanelli D+, *Arch Dermatol* 88, 419
  (1959): Dall JLC+, *BMJ* 1, 1387
Polymorphous light eruption
  (1968): Reed WB+, *Arch Dermatol* 98, 327
Pruritus
  (2000): Ademowo OG+, *Clin Pharm Ther* 67, 237
  (1999): Millard TP+, *Clin Exp Dermatol* 24, 263
  (1997): Adebayo RA+, *Br J Clin Pharmacol* 44, 157
  (1997): Sowunmi A+, *Trans R Trop Med Hyg* 91, 63
  (1996): George AO, *Int J Dermatol* 35, 323
  (1995): Osifo NG, *Afr J Med Sci* 24, 67
  (1992): Ogunranti JO+, *Eur J Clin Pharmacol* 43, 323
  (1991): Ajayi AA+, *Eur J Clin Pharmacol* 41, 383
  (1991): Ezeamuzie IC+, *J Trop Med Hyg* 94, 184
  (1991): Mnyika KS, *East Afr Med J* 68, 139
  (1991): Mnyika KS+, *J Trop Med Hyg* 94, 27 (47%)
  (1991): Okor RS, *J Clin Pharm Ther* 16, 463
  (1990): Abdulkadir SA+, *Trans Roy Soc Trop Med Hyg* 84, 898
  (1990): Okor RS, *J Clin Pharm Ther* 15, 147
  (1990): Simoneaux PW, *Curr Concept Skin Dis* Winter, 15
  (1989): Abila B+, *J Trop Med Hyg* 92, 356
  (1989): Burnham G+, *Trans R Soc Trop Med Hyg* 83, 527
  (1989): Hallwood PM+, *Lancet* 2, 397
  (1989): Osifo NG, *Afr J Med Sci* 18, 121
  (1989): Soro B+, *Bull Soc Pathol Exot Filiales* (French) 82, 88
  (1989): Sowunmi A+, *Lancet* 2, 213
  (1987): Spencer HC+, *Ann Trop Med Parasitol* 81, 124
  (1986): Harries AD+, *Ann Trop Med Parasitol* 80, 479
  (1984): Bhasin V+, *J Indian Med Assoc* 82, 447
  (1984): Caussade P, *Arch Fr Pediatr* (French) 41, 727
  (1984): Osifo NG, *Arch Dermatol* 120, 80
  (1982): Spencer HC+, *BMJ* 285, 1703

(1977): Olatunde A, *Afr J Med Sci* 6, 27
(1969): Olatunde IA, *J Nigerian Med Assoc* 6, 23
(1964): Ekpechi OL+, *Arch Dermatol* 120, 80
Psoriasis
(1993): Schopt RE+, *Dermatology* 187, 100
(1992): Vestey JP+, *J Infect* 24, 211
(1991): Damstra RJ+, *Ned Tijdschr Geneeskd* (Dutch) 135, 671
(1990): Abdulkadir SA+, *Trans R Soc Trop Med Hyg* 84, 898
(1990): Katugampola G+, *Int J Dermatol* 29, 153
(1990): Okor RS, *J Clin Pharm Ther* 15, 147
(1989): Mallett R+, *BMJ* 299, 1400
(1988): Nicolas J-F+, *Ann Dermatol Venereol* (French) 115, 289
(1985): Stone OJ, *Int J Dermatol* 24, 539
(1982): Abel EA+, *J Am Acad Dermatol* 15, 2007
(1982): Luzar MJ, *J Rheumatol* 9, 462
(1981): Olsen TG, *Ann Intern Med* 94, 546
(1980): Kuflik EG, *Cutis* 26, 153
(1966): Baker H, *Br J Dermatol* 78, 161
(1957): Cornbleet T+, *Arch Dermatol* 75, 286
Pustular psoriasis
(1999): Capper N, Mobile, AL (from Internet) (observation)
(1998): Wilairatana P+, *Int J Dermatol* 37, 713
(1997): Wilairatana P+, *Int J Dermatol* 36, 634
(1987): Friedman SJ, *J Am Acad Dermatol* 16, 1256
Pustules
(1990): Lotem M+, *Acta Derm Venereol* (Stockh) 70, 250
Stevens–Johnson syndrome
(2000): Madnani N, Mumbai, India (from Internet) (observation)
(1989): Ortel B+, *Dermatologica* 178, 39
(1987): Lenox-Smith I, *J Infect* 14, 90 (fatal)
(1986): Bamber MG+, *J Infect* 13, 31 (fatal)
Toxic epidermal necrolysis (<1%)
(1994): Boffa MJ+, *Br J Dermatol* 131, 444
(1988): Phillips-Howard PA+, *Br Med J Clin Res Ed* 296, 1605
(1979): Bazarnaia NS+, *Ter Arkh* (Russian) 51, 99
(1976): Kanwar AJ+, *Indian J Dermatol* 21, 73
(1972): Shul'tsev GP+, *Sov Med* (Russian) 35, 133
Urticaria
(2002): Pages F+, *Trop Med Int Health* 7(11), 919 (with proguanil)
(1990): Simoneaux PW, *Curr Concept Skin Dis* Winter, 15
(1980): Koranda FC, *J Am Acad Dermatol* 4, 650 (passim)
(1973): Rees RB+, *Arch Dermatol* 88, 280 (passim)
Vasculitis
Vitiligo
(2003): Martin-Garcia RF+, *J Am Acad Dermatol* 48(6), 981
(2002): Martin R+, *World Congress Dermatol* Poster, 0114
(1997): Selvaag E, *Ann Trop Pediatr* 17, 45
(1996): Selvaag E, *Acta Derm Venereol* 76, 166
(1996): Selvaag E, *Trans R Trop Med Hyg* 90, 683
(1995): Selvaag E+, American Academy of Dermatology Meeting, New Orleans (observation)
(1992): Gonggryp LA+, *Br J Rheumatol* 31, 790
(1980): Bentsi-Enchill KO, *Trop Geogr Med* 32, 216

Hair

Hair – alopecia
Hair – pigmentation (<1%)
(1997): Asch PH+, *Ann Dermatol Venereol* (French) 124, 552
(1992): Bublin JG+, *J Clin Pharm Ther* 17, 297
(1991): Ochsendorf FR+, *Hautarzt* (German) 42, 140
(1981): Koranda FC, *J Am Acad Dermatol* 4, 650 (passim)
(1978): Dubois EL, *Semin Arthritis Rheum* 8, 33
(1976): Sams WM, *Int J Dermatol* 15, 99
(1973): Rees RB+, *Arch Dermatol* 88, 280 (passim)
(1965): Rook A, *Br J Dermatol* 77, 115
Hair – poliosis
(1985): Dupre A+, *Arch Dermatol* 121, 1164
(1968): Pasykowa K+, *Pol Tyg Lek* (Polish) 23, 2014
(1966): Fraga S+, *An Bras Dermatol* (Portuguese) 41, 57

Nails

Nails – discoloration
(1991): Zic JA+, *Arch Dermatol* 127, 1037
Nails – pigmentation
(1981): Koranda FC, *J Am Acad Dermatol* 4, 650 (passim)
(1963): Tuffanelli D+, *Arch Dermatol* 88, 419
Nails – shoreline
(1993): Pavithran K, *Indian J Lepr* 65, 225

Other

Acute intermittent porphyria
(1996): Puri AS+, *Indian Pediatr* 33, 241
Death
Gingival pigmentation
(1992): Veraldi S+, *Cutis* 49, 281
Headache
Myalgia
(1998): Guedira N+, *Rev Rhum Engl Ed* 65, 58
Myopathy
(1969): Chapman RS+, *Br J Dermatol* 81, 217
Necrotizing vasculitis
(2003): Luong MS+, *Acta Derm Venereol* 83(2), 141
Oral mucosal pigmentation
(1992): Veraldi S+, *Cutis* 49, 281
(1991): Zic JA+, *Arch Dermatol* 127, 1037
(1990): Wollina U+, *Dtsch Z Mund Kiefer Gesichtschir* (German) 14, 104
(1981): Koranda FC, *J Am Acad Dermatol* 4, 650 (passim)
(1980): Bentsi-Enchill KO, *Trop Geogr Med* 32, 216
(1971): Giansanti JS+, *Oral Surg* 31, 66
(1970): Brynolf I, *Sven Tandlak Tidskr* (Swedish) 63, 585
Oral mucosal ulceration
Oral ulceration
(2002): Pages F+, *Trop Med Int Health* 7(11), 919 (with proguanil)
Porphyria
(1980): Gerwel M, *Pol Tyg Lek* (Polish) 35, 1351
(1974): Kordac V+, *Br J Dermatol* 90, 95
(1973): Knutsson F+, *Lakartidningen* (Swedish) 70, 1547
(1962): Cripps DL+, *Arch Dermatol* 86, 575
(1959): Marsden CW, *Br J Dermatol* 71, 219
(1957): Davis MJ+, *Arch Dermatol* 75, 796
(1954): Linden IH+, *Calif Med* 81, 235
Porphyria cutanea tarda
(1985): Handa F+, *Indian J Dermatol* 30, 49
Stomatitis (<1%)
Stomatopyrosis
Tinnitus

CHLOROTHIAZIDE

Trade names: Aldochlor (Merck); Diuril (Merck)
Other common trade names: *Azide; Chlothin; Chlotride; Diurazide; Diuret; Saluretil; Saluric*
Indications: Hypertension, edema
Category: Antihypertensive; Thiazide diuretic
Half-life: 1–2 hours
Clinically important, potentially hazardous interactions with: digoxin, lithium

Reactions

Skin

Bullous eruption
Erythema multiforme

Exanthems
  (1972): Kuokannen K, *Acta Allergol* 27, 407
  (1966): Sherlock S+, *Lancet* 1, 1049 (10%)
  (1966): Smith JW+, *Ann Intern Med* 65, 629 (1.3%)
  (1960): Smirk H+, *BMJ* 1, 515
  (1959): Kirkendall WM, *Circulation* 19, 933 (1.1%)
  (1958): Rogin JR, *Arch Dermatol* 78, 504
Exfoliative dermatitis
Fixed eruption
  (1984): Chan HL, *Int J Dermatol* 23, 607
Lichenoid eruption
  (1986): Gonzalez JG+, *J Am Acad Dermatol* 15, 87
  (1971): Almeyda J+, *Br J Dermatol* 85, 604
  (1959): Harber LC+, *J Invest Dermatol* 33, 83
  (1959): Harber LC+, *N Engl J Med* 261, 1378
Lupus erythematosus
  (1966): Cohen P+, *JAMA* 197, 817
Photosensitivity (<1%)
  (1994): Enta T, *Can Fam Physicians* 40, 1269
  (1993): Iwamoto Y, *Nippon Saikingaku Zasshi* (Japanese) 48, 523
  (1984): Horio T, *Int J Dermatol* 23, 376
  (1980): Stern RS+, *Arch Dermatol* 116, 1269
  (1973): Stern WK, *Acta Derm Venereol* 53, 321
  (1970): Zurcher K+, *Dermatologica* 141, 119
  (1969): Kalivas J, *JAMA* 209, 1706
  (1965): Jung EG+, *Int Arch Allergy Appl Immunol* 27, 313
  (1959): Harber LC+, *J Invest Dermatol* 33, 83
  (1959): Harber LC+, *N Engl J Med* 261, 1378
  (1959): Norins AL, *Arch Dermatol* 79, 592
Pruritus
  (1969): Kalivas J, *JAMA* 209, 1706
  (1959): Norins AL, *Arch Dermatol* 79, 592
  (1958): Rogin JR, *Arch Dermatol* 78, 504
Purpura
  (1992): Breathnach SM+, *Adverse Drug Reactions and the Skin*
      Blackwell, Oxford, 46
  (1980): Miescher PA+, *Clin Haematol* 9, 505
  (1960): Ball P, *JAMA* 173, 663
  (1959): Horowitz HI+, *N Y State J Med* 59, 1117
  (1959): Nordquist P+, *Lancet* 1, 271
  (1958): Jaffe MO+, *JAMA* 168, 2264
Rash (sic) (<1%)
Stevens–Johnson syndrome
Toxic epidermal necrolysis
Urticaria
  (1960): Smirk H+, *BMJ* 1, 515
Vasculitis
  (1965): Björnberg A+, *Lancet* 2, 982
  (1960): Fitzgerald EW, *Arch Intern Med* 105, 305
  (1958): Jaffe MO+, *JAMA* 168, 2264

Hair

Hair – alopecia

Other

Anaphylactoid reactions
Dysgeusia
Oral mucosal lesions
Paresthesias (<1%)
Xanthopsia

*Note: Chlorothiazide is a sulfonamide and can be absorbed systemically. Sulfonamides can produce severe, possibly fatal, reactions such as toxic epidermal necrolysis and Stevens–Johnson syndrome

CHLOROTRIANISENE

Trade name: Tace (Aventis)
Other common trade names: *Estregur; Merbentul*
Indications: Inoperable prostate cancer, atrophic vaginitis
Category: Estrogen replacement
Half-life: N/A

Reactions

Skin

Acne pustulosa
  (1964): Sneddon IB+, *Br J Dermatol* 76, 491
Candidiasis
Chloasma (<1%)
Dermatitis (sic)
Edema (>1%)
Erythema
Erythema multiforme
Erythema nodosum
Melasma (<1%)
Peripheral edema (>10%)
Photosensitivity
Rash (sic) (<1%)
Urticaria

Hair

Hair – alopecia
Hair – hirsutism

Other

Acute intermittent porphyria
Gynecomastia (>10%)
Mastodynia (>10%)
Porphyria cutanea tarda
  (1970): Domonkos AN, *Arch Dermatol* 102, 229
  (1970): Roenigk HH+, *Arch Dermatol* 102, 260
Vaginal candidiasis
Vaginitis

CHLORPHENIRAMINE

Trade names: AL-R; Aller-Chlor (Rugby); Chlo-Amine; Chlor-Pro; Chlor-Trimeton (Schering); Chlorate (Major); Ornade (GSK); Phenetron (Lannett); Telachlor (Major); Teldrin (GSK); Triaminic (Novartis)
Other common trade name: *Chlor-Tripolon*
Indications: Allergic rhinitis, urticaria
Category: Antihistamine H$_1$-blocker
Half-life: 20–40 hours
Clinically important, potentially hazardous interactions with: alcohol, anticholinergics, barbiturates, benzodiazepines, butabarbital, chloral hydrate, chlordiazepoxide, chlorpromazine, clonazepam, clorazepate, diazepam, ethchlorvynol, fluphenazine, flurazepam, hypnotics, lorazepam, MAO inhibitors, mephobarbital, mesoridazine, midazolam, narcotics, oxazepam, pentobarbital, phenobarbital, phenothiazines, primidone, prochlorperazine, promethazine, quazepam, secobarbital, sedatives, temazepam, thioridazine, tranquilizers, trifluoperazine, zolpidem

Reactions

Skin

Angioedema (1–10%)

Dermatitis (sic) (1–10%)
  (2001): Hayashi K+, *Contact Dermatitis* 44(1), 38
  (1990): Tosti A+, *Contact Dermatitis* 22, 55 (eye-drops)
Diaphoresis
Photosensitivity (1–10%)

Other

Hypersensitivity
Myalgia (<1%)
Paresthesias (<1%)
Tardive dyskinesia
  (1990): Miller LG+, *South Med J* 83(5), 525 (20%)
Tinnitus
Xerostomia (1–10%)

CHLORPROMAZINE

Trade name: Thorazine (GSK)
Other common trade names: *Chloractil; Chlorazin; Chlorpromanyl; Esmino; Largactil; Novo-Chlorpromazine; Ormazine; Propaphenin; Prozin*
Indications: Psychosis, manic-depressive disorders
Category: Phenothiazine antipsychotic
Half-life: initial: 2 hours; terminal: 30 hours
Clinically important, potentially hazardous interactions with: alcohol, antihistamines, arsenic, chlorpheniramine, dofetilide, epinephrine, guanethidine, quinolones, sparfloxacin

Note: The prolonged use of chlorpromazine can produce a gray-blue or purplish pigmentation over light-exposed areas. This is a result of either dermal deposits of melanin, a chlorpromazine metabolite, or to a combination of both. Chlorpromazine melanosis is seen more often in women

Reactions

Skin

Actinic reticuloid
  (1982): Amblard P+, *Ann Dermatol Venereol* (French) 109, 225
Angioedema (<1%)
  (1958): Hine FR, *Am J Psychiatry* 114, 942
Bullous eruption (<1%)
  (1979): Matsuo I+, *Dermatologica* 159, 46
Dermatitis (sic)
  (1955): Lewis GM+, *JAMA* 157, 909
Erythema multiforme (<1%)
  (1961): Baer RL+, *Year Book of Dermatology* Chicago, 9–37
Exanthems (>5%)
  (1969): Török H, *Dermatol Int* 8, 57
  (1968): Raskin A, *J Nerv Ment Dis* 147, 184 (5%)
  (1967): Lockey SD, *Med Sci* 18, 43
  (1966): Zelickson AS, *JAMA* 198, 341
  (1961): Stevanovic DV, *Br J Dermatol* 73, 233
  (1957): Bernstein C+, *JAMA* 163, 930 (7–14%)
  (1956): Mullins JF+, *JAMA* 162, 946
  (1955): Margolis LH+, *Arch Dermatol* 72, 72 (13%)
Exfoliative dermatitis
  (1961): Baer RL+, *Year Book of Dermatology* Chicago, 9–37
Fixed eruption (<1%)
Hypohidrosis (>10%)
Lichenoid eruption
  (1979): Matsuo I+, *Dermatologica* 159, 46
Lupus erythematosus
  (1996): Matsukawa Y+, *J Int Med Res* 24, 147
  (1995): Price EJ+, *Drug Saf* 12(4), 283
  (1994): Yung RL+, *Rheum Dis Clin North Am* 20, 61

(1990): Roche-Bayard P, *Chest* 98, 1545
  (1985): Pavlidakey GP+, *J Am Acad Dermatol* 13, 109
  (1981): Grossman J+, *Arthritis Rheum* 24, 927
  (1980): Condemi JJ, *Geriatrics* 35(3), 81
  (1980): Goldman LS+, *Am J Psychiatry* 137, 1613
  (1973): Ananth JV+, *Can Med Assoc J* 108, 680
  (1972): Dubois EL+, *JAMA* 221, 595
  (1963): Shulman LE+, *Arthritis Rheum* 6, 558
Miliaria
  (1956): Mullins JF+, *JAMA* 162, 946
Peripheral edema
Photodermatitis
  (1962): Calnan CD+, *Trans St. Johns Hosp Derm Soc* 48, 49
Photosensitivity (1–10%)
  (1995): Kim TH+, *Photodermatol Photoimmunol Photomed* 11, 170
  (1993): Jeanmougin M+, *Ann Dermatol Venereol* (French) 120, 840
  (1993): Wolf ME+, *Int J Clin Pharmacol* 31, 365
  (1989): Hoshino T+, *Arch Dermatol Res* 281, 60
  (1989): Rosen C, *Semin Dermatol* 8, 149
  (1986): Lovell CR+, *Contact Dermatitis* 14, 290
  (1982): Amblard P+, *Ann Dermatol Venereol* (French) 109, 225
  (1979): Matsuo I+, *Dermatologica* 159, 46
  (1975): Horio T, *Arch Dermatol* 111, 1469
  (1974): Johnson BE, *Proc R Soc Med* 67, 871
  (1973): Johnson BE, *Br J Dermatol* 89, 16
  (1971): Hägermark O+, *Br J Dermatol* 84, 605
  (1969): Kalivas J, *JAMA* 209, 1706 (3%)
  (1968): Prien RF+, *Arch Gen Psychiatry* 18, 482 (1–22%)
  (1967): Lockey SD, *Med Sci* 18, 43
  (1967): Satanove A+, *JAMA* 200, 121
  (1961): Stevanovic DV, *Br J Dermatol* 73, 233
  (1958): Calnan CD+, *Trans St. Johns Hosp Derm Soc* 44, 26
  (1957): Epstein JH+, *J Invest Dermatol* 28, 329
  (1957): Winkelmann NR, *Am J Psychiatry* 113, 961 (3%)
  (1956): Mullins JF+, *JAMA* 162, 946
  (1955): Margolis LH+, *Arch Dermatol* 72, 72
Phototoxicity
  (1997): Eberlein-Konig B+, *Dermatology* 194, 131
  (1979): Matsuo I+, *Dermatologica* 159, 46
  (1977): Ljunggren B, *J Invest Dermatol* 69, 383
  (1975): Raffle EJ+, *Arch Dermatol* 111, 1364
  (1967): Satanove A+, *JAMA* 200, 121
  (1964): Greiner AC+, *Can Med Assoc J* 90, 663
Pigmentation (<1%)
  (2001): Kass J+, *Cutis* 68(4), 260
  (2000): Lal+, *J Psychiatry Neurosci* 25, 281
  (1993): Bloom D+, *Acta Psychiatr Scand* 87, 223
  (1993): Lal S+, *J Psychiatry Neurosci* 18, 173
  (1993): Wolf ME+, *Int J Clin Pharmacol* 31, 365 (blue-gray)
  (1988): Benning TL+, *Arch Dermatol* 124, 1541
  (1988): Thompson TR+, *Acta Psychiatr Scand* 78, 763
  (1975): Robins AH, *S Afr Med J* 49, 1521
  (1967): Satanove A+, *JAMA* 200, 209
  (1966): Hashimoto K+, *J Invest Dermatol* 47, 296
  (1966): Zelickson AS, *JAMA* 198, 341
  (1964): Greiner AC+, *Can Med Assoc J* 90, 663
  (1964): Hays GB+, *Arch Dermatol* 90, 471
  (1964): Zelickson AS+, *JAMA* 188, 394
Pruritus (1–10%)
  (1968): Prien RF+, *Arch Gen Psychiatry* 18, 482 (1–22%)
  (1957): Bernstein C+, *JAMA* 163, 930 (4%)
Purpura
  (1987): Aram H, *J Am Acad Dermatol* 17, 139
  (1967): Lockey SD, *Med Sci* 18, 43
  (1965): Horowitz HI+, *Semin Hematol* 2, 287
  (1957): Shannon J+, *Dermatologica* 114, 101
  (1956): Mullins JF+, *JAMA* 162, 946
  (1956): Wintrobe MM+, *Arch Intern Med* 98, 559

Pustules
  (1994): Burrows NP+, *BMJ* 309, 97
Rash (sic) (1–10%)
Seborrheic dermatitis
  (1983): Binder RL+, *Arch Dermatol* 119, 473 (1–5%)
  (1981): Kanwar AJ+, *Arch Dermatol* 117, 65 (passim)
  (1965): Fellner MJ+, *Int J Dermatol* 19, 392
  (1956): Mullins JF+, *JAMA* 162, 946
Toxic epidermal necrolysis (<1%)
  (1996): Purcell P+, *Postgrad Med J* 72, 186
  (1990): Ward DJ+, *Burns* 16, 97
Urticaria
  (1992): Loesche C+, *Contact Dermatitis* 26, 278
  (1986): Lovell CR+, *Contact Dermatitis* 14, 290
  (1967): Lockey SD, *Med Sci* 18, 43
  (1961): Baer RL+, *Year Book of Dermatology* Chicago, 9–37
  (1956): Mullins JF+, *JAMA* 162, 946
Vasculitis
  (1987): Aram H, *J Am Acad Dermatol* 17, 139
  (1969): Peterkin GAG+, *Practitioner* 202, 117
  (1957): Shannon J+, *Dermatologica* 114, 101
Xerosis

Nails

Nails – photo-onycholysis
  (1985): Kechijian P, *J Am Acad Dermatol* 12, 552
Nails – pigmentation
  (1971): Hägermark O+, *Br J Dermatol* 84, 605
  (1966): Zelickson AS, *JAMA* 198, 341
  (1965): Satanove A+, *JAMA* 200, 209
  (1964): Greiner AC+, *Can Med Assoc J* 90, 663

Other

Anaphylactoid reactions (<1%)
  (2001): Nikolic S+, *Srp Arh Celok Lek* 129(7), 203
Cataract
  (2002): Shahzad S+, *Psychosomatics* 43(5), 354
Death
  (2001): Nikolic S+, *Srp Arh Celok Lek* 129(7), 203
Galactorrhea (1–10%)
Gynecomastia (1–10%)
Headache
Injection-site aseptic necrosis
Mastodynia (1–10%)
Oral mucosal eruption
Oral mucosal pigmentation
Oral ulceration
Polyarteritis nodosa
  (1960): Meyler L+, *Acta Med Scand* 167, 95
Priapism (<1%)
  (2001): Compton MT+, *J Clin Psychiatry* 62(5), 362 (passim)
  (1999): Mutlu N+, *Int J Clin Pract* 53, 152
Pseudolymphoma
  (1995): Magro CM+, *J Am Acad Dermatol* 32, 419
Tremor
  (2001): Chetty M+, *Ther Drug Monit* 23(5), 556 (with oral
    contraceptives)
Xerostomia (1–10%)

CHLORPROPAMIDE

Trade name: Diabinese (Pfizer)
Other common trade names: *Apo-Chlorpropamide; Arodoc C;
Chlormide; Diabemide; Diabenese; Insogen; Melormin; Tesmel*
Indications: Diabetes
Category: First generation sulfonylurea
Half-life: 30–42 hours
**Clinically important, potentially hazardous interactions
with: alcohol**, phenylbutazones

Reactions

Skin

Angioedema
  (1991): Chinchmanian RM+, *Therapie* (French) 46, 163
Bullous eruption (<1%)
Dermatitis
  (1982): Fisher AA, *Cutis* 29, 551
Edema (<1%)
Erythema multiforme (<1%)
  (1980): Kanefsky TM+, *Arch Intern Med* 140, 1543
  (1971): Harris EL, *BMJ* 3, 29
  (1966): Tullett GL, *BMJ* 1, 148 (fatal)
  (1960): Rothfeld EL+, *JAMA* 172, 54 (passim)
  (1960): Yaffee HS, *Arch Dermatol* 82, 636
  (1959): Greenhouse B, *Ann N Y Acad Sci* 74, 643
  (1959): Stewart RC+, *N Engl J Med* 261, 427
Erythema nodosum (<1%)
  (1971): Harris EL, *BMJ* 3, 29
  (1966): Tullett GL, *BMJ* 1, 148
Exanthems (1–5%)
  (1970): Almeyda J+, *Br J Dermatol* 82, 634 (1–5%)
  (1960): Rothfeld EL+, *JAMA* 172, 54 (passim)
  (1959): Hamff LH+, *Ann N Y Acad Sci* 74, 820
Exfoliative dermatitis
  (1971): Harris EL, *BMJ* 3, 29
  (1967): Coleman WP, *Med Clin North Am* 51, 1073
  (1966): Tullett GL, *BMJ* 1, 148
  (1962): Hitselberger JF+, *JAMA* 180, 62
  (1960): Rothfeld EL+, *JAMA* 172, 54 (passim)
  (1959): Reyes JAG+, *Ann N Y Acad Sci* 74, 1012
  (1959): Stewart RC+, *N Engl J Med* 261, 427
Fixed eruption
  (1979): Rupp T, *Int J Dermatol* 18, 590
Flushing
  (1992): Shelley WB+, *Advanced Dermatologic Diagnosis* WB
    Saunders, 582 (passim)
  (1983): Fui SNT+, *N Engl J Med* 309, 93 (alcohol flush)
  (1983): Jerntorp P+, *Eur J Clin Pharmacol* 24, 237
  (1982): Ohlin H+, *Br Med J Clin Res Ed* 285, 838
  (1981): Barnett AH+, *Br Med J Clin Res Ed* 283, 939
  (1981): Capretti L+, *Br Med J Clin Res Ed* 283, 1361
  (1981): Jentorp P+, *Acta Med Scand Suppl* 656, 33
  (1981): Medback S+, *BMJ* 283, 937 (alcohol flush)
  (1981): Wilkin JK, *Ann Intern Med* 95, 468
  (1980): Strakosch CR+, *Lancet* 1, 394
  (1979): Leslie RDG+, *Lancet* 1, 997
  (1978): Leslie RDG+, *BMJ* 2, 1519 (35%)
  (1978): Pyke DA+, *BMJ* 2, 1521
  (1971): Fairman MJ+, *BMJ* 4, 297 (40%)
  (1971): Harris EL, *BMJ* 3, 29
  (1966): Muller SA, *Proc Staff Meet Mayo Clin* 41, 689 (10–30%)
  (1962): FitzGerald MG+, *Diabetes* 11, 40
  (1962): Larsen JA+, *Proc Soc Exp Biol Med* 109, 120
  (1959): Signorelli S, *Ann NY Acad Sci* 74, 900
Granulomas

(1976): Rigberg LA+, *JAMA* 235, 409
Lichenoid eruption
  (1990): Franz CB+, *J Am Acad Dermatol* 22, 128
  (1984): Barnett JH+, *Cutis* 34, 542
  (1971): Almeyda J+, *Br J Dermatol* 85, 604
  (1968): Dinsdale RCW+, *BMJ* 1, 100
Lupus erythematosus
  (1979): Rupp T, *Int J Dermatol* 18, 590
Photosensitivity (1–10%)
  (1973): Feuerman E+, *Dermatologica* 146, 25
  (1971): Harris EL, *BMJ* 3, 29
  (1962): Hitselberger JF+, *JAMA* 180, 62
Pruritus (<3%)
  (1971): Harris EL, *BMJ* 3, 29
  (1962): Hitselberger JF+, *JAMA* 180, 62
Purpura
  (1977): Cunliffe DJ, *Postgrad Med* 53, 87
  (1971): Harris EL, *BMJ* 3, 29
  (1965): Horowitz HI+, *Semin Hematol* 2, 287
  (1963): FitzPatrick WJ, *Diabetes* 12, 457
  (1960): Rothfeld EL+, *JAMA* 172, 54 (passim)
  (1959): Grace WJ, *N Engl J Med* 260, 711
  (1959): Haynes WS, *BMJ* 2, 1403
  (1959): Yuen H, *Ann N Y Acad Sci* 74, 918
Rash (sic) (1–10%)
  (1985): Baciewicz AM+, *Diabetes Care* 8, 200
Side effects (sic)
  (1967): McKiddie MT+, *Scott Med J* 12, 6 (1.65%)
  (1965): Cervantes-Amezcua A+, *JAMA* 193, 759 (1.4%)
  (1960): Duncan LJP+, *Pharmacol Rev* 12, 91 (5%)
Stevens–Johnson syndrome
  (1980): Kanefsky TM+, *Arch Intern Med* 140, 1543
  (1966): Coursin DB, *JAMA* 198, 113
  (1960): Rothfeld EL+, *JAMA* 172, 54 (passim)
  (1960): Yaffee HS, *Arch Dermatol* 82, 636
  (1959): Stewart RC+, *N Engl J Med* 261, 427
Toxic epidermal necrolysis
  (1989): Stern RS+, *J Am Acad Dermatol* 21, 317
  (1966): Tullett GL, *BMJ* 1, 148 (fatal)
Urticaria (1–10%)
  (1991): Chinchmanian RM+, *Therapie* (French) 46, 163
  (1973): Feuerman E+, *Dermatologica* 146, 25
  (1960): Rothfeld EL+, *JAMA* 172, 54 (passim)
Vasculitis
  (1983): Batko B, *Wiad Lek* (Polish) 36, 761
  (1973): Feuerman E+, *Dermatologica* 146, 25

Hair
Hair – alopecia
  (1971): Harris EL, *BMJ* 3, 29

Other
Acute intermittent porphyria
Death
Oral lichenoid eruption
  (1988): Zain RB+, *Dent J Malays* 10, 15
  (1984): Barnett J+, *Cutis* 34, 542
  (1968): Dinsdale RCW+, *BMJ* 1, 100
Paresthesias
Porphyria
  (1965): Zarowitz H+, *N Y State J Med* 65, 2385
Porphyria cutanea tarda
  (1965): Zarowitz H+, *N Y State J Med* 65, 2385
Tongue ulceration
  (1984): Barnett J+, *Cutis* 34, 542

*Note: Chlorpropamide is a sulfonamide and can be absorbed systemically. Sulfonamides can produce severe, possibly fatal, reactions such as toxic epidermal necrolysis and Stevens–Johnson syndrome

CHLORTETRACYCLINE

Trade name: Aureomycin (Proter Spa)
Other common trade name: *Aureomicina*
Indications: Various infections due to susceptible organisms
Category: Topical ophthalmic tetracycline antibiotic
Half-life: N/A

Reactions

Skin
Burning (topical) (ophthalmic)
Edema (topical)
Erythema (topical)
Irritation (topical)
Photosensitivity
  (1965): Verhagen AR, *Dermatologica* 130, 439
Pruritus (topical)
Rash (sic) (topical)
Stinging (topical) (ophthalmic)
Xerosis (topical)

Other
Xerostomia (ophthalmic)

CHLORTHALIDONE

Trade names: Combipres (Boehringer Ingelheim); Hygroton (Aventis); Tenoretic (AstraZeneca); Thalitone (Monarch)
Other common trade names: *Higroton; Hydro-Long; Hypertol; Igroton; Thalidone; Uridon*
Indications: Hypertension
Category: Antihypertensive; Thiazide diuretic
Half-life: 35–50 hours
Clinically important, potentially hazardous interactions with: digoxin, lithium

Combipres is chlorthalidone and clonidine

Reactions

Skin
Erythema multiforme
Exanthems
Exfoliative dermatitis
Lupus erythematosus
Necrotizing angiitis
Photosensitivity (1–10%)
  (1989): Baker EJ+, *J Am Acad Dermatol* 21, 1026
  (1988): Lehmann P+, *Hautarzt* (German) 39, 38
Psoriasis
  (1987): Wolf R+, *Cutis* 40, 162
Purpura (<1%)
Rash (sic) (<1%)
Stevens–Johnson syndrome
Toxic epidermal necrolysis
  (1999): Egan CA+, *J Am Acad Dermatol* 40(3), 458
Urticaria (<1%)
  (1993): Neaton JD+, *JAMA* 279, 713 (passim)
Vasculitis (<1%)
  (1965): Björnberg A+, *Lancet* 2, 982

Hair
Hair – alopecia

Other
Headache
Paresthesias (<1%)
Pseudoporphyria
(1989): Baker EJ+, *J Am Acad Dermatol* 21, 1026
Xanthopsia

*Note: Chlorthalidone is a sulfonamide and can be absorbed systemically. Sulfonamides can produce severe, possibly fatal, reactions such as toxic epidermal necrolysis and Stevens–Johnson syndrome

CHLORZOXAZONE

Trade names: Paraflex (Ortho-McNeil); Parafon Forte DSC (Ortho-McNeil)
Other common trade names: *Escoflex; Flexaphen; Klorzoxazon; Muscol; Prolax; Remular-S; Solaxin*
Indications: Painful musculoskeletal conditions
Category: Skeletal muscle relaxant
Half-life: 1–2 hours

Reactions

Skin
Angioedema (1–10%)
Ecchymoses
Erythema multiforme (<1%)
(1979): Lindholm L, *Lakartidningen* (Swedish) 76, 2795
Exanthems
Flushing (1–10%)
Petechiae
Pruritus
Rash (sic) (<1%)
Urticaria (<1%)

Other
Anaphylactoid reactions
Hypersensitivity
Trembling (sic) (1–10%)

CHOLESTYRAMINE

Trade names: Lo-Cholest; Questran (Par)
Other common trade names: *Chol-Less; Colestrol; Lismol; PMS-Cholestyramine; Prevalite; Quantalan; Questran Lite*
Indications: Pruritus associated with biliary obstruction, primary hypercholesterolemia
Category: Antidiarrheal; Antihyperlipidemic; Antipruritic (cholestasis)
Half-life: N/A
Clinically important, potentially hazardous interactions with: acetaminophen, acitretin, aspirin, chloroquine, cyclosporine, digoxin, doxepin, fat-soluble vitamins A D E K, hydroxychloroquine, isotretinoin, lovastatin, mycophenolate, raloxifene, sulfasalazine, sulfonylureas, tetracycline, tricyclic antidepressants, valproic acid

Reactions

Skin
Ecchymoses

Edema
Exanthems
Rash (sic) (<1%)
Urticaria

Other
Dysgeusia
Paresthesias
Tinnitus
Tongue irritation (sic) (<1%)

CHONDROITIN

Scientific names: *Chondroitin 4-sulfate; chondroitin 4- and 6-sulfate*
Family: None
Trade and other common names: CDS; Chondroitin Sulfate C; CSA; CSC; GAG
Category: Food supplement
Purported indications and other uses: Osteoarthritis (often with glucosamine), ischemic heart disease, osteoporosis, hyperlipidemia, keratoconjunctivitis, agent in cataract surgery
Half-life: N/A

Reactions

Skin
Allergic reactions (sic)
Eyelid edema
(2000): Leeb BF+, *J Rheumatology* 27, 205
Peripheral edema

Hair
Hair – alopecia

CIDOFOVIR

Trade names: Forvade; Vistide (Gilead)
Indications: Cytomegalovirus (CMV) retinitis in patients with AIDS
Category: Antiviral (nucleotide analog)
Half-life: ~2.6 hours
Clinically important, potentially hazardous interactions with: amphotericin B, tenofovir

Reactions

Skin
Acne (>10%)
Allergic reactions (sic) (1–10%)
Chills (24%)
Diaphoresis (1–10%)
Edema
Facial edema
Herpes simplex
Local irritation (sic)
(1998): Zabawski EJ+, *J Am Acad Dermatol* 39, 741
Pallor (1–10%)
Pigmentation (>10%)
Pruritus (1–10%)
Rash (sic) (27%)
Urticaria (1–10%)
Xerosis

Hair
Hair – alopecia (22%)

Other
Aphthous stomatitis
Application-site reactions (sic) (39%)
  (1998): Zabawski EJ+, J Am Acad Dermatol 39, 741
Dysgeusia (1–10%)
Headache
Myalgia
Oral candidiasis
Oral ulceration
Paresthesias (>10%)
Stomatitis (1–10%)
Tongue discoloration
Xerostomia

CILOSTAZOL

Synonym: OPC13013
Trade name: Pletal (Otsuka) (Pharmacia)
Indications: Peripheral vascular disease, intermittent claudication
Category: Platelet aggregation inhibitor
Half-life: 11–13 hours
Clinically important, potentially hazardous interactions with: fondaparinux

Reactions

Skin
Chills (<2%)
Ecchymoses (<2%)
Edema (<2%)
Facial edema (<2%)
Furunculosis (<2%)
Hypertrophy (sic)
Infections (sic)
Peripheral edema (7–9%)
Pruritus
Purpura (<2%)
Rash (sic) (2%)
Urticaria (<2%)
Xerosis (<2%)

Other
Headache
Hyperesthesia (2%)
Myalgia (2–3%)
Paresthesias (2%)
Tongue edema (<2%)
Vaginitis (<2%)

CIMETIDINE

Trade name: Tagamet (GSK)
Other common trade names: Apo-Cimetidine; Azucimet; Blocan; Cimedine; Cimehexal; Ciuk; Dyspamet; Novocimetine; Nu-Cimet; Peptol; Stomedine; Ulcedine; Zymerol
Indications: Duodenal ulcer
Category: Antihistamine H$_2$-blocker
Half-life: 2 hours
Clinically important, potentially hazardous interactions with: aminophylline, anisindione, anticoagulants, buprenorphine, butorphanol, **caffeine**, carmustine, dicumarol, dofetilide, epirubicin, fentanyl, floxuridine, fluorouracil, galantamine, hydromorphone, itraconazole, ketoconazole, lidocaine, midazolam, morphine, narcotic analgesics, oxycodone, pentazocine, phenytoin, propranolol, sufentanil, theophylline, warfarin, xanthines

Reactions

Skin
Acne
Angioedema (<1%)
  (1985): Whelan JP, J Clin Pharmacol 25, 610
  (1982): Sandhu BS+, Ann Intern Med 97, 138
  (1979): Delaunois L, N Engl J Med 300, 1216
Baboon syndrome
  (1998): Helmbold P+, Dermatology 197, 402
Erythema annulare centrifugum
  (1982): Merrett AC+, N Z J Med 12, 107
  (1981): Merrett AC+, BMJ 283, 698
Erythema multiforme (<1%)
  (1987): Talvard O+, Presse Med (French) 16, 825
  (1983): Guan R+, Aust N Z J Med 13, 182
  (1982): Wallach D+, Dermatologica 165, 197
  (1981): Bjaeldager PA, Ugeskr Laeger (Danish) 143, 1406
  (1978): Ahmed AH+, Lancet 2, 433
Erythroderma
Erythrosis-like lesions (sic)
  (1979): Angelini G+, BMJ 1, 1147
Exanthems
  (1986): Peters K, Contact Dermatitis 15, 190
  (1982): Freston JW, Ann Intern Med 97, 728
  (1979): Hadfield WA, Ann Intern Med 91, 128
Exfoliative dermatitis
  (1983): Mitchell GG, Am J Med 75, 875
  (1980): Yantis PL+, Dig Dis Sci 25, 73
Fixed eruption
  (1998): Helmbold P+, Dermatology 197, 402 (baboon syndrome)
  (1995): Inoue A+, Acta Derm Venereol 75, 250
Ichthyosis
  (1984): Aram H, Int J Dermatol 23, 458
Id reaction
  (1987): Sander-Jensen K+, Dermatologica 174, 103
Lupus erythematosus
  (1982): Davidson BL+, Arch Intern Med 142, 166 (exacerbation)
  (1979): Littlejohn GO+, Ann Intern Med 91, 317
Pruritus (<1%)
  (1994): Warner DMc+, J Am Acad Dermatol 31, 677 (passim)
  (1982): Freston JW, Ann Intern Med 97, 728
  (1982): Sandhu BS+, Ann Intern Med 97, 138
  (1982): Wallach D+, Dermatologica 165, 197
  (1981): Taillandier J+, Nouv Presse Med (French) 10, 258
  (1979): Matthews CNA+, Br J Dermatol 101, 57
Psoriasis
  (1991): Andersen M, Ugeskr Laeger (Danish) 153, 132

(1986): Peters K, *Contact Dermatitis* 15, 190
(1983): Mitchell GG, *Am J Med* 75, 875
(1982): Wallach D+, *Dermatologica* 165, 197
(1980): Yates VM+, *BMJ* 280, 1453
(1979): Rai GS+, *Lancet* 1, 50
Purpura
Pustular psoriasis
(1979): Rai GS+, *Lancet* 1, 50
Rash (sic) (<2%)
(1991): Marshall J+, *Chest* 99, 1016
Seborrheic dermatitis
(1981): Kanwar AJ, *Arch Dermatol* 117, 65
Side effects (sic) (0.4%)
(1982): Freston JW, *Ann Intern Med* 97, 728
Stevens–Johnson syndrome
(1987): Talvard O+, *Presse Med* (French) 16, 825
(1983): Guan R+, *Aust N Z J Med* 13, 182
(1978): Ahmed AH+, *Lancet* 2, 433
Toxic dermatitis (sic)
(1981): Pasquier P+, *Nouv Presse Med* (French) 10, 2994
Toxic epidermal necrolysis (<1%)
(1998): Tidwell BH+, *Am J Health Syst Pharm* 55, 163
(1983): Dabadie H+, *Gastroenterol Clin Biol* (French) 7, 425
Urticaria
(1985): Goolamali SK, *Postgrad Med J* 61, 925
(1983): Mitchell GG, *Am J Med* 75, 875
(1982): Freston JW, *Ann Intern Med* 97, 728
(1982): Sandhu BS+, *Ann Intern Med* 97, 138
(1981): Brandrup E, *Ugeskr Laeger* (Danish) 143, 1715
(1979): Hadfield WA, *Ann Intern Med* 91, 128
Vasculitis
(1983): Mitchell GG, *Am J Med* 75, 875
(1982): Wallach D+, *Dermatologica* 165, 197
(1981): Dernbach WK+, *JAMA* 246, 331
Xerosis
(1982): Greist MC+, *Arch Dermatol* 118, 253

Hair

Hair – alopecia
(1985): Tullio CJ+, *Clin Pharm* 4, 145
(1983): Khalsa JH+, *Int J Dermatol* 22, 202
(1981): Vircburger MI+, *Lancet* 1, 1160
(1979): Ahmad S, *Ann Intern Med* 91, 930

Other

Anaphylactoid reactions
(1982): Knapp AB+, *Ann Intern Med* 97, 374
Galactorrhea
(1977): Bateson MC+, *Lancet* 2, 247
Gynecomastia (<1%)
(2000): Hugues FC+, *Ann Med Interne (Paris)* (French) 151, 10 (passim)
(1994): Garcia-Rodriguez LA+, *BMJ* 308, 503
(1991): Barth JA, *Zentralbl Gynakol* (German) 113, 667
(1983): Jensen RT+, *N Engl J Med* 308, 883
(1982): Peden NR+, *Br J Clin Pharmacol* 14, 565
(1979): Spence RW+, *Gut* 20, 154
(1977): Della-Fave GF+, *Lancet* 1, 1319
(1976): Hall WH, *N Engl J Med* 841, 295 (letter)
Headache
Hypersensitivity
(2000): Evans RD+, *Clin Podiatr Med Surg* 17, 371
(1986): Peters K, *Contact Dermatitis* 15, 190
(1985): Whalen JP, *J Clin Pharmacol* 25, 610
Injection-site pain
Myalgia (<1%)
Myopathy
(1982): Kaplinsky N+, *J Rheumatol* 9, 156
(1980): Feest TG+, *BMJ* 281, 1284

Porphyria
(1985): Singh R+, *J Assoc Physicians India* 33, 187
Pseudolymphoma
(1995): Magro CM+, *J Am Acad Dermatol* 32, 419
(1988): Kardaun SH+, *Br J Dermatol* 118(4), 545
Xerostomia

CINOXACIN

Trade name: Cinobac (Watson)
Other common trade names: *Cerexin; Cinobact; Cinobactin; Gugecin; Nossacin; Noxigram; Uronorm*
Indications: Various urinary tract infections caused by susceptible organisms
Category: Quinolone antibiotic
Half-life: 1.5 hours

Reactions

Skin

Allergic reactions (sic)
Angioedema (<3%)
Edema (<3%)
Erythema multiforme
Photosensitivity
Pruritus (<3%)
Rash (sic)
Stevens–Johnson syndrome
Toxic epidermal necrolysis
Urticaria (<3%)

Other

Anaphylactoid reactions
(2003): Quercia O+, *Allerg Immunol* (Paris) 35(2), 61
(1988): Stricker BH+, *BMJ* 297, 1434
Dysgeusia (<1%)
Hypersensitivity
(1982): Scavone JM+, *Pharmacotherapy* 2, 266
Paresthesias (<1%)
Tinnitus

CIPROFLOXACIN

Trade names: Ciloxan Ophthalmic (Alcon); Cipro (Bayer) (Alcon)
Other common trade names: *Ciflox; Cimogal; Ciplox; Ciprobay Uro; Cipromycin; Ciproxin; Italnik; Kenzoflex; Uniflox*
Indications: Various infections caused by susceptible organisms
Category: Synthetic fluoroquinolone antibiotic
Half-life: 4 hours
Clinically important, potentially hazardous interactions with: amiodarone, antacids, antineoplastics, arsenic, bepridil, bismuth subsalicylate, bretylium, calcium salts, didanosine, disopyramide, erythromycin, iron, magnesium salts, methylxanthines, NSAIDs, phenothiazines, procainamide, quinidine, sotalol, sucralfate, theophylline, tricyclic antidepressants, zinc

Ciprofloxacin is chemically related to nalidixic acid

Reactions

Skin

Acne

(1989): Rahm V+, *Scand J Infect Dis* 60, 120
(1988): Campoli-Richards DM+, *Drugs* 35, 373
(1988): Schacht P+, *Infection* 16, S29

Allergic reactions (sic)
(2000): Burke P+, *BMJ* 320, 679

Angioedema (<1%)
(1995): Vidal C+, *Postgrad Med J* 71, 318
(1989): Davis H+, *Ann Intern Med* 111, 1041
(1989): Rahm V+, *Scand J Infect Dis* 60, 120
(1989): Schacht P+, *Am J Med* 87, 98S
(1988): Campoli-Richards DM+, *Drugs* 35, 373
(1988): Schacht P+, *Infection* 16, S29

Bullous eruption
(1988): Kaufmann I+, *Z Hautkr* (German) 63, 679

Bullous pemphigoid
(2000): Kimyadi-Asadi A+, *J Am Acad Dermatol* 42, 847

Candidiasis (<1%)
(1997): Litt JZ, Beachwood, OH (penile) (personal case)
(observation)
(1989): Yangco BG+, *Clin Ther* 11, 503
(1988): Schacht P+, *Infection* 16, S29

Diaphoresis
(1990): Karimi K, *Indiana Med* 83, 266
(1989): Rahm V+, *Scand J Infect Dis* 60, 120
(1988): Campoli-Richards DM+, *Drugs* 35, 373 (0.05%)
(1988): Schacht P+, *Infection* 16, S29

Edema (<1%)
(1995): Shelley ED, Toledo, OH (personal case) (observation)

Elastolysis
(1993): Lien YH+, *Am J Kidney Dis* 22, 598

Erythema multiforme
(1994): Win A+, *Int J Dermatol* 33, 512
(1993): Imrie K+, *Am J Hematol* 43, 159

Erythema nodosum (<1%)

Erythroderma (<1%)
(1989): Wurtz RM+, *Lancet* 1, 955

Exanthems
(2002): Litt JZ, Beachwood, OH (personal case) (observation)
(2000): Litt JZ, Beachwood, OH (personal case) (observation)
(1999): Litt JZ, Beachwood, OH (anecdote from lay person on
the Internet)
(1999): Litt JZ, Beachwood, OH (personal case) (observation)
(1997): Bircher AJ+, *Allergy* 52, 1246
(1996): McCarty JR, Fort Worth, TX (from Internet)
(observation)
(1989): Gaut PL+, *Am J Med* 87 (Suppl 5A), 169S
(1988): Campoli-Richards DM+, *Drugs* 35, 373 (0.7%)

Exfoliative dermatitis (<1%)

Fixed eruption
(2001): Hamamoto Y+, *Clin Exp Dermatol* 26(1), 48
(2001): Rodriguez-Morales A+, *Contact Dermatitis* 44(4), 255
(2001): Sharma R, Aligarh, India (from Internet) (observation)
(recurrence after fixed eruption from sparfloxacin)
(1998): Litt JZ, Beachwood, OH (personal case) (observation)
(1998): Maquirriain Gorriz MT+, *Aten Primaria* (Spanish) 21, 585
(1996): Dhar S+, *Br J Dermatol* 134, 156
(1995): Lozano-Ayllon M+, *Allergy* 50, 598
(1994): Kawada A+, *Contact Dermatitis* 31, 182
(1993): Alonso MD+, *Allergy* 48, 296
(1992): Alonso MD+, *Allergy* 47, 194

Flushing (<1%)
(1988): Campoli-Richards DM+, *Drugs* 35, 373

Linear IgA bullous dermatosis
(2001): Wiadrowski TP+, *Austral J Dermatol* 42, 196 (with
vancomycin)

Livedo reticularis
(1999): Verros CD, Tripolis, Greece (from Internet)
(observation) (recurred on rechallenge)

Photosensitivity (<1%)

(2000): Ferguson J+, *J Antimicrob Chemother* 45, 503
(1998): Kimura M+, *Contact Dermatitis* 38, 180
(1997): Ferguson J+, *J Antimicrob Chemother* 40, 93
(1995): Burdge DR+, *Antimicrob Agents Chemother* 39, 793
(1993): Shelley WB+, *Cutis* 51, 154 (observation)
(1993): Shelley WB+, *Cutis* 52, 27 (observation)
(1990): Ferguson J+, *Br J Dermatol* 123, 9
(1989): Granowitz EV, *J Infect Dis* 160, 910
(1989): Nedorost ST+, *Arch Dermatol* 125, 433
(1989): Rahm V+, *Scand J Infect Dis* 60, 120
(1988): Campoli-Richards DM+, *Drugs* 35, 373
(1988): Kaufmann I+, *Z Hautkr* (German) 63, 679
(1988): Schacht P+, *Infection* 16, S29
(1987): Jensen T+, *J Antimicrob Chemother* 20, 585
(1986): Ball P, *J Antimicrob Chemother* 18 (Suppl D), 187

Phototoxicity
(2000): Traynor NJ+, *Toxicol Vitr* 14, 275
(1998): Martinez LJ+, *Photochem Photobiol* 67, 399
(1993): Ferguson J+, *Br J Dermatol* 128, 285

Pigmentation (<1%)

Pruritus (<1%)
(2002): Litt JZ, Beachwood, OH (personal case) (observation)
(1999): Litt JZ, Beachwood, OH (2 personal cases) (observation)
(1989): Davis H+, *Ann Intern Med* 111, 1041
(1989): Gaut PL+, *Am J Med* 87 (Suppl 5A), 169S
(1989): Rahm V+, *Scand J Infect Dis* 60, 120
(1989): Schacht P+, *Am J Med* 87, 98S
(1989): Yangco BG+, *Clin Ther* 11, 503
(1988): Campoli-Richards DM+, *Drugs* 35, 373 (0.3%)
(1988): Sanders WE, *Rev Infect Dis* 10, 528
(1988): Schacht P+, *Infection* 16, S29
(1988): Thorsteinsson SB+, *Chemotherapy* 34, 256

Purpura
(1999): Goldberg EI+, *J Clin Dermatol* 2, 25
(1997): Sapadin A+, New York, American Academy of
Dermatology Meeting (SF), Poster #110
(1994): Gamboa F+, *Ann Pharmacol* 29, 84

Radiation recall
(2001): Krishnan RS+, *J Am Acad Dermatol* 44, 1045 (with
piperacillin & tobramycin)

Rash (sic) (1–10%)
(2000): Johansson A+, *Pediatr Infect Dis J* 19, 449
(2000): Talan DA+, *JAMA* 283, 1583 (4%)
(1995): Chaisson RE, *Infections in Medicine* 12, 48
(1989): Fass RJ+, *Am J Med* 87, 164S
(1989): Modai J, *Am J Med* 87, 243S
(1989): Rahm V+, *Scand J Infect Dis* 60, 120
(1989): Schacht P+, *Am J Med* 87, 98S
(1988): Sanders WE, *Rev Infect Dis* 10, 528
(1988): Schacht P+, *Infection* 16, S29

Stevens–Johnson syndrome (<1%)
(1994): Bhatia RS, *J Assoc Physicians India* 42, 344
(1994): Gohel DR+, *J Assoc Physicians India* 42, 665
(1994): Kamili MA+, *J Assoc Physicians India* 42, 755
(1994): Win A+, *Int J Dermatol* 33, 512

Thrombocytopenic purpura
(2002): Mouraux A+, *Rev Neurol* (Paris) 158(11), 1115

Toxic epidermal necrolysis (<1%)
(1997): Livasy CA+, *Dermatology* 195, 173 (fatal)
(1997): Yerasi AB+, *Ann Pharmacother* 30, 297
(1993): Moshfeghi M+, *Ann Pharmacother* 27, 1467
(1991): Sakellariou G+, *Int J Artif Organs* 14, 634
(1991): Tham TC+, *Lancet* 338, 522

Urticaria (<1%)
(1999): Litt JZ, Beachwood, OH (personal case) (observation)
(1994): Guharoy SR, *Vet Hum Toxicol* 36, 540
(1993): Litt JZ, Beachwood, OH (personal case) (observation)
(1989): Davis H+, *Ann Intern Med* 111, 1041
(1989): Rahm V+, *Scand J Infect Dis* 60, 120

(1989): Schacht P+, *Am J Med* 87, 98S
(1988): Campoli-Richards DM+, *Drugs* 35, 373 (0.05%)
(1988): Schacht P+, *Infection* 16, S29
(1986): Ball P, *J Antimicrob Chemother* 18 (Suppl D), 187
Vasculitis (<1%)
(2000): Perez Vazquez A+, *An Med Interna* (Spanish) 17, 225
(1999): Goldberg EI+, *J Clin Dermatol* 2, 25
(1997): Lieu PK+, *Allergy* 52, 593
(1997): Reano M+, *Allergy* 52, 599
(1994): Beuselinck B+, *Acta Clin Belg* 49, 173
(1993): Wagh SS+, *Indian J Pediatr* 60, 610
(1992): Stubbings J+, *BMJ* 305, 29
(1991): Kanuga J+, *Ann Allergy* 66, 76
(1989): Choe U+, *N Engl J Med* 320, 257

Other

Anaphylactoid reactions (<1%)
(2003): Ho DY+, *Ann Pharmacother* 37(7), 1018
(1999): Corcoy M+, *Rev Esp Anestesiol Reanim* (Spanish) 46, 419
(1999): Erdem G+, *Pediatr Infect Dis J* 18, 563
(1997): Clutterbuck DJ+, *Int J STD AIDS* 8, 707
(1997): Salon EJ+, *Ann Pharmacother* 31, 119
(1995): Assouad M+, *Ann Intern Med* 122, 396
(1994): Beuselinck B+, *Acta Clin Belg* (Dutch; French) 49, 173
(1993): Soetikno RM+, *Ann Pharmacother* 27, 1404 (in AIDS)
(1992): Berger TG+, *J Am Acad Dermatol* 26, 256
(1992): Deamer RL+, *Ann Pharmacother* 26, 1081
(1989): Davis H+, *Ann Intern Med* 111, 1041
(1989): Wurtz RM+, *Lancet* 1, 955
Anosmia
Arthralgia
(1991): Chysky V+, *Infection* 19, 289
Death
Dysesthesia (<1%)
(1995): Zehnder D+, *BMJ* 311, 1204
Dysgeusia (<1%)
(1988): Schacht P+, *Infection* 16, S29
Gynecomastia (<1%)
(1991): MacGowan AP+, *J Infect* 22, 100
Headache
Hypersensitivity
(2001): Scala E+, *Int J Dermatol* 40(9), 603
(1992): Deamer RL+, *Ann Pharmacother* 26, 1081
(1991): Bhatia RS, *J Assoc Physicians India* 39, 972
Injection-site pain
(1988): Thorsteinsson SB+, *Chemotherapy* 34, 256
(1987): Thorsteinsson SB+, *Chemotherapy* 33, 448 (with itching and burning)
Lobular panniculitis (erythematous tender nodules of extremities)
(1990): Rodriguez E+, *BMJ* 300, 1468
Oral candidiasis
(1988): Esposito S+, *Infection* 16, S57
Oral mucosal lesions
(1988): Campoli-Richards DM+, *Drugs* 35, 373
Paresthesias
(1989): Rahm V+, *Scand J Infect Dis* 60, 120
Seizures
(2003): Orr CF+, *Med J Aust* 178(7), 343
(2001): Kushner JM+, *Ann Pharmacother* 35(10), 1194
Serum sickness
(1994): Guharoy SR, *Vet Hum Toxicol* 36, 540
(1990): Slama TG, *Antimicrob Agents Chemother* 34, 904
Stomatitis
(1989): Rahm V+, *Scand J Infect Dis* 60, 120
(1989): Schacht P+, *Am J Med* 87, 98S
(1988): Schacht P+, *Infection* 16, S29
Tendinitis
(1999): Harrell RM, *South Med J* 92, 622 (passim)

(1998): Blanco Andres C+, *Aten Primaria* (Spanish) 21, 184 (bilateral)
(1998): West MB+, *N Z Med J* 111, 18 (bilateral)
(1997): Carrasco JM+, *Ann Pharmacother* 31, 120
Tendinopathy
(2003): Khaliq Y+, *Clin Infect Dis* 36(11), 1404
Tendon disorder
(2002): Corps AN+, *Arthritis Rheum* 46(11), 3034
Tendon rupture
(2001): Malaguti M+, *J Nephrol* 14(5), 431
(2000): Casparian JM+, *South Med J* 93, 488 (2 cases)
(1998): Petersen W+, *Umfallchirurg* (German) 101, 731 (bilateral)
(1998): West MB+, *N Z Med J* 111, 18
(1997): Movin T+, *Foot Ankle Int* 18, 297 (2 cases)
(1997): Peyrade F+, *Presse Med* (French) 26, 1489
(1997): Poon CC+, *Med J Aust* 166, 665
(1997): Shinohara YT+, *J Rheumatol* 24, 238
(1996): Hugo-Persson M, *Lakartidningen* (Swedish) 93, 1520
(1996): Jagose JT+, *N Z Med J* 109, 471
(1996): McGarvey WC+, *Foot Ankle Int* 17, 496
(1993): Boulay I+, *Ann Med Interne (Paris)* (French) 144, 493
(1992): Lee TW+, *Aust N Z J Med*, 22, 500
Tinnitus
Tremor
Vaginitis (<1%)
(1990): Karimi K, *Indiana Med* 83, 266
(1987): Arcieri G+, *Am J Med* 82, 381
Xerostomia
(1989): Rahm V+, *Scand J Infect Dis* 60, 120
(1988): Campoli-Richards DM+, *Drugs* 35, 373
(1988): Schacht P+, *Infection* 16, S29

CISATRACURIUM

Trade name: Nimbex (Abbott)
Indications: Adjunct to general anesthesia, relaxes skeletal muscle
Category: Nondepolarizing neuromuscular blocker (skeletal muscle relaxant)
Half-life: 22 minutes
Clinically important, potentially hazardous interactions with: aminoglycosides, clindamycin, cyclopropane, enflurane, halothane, isoflurane, methoxyflurane, piperacillin

Reactions

Skin

Flushing (0.2%)
Rash (sic) (0.1%)

Other

Anaphylactoid reactions
(2003): Rieder J+, *Anesth Analg* 96(1), 301
(2002): Iannuzzi E+, *Eur J Anaesthesiol* 19(9), 691
(2001): Krombach J+, *Anesth Analg* 93(5), 1257
(2001): Legros CB+, *Anesth Analg* 92(3), 648
(2000): Briassoulis G+, *Paediatr Anaesth* 10(4), 429
(1999): Toh KW+, *Anesth Analg* 88(2), 462
(1997): Clendenen SR+, *Anesthesiology* 87(3), 690
Hypersensitivity
Myopathy
(1998): Davis NA+, *Crit Care Med* 26(7), 1290

CISPLATIN

Synonym: CDDP
Trade name: Platinol (Bristol-Myers Squibb)
Other common trade names: *Cisplatyl; Plasticin; Platiblastin; Platinex; Platinol-AQ; Platistil*
Indications: Carcinomas, lymphomas
Category: Antineoplastic
Half-life: α phase: 25–49 minutes; β phase: 58–73 hours
Clinically important, potentially hazardous interactions with: aldesleukin, methotrexate, selenium

Reactions

Skin

Acral erythema
 (1998): Vakalis D+, *Br J Dermatol* 139, 750
Actinic keratoses
 (1987): Johnson TM+, *J Am Acad Dermatol* 17(2 Pt 1), 192
Allergic reactions (sic)
 (2002): Cantu MG+, *J Clin Oncol* 20(5), 1232 (2%) (with cyclophosphamide and doxorubicin)
Angioedema
 (1984): Loehrer PJ+, *Ann Intern Med* 100, 704
 (1983): Bronner AK+, *J Am Acad Dermatol* 9, 645 (1–5%)
 (1981): Weiss RB+, *Ann Intern Med* 94, 66 (1–5%)
 (1977): Rozencweig M+, *Ann Intern Med* 86, 803
Dermatitis
 (1996): Schena D+, *Contact Dermatitis* 34, 220
Diaphoresis
 (1983): Bronner AK+, *J Am Acad Dermatol* 9, 645
Erythema
 (2001): Robinson JB+, *Gynecol Oncol* 82(3), 550
 (1983): Bronner AK+, *J Am Acad Dermatol* 9, 645
 (1980): Vogl SE+, *Cancer* 45, 11
Exanthems
 (1984): Loehrer PJ+, *Ann Intern Med* 100, 704
 (1981): Weiss RB+, *Ann Intern Med* 94, 66 (1–5%)
 (1980): Vogl SE+, *Cancer* 45, 11
Exfoliative dermatitis
 (1994): Lee TC+, *Mayo Clin Proc* 69, 80
Facial edema
 (1994): Lee TC+, *Mayo Clin Proc* 69, 80
Flushing
 (2001): Robinson JB+, *Gynecol Oncol* 82(3), 550
 (1998): Kempf W+, *Arch Dermatol* 134, 1343
 (1984): Loehrer PJ+, *Ann Intern Med* 100, 704
 (1983): Bronner AK+, *J Am Acad Dermatol* 9, 645
 (1980): Vogl SE+, *Cancer* 45, 11
Necrosis
 (1983): Leyden M+, *Cancer Treat Rep* 67, 199
Pigmentation
 (2002): Kim KJ+, *Clin Exp Dermatol* 27(2), 118
 (1996): Al-Lamki Z+, *Cancer* 77, 1578
Pruritus
 (2002): Koren C+, *Am J Clin Oncol* 25(6), 625
 (2001): Robinson JB+, *Gynecol Oncol* 82(3), 550
 (1994): Lee TC+, *Mayo Clin Proc* 69, 80 (passim)
 (1983): Bronner AK+, *J Am Acad Dermatol* 9, 645 (1–5%)
 (1981): Weiss RB+, *Ann Intern Med* 94, 66 (1–5%)
Pyoderma (verrucous)
 (1982): Person JR+, *Arch Dermatol* 118, 336
Rash (sic)
 (2002): Koren C+, *Am J Clin Oncol* 25(6), 625
Raynaud's phenomenon
 (1992): Doll DC+, *Semin Oncol* 19(5), 580

(1984): Loehrer PJ+, *Ann Intern Med* 100, 704
(1981): Vogelzang NJ+, *Ann Intern Med* 95, 288
Stevens–Johnson syndrome
 (1989): Brodsky A+, *J Clin Pharmacol* 29, 821
Urticaria
 (1996): Schena D+, *Contact Dermatitis* 34, 220
 (1994): Lee TC+, *Mayo Clin Proc* 69, 80 (passim)
 (1983): Bronner AK+, *J Am Acad Dermatol* 9, 645 (1–5%)
 (1981): Weiss RB+, *Ann Intern Med* 94, 66 (1–5%)
 (1980): Vogl SE+, *Cancer* 45, 11

Hair

Hair – alopecia (>10%)
 (2001): Sakai H+, *Cancer Chemother Pharmacol* 48(6), 499 (with paclitaxel)
 (1996): Planting AS+, *Eur J Cancer* 32A, 2026
 (1992): Zaun H+, *Hautarzt* (German) 43, 215
 (1989): Umeki S+, *Chemotherapy* 35, 54

Nails

Nails – Beau's lines (transverse nail bands)
 (1994): Ben-Dyan D+, *Acta Haematol* 91, 89
Nails – hypomelanosis
 (1983): James WD+, *Arch Dermatol* 119, 334

Other

Ageusia
Anaphylactoid reactions (<1%)
 (2002): Basu R+, *Int J Clin Oncol* 7(6), 365
 (1999): Ozguroglu M+, *Am J Clin Oncol* 22, 172 (intraperitoneal infusion)
 (1997): Ciesielski-Carlucci C+, *Am J Clin Oncol* 20(4), 373 (with paclitaxel)
 (1994): Lee TC+, *Mayo Clin Proc* 69, 80 (passim)
 (1983): Bronner AK+, *J Am Acad Dermatol* 9, 645
 (1982): Dunagin WG, *Semin Oncol* 9, 14
 (1980): Vogl SE+, *Cancer* 45, 11
 (1977): Rozencweig M+, *Ann Intern Med* 86, 803
Digital necrosis
 (2000): Marie I+, *Br J Dermatol* 142, 833
Extravasation
Fatigue
 (2002): Ishii K+, *Gynecol Oncol* 87(1), 150
Gingival pigmentation
 (1982): Dunagin WG, *Semin Oncol* 9, 14
Hypersensitivity
 (2002): Koren C+, *Am J Clin Oncol* 25(6), 625
 (2001): Robinson JB+, *Gynecol Oncol* 82(3), 550
Injection-site cellulitis
 (1994): Lee TC+, *Mayo Clin Proc* 69, 80 (passim)
 (1990): Fields S+J, *Natl Cancer Inst* 82, 1649
 (1989): Kerker BJ+, *Semin Dermatol* 8, 173
 (1980): Lewis KP+, *Cancer Treat Rep* 64, 1162
Injection-site pain
 (1998): Kempf W+, *Arch Dermatol* 134, 1343
Injection-site thrombophlebitis
Myalgia
 (2002): Cantu MG+, *J Clin Oncol* 20(5), 1232 (4%) (with cyclophosphamide and doxorubicin)
Oral mucosal lesions (<1%)
 (1997): Herlofson BB+, *Eur J Oral Sci* 105, 523
 (1990): Al-Sarraf M+, *J Clin Oncol* 8, 1342 (>5%)
Oral ulceration (<1%)
Phlebitis
Porphyria
 (1986): Aramburo-Gonzalez P+, *Med Clin (Barc)* (Spanish) 87, 738
Rhabdomyolysis
 (1995): Anderlini P+, *Cancer* 76(4), 678
Tinnitus

CITALOPRAM

Synonym: nitalapram
Trade name: Celexa (Forest)
Indications: Depression, obsessive-compulsive disorder, panic disorder
Category: Selective serotonin reuptake inhibitor (SSRI)
Half-life: 33 hours
Clinically important, potentially hazardous interactions with: isocarboxazid, MAO inhibitors, phenelzine, selegiline, **St John's wort**, sumatriptan, tramadol, tranylcypromine, trazodone

Reactions

Skin
Cellulitis
Dermatitis (sic)
Diaphoresis (11%)
    (2001): Bostic JQ+, *J Child Adole Pyschopharmacol* 11(2), 159
    (1999): Feighner JP+, *J Clin Psychiatry* 60(12), 824
Eczema (sic)
Exanthems
    (2001): Richard MA+, *Ann Dermatol Venereol* 128(6), 759
Facial edema
Hot flashes
Hypohidrosis
Neuroleptic malignant syndrome
    (2000): Aydin N+, *Can J Psychiatry* 45(10), 941
Photopigmentation
    (2001): Inaloz HS+, *J Dermatol* 28(12), 742
Photosensitivity
Pigmentation
    (2001): Inaloz HS+, *J Dermatol* 28(12), 742
Pruritus (<10%)
    (2001): Richard MA+, *Ann Dermatol Venereol* 128(6), 759
Pruritus ani
Psoriasis
    (2000): Elliott P, Logan Central, Australia (from Internet) (observation)
Purpura
    (2001): Robinson MJ, *Can Psychiatry* 46, 286
Rash (sic) (<10%)
Urticaria
Vasculitis
    (2001): Richard MA+, *Ann Dermatol Venereol* 128(6), 759
Xerosis

Hair
Hair – alopecia
Hair – hypertrichosis

Other
Bruxism
    (2001): Wise M, *Br J Psychiatry* 178, 182
Death
    (2002): Jonasson B+, *Forensic Sci Int* 126(1), 1 (5 cases)
    (2001): Dams R+, *J Anal Toxicol* 25(2), 147 (with moclobemide)
    (2001): Isbister GK+, *J Anal Toxicol* 25(8), 716 (with moclobemide)
    (1999): Musshoff F+, *Forensic Sci Int* 106(2), 125
Dysgeusia
Galactorrhea
    (2001): Gonzalez Pablos E+, *Actas Esp Psiquiatr* 29(6), 414
Gingivitis
Gynecomastia
Headache

    (2003): Barak Y+, *Prog Neuropsychopharmacol Biol Psychiatry* 27(3), 545
Hyperesthesia
Mastodynia
Myalgia (>2%)
Paresthesias
Parkinsonism
    (2000): Stadtland C+, *Pharmacopsychiatry* 33(5), 194
Priapism (clitoral)
    (2002): Baptista T, *J Clin Psychiatry* 63(3), 245 (with risperidone)
    (2002): Dent LA+, *Pharmacotherapy* 22(4), 538
    (2002): Freudenreich O, *J Clin Psychiatry* 63(3), 249 (with risperidone)
    (1997): Berk M+, *Int Clin Psychopharmacol* 12, 121 (3 cases)
Serotonin syndrome
    (2003): Bernard L+, *Clin Infect Dis* 36(9), 1197
    (2002): Chechani V, *Crit Care Med* 30(2), 473
    (2001): Dams R+, *J Anal Toxicol* 25(2), 147 (with moclobemide)
    (2000): Voirol P+, *J Clin Psychopharmacol* 20(6), 713
Sialorrhea
Stomatitis
Torsades de pointes
    (2001): Meuleman C+, *Arch Mal Coeur Vaiss* 94(9), 1021
Tremor (<10%)
Twitching
    (2001): Rojas VM+, *J Child Adolesc Psychopharmacol* 11(3), 295
Xerostomia (20%)
    (1999): Feighner JP+, *J Clin Psychiatry* 60(12), 824

CLADRIBINE

Synonyms: 2-CdA; 2-chlorodeoxyadenosine
Trade name: Leustatin (Ortho)
Indications: Leukemias
Category: Antimetabolite; Antineoplastic
Half-life: α phase: 25 minutes; β phase: 6.7 hours

Reactions

Skin
Allergic reactions (sic)
    (1997): Robak T+, *J Med* 28, 199
Diaphoresis (1–10%)
Edema (6%)
Erythema (6%)
Exanthems (27–50%)
    (1996): Meunier P+, *Acta Derm Venereol* 76, 385 (21%)
Halogenoderma (sic)
    (1996): Zevin S+, *Am J Hematol* 53, 209
Herpes
    (2002): Robak T+, *Eur J Haematol* 69(1), 27 (10 cases)
Infections
    (2003): Byrd JC+, *Leukemia* 17(2), 323 (43%)
Petechiae (8%)
Pruritus (6%)
Purpura (10%)
Rash (sic) (27%)
    (2000): Grey MR+, *Clin Lab Haematol* 22, 111
Toxic epidermal necrolysis
    (1996): Meunier P+, *Acta Derm Venereol* 76, 385
Transient acantholytic dermatosis (sic)
    (1997): Cohen PR+, *Acta Derm Venereol* 77, 412
Vasculitis
    (2002): Tousi B+, *Clin Lab Haematol* 24(4), 259 (1 case)

Other
Gynecomastia
  (2001): Abhyankar D+, *Leuk Lymphoma* 42(1), 243
Headache
Injection-site edema (9%)
Injection-site erythema (9%)
Injection-site pain (9%)
Injection-site phlebitis (2%)
Injection-site thrombosis (2%)
Myalgia (7%)
Pneumonia
  (2002): Robak T+, *Eur J Haematol* 69(1), 27 (10 cases)
Thrombocytopenia
  (2002): Tousi B+, *Clin Lab Haematol* 24(4), 259 (1 case)

CLARITHROMYCIN

Synonym: Cla
Trade names: Biaxin (Abbott); Prevpac (TAP)
Other common trade names: *Biaxin HP; Clacine; Clarith; Klacid; Klaricid; Macladin; Veclam*
Indications: Various infections caused by susceptible organisms
Category: Macrolide antibiotic
Half-life: 5–7 hours
Clinically important, potentially hazardous interactions with: alprazolam, aprepitant, atorvastatin, benzodiazepines, carbamazepine, chlordiazepoxide, clonazepam, clorazepate, cyclosporine, diazepam, digoxin, dihydroergotamine, disopyramide, ergot alkaloids, fluoxetine, flurazepam, fluvastatin, imatinib, lorazepam, lovastatin, methysergide, midazolam, oxazepam, paroxetine, pimozide, pravastatin, quazepam, sertraline, simvastatin, temazepam, triazolam, warfarin, zidovudine

Reactions

Skin
Exanthems
Fixed eruption
  (2001): Hamamoto Y+, *Clin Exp Dermatol* 26(1), 48
  (1988): Rosina P+, *Contact Dermatitis* 38, 105
Henoch-Schonlein purpura
  (2003): Borras-Blasco J+, *Int J Clin Pharmacol Ther* 41(5), 213
Phototoxicity
  (2002): Parkash P+, *J Assoc Physicians India* 50, 1192
Pruritus
  (1991): Poirier R, *J Antimicrob Chemother* 27 (Suppl A), 109
Psoriasis
  (1994): Ellerin P, *The Schoch Letter* 44, 47 (#185) (observation)
Purpura
  (2002): Alexopoulou A+, *Eur J Haematol* 69(3), 191
Pustules
Rash (sic) (3%)
Stevens–Johnson syndrome (<1%)
Thrombocytopenic purpura
  (2002): Alexopoulou A+, *Eur J Haematol* 69(3), 191
Toxic epidermal necrolysis
  (2002): Masia M+, *Arch Intern Med* 162(4), 474 (with disulfiram)
Urticaria
Vasculitis
  (1998): Gavura SR+, *Ann Pharmacol* 32, 543
  (1993): de Vega T+, *Eur J Clin Microbiol Infect Dis* 12, 563

Other
Anaphylactoid reactions (<1%)
Black tongue
  (1997): Greco S+, *Ann Pharmacother* 31, 1548
Death
  (2002): Masia M+, *Arch Intern Med* 162(4), 474
Dysgeusia (3%)
  (2001): Litt JZ, Beachwood, OH (personal case)
  (2001): McCarty JM+, *Ann Allergy Asthma Immunol* 87(4), 327
  (1997): Saluja A+, *Derm Surg* 23, 539
Ergotism
  (2001): Ausband SC+, *J Emerg Med* 21(4), 411
Glossitis
  (1997): Greco S+, *Ann Pharmacother* 31, 1548
Headache
Hypersensitivity
  (1998): Igea JM+, *Allergy* 53, 107
  (1998): Kruppa A+, *Dermatology* 196(3), 335
Injection-site extravasation
  (2001): Zimmerman T+, *Clin Drug Invest* 21, 527 (8%)
Injection-site pain
  (2001): Zimmerman T+, *Clin Drug Invest* 21, 527 (100%)
  (1996): Peck KD+, *Pharm Res* 13, PT6028 (9 Suppl)
Oral candidiasis
Parosmia
Phlebitis
  (2001): De Dios Garcia-Diaz J+, *Med Clin* (Barc) 116(4), 133 (from intravenous administration)
Pseudolymphoma
  (1995): Magro CM+, *J Am Acad Dermatol* 32, 419
Rhabdomyolysis
  (2003): Mah Ming+, *AIDS Patient Care STDS* 17(5), 207 (with atorvastatin, and lopinavir/ritonavir)
  (2003): Sipe BE+, *Ann Pharmacother* 37(6), 808 (with atorvastatin and esomeprazole)
  (2001): Lee AJ, *Ann Pharmacother* 35(1), 26 (with simvastatin)
  (1999): Shimada N+, *Nippon Jinzo Gakkai Shi* 41(4), 460 (with theophylline)
Stomatitis
  (1997): Greco S+, *Ann Pharmacother* 31, 1548
Torsades de pointes
  (2003): Yamaguchi S+, *Nippon Naika Gakkai Zasshi* 92(1), 143
  (2002): Shaffer D+, *Clin Infect Dis* 35(2), 197
Tremor (<1%)
Xerostomia
  (2001): McCarty JM+, *Ann Allergy Asthma Immunol* 87(4), 327

CLEMASTINE

Trade name: Tavist (Novartis)
Other common trade names: *Aller-Eze; Antihist-1; Clema; Darvine; Tavegil; Tavegyl*
Indications: Allergic rhinitis, urticaria
Category: Antihistamine H$_1$-blocker
Half-life: 4–6 hours
Clinically important, potentially hazardous interactions with: barbiturates, chloral hydrate, ethchlorvynol, phenothiazines, zolpidem

Reactions

Skin
Angioedema (<1%)
Diaphoresis
Edema (<1%)

Exanthems
  (1975): Todd G+, *Curr Med Res Opin* 3, 126
Flushing
  (1975): Todd G+, *Curr Med Res Opin* 3, 126
Photosensitivity (<1%)
  (1962): Schreiber M+, *Arch Dermatol* 86, 58
Purpura
Rash (sic) (<1%)
Toxic pustuloderma
  (1996): Feind-Koopmans A+, *Clin Exp Dermatol* 21, 293
Urticaria
  (1984): Savchak VI, *Vestn Dermatol Venerol* (Russian) 1, 47

Other
Anaphylactoid reactions
Hypersensitivity
Myalgia (<1%)
Paresthesias (<1%)
Tinnitus
Xerostomia (1–10%)
  (1990): Frolund L+, *Allergy* 45, 254

CLIDINIUM

Trade names: Librax (ICN); Quarzan (Roche)
Other common trade names: *Bralix; Diporax; Epirax; Libraxin; Librocol; Nirvaxal; Spasmoten*
Indications: Duodenal and gastric ulcers
Category: Anticholinergic
Half-life: N/A
Clinically important, potentially hazardous interactions
with: anticholinergics, arbutamine

Librax is clidinium and chlordiazepoxide (see chlordiazepoxide)

Reactions

Skin
Flushing
Hypohidrosis
Purpura
  (2001): Alexopoulou A+, *Arch Intern Med* 161(14), 1778 (with chlordiazepoxide)
Urticaria

Other
Ageusia
Anaphylactoid reactions
Dysgeusia
Xerostomia

CLINDAMYCIN

Trade names: Benzaclin (cream) (Dermik); Cleocin (Pharmacia); Cleocin-T (Pharmacia); Clindagel (Galderma); Clindets (Stiefel)
Other common trade names: *Aclinda; BB; Clindacin; Dalacin; Dalacin C; Dalacine; Galecin; Sobelin*
Indications: Various serious infections caused by susceptible organisms
Category: Lincosamide antibiotic
Half-life: 2–3 hours
Clinically important, potentially hazardous interactions
with: cisatracurium, erythromycin, kaolin, saquinavir

Reactions

Skin
Acute generalized exanthematous pustulosis (AGEP)
  (2000): Schwab RA+, *Cutis* 65, 391
Allergic reactions (sic)
  (1996): Garcia R+, *Contact Dermatitis* 35, 116
Dermatitis (from topical preparations)
  (1995): Vejlstrup E+, *Contact Dermatitis* 32, 110
  (1994): Rietschel RL, *Infect Dis Clin North Am* 8, 607
  (1992): de Groot AC, *Contact Dermatitis* 8, 428
  (1991): Yokayama R+, *Contact Dermatitis* 25, 125
  (1983): Conde-Salazar L, *Contact Dermatitis* 9, 225
  (1978): Coskey RJ, *Arch Dermatol* 114, 446
  (1978): Herstoff JK, *Arch Dermatol* 114, 1402
Eczema (sic)
  (1991): Yokoyama R+, *Contact Dermatitis* 25, 125
Edema of lip
  (1993): Segars LW+, *Ann Pharmacother* 27, 885
Erythema multiforme (<1%)
  (1996): Munoz D+, *Contact Dermatitis* 34, 227
  (1973): Fulghum DD+, *JAMA* 223, 318
Erythroderma
  (2002): Horiuchi Y+, *J Dermatol* 29(2), 115
Exanthems
  (2002): Lammintausta K+, *Br J Dermatol* 146, 643 (6 cases)
  (1999): Mazur N+, *Ann Allergy Asthma Immunol* 82, 443
  (1984): Brenner S+, *Harefuah* (Hebrew) 106, 570
  (1970): Geddes AM+, *BMJ* 2, 703 (>5%)
Facial edema
  (1999): Mazur N+, *Ann Allergy Asthma Immunol* 82, 443
Fixed eruption
  (1998): Mahboob A+, *Int J Dermatol* 37, 833
Leukocytoclastic angiitis
  (1982): Lamber WC+, *Cutis* 30, 615
Pruritus (<1%)
  (1973): Fass RJ+, *Ann Intern Med* 78, 853 (10%)
Pruritus ani
Purpura
Rash (sic) (1–10%)
  (2002): Maraqa NF+, *Clin Infect Dis* 34(1), 50 (1.4%)
Rosacea
  (1989): de Kort WJ+, *Contact Dermatitis* 20, 72
Stevens–Johnson syndrome (<1%)
  (1974): Maulide T+, *Pneumologica* (Lisbon) 5, 79
  (1973): Fulghum DD+, *JAMA* 223, 318
  (1973): Pickering LK, *JAMA* 223, 1392
Toxic epidermal necrolysis
  (1995): Paquet P+, *Br J Dermatol* 132, 665
  (1993): Correia O+, *Dermatology* 186, 32
  (1992): Saiag P+, *J Am Acad Dermatol* 26, 567
Urticaria (<1%)
  (1973): Fulghum DD+, *JAMA* 223, 31

(1972): Meyler L+, *Side Effects of Drugs* Vol 7, Excerpta Medica, 389
(1970): Newell AC, *Med J Aust* 2, 321
(1969): Lattanzi WE+, *Int Med Dig* 4, 29
Vasculitis
(1982): Lambert WC+, *Cutis* 30, 615
Xerosis (from topical preparations)

Other

Anaphylactoid reactions
(1977): Lochmann O+, *J Hyg Epiderm Microbiol Immunol* 21, 441
Dysgeusia
Hypersensitivity
(2002): Kim P+, *Clin Experiment Ophthalmol* 30(2), 147
(2002): Lammintausta K+, *Br J Dermatol* 146(4), 643
Injection-site phlebitis (<1%)
Lymphadenitis
(1997): Southern PM, *Am J Med* 103, 164
Thrombophlebitis

CLOFAZIMINE

Trade name: Lamprene (Novartis)
Other common trade names: *Clofozine; Hansepran; Lampren; Lapren*
Indications: Leprosy
Category: Antileprotic
Half-life: 10 days after a single dose

Reactions

Skin

Acne (<1%)
(1992): Breathnach SM+, *Adverse Drug Reactions and the Skin* Blackwell, Oxford, 161 (passim)
Acute febrile neutrophilic dermatosis (Sweet's syndrome)
(1994): Tacke J+, *Hautarzt* (German) 45, 184
Ankle edema (<1%)
(1990): Oommen T, *Leprosy Review* 61, 289
Cheilitis (candidal) (<1%)
Discoloration (sic)
(1979): Thomsen K+, *Arch Dermatol* 115, 851
Erythroderma (<1%)
Exanthems
Exfoliative dermatitis
(1985): Pavithran K, *Int J Lepr* 53, 645
Ichthyosis (8–28%)
(1989): Patki AH+, *Indian J Lepr* 61, 92
(1987): Kumar B+, *Indian J Lepr* 59, 63
(1984): Aram H, *Int J Dermatol* 23, 458
(1982): Caver CV, *Cutis* 29, 341
(1979): Thomsen K+, *Arch Dermatol* 115, 851
Nodules
(1993): Tyagi PY+, *Int J Lepr Other Mycobact Dis* 61, 636
Photosensitivity (<1%)
(1992): Breathnach SM+, *Adverse Drug Reactions and the Skin* Blackwell, Oxford, 161 (passim)
Pigmentation (pink to brownish-black) (75–100%)
(1993): Krop LC+, *N Engl J Med* 329, 1582
(1992): Fitzpatrick JE, *Derm Clinics* 10, 19
(1992): Gallais V+, *Ann Dermatol Venereol* (French) 119, 471
(1991): Garrelts JC, *Ann Pharmacother* 25, 525 (orange-pink)
(1990): Job CK+, *J Am Acad Dermatol* 23, 236
(1989): Langford A+, *Oral Surg Oral Med Oral Pathol* 67, 301 (oral)
(1989): Patki AH+, *Indian J Lepr* 61, 92 (oral)

(1989): Zhang X+, *J Oral Pathol Med* 18, 471
(1988): Mensing H, *Dermatologica* 177, 232
(1987): Kossard S+, *J Am Acad Dermatol* 17, 867 (reddish-blue)
(1987): Kumar B+, *Indian J Lepr* 59, 63
(1983): Burte NP+, *Lepr India* 55, 265
(1983): Moore VJ, *Lepr Rev* 54, 327
(1981): Granstein RD+, *J Am Acad Dermatol* 5, 1 (red)
(1978): Chuaprapaisilp T+, *Br J Dermatol* 99, 303 (deep-red)
(1978): Pettit JH, *Int J Lepr Other Mycobact Dis* 46, 227
(1971): Karat ABA+, *BMJ* 4, 514
(1969): Levy L+, *Int J Lepr* 38, 404
Pruritus (1–5%)
(1992): Breathnach SM+, *Adverse Drug Reactions and the Skin* Blackwell, Oxford, 161 (passim)
Rash (sic) (1–5%)
(1995): Chaisson RE, *Infections in Medicine* 12, 48
(1992): Breathnach SM+, *Adverse Drug Reactions and the Skin* Blackwell, Oxford, 161 (passim)
Urticaria
Vitiligo
(1996): Brown-Harrell V+, *Clin Infect Dis* 22, 581
Xerosis (8–28%)
(1992): Breathnach SM+, *Adverse Drug Reactions and the Skin* Blackwell, Oxford, 161 (passim)

Nails

Nails – discoloration
(1989): Dixit VB+, *Indian J Lepr* 61, 476
(1982): Caver CV, *Cutis* 29, 341
Nails – onycholysis
(1989): Dixit VB+, *Indian J Lepr* 61, 476
Nails – subungual hyperkeratosis
(1989): Dixit VB+, *Indian J Lepr* 61, 476

Other

Chromhidrosis (red sweat) (1–10%)
(1987): Kumar B+, *Indian J Lepr* 59, 63
(1979): Thomsen K+, *Arch Dermatol* 115, 851
(1979): Yawalkar SJ+, *Lepr Rev* 50, 135
Dysgeusia (<1%)

CLOFIBRATE

Trade names: Abitrate; Claripex; Col; Lipavlon; Novo-Fibrate; Regelan N; Skleromexe
Indications: Type III hyperlipidemia
Category: Antihyperlipidemic
Half-life: 6–25 hours after a single dose
Clinically important, potentially hazardous interactions with: anisindione, anticoagulants, dicumarol, warfarin

Reactions

Skin

Dermatitis (sic)
(1988): Murata Y+, *J Am Acad Dermatol* 18, 381
(1972): Inman WHW+, *BMJ* 3, 746
(1972): Krasno LR+, *JAMA* 219, 845
Diaphoresis
Erythema multiforme
(1988): Murata Y+, *J Am Acad Dermatol* 18, 381
Exanthems
(1988): Murata Y+, *J Am Acad Dermatol* 18, 381
(1980): Cumming A, *BMJ* 281, 1529
(1977): Heid E+, *Ann Dermatol Venereol* (French) 104, 494
(1975): Arif MA+, *Lancet* 2, 1202 (7%)
(1971): Five Year Study, *BMJ* 4, 767 (0.8%)

(1965): Hollander W, *Cardiovascular Drug Therapy* 339
Exfoliative dermatitis
  (1972): Inman WHW+, *BMJ* 3, 746
Facial dermatitis
  (1967): Orgain ES+, *Arch Intern Med* 119, 80
Lupus erythematosus
  (1973): Howard EJ+, *JAMA* 226, 1358
Photosensitivity
  (1990): Leroy D+, *Photodermatology* 7, 136
  (1988): Murata Y+, *J Am Acad Dermatol* 18, 381
  (1977): Heid E+, *Ann Dermatol Venereol* (French) 104, 494
  (1967): Orgain ES+, *Arch Intern Med* 119, 80
Pruritus (<1%)
Purpura
  (1975): Arif MA+, *Lancet* 2, 1202
Rash (sic) (<1%)
Sarcoidosis
  (1986): Yamada S+, *J Dermatol* (Tokio) 13, 217
Stevens–Johnson syndrome
  (1994): Wong SS, *Acta Derm Venereol* 74, 475
Toxic epidermal necrolysis
Urticaria (<1%)
Vesiculobullous eruption
  (1977): Heid E+, *Ann Dermatol Venereol* (French) 104, 494
Xerosis

Hair
Hair – alopecia (<1%)
  (1971): Five Year Study, *BMJ* 4, 767 (0.8%)
Hair – dry (<1%)

Other
Dysgeusia
Gynecomastia
Hypogeusia
Myalgia
Myopathy (<1%)
  (1976): Rumpf KW+, *Lancet* 1, 249
  (1975): Pierides AM+, *Lancet* 2, 1279
  (1968): Langer T+, *N Engl J Med* 279, 856
Oral ulceration
  (1973): Howard EJ+, *JAMA* 226, 1358
Rhabdomyolysis
  (1977): Smals AG+, *N Engl J Med* 296(16), 942
Stomatitis

CLOMIPHENE

Trade names: Clomid (Aventis); Serophene (Serono)
Other common trade names: *Clom 50; Clomifen; Dyneric; Milophene; Omifin; Pergotime; Phenate; Serophene*
Indications: Ovulatory failure
Category: Infertility therapy adjunct; Ovulation stimulator
Half-life: 5–7 days

Reactions

Skin
Acne
  (2001): Guzick ND, Houston, TX (from Internet) (several observations)
Allergic reactions (sic)
Dermatitis (sic) (<1%)
Diaphoresis
Edema

Erythema
Erythema multiforme
Erythema nodosum
  (1980): Salvatore MA+, *Arch Dermatol* 116, 557
Exanthems
  (1996): Coots NV+, *Cutis* 57, 91
  (1966): Johnson JE+, *Pacif Med Surg* 74, 153 (0.8%)
Flushing (10%)
  (1966): Johnson JE+, *Pacif Med Surg* 74, 153 (14%)
Hot flashes (>10%)
Melanoma
  (1999): Fuller PN, *Am J Obstet Gynecol* 180, 1499
  (1995): Rossing MA+, *Melanoma Res* 5, 123
  (1992): Kuppens E+, *Melanoma Res* 2, 71
Pruritus
Purpura (palpable)
  (1996): Coots NV+, *Cutis* 57, 91
Rash (sic) (<1%)
Urticaria
  (1969): *Drug and Therapeutic Bulletin* (London) 7, 34

Hair
Hair – alopecia (<1%)
  (1969): *Drug and Therapeutic Bulletin* (London) 7, 34 (0.4%)
  (1966): Johnson JE+, *Pacif Med Surg* 74, 153 (0.3%)
Hair – hypertrichosis
  (2001): Smith KC, Niagara Falls, ON, Canada (from Internet) (several observations)

Other
Gynecomastia (1–10%)
  (1978): Check JH+, *Fertility and Sterility* 30, 713
Headache
Mastodynia (1–10%)
Myalgia

CLOMIPRAMINE

Trade name: Anafranil (Mallinckrodt)
Other common trade names: *Anafranil Retard; Apo-Clomipramine; Clofranil; Clopress; Placil*
Indications: Obsessive-compulsive disorder
Category: Tricyclic antidepressant
Half-life: 21–31 hours
Clinically important, potentially hazardous interactions with: amprenavir, arbutamine, clonidine, epinephrine, formoterol, guanethidine, isocarboxazid, linezolid, MAO inhibitors, phenelzine, quinolones, sparfloxacin, tranylcypromine

Reactions

Skin
Acne (2%)
Allergic reactions (sic) (<3%)
Cellulitis (2%)
Cheilitis
Chloasma
Dermatitis (sic) (2%)
  (1991): Ljunggren B+, *Contact Dermatitis* 24, 259
Diaphoresis (29%)
  (1992): Guelfi JD+, *Br J Psychiatry* 160, 519
  (1990): McTavish D+, *Drugs* 38, 19 (43%)
Edema (2%)
Erythema
Exanthems

Flushing (8%)
Folliculitis
Photosensitivity (<1%)
   (1991): Ljunggren B+, *Contact Dermatitis* 24, 259
   (1989): Tunca Z+, *Am J Psychiatry* 146, 552
   (1979): Parkes JD+, *Lancet* 2, 1085
Pigmentation (pseudocyanotic)
   (1989): Tunca Z+, *Am J Psychiatry* 146, 552
Pruritus (6%)
Psoriasis
Purpura (3%)
Pustules
Rash (sic) (8%)
Seborrhea
Urticaria (1%)
Vasculitis
Xerosis (2%)

Hair
Hair – alopecia (<1%)
Hair – alopecia areata
   (1993): Kubota T+, *Acta Neurol Napoli* (Italian) 15, 200
Hair – hypertrichosis

Other
Ageusia
Black tongue
Dysgeusia (8%)
Galactorrhea (<1%)
Gingivitis
Glossitis
Gynecomastia (2%)
Headache
Mastodynia (1%)
Myalgia (13%)
Paresthesias
Sialorrhea
Stomatitis
Tongue ulceration
Vaginitis (2%)
Xerostomia (84%)
   (1992): Cohen DJ+, *Psychiatr Clin North Am* 15, 109
   (1992): DeVeaugh-Geiss J+, *J Am Acad Child Adolesc Psychiatry*
      31, 45
   (1992): Guelfi JD+, *Br J Psychiatry* 160, 519
   (1990): McTavish D+, *Drugs* 38, 19

   (1976): Pinder RM+, *Drugs* 12, 321
Ankle edema
Dermatitis (sic) (1–10%)
Diaphoresis (>10%)
Erythema multiforme
   (1998): Amichai B+, *Clin Exp Dermatology* 23, 206
Exanthems
   (1976): Pinder RM+, *Drugs* 12, 321
Facial edema
Hypermelanosis
   (1976): Pinder RM+, *Drugs* 12, 321
Pruritus
Pseudo-mycosis fungoides
   (1996): Gordon KB+, *J Am Acad Dermatol* 34, 304
Purpura
   (1976): Pinder RM+, *Drugs* 12, 321
Rash (sic) (>10%)
Urticaria

Hair
Hair – alopecia
   (2000): Mercke Y+, *Ann Clin Psychiatry* 12, 35
Hair – hirsutism

Other
Black tongue
   (2000): Heymann WR, *Cutis* 66, 25
Burning mouth syndrome
   (2001): Culhane NS+, *Ann Pharmacother* 35(7), 874
Dysgeusia
   (2000): Heymann WR, *Cutis* 66, 25
Gingivitis
Headache
Injection-site phlebitis
Injection-site thrombosis
Oral mucosal eruption
   (1986): Bernard K, *Lijec Vjesn* (Serbo-Croatian-Roman) 108, 235
Oral ulceration
Paresthesias
Pseudolymphoma
   (1995): Magro CM+, *J Am Acad Dermatol* 32, 419
   (1988): Kardaun SH+, *Br J Dermatol* 118(4), 545
Sialopenia (>10%)
Sialorrhea (1–10%)
Xerostomia (>10%)
   (2000): Heymann WR, *Cutis* 66, 25

CLONAZEPAM

Trade name: Klonopin (Roche)
Other common trade names: *Clonex; Iktorivil; Landsen; Lonazep; Rivotril*
Indications: Petit mal and myoclonic seizures
Category: Benzodiazepine anticonvulsant
Half-life: 18–50 hours
Clinically important, potentially hazardous interactions with: amprenavir, chlorpheniramine, clarithromycin, efavirenz, esomeprazole, imatinib, indinavir, nelfinavir

Reactions

Skin
Allergic reactions (sic) (1–10%)
Angioedema

CLONIDINE

Trade names: Catapres (Boehringer Ingelheim); Combipres (Boehringer Ingelheim)
Other common trade names: *Barclyd; Catapresan; Daipres; Dixarit; Duraclon; Haemiton; Nu-Clonidine; Sulmidine*
Indications: Hypertension
Category: Alpha-2-adrenoceptor blocker; Antihypertensive
Half-life: 6–24 hours
Clinically important, potentially hazardous interactions with: acebutolol, amitriptyline, amoxapine, atenolol, betaxolol, carteolol, clomipramine, desipramine, doxepin, esmolol, imipramine, metoprolol, nadolol, nortriptyline, penbutolol, pindolol, propranolol, protriptyline, timolol, tricyclic antidepressants, trimipramine, verapamil

Combipres is clonidine and chlorthalidone

Reactions

Skin
Angioedema (<1%)
 (1995): Waldfahrer F+, *HNO* (German) 43, 35
Depigmentation
 (2002): Prisant LM, *J Clin Hypertens* (Greenwich) 4(2), 136
 (1995): Doe N+, *Arch Intern Med* 155, 2129 (from patch)
Dermatitis (from patch) (20%)
 (2002): Prisant LM, *J Clin Hypertens* (Greenwich) 4(2), 136
 (1999): Polster AM+, *Cutis* 63, 154
 (1997): Shelley ED+, *J Geriatr Dermatol* 4, 192
 (1995): Corazza M+, *Contact Dermatitis* 32, 246
 (1994): Tom GR+, *Ann Pharmacother* 28, 889
 (1992): Breathnach SM+, *Adverse Drug Reactions and the Skin*
    Blackwell, Oxford, 226 (passim)
 (1991): Ito MK+, *Am J Med* 91, 42S
 (1991): McChesney JA, *West J Med* 154, 736
 (1990): Hogan DJ+, *J Am Acad Dermatol* 22, 811
 (1990): Scheper RJ+, *Contact Dermatitis* 23, 81
 (1989): Fillingim JM+, *Clin Ther* 11, 398
 (1989): Holdiness MR, *Contact Dermatitis* 20, 3
 (1988): Horning JR+, *Chest* 93, 941
 (1987): Bigby M+, *JAMA* 258, 1819 (letter)
 (1987): Maibach HI, *Contact Dermatitis* 16, 1
 (1986): Hollifield J, *Am Heart J* 112, 900
 (1986): Weber MA, *Am Heart J* 112, 906
 (1986): White TM+, *West J Med* 145, 104
 (1985): Grattan CEH+, *Contact Dermatitis* 2, 225
 (1985): Maibach H, *Contact Dermatitis* 12, 192
 (1984): van Ketel WG, *Ned Tijdschr Geneeskd* (Dutch) 128, 34
 (1983): Boekhorst JC, *Lancet* 2, 1031
 (1983): Groth H+, *Lancet* 2, 850
Diaphoresis
 (1990): Leeman CP, *J Clin Psychiatry* 51, 258
Eczema (sic)
 (1987): Dick JBC+, *Lancet* 1, 516
 (1985): Grattan CEH+, *Contact Dermatitis* 12, 225
Edema
Erythema
 (2002): Prisant LM, *J Clin Hypertens* (Greenwich) 4(2), 136
 (1987): Dick JBC+, *Lancet* 1, 516
Exanthems
Excoriations
 (2002): Prisant LM, *J Clin Hypertens* (Greenwich) 4(2), 136
Herpes simplex
 (1987): Wiser TH+, *J Am Acad Dermatol* 17, 143
Irritation (from patch)
 (1999): Dias VC+, *Am J Ther* 6, 19

Lupus erythematosus
 (1994): Heilmann G+, *Dtsch Med Wochenschr* (German) 119, 858
 (1994): Yung RL+, *Rheum Dis Clin North Am* 20, 61
 (1992): Breathnach SM+, *Adverse Drug Reactions and the Skin*
    Blackwell, Oxford, 226 (passim)
 (1981): Witman G+, *R I Med J* 64, 147
Pemphigus (anogenital and cicatricial)
 (1980): van Joost T+, *Br J Dermatol* 102, 715
Peripheral edema
Pigmentation
 (2002): Prisant LM, *J Clin Hypertens* (Greenwich) 4(2), 136
 (1987): Wiser TH+, *J Am Acad Dermatol* 17, 143 (from patch)
Pityriasis rosea
 (1998): Reed BR, Denver, CO (2 cases – in siblings) (from Internet) (observation)
 (1992): Breathnach SM+, *Adverse Drug Reactions and the Skin*
    Blackwell, Oxford, 226 (passim)
Pruritus (>5%)
 (1999): Dias VC+, *Am J Ther* 6, 19
 (1987): Dick JBC+, *Lancet* 1, 516
 (1984): Weber MA+, *Arch Intern Med* 144, 1211
 (1984): Weber MA+, *Lancet* 1, 9
 (1983): Boekhorst JC, *Lancet* 2, 1031
Psoriasis
 (1981): Wilkin J, *Arch Dermatol* 117, 4
Rash (sic) (1–10%)
 (1988): Glassman AH, *JAMA* 259, 2863
Raynaud's phenomenon (<1%)
Scaling
 (2002): Prisant LM, *J Clin Hypertens* (Greenwich) 4(2), 136
Ulcerations (1–10%)
Urticaria (<1%)
Vesiculation
 (2002): Prisant LM, *J Clin Hypertens* (Greenwich) 4(2), 136

Hair
Hair – alopecia (<1%)

Other
Acute intermittent porphyria
Application-site vesicles
 (1987): Dick JBC+, *Lancet* 1, 516
Dysgeusia (from patch)
Gynecomastia (<1%)
Headache
Hyperesthesia (1–10%)
Immune complex disease
 (1989): Petersen HH+, *Acta Derm Venereol* (Stockh) 69, 519
Induration
 (2002): Prisant LM, *J Clin Hypertens* (Greenwich) 4(2), 136
Pseudolymphoma
 (1997): Shelley WB+, *Lancet* 350, 1223 (at site of patch)
Xerostomia (40%)
 (2000): Geyer O+, *Graefes Arch Clin Exp Ophthalmol* 238, 149
 (2000): Litt JZ, Beachwood, OH (personal case) (observation)
 (1999): Dias VC+, *Am J Ther* 6, 19
 (1988): Glassman AH, *JAMA* 259, 2863
 (1984): Weber MA+, *Arch Intern Med* 144, 1211
 (1984): Weber MA+, *Lancet* 1, 9
 (1983): Boekhorst JC, *Lancet* 2, 1031

CLOPIDOGREL

Trade name: Plavix (Bristol-Myers Squibb) (Sanofi-Synthelabo)
Indications: Atherosclerotic events
Category: Antiplatelet (thienopyridine derivative)
Half-life: ~8 hours
**Clinically important, potentially hazardous interactions
with:** anisindione, anticoagulants, dicumarol, fondaparinux,
warfarin

Reactions

Skin
Allergic reactions (sic) (1–2.5%)
Angioedema
  (2003): Fischer TC+, *Am J Med* 114(1), 77
Bullous eruption (1–2.5%)
Cellulitis
  (2003): Wolf I+, *Mayo Clin Proc* 78(5), 618
Eczema (sic) (1–2.5%)
Edema (3–5%)
Exanthems (1–2.5%)
  (2001): Blumenthal HL, Beachwood, OH (personal
    communication)
  (1999): Smith JG, Mobile, AL (from Internet) (observation)
    (generalized)
Flu-like syndrome (sic) (7.5%)
Lichenoid eruption
  (2003): Dogra S+, *Br J Dermatol* 148(3), 609
Photosensitivity (lichenoid)
  (2003): Dogra S+, *Br J Dermatol* 148(3), 609
Pruritus (3.3%)
  (1999): Smith JG, Mobile, AL (from Internet) (observation)
Purpura (5.3%)
  (2002): Paradiso-Hardy FL+, *Can J Cardiol* 18(7), 771 (5 cases)
  (2001): Nara W+, *Am J Med Sci* 322(3), 170
  (2000): Brooker JZ, *N Engl J Med* 343(16), 1192
  (2000): Cheung RT, *N Engl J Med* 343(16), 1192
  (2000): Goldstein MR, *N Engl J Med* 343(16), 1192
  (2000): Salliere D+, *N Engl J Med* 343(16), 1191
  (2000): Trontell AE+, *N Engl J Med* 343(16), 1191
Rash (sic) (4.2%)
Thrombocytopenic purpura
  (2002): Paradiso-Hardy FL+, *Can J Cardiol* 18(7), 771
  (2001): Briguori C+, *Ital Heart J* 2(12), 935
  (2001): Medina PJ+, *Curr Opin Hematol* 8(5), 286
  (2001): Nara W+, *Am J Med Sci* 322(3), 170
  (2000): Bennett CL+, *N Engl J Med* 342, 1773 (11 patients)
  (2000): Chinnakotla S+, *Transplantation* 70, 550
  (2000): SoRelle R, *Circulation* 101, E9036
  (1999): Carwile JM+, *Blood* 94, 1:78
  (1999): Connors JM+, *Transfusion* 39, 56S
Toxic skin reaction (sic)
  (2001): El-Majjaoui S+, *J Mal Vasc* 26(3), 207
Ulcerations (1–2.5%)
Urticaria (1–2.5%)
  (1997): Coukell AJ+, *Drugs* 54, 745

Other
Ageusia
  (2000): Golka K+, *Lancet* 355, 465
Fever
  (2003): Wolf I+, *Mayo Clin Proc* 78(5), 618
Headache
Hyperesthesia (1–2.5%)
Hypersensitivity
  (2001): Sarrot-Reynauld F+, *Ann Intern Med* 135(4), 305
Leukopenia
  (2003): Wolf I+, *Mayo Clin Proc* 78(5), 618
Paresthesias (1–2.5%)
Rhabdomyolysis
  (2003): Uber PA+, *J Heart Lung Transplant* 22(1), 107

CLORAZEPATE

Trade name: Tranxene (Ovation) (Abbott)
Other common trade names: *Gen-XENE; Novoclopate;
Transene; Tranxal; Tranxen; Tranxilen; Tranxilium*
Indications: Anxiety and panic disorders
Category: Anxiolytic; Benzodiazepine sedative-hypnotic
Half-life: 48–96 hours
**Clinically important, potentially hazardous interactions
with:** amprenavir, antacids, carbamazepine, carmustine,
chlorpheniramine, clarithromycin, efavirenz, esomeprazole,
imatinib, indinavir, itraconazole, ketoconazole, MAO inhibitors,
midazolam, moclobemide, nelfinavir, phenytoin, sucralfate,
theophylline, warfarin

Reactions

Skin
Blistering (sic)
  (1979): Herschthal D+, *Arch Dermatol* 115, 499
Dermatitis (sic) (1–10%)
Diaphoresis (>10%)
Exanthems
  (2001): Sachs B+, *Br J Dermatol* 144(2), 316 (generalized)
Photosensitivity
  (1989): Torras H+, *J Am Acad Dermatol* 21, 1304
Pruritus
Purpura
Rash (sic) (>10%)
Urticaria
  (1981): Bonnetblanc JM+, *Ann Dermatol Venereol* (French)
    108, 177
Vasculitis
  (1985): Sanchez NP+, *Arch Dermatol* 121, 220

Nails
Nails – photo-onycholysis
  (1989): Torras H+, *J Am Acad Dermatol* 21, 1304

Other
Headache
Oral ulceration
Paresthesias
Porphyria
  (2001): Rassiat E+, *Gastroenterol Clin Biol* 25(8), 832
Sialopenia (>10%)
Sialorrhea (1–10%)
Tremor
Xerostomia (>10%)

CLOTRIMAZOLE

Trade names: Gyne-Lotrimin (Schering); Lotrimin (Schering); Lotrisone (Schering), Mycelex (Bayer)
Other common trade names: *Agisten; Candid; Canestene; Imazol; Taon*
Indications: Candidiasis, dermatophyte infections of the skin
Category: Imidazole antifungal
Half-life: N/A

Reactions

Skin
Burning
  (1994): Binet O+, *Mycoses* 37, 455
  (1983): Higashide K+, *J Int Med Res* 11, 21 (from vaginal tablets)
Dermatitis
  (1999): Cooper SM+, *Contact Dermatitis* 41, 168
  (1999): Erdmann S+, *Contact Dermatitis* 40, 47
  (1997): Dharmagunawardena B+, *Contact Dermatitis* 32, 187
  (1995): Baes H, *Contact Dermatitis* 32, 187
  (1994): Valsecchi R+, *Contact Dermatitis* 30, 248
  (1987): Raulin C+, *Derm Beruf Umwelt* (German) 35, 64
  (1985): Balato N+, *Contact Dermatitis* 12, 110
  (1985): Kalb RE+, *Cutis* 36, 240
  (1978): Roller JA, *Br Med J* 2, 737
Edema
Erythema
Exfoliation
Irritation (sic)
  (1994): Binet O+, *Mycoses* 37, 455
Pruritus
Stinging
Urticaria
Vesiculation

Other
Dysgeusia

CLOXACILLIN

Trade names: Cloxapen (GSK); Tegopen (Bristol-Myers Squibb)
Other common trade names: *Alclox; Apo-Cloxi; Ekvacillin; Loxavit; Nu-Cloxi; Orbenin; Orbenine*
Indications: Various infections caused by susceptible organisms
Category: Penicillinase-resistant penicillin
Half-life: 0.5–1.1 hours
Clinically important, potentially hazardous interactions with: anticoagulants, cyclosporine, demeclocycline, doxycycline, methotrexate, minocycline, oxytetracycline, tetracycline

Reactions

Skin
Angioedema
Dermatitis
  (1996): Gamboa P+, *Contact Dermatitis* 34, 75
Ecchymoses
Erythema multiforme
Exanthems
Exfoliative dermatitis
Hematomas
Jarisch–Herxheimer reaction
Pruritus

Rash (sic) (<1%)
  (1979): Puri V+, *Indian Pediatr* 16, 1153
Stevens–Johnson syndrome
Urticaria

Nails
Nails – loss
  (1984): Daniel CR, *J Am Acad Dermatol* 10, 250
  (1969): Eastwood JB+, *Br J Dermatol* 81, 750
Nails – onycholysis

Other
Anaphylactoid reactions
Black tongue
Glossitis
Glossodynia
Hypersensitivity
Injection-site pain
Oral candidiasis
Serum sickness (<1%)
Stomatitis
Vaginitis

CLOZAPINE

Trade name: Clozaril (Novartis)
Other common trade names: *Entumin; Entumine; Leponex; Lozapin; Sizopin*
Indications: Schizophrenia
Category: Tricyclic antipsychotic
Half-life: 8–12 hours
Clinically important, potentially hazardous interactions with: caffeine, carbamazepine, fluoxetine, risperidone, ritonavir, selenium

Reactions

Skin
Acute febrile neutrophilic dermatosis (Sweet's syndrome)
  (2002): Schonfeldt-Lecuona C+, *Am J Psychiatry* 159(11), 1947
Acute generalized exanthematous pustulosis (AGEP)
  (1997): Bosonnet S+, *Ann Dermatol Venereol* (French) 124, 547
Dermatitis (sic) (<1%)
Diaphoresis (6%)
  (2001): Kane JM+, *Arch Gen Psychiatry* 58(10), 965
  (2001): Richardson C+, *Am J Psychiatry* 158(8), 1329
  (1991): Safferman A+, *Schizophr Bull* 17, 247 (31%)
  (1990): Fitton A+, *Drugs* 40, 722
Eczema (sic) (<1%)
  (1994): Shelley WB+, *Cutis* 53, 33 (observation)
Edema (<1%)
Erythema (<1%)
Erythema multiforme (<1%)
Exanthems
Facial erosions
  (1994): Shelley WB+, *Cutis* 53, 33 (observation)
Lupus erythematosus
  (1994): Wickert WA+, *Postgrad Med J* 70, 940
Neuroleptic malignant syndrome
  (2003): Spivak M+, *Can J Psychiatry* 48(1), 66 (with haloperidol)
  (2002): Baciewicz AM+, *Ann Intern Med* 137(5), 374
  (2002): Beauchemin MA+, *Can J Psychiatry* 47(9), 886
  (2002): Bottlender R+, *Pharmacopsychiatry* 35(3), 119
Nodules
  (2000): Durst R+, *Isr Med Assoc* 2, 485

Periorbital edema (<1%)
Petechiae (<1%)
  (1994): Shelley WB+, *Cutis* 53, 33 (observation)
Photosensitivity
  (1995): Howanitz E+, *J Clin Psychiatry* 56, 589
Pruritus (<1%)
Purpura (<1%)
Rash (sic) (2%)
Stevens–Johnson syndrome (<1%)
Urticaria (<1%)
Vasculitis (<1%)

Other
Death
  (2002): Levin TT+, *Psychosomatics* 43(1), 71
  (2001): Gillespie JA, *Ann Pharmacother* 35(12), 1671
  (2001): Hoehns JD+, *Ann Pharmacother* 35(7), 862 (with
    sertraline)
  (2001): Tie H+, *J Clin Psychopharmacol* 21(6), 630
Dysgeusia (<1%)
Fever
  (2002): Jeong SH+, *Schizophr Res* 56(1), 191
Glossodynia (1%)
Headache
Mastodynia (<1%)
Priapism
  (2001): Bongale RN+, *Am J Psychiatry* 158(12), 2087
  (2001): Compton MT+, *J Clin Psychiatry* 62(5), 363 (passim)
  (2000): Compton MT+, *Am J Psychiatry* 157, 659
  (1994): Barbieri NB+, *Can J Psychiatry* 39, 128
Rhabdomyolysis
  (2002): Jung HH+, *Muscle Nerve* 26(3), 424
  (1996): Meltzer HY+, *Neuropsychopharmacology* 15(4), 395
Seizures
  (2002): Duggal HS+, *Am J Psychiatry* 159(2), 315
  (2001): Landry P, *Am J Psychiatry* 158(11), 1930
  (2001): Navarro V+, *Am J Psychiatry* 158(6), 968
Sialorrhea (31%)
  (2002): Tuunainen A+, *Schizophr Res* 56(1-2), 1
  (2001): Bai YM+, *J Clin Psychopharmacol* 21(6), 608
  (2001): Kane JM+, *Arch Gen Psychiatry* 58(10), 965
  (2000): Miller DD, *J Clin Psychiatry* 61, 14
  (2000): Wahlbeck K+, *Cochran Database Syst Rev* (2):CD000059
  (1999): Antonello C+, *J Psychiatry Neurosci* 24, 250
  (1999): Campbell M+, *Br J Clin Pharmacol* 47, 13
  (1998): Young CR+, *Schizophr Bull* 24, 381
  (1997): Spivak B+, *Int Clin Psychopharmacol* 12, 213
  (1995): Fritze J+, *Lancet* 346, 1034
  (1991): Bourgeois JA+, *Hosp Community Psychiatry* 42, 1174
  (1991): Calabrese JR+, *J Clin Psychopharmacol* 11, 396
  (1991): Copp PJ+, *Br J Psychiatry* 159, 166
  (1991): Goumeniouk AD+, *Can J Psychiatry* 36, 234
  (1991): Kahn N+, *Neurology* 41, 1699
  (1991): Ogle MR+, *Indiana Med* 84, 606
  (1991): Safferman A+, *Schizophr Bull* 17, 247
  (1990): Fitton A+, *Drugs* 40, 722
Tardive dyskinesia
  (2003): Miller del, *Am J Psychiatry* 160(3), 588
Tremor (1–10%)
Xerostomia (6%)
  (2001): Kane JM+, *Arch Gen Psychiatry* 58(10), 965
  (1991): Safferman A+, *Schizophr Bull* 17, 247 (6%)
  (1990): Fitton A+, *Drugs* 40, 722

CO-TRIMOXAZOLE

Synonyms: sulfamethoxazole-trimethoprim; SMX-TMP; SMZ-TMP; TMP-SMX; TMP-SMZ
Trade names: Bactrim (Women First); Cotrim (Teva); Septra (Monarch); Septrin (GSK)
Other common trade names: *Anitrim; Apo-Sulfatrim; Bactelan; Batrizol; Ectaprim; Esteprim; Isobac; Pro-Trin; Roubac; Sulfatrim; Trimzol; Trisulfa*
Indications: Various infections caused by susceptible organisms
Category: Antiprotozoal sulfonamide
Half-life: 6–10 hours
Clinically important, potentially hazardous interactions with: anticoagulants, cyclosporine, dofetilide, isotretinoin, methotrexate, warfarin

Co-trimoxazole is sulfamethoxazole* and trimethoprim

Reactions

Skin
Acute febrile neutrophilic dermatosis (Sweet's syndrome)
  (1996): Walker DC+, *J Am Acad Dermatol* 34, 918
  (1989): Cobb MW, *J Am Acad Dermatol* 21, 339 (passim)
  (1986): Su WPD+, *Cutis* 37, 167
Acute generalized exanthematous pustulosis (AGEP)
  (1995): Moreau A+, *Int J Dermatol* 34, 263 (passim)
Allergic reactions (sic)
  (1999): ter Hofstede HJ+, *Br Clin Pharmacol* 47, 571
Angioedema
  (1988): Fihn SD+, *Ann Intern Med* 108, 350 (1–5%)
Bullous eruption
  (1989): Caumes E+, *Presse Med* (French) 18, 1708
Dermatitis (sic)
  (1989): Atahan IL+, *Br J Radiol* 62, 1107 (at previously irradiated
    area)
  (1987): Vukelja SJ+, *Cancer Treat Rep* 71, 668 (at previously
    irradiated area)
  (1984): Shelley WB+, *J Am Acad Dermatol* 11, 53 (at site of
    previous sunburn)
  (1971): Cotterill JA+, *Br J Dermatol* 84, 366
Erythema multiforme
  (1999): Lehman DF+, *J Clin Pharmacol* 39, 533
  (1998): Siegfried EC+, *J Am Acad Dermatol* 39, 797 (passim)
  (1997): Rieder MJ+, *Pediatr Infect Dis J* 16, 1028 (70% in
    children with HIV)
  (1995): Jick H+, *Pharmacotherapy* 15, 428
  (1991): Tilden ME+, *Arch Ophthalmol* 109, 67
  (1990): Chan HL+, *Arch Dermatol* 126, 43
  (1989): Alanko K+, *Acta Derm Venereol* (Stockh) 69, 223
  (1988): Hira SK+, *J Am Acad Dermatol* 19, 451
  (1988): Platt R+, *J Infect Dis* 158, 474
  (1987): Penmetcha M, *BMJ* 295, 556
  (1987): Schöpf E, *Infection* 15 (Suppl 5P), S254
  (1985): Heer M+, *Gastroenterology* 88, 1954
  (1982): Brettle RP+, *J Infect* 4, 149
  (1979): Beck MH+, *Clin Exp Dermatol* 4, 201
  (1978): Assaad D+, *Can Med Assoc J* 118, 154
  (1978): Azinge NO+, *J Allergy Clin Immunol* 62, 125
  (1975): Bernstein LS, *Can Med Assoc J* 112 (Suppl), 96
  (1971): Koch-Weser J+, *Arch Intern Med* 128, 399 (0.15%)
Erythema nodosum
  (1974): Delaney TJ+, *Br J Dermatol* 90, 205
  (1971): Koch-Weser J+, *Arch Intern Med* 128, 399
Erythroderma
  (1979): Kennedy C+, *BMJ* 1, 1356
Exanthems

(1999): Iborra C+, *Arch Dermatol* 135, 350
(1998): Blumenthal HL, Beachwood, OH (personal case)
(observation)
(1998): Hattori N+, *J Dermatol* 25, 269
(1998): Litt JZ, Beachwood, OH (personal case) (observation)
(1997): Blumenthal HL, Beachwood, OH (personal case)
(observation)
(1997): Palau LA+, *Infect Med* 14, 846
(1996): Caumes E, *Rev Mal Respir* (French) 13, 101 (passim)
(1995): Hertl M+, *Br J Dermatol* 132, 215
(1995): Wolkenstein P+, *Arch Dermatol* 131, 544
(1994): Litt JZ, Beachwood, OH (personal case) (observation)
(1993): Agarwal BR+, *Indian Pediatr* 30, 1026
(1993): Litt JZ, Beachwood, OH (personal case) (observation)
(1993): Malnick SDH+, *Ann Pharmacotherapy* 27, 1139
(1990): Medina I+, *N Engl J Med* 323, 776 (47% in AIDS)
(1988): DeRaeve L+, *Br J Dermatol* 119, 521
(1988): Fihn SD+, *Ann Intern Med* 108, 350 (1–5%)
(1988): Sattler FR+, *Ann Intern Med* 109, 280 (44% in AIDS)
(1988): Weinke T+, *Dtsch Med Wochenschr* (German) 113, 1129
(25% in AIDS)
(1987): Goa KL+, *Drugs* 33, 242 (65% in AIDS)
(1987): Schöpf E, *Infection* 15 (Suppl 5P), S254
(1986): Sonntag MR+, *Schweiz Med Wochenschr* (German)
116, 142
(1985): DeHovitz JA+, *Ann Intern Med* 103, 479
(1985): Maayan S+, *Arch Intern Med* 145, 1607
(1984): Gordon FM+, *Ann Intern Med* 100, 495 (51% in AIDS)
(1984): Kovacs JA+, *Ann Intern Med* 100, 663 (29% in AIDS)
(1983): Mitsuyasu R+, *N Engl J Med* 308, 1535 (69% in AIDS)
(1982): Goetz MB+, *JAMA* 247, 3118
(1980): Fennell RS+, *Clin Pediatr* 19, 124
(1979): Abengowe CU, *Curr Med Res Opin* 5, 749 (3.2%)
(1977): Taylor B+, *BMJ* 2, 552 (12%)
(1976): Arndt KA+, *JAMA* 235, 918 (5.9%)
(1976): Gower PE+, *BMJ* 1, 684 (>5%)
(1975): Bernstein LS, *Can Med Assoc J* 112 (Suppl), 96 (1.9%)
(1975): Gleckman RA, *JAMA* 233, 427 (0.84%)
(1975): Sallam MA+, *Curr Med Res Opin* 3, 229 (3.4%)
(1972): Halpern GM, *BMJ* 1, 691
(1971): Koch-Weser J+, *Arch Intern Med* 128, 399 (1%)

Exfoliative dermatitis
(1990): Ponte CD+, *Drug Intell Clin Pharm* 24, 140 (feet)
(1975): Bernstein LS, *Can Med Assoc J* 112 (Suppl), 96
(1971): Koch-Weser J+, *Arch Intern Med* 128, 399

Fixed eruption
(2002): Litt JZ, Beachwood, OH (personal case) (glans penis)
(recurrent)
(2001): Bayazit-Ozkaya E+, *J Am Acad Dermatol* 45(5), 712
(2000): Ozkaya-Bayazit E+, *Eur J Dermatol* 10, 288
(1999): Mohamed KB, *J Pediatr* 135, 396
(1999): Morelli JG+, *J Pediatr* 134, 365
(1998): Lee AY, *Contact Dermatitis* 38(5), 258
(1998): Mahboob A+, *Int J Dermatol* 37, 833
(1998): Ozkaya-Bayazit E+, *Contact Dermatitis* 39, 87
(trimethoprim)
(1997): Gruber F+, *Clin Exp Dermatol* 22, 144
(1997): Ozkaya-Bayazit E+, *Br J Dermatol* 137, 1028 (linear)
(trimethoprim)
(1996): Sharma VK+, *J Dermatol* 23, 530
(1995): Wolkenstein P+, *Arch Dermatol* 131, 544
(1993): Oleaga JM+, *Contact Dermatitis* 29, 155
(1993): Ramam M+, *Indian Pediatr* 30, 110 (in an infant)
(1992): Lim JT+, *Ann Acad Med Singapore* 21, 408
(1991): Jain VK+, *Ann Dent* 50, 9 (oral mucous membrane)
(1991): Smoller BR+, *J Cutan Pathol* 18, 13
(1991): Thankappen TP+, *Int J Dermatol* 30, 867 (36.3%)
(1990): Gaffoor PMA+, *Cutis* 45, 242 (genitalia)
(1989): Basomba A+, *J Allergy Clin Immunol* 84, 409
(1989): Bharija SC+, *Australas J Dermatol* 30, 43

(1989): Gupta R, *Indian J Dermatol* 55, 181 (in an infant)
(1989): Varsano I+, *Dermatologica* 178, 232
(1988): Baird BJ+, *Int J Dermatol* 27, 170 (bullous and
generalized)
(1988): Bharija SC+, *Dermatologica* 176, 108 (in an infant)
(1987): Amir J+, *Drug Intell Clin Pharm* 21, 41
(1987): Hughes BR+, *Br J Dermatol* 116, 241
(1987): Van Voorhees A+, *Am J Dermatopathol* 9, 528
(1986): Kanwar AJ+, *Dermatologica* 172, 230
(1985): Gomez B+, *Allergol Immunopathol Madr* (Spanish) 13, 87
(1984): Pandhi RK+, *Sex Transm Dis* 11, 164
(1982): Gibson JR, *BMJ* 284, 1529
(1980): Talbot MD, *Practitioner* 224, 823
(1978): Verbov J, *Arch Dermatol* 114, 963
(1972): Aoyama H+, *Jpn J Dermatol* B 82, 16

Flushing
(1984): Jick SS+, *Lancet* 2, 631

Genital ulceration
(2001): Cherian G, *Int J Clin Pract* 55(2), 151

Jarisch–Herxheimer reaction
(2001): Peschard S+, *Presse Med* 30(31), 1549

Lichenoid eruption
(1994): Berger TG+, *Arch Dermatol* 130, 609

Linear IgA bullous dermatosis
(2002): Cohen LM+, *J Am Acad Dermatol* 46, S32 (passim)
(1997): Paul C+, *Br J Dermatol* 136, 406
(1994): Kuechle MK+, *J Am Acad Dermatol* 30, 187

Lupus erythematosus
(1985): Stratton MA, *Clin Pharm* 4, 657
(1975): Grennan DM+, *BMJ* 4, 385

Photosensitivity
(1994): Berger TG+, *Arch Dermatol* 130, 609 (in HIV-infected)
(4 cases)
(1994): Shelley WB+, *Cutis* 53, 162 (observation)
(1987): Schöpf E, *Infection* 15 (Suppl 5P), S254
(1986): Chandler MJ, *J Infect Dis* 153, 1001

Pruritus
(1997): Caumes E+, *Arch Dermatol* 133, 465
(1997): Thaler D, Monona, WI (from internet) (observation)
(1996): Litt JZ, Beachwood, OH (from Internet) (observation)
(1990): Medina I+, *N Engl J Med* 323, 776 (1–5%)
(1987): Colebunders R+, *Ann Intern Med* 107, 599 (4% in AIDS)
(1986): Sher MR, *J Allergy Clin Immunol* 77, 133
(1984): Kramer BS+, *Cancer* 53, 329
(1975): Gleckman RA, *JAMA* 233, 427 (0.84%)
(1971): Koch-Weser J+, *Arch Intern Med* 128, 399 (0.15%)

Pruritus vulvae
(1981): *Modern Medicine* 49, 111

Psoriasis
(1979): Kennedy C+, *BMJ* 1, 1356

Purpura
(1993): Kaufman DW+, *Blood* 82, 2714
(1989): Saxena SK, *J Assoc Physicians India* 37, 479
(1971): Koch-Weser J+, *Arch Intern Med* 128, 399

Purpuric "gloves and socks syndrome"
(1999): van Rooijen MM+, *Hautarzt* (German) 50, 280

Pustules
(1994): Spencer JM+, *Br J Dermatol* 130, 514
(1990): Guy C+, *Nouv Dermatol* (French) 9, 540
(1989): Grattan CEH, *Dermatologica* 179, 57 (passim)
(1986): Macdonald KJS+, *BMJ* 293, 1279
(1978): Braun-Falco O+, *Hautarzt* (German) 29, 371
(1977): Knudsen L+, *Ugeskr Laeger* (Danish) 139, 1007

Radiation recall
(1990): Leslie MD+, *Br J Radiol* 63, 661
(1987): Vukelja SJ+, *Cancer Treat Rep* 71, 668 (at previously
irradiated area)
(1984): Shelley WB+, *J Am Acad Dermatol* 11, 53 (at site of
previous sunburn)

Rash (sic) (>10%)
  (2001): Meyers B+, *Liver Transpl* 7(8), 750
  (2000): Talan DA+, *JAMA* 283, 1583 (14%)
  (1995): Williams JW+, *JAMA* 273, 1015
  (1993): Malnick SD+, *Ann Pharmacother* 27, 1139
  (1984): Gordin FM+, *Ann Intern Med* 100, 495
  (1978): Lawson DH+, *Am J Med Sci* 275, 53
Side effects (sic)
  (1994): Roudier C+, *Arch Dermatol* 130, 1383 (48% in AIDS
    patients)
  (1971): Koch-Weser J+, *Arch Intern Med* 128, 399. (2.1%)
Stevens–Johnson syndrome (1–10%)
  (2001): Brett AS+, *South Med J* 94, 342
  (1998): Arola O+, *Lancet* 351, 1102 (trimethoprim)
  (1998): Siegfried EC+, *J Am Acad Dermatol* 39, 797 (passim)
  (1997): Douglas R+, *Clin Infect Dis* 25, 1480 (2 cases)
  (1997): Rieder MJ+, *Pediatr Infect Dis J* 16, 1028 (10% in
    children with HIV)
  (1996): Caumes E, *Rev Mal Respir* (French) 13, 101
  (1996): Eastham JH+, *Ann Pharmacother* 30, 606
  (1996): McCarty J, Fort Worth, TX (from Internet) (observation)
  (1995): Kuper K+, *Ophthalmologe* (German) 92, 823
  (1995): Lewis RJ, *Br J Rheumatol* 34, 84
  (1995): Sharma VK+, *Pediatr Dermatol* 12, 178
  (1995): Wolkenstein P+, *Arch Dermatol* 131, 544
  (1994): Shelley WB+, *Cutis* 53, 159 (observation)
  (1993): Litt JZ, Beachwood, OH (personal case) (observation)
  (1990): Chan HL+, *Arch Dermatol* 126, 43
  (1988): Platt R+, *J Infect Dis* 158, 474
  (1985): Heer M+, *Gastroenterology* 88, 1954
  (1982): Brettle RP+, *J Infect* 4, 149
  (1979): Beck MH+, *Clin Exp Dermatol* 4, 201
  (1978): Assaad D+, *Can Med Assoc* 118, 154
  (1978): Azinge NO+, *J Allergy Clin Immunol* 62, 125
  (1978): Kikuchi S+, *Lancet* 2, 580
  (1978): Thorpe JA+, *Lancet* 1, 276 (fatal)
  (1975): Bernstein LS, *Can Med Assoc J* 112 (Suppl), 96
  (1970): Shaw DJ+, *Johns Hopkins Med J* 126, 130
Toxic epidermal necrolysis (1–10%)
  (2002): Correia O+, *Arch Dermatol* 138, 29 (three cases)
  (2002): John T+, *Ophthalmology* 109(2), 351
  (2002): Nassif A+, *J Invest Dermatol* 118(4), 728
  (2001): Paquet P+, *Burns* 27(6), 652
  (2001): See S+, *Ann Pharmacother* 35(6), 694
  (2001): Spies M+, *Pediatrics* 108, 1162
  (2000): Moussala M+, *J Fr Ophtalmol* (French) 23, 229
  (2000): Yang CH+, *Int J Dermatol* 39, 621 (with methotrexate)
  (1999): Egan CA+, *J Am Acad Dermatol* 40, 458 (6 cases)
  (1998): Arora VK+, *Indian J Chest Dis Allied Sci* 40, 125
  (1998): Rademaker M+, *New Zealand Adverse Drug Reactions
    Committee*, April, 1998 (from Internet)
  (1998): Siegfried EC+, *J Am Acad Dermatol* 39, 797 (passim)
  (1996): Caumes E, *Rev Mal Respir* (French) 13, 101
  (1996): Rehbein H, Jacksonville, FL (from Internet) (observation)
  (1996): Wagner FF+, *N Engl J Med* 334, 922
  (1995): Jick H+, *Pharmacotherapy* 15, 428
  (1995): Sharma VK+, *Pediatr Dermatol* 12, 178
  (1995): Wolkenstein P+, *Arch Dermatol* 131, 544 (7 cases)
  (1993): Correia O+, *Dermatology* 186, 32
  (1990): Chan HL+, *Arch Dermatol* 126, 43
  (1990): Kobza Black A+, *Br J Dermatol* 123, 277
  (1990): Roujeau JC+, *Arch Dermatol* 126, 37
  (1990): Ward DJ+, *Burns* 16, 97
  (1989): Carmichael AJ+, *Lancet* 2, 808
  (1989): Whittington RM, *Lancet* 2, 574
  (1988): De Raeve L+, *Br J Dermatol* 119, 521 (passim)
  (1987): Guillaume JC+, *Arch Dermatol* 123, 1166
  (1987): Schöpf E, *Infection* 15 (Suppl 5P), S254
  (1986): Miller KD+, *Am J Trop Med Hyg* 33, 451
  (1986): Revuz J, *J Dermatol Paris* 153 (abstract)

  (1986): Roman O+, *Rev Pediatr Obstet Ginecol Pediatr*
    (Romanian) 35, 261
  (1984): Fong PH+, *Singapore Med J* 25, 184
  (1984): Westly ED+, *Arch Dermatol* 120, 721
  (1983): Petersen P+, *Ugeskr Laeger* (Danish) 145, 3345
  (1982): Ortiz JE+, *Ann Plast Surg* 9, 249
  (1978): Anhalt G+, *Plastic Reconstr Surg* 61, 905
  (1978): Assaad D+, *Can Med Assoc J* 118, 154
  (1978): Petricevic I+, *Lijec Vjesn* (Serbo-Croatian-Roman)
    100, 596
  (1975): Bernstein LS, *Can Med Assoc J* 112 (Suppl), 96
  (1973): Beyvin AJ+, *Anesth Analg Paris* (French) 30, 767
  (1972): Chanial G+, *J Med Lyon* (French) 53, 859
  (1971): Chanial G+, *Bull Soc Fr Dermatol Syphiligr* (French)
    78, 565
Urticaria
  (1994): Blumenthal HL, Beachwood, OH (personal case)
    (observation)
  (1993): Litt JZ, Beachwood, OH (personal case) (observation)
  (1991): Greenberger PA, *JAMA* 265, 458
  (1987): Schöpf E, *Infection* 15 (Suppl 5P), S254
  (1985): Goolamali SK, *Postgrad Med J* 61, 925
  (1985): Maayan S+, *Arch Intern Med* 145, 1607
  (1984): Kramer BS+, *Cancer* 53, 329
  (1981): Abi-Mansur P+, *Am J Gastroenterol* 76, 356
  (1971): Koch-Weser J+, *Arch Intern Med* 128, 399
Vasculitis
  (1998): Tonev S+, *J Eur Acad Dermatol Venereol* 11, 165
  (1995): Lewis RJ, *Br J Rheumatol* 34, 84
  (1989): Verne-Pignatelli J+, *Postgrad Med J* 65, 51
  (1987): Schöpf E, *Infection* 15 (Suppl 5P), S254
  (1978): Braun-Falco O+, *Hautarzt* (German) 29, 371
  (1978): Coquin Y+, *Nouv Presse Med* (French) 7, 3145
  (1976): Wåhlin A+, *Lancet* 2, 1415
  (1971): Koch-Weser J+, *Arch Intern Med* 128, 399
Vulvovaginitis
  (1985): Wong ES+, *Ann Intern Med* 102, 302

Hair
Hair – straight
  (1999): Oakley A, Hamilton, New Zealand (from Internet)
    (observation)

Nails
Nails – loss
  (2000): Canning DA, *J Urol* 163, 1386

Other
Anaphylactoid reactions
  (1998): Bijl AM+, *Clin Exp Allergy* 28, 510 (trimethoprim)
  (1998): Siegfried EC+, *J Am Acad Dermatol* 39, 797 (passim)
  (1988): Arnold PA+, *Drug Intell Clin Pharm* 22, 43
  (1985): Gossius G+, *Scand J Infect Dis* 16, 373
Aphthous stomatitis
  (1981): *J Antimicrob Chemother* 7, 179
Black tongue
  (1993): Blumenthal HL, Beachwood, OH (personal case)
    (observation)
Dysgeusia
  (1988): Fischl MA+, *JAMA* 259, 1185
Gingival hyperplasia
  (1997): Caron F+, *Therapie* (French) 52, 73
Glossitis
Hypersensitivity
  (2001): Moran KA+, *South Med J* 94(3), 350 ('sepsis-like')
  (2000): Pirmohamed M+, *Pharmacogenetics* 10(8), 705
  (1999): Lehman DF+, *J Clin Pharmacol* 39, 533
  (1999): Pakianathan MR+, *AIDS* 13, 1787
  (1998): Mohanasundaram J+, *J Indian Med Assoc* 96, 21
  (1998): Ryan C+, *WMJ* 97, 23

(1997): Hicks ME+, *Ann Pharmacother* 31, 1259
(1994): Carr A+, *AIDS* 8, 333
(1993): Marinac JS+, *Clin Infect Dis* 16, 178
(1993): Martin GJ+, *Clin Infect Dis* 16, 175
(1993): Mathelier-Fusade P+, *Presse Med* (French) 22, 1363
(1993): Mehta J+, *J Assoc Physicians India* 41, 235
Mucocutaneous syndrome
  (1982): Brettle RP+, *J Infect* 4, 149
Myalgia
Oral mucosal eruption
  (1991): Tilden ME+, *Arch Ophthalmol* 109, 67
  (1988): Fihn SD+, *Ann Intern Med* 108, 350 (1–5%)
Oral ulceration
  (1987): Hughes WT+, *N Engl J Med* 316, 1627
  (1981): Orenstein WA+, *Am J Med Sci* 282, 27
Pseudolymphoma
  (1978): Laugier P+, *Z Hautkr* (German) 53, 353
Rhabdomyolysis
  (1988): Arnold PA+, *Drug Intell Clin Pharm* 22, 43
Serum sickness (<1%)
  (1988): Platt R+, *J Infect Dis* 158, 474
Stomatitis (<1%)
  (1999): Iborra C+, *Arch Dermatol* 135, 350
Tinnitus
Tongue ulceration
  (1981): *J Antimicrob Chemother* 7, 179
Tremor
  (1999): Patterson RG+, *Pharmacotherapy* 19, 1456

*Note: Co-trimoxazole is a sulfonamide and can be absorbed systemically. Sulfonamides can produce severe, possibly fatal, reactions such as toxic epidermal necrolysis and Stevens–Johnson syndrome

COCAINE

Trade name: Cocaine
Indications: Topical anesthesia
Category: Substance abuse drug; Topical anesthetic
Half-life: 75 minutes
Clinically important, potentially hazardous interactions with: epinephrine

Note: Cocaine is a benzoylmethylecogonine alkaloid derived from the leaves of the *Erythroxylon coca* tree. Street names for cocaine include: coke; flake; snow; toot, etc. Crack cocaine is a highly potent smokable form of cocaine

Reactions

Skin
Angioedema
  (2003): Kestler A+, *N Engl J Med* 349(9), 867
  (1999): Castro-Villamor MA+, *Ann Emerg Med* 34, 296
Bullous eruption
  (1985): Tomecki KJ+, *J Am Acad Dermatol* 12, 585
Diaphoresis
Formication
Granulomas (foreign body)
  (1985): Posner DI+, *J Am Acad Dermatol* 13, 869
Hyperkeratosis (fingers and palms)
  (1992): Feeney CM+, *Cutis* 50, 193 (from crack cocaine)
Necrosis
  (2000): Carter EL+, *Cutis* 65, 73 (mid-facial)
  (1988): Zamora-Quezada JC+, *Ann Intern Med* 108, 564
Nodules (sic)
  (1989): Heng MCY+, *J Am Acad Dermatol* 21, 570

Scleroderma (reversible)
  (1992): Lam M+, *N Engl J Med* 326, 1435
  (1991): Bourgeois P+, *Baillieres Clin Rheumatol* 5, 13
  (1989): Kerr HD, *South Med J* 82, 1275
Urticaria
  (1999): Castro-Villamor MA+, *Ann Emerg Med* 34, 296
Vasculitis
  (1999): Hofbauer GF+, *Br J Dermatol* 141, 600
Warts (snorters' warts)
  (1987): Schuster DS, *Arch Dermatol* 123, 571

Other
Ageusia (>10%)
Anosmia (>10%)
Black tongue
  (1999): Burnett LB+, *Online Textbook of Emergency Medicine* (from crack cocaine)
Bruxism
  (1999): Fazzi M+, *Minerva Stomatol* (Italian) 48, 485
Gingival ulceration
  (1999): Fazzi M+, *Minerva Stomatol* (Italian) 48, 485
Injection-site scarring
  (1968): Yaffee HS, *Cutis* 4, 286
Nasal septal perforation
  (2001): Millard DR+, *Plast Reconstr Surg* 107(2), 419
  (2000): Patel R+, *J Natl Med Assoc* 92, 39
  (1986): Schwartz RH+, *Am Fam Physician* 43, 187
Necrosis of palate
  (1999): Fazzi M+, *Minerva Stomatol* (Italian) 48, 485
Porphyria
  (1987): Dick AD+, *Lancet* 2, 1150
Priapism
  (1999): Altman AL+, *J Urol* 161, 1817
  (1998): Myrick H+, *Ann Clin Psychiatry* 10, 8 (with trazodone)
Rhabdomyolysis
  (2003): Doctora JS+, *J Oral Maxillofac Surg* 61(8), 964
  (2000): Richards JR, *J Emerg Med* 19(1), 51
  (1999): Hedetoft C+, *Ugeskr Laeger* 161(50), 6907
  (1996): Bakir AA+, *Curr Opin Nephrol Hypertens* 5(2), 122
  (1996): Lampley EC+, *Obstet Gynecol* 87(5), 804
  (1994): Villalba Garcia MV+, *An Med Interna* 11(3), 119
  (1992): Garcia Castano J+, *An Med Interna* 9(7), 340 (13 cases)
  (1992): Zele I+, *Minerva Med* 83(12), 847 (24%)
  (1991): Horst E+, *South Med J* 84(2), 269
  (1989): Loper KA, *Med Toxicol Adverse Drug Exp* 4(3), 174
  (1989): VanDette JM+, *Clin Pharm* 8(6), 401
Thrombophlebitis
  (1987): Heng MC+, *J Am Acad Dermatol* 16, 462
Tremor (1–10%)

CODEINE

Synonym: methylmorphine
Trade names: Calcidrine; Cheracol; Guaituss AC; Halotussin (Watson); Novahistine DH; Nucofed (Monarch); Robitussin AC (Wyeth); Tussar-2; Tussi-Organidin (Wallace)
Other common trade names: *Actacode; Codicept; Codiforton; Paveral; Solcodein; Tricodein*
Indications: Pain, cough suppressant
Category: Antitussive; Opioid (narcotic) analgesic
Half-life: 2.5–4 hours
Clinically important, potentially hazardous interactions with: alcohol, CNS depressants, MAO inhibitors, **raspberry leaf**

Reactions

Skin

Acute generalized exanthematous pustulosis (AGEP)
  (1995): Lee S+, *Australas J Dermatol* 36, 25
Angioedema
  (1992): Breathnach SM+, *Adverse Drug Reactions and the Skin*
    Blackwell, Oxford, 211 (passim)
  (1960): Schoenfeld MR, *N Y State J Med* 60, 2591
Bullous eruption
  (1992): Breathnach SM+, *Adverse Drug Reactions and the Skin*
    Blackwell, Oxford, 211 (passim)
Dermatitis
  (1995): Waclawski ER+, *Contact Dermatitis* 33, 51
  (1983): Romaguera C+, *Contact Dermatitis* 9, 170
Diaphoresis
Edema
  (2001): Estrada JL+, *Contact Dermatitis* 44(3), 185 (generalized)
Erythema multiforme (<1%)
  (1992): Breathnach SM+, *Adverse Drug Reactions and the Skin*
    Blackwell, Oxford, 211 (passim)
  (1983): Ponte CD, *Drug Intell Clin Pharm* 17, 128
  (1975): Vanderveen TW+, *Am J Hosp Pharm* 32, 1149
  (1968): Bianchine JR+, *Am J Med* 7, 390
Erythema nodosum (<1%)
  (1992): Breathnach SM+, *Adverse Drug Reactions and the Skin*
    Blackwell, Oxford, 211 (passim)
Exanthems
  (1985): Hunskaar S+, *Ann Allergy* 54, 240
  (1980): Voorhorst R+, *Ann Allergy* 44, 116
  (1976): Nishioka K+, *Nippon Rinsho* (Japanese) 34, 3123
  (1969): Török H, *Int J Dermatol* 8, 57
  (1960): Heijer A, *Acta Derm Venereol* (Stockh) 40, 35
  (1934): Scheer M+, *JAMA* 102, 908
Exfoliative dermatitis
  (1995): Rodriguez F+, *Contact Dermatitis* 32, 120
Facial edema
Fixed eruption (<1%)
  (1996): Gonzalo-Garijo MA+, *Br J Dermatol* 135, 498
  (1992): Breathnach SM+, *Adverse Drug Reactions and the Skin*
    Blackwell, Oxford, 211 (passim)
  (1990): Gaffoor PMA+, *Cutis* 45, 242 (passim)
  (1974): Kuokkanen K, *Int J Dermatol* 13, 4
  (1969): Török H, *Int J Dermatol* 8, 57
  (1960): Heijer A, *Acta Derm Venereol* (Stockh) 40, 35
Flushing
  (1983): Shanahan EC+, *Anaesthesia* 38, 40
Pityriasis rosea
  (1993): Yosipovitch G+, *Harefuah* (Hebrew) 124, 198; 247
Pruritus (<1%)
  (1986): de Groot AC+, *Contact Dermatitis* 14, 209

(1976): von Muhlendahl KE+, *Lancet* 2, 303
(1934): Scheer M+, *JAMA* 102, 908
Radiation recall (sunlight and electronic beam)
  (1984): Shelley WB+, *J Am Acad Dermatol* 11, 53
Rash (sic) (1–10%)
  (1976): von Muhlendahl KE+, *Lancet* 2, 303
Toxic epidermal necrolysis (<1%)
  (1973): Steigleder GK, *Hautarzt* (German) 24, 261
  (1972): Monnat A, *Schweiz Med Wochenschr* (French) 102, 1876
Urticaria (1–10%)
  (2000): Vidal C+, *Allergy* 55, 416
  (1986): de Groot AC+, *Contact Dermatitis* 4, 209
  (1986): Rosenstreich DL, *J Allergy Clin Immunol* 78, 1099
  (1985): Hunskaar S+, *Ann Allergy* 54, 240
  (1976): von Muhlendahl KE+, *Lancet* 2, 303
  (1960): Heijer A, *Acta Derm Venereol* (Stockh) 40, 35
  (1960): Schoenfeld MR, *N Y State J Med* 60, 2591

Nails

Nails – shoreline
  (1985): Shelley WB+, *Cutis* 35, 220

Other

Anaphylactoid reactions
Dysgeusia
Headache
Injection-site pain (1–10%)
Oral ulceration
Paresthesias
Priapism
  (2002): Goldmeier D+, *BMJ* 324(7353), 1555
Seizures
  (2001): Zolezzi M+, *Ann Pharmacother* 35(10), 1211
Trembling (sic) (<1%)
Xerostomia (1–10%)

COENZYME Q-10

Scientific names: *Mitoquinone; Ubidecarenone; Ubiquinone*
Family: None
Trade and other common names: Co Q10; Co-Q10; CoQ; CoQ-10; Q10
Category: Food supplement
Purported indications and other uses: Congestive heart failure, angina, diabetes, hypertension, breast cancer, increasing exercise tolerance, muscular dystrophy, chronic fatigue
Half-life: N/A
Clinically important, potentially hazardous interactions with: warfarin

Reactions

Skin

None

Note: CoQ-10 was first identified in 1957. It is widely used in Japan where millions of Japanese patients receive CoQ-10 as part of their treatment for congestive heart failure

COLCHICINE

Trade name: ColBenemid* (Merck)
Other common trade names: *Cochiquim; Colchineos; Colgout; Goutnil; Kolkicin; Konicine*
Indications: Gouty arthritis
Category: Antigout anti-inflammatory; Uricosuric
Half-life: 20 minutes
Clinically important, potentially hazardous interactions with: erythromycin, troleandomycin

ColBenemid is colchicine and probenecid

Reactions

Skin

Allergic reactions (sic)
(2001): Vittori F+, *Therapie* 56(1), 63
Angioedema
Behçet's disease
(2003): Fujii Y+, *Ryumachi* Feb 43(1), 44
Bullous eruption (<1%)
(1957): Ott H+, *Dtsch Med Wochenschr* (German) 82, 1163
Erythema nodosum
(2002): Guven AG+, *Pediatrics* 109(5), 971
Erythroderma
(1971): Durkalec J+, *Pol Tyg Lek* (Polish) 26, 1048
Exanthems
Fixed eruption
(1996): Mochida K+, *Dermatology* 192, 61
Flushing
Lichenoid eruption
(1974): Sayag J+, *Bull Soc Fr Dermatol Syphiligr* (French) 81, 94
Necrosis
Photodermatitis
(1992): Foti C+, *Contact Dermatitis* 27, 201
Pruritus (<1%)
(1957): Hollander L, *Arch Dermatol* 75, 872
(1957): Ott H+, *Dtsch Med Wochenschr* (German) 82, 1163
Purpura
Pyoderma
(1957): Ott H+, *Dtsch Med Wochenschr* (German) 82, 1163
Rash (sic) (<1%)
Side effects (sic) (14%)
(1957): Ott H+, *Dtsch Med Wochenschr* (German) 82, 1163
Staphylococcal scalded skin syndrome
(1993): Khuong MA+, *Dermatology* 186, 153
(1967): Halprin KM, *JAMA* 202, 137
Toxic epidermal necrolysis
(1994): Alfandari S+, *Infection* 22, 365
(1990): Roujeau JC+, *Arch Dermatol* 126, 37
Urticaria
(1991): Anderson MH+, *Ann Allergy* 66, 207
Vasculitis
(1993): Barash J+, *Isr J Med Sci* 29, 310
(1964): Sinaly NP, *Ann Intern Med* 60, 470
Vesicular eruptions (palms)
(1957): Hollander L, *Arch Dermatol* 75, 872

Hair

Hair – alopecia (1–10%)
(2002): Guven AG+, *Pediatrics* 109(5), 971
(1980): Harms M, *Hautarzt* (German) 31, 161 (20–50%)
(1977): Naidus RM+, *Arch Intern Med* 137, 394
(1970): Wallace S+, *Am J Med* 48, 443
(1967): Spanopoulos GJ, *Practitioner* 198, 426

Other

Anaphylactoid reactions
Death
(2002): Maxwell MJ+, *Emerg Med J* 19(3), 265 (overdose)
(2002): Sannohe S+, *J Forensic Sci* 47(6), 1391 (overdose)
Hypersensitivity
Injection-site thrombophlebitis
Musculoskeletal pain
(2002): Guven AG+, *Pediatrics* 109(5), 971
Myalgia
(2002): Atmaca H+, *Ann Pharmacother* 36(11), 1719 (with gemfibrozil)
(2002): Fernandez C+, *Acta Neuropathol* (Berlin) 103(2), 100
Myopathy (<1%)
(2002): Ayllon-Munoz JA+, *Rev Neurol* 35(2), 195
(2002): Caglar K+, *Nephron* 92(4), 922
(2002): Hsu WC+, *Clin Neuropharmacol* 25(5), 266 (with simvastatin)
(1999): Gruberg L+, *Transplant Proc* 31, 2157
(1998): Duarte J+, *Muscle Nerve* 21, 550
(1997): Ducloux D+, *Nephrol Dial Transplant* 12, 2389
(1997): Sinsawaiwong S+, *J Med Assoc Thai* 80, 667
(1992): Himmelmann F+, *Acta Neuropathologica* 83, 440
Porphyria cutanea tarda
(1971): Kuokkanen K, *Acta Derm Venereol* (Stockh) 51, 318
Rhabdomyolysis
(2003): Phanish MK+, *Am J Med* 114(2), 166
(2003): Vasudevan AR+, *Am J Med* 115(3), 249
(2002): Atmaca H+, *Ann Pharmacother* 36(11), 1719 (with gemfibrozil)
(2001): Chattopadhyay I+, *Postgrad Med J* 77(905), 191
(1997): Dawson TM+, *J Rheumatol* 24(10), 2045

*****Note:** Colchicine, by itself, is generic

COLESEVELAM

Trade name: Welchol (Sankyo)
Indications: Hypercholesterolemia
Category: Antilipemic; Bile acid sequestrant
Half-life: N/A

Reactions

Skin

Flu-like syndrome (sic)

Other

Myalgia (2%)
Oral ulceration

COLESTIPOL

Trade name: Colestid (Pharmacia)
Other common trade names: *Cholestabyl; Lestid*
Indications: Primary hypercholesterolemia
Category: Antilipidemic
Half-life: N/A

Reactions

Skin

Dermatitis (sic) (<1%)
Edema

Exanthems (<1%)
Urticaria (<1%)

COLLAGEN*

Synonym: gluteraldehyde cross-linked (GAX) collagen
Trade names: Artecoll (contains polymethyl-methacrylate microspheres); Autologen; Avitene; Contigen (Bard); Dermalogen; Fibrel (Mentor); Zyderm-1 (Collagen Biomedical); Zyplast (Collagen Biomedical)
Indications: Cataract surgery (collagen shields), depressed cutaneous scars, facial lines, wrinkles, glottic insufficiency, phonosurgey, urinary incontinence
Category: Bovine, porcine or human protein
Half-life: Several months to years

Reactions

Skin

Abscess
 (1999): Sweat SD+, *J Urol* 161(1), 93
 (1998): McLennan MT+, *Obstet Gynecol* 92(4 Pt 2), 650
Adverse effects (sic)
 (2001): Klein AW, *Facial Plast Surg Clin North Am* 9(2), 205
 (2000): Moody BR+, *Dermatol Surg* 26(10), 936
 (1999): Constantinides M+, *Otolaryngol Head Neck Surg* 120(4), 557
 (1998): Stothers L+, *J Urol* 159(3), 806 (0.9%)
 (1995): Gold MH, *Dermatol Clin* 13(2), 353
 (1994): Moscona R+, *Plast Reconstr Surg* 93(7), 1525
 (1989): Clark DP+, *J Am Acad Dermatol* 21(5 Pt 1), 992
 (1989): Elson ML, *J Am Acad Dermatol* 20(5 Pt 1), 861
 (1986): Vanderveen EE+, *Arch Dermatol* 122(6), 650
 (1985): Cooperman LS+, *Aesthetic Plast Surg* 9(2), 145 (1.3%)
 (1985): Klein AW+, *J Dermatol Surg Oncol* 11(3), 337
Allergic reactions (sic)
 (2002): Echols KT+, *Int Urogynecol J Pelvic Floor Dysfunct* 13(1), 52
 (1999): Gorton E+, *BJU Int* 84(9), 966
 (1999): Su TH+, *Int Urogynecol J Pelvic Floor Dysfunct* 10(3), 200
 (1998): Stothers L+, *J Urol* 159(5), 1507
 (1985): Pieyre JM, *Aesthetic Plast Surg* 9(2), 153 (4 cases)
 (1985): Robinson JK+, *J Dermatol Surg Oncol* 11(2), 124
 (1984): Webster RC+, *Arch Otolaryngol* 110(10), 652
Autoimmune disease
 (1994): Lewy RI, *Ann Intern Med* 120(6), 525
Bruising
Dermatomyositis
 (1993): Cukier J+, *Ann Intern Med* 118(12), 920
 (1993): Elson ML, *J Dermatol Surg Oncol* 19(2), 165
Discoloration
 (1999): Davis PK, *Br J Plast Surg* 52(1), 81
Edema
 (1985): Cooperman L+, *J Int Med Res* 13(2), 109 (localized)
 (1985): Cooperman LS+, *Aesthetic Plast Surg* 9(2), 145 (localized)
Erythema
 (1987): DeLustro F+, *Plast Reconstr Surg* 79(4), 581
 (1985): Cooperman L+, *J Int Med Res* 13(2), 109
 (1985): Cooperman LS+, *Aesthetic Plast Surg* 9(2), 145
Erythematous nodules
 (1993): Moscona RR+, *Plast Reconstr Surg* 92(2), 331
Erythematous plaques
 (1993): Moscona RR+, *Plast Reconstr Surg* 92(2), 331
Flu-like syndrome
 (1999): Gorton E+, *BJU Int* 84(9), 966

Granuloma annulare
 (1984): Rapaport MJ, *Arch Dermatol* 120(7), 837
Granulomas
 (2001): Heise H+, *J Craniomaxillofac Surg* 29(4), 238
 (2000): Garcia-Domingo MI+, *J Investig Allergol Clin Immunol* 10(2), 107
 (1986): Schurig V+, *Hautarzt* 37(1), 42
 (1982): Barr RJ+, *J Am Acad Dermatol* 6(5), 867
Herpes simplex
Infections
 (1998): Faerber GJ+, *Tech Urol* 4(3), 124
Inflammation
 (1995): Gold MH, *Dermatol Clin* 13(2), 353
Itching
Rash (sic)
Scar
 (1995): Lemperle G+, *Plast Reconstr Surg* 1995 Sep; 96(3), 627
Urticaria

Other

Arthralgia
 (1998): Stothers L+, *J Urol* 159(3), 806
 (1998): Stothers L+, *J Urol* 159(5), 1507
Asthenia
Death
 (2003): McCarthy DM+, *Arch Pathol Lab Med* 127(2), E67
Hypersensitivity
 (2002): Echols KT+, *Int Urogynecol J Pelvic Floor Dysfunct* 13(1), 52
 (2000): Garcia-Domingo MI+, *J Investig Allergol Clin Immunol* 10(2), 107
 (1993): Cukier J+, *Ann Intern Med* 118(12), 920
 (1991): Frank DH+, *Plast Reconstr Surg* 87(6), 1080
 (1991): Schnitzler L, *Rev Fr Gynecol Obstet* 86(6), 469
 (1989): Elson ML, *J Dermatol Surg Oncol* 15(3), 301 (2.5%)
 (1988): Elson ML, *J Am Acad Dermatol* 18(4), 707 (3%)
 (1987): DeLustro F+, *Plast Reconstr Surg* 79(4), 581
 (1984): Kamer FM+, *Arch Otolaryngol* 110(2), 93
Induration
 (1987): DeLustro F+, *Plast Reconstr Surg* 79(4), 581
 (1985): Cooperman L+, *J Int Med Res* 13(2), 109
Joint pains
Musculoskeletal pain
Panniculitis
 (2000): Garcia-Domingo MI+, *J Investig Allergol Clin Immunol* 10(2), 107
 (1999): Biasi D+, *Clin Rheumatol* 18(4), 328
Panniculitis (nodular nonsuppurative)
Polyarthralgia
Polymyositis
 (1993): Cukier J+, *Ann Intern Med* 118(12), 920
 (1993): Elson ML, *J Dermatol Surg* 19(2), 165
Shock

*__Note:__ A reaction to the anesthesic, lidocaine, in liquid collagen injections may occur

COMFREY

Scientific names: *Symphytum asperum; Symphytum officinale; Symphytum. peregrinum; Symphytum x uplandicum*
Family: *Boraginaceae*
Trade and other common names: Ass ear; Blackwort; Boneset ; Bruisewort; consolida; consormol; consound; gum plant; knitback; Knitback; Knitbone; nipbone; Russian comfrey; Slippery Root; Wallwort
Category: Carminative
Purported indications and other uses: Leaf : Gastric and duodenal ulcer, rheumatic pain, gout, arthritis. Topical: poultice for bruises, sprains, athlete's foot, crural ulcers, mastitis, varicose ulcers. **Root**: Gastric and duodenal ulcers, hematemesis, colitis, diarrhea, Topical: ulcers, wounds, fractures, hernia
Half-life: N/A

Reactions

Skin
None

Other
Budd–Chiari syndrome
(2002): Ramlau J, *Ugeskr Laeger* 164(34), 3979
(1990): McDermott WV+, *Arch Surg* 125(4), 525
(1985): Ridker PM+, *Gastroenterology* 88(4), 1050
Death
(2003): Dasgupta A, *Am J Clin Pathol* 120(1), 127
(1990): Yeong ML+, *J Gastroenterol Hepatol* 5(2), 211
Toxicity (sic)
(2002): Rode D, *Trends Pharmacol Sci* 23(11), 497
Tumors
(1988): Abbott PJ, *Med J Aust* 149(11–12), 678

Note: The FDA warns that comfrey contains pyrrolizidine alkaloids that can cause cirrhosis and liver failure when taken orally in high doses. It is banned in Germany and Canada. Topical application is safer and more effective; allantoin in comfrey stimulates cell proliferation, accelerating wound healing

CORTICOSTEROIDS

Generic names:
Alclometasone [Al]
Trade name: Aclovate (GSK)
Topical
Amcinonide [A]
Trade name: Cyclocort (Fujisawa)
Topical
Beclomethasone [Be]
Trade names: Beclovent (GSK), Vanceril, Beconase (GSK), Vancenase (Schering)
Systemic
Betamethasone [B]
Trade names: Celestone (Schering), Betaderm (Stiefel), Diprosone (Schering), Luxiq (Connetics)
Systemic/Topical
Budesonide [Bu]
Trade name: Rhinocort (AstraZeneca)
Systemic
Clobetasol
Trade names: Temovate (GSK), Embeline (HealthPoint), Olux (Connetics)
Topical/Systemic

Cortisone [C]
Trade name: Cortone (Merck)
Systemic
Desonide
Trade name: DesOwen (Galderma)
Topical
Desoximetasone
Trade names: Topicort (Medicis)
Topical
Dexamethasone [D]
Trade name: Decadron (Merck); Maxidex (Alcon); Maxitrol (Alcon)
Systemic/Topical
Fludrocortisone
Trade name: Florinef (Monarch)
Systemic
Flumetasone
Trade names: Locacorten (Bioglan), Locasalen (Bioglan)
Topical
Flunisolide
Trade names: Aerobid (Forest), Nasalide (Dura)
Systemic
Fluocinolone
Trade names: Capex (Galderma), Synalar (Bioglan), Synemol (Medicis)
Topical
Fluocinonide
Topical
Flurandrenolide
Trade name: Cordan (Watson)
Topical
Fluticasone [Ft]
Trade names: Cutivate (GSK); Flonase (GSK)
Topical/Systemic
Halcinonide
Trade name: Halog (Bristol-Myers Squibb)
Topical
Halobetasol
Trade name: Ultravate (Bristol-Myers Squibb)
Topical
Halomethasone
Trade name: Sicorten (Bioglan)
Topical
Hydrocortisone [H]
Trade names: Hytone (Dermik); Cortef (Pharmacia); Solu-Cortef (Pharmacia)
Systemic/Topical
Methylprednisolone [M]
Trade names: Medrol (Pharmacia); Depo-Medrol (Pharmacia); Solu-Medrol (Pharmacia)
Systemic
Mometasone
Trade names: Elocon (Schering); Nasonex (Schering)
Topical
Prednicarbate
Trade name: Dermatop (Dermik)
Topical
Prednisolone [Prl]
Trade names: Delta-Cortef; Hydeltra (Merck); Hydeltrasol (Merck); Poly-Pred (Allergan); Pred Mild (Allergan); Pred-G (Allergan); Vasocidin (Novartis)
Prednisone [Pr]
Trade names: Deltasone (Pharmacia); Meticorten (Schering); Orasone
Systemic
Triamcinolone [T]
Trade names: Aristocort (Fujisawa); Azmacort (Aventis); Kenalog (Apothecon), Nasocort (Fujisawa) (Aventis)
Topical/Systemic

Tixocortol [Tx}
Trade name: (not available in USA)
Topical
Category: anti-inflammatory
**Clinically important, potentially hazardous interactions
with:** acitretin, aldesleukin, anticholinesterases, **cascara,**
cyclosporine, didanosine, doxycycline, **echinacea,**
imatinib, isotretinoin, **mistletoe,** mycophenolate, physostigmine,
rifabutin, rifampin, rifapentine, **smallpox vaccine,** tetracycline,
varicella vaccine

Reactions

Skin
Acanthosis nigricans
   (1982): Bailin PL+, *Clin Rheum Dis* 8, 493 (passim)
   (1980): Gottlieb NL+, *JAMA* 243, 1260 ([Pr])
   (1968): Brown J+, *Medicine* 47, 33
Acne
   (2002): Guillot B, *Expert Opin Drug Saf* 1(4), 325
   (2001): Werth V, *Dermatology Times* 18
   (2000): Fung MA+, *Dermatology* 200, 43
   (2000): Stein RB+, *Drug Saf* 23, 429
   (1993): Monk B+, *Clin Exp Dermatol* 18, 148
   (1982): Bailin PL+, *Clin Rheum Dis* 8, 493 (passim)
   (1953): Smith RC+, *Arch Dermatol* 67, 630
Acute generalized exanthematous pustulosis (AGEP)
   (1996): Demitsu T+, *Dermatology* 193, 56 ([D])
Allergic reactions (sic)
   (2002): Guillot B, *Expert Opin Drug Saf* 1(4), 325
   (2002): Rocha N+, *Contact Dermatitis* 47(6), 362
   (1999): Alexiou C+, *Laryngorhinootologie* (German) 78, 573 ([Pr])
Angioedema
   (1980): Ashord RFU+, *Postgrad Med J* 56, 437 ([H])
Atrophy
   (1990): Ford MD+, *Ophthalmic Surg* 21, 215 ([T])
   (1978): Gottlieb NL+, *JAMA* 240, 559 ([Pr])
   (1975): Kikuchi I+, *Arch Dermatol* 111, 795
   (1974): Kikuchi I+, *Arch Dermatol* 109, 558
   (1974): Rimbaud P+, *Presse Med* (French) 3, 665
   (1972): Di Stefano V+, *Clin Orthop* 87, 254
   (1966): Cassidy JT+, *Ann Intern Med* 65, 1008
   (1964): Ayres S, *Arch Dermatol* 90, 242
Bacterial infections
Bruising
   (2002): Guillot B, *Expert Opin Drug Saf* 1(4), 325
Bullous eruption
   (1999): Lew DB+, *Pediatr Dermatology* 16, 146 ([P])
Calcification
   (1979): Leigh IM+, *Br J Dermatol* 101, 71
Candidiasis
   (2002): Guillot B, *Expert Opin Drug Saf* 1(4), 325
Depigmentation
   (1974): Rimbaud P+, *Presse Med* (French) 3, 665
   (1972): Bloomfield E, *BMJ* 3, 766
   (1972): Glick EN, *BMJ* 4, 300
Dermal thinning
   (1992): Breathnach SM+, *Adverse Drug Reactions and the Skin*
      Blackwell, Oxford, 267 (passim)
   (1990): Capewell S+, *BMJ* 300, 1548 ([Pr])
Dermatitis (sic)
   (2001): Weber F+, *Contact Dermatitis* 44(2), 105
   (2000): Chew AL+, *Cutis* 65, 307 ([T, Pr, D, P])
   (2000): Harris A+, *Australas J Dermatol* 41, 124 ([Pr])
   (1997): Murata Y+, *Arch Dermatol* 133, 1053
   (1997): Vestergaard L+, *Ugeskr Laeger* (Danish) 159, 5662 ([Bu,
      H, Tx])

   (1995): Bircher AJ+, *Acta Derm Venereol* 75, 490 ([P, B])
   (1995): Lepoittevin J-P+, *Arch Dermatol* 131, 31
   (1994): Whitmore SE, *Br J Dermatol* 131, 296 ([D]) (generalized)
   (1993): Elsner P, *Curr Prob Dermatol* 21, 170
   (1993): Fedler R+, *Hautarzt* (German) 44, 91 ([A])
   (1993): Hisa T+, *Contact Dermatitis* 28, 174 ([B, Bu, F, A, H])
   (1985): Hayakawa R+, *Contact Dermatitis* 12, 213 ([A])
   (1985): Yoshikawa K+, *Contact Dermatitis* 12, 55 ([H])
Dermatofibromas
   (1991): Cohen PR, *Int J Dermatol* 30, 266
   (1991): Margolis DJ, *Int J Dermatol* 30, 750
Diaphoresis
   (1999): Alexiou C+, *Laryngorhinootologie* (German) 78, 573 ([Pr])
Ecchymoses
   (1992): Breathnach SM+, *Adverse Drug Reactions and the Skin*
      Blackwell, Oxford, 267 (passim)
   (1991): Anderson B+, *Intern Med* 151, [M, T] ([M, T])
Eczema (sic)
   (1993): Belsito DV, *Cutis* 52, 291
   (1993): Torres V+, *Contact Dermatitis* 29, 106 ([H])
   (1992): Lauerma AI+, *Arch Dermatol* 128, 275 ([H])
   (1988): Lindehof B, *Contact Dermatitis* 18, 309
Erythema (diffuse and widespread)
   (1999): Alexiou C+, *Laryngorhinootologie* (German) 78, 573 ([Pr])
   (1995): Saff DM+, *Arch Dermatol* 131, 742 ([T]) (localized)
      (intralesional triamcinolone)
   (1993): Fedler R+, *Hautarzt* 44, 91 ([A])
   (1993): Räsänen L+, *Br J Dermatol* 128, 407
Erythema multiforme
   (1999): Lew DB+, *Pediatr Dermatol* 16, 146 ([P])
Exanthems
   (1995): Ijsselmuiden O+, *Acta Derm Venereol* (Stockh) 75, 57
      ([T]) (intraarticular triamcinolone)
   (1995): Whitmore SE, *Contact Dermatitis* 32, 193
   (1987): Maucher OM+, *Hautarzt* (German) 38, 577 ([B,D])
Facial edema
   (2001): Werth V, *Dermatology Times* 18
   (1995): Whitmore SE, *Contact Dermatitis* 32, 193
Fixed eruption
   (2001): Sener O+, *Ann Allergy Asthma* 86(3), 335 (solitary, non-
      pigmenting) ([T])
Flushing
   (1999): Alexiou C+, *Laryngorhinootologie* (German) 78, 573 ([P])
   (1980): Gottlieb NL+, *JAMA* 243, 1547
Fungal infections
Herpes simplex
Herpes zoster
Infections (sic)
   (2002): Beeh KM+, *Pneumologie* 56(2), 91 (2.7%)
Kaposi's sarcoma
   (1993): Trattner A+, *J Am Acad Dermatol* 29, 890
   (1991): Soria C+, *J Am Acad Dermatol* 24, 1027
   (1981): Ilie B+, *Dermatologica* 163, 455
   (1981): Leung F+, *Am J Med* 71, 320
Leucoderma acquisitum
   (1972): Cahn BJ+, *Cutis* 9, 509
Linear atrophy
   (1988): Friedman SJ+, *J Am Acad Dermatol* 19, 537
   (1988): Jemec GBE, *J Dermatol Surg Oncol* 14, 88
   (1987): Gupta A+, *Pediatr Dermatol* 4, 259
   (1985): Litt JZ, *Arch Dermatol* 121, 26
Linear hypopigmentation
   (1999): George WM+, *Cutis* 64, 61 (also perilinear)
   (1988): Friedman SJ+, *J Am Acad Dermatol* 19, 537
   (1985): Litt JZ, *Arch Dermatol* 121, 26
   (1984): McCormack PC+, *Arch Dermatol* 120, 708
   (1980): Gottlieb L+, *Arch Dermatol* 140, 1507 ([Pr])
   (1962): Goldman L, *JAMA* 182, 614

Lupus erythematosus
  (1973): Hardin JG, *Ann Intern Med* 78, 558
Mycotic infection
Necrosis
  (1974): Rimbaud P+, *Presse Med* (French) 3, 665
Perianal ulcerations
  (2002): Adams BB+, *Cutis* 69, 67 (Be for 3 months)
Perioral dermatitis
  (2002): Guillot B, *Expert Opin Drug Saf* 1(4), 325
  (1992): Breathnach SM+, *Adverse Drug Reactions and the Skin*
      Blackwell, Oxford, 267 (passim)
Photodermatitis
  (1978): Rietchel RL, *Contact Dermatitis* 4, 334
Pigmentation (sic)
  (1992): Breathnach SM+, *Adverse Drug Reactions and the Skin*
      Blackwell, Oxford, 267 (passim)
  (1982): Bailin PL+, *Clin Rheum Dis* 8, 493 (passim)
Pityriasis rosea
  (1981): Leonforte JF, *Dermatologica* 163, 480
Porokeratosis
  (1980): Feuerman EJ+, *Acta Derm Venereol* (Stockh) 85, 59
Pruritus
  (1999): Alexiou C+, *Laryngorhinootologie* (German) 78, 573 ([Pr])
  (1999): Lew DB+, *Pediatr Dermatology* 16, 146 ([P])
  (1998): Klein-Gitelman MS+, *J Rheumatol* 25, 1995
  (1995): Saff DM+, *Arch Dermatol* 131, 742 ([T]) (localized)
      (intralesional T)
Pseudoxanthoma elasticum
  (1982): Miki Aso+, *J Dermatol* (Tokio) 9, 207
Purpura
  (2000): Rosen R, Sydney, Australia (from Internet) (observation)
      (from inhaled steroid)
  (1990): Capewell S+, *BMJ* 300, 1548 ([Pr])
  (1982): Bailin PL+, *Clin Rheum Dis* 8, 493 (passim)
  (1980): Gottlieb NL+, *JAMA* 243, 1260
Pustular psoriasis
  (1982): Bailin PL+, *Clin Rheum Dis* 8, 493 (passim)
Rash (sic)
  (2002): Butani L, *Ann Allergy Asthma Immunol* 89(5), 439
Redness of face (sic)
Staphylococcal scalded skin syndrome
  (1998): Shirin S+, *Cutis* 62, 223 ([Pr]) (in an adult)
Striae
  (2001): Werth V, *Dermatology Times* 18
  (1982): Bailin PL+, *Clin Rheum Dis* 8, 493 (passim)
  (1975): Nikolowski W, *Akt Dermatol* (German) 1, 9
Telangiectasia
  (1989): Hogan DJ+, *J Am Acad Dermatol* 20, 1129
  (1982): Bailin PL+, *Clin Rheum Dis* 8, 493 (passim)
  (1972): DiStefano V+, *Clin Orthop* 87, 254
Thinning
  (2002): Guillot B, *Expert Opin Drug Saf* 1(4), 325
Urticaria
  (2001): Borja JM+, *Allergy* 56(8), 802 ([H])
  (2001): Nettis E+, *Allergy* 56(8), 791 ([H])
  (2001): Pollack B+, *Br J Dermatol* 144, 1228 ([M])
  (2001): Rasanen L+, *Allergy* 56, 352 ([H])
  (2001): Werth V, *Dermatology Times* 18
  (1995): Ijsselmuiden OE+, *Acta Derm Venereol* 75, 57 ([T])
  (1995): Whitmore SE, *Contact Dermatitis* 32, 193
  (1993): Fedler R+, *Hautarzt* 44, 91 ([A])
  (1980): Ashford RF+, *Postgrad Med J* 56, 437 ([Pr])
Vasculitis
  (1995): Wolkenstein P+, *Drug Saf* 13, 56
  (1982): Bailin PL+, *Clin Rheum Dis* 8, 493 (passim)
  (1969): Rosenberg AL+, *Arthritis Rheum* 12, 317
  (1967): Main RA, *Br J Dermatol* 79, 68
Viral infections

Hair

Hair – alopecia
  (2001): Werth V, *Dermatology Times* 18
Hair – hirsutism
Hair – hypertrichosis
  (1988): Holman GA+, *Pediatrics* 81, 452
  (1982): Bailin PL+, *Clin Rheum Dis* 8, 493 (passim)

Other

Anaphylactoid reactions
  (2001): Werth V, *Dermatology Times* 18
  (2000): Alexander J, Tulsa, OK [T] (from Internet) (observation)
      (triamcinolone)
  (2000): Heeringa M+, *BMJ* 321(7266), 927 ([Bu])
  (2000): Vedamurthy M, Chennai, India, [T] (from Internet)
      (observation) (triamcinolone)
  (1999): Kamm GL+, *Ann Pharmacother* 33, 451
  (1998): Klein-Gitelman MS+, *J Rheumatol* 25, 1995
  (1995): Jacqz-Aigrain E+, *Arch Pediatr* (French) 2, 353 ([P, Pr, B])
  (1992): Coronminas N+, *Pharm Weekbl Sci* 14, 93 ([H])
  (1985): Peller JS+, *Ann Allergy* 54, 302 ([H])
  (1981): Dajani BM+, *J Allergy Clin* 68, 201 ([H])
  (1974): Mendelson LM+, *J Allergy Clin Immunol* 54, 125
  (1960): King RA, *Lancet* 2, 1093
Black tongue
Buffalo hump
  (1982): Bailin PL+, *Clin Rheum Dis* 8, 493 (passim)
Embolia cutis medicamentosa (Nicolau syndrome)
  (2003): Reding EL+, *J Am Acad Dermatol* 48(3), 472 (passim)
Hypersensitivity
  (2002): Butani L, *Ann Allergy Asthma Immunol* 89(5), 439
  (2000): Brancaccio RR+, *Cutis* 65, 31 ([T]) (at injection site)
  (1993): Chan AT, *BMJ* 306, 109 ([D])
Impaired wound healing
  (1992): Breathnach SM+, *Adverse Drug Reactions and the Skin*
      Blackwell, Oxford, 267 (passim)
Injection-site aseptic necrosis
Injection-site lipoatrophy
  (2000): Anderson B+, *Arch Intern Med* 151, 153 ([M, T])
  (1975): Nikolowski W, *Akt Dermatol* (German) 1, 9
  (1974): Kikuchi I+, *Arch Dermatol* 109, 558
  (1974): Rimbaud P+, *Presse Med* (French) 3, 665
  (1963): Schetman D+, *Arch Dermatol* 88, 820
Moon face
  (1982): Bailin PL+, *Clin Rheum Dis* 8, 493 (passim)
Mucocutaneous eruption
  (2002): Guillot B, *Expert Opin Drug Saf* 1(4), 325
Myopathy
  (2003): Genel F+, *Panminerva Med* 45(1), 75
  (2002): Polsonetti BW+, *Ann Pharmacother* 36(11), 1741
  (1992): Decramer M+, *Am Rev Resp Dis* 146, 800
  (1990): Shee CD, *Respiratory Medicine* 84, 229 ([H])
  (1986): Knox AJ+, *Thorax* 41, 411 ([H])
  (1985): Bowyer SL+, *J Allerg Clin Immunol* 2, 234
  (1982): Mastaglia FL, *Drugs* 24, 304
  (1980): Van Marle W+, *BMJ* 281, 271 ([H])
Oral candidiasis
  (2002): Beeh KM+, *Pneumologie* 56(2), 91
  (1998): Reed CE+, *J Allergy Clin Immunol* 101, 14 ([Be])
  (1984): Clissold SP+, *Drugs* 28, 485 ([Bu])
Panniculitis
  (1988): Saxena AK+, *Cutis* 43, 241
Stomatitis
  (1990): Yamaguchi M+, *Kyobu Shikkan Gakkai Zasshi* (Japanese)
      28, 1410 ([Be])

CRANBERRY

Scientific name: *Vaccinium oxycoccus*
Family: Ericaceae
Trade and other common names: Kranbeere;
Ronce d'Amerique; Tsuru-kokemomo
Category: Antipyretic; Antiseptic; Bacteriostat; Diuretic
Purported indications and other uses: Erythema, hyperplasia,
thrush, cystitis, prevention of urinary tract infections, tumor
inhibition, influenza, common cold, scurvy, pleurisy
Half-life: N/A

Reactions

Skin
None

Other
Astrocytoma
  (1996): Aschengrau A+, *Am J Public Health* 86(9), 1289
Toxicity
  (2002): Garcia-Calatayud S+, *An Esp Pediatr* 56(1), 72

Note: Cranberry juice contains oxalates, a common component of
kidney stones, and should be limited in patients with a history of
nephrolithiasis

CREATINE

Scientific names: *N-(aminoiminomethyl)-N methyl glycine; N-
amidinosarcosine*
Family: None
Trade and other common names: Cr; Creatine monohydrate
Category: Food supplement
Purported indications and other uses: Improve exercise
performance, increase muscle mass, heart failure, neuromuscular
disease, cholesterol-lowering, amyotrophic lateral sclerosis (ALS),
rheumatoid arthritis, cardiac surgery (IV)
Half-life: N/A

Reactions

Skin
Acne
  (1998): Gregg LJ, Tulsa, OK (from Internet) (2 observations)
Facial rash (sic)
  (1998): US Food & Drug Administration
Periorbital edema
  (1998): US Food & Drug Administration

Other
Anaphylactoid reactions
  (1998): US Food & Drug Administration
Myalgia
  (1998): US Food & Drug Administration
Polymyositis
  (1998): US Food & Drug Administration
Rhabdomyolysis
  (2001): Ray TR+, *South Med J* 94(6), 608
  (2000): Robinson SJ, *J Am Board Fam Pract* 13(2), 134
  (1998): US Food & Drug Administration
Side effects (sic)

  (2002): Lawrence ME+, *J Clin Gastroenterol* 35(4), 299

*Note: Creatine is found primarily in skeletal muscle (95%), also in
heart, brain, testes & other tissues. The body synthesizes 1 to 2
grams of creatine a day

**Note: Creatine use is widespread among amateur and professional
athletes including, Mark McGuire, Sammy Sosa, John Elway and
others. The annual consumption of creatine in the US exceeds 10
million pounds

CROMOLYN

Synonyms: cromolyn sodium; disodium cromoglycate
Trade names: Crolom (Bausch & Lomb); Gastrocrom
(Celltech); Intal (Monarch); Nasalcrom (Pharmacia); Opticrom
(Allergan)
Other common trade names: *Colimune; Cromlom; Cromoptic;
Fivent; Nalcrom; Opticrom; Rynacrom*
Indications: Allergic rhinitis, asthma, mastocytosis
Category: Mast cell stabilizer
Half-life: 80 minutes

Reactions

Skin
Angioedema (1–10%)
  (1992): Breathnach SM+, *Adverse Drug Reactions and the Skin*
    Blackwell, Oxford, 235 (passim)
  (1979): Settipane GA+, *JAMA* 241, 811
  (1975): Sheffer AL+, *N Engl J Med* 293, 1220
  (1974): Crisp J+, *JAMA* 229, 787
Dermatitis (sic) (generalized)
  (1997): Camarasa JG+, *Contact Dermatitis* 36, 160 (from eye
    drops)
  (1993): Lewis FM+, *Contact Dermatitis* 28, 246
  (1988): Kudo H+, *Contact Dermatitis* 19, 312
  (1979): Settipane GA+, *JAMA* 241, 811
Eczema (sic)
Edema
Erythema
Exanthems
Exfoliative dermatitis
Facial dermatitis (sic)
  (1979): Settipane GA+, *JAMA* 241, 811
  (1974): Brogden RN+, *Drugs* 7, 164
Flushing
Photosensitivity
Pruritus
  (1975): Sheffer AL+, *N Engl J Med* 293, 1220
Rash (sic) (<1%)
Rosacea
  (1979): Mayberry JF+, *BMJ* 2, 1366
Urticaria (<1%)
  (1992): Breathnach SM+, *Adverse Drug Reactions and the Skin*,
    Blackwell, Oxford, 235 (passim)
  (1977): Menon MP+, *Scand J Respir Dis* 58, 145
  (1975): Sheffer AL+, *N Engl J Med* 293, 1220
Vasculitis
  (1978): Rosenberg JL+, *Arch Intern Med* 138, 989

Other
Anaphylactoid reactions (<1%)
  (1996): Ibanez MD+, *Ann Allergy Asthma Immunol* 77, 185
  (1996): Shearer WT, *Ann Allergy Asthma Immunol* 77, 165
  (1992): Breathnach SM+, *Adverse Drug Reactions and the Skin*
    Blackwell, Oxford, 235 (passim)

(1983): Ahmad S, *Ann Intern Med* 99, 882
(1975): Sheffer AL+, *N Engl J Med* 293, 1220
Anosmia
(1998): Graedon J+Newspaper anecdote from, *People's Pharmacy* column
Dysgeusia (>10%)
Hypersensitivity (immediate type)
(1987): Skarpass IJK, *Allergy* 42, 318
Myalgia
Myopathy
(1979): Settipane GA+, *JAMA* 241, 811
Paresthesias
Serum sickness
Xerostomia (1–10%)

CYANOCOBALAMIN

Synonym: vitamin B$_{12}$
Trade names: Berubigen; Crysti-12; Cyanoject (Mayrand); Cyomin (Forest); Ener-B; Nascobal (Nastech); Rubramin (Bristol-Myers Squibb); Vitamin B$_{12}$
Other common trade names: *Anacobin; Betolvex; Cobex; Crystamine; Cytamen; Dobetin; Lifaton B$_{12}$; Redisol; Rubesol-1000; Sytobex; Vicapan N*
Indications: Vitamin B$_{12}$ deficiency, pernicious anemia
Category: Water-soluble nutritional supplement
Half-life: 6 days

Reactions

Skin
Acne
(1991): Sherertz EF, *Cutis* 48, 119
(1979): Dupre A+, *Cutis* 24, 210
(1976): Braun-Falco O+, *Münch Med Wochenschr* (German) 118, 155
(1969): Dugois P+, *Bull Soc Fr Dermatol Syphiligr* (French) 76, 382
(1969): Dugois P+, *Lyon Med* (French) 221, 1165
(1967): Puissant A+, *Bull Soc Fr Derm Syphiligr* (French) 74, 813
(1966): Goldblatt S, *Hautarzt* (German) 17, 106
Allergic reactions (sic)
(1986): Bigby M+, *JAMA* 256, 3358 (1.79%)
Angioedema
(1952): Bedford PD, *BMJ* 1, 690
Bullous eruption (<1%)
(1977): Pevny I+, *Hautarzt* (German) 28, 600
Cheilitis
(1981): Price ML+, *Contact Dermatitis* 7, 352
Dermatitis
(1994): Rodriguez A+, *Contact Dermatitis* 31, 271
(1975): Malten KE, *Contact Dermatitis* 1, 325
Eczema (sic)
(1977): Pevny I+, *Hautarzt* (German) 28, 600
Exanthems
(1986): Woodliff HJ, *Med J Aust* 144, 223
(1977): Pevny I+, *Hautarzt* (German) 28, 600
(1976): Arndt KA+, *JAMA* 235, 918
Folliculitis
(1989): Gallastegui C+, *Drug Intell Clin Pharm* 23, 1033
Pruritus (1–10%)
(1974): Nalivko F+, *Vestn Dermatol Venerol* (Russian) 8, 66
Rosacea fulminans
(2001): Jansen T+, *J Eur Acad Dermatol Venereol* 15(5), 484
Systemic eczematous contact dermatitis

Urticaria (<1%)
(1996): Denis R+, *Clin Lab Haematol* 18, 129
(1986): Woodliff HJ, *Med J Aust* 144, 223
(1977): Pevny I+, *Hautarzt* (German) 28, 600
(1974): Nalivko F+, *Vestn Dermatol Venerol* (Russian) 8, 66
(1971): James J+, *BMJ* 2, 262
(1969): Meyer de Schmid JJ+, *Bull Soc Fr Dermatol Syphiligr* (French) 76, 670
(1952): Bedford PD, *BMJ* 1, 690

Other
Anaphylactoid reactions (<1%)
(1998): Tordjman R+, *Eur J Haematol* 60, 269
(1984): Sobolevskii AI+, *Vestn Dermatol Venerol* (Russian) April, 66
(1977): Pevny I+, *Hautarzt* (German) 28, 600
(1971): James J+, *BMJ* 2, 262
(1968): Hovding G, *BMJ* 3, 102
Embolia cutis medicamentosa (Nicolau syndrome)
(2002): Poletti E+, *World Congress Dermatol* Poster, 0124
(1995): Kunzi T+, *Schweiz Rundsch Med Prax* (German) 84, 640
Headache
Hypersensitivity
(1974): Nalivko SN+, *Vestn Dermatol Venerol* (Russian) August, 66
Injection-site aseptic necrosis
(1995): Kunzi T+, *Schweiz Rundsch Med Prax* (German) 84, 640
Injection-site pain
Paresthesias
Porphyria cutanea tarda
(1965): DeFeo CP, *Arch Dermatol* 92, 330

CYCLAMATE

Trade name: Sucaryl (Abbott)
Indications: Sweetening
Category: Sulfonamide sweetener
Half-life: N/A

Reactions

Skin
Angioedema
(1968): Feingold BF, *Ann Allergy* 26, 309
Bullous eruption
(1968): Feingold BF, *Ann Allergy* 26, 309
Exanthems
(1965): Boros E, *JAMA* 194, 571
Photosensitivity
(1981): Fujita M+, *Arch Dermatol* 117, 246 (passim)
(1972): Jung EG, *Z Haut Geschlechtskr* (German) 47, 329
(1970): *Nutr Rev* 28, 122
(1969): Yong JM+, *Lancet* 2, 1273
(1968): Feingold BF, *Ann Allergy* 26, 309
(1968): Turk JL+, *Br J Dermatol* 80, 200
(1966): Kobori T+, *J Asthma Res* 3, 213
Pruritus
(1968): Feingold BF, *Ann Allergy* 26, 309
(1967): Lamberg SI, *JAMA* 201, 747
(1965): Boros E, *JAMA* 194, 571
Urticaria
(1981): Fujita M+, *Arch Dermatol* 117, 246
(1968): Feingold BF, *Ann Allergy* 26, 309

Other
Hypersensitivity (nonallergic)
(1998): Ehlers I+, *Allergy* 53, 1074

Paresthesias
(1992): Shelley WB+, *Advanced Dermatologic Diagnosis* WB Saunders, 1039

*Note: Cyclamate is a sulfonamide and can be absorbed systemically. Sulfonamides can produce severe, possibly fatal, reactions such as toxic epidermal necrolysis and Stevens–Johnson syndrome

CYCLOBENZAPRINE

Trade name: Flexeril (McNeil) (Merck)
Other common trade names: *Benzamin; Cloben; Cyben; Flexiban; Novo-Cycloprine; Yurelax*
Indications: Muscle spasms
Category: Skeletal muscle relaxant
Half-life: 1–3 days

Reactions

Skin
Allergic reactions (sic)
Angioedema (<1%)
Dermatitis (sic) (<1%)
Diaphoresis
(1984): Heckerling PS+, *Ann Intern Med* 101, 881
Facial edema (<1%)
Flushing
Photosensitivity
Pruritus (<1%)
Purpura
Rash (sic) (<1%)
Urticaria (<1%)

Hair
Hair – alopecia

Other
Ageusia (<1%)
Anaphylactoid reactions (<1%)
Dysgeusia (3%)
Galactorrhea
Gynecomastia
Headache
Paresthesias (<1%)
Stomatitis
Tinnitus
Tongue edema (<1%)
Tongue pigmentation
Xerostomia (27%)
(1988): Bennett RM+, *Arthritis Rheum* 31, 1535
(1988): Katz WA+, *Clin Ther* 10, 216

CYCLOPHOSPHAMIDE

Synonyms: CPM; CTX; CYT
Trade names: Cytoxan (Bristol-Myers Squibb); Neosar (Pharmacia)
Other common trade names: *Cycloblastin; Cyclostin; Endoxan; Endoxana; Genoxal; Ledoxina; Procytox; Sendoxan*
Indications: Lymphomas
Category: Antineoplastic immunosuppressant
Half-life: 4–7 hours
Clinically important, potentially hazardous interactions with: aldesleukin, azathioprine, cyclosporine, mycophenolate, vaccines

Reactions

Skin
Acral erythema
(1995): Komamura H+, *J Dermatol* 22(2), 116 (with vincristine, doxorubicin and GCSF)
(1993): Vukelja SJ+, *Cutis* 52, 89
(1986): Crider MK+, *Arch Dermatol* 122, 1023
Allergic reactions (sic) (sic)
(2002): Cantu MG+, *J Clin Oncol* 20(5), 1232 (2%) (with doxorubicin and cisplatin)
(2001): Stratton J+, *Nephrol Dial Transplant* 16(8), 1724
Angioedema
(1977): Ross WE+, *Cancer Treat Rep* 61, 495
Condylomata acuminata
(1996): D'Hondt L+, *Acta Gastroenterol Belg* (French) 59, 254
Dermatitis
(1967): Maguire HC, *J Invest Dermatol* 48, 39
Dermatitis herpetiformis
(1986): Gottlieb D+, *Med J Aust* 145, 241
Dermatofibromas
(1986): Bargman HB+, *J Am Acad Dermatol* 14, 351
Diaphoresis
Eccrine squamous syringometaplasia
(1997): Valks R+, *Arch Dermatol* 133, 873
Erythema multiforme (<1%)
Erythrodysesthesia
(1989): Matsuyama JR+, *Drug Intell Clin Pharm* 23, 776
Exanthems
(1992): Breathnach SM+, *Adverse Drug Reactions and the Skin* Blackwell, Oxford, 289 (passim)
(1992): Hann SK+, *J Dermatol* 20, 94
(1982): Bailin PL+, *Clin Rheum Dis* 8, 493 (passim)
Facial burning
(1994): Kosirog-Glowacki JL+, *Ann Pharmacother* 28, 197
Flushing (1–10%)
(1994): Dhar S+, *Dermatology* 188, 332
Graft-versus-host reaction
(2001): Valks R+, *Arch Dermatol* 137, 61 (3 cases)
Keratoacanthoma
(1972): Lowney ED, *Arch Dermatol* 105, 924
Lupus erythematosus
(2001): McClain S, New York, NY (from Internet) (observation)
Lymphoma
(1992): Pandya AG+, *Arch Dermatol* 128, 1626 (passim)
(1983): Goslen JB+, *Arch Dermatol* 119, 326
Myxedema
(1971): Coffey VJ, *BMJ* 4, 682
Palmar–plantar erythema
(1990): Pagliuca A+, *Postgrad Med J* 66, 242
Pigmentation (<1%)

(2001): Viana G, *Belo Horizonte* (Brazil) (from Internet) (observation)
(1993): Pai BH, *J Assoc Physicians India* 41, 124
(1992): Babu KG, *J Assoc Physicians India* 40, 211
(1992): Pandya AG+, *Arch Dermatol* 128, 1626 (passim)
(1991): Dutta TK+, *J Assoc Physicians India* 39, 230
(1991): Singal R+, *Pediatr Dermatol* 8, 231
(1981): Nixon DW+, *Cutis* 27, 181
(1975): No Author, *Lancet* 2, 128
(1975): Shah PC+, *Lancet* 2, 548 (palmar)
(1974): Romankiewicz JA, *Am J Hosp Pharm* 31, 1074
(1973): Levantine A+, *Br J Dermatol* 89, 105
(1973): Mani MK+, *J Assoc Physicians India* 21, 799
(1972): Amar Inalsingh CH, *Arch Dermatol* 106, 765 (palmar)
(1972): Harrison BM+, *BMJ* 2, 352
(1966): Solidoro A+, *Cancer Chemotherapy* 50, 265

Pruritus
(1978): Krutchik AN+, *Arch Intern Med* 138, 1725

Purpura

Rash (sic) (1–10%)

Squamous cell carcinoma
(1992): Pandya AG+, *Arch Dermatol* 128, 1626 (passim)
(1972): Lowney ED, *Arch Dermatol* 105, 924

Stevens–Johnson syndrome
(1996): Assier-Bonnet H+, *Br J Dermatol* 135, 864
(1985): Leititis JU+, *Klin Padiatr* (German) 197, 441

Toxic epidermal necrolysis (<1%)

Ultraviolet light recall
(1993): Williams BJ+, *Clin Exp Dermatol* 18, 452
(1984): Andersen KE+, *Photodermatol* 1, 129

Urticaria
(1992): Breathnach SM+, *Adverse Drug Reactions and the Skin* Blackwell, Oxford, 289 (passim)
(1987): Grosbois B+, *Rev Med Interne* (French) 8, 208
(1982): Anku V, *Cancer Treat Rep* 66, 2106
(1980): Diaz-Rubio E+, *Rev Clin Esp* (Spanish) 156, 461
(1978): Krutchik AN+, *Arch Intern Med* 138, 1725
(1978): Legha SS+, *Cancer Treat Rep* 62, 180
(1977): Ross WE+, *Cancer Treat Rep* 61, 495
(1976): Lakin JD+, *J Allergy Clin Immunol* 58, 160

Vasculitis
(1989): Green RM+, *Aust N Z J Med* 19, 55

Hair

Hair – alopecia (universal and severe in one-third)
(2002): de Jonge ME+, *Bone Marrow Transplantation* 30(9), 593 (permanent) (with carboplatin and thiotepa)
(2002): Klasa RJ+, *J Clin Oncol* 20(24), 4649 (with vincristine and prednisone)
(2001): Viana G, *Belo Horizonte* (Brazil) (from Internet) (observation)
(2000): Tran D+, *Australas J Dermatology* 41, 106
(1996): Infanti L+, *Haematologica* 81, 521
(1992): Pandya AG+, *Arch Dermatol* 128, 1626 (passim)
(1987): David J+, *Nurs Times* 83, 36
(1987): Parker R, *Oncol Nurs Forum* 14, 49
(1985): Middleton J+, *Cancer Treat Rep* 69, 373
(1984): Ahmed AR+, *J Am Acad Dermatol* 11, 1115
(1984): Cline BW, *Cancer Nurs* 7, 221
(1982): Bailin PL+, *Clin Rheum Dis* 8, 493 (passim)
(1980): Maxwell MB, *Am J Nursing* 80, 900
(1979): Holmes W, *ANA Publ* (NP-59), 223
(1972): Harrison BM+, *BMJ* 2, 352
(1966): Herzberg JJ, *Arch Klin Exp Dermatol* (German) 227, 452
(1966): Simister JM, *BMJ* 2, 1138

Nails

Nails – Beau's lines (transverse nail bands)
(1994): Ben-Dyan D+, *Acta Haematol* 91, 89

Nails – dystrophy

(1992): Breathnach SM+, *Adverse Drug Reactions and the Skin* Blackwell, Oxford, 289 (passim)

Nails – leukonychia (Muehrcke's lines)
(1992): Bianchi L+, *Dermatology* 185, 216 (longitudinal)
(1990): Bader-Meunier B+, *Ann Pediatr Paris* (French) 37, 337
(1983): James WD+, *Arch Dermatol* 119, 334

Nails – onychodermal band
(1993): Kowal-Vern A+, *Cutis* 52, 43

Nails – pigmentation (<1%)
(2002): Srikant M+, *Br J Haematol* 117(1), 2
(2001): Viana G, *Belo Horizonte* (Brazil) (from Internet) (observation)
(1992): Bianchi L+, *Dermatology* 185, 216 (longitudinal)
(1983): Manigand G+, *Sem Hop* (French) 59, 1840
(1982): Bailin PL+, *Clin Rheum Dis* 8, 493 (passim)
(1981): Adam BA, *Singapore Med J* 22, 35
(1980): Daniel CR+, *Cutis* 25, 595
(1980): Sulis E+, *Eur J Cancer* 16, 1517
(1978): Shah PC+, *Br J Dermatol* 98, 675
(1975): Markenson AL+, *Lancet* 2, 128 (pigmented banding)
(1975): Shah PC+, *Lancet* 2, 548
(1973): Mani MK+, *J Assoc Physicians of India* 21, 799
(1972): Amar Inalsingh CH, *Arch Dermatol* 106, 765
(1966): Solidoro A+, *Cancer Chemother* 50, 265

Other

Acute intermittent porphyria

Anaphylactoid reactions (<1%)
(1992): Breathnach SM+, *Adverse Drug Reactions and the Skin* Blackwell, Oxford, 289 (passim)
(1979): Murti L+, *J Pediatr* 94, 844
(1977): Karchmer RK+, *JAMA* 237, 475

Gingival pigmentation
(1979): Krutchik AN+, *South Med J* 72, 1615
(1972): Harrison BM+, *BMJ* 2, 352

Hypersensitivity
(1996): Popescu NA+, *J Allergy Clin Immunol* 97, 26
(1992): Weiss RB, *Semin Oncol* 19, 458
(1978): Legha SS+, *Cancer Treat Rep* 62, 180

Injection-site pain

Myalgia
(2002): Cantu MG+, *J Clin Oncol* 20(5), 1232 (4%) (with doxorubicin and cisplatin)

Oral mucosal ulceration
(1992): Pandya AG+, *Arch Dermatol* 128, 1626 (passim)
(1982): Bailin PL+, *Clin Rheum Dis* 8, 493 (passim)

Oral mucositis
(2000): Wardley AM+, *Br J Haematol* 110, 292

Polyarteritis nodosa
(1983): Goslen JB+, *Arch Dermatol* 119, 326

Porphyria cutanea tarda
(1988): Manzione NC+, *Gastroenterology* 95, 1119

Rhabdomyolysis

Scalp burning
(1994): Kosirog-Glowacki JL+, *Ann Pharmacother* 28, 197

Stomatitis (10%)
(1982): Bailin PL+, *Clin Rheum Dis* 8, 493 (passim)
(1975): Carter SK, *Cancer Treat Rev* 2, 295

Tooth discoloration
(1972): Harrison BM+, *BMJ* 2, 352

CYCLOSERINE

Trade name: Seromycin (Dura)
Other common trade names: *Closerin; Closerina; Cyclomycin; Cyclorine; Cycosin; Orientomycin*
Indications: Tuberculosis
Category: Tuberculostatic
Half-life: 10 hours

Reactions

Skin
Allergic reactions (sic)
Dermatitis (sic)
  (1972): Levantine A+, *Br J Dermatol* 86, 651
  (1971): Nava C, *Med Lav* (Italian) 62, 351
Exanthems
  (1985): Holdiness R, *Int J Dermatol* 24, 280
  (1973): Mühlberger F, *Schweiz Med Wochenschr* (German) 103, 126
  (1969): Agrawal R, *BMJ* 4, 540
  (1959): Bereston ES, *J Invest Dermatol* 33, 427
Lichenoid eruption
  (1995): Shim JH+, *Dermatology* 191, 142
Pruritus
Rash (sic) (<1%)
Stevens–Johnson syndrome
  (1997): Akula SK+, *Int J Tuberc Lung Dis* 1, 187 (in AIDS)
Urticaria
  (1959): Bereston ES, *J Invest Dermatol* 33, 427

Other
Headache
Oral mucosal lesions
Paresthesias

CYCLOSPORINE

Synonyms: CsA; CyA; cyclosporin A
Trade names: Neoral (Novartis); Sandimmune (Novartis)
Other common trade names: *Ciclosporin; Consupren; Implanta; Sandimmun*
Indications: Prophylaxis of organ rejection in transplants
Category: Immunosuppressant
Half-life: 10–27 hours (adults)
Clinically important, potentially hazardous interactions with: amiloride, aminoglycosides, amphotericin B, ampicillin, anisindione, anticoagulants, atorvastatin, azathioprine, azithromycin, bacampicillin, basiliximab, bosentan, carbenicillin, caspofungin, cholestyramine, clarithromycin, cloxacillin, co-trimoxazole, corticosteroids, cyclophosphamide, danazol, dicloxacillin, dicumarol, digoxin, diltiazem, disulfiram, **echinacea**, erythromycin, ethotoin, etoposide, ezetimibe, fluoxymesterone, fluvastatin, foscarnet, fosphenytoin, gemfibrozil, imatinib, imipenem/cilastin, ketoconazole, lovastatin, mephenytoin, methicillin, methoxsalen, methyltestosterone, mezlocillin, mycophenolate, nafcillin, NSAIDs, orlistat, oxacillin, penicillins, phenytoin, pravastatin, rifabutin, rifampin, rifapentine, ritonavir, simvastatin, spironolactone, **St John's wort**, sulfacetamide, sulfadiazine, sulfamethoxazole, sulfisoxazole, sulfonamides, tacrolimus, testosterone, ticarcillin, triamterene, troleandomycin, **vaccines**, warfarin

Note: A good discussion of cyclosporine in dermatology can be found in (1989): Gupta AK+, *J Am Acad Dermatol* 21, 1245

Reactions

Skin
Acne
  (2001): Reitamo S+, *Br J Dermatol* 145(3), 438 (13%) (with sirolimus)
  (2001): Werth V, *Dermatology Times* 15
Acne keloid
  (2001): Carnero L+, *Br J Dermatol* 144(2), 429 (nuchal scalp)
Angioedema
  (1980): Isenberg DA+, *N Engl J Med* 303, 754
Angiomas
  (1998): De Felipe I+, *Arch Dermatol* 134, 1487
Ankle edema
  (1997): Berthe-Jones J+, *Br J Dermatol* 136, 76
Basal cell carcinoma
  (2001): Otley CC+, *Arch Dermatol* 137, 459
  (1992): Pakula A+, *J Am Acad Dermatol* 26, 139
  (1987): Penn I, *Transplantation* 43, 32
Bullous eruption (1%)
  (1990): Petit D+, *J Am Acad Dermatol* 22, 851
Burning
  (2002): Pucci N+, *Ann Allergy Asthma Immunol* 89(3), 298 (topical)
Buschke–Lowenstein penile carcinoma
  (1993): Piepkorn M+, *J Am Acad Dermatol* 29, 321
Cyst
  (1993): Richter A+, *Hautarzt* (German) 44, 521
  (1993): Valicenti JMK+, *Arch Dermatol* 129, 794 (passim)
  (1992): Schoendorff C+, *Cutis* 50, 36 (epidermoid)
  (1986): Bencini PL+, *Dermatologica* 172, 24
Dyshidrosis
  (2002): Sharma AK+, *Transpl Int* 15(9), 519
Eccrine squamous syringometaplasia
  (1997): Valks R+, *Arch Dermatol* 133, 873
Edema

(1997): Shapiro J+, *J Am Acad Dermatol* 36, 114

Erythema
  (2001): Takamatsu Y+, *Bone Marrow Transplant* 28(4), 421

Exanthems
  (1985): Chapius B+, *N Engl J Med* 312, 1259

Facial edema
  (1986): Schmitz-Schumann M, *Prog Allergy* 38, 436

Fixed eruption
  (2002): Verma SB (Baroda) (India) (from Internet) (observation)

Flushing (>3%)
  (2000): Ramsay HM+, *Br J Dermatol* 142, 832
  (1992): Goodman MM+, *J Am Acad Dermatol* 27, 594
  (1992): Shelley WB+, *Advanced Dermatologic Diagnosis* WB
    Saunders, 583 (passim)
  (1990): Gupta AK+, *J Am Acad Dermatol* 22, 242
  (1986): Kahan BD+, *World J Surg* 10, 348

Folliculitis
  (2003): Harman KE+, *Clin Exp Dermatol* 28(3), 341
  (2001): Werth V, *Dermatology Times* 15
  (1995): Ojeda-Vargas M+, *Enferm Infecc Microbiol Clin* (Spanish)
    13, 637
  (1993): Richter A+, *Hautarzt* (German) 44, 521
  (1993): Sepp N+, *Br J Dermatol* 128, 213
  (1993): Valicenti JMK+, *Arch Dermatol* 129, 794 (passim)
  (1986): Bencini PL+, *Dermatologica* 172, 24

Granulomas
  (2002): Kim SS+, *J Korean Med Sci* 17(5), 704

Herpes simplex
  (1993): Sepp N+, *Br J Dermatol* 128, 213
  (1993): Valicenti JMK+, *Arch Dermatol* 129, 794 (passim)
  (1986): Bencini PL+, *Dermatologica* 172, 24

Herpes zoster
  (1986): Bencini PL+, *Dermatologica* 172, 24

Hidradenitis
  (1984): Palestine AG+, *Am J Med* 4:77, 652

Hot flashes
  (2001): Reitamo S+, *Br J Dermatol* 145(3), 438 (12%) (with
    sirolimus)

Hyperkeratosis (follicular spiny)
  (1995): Izakovic J+, *Hautarzt* (German) 46, 841

Hypohidrosis
  (1990): Gupta AK+, *Arch Dermatol* 126, 339

Ichthyosis
  (1986): Bencini PL+, *Dermatologica* 172, 24

Kaposi's sarcoma
  (1997): Vella JP+, *N Engl J Med* 336, 1761
  (1996): Ozen S+, *Nephrol Dial Transplant* 11, 1162
  (1988): Bencini PL+, *Br J Dermatol* 118, 709
  (1987): Penn I, *Transplantation* 43, 32

Keratoses
  (1995): Yamamoto T+, *J Dermatol* 22, 298
  (1993): Piepkorn M+, *J Am Acad Dermatol* 29, 321
  (1992): Ross M+, *J Am Acad Dermatol* 26, 128

Keratosis pilaris
  (1993): Valicenti JMK+, *Arch Dermatol* 129, 794 (passim)
  (1986): Bencini PL+, *Dermatologica* 172, 24

Lichenoid eruption
  (1995): Shim JH+, *Dermatology* 191, 142

Linear IgA bullous dermatosis
  (1990): Petit D+, *J Am Acad Dermatol* 22, 851

Lupus erythematosus
  (1990): Cooper KD, *Dermatology* 1(2), 3

Lymphocytic infiltration
  (1992): Bagot M+, *J Am Acad Dermatol* 26, 283
  (1991): Sabourin JC, *Ann Pathol* 11, 208
  (1990): Gupta AK+, *J Am Acad Dermatol* 22, 242
  (1990): Gupta AK+, *J Am Acad Dermatol* 23, 1137
  (1988): Brown MD+, *Arch Dermatol* 124, 1097

Lymphoma
  (2002): Kirby B+, *J Am Acad Dermatol* 47(2 Suppl), S165
  (1993): Masouye I+, *Arch Dermatol* 129, 914
  (1992): Koo JY+, *J Am Acad Dermatol* 26, 836
  (1992): Zijlmans JM+, *N Engl J Med* 326, 1363
  (1991): Tomson CR+, *Nephrol Dial Transplant* 6, 896
  (1989): Walker RJ+, *Aust N Z J Med* 19, 154
  (1987): Penn I, *Transplantation* 43, 32
  (1984): Beveridge T+, *Lancet* 1, 788
  (1983): Inglehart JK, *N Engl J Med* 309, 123

Melanoma
  (1990): Merot Y+, *Br J Dermatol* 123, 237

Mycosis fungoides
  (2002): Zackheim HS+, *J Am Acad Dermatol* 47(1), 155
  (1990): Fradin MS+, *J Am Acad Dermatol* 23, 1265

Neoplasms (sic)
  (1995): Kohler LD+, *Hautarzt* (German) 46, 638

Nodular cutaneous T-lymphocyte infiltrate
  (1988): Brown MD+, *Arch Dermatol* 124, 1097

Papillomas (facial)
  (1993): Valicenti JMK+, *Arch Dermatol* 129, 794

Papulo-vesicular eruptions (sic)
  (1988): Frosch PJ+, *Hautarzt* (German) 39, 611

Pigmentation
  (1997): Oakley A, Hamilton, New Zealand (from Internet)
    (observation)

Poikiloderma
  (1986): Bencini PL+, *Dermatologica* 172, 24

Porokeratosis (superficial actinic)
  (1997): Matsushita S+, *J Dermatol* 24, 110

Pruritus (<2%)
  (1992): Goodman MM+, *J Am Acad Dermatol* 27, 594

Psoriasis
  (1986): Bencini PL+, *Dermatologica* 172, 24

Purpura (3%)
  (1998): Roberts P+, *Transplant Proc* 30, 1512
  (1986): Bencini PL+, *Dermatologica* 172, 24

Pustular psoriasis
  (1998): Mahendran R+, *Br J Dermatol* 139, 934
  (1997): Drugge R, Stamford, CT (from Internet) (observation)

Pyogenic granuloma
  (2001): al-Zayer M+, *Spec Care Dentist* 21(5), 187

Rash (sic) (10%)
  (1992): Goodman MM+, *J Am Acad Dermatol* 27, 594

Raynaud's phenomenon
  (2002): Sharma AK+, *Transpl Int* 15(9), 517
  (1986): Deray G+, *Lancet* 2, 1092

Sebaceous hyperplasia
  (1998): Walther T+, *Dtsch Med Wochenschr* 123, 798
  (1993): Valicenti JMK+, *Arch Dermatol* 129, 794 (passim)
  (1992): Pakula A+, *J Am Acad Dermatol* 26, 139
  (1986): Bencini PL+, *Dermatologica* 172, 24

Shivering (sic)
  (2000): Lepine EM, Rock Hill, SC (from Internet) (observation)

Squamous cell carcinoma
  (2001): Marcil I+, *Lancet* 358(9287), 1042
  (2001): Otley CC+, *Arch Dermatol* 137, 459
  (1997): van de Kerkhof PC+, *Br J Dermatol* 136, 275
  (1996): Cox NH, *Clin Exp Dermatol* 21, 323
  (1993): Piepkorn M+, *J Am Acad Dermatol* 29, 321 (penis)
  (1990): Fradin MS+, *J Am Acad Dermatol* 23, 1265 (passim)
  (1989): Bos JD+, *J Am Acad Dermatol* 21, 1305
  (1985): Bencini PL+, *Br J Dermatol* 113, 373
  (1985): Price ML+, *N Engl J Med* 313, 1420
  (1985): Thompson JF+, *Lancet* 1, 158
  (1983): Mortimer PS+, *J R Soc Med* 76, 786

Striae
  (1986): Bencini PL+, *Dermatologica* 172, 24

Thrombocytopenic purpura
 (2001): Medina PJ+, *Curr Opin Hematol* 8(5), 286
Toxic epidermal necrolysis
 (1997): Jarrett P+, *Clin Exp Dermatol* 22, 254
Ulcerations (1%)
Urticaria
 (2001): Takamatsu Y+, *Bone Marrow Transplant* 28(4), 421 (with
  tacrolimus)
 (1985): Ptachcinski RJ+, *Lancet* 1, 636
Vasculitis
 (2000): Gupta MN+, *Ann Rheum Dis* 59, 319
 (1994): Henckes M+, *Transpl Int* 7, 292
Verruca vulgaris
 (1998): Irimajiri J+, *J Dermatol* 25, 688
Vitiligo
 (1986): Bencini PL+, *Dermatologica* 172, 24

Hair

Hair – alopecia (3%)
 (1998): Hunt M, *Cosmetic Dermatology* 23
 (1987): Keown PA+, *Hospital Practice* 22, 207
Hair – alopecia areata
 (1999): Cerottini JP+, *Dermatology* 198, 415
 (1996): Misciali C+, *Arch Dermatol* 132, 843 (universalis)
 (1996): Parodi A+, *Br J Dermatol* 135, 657 (universalis)
 (1995): Davies MG+, *Br J Dermatol* 132, 835
 (1994): Roger D+, *Acta Derm Venereol* 74, 154
Hair – brittle
Hair – growth
 (1995): Mannes GP+, *Transpl Int* 8, 247 ("delightful")
 (1994): Yamamoto S+, *J Dermatol Sci* 7 s47
Hair – hypertrichosis (19%)
 (2001): Werth V, *Dermatology Times* 15
 (2000): Ionnides D+, *Arch Dermatol* 136, 868
 (1997): Avci O+, *J Am Acad Dermatol* 36, 796
 (1997): Brehler R+, *J Am Acad Dermatol* 36, 983 (passim)
 (1997): Ellis CN, *Int J Dermatol* 36 (Supplement), 7 (passim)
 (1997): Shapiro J+, *J Am Acad Dermatol* 36, 114
 (1997): Shupack J+, *J Am Acad Dermatol* 36, 423
 (1996): el Shahawy MA+, *Nephron* 72, 679
 (1996): Jayamanne DG+, *Nephrol Dial Transplant* 11, 1159
  (eyelashes)
 (1995): Honeyman JF+, *Int J Dermatol* 34, 583
 (1993): Sepp N+, *Br J Dermatol* 128, 213
 (1993): Valicenti JMK+, *Arch Dermatol* 129, 794 (passim)
 (1992): Humphreys TR+, *J Am Acad Dermatol* 29, 490 (passim)
 (1990): Fradin MS+, *J Am Acad Dermatol* 23, 1265
 (1988): Frosch PJ+, *Hautarzt* (German) 39, 611
 (1988): Penmetcha M+, *Int J Dermatol* 27, 53
 (1987): Keown PA+, *Hospital Practice* 22, 207
 (1987): Wysocki GP+, *Clin Exp Dermatol* 12, 191
 (1986): Bencini PL+, *Br J Dermatol* 114, 396
 (1986): Kahan BD+, *World J Surg* 10, 348
 (1984): Harper JL+, *Br J Dermatol* 110, 469
Hair – perifolliculitis barbae
 (2002): Moderer M+, *World Congress Dermatol* Poster, 0117
Hair – pseudofolliculitis barbae
 (1997): Lear J+, *Br J Dermatol* 136, 132

Nails

Nails – abnormal growth
 (1986): Gratwohl A+, *Prog Allergy* 38, 404
Nails – brittle (<2%)
Nails – changes (sic)
 (1994): Wakelin SH+, *Br J Dermatol* 131, 147
Nails – ingrown
 (1993): Olujohungbe A+, *Lancet* 342, 1111
Nails – leukonychia
 (1986): Bencini PL+, *Dermatologica* 172, 24

Nails – periungual granuloma
 (1995): Higgins EM+, *Br J Dermatol* 132, 829

Other

Acromegaloid features
 (1987): Reznik VM, *Lancet* 1, 1405
Anaphylactoid reactions (<1%)
 (2001): Ebo DG+, *Ann Allergy Asthma Immunol* 87(3), 243
 (2001): Riegert-Johnson DL+, *Bone Marrow Transplant*
  28(12), 1176
 (2001): Takamatsu Y+, *Bone Marrow Transplant* 28(4), 421
 (1989): Gupta AK+, *J Am Acad Dermatol* 21, 1245
 (1985): Chapuis B+, *N Engl J Med* 312, 1259
 (1985): Leunissen KML+, *Lancet* 1, 636
 (1985): Ptachcinski RJ+, *Lancet* 1, 636
Angiosarcoma (fatal)
 (2001): Schulze R+, *Internist* 42, 119
Aphthous stomatitis
 (2001): Reitamo S+, *Br J Dermatol* 145(3), 438 (9%) (with
  sirolimus)
 (1986): Bencini PL+, *Dermatologica* 172, 24
Breast lumps (sic)
 (1980): Rolles K+, *Lancet* 2, 795
Death
 (2002): Zackheim HS+, *J Am Acad Dermatol* 47(1), 155
Dysesthesia
 (2000): Capper N, Mobile, AL (from Internet) (observation)
 (1990): Gupta AK+, *J Am Acad Dermatol* 22, 242
Erythromelalgia
 (2003): Thami GP+, *BMJ* 326(7395), 910
Facial numbness
 (2002): Ozkaya O+, *Pediatr Nephrol* 17(7), 544
Fibroadenoma
 (2001): Muttarak M+, *Australas Radiol* 45(4), 517
 (2001): Weinstein SP+, *Radiology* 220(2), 465
Gingival hyperplasia (>10%)
 (2003): Afonso M+, *J Periodontol* 74(1), 51
 (2003): Guelmann M+, *J Clin Pediatr Dent* 27(2), 123
 (2003): Hyland PL+, *J Periodontol* 74(4), 437
 (2003): Perez-Espana L+, *Nefrologia* 23(2), 179
 (2002): Bulut S+, *J Periodontol* 73(8), 892
 (2002): Das SJ+, *J Dent Res* 81(10), 683
 (2002): Hosey MT+, *Int J Paediatr Dent* 12(4), 236
 (2002): Keglevich T+, *Fogorv Sz* 95(1), 15
 (2002): McKaig SJ+, *Int J Paediatr Dent* 12(6), 398
 (2002): Voulgari PV+, *J Rheumatol* 29(11), 2466
 (2001): Brennan MT+, *Oral Surg Oral Med Oral Pathol Oral Radiol*
  Endod 92(5), 503
 (2001): Buduneli N+, *Acta Odontol Scand* 59(6), 367
 (2001): Bustos DA+, *J Periodontol* 72(6), 741
 (2001): Irshied J+, *J Clin Pediatr Dent* 26(1), 93
 (2001): Oettinger-Barak O+, *J Periodontol* 72(9), 1236
 (2001): Thomas DW+, *J Clin Periodontol* 28(7), 706
 (2001): Uzel MI+, *J Periodontol* 72(7), 921
 (2001): Vallejo C+, *Haematologica* 86(1), 110
 (2001): Werth V, *Dermatology Times* 15
 (2001): Wondimu B+, *Int J Paediatr Dent* 11(6), 424
 (2000): Czech W+, *J Am Acad Dermatol* 42, 653
 (2000): Hernandez G+, *J Periodontol* 71(10), 1630
 (2000): Kirby B+, *Clin Exp Dermatol* 25, 97
 (2000): Oettinger-Barak O+, *J Periodontol* 71, 650
 (2000): Thomas DW+, *Transplantation* 69, 522
 (1999): Spratt H+, *Oral Dis* 5, 27
 (1999): Wirnsberger GH+, *Transplantation* 67, 1289
 (1998): Cebeci I+, *J Periodontol* 69, 1435
 (1998): Desai P+, *J Can Dent Assoc* 64, 263
 (1998): Jucgla A+, *Br J Dermatol* 138, 198
 (1998): Kohnle M+, *Transplant Proc* 30, 2122
 (1998): Mattson JS+, *J Am Dent Assoc* 129, 78
 (1998): Nash MM+, *Transplantation* 65, 1611

(1998): Nohl F+, *Ther Umsch* (German) 55, 573
(1998): Nowicki M+, *Ann Transplant* 3, 25
(1998): Pilloni A+, *J Periodontol* 69, 791
(1998): Varga E+, *J Clin Periodontol* 25, 225
(1998): Wirnsberger GH+, *Transplant Proc* 30, 2117
(1997): Avci O+, *J Am Acad Dermatol* 36, 796
(1997): Brehler R+, *J Am Acad Dermatol* 36, 983 (passim)
(1997): Cecchin E+, *Ann Intern Med* 126, 409
(1997): Dodd DA, *J Heart Lung Transplant* 16, 579
(1997): Ellis CN, *Int J Dermatol* 36 (Supplement), 7 (passim)
(1997): Gómez E+, *Nephrol Dial Transplant* 12, 2694
(1997): Hall EE, *Curr Opin Peridontology* 4, 59 (passim)
(1997): Iacopino AM+, *J Periodontol* 68, 73
(1997): Jackson C+, *N Y State Dent J* 63, 46
(1997): Puig JM+, *Transplant Proc* 29, 2379
(1997): Silverstein LH+, *Gen Dent* 45, 371
(1996): Ashrafi SH+, *Scanning Microsc* 10, 219
(1996): Boran M+, *Transplant Proc* 28, 2316
(1996): Cebeci I+, *J Periodontol* 67, 1201
(1996): Darbar UR+, *J Clin Periodontol* 23, 941
(1996): Montebugnoli L+, *J Clin Periodontol* 23, 868
(1996): Somacarrera ML+, *Spec Care Dent* 16, 18
(1995): Moghadam BKH+, *Cutis* 56, 46 (passim)
(1995): Wahlstrom E+, *N Engl J Med* 332, 753
(1994): Wong W+, *Lancet* 343, 986
(1993): King GN+, *J Clin Periodontol* 20, 286
(1993): Seymour RA, *Adverse Drug React Toxicol Rev* 12, 215
(1993): Seymour RA+, *J R Coll Surg Edinb* 38, 328
(1993): Thomason JM+, *J Clin Periodontol* 20, 37
(1993): Valicenti JMK+, *Arch Dermatol* 129, 794 (passim)
(1992): Humphreys TR+, *J Am Acad Dermatol* 29, 490 (passim)
(1992): Mastrolonardo M+, *Dermatol Clin* (Italian) 4, 246
(1992): Seymour RA+, *J Clin Periodontol* 19, 1
(1991): Puelacher W+, *Z Stomatol* (German) 88, 7
(1990): Cooper KD, *Dermatology* 1(2), 3
(1989): Ross PJ+, *J Dent Child* 56, 56
(1988): Frosch PJ+, *Hautarzt* (German) 39, 611
(1988): Veraldi S+, *Int J Dermatol* 27, 730
(1987): Keown PA+, *Hospital Practice* 22, 207
(1987): Reznik VM, *Lancet* 1, 1405
(1986): Kahan BD+, *World J Surg* 10, 348

Gingivitis
Glossitis (atrophic)
(1986): Bencini PL+, *Dermatologica* 172, 24
Gynecomastia (>3%)
(1998): Kollias J+, *Aust N Z J Surg* 68, 679
(1994): Jacobs U+, *Transplant Proc* 26, 3122
(1987): Beris P+, *Schweiz Med Wochenschr* (German) 117, 1751
Headache
Hyperesthesia
(1987): Keown PA+, *Hospital Practice* 22, 207
Hypersensitivity
(2001): Sumpton JE+, *Transplant Proc* 33(6), 3015
Lingual fungiform papillae hypertrophy (sic)
(1996): Silverberg NB+, *Lancet* 348, 967
Lymphoproliferative disease
(1989): Walker RJ+, *Aust N Z J Med* 19, 154
(1988): Brown MD+, *Arch Dermatol* 124, 1097
Myalgia
(2001): Kappers-Klunne MC+, *Br J Haematol* 114(1), 121
(1988): Brown MD+, *Arch Dermatol* 124, 1097 (passim)
Myopathy
(1990): Fernandez-Sola J+, *Lancet* 335, 362
(1989): Chassagne P+, *Lancet* 2, 1104
Oral ulceration
(1986): Bencini PL+, *Dermatologica* 172, 24
Paresthesias (>8%)
(2001): Capper RN, Mobile, AL (from Internet) (observation) (tingling lips & fingers)

(2001): Laws RA, Providence, RI (from Internet) (observation) (hands & feet)
(2001): Thaler D, Monona, WI (from Internet) (observation) (numb lips)
(2000): Baumgaertnet J, LaCrosse, WI (from Internet) (3 observations)
(2000): Lepine EM, Rock Hill, SC (from Internet) (observation)
(2000): Thaler D, Monona, WI (from internet) (observation)
(1997): Berthe-Jones J+, *Br J Dermatol* 136, 76
(1997): Ellis CN, *Int J Dermatol* 36 (Supplement), 7 (passim)
(1997): Shupack J+, *J Am Acad Dermatol* 36, 423
(1992): Goodman MM+, *J Am Acad Dermatol* 27, 594
(1990): Cooper KD, *Dermatology* 1(2), 3
(1988): Bennett WM+, *Ann Rev Med* 37, 215 (passim)
(1987): Dougados M+, *Arthritis Rheum* 30, 83
Parkinsonism
(2002): Kim HC+, *Nephrol Dial Transplant* 17(2), 319
Pseudolymphoma
(1993): Kerl H+, *Dermatology in General Medicine* McGraw-Hill New York
(1990): Gupta AK+, *J Am Acad Dermatol* 23(6), 1137
(1988): Brown MD+, *Arch Dermatol*

PG 124(7), 1097
(1988): Thestrup-Pedersen K+, *Dermatologica* 177, 376
Rhabdomyolysis
(2002): Cassidy JV+, *Paediatr Anaesth* 12(8), 729
(1999): Maltz HC+, *Ann Pharmacother* 33(11), 1176 (with atorvastatin)
(1995): Meier C+, *Schweiz Med Wochenschr* 125(27), 1342 (with simvastatin)
(1992): Blaison G+, *Rev Med Interne* 13(1), 61 (with simvastatin)
(1988): Tobert JA, *Am J Cardiol* 62, 28J (with lovastatin)
Stomatitis (7%)
Tinnitus
Tremor (>10%)
Tumors
(2001): Werth V, *Dermatology Times* 15

CYCLOTHIAZIDE

Trade name: Anhydron (Lilly)
Other common trade names: *Doburil; Valmiran*
Indications: Edema, hypertension
Category: Thiazide diuretic
Half-life: N/A
Clinically important, potentially hazardous interactions with: digoxin

Reactions

Skin
Exanthems (<1%)
Photosensitivity
Purpura
Rash (sic)
Urticaria
Vasculitis

Other
Paresthesias

*Note: Cyclothiazide is a sulfonamide and can be absorbed systemically. Sulfonamides can produce severe, possibly fatal, reactions such as toxic epidermal necrolysis and Stevens–Johnson syndrome

CYPROHEPTADINE

Trade name: Periactin (Merck)
Other common trade names: *Ciplactin; Ciproral; Nuran; Periactine; Periactinol; Peritol; Sigloton*
Indications: Allergic rhinitis, urticaria
Category: Antihistamine H₁-blocker
Half-life: 1–4 hours
Clinically important, potentially hazardous interactions with: anticholinergics, MAO inhibitors, phenelzine, tranylcypromine

Reactions

Skin

Allergic reactions (sic) (<1%)
Angioedema (<1%)
Dermatitis (sic)
  (1995): Li LF+, *Contact Dermatitis* 33, 50
Diaphoresis
Edema (<1%)
Erythema
Exanthems
  (1964): Gould AH+, *Med Clin North Am* 48, 411
Flushing
Lichenoid eruption
  (1971): Baer RL+in Fitzpatrick, *Dermatology in General Medicine* McGraw-Hill 1281
Lupus erythematosus
Peripheral edema
Photosensitivity
  (1971): Kalivas J, *JAMA* 216, 526
Purpura
Rash (sic) (<1%)
Urticaria
Vasculitis
  (1984): Ekenstam E+, *Arch Dermatol* 120, 484

Other

Anaphylactoid reactions
Dysgeusia
  (1997): Neufeld-Kaiser W+, *Arch Dermatol* 133, 251
Myalgia (<1%)
Paresthesias (<1%)
Tinnitus
Xerostomia (1–10%)
  (1990): Kardinal CG+, *Cancer* 65, 2657
  (1990): Pontius EB, *J Clin Psychopharmacol* 8, 230

CYTARABINE

Synonyms: arabinosylcytosine; ara-C
Trade names: Cytosar-U (Pharmacia); Tarabine (Pharmacia)
Other common trade names: *Alexan; Arabitin; Arace; Aracytine; Cytarbel; Cytosar; Uducil*
Indications: Leukemias
Category: Antimetabolite; Antineoplastic
Half-life: initial: 10–15 minutes
Clinically important, potentially hazardous interactions with: aldesleukin

Reactions

Skin

Acral erythema
  (2002): Cetkovska P+, *J Eur Acad Dermatol Venereol* 16(5), 481
  (2001): Takeuchi M+, *Rinsho Ketsueki* 42(3), 216
  (1999): Azurdia RM+, *Clin Exp Dermatol* 24, 64
  (1998): Calista D+, *J Eur Acad Dermatol Venereol* 10, 274
  (1997): Arranz FR+, *Arch Dermatol* 133, 499
  (1997): Demircay Z+, *Int J Dermatol* 36, 593
  (1995): Dechaufour F+, *Ann Dermatol Venereol* (French) 120, 219
  (1992): Doll DC+, *Semin Oncol* 19(5), 580
  (1992): Rongioletti F+, *J Am Acad Dermatol* 26, 284
  (1991): Brown J+, *J Am Acad Dermatol* 24, 1023
  (1991): Rongioletti F+, *J Cutan Pathol* 18, 453
  (1989): Alexander J, *Oncol Nurs Forum* 16, 829
  (1989): Kroll SS+, *Ann Plast Surg* 23, 263
  (1989): Oksenhendler E+, *Eur J Cancer Clin Oncol* 25, 1181
Acral erythrodysesthesia syndrome (hand–foot syndrome)
  (1993): Waltzer JF+, *Arch Dermatol* 129, 43 (bullous variety)
  (1991): Baack BR+, *J Am Acad Dermatol* 24, 457
  (1989): Kampmann KK+, *Cancer* 63, 2482 (bullous variety)
  (1988): Shall L+, *Br J Dermatol* 119, 249
  (1986): Crider MK+, *Arch Dermatol* 122, 1023 (>5%)
  (1985): Baer MR+, *Ann Intern Med* 102, 556 (bullous variety)
  (1985): Cardonnier C+, *Ann Intern Med* 97, 783
  (1985): Levine LE+, *Arch Dermatol* 121, 102
  (1985): Peters WG+, *Ann Intern Med* 103, 805 (bullous variety)
  (1985): Walker IR+, *Arch Dermatol* 121(10), 1240 (10–67%) (dose-related)
  (1983): Herzig RH+, *Blood* 62, 361 (1–5%)
  (1982): Burgdorf WHC+, *Ann Intern Med* 97, 61
Actinic keratoses (with pruritus and erythema)
  (1989): Kerker BJ+, *Semin Dermatol* 8, 173
Acute febrile neutrophilic dermatosis (Sweet's syndrome)
  (1993): Torri O+, *Ann Dermatol Venereol* (French) 120, 884
Bullous eruption
  (1992): Richards C+, *Oncol Nurs Forum* 19, 1191
Desquamation
  (1992): Richards C+, *Oncol Nurs Forum* 19, 1191
Edema (sic)
Erythema
  (2002): Tay J, *CMAJ* 167(6), 672
  (1998): Taverna C+, *Schweiz Med Wochenschr* (German) 128, 1117
  (1992): Richards C+, *Oncol Nurs Forum* 19, 1191
Erythema
  (1990): Krulder JWM+, *Eur J Cancer* 26, 649
Erythroderma (generalized)
  (1988): Benson PM+, *J Assoc Military Derm* XIV, 28 (passim)
Exanthems
  (2002): Cetkovska P+, *J Eur Acad Dermatol Venereol* 16(5), 481 (44.4%)
  (2002): Chiu A+, *J Am Acad Dermatol* 47(4), 633

(1988): Benson PM+, *J Assoc Military Derm* XIV, 28
(1986): Morant R+, *Schweiz Med Wochenschr* (German) 116, 1415 (60%)
(1983): Herzig RH+, *Blood* 62, 361 (1–5%)
(1983): Shah SS+, *Cancer Treat Rep* 67, 405*

Exfoliative dermatitis
(1989): Williams SF+, *Br J Haematol* 73, 274

Freckles (1–10%)

Herpes zoster
(1973): Stevens DA+, *N Engl J Med* 289, 873

Neutrophilic eccrine hidradenitis
(1997): Jegasothy SM+, Pittsburgh, American Academy of Dermatology Meeting (SF) (gross and microscopic)
(1995): Kanzaki H+, *J Dermatol* 22, 137
(1993): Thorisdottir K+, *J Am Acad Dermatol* 28, 775
(1992): Bernstein EF+, *Br J Dermatol* 127, 529 (recurrent)
(1991): Vion B+, *Dermatologica* 183, 70
(1990): Hurt MA+, *Arch Dermatol* 126, 73
(1989): Bailey DL+, *Pediatr Dermatol* 6, 33
(1989): Kerker BJ+, *Semin Dermatol* 8, 173
(1987): Katsanis E+, *Am J Pediatr Hematol Oncol* 9, 204
(1984): Flynn TC+, *J Am Acad Dermatol* 11, 584

Palmar–plantar erythrodysesthesia
(2002): Crawford JH+, *Eur J Haematol* 69(5), 315

Petechiae
(1998): Taverna C+, *Schweiz Med Wochenschr* (German) 128, 1117

Pruritus (1–10%)

Rash (sic) (>10%)
(2002): Cetkovska P+, *J Eur Acad Dermatol Venereol* 16(5), 481 (40–73%)

Seborrheic keratoses (inflammation of) (Leser–Trélat syndrome)
(1999): Williams JV+, *J Am Acad Dermatol* 40, 643
(1979): Kechijian P+, *Ann Intern Med* 91, 868

Syringosquamous metaplasia (sic)
(1990): Bhawan J+, *Am J Dermatopathol* 12, 1

Toxic epidermal necrolysis
(2001): Özkan A+, *Pediatr Dermatol* 18(1), 38
(1998): Figueiredo MS+, *Rev Assoc Med Bras* (Portuguese) 44, 53

Ulcerations
(1969): Bodey GP+, *Cancer Chemother Rep* 53, 59

Urticaria
(2002): Cetkovska P+, *J Eur Acad Dermatol Venereol* 16(5), 481

Vasculitis*
(1998): Ahmed I+, *Mayo Clin Proc* 73, 239
(1989): Kerker BJ+, *Semin Dermatol* 8, 173

(1989): Williams SF+, *Br J Haematol* 73, 274

Hair

Hair – alopecia (1–10%)
(1988): Benson PM+, *J Assoc Military Derm* XIV, 28 (passim)
(1986): Morant R+, *Schweiz Med Wochenschr* (German) 116, 1415 (100%)
(1970): Upjohn Company, *Clin Pharmacol Ther* 11, 155
(1969): Bodey GP+, *Cancer Chemother Rep* 53, 59

Nails

Nails – leukonychia
(1990): Bader-Meunier B+, *Ann Pediatr Paris* (French) 37, 337
Nails – Mees' lines
(1982): Jeanmougin M+, *Ann Dermatol Venereol* (French) 109, 169

Other

Anal ulceration (>10%)
Anaphylactoid reactions
(1997): Blanca M+, *Allergy* 52, 1009
(1989): Williams SF+, *Br J Haematol* 73, 274
(1980): Rassiga AL+, *Arch Intern Med* 104, 425
Headache
Hypersensitivity
(1992): Weiss RB, *Semin Oncol* 19, 458
Injection-site cellulitis (1–10%)
Myalgia (1–10%)
Oral mucosal lesions
(1986): Morant R+, *Schweiz Med Wochenschr* (German) 116, 1415 (1–5%)
(1978): Levine N+, *Cancer Treat Rev* 5, 67
(1974): Levantine A+, *Br J Dermatol* 90, 239 (66%)
(1971): Lang HN+, *Med J Aust* 2, 187
(1968): Howard JP+, *Cancer* 21, 341
Oral ulceration (>10%)
Pseudotumor cerebri
(1999): Fort JA+, *Ann Pharmacother* 33, 576
Rhabdomyolysis
(2002): Truica CI+, *Am J Hematol* 70(4), 320
Stomatitis
(1988): Benson PM+, *J Assoc Military Derm* XIV, 28 (passim)
Thrombophlebitis (>10%)

*Note: Vasculitis, a part of the cytarabine syndrome, consists of fever, malaise, myalgia, conjunctivitis, arthralgia and a diffuse erythematous maculopapular eruption that occurs from 6 to 12 hours following the administration of the drug

DACARBAZINE

Synonym: DIC
Trade name: DTIC-Dome (Bayer)
Other common trade names: *D.T.I.C; Dacatic; Deticene; Detimedac*
Indications: Malignant melanoma, carcinomas
Category: Antineoplastic
Half-life: initial: 20–40 minutes
Clinically important, potentially hazardous interactions with: aldesleukin

Reactions

Skin
Actinic keratoses
  (1987): Johnson TM+, *J Am Acad Dermatol* 17(2 Pt 1), 192
Angioedema
  (1981): Wassilew SW+, *Hautarzt* (German) 32 (Suppl 5), 453
Erythema
Exanthems
  (1981): Wassilew SW+, *Hautarzt* (German) 32 (Suppl 5), 453
Fixed eruption
  (1982): Koehn GG+, *Arch Dermatol* 118, 1018
Flushing (1–10%)
  (1982): Dunagin WG, *Semin Oncol* 9, 14
  (1978): Levine N+, *Cancer Treat Rev* 5, 67 (100%)
Photosensitivity (<1%)
  (1989): Serrano G+, *Photodermatol* 6, 140
  (1982): Koehn GG+, *Arch Dermatol* 118, 1018
  (1981): Bonifazi E+, *Contact Dermatitis* 7, 161
  (1981): Wassilew SW+, *Hautarzt* (German) 32 (Suppl 5), 453
  (1981): Yung CW+, *J Am Acad Dermatol* 4, 541
  (1980): Beck TM+, *Cancer Treat Rep* 64, 725
  (1980): Bolling R+, *Hautarzt* (German) 31, 602
  (1980): Ippen H, *Dtsch Med Wochenschr* (German) 105, 531
  (1980): Kunze J+, *Z Hautkr* (German) 55, 100
Rash (sic) (1–10%)
Urticaria
  (1995): Bourry C+, *Therapie* (French) 50, 588
  (1981): Wassilew SW+, *Hautarzt* (German) 32 (Suppl 5), 453
Vasculitis

Hair
Hair – alopecia (1–10%)
  (1978): Levine N+, *Cancer Treat Rev* 5, 67

Nails
Nails – pigmentation
  (1984): Daniel CR+, *J Am Acad Dermatol* 10, 250

Other
Anaphylactoid reactions (1–10%)
Death
  (2001): Ramanathan RK+, *Ann Oncol* 12(8), 1139
Depression
  (2001): Ramanathan RK+, *Ann Oncol* 12(8), 1139
Dysgeusia (1–10%) (metallic taste)
Headache
Hypersensitivity
  (1992): Weiss RB, *Semin Oncol* 19, 458
Injection-site burning (>10%)
Injection-site cellulitis
  (1989): Kerker BJ+, *Semin Dermatol* 8, 173
Injection-site dermatitis
  (1987): Dufresne RG, *Cutis* 39, 197
Injection-site necrosis (>10%)

  (1987): Dufresne RG, *Cutis* 39, 197
Injection-site pain (>10%)
Injection-site phlebitis
  (1989): Kerker BJ+, *Semin Dermatol* 8, 173
Myalgia (1–10%)
Paresthesias (facial)
Rhabdomyolysis
  (1995): Anderlini P+, *Cancer* 76(4), 678
Stomatitis (<1%)

DACTINOMYCIN

Synonyms: ACT; actinomycin D
Trade name: Cosmegen (Merck)
Other common trade names: *Ac-De; Cosmegen Lyovac; Lyovac*
Indications: Melanonas, sarcomas
Category: Antineoplastic antibiotic
Half-life: 36 hours
Clinically important, potentially hazardous interactions with: aldesleukin

Reactions

Skin
Acne (>10%)
  (1993): Blatt J+, *Med Pediatr Oncol* 21, 373
  (1983): Bronner AK+, *J Am Acad Dermatol* 9, 645
  (1982): Dunagin WG, *Semin Oncol* 9, 14
  (1974): Levantine A+, *Br J Dermatol* 90, 239 (>5%)
  (1969): Epstein EH+, *N Engl J Med* 281, 1094
Actinic keratoses
  (1987): Johnson TM+, *J Am Acad Dermatol* 17(2 Pt 1), 192
Bullous pemphigoid
  (1982): Amer MH+, *Int J Dermatol* 21, 32
Cellulitis
  (1989): Kerker BJ+, *Semin Dermatol* 8, 173
Cheilitis
Dermatitis (sic)
  (1975): Cassady JR+, *Radiology* 115, 171
Erythema
  (1997): Coppes MJ+, *Med Pediatr Oncol* 29, 226
Erythema multiforme
Exanthems
Folliculitis
  (1981): Henkes J+, *Actas Dermosifiliogr* (Spanish) 72, 469
  (1969): Epstein EH+, *N Engl J Med* 281, 1094
Keratoses (reactivation of)
  (1989): Kerker BJ+, *Semin Dermatol* 8, 173
Pigmentation
  (1995): Kanwar VS+, *Med Pediatr Oncol* 24, 329
  (1978): Levine N+, *Cancer Treat Rev* 5, 67 (100%)
  (1971): Ma HK+, *J Obstet Gynaecol Br Commonw* 78, 166
Pruritus
  (1989): Kerker BJ+, *Semin Dermatol* 8, 173
Pustules
  (1983): Bronner AK+, *J Am Acad Dermatol* 9, 645
  (1969): Epstein EH+, *N Engl J Med* 281, 1094
Radiation recall (>10%)
  (1997): Coppes MJ+, *Med Pediatr Oncol* 29, 226
  (1978): Levine N+, *Cancer Treat Rev* 5, 67 (50%)
  (1975): Dreizen S+, *Postgrad Med* 58, 150
  (1974): Levantine A+, *Br J Dermatol* 90, 239 (>5%)
Serpentine supravenous hyperpigmentation (sic)
  (2000): Marcoux D+, *J Am Acad Dermatol* 43, 540 (with vincristine)

Toxic epidermal necrolysis
Urticaria

Hair

Hair – alopecia (>10%)
  (1964): Falkson G+, *Br J Dermatol* 76, 309

Other

Anaphylactoid reactions (<1%)
Injection-site extravasation (>10%)
  (1997): Coppes MJ+, *Med Pediatr Oncol* 29, 226
Injection-site necrosis (>10%)
  (1987): Dufresne RG, *Cutis* 39, 197
Injection-site phlebitis (>10%)
Myalgia
Oral mucosal lesions
  (1983): Bronner AK+, *J Am Acad Dermatol* 9, 645 (>5%)
  (1975): Dreizen S+, *Postgrad Med* 58, 150
  (1972): Cridland MD, *Drugs* 3, 352
Phlebitis
  (1989): Kerker BJ+, *Semin Dermatol* 8, 173
Stomatitis (ulcerative) (>5%)

DALTEPARIN

Trade name: Fragmin (Pfizer)
Other common trade name: *Fragmine*
Indications: Prophylaxis of deep vein thrombosis
Category: Anticoagulant; Low-molecular weight heparin
Half-life: 4–8 hours
Clinically important, potentially hazardous interactions with: butabarbital, danaparoid

Reactions

Skin

Allergic reactions (sic) (1–10%)
Bullous eruption (1–10%)
  (1999): Tong, M, Kota Kinabalu, Malaysia (from Internet)
    (observation)
Exanthems (<1%)
Lesions
  (2003): Payne SM+, *Ann Pharmacother* 37(5), 655
Necrosis
Pruritus (1–10%)
Rash (sic) (1–10%)

Hair

Hair – alopecia
  (2001): Apsner R+, *Blood* 97(9), 2914–5
  (2000): Barnes C, *Blood* 96, 1618

Other

Anaphylactoid reactions (1–10%)
  (2001): Ueda A+, *Nephron* 87(1), 93
Injection-site edema
  (2000): Szolar-Platzer C+, *J Am Acad Dermatol* 43, 920
Injection-site hematoma (1–10%)
Injection-site pain (1–10%)
Injection-site pruritus
  (2000): Szolar-Platzer C+, *J Am Acad Dermatol* 43, 920

DAN-SHEN

Scientific name: *Salvia miltiorrhiza*
Family: Labiatae; Lamiaceae
Trade and other common names: Huang Ken; Red Rooted Sage; Red Sage; Salvia Root; Tzu Tan-Ken
Category: Cardiovascular stimulant
Purported indications and other uses: Circulation problems, ischemic stroke, angina pectoris, menstrual problems, chronic hepatitis, abdominal masses, insomnia, acne, psoriasis, eczema, bruising, hearing loss
Half-life: N/A
Clinically important, potentially hazardous interactions with: warfarin

Reactions

Skin

Pruritus

DANAPAROID

Trade name: Orgaran (Organon)
Indications: Prevention of postoperative deep thrombosis
Category: Anticoagulant
Half-life: ~24 hours
Clinically important, potentially hazardous interactions with: butabarbital, dalteparin, enoxaparin, heparin

Reactions

Skin

Allergic reactions (sic) (<1%)
  (2000): de Saint-Blanquat L+, *Ann Fr Anesth Reanim* 19, 751
Edema (2.6%)
Infections (sic) (2.1%)
Peripheral edema (3.3%)
Pruritus (3.9%)
Purpura
Rash (sic) (2.1–4.8%)
  (1999): Wutschert R+, *Drug Saf* 20, 515

Other

Injection-site hematoma (5%)
Injection-site infiltrated plaques
  (2000): Koch P+, *J Am Acad Dermatol* 42, 612
  (2000): Martin L+, *Contact Dermatitis* 42, 295
  (2000): Szolar-Platzer C+, *J Am Acad Dermatol* 43, 920
Injection-site pain (7.6–13.7%)
Injection-site reactions
  (2001): Figarella I+, *Ann Dermatol Venereol* 128, 35
Paresthesias

DANAZOL

Trade name: Danocrine (Sanofi-Synthelabo)
Other common trade names: *Azol; Bonzol; Cyclomen; D-Zol; Danol; Ladogal; Winobanin; Zoldan-A*
Indications: Endometriosis, fibrocystic breast disease
Category: Synthetic pituitary gonadotropin inhibitor
Half-life: ~4.5 hours
Clinically important, potentially hazardous interactions with: acitretin, cyclosporine, oral contraceptives, tacrolimus, warfarin

Reactions

Skin

Acne (>10%)
  (1982): Madanes AE+, *Ann Intern Med* 96, 625 (20%)
  (1980): Hosea SW+, *Ann Intern Med* 93, 809 (8%)
  (1979): Greenberg RD, *Cutis* 24, 431
  (1977): Spooner JB+, *J Int Med Res* 5 (Suppl 3), 15
Angioedema
  (1993): Litt JZ, Beachwood, OH (personal case) (observation)
  (1988): Guillet G+, *Dermatologica* 177, 370
Diaphoresis (3%)
  (1977): Spooner JB+, *J Int Med Res* 5 (Suppl 3), 15
Edema (>10%)
  (1977): Spooner JB+, *J Int Med Res* 5 (Suppl 3), 15
Erythema multiforme
  (1992): Reynolds NJ+, *Clin Exp Dermatol* 17, 140
  (1988): Gately LE+, *Ann Intern Med* 109, 85
Exanthems
  (1993): Litt JZ, Beachwood, OH (personal case) (observation)
  (1989): Ahn YS+, *Ann Intern Med* 111, 723 (6%)
  (1982): Madanes AE+, *Ann Intern Med* 96, 625
  (1975): 13, 94
Flushing
  (1988): Henzl MR+, *N Engl J Med* 318, 485 (68%)
  (1980): Hosea SW+, *Ann Intern Med* 93, 809 (12%)
  (1977): Spooner JB+, *J Int Med Res* 5 (Suppl 3), 15
  (1975): 13, 94
Lupus erythematosus
  (1994): Yung RL+, *Rheum Dis Clin North Am* 20, 61
  (1991): Sassolas B+, *Br J Dermatol* 125, 190
  (1988): Guillet G+, *Dermatologica* 177, 370
  (1982): Fretwell MD, *Allergy Clin Immunol* 69, 306
Lymphomatoid papulosis
  (1985): Wise C+, *Fertil Steril* 44, 702
Petechiae
Photosensitivity (<1%)
Pruritus
  (1989): Ahn YS+, *Ann Intern Med* 111, 723 (3.5%)
Purpura
  (1990): Taillan B+, *Presse Med* (French) 19, 721
Rash (sic) (3%)
  (1977): Spooner JB+, *J Int Med Res* 5 (Suppl 3), 15
Seborrhea
  (1989): Ahn YS+, *Ann Intern Med* 111, 723
  (1982): Madanes AE+, *Ann Intern Med* 96, 625 (30%)
  (1981): Duff P+, *Am J Obstet Gynecol* 141, 349 (passim)
  (1977): Spooner JB+, *J Int Med Res* 5 (Suppl 3), 15
Stevens–Johnson syndrome
Urticaria

Hair

Hair – alopecia
  (1989): Ahn YS+, *Ann Intern Med* 111, 723 (3.5%)
  (1981): Duff P+, *Am J Obstet Gynecol* 141, 349

  (1980): Hosea SW+, *Ann Intern Med* 93, 809 (17%)
Hair – hirsutism (<10%)
  (1991): Bates GW+, *Clin Obstet Gynecol* 34, 848
  (1989): Ahn YS+, *Ann Intern Med* 111, 723 (3.5%)
  (1982): Madanes AE+, *Ann Intern Med* 96, 625 (7%)
  (1980): Hosea SW+, *Ann Intern Med* 93, 809 (8%)

Other

Acute intermittent porphyria
Breast changes (sic)
  (1977): Spooner JB+, *J Int Med Res* 5 (Suppl 3), 15
Candidal vaginitis (<1%)
  (1977): Spooner JB+, *J Int Med Res* 5 (Suppl 3), 15
Death
  (2001): Hayashi T+, *J Gastroenterol* 36(11), 783
Gingivitis
Guillain–Barré syndrome
  (1985): Hory B+, *Am J Med* 79, 111
Paresthesias
Rhabdomyolysis
  (1994): Dallaire M+, *CMAJ* 150(12), 1991 (with lovastatin)
Vaginal dryness (sic)

DANTROLENE

Trade name: Dantrium (Procter & Gamble)
Other common trade names: *Dantamacrin; Dantrolen*
Indications: Spasticity, malignant hyperthermia
Category: Skeletal muscle relaxant
Half-life: 8.7 hours
Clinically important, potentially hazardous interactions with: verapamil

Reactions

Skin

Acne
  (1981): Pembroke AC+, *Br J Dermatol* 104, 465
  (1980): Dykes MHM, *JAMA* 231, 862
Chills (1–10%)
Dermatitis (sic)
Diaphoresis
Erythema
Exanthems
  (1980): Dykes MHM, *JAMA* 231, 862
Photosensitivity
Pruritus
Rash (sic) (>10%)
Urticaria

Hair

Hair – growth

Other

Anaphylactoid reactions
Dysgeusia
Headache
Malignant lymphoma
  (1980): Wan HH+, *Postgrad Med J* 56, 261
Myalgia
Thrombophlebitis
Tremor

DAPSONE

Trade name: Dapsone (Jacobus)
Other common trade names: *Avlosulfon; Dapson; Dapson-Fatol; Protogen; Sulfona*
Indications: Leprosy, dermatitis herpetiformis
Category: Antileprotic; Dermatitis herpetiformis suppressant
Half-life: 10–50 hours
Clinically important, potentially hazardous interactions with: chloroquine, didanosine, furazolidone, ganciclovir, hydroxychloroquine, methotrexate, pyrimethamine, rifabutin, rifampin, sulfonamides

Reactions

Skin

Bullous eruption (<1%)
  (1984): Alarcon GS+, *Arthritis Rheum* 27, 1071
Cyanosis
  (1981): Editorial, *Lancet* 2, 184
Dapsone syndrome*
  (1998): Kumar RH+, *Indian J Lepr* 70, 271 (17 cases)
  (1997): McKenna KE+, *Br J Dermatol* 137, 657
  (1994): Barnard GF+, *Am J Gastroenterol* 89, 2057
  (1994): Hiran S+, *J Assoc Physicians India* 42, 497
  (1994): Risse L+, *Ann Dermatol Venereol* (French) 121, 242
  (1994): Saito S+, *Clin Exp Dermatol* 19, 152
  (1994): Stephen G+, *J Assoc Physicians India* 42, 72
  (1992): Kraus A+, *J Rheumatol* 19, 178
  (1991): Ramanan C+, *Indian J Lepr* 63, 226
  (1988): Grayson ML+, *Lancet* 1, 531
  (1987): Khare AK+, *Indian J Lepr* 59, 106
  (1985): Sharma VK+, *Indian J Lepr* 57, 807
  (1982): Kromann NP+, *Arch Dermatol* 118, 531
  (1981): Tomecki KJ+, *Arch Dermatol* 117, 38
Epidermolysis bullosa
  (1992): Kong LN, *Chung Hua Li Tsa Chih* (Chinese) 27, 495
Erythema multiforme (<1%)
  (2001): Werth V, *Dermatology Times* 15
  (1994): Pertel P+, *Clin Infect Dis* 18, 630
  (1993): Stern RS, *Arch Dermatol* 129, 301 (passim)
  (1981): Frey HM+, *Ann Intern Med* 94, 777
  (1980): Dutta RK, *Lepr India* 52, 306
  (1970): Millikan LE+, *Arch Dermatol* 102, 220
  (1961): Browne SG+, *BMJ* 1, 550 (passim)
Erythema nodosum
  (1993): Stern RS, *Arch Dermatol* 129, 301 (passim)
  (1981): Editorial, *Lancet* 2, 184
  (1970): Millikan LE+, *Arch Dermatol* 102, 220
Erythroderma
  (1989): Patki AH+, *Lepr Rev* 60, 274
Exanthems (1–5%)
  (2002): Thong BY+, *Ann Allergy Asthma Immunol* 88(5), 527 (with pyrimethamine)
  (2001): Werth V, *Dermatology Times* 15
  (1993): Stern RS, *Arch Dermatol* 129, 301 (passim)
  (1986): Lindskov R+, *Dermatologica* 172, 214 (6%)
  (1981): Frey HM+, *Ann Intern Med* 94, 777
  (1981): Tomecki KJ+, *Arch Dermatol* 117, 38
  (1970): Millikan LE+, *Arch Dermatol* 102, 220
  (1968): Ramanujam K+, *Lepr India* 40, 6
  (1965): Rosenthal AL+, *Arch Intern Med* 115, 73 (1–5%)
  (1964): Browne SG, *BMJ* 2, 1041
  (1963): Browne SG, *BMJ* 2, 664 (2%)
Exfoliative dermatitis (<1%)
  (1993): Stern RS, *Arch Dermatol* 129, 301 (passim)
  (1981): Frey HM+, *Ann Intern Med* 94, 777

  (1981): Tomecki KJ+, *Arch Dermatol* 117, 38
  (1980): Lal S+, *Lepr India* 52, 302
  (1971): Browne SG, *BMJ* 2, 558 (passim)
  (1970): Millikan LE+, *Arch Dermatol* 102, 220
  (1963): Browne SG, *BMJ* 2, 664
  (1961): Browne SG+, *BMJ* 1, 550 (passim)
Fixed eruption
  (1988): Tham SN+, *Singapore Med J* 29, 300
  (1982): Sinha MR, *Lepr India* 54, 152
  (1964): Browne SG, *BMJ* 2, 1041 (1–5%)
Flu-like syndrome
  (2001): Werth V, *Dermatology Times* 15
Lichenoid eruption
Lupus erythematosus (<1%)
  (1992): Kraus A+, *J Rheumatol* 19, 178
  (1984): Alarcon GS+, *Arthritis Rheum* 27, 1071 (bullous)
  (1979): Fine RM, *Int J Dermatol* 18, 811
  (1979): Lang PG, *J Am Acad Dermatol* 1, 479
  (1974): Vandersteen PR+, *Arch Dermatol* 110, 95
Photosensitivity (<1%)
  (2001): Stockel S+, *Eur J Dermatol* 11(1), 50
  (1994): Berger TG+, *Arch Dermatol* 130, 609 (in HIV-infected) (4 cases)
  (1989): Dhanapaul S, *Lepr Rev* 60, 147
  (1988): Fumey SM+, *Z Hautkr* (German) 63, 53
  (1987): Joseph MS, *Lepr Rev* 58, 425
  (1979): Lang PG, *J Am Acad Dermatol* 1, 479
Pigmentation
  (1997): David KP+, *Trans R Soc Trop Med Hyg* 91, 204 ("hyperpigmented dermal macules")
  (1977): Sakurai I+, *Int J Lepr Other Mycobact Dis* 45, 343
  (1976): Shelley WB+, *Br J Dermatol* 95, 79 (bluish-gray)
  (1964): Browne SG, *BMJ* 2, 1041
  (1963): Browne SG, *BMJ* 2, 664
  (1961): Browne SG+, *BMJ* 1, 550
Pruritus
  (1964): Browne SG, *BMJ* 2, 1041
Purpura
  (1968): Ramanujam K+, *Lepr India* 40, 6
Rash (sic)
  (2000): Chogle A+, *Indian J Gastroenterol* 19, 85
  (1996): Beumont MG+, *Am J Med* 100, 611
Scleroderma
  (1990): May DG+, *Clin Pharm Ther* 48, 286
Stevens–Johnson syndrome
  (1994): Pertel P+, *Clin Infect Dis* 18, 630
  (1961): Browne SG+, *BMJ* 1, 550 (passim)
Subcorneal pustular dermatosis
  (1983): Halevy S+, *Acta Derm Venereol* (Stockh) 63, 441
Toxic epidermal necrolysis (<1%)
  (1993): Fitzpatrick TB+, *Dermatologic Capsule and Comment* 15, 10 (observation)
  (1993): Stern RS, *Arch Dermatol* 129, 301 (passim)
  (1988): Phillips-Howard PA+, *Br Med J Clin Res Ed* 296, 1605
  (1983): Katoch K+, *Lepr India* 55, 133
  (1981): Editorial, *Lancet* 2, 184
  (1961): Browne SG+, *BMJ* 1, 550
Toxic erythema (sic)
  (1993): Stern RS, *Arch Dermatol* 129, 301 (passim)
Urticaria
  (1970): Millikan LE+, *Arch Dermatol* 102, 220

Nails

Nails – Beau's lines (transverse nail bands)
  (1989): Patki AH+, *Lepr Rev* 60, 274
  (1988): Grayson ML+, *Lancet* 1, 531
  (1984): Daniel CR+, *J Am Acad Dermatol* 10, 250

Other

Acute intermittent porphyria
Agranulocytosis
  (2003): Bhat RM+, *Lepr Rev* 74(2), 167
Headache
Hypersensitivity*
  (2002): Thong BY+, *Ann Allergy Asthma Immunol* 88(5), 527
    (with pyrimethamine)
  (2001): Rao PN+, *Lepr Rev* (72(1) (57)
  (2001): Werth V, *Dermatology Times* 15
  (2000): Chogle A+, *Indian J Gastroenterol* 19, 85
  (1998): Holtzer CD+, *Pharmacotherapy* 18(4), 831
  (1998): Pei-Lin Ng P+, *J Am Acad Dermatol* 39, 646
  (1998): Schlienger RG+, *Epilepsia* 39, S3 (passim)
  (1998): Siegfried EC+, *J Am Acad Dermatol* 39, 797 (passim)
  (1996): Prussick R+, *J Am Acad Dermatol* 35, 346
  (1995): Bocquet H+, *Ann Dermatol Venereol* (French) 122, 514
  (1984): Mohamed KN, *Lepr Rev* 55, 385
Nodular panniculitis
  (1986): Uplekar MW+, *Indian J Lepr* 58, 286
Oral mucosal eruption
  (1981): Frey HM+, *Ann Intern Med* 94, 777
Oral mucosal pigmentation
  (1964): Browne SG, *BMJ* 2, 1041
Porphyria cutanea tarda
  (1992): Shelley WB+, *Advanced Dermatologic Diagnosis* WB
    Saunders, 414 (passim)
Pseudolymphoma
  (1993): Kerl H+, *Dermatology In General Medicine* McGraw-Hill
    New York
Sulfone syndrome
  (2003): Lee KB+, *Ann Pharmacother* 37(7), 1044
Tinnitus

*Note: A hypersensitivity reaction – termed the "sulfone syndrome"
or "dapsone syndrome" – may infrequently develop during the first
six weeks of treatment. This syndrome consists of exfoliative
dermatitis, fever, malaise, nausea, anorexia, hepatitis, jaundice,
lymphadenopathy and hemolytic anemia. See (1982): Kromann NP+,
Arch Dermatol 118, 531

DARBEPOETIN ALFA

Synonym: Erythropoesis stimulating protein
Trade name: Aranesp (Amgen)
Indications: Anemia associated with renal failure and
chemotherapy
Category: Colony stimulating factor; Growth factor; Long-acting
Erythropoetin; Recombinant human erythropoetin
Half-life: Terminal: I.V. = 21 Hours

Reactions

Skin

Edema (21%)
Flu-like syndrome (6%)
Infections
Peripheral edema (11%)
Pruritus (8%)
Rash (sic) (7%)
Upper respiratory infection (14%)
Urticaria

Other

Abdominal pain (12%)
Arthralgia (11–13%)

Back pain (8%)
Cough (10%)
Death (7%)
Dizziness (8–14%)
Fatigue (9–33%)
Fever (9–19%)
Headache
Injection-site pain (7%)
Limb pain (sic) (10%)
Myalgia (21%)
Seizures (<1%)

DAUNORUBICIN

Synonyms: daunomycin; DNR; rubidomycin
Trade name: Cerubidine (Bedford)
Other common trade name: *Daunoxome*
Indications: Acute leukemias
Category: Antineoplastic
Half-life: 14–20 hours
**Clinically important, potentially hazardous interactions
with:** aldesleukin

Reactions

Skin

Angioedema
  (1983): Bronner AK+, *J Am Acad Dermatol* 9, 645
  (1981): Weiss RB+, *Ann Intern Med* 94, 66 (1–5%)
  (1978): Levine N+, *Cancer Treat Rev* 5, 67
  (1970): Freeman AI, *Cancer Chemother Rep* 54, 475
Chills (<1%)
Dermatitis
  (1986): Eddy JL+, *Oncol Nurs Forum* 13, 9
  (1975): Reich SD+, *Cancer Chemother Rep* 59, 677
Erythema
Exanthems
  (1978): Levine N+, *Cancer Treat Rev* 5, 67 (2%)
  (1970): Zanoni G+, *Blut* (German) 25, 20
Flushing
Folliculitis
  (1997): Fournier S+, *Arch Dermatol* 133, 918 (disseminated)
Hypopigmentation
  (1975): Dreizen S+, *Postgrad Med* 58, 150
Neutrophilic eccrine hidradenitis
  (1993): Thorisdottir K+, *J Am Acad Dermatol* 28, 775
Pigmentation
  (2002): Kroumpouzos G+, *J Am Acad Dermatol* 46(2), S1
    (generalized)
  (1992): Anderson LL+, *J Am Acad Dermatol* 26, 255
  (1984): Kelly TM+, *Arch Dermatol* 120, 262
Pruritus
Rash (sic) (<1%)
Urticaria (<1%)
  (1983): Bronner AK+, *J Am Acad Dermatol* 9, 645
  (1981): Weiss RB+, *Ann Intern Med* 94, 66 (1–5%)
  (1970): Freeman AI, *Cancer Chemother Rep* 54, 475

Hair

Hair – alopecia (>10%)
  (1997): Fournier S+, *Arch Dermatol* 133, 918
  (1972): Cridland MD, *Drugs* 3, 352
  (1972): Jacquillat C+, *BMJ* 4, 468
  (1969): Bonadonna G+, *BMJ* 3, 503

Nails

Nails – pigmentation (<1%)
  (1983): James WD+, *Arch Dermatol* 119, 334
  (1982): Daniel CR+, *Cutis* 30, 348
  (1979): Hanada T+, *Nippon Naika Gakkai Zasshi* (Japanese) 68, 1319 (bands)
  (1978): de Marinis M+, *Ann Intern Med* 89, 516

Other

Anaphylactoid reactions
Death
  (2002): Fassas A+, *Br J Haematol* 116(2), 308
Headache
Injection-site cellulitis
  (1989): Kerker BJ+, *Semin Dermatol* 8, 173
Injection-site extravasation
  (2000): Kassner E, *J Pediatr Oncon Nurs* 17, 135
Injection-site necrosis (1–10%)
  (1987): Dufresne RG, *Cutis* 39, 197
  (1979): Dragon LH+, *Ann Intern Med* 91, 58
Injection-site phlebitis
  (1989): Kerker BJ+, *Semin Dermatol* 8, 173
Injection-site ulceration (1–10%)
  (1984): Cox RF, *Am J Hosp Pharm* 41, 2410
Mucositis
  (2002): Fassas A+, *Br J Haematol* 116(2), 308
Oral mucosal lesions
  (1983): Bronner AK+, *J Am Acad Dermatol* 9, 645 (>5%)
  (1975): Dreizen S+, *Postgrad Med* 58, 75
Stomatitis (>10%)
  (1969): Bonadonna G+, *BMJ* 3, 503

DEFEROXAMINE

Trade name: Desferal (Novartis)
Other common trade name: *Desferin*
Indications: Hemochromatosis, acute iron overload
Category: Antidote; Chelating agent
Half-life: 6.1 hours
Clinically important, potentially hazardous interactions with: ascorbic acid

Reactions

Skin

Acne
Angioedema
  (1984): Romeo MA+, *J Inherited Metab Dis* 7, 121
Depigmentation
  (2001): Lopez L+, *Dermatol Surg* 27(9), 795
Dermatitis (sic)
  (1988): Venencie PY+, *Ann Dermatol Venereol* (French) 115, 1174
Edema (<1%)
Erythema (<1%)
Erythema multiforme
Exanthems
Flushing (<1%)
Pigmentation
Pruritus (<1%)
  (1984): Romeo MA+, *J Inherited Metab Dis* 7, 121
Purpura
Rash (sic) (<1%)
Toxic epidermal necrolysis
Urticaria (<1%)

Other

Anaphylactoid reactions (<1%)
Arthralgia
  (2001): Taher A+, *Eur J Haematol* 67(1), 30
Injection-site erythema
Injection-site inflammation (1–10%)
Injection-site pain (1–10%)
Oral mucosal lesions
Tinnitus

DELAVIRDINE

Synonym: U-90152S
Trade name: Rescriptor (Agouron)
Indications: HIV-1 infection
Category: Antiretroviral; Non-nucleoside reverse transcriptase inhibitor
Half-life: 5.8 hours
Clinically important, potentially hazardous interactions with: adefovir, alprazolam, amprenavir, anisindione, anticoagulants, dicumarol, dihydroergotamine, ergot, indinavir, methysergide, midazolam, phenytoin, quinidine, rifampin, triazolam, warfarin

Reactions

Skin

Allergic reactions (sic) (<2%)
Angioedema (<2%)
Cyst (<2%)
Dermatitis (sic) (<2%)
Desquamation (<2%)
Diaphoresis (<2%)
Ecchymoses (<2%)
Edema of lip (<2%)
Erythema (<2%)
Erythema multiforme (<2%)
Exanthems (6.6%)
Folliculitis (<2%)
Fungal dermatitis (sic) (<2%)
Nodules (sic) (<2%)
Peripheral edema (<2%)
Petechiae (<2%)
Pruritus (<2%)
Purpura (<2%)
Rash (sic) (9.8%)
  (2003): Justesen US+, *Br J Clin Pharmacol* 55(1), 100 (with amprenavir)
Seborrhea (<2%)
Stevens–Johnson syndrome (<2%)
Urticaria (<2%)
Vasculitis (<2%)
Vesiculobullous eruption (<2%)
Xerosis (<2%)

Hair

Hair – alopecia (<2%)

Nails

Nails – changes (sic) (<2%)

Other

Aphthous stomatitis (<2%)
Dysgeusia (<2%)

Gingivitis (<2%)
Gynecomastia (<2%)
Headache
Hyperesthesia (<2%)
Myalgia (<2%)
Oral ulceration (<2%)
Paresthesias (<2%)
Rhabdomyolysis
  (2002): Castro JG+, Am J Med 112(6), 505 (with atorvastatin)
Sialorrhea (<2%)
Stomatitis (<2%)
Tingling (<2%)
Tongue edema (<2%)
Vaginal candidiasis (<2%)
Xerostomia (<2%)

DEMECLOCYCLINE

Trade name: Declomycin (Wyeth)
Other common trade names: *Ledermicina; Ledermycin; Rynabron*
Indications: Various infections caused by susceptible organisms
Category: Tetracycline antibiotic
Half-life: 10–17 hours
Clinically important, potentially hazardous interactions with: amoxicillin, ampicillin, antacids, bacampicillin, calcium carbonate, carbenicillin, cloxacillin, digoxin, methotrexate, methoxyflurane, mezlocillin, nafcillin, oxacillin, penicillins, piperacillin, ticarcillin

Reactions

Skin
Acne
  (1969): Weary PE+, Arch Dermatol 100, 179
Angioedema
Bullous eruption
Candidiasis
Exanthems
Exfoliative dermatitis (<1%)
Fixed eruption
  (1978): Jolly HW+, Arch Dermatol 114, 1484
  (1970): Delaney TJ, Br J Dermatol 83, 357
  (1970): Savin JA, Br J Dermatol 83, 546
  (1968): Sarkany I, Proc R Soc Med 61, 891
Lichenoid eruption
  (1972): Jones HE+, Arch Dermatol 106, 58
Lupus erythematosus
Perianal rash
Photosensitivity (1–10%)
  (1984): Kromann N+, Ugeskr Laeger (Danish) 146, 515
  (1980): Stern RS+, Arch Dermatol 116, 1269
  (1974): Maibach HI+, Arch Dermatol 109, 97 (1.5%) (lichenoid)
  (1972): Jones HE+, Arch Dermatol 106, 58 (lichenoid)
  (1971): Frost P+, JAMA 216, 326 (90%)
  (1971): Ippen H, Hautarzt (German) 22, 549
  (1971): Kahn G+, Arch Dermatol 103, 94
  (1968): Stratigos JD+, Br J Dermatol 80, 391
  (1967): Kotani Y, Acta Dermatol Kyoto Engl Ed (Japanese) 62, 188
  (1965): Clendenning WE, Arch Dermatol 91, 628 (20%)
  (1962): de Veber LL, Can Med Assoc J 86, 168
  (1962): Hicks JH, South Med J 55, 357
  (1961): Orentreich N+, Arch Dermatol 83, 68
  (1961): Shapiro JL+, JAMA 176, 596

  (1960): Carey BW, JAMA 172, 1196 (1.5%)
  (1960): Falk MS, JAMA 172, 1156
  (1960): Fuhrman DL+, Arch Dermatol 82, 244
  (1960): Morris WE, JAMA 172, 1155
Phototoxicity
  (1968): Blank H+, Arch Dermatol 97, 1 (90%)
  (1961): Cahn MM+, Arch Dermatol 84, 485
  (1961): Saslaw S, N Engl J Med 264, 1301
Pigmentation
Pruritus (<1%)
Pruritus ani
Purpura
Stevens–Johnson syndrome
Toxic epidermal necrolysis
  (1988): Massullo RE+, J Am Acad Dermatol 19, 358
Urticaria

Nails
Nails – onycholysis
Nails – photo-onycholysis
  (1977): Bethell HJN, BMJ 2, 96
  (1974): Bettley FR+, Proc R Soc Med 67, 600
  (1973): Verma KC+, Indian J Dermatol 18, 23
  (1972): Cabre J+, Actas Dermosifiliogr (Spanish) 63, 211
  (1962): de Veber LL, Can Med Assoc J 86, 168
  (1961): Orentreich N+, Arch Dermatol 83, 68
Nails – pigmentation (<1%)

Other
Anaphylactoid reactions (<1%)
Glossitis
Mucous membrane pigmentation
Oral mucosal eruption
  (1964): Martin WJ, Med Clin North Am 48, 255
Paresthesias (<1%)
Porphyria
  (1979): Boissonnas A+, Nouv Presse Med (French) 8, 210
Pseudotumor cerebri
Tongue pigmentation
Tooth discoloration

DENILEUKIN

Trade name: Ontak (Ligand)
Indications: Cutaneous T-cell lymphoma
Category: Antineoplastic
Half-life: distribution: 2–5 minutes; terminal: 70–80 minutes

Reactions

Skin
Allergic reactions (sic) (1%)
Bullous eruption
Chills (81%)
Diaphoresis (10%)
Ecchymoses
Edema (47%)
Exanthems
Flushing
Infections (sic) (48%)
Petechiae
Pruritus (20%)
Purpura
Rash (sic) (34%)
Urticaria
Vesicular eruptions

Other

Anaphylactoid reactions (1%)
Headache
Hypersensitivity (69%)
Injection-site reactions (sic) (8%)
Myalgia (18%)
Paresthesias (13%)
Phlebitis
Thrombophlebitis

DESFLURANE

Trade name: Suprane (Baxter)
Other common trade name: *Sulorane*
Indications: Induction or maintenance of anesthesia
Category: General anesthetic
Half-life: Onset of action: 1–2 minutes
**Clinically important, potentially hazardous interactions
with:** tramadol

Reactions

Skin

Pruritus
Shivering
(1998): Horn EP+, *Anesthesiology* 89(4), 878

Other

Cough (34%)
Death
(1998): Murray JM+, *Can J Anaesth* 45(12), 1200 (4 cases)
Malignant hyperthermia
(2000): Lane JE+, *Anesth Analg* 91(4), 1032
(1999): Garrido S+, *Anesthesiology* 90(4), 1208
(1998): Allen GC+, *Anesth Analg* 86(6), 1328
(1998): Celebioglu B, *Anesth Analg* 86(4), 916
(1998): Lowes R+, *Anesth Analg* 86(2), 449
(1997): Michalek-Sauberer A+, *Anesth Analg* 85(2), 461
(1996): Fu ES+, *Can J Anaesth* 43(7), 687
Myalgia
Pharyngitis (3–10%)

DESIPRAMINE

Trade name: Norpramin (Aventis)
Other common trade names: *Deprexan; Nebril; Nortimil;
Pertofran; Pertofrane; Petylyl; PMS-Desipramine*
Indications: Depression
Category: Tricyclic antidepressant
Half-life: 7–60 hours
**Clinically important, potentially hazardous interactions
with:** amprenavir, arbutamine, clonidine, epinephrine, fluoxetine,
formoterol, guanethidine, isocarboxazid, linezolid, MAO
inhibitors, phenelzine, quinolones, sparfloxacin, tranylcypromine

Reactions

Skin

Acne
Allergic reactions (sic) (<1%)
(1987): Joffe RT+, *Can J Psychiatry* 32, 695
(1987): Richter MA+, *Am J Psychiatry* 144, 526

Angioedema
(1963): Mann AM+, *Can Med Assoc J* 88, 1102
Diaphoresis (1–10%)
(1965): Editorial, *JAMA* 194, 82
Ecchymoses
(1968): Rachmilewitz EA+, *Blood* 32, 524
Edema
Erythema
Exanthems
(1988): Biederman J+, *J Clin Psychiatry* 49, 178 (5.8%)
(1988): McLean JD, *Can J Psychiatry* 33, 331
(1987): Ellsworth A+, *Drug Intell Clin Pharm* 21, 510
(1987): Joffe RT+, *Can J Psychiatry* 32, 695 (6.2%)
(1968): Powell WJ+, *JAMA* 206, 642
Exfoliative dermatitis
(1968): Powell WJ+, *JAMA* 206, 642
Flushing
(1965): Editorial, *JAMA* 194, 82
Petechiae
(1968): Rachmilewitz EA+, *Blood* 32, 524
Photosensitivity (1.4%)
(1965): Editorial, *JAMA* 194, 82
Pigmentation (blue-gray) (photosensitive)
(1993): Narurkar V+, *Arch Dermatol* 129, 474
(1993): Steele TE+, *J Clin Psychopharmacol* 13, 76
Pruritus
(1988): Biederman J+, *J Clin Psychiatry* 49, 178
(1987): Ellsworth A+, *Drug Intell Clin Pharm* 21, 510
(1987): Pohl R+, *Am J Psychiatry* 144, 237
(1968): Powell WJ+, *JAMA* 206, 642
Purpura
(1980): Miescher PA+, *Clin Haematol* 9, 505
(1968): Rachmilewitz EA+, *Blood* 32, 524
Rash (sic)
(1965): Editorial, *JAMA* 194, 82
Side effects (sic)
(2002): Galanter CA+, *J Child Adolesc Psychopharmacol*
12(2), 137
Urticaria
(1991): Bajwa WK+, *J Nerv Ment Dis* 179, 108
(1988): Biederman J+, *J Clin Psychiatry* 49, 178
(1987): Pohl R+, *Am J Psychiatry* 144, 237
Vasculitis
Xerosis

Hair

Hair – alopecia (<1%)
(1991): Warnock JK+, *J Nerv Ment Dis* 179, 441

Other

Black tongue
Bromhidrosis
Dry mouth
(2002): Galanter CA+, *J Child Adolesc Psychopharmacol*
12(2), 137
Dysgeusia (>10%)
Galactorrhea (<1%)
Gynecomastia (<1%)
Hypersensitivity
Mucous membrane desquamation
(1968): Powell WJ+, *JAMA* 206, 642
Paresthesias
Pseudolymphoma
(1995): Magro CM+, *J Am Acad Dermatol* 32, 419
(1988): Kardaun SH+, *Br J Dermatol* 118(4), 545
Stomatitis
Tinnitus
Xerostomia (>10%)

(2002): Galanter CA+, *J Child Adolesc Psychopharmacol*
12(2), 137
(1993): Pataki CS+, *J Am Acad Child Adolesc Psychiatry* 32, 1065
(1965): Editorial, *JAMA* 194, 82

DESLORATADINE

Trade name: Clarinex (Schering)
Indications: Allergic rhinitis, urticaria
Category: Antihistamine
Half-life: 27 hours

Reactions

Skin
None

Other
Anaphylactoid reactions
Hypersensitivity
Myalgia
Xerostomia

DESMOPRESSIN

Trade names: DDAVP (Aventis); Stimate (Aventis)
Other common trade names: *Defirin; Desmospray; Minirin; Minurin; Octostim*
Indications: Primary nocturnal enuresis
Category: Antidiuretic pituitary hormone; Antihemophilic; Antihemorrhagic
Half-life: 75 minutes

Reactions

Skin
Allergic reactions (sic)
(1982): Yokota M+, *Endocrinol Jpn* 29, 475
Diaphoresis
(1985): Richardson DW+, *Ann Intern Med* 103, 228
Edema
Flushing (1–10%)
(1985): Richardson DW+, *Ann Intern Med* 103, 228 (1–5%)
Rash (sic)

Other
Headache
Injection-site edema
Injection-site erythema
Injection-site pain (1–10%)
Seizures
(2002): Pruthi RS+, *J Urol* 168(1), 187
Syndrome of inappropriate antidiuretic hormone secretion (SIADH)
(2002): Pruthi RS+, *J Urol* 168(1), 187

DEVIL'S CLAW

Scientific names: *Harpagophytum procumbens; Harpagophytum zeyheri*
Family: Pedaliaceae
Trade and other common names: Doloteffin; Grapple plant; Griffe du diable; Harpadol; wood spider
Trade names: Doloteffin, Harpadol
Category: Analgesic; Anti-inflammatory; Antioxidant; Antiviral; Diuretic
Purported indications and other uses: Oral: anorexia, arteriosclerosis, rheumatoid arthritis, GI disorders, fibromyalgia, loss of appetite, headache, fever, high cholesterol, menstrual complaints, liver and gallbladder problems. Topical: rash, ulcers
Half-life: 3–6 hours
Clinically important, potentially hazardous interactions with: anesthetics, antacids, antiarrhythmic drugs, anticoagulants, aspirin, beta blockers, digoxin, histamine 2 blockers (e.g ranitidine and famotidine), hypoglycemics, NSAIDs, sympathomimetics, terfenadine, warfarin

Reactions

Skin
Adverse effects (sic)
(2003): Chrubasik S+, *Rheumatology* (Oxford) 42(1), 141
(2002): Chrubasik S+, *Phytomedicine* 9(3), 181
(2001): Gobel H+, *Schmerz* 15(1), 10
(2000): Chantre P+, *Phytomedicine* 7(3), 177

Other
Dysgeusia
(1981): Grahame R+, *Ann Rheum Dis* 40, 632
Tinnitus
(1981): Grahame R+, *Ann Rheum Dis* 40, 632

Note: Devil's claw stimulates stomach acid production, and should be avoided by those with stomach or duodenal ulcers. It should not be taken by people with cardiac arrhythmias or other heart problems

DEXCHLORPHENIRAMINE

Trade names: Poladex; Polaramine (Schering); Tanafed (First Horizon)
Other common trade names: *Delamin; Polaramin; Polaronil; Polazit; Trenolone*
Indications: Allergic rhinitis, urticaria
Category: Antihistamine H_1-blocker
Half-life: 20–24 hours
Clinically important, potentially hazardous interactions with: barbiturates, chloral hydrate, ethchlorvynol, glutethimide, phenothiazines, zolpidem

Reactions

Skin
Angioedema (<1%)
Chills
Dermatitis
(1989): Cusano F+, *Contact Dermatitis* 21, 340
Diaphoresis
Edema (<1%)
Photosensitivity (<1%)
Rash (sic) (<1%)
Urticaria

Other
Anaphylactoid reactions
Headache
Myalgia (<1%)
Paresthesias (<1%)
Xerostomia (1–10%)

DEXMEDETOMIDINE

Trade name: Precedex (Abbott)
Indications: Sedation for intensive care unit intubation
Category: Alpha-adrenoceptor blocker; Sedative
Half-life: 2 hours

Reactions

Skin
Diaphoresis (<1%)
Infections (sic) (2%)
Photopsia (<1%)
Xerosis

Other
Pain (3%)
Sialopenia
(1990): Aantaa RE+, *Anesth Analg* 70, 407

DEXTROAMPHETAMINE

Trade names: Adderall (Shire); Dexedrine (GSK)
Other common trade names: *Dexamphetamine; Dexamphetamini; Dextrostat; Ferndex; Oxydess*
Indications: Narcolepsy, attention deficit disorder (ADD)
Category: Amphetamine; Central nervous system stimulant
Half-life: 10–12 hours
Clinically important, potentially hazardous interactions with: fluoxetine, fluvoxamine, MAO inhibitors, paroxetine, phenelzine, sertraline, tranylcypromine

Reactions

Skin
Chills
Diaphoresis (1–10%)
Rash (sic) (<1%)
Toxic epidermal necrolysis
(1975): Giallorenzi AF+, *Oral Surg Oral Med Oral Pathol* 40, 611
Urticaria (<1%)

Other
Dysgeusia
Headache
Rhabdomyolysis
(2000): Richards JR, *J Emerg Med* 19(1), 51
(1999): Hedetoft C+, *Ugeskr Laeger* 161(50), 6907
(1998): Robertsen A+, *Tidsskr Nor Laegeforen* 118(28), 4340
(1996): Hofland E+, *Ned Tijdschr Geneeskd* 140(12), 681
(1996): Roebroek RM+, *Ned Tijdschr Geneeskd* 140(29), 1519
(1996): Roebroek RM+, *Ned Tijdschr Geneeskd* 140(4), 205
(1996): Sultana SR+, *J R Coll Surg Edinb* 41(6), 419
(1992): Kao CH+, *Clin Nucl Med* 17(2), 101
(1990): Yamazaki F+, *Nippon Naika Gakkai* 79(1), 100
(1977): Kendrick WC+, *Ann Intern Med* 86(4), 381 (5 cases)
Xerostomia (1–10%)

DEXTROMETHORPHAN

Trade names: Benylin (Warner Lambert); Cheracol-D; Pertussin; Robitussin (Wyeth); Sucrets; Suppress; Trocal; Vicks Formula 44 (Procter & Gamble)
Other common trade names: *Balminil; Delsym; Koffex; Triaminic DM*
Indications: Nonproductive cough
Category: Antitussive (nonnarcotic)
Half-life: N/A
Clinically important, potentially hazardous interactions with: linezolid, phenelzine, sibutramine, tranylcypromine, valdecoxib

Reactions

Skin
Bullous eruption
(1999): Sahn EE, *Dermatology Times* April, 5 (infant with urticaria pigmentosa)
(1996): Cook J+, *Pediatr Dermatol* 13, 410 (infant with urticaria pigmentosa)
Fixed eruption
(1991): Smoller BR+, *J Cutan Pathol* 18, 13
(1990): Stubb S+, *Arch Dermatol* 126, 970

Other
Anaphylactoid reactions
(1998): Knowles SR+, *J Allergy Clin Immunol* 102, 316
Headache

DIACETYLMORPHINE

(See HEROIN)

DIAZEPAM

Trade names: Diastat (Elan); Dizac; Valium (Roche)
Other common trade names: *Assival; Dialar; Diapax; Diazemuls; Ducene; E-Pam; Meval; Novazam; Solis; Vivol*
Indications: Anxiety
Category: Anxiolytic; Benzodiazepine sedative-hypnotic
Half-life: 20–70 hours
Clinically important, potentially hazardous interactions with: alcohol, amprenavir, barbiturates, chlorpheniramine, clarithromycin, CNS depressants, efavirenz, esomeprazole, fluoroquinolones, imatinib, indinavir, ivermectin, macrolide antibiotics, MAO inhibitors, methadone, nalbuphine, narcotics, nelfinavir, phenothiazines, ritonavir, SSRIs

Reactions

Skin
Acne
(1962): Grayson LD, *Gen Pract* 25, 9
Allergic reactions (sic)
(1982): Allin DM, *Curr Med Res Opin* 8, 33
(1977): Padfield A+, *BMJ* 1, 575
Angioedema
(1974): Felix RH+, *Lancet* 1, 1017
Bullous eruption
(1977): Varma AJ+, *Arch Intern Med* 137, 1207
Dermatitis (sic) (1–10%)

(1995): Fisher AA, *Cutis* 55, 327 (systemic)
(1995): Kampgen E+, *Contact Dermatitis* 33, 356
(1994): Garcia-Bravo B+, *Contact Dermatitis* 30, 40
Diaphoresis (>10%)
Eczema (sic)
(1974): Felix RH+, *Lancet* 1, 1017
Edema of foot
(1982): Stadler R+, *Hautarzt* (German) 33, 276
Exanthems
(1986): Bigby M+, *JAMA* 256, 3358 (0.04%)
(1981): Adverse Drug Reaction List, *Jpn Med Gaz* (Japanese)
18:6–7, 16
(1976): Arndt KA+, *JAMA* 235, 918 (0.38%)
(1967): Jenner FA+, *Dis Nerv Syst* 28, 245
(1964): Holt KS, *Ann Physiol Med* (Suppl) 16
(1963): Love J, *Dis Nerv Syst* 24, 674
Exfoliative dermatitis
(1967): Satyadas JS+, *J Indian Med Assoc* 3, 49
(1963): Love J, *Dis Nerv Syst* 24, 674
Fixed eruption (<1%)
(1979): Olumide F, *Int J Dermatol* 18, 818
(1966): Jadassohn W+, *Dermatologica* 133, 91
Flushing
(1964): Holt KS, *Ann Physiol Med* (Suppl) 16
Granuloma disciformis (Miescher)
(1969): Clarke DM, *Australas J Dermatol* 10, 194
Melanoma
(1981): Adam S+, *Lancet* 2, 1344
Pigmentation
(2002): Viale PH+, *Clin J Oncol Nurs* 6(5), 310
(1980): Ferreira JA, *Aesthetic Plast Surg* 4, 343
Pruritus
(1995): Kampgen E+, *Contact Dermatitis* 33, 356
Purpura
(1985): Ambriz-Fernandez R+, *Rev Invest Clin* (Spanish) 37, 347
(1980): Miescher PA+, *Clin Haematol* 9, 505
(1977): Cimo PL+, *Am J Hematol* 2, 65
(1977): Ghosh JS, *BMJ* 1, 902
Rash (sic) (>10%)
(1983): O'Brien JE+, *Curr Ther Res* 34, 825
Urticaria
(1987): Deardon DJ+, *Br J Anaesth* 59, 391
Vasculitis
(1999): Olcina GM+, *Am J Psychiatry* 156, 972

Nails
Nails – parrot-beak
(1971): Kandil E, *J Med Liban* 24, 433

Other
Anaphylactoid reactions
(1987): Deardon DJ+, *Br J Anaesth* 59, 391
Dizziness
(2002): Cereghino JJ+, *Arch Neurol* 59(12), 1915
Gynecomastia
(2000): Hugues FC+, *Ann Med Interne (Paris)* (French) 151, 10 (passim)
(1994): Llop R+, *Ann Pharmacother* 28, 671
(1979): Moerck HJ+, *Lancet* 1, 1344 (letter)
Headache
Hypersensitivity
(2002): Asero R, *Allergy* 57(12), 1209
Injection-site pain
(2002): Majedi H+, *Anesth Analg* 95(5), 1297
Injection-site phlebitis (>10%)
(1981): Clarke RSJ, *Drugs* 22, 26 (39%)
(1980): Schou-Olesen A+, *Br J Anaesth* 52, 609
Paresthesias
Porphyria

(1979): Stone DR+, *Br J Anaesth* 51, 809
(1978): Mees DE+, *South Med J* 68, 29
Porphyria variegata
Rhabdomyolysis
(1982): Bogaerts Y+, *Clin Nephrol* 17(4), 206
Sialorrhea
Tongue furry
Xerostomia (>10%)

DIAZOXIDE

Trade name: Hyperstat (Schering)
Other common trade names: *Eudimine; Proglicem; Proglycem; Sefulken*
Indications: Hypoglycemia, hypertension
Category: Antihypertensive; Antihypoglycemic
Half-life: 20–36 hours
Clinically important, potentially hazardous interactions with: phenytoin

Reactions

Skin
Candidiasis
Cellulitis (<1%)
Diaphoresis
Edema
Exanthems
Flushing (<1%)
Herpes (sic)
Leukomelanosis (sic)
(1967): Saito T+, *Acta Dermatol* (Kyoto) 61, 207
Lichenoid eruption
(1975): Burton JL+, *Br J Dermatol* 93, 707
(1973): Menter MA, *Proc R Soc Med* 66, 326
Photosensitivity
(1967): Saito T+, *Acta Dermatol* (Kyoto) 61, 207
Pruritus
Purpura
Rash (sic) (<1%)
Urticaria
Xerosis
(1975): Burton JL+, *Br J Dermatol* 93, 707

Hair
Hair – alopecia
(1975): Burton JL+, *Br J Dermatol* 93, 707
(1972): Milner RD+, *Arch Dis Child* 47, 537
Hair – hypertrichosis (<1%)
(1989): Rousseau C+, *Dermatologica* 179, 221
(1988): Prigent F+, *Ann Dermatol Venereol* (French) 115, 191
(1987): Turpin G+, *Presse Med* (French) 16, 398
(1983): Schiazza L+, *G Ital Dermatol Venereol* (Italian) 118, 113
(1981): Perez-Mijares R+, *Rev Clin Esp* (Spanish) 162, 225
(1975): Burton JL+, *Br J Dermatol* 93, 707 (>5%)
(1973): Menter MA, *Proc R Soc Med* 66, 326
(1972): Leng JJ+, *Pediatr Clin North Am* 19, 681
(1972): Milner RD+, *Arch Dis Child* 47, 537
(1968): Koblenzer PJ+, *Ann N Y Acad Sci* 150, 373

Other
Ageusia
Dysgeusia
Headache
Hypersensitivity
Injection-site pain (<1%)

Injection-site phlebitis (<1%)
Paresthesias
Sialorrhea
Tinnitus
Xerostomia

DICLOFENAC

Trade names: Arthrotec (Pharmacia); Solaraze Gel (Bioglan); Voltaren (Novartis)
Other common trade names: *Allvoran; Apo-Diclo; Fenac; Galedol; Liroken; Monoflam; Nu-Diclo; Remethan; Taks; Voltarene; Voltarol*
Indications: Rheumatoid and osteoarthritis
Category: Nonsteroidal anti-inflammatory (NSAID)
Half-life: 1–2 hours
Clinically important, potentially hazardous interactions with: methotrexate

Arthrotec is diclofenac and misoprostol

Reactions

Skin

Adverse effects (sic)
   (1986): Catalano MA, *Am J Med* 80, 81
Allergic reactions (sic)
   (1992): Schiavino D+, *Contact Dermatitis* 26, 357
   (1979): Ciucci AG, *Rheum Rehab* 18 (Suppl 2), 116
Angioedema (1–3%)
   (2000): Hadar A+, *Harefuah* (Hebrew) 138, 211 (from suppository)
Bullous eruption (1–3%)
   (1982): Valsecchi R+, *G Ital Derm Venereol* (Italian) 117, 221
   (1981): Gabrielsen TO+, *Acta Derm Venereol* (Stockh) 61, 439
Dermatitis (sic) (1–3%)
   (2002): Bohannon JS, Midlothian, VA (from Internet) (observation)
   (2002): Kerr OA+, *Contact Dermatitis* 47(3), 175
   (2002): Sorkin M, Denver, CO (from Internet) (observation)
   (1998): Ueda K+, *Contact Dermatitis* 39, 323
   (1996): Gonzalo MA+, *Dermatology* 193, 59
   (1996): Valsecchi R+, *Contact Dermatitis* 34, 150
   (1994): Gebhardt M+, *Contact Dermatitis* 30, 183
   (1994): Romano A+, *Allergy* 49, 57
Dermatitis herpetiformis
   (1989): Grob JJ+, *Dermatologica* 178, 58
   (1981): Gabrielsen TO+, *Acta Derm Venereol* (Stockh) 61, 439
Dermatomyositis
   (1989): Grob JJ+, *Dermatologica* 178, 58
Diaphoresis (<1%)
Eczema (sic) (1–3%)
Edema
Eruptions
   (1998): Schaad HJ+, *Ther Umsch* (German) 55, 586
Erythema (sic)
   (1998): Schaad HJ+, *Ther Umsch* (German) 55, 586 (generalized)
   (1992): Barrett PJ+, *Anaesthesia* 47, 83
   (1979): Ciucci AG, *Rheum Rehab* 18 (Suppl 2), 116
Erythema multiforme (<1%)
   (1999): Emmett SD, Solana Beach, CA (from internet) (observation)
   (1996): Delrio FG+, *Am J Med Sci* 312(2), 95
   (1995): Dhar S+, *Dermatology* 191, 76
   (1993): Khalil H+, *Arch Intern Med* 153, 1649
   (1988): Todd PA+, *Drugs* 35, 244

   (1985): Morris BAP+, *Can Med Assoc J* 133, 665
   (1982): Seigneuric C+, *Ann Dermatol Venereol* (French) 109, 287
Erythema nodosum (<1%)
Exanthems (1–5%)
   (1994): Romano A+, *Allergy* 49, 57
   (1992): Breathnach SM+, *Adverse Drug Reactions and the Skin* Blackwell, Oxford, 188 (passim)
   (1988): Todd PA+, *Drugs* 35, 244
   (1986): Halevy S+, *Harefuah* (Hebrew) 110, 30
   (1985): Morris BAP+, *Can Med Assoc J* 133, 665
   (1979): Ciucci AG, *Rheum Rehab* 18 (Suppl 2), 116
Exfoliative dermatitis (<1%)
Fixed eruption
   (1998): Mahboob A+, *Int J Dermatol* 37, 833
Flushing (<1%)
Lichenoid eruption
   (1999): Fetterman M, Miami, FL (from Internet) (observation)
Linear IgA bullous dermatosis
   (2002): Cohen LM+, *J Am Acad Dermatol* 46, S32 (passim)
   (1997): Paul C+, *Br J Dermatol* 136, 406
   (1982): Valsecchi R+, *G Ital Derm Venereol* (Italian) 117, 221
   (1981): Gabrielsen TO+, *Acta Derm Venereol* (Stockh) 61, 439
Lupus erythematosus
Necrotizing fasciitis
   (2002): Verfaillie G+, *Eur J Emerg Med* 9(3), 270
Pemphigus
   (1997): Matz H+, *Dermatology* 195, 48
Peripheral edema
   (2002): Chan FK+, *N Engl J Med* 347(26), 2104 (with omeprazole)
Photoallergic reaction
   (2003): Montoro J+, *Contact Dermatitis* 48(2), 115
Photosensitivity (1–3%)
   (1998): Encinas S+, *Chem Res Toxicol* 11, 946
   (1997): O'Reilly FM+, American Academy of Dermatology Meeting, Poster #14
   (1996): Becker L+, *Acta Derm Venereol* (Stockh) 76, 337
   (1992): Le Corre Y+, *Ann Dermatol Venereol* (French) 119, 923 (granuloma annulare type)
   (1988): Todd PA+, *Drugs* 35, 244
Pruritus (1–10%)
   (1995): Litt JZ, Beachwood, OH (personal case) (observation)
   (1994): Litt JZ, Beachwood, OH (personal case) (observation)
   (1992): Breathnach SM+, *Adverse Drug Reactions and the Skin* Blackwell, Oxford, 188 (passim)
   (1988): Todd PA+, *Drugs* 35, 244
   (1981): Gabrielsen TO+, *Acta Derm Venereol* (Stockh) 61, 439
   (1979): Ciucci AG, *Rheum Rehab* 18 (Suppl 2), 116
Pseudoreactions (sic)
   (1991): VanArsdel PP, *JAMA* 266, 3343
Psoriasis
   (1999): Dintiman B, Fairfax, VA (from Internet) (observation)
   (1999): Fetterman M, Miami, FL (from Internet) (observation)
   (1987): Sendagorta E+, *Dermatologica* 175, 300 (pustular)
Purpura (1–3%)
   (1988): Todd PA+, *Drugs* 35, 244
   (1979): Ciucci AG, *Rheum Rehab* 18 (Suppl 2), 116
Purpura fulminans
   (2002): Hengge UR+, *Hautarzt* 53(7), 483
Pustular psoriasis
   (1999): Dintiman B, Fairfax, VA (from Internet) (observation)
   (1999): Fetterman M, Miami, FL (from Internet) (observation)
   (1987): Sendagorta E+, *Dermatologica* 175, 300
Rash (sic) (>10%)
   (1978): Abrams GJ+, *S Afr Med J* 53, 442
Stevens–Johnson syndrome (1–3%) (1 fatal case)
   (1988): Todd PA+, *Drugs* 35, 244
   (1979): Ciucci AG, *Rheum Rehab* 18 (Suppl 2), 116
Toxic epidermal necrolysis

(1998): Choi KL, Toronto, Canada (from Internet) (observation)
(1993): Correia O+, *Dermatology* 186, 32
(1985): Kamanabroo D+, *Arch Dermatol* 121, 1548
Urticaria (1–3%)
(1998): Gala G+, *Allergy* 53, 623
(1995): Litt JZ, Beachwood, OH (personal case) (observation)
(1995): Rademaker M, *N Z Med J* 108, 165
(1992): Breathnach SM+, *Adverse Drug Reactions and the Skin*
Blackwell, Oxford, 188 (passim)
(1988): Todd PA+, *Drugs* 35, 244
(1979): Ciucci AG, *Rheum Rehab* 18 (Suppl 2), 116
Vasculitis
(1999): Emmet S, Solana Beach, CA (from Internet) (from
ophthalmic solution) (observation)
(1997): Morros R+, *Br J Rheumatol* 36, 503
(1992): Breathnach SM+, *Adverse Drug Reactions and the Skin*
Blackwell, Oxford, 188 (passim)
(1982): Bonafe JL+, *Ann Dermatol Venereol* (French) 109, 283

Hair

Hair – alopecia (1–3%)

Other

Acute intermittent porphyria
Anaphylactoid reactions (1–3%)
(2000): Hadar A+, *Harefuah* (Hebrew) 138, 211 (from
suppository)
(2000): Ray M+, *Indian Pediatr* 36, 1067 (fatal)
(1999): Enrique E+, *Allergy* 54, 529
(1996): Levy JH+, *N Engl J Med* 335, 1925
(1993): Alkhawajah AM+, *Forensic Sci Int* 60, 107
(1993): van der Klauw MM+, *Br J Clin Pharmacol* 35, 400
(1992): *Australian Adverse Drug Reactions Bulletin* 11, 7
Aphthous stomatitis
(1988): Todd PA+, *Drugs* 35, 244
Death
(2002): Hengge UR+, *Hautarzt* 53(7), 483
(2002): Verfaillie G+, *Eur J Emerg Med* 9(3), 270
Dysgeusia (1–3%)
Embolia cutis medicamentosa (Nicolau syndrome)
(2003): Reding EL+, *J Am Acad Dermatol* 48(3), 472 (passim)
(2002): Poletti E+, *World Congress Dermatol* Poster, 0124
(1999): Forsbach Sanchez G+, *Rev Invest Clin* (Spanish) 51, 71
(1992): Stricker BH+, *Ann Intern Med* 117(12), 1058
Headache
Hypersensitivity
(2000): del Pozo MD+, *Allergy* 55, 412
(1998): Romano A+, *Ann Allergy Asthma Immunol* 81, 373
Injection-site necrosis
(1989): Tweedie DG, *Anaesthesia* 44, 932
Injection-site pain
(1998): Schaad HJ+, *Ther Umsch* (German) 55, 586
Oral ulceration
(2000): Madinier I+, *Ann Med Interne (Paris)* (French) 151, 248
Paresthesias (<1%)
Pseudolymphoma
(2001): Werth V, *Dermatology Times* 18
Rhabdomyolysis
(2002): Hengge UR+, *Hautarzt* 53(7), 483
(1996): Delrio FG+, *Am J Med Sci* 312(2), 95
Serum sickness
Still's disease
(1985): Wouters JM+, *J Rheumatol* 12, 791
Stomatitis (<1%)
Tinnitus
Tongue edema (1–3%)
Xerostomia (1–3%)
(1988): Todd PA+, *Drugs* 35, 244

DICLOXACILLIN

Trade names: Dycill (GSK); Dynapen (Bristol-Myers Squibb)
Other common trade names: *Brispen; Dichlor-Stapenor; Diclo;
Diclocil; Diclocillin; Diclox; Novapen; Pathocil; Posipen*
Indications: Infections due to penicillinase-producing
staphylococci
Category: Penicillinase-resistant penicillin
Half-life: 0.5–1.0 hours
**Clinically important, potentially hazardous interactions
with:** anticoagulants, cyclosporine, methotrexate, tetracycline

Reactions

Skin

Angioedema
Bullous eruption
Dermatitis (sic)
Ecchymoses
Erythema multiforme
(1991): Porteous DM+, *Arch Dermatol* 127, 740
Erythema nodosum
Erythroderma
(1985): Shelley WB+, *Cutis* 220, 224
Exanthems (<1%)
Exfoliative dermatitis (<1%)
Hematomas
Jarisch–Herxheimer reaction
Pruritus
(1998): Siegfried EC+, *J Am Acad Dermatol* 39, 797 (passim)
Purpura
Rash (sic) (<1%)
Stevens–Johnson syndrome
(1991): Porteous DM+, *Arch Dermatol* 127, 740
Toxic epidermal necrolysis
Urticaria
(1998): Siegfried EC+, *J Am Acad Dermatol* 39, 797 (passim)
(1985): Green RL+, *JAMA* 254, 531 (postcoital)
Vasculitis
Vesicular eruptions

Nails

Nails – shoreline
(1985): Shelley WB+, *Cutis* 220, 224

Other

Anaphylactoid reactions
(1998): Siegfried EC+, *J Am Acad Dermatol* 39, 797 (passim)
Black tongue
Dysgeusia
Glossitis
Glossodynia
Hypersensitivity (<1%)
Injection-site pain
Myalgia
Oral candidiasis
Serum sickness (<1%)
Stomatitis
Stomatodynia
Vaginitis (<1%)
Xerostomia

DICUMAROL

Synonym: bishydroxycoumarin
Trade name: Dicumarol (Abbott)
Other common trade names: *Apekumarol; Dicumol; Embolin*
Indications: Atrial fibrillation, pulmonary embolism, venous thrombosis
Category: Anticoagulant
Half-life: 1–4 days
Clinically important, potentially hazardous interactions with: allopurinol, amiodarone, amobarbital, anabolic steroids, anti-thyroid agents, aprobarbital, aspirin, barbiturates, bivalirudin, butabarbital, butalbital, cimetidine, clofibrate, clopidogrel, cyclosporine, delavirdine, disulfiram, fenofibrate, fluconazole, gemfibrozil, glutethimide, imatinib, itraconazole, ketoconazole, levothyroxine, liothyronine, mephobarbital, methimazole, metronidazole, miconazole, penicillins, pentobarbital, phenobarbital, phenylbutazones, piperacillin, primidone, propylthiouracil, quinidine, quinine, rifabutin, rifampin, rifapentine, rofecoxib, salicylates, secobarbital, sulfinpyrazone, sulfonamides, testosterone, thyroid, zileuton

Reactions

Skin

Acral purpura
  (1986): Stone MS+, *J Am Acad Dermatol* 14, 796
Angioedema (<1%)
Bullous eruption
  (1986): Stone MS+, *J Am Acad Dermatol* 14, 796 (passim)
Dermatitis (sic)
  (1992): Breathnach SM+, *Adverse Drug Reactions and the Skin*
    Blackwell, Oxford, 248 (passim)
  (1991): Quintavalla R+, *Int Angiol* 10, 103
Ecchymoses
  (1988): Cole MS+, *Surgery* 103, 271 (passim)
Exanthems
  (1989): Kruis-de Vries MH+, *Dermatologica* 178, 109
  (1988): Cole MS+, *Surgery* 103, 271 (passim)
  (1978): Kwong P+, *JAMA* 239, 1884
  (1968): Schiff BL+, *Arch Dermatol* 98, 136
  (1960): Adams CW+, *Circulation* 22, 947
Hemorrhage
  (1989): Geoghegan+, *BMJ* 298, 902
  (1988): Cole MS, *Surgery* 103, 271
  (1980): Schleicher SM+, *Arch Dermatol* 116, 444
Necrosis
  (2002): Cirafici P+, *Dermatology* 204(2), 157
  (1992): Sharafuddin MA+, *Arch Dermatol* 128, 105
  (1989): Grimaudo V+, *BMJ* 289, 233
  (1988): Cole MS+, *Surgery* 103, 271
  (1987): Gladson CL+, *Arch Dermatol* 123, 1701a
  (1984): Slutzki S+, *Int J Dermatol* 23, 117
  (1982): Faraci PA, *Int J Dermatol* 21, 329
  (1981): Horn JR+, *Am J Hosp Pharm* 38, 1763
  (1976): Kirby JD+, *Br J Dermatol* 94, 97
  (1971): Danilov B+, *Rev Med Chir Soc Med Nat Iasi* (Romanian)
    75, 479
Pigmentation
  (1978): Rebhun J, *Ann Allergy* 40, 44
Pruritus (<1%)
Purplish erythema (sic) (feet and toes)
  (1978): Kwong P+, *JAMA* 239, 1884
  (1961): Feder W+, *Ann Intern Med* 55, 911
Purpura
  (1988): Cole MS+, *Surgery* 103, 271 (passim)

  (1965): Selye H+, *Arch Klin Exp Dermatol* (German) 223, 527
Rash (sic)
Urticaria
  (1988): Cole MS+, *Surgery* 103, 271 (passim)
  (1986): Stone MS+, *J Am Acad Dermatol* 14, 796 (passim)
  (1959): Sheps ES+, *Am J Cardiol* 3, 118
Vesicular eruptions
  (1986): Stone MS+, *J Am Acad Dermatol* 14, 796 (passim)

Hair

Hair – alopecia (1–10%)
  (1989): Kruis-de Vries MH+, *Dermatologica* 178, 109 (passim)
  (1988): Umlas J+, *Cutis* 42, 63
  (1986): Stone MS+, *J Am Acad Dermatol* 14, 796 (passim)
  (1969): Baker H+, *Br J Dermatol* 81, 236
  (1957): Cornbleet T+, *Arch Dermatol* 75, 440

Other

Hypersensitivity
Oral ulceration
Priapism

DICYCLOMINE

Trade names: Antispaz; Bemote; Bentyl (Aventis); Byclomine; Di-Spaz; Dibent; Neoquess; OrTyl; Spasmoject
Other common trade names: *Bentylol; Formulex; Lomine; Merbentyl; Notensyl; Panakiron; Spasmoban; Swityl*
Indications: Irritable bowel syndrome
Category: Anticholinergic; Antispasmodic
Half-life: initial: 1.8 hours; terminal: 9–10 hours
Clinically important, potentially hazardous interactions with: anticholinergics, arbutamine

Reactions

Skin

Exanthems
  (1987): Castleden CM+, *J Clin Exp Gerontol* 9, 265
  (1952): Pakula SF, *Postgrad Med* 11, 123
Flushing
Hypohidrosis (>10%)
Pruritus
  (1951): Ausman DC+, *Wisconsin Med J* 50, 1089
Rash (sic) (<1%)
  (1975): Hennessy WB, *Med J Aust* 2, 421
  (1951): Chamberlain DT, *Gastroenterology* 17, 224
Urticaria
Xerosis (>10%)

Other

Ageusia
Anaphylactoid reactions
Dysgeusia
Headache
Injection-site reactions (sic) (>10%)
Tremor
Xerostomia (>10%)
  (1975): Hennessy WB, *Med J Aust* 2, 421

DIDANOSINE

Trade name: Videx (Bristol-Myers Squibb)
Indications: Advanced HIV infection
Category: Antiretroviral; Nucleoside reverse transcriptase inhibitor (NRTI)
Half-life: 1.5 hours
Clinically important, potentially hazardous interactions with: acetaminophen, ciprofloxacin, corticosteroids, dapsone, itraconazole, ketoconazole, lomefloxacin, sulfones, tenofovir, tetracycline

Reactions

Skin
Acral erythema
   (1993): Pedailles S+, *Ann Dermatol Venereol* (French) 120, 837
Chills
Diaphoresis
Erythema multiforme
   (2001): Scully C+, *Oral Dis* 7(4), 205 (passim)
   (1992): Parneix-Spake A+, *Lancet* 340, 847
Exanthems
Pruritus (9%)
Purpura
Rash (sic) (9%)
Stevens–Johnson syndrome
   (1992): Parneix-Spake A+, *Lancet* 340, 847
Urticaria
Vasculitis
   (1994): Herranz P+, *Lancet* 344, 680

Hair
Hair – alopecia (<1%)

Other
Anaphylactoid reactions (<1%)
Death
   (2001): Hwang SW+, *Singapore Med J* 42(6), 247 (2 cases) (with stavudine)
Gynecomastia
   (2001): Aquilina C+, *Int J STD AIDS* 12(7), 481 (with stavudine)
   (2001): Manfredi R+, *Ann Pharmacother* 35(4), 438 (with stavudine)
Headache
Hypersensitivity (<1%)
Lipodystrophy
   (2001): Aquilina C+, *Int J STD AIDS* 12(7), 481 (with didanosine)
Myalgia
Myopathy
Paresthesias
Xerostomia
   (2001): Scully C+, *Oral Dis* 7(4), 205 (up to 33%) (passim)

DIDEOXYCYTIDINE (ddC)

(See ZALCITABINE)

DIETHYLPROPION

Synonym: amfepramone
Trade name: Tenuate (Aventis)
Other common trade names: *Anorex; Linea; Nobesine; Prefamone; Regenon; Tenuate Retard; Tepanil*
Indications: Weight reduction
Category: Anorexiant; CNS stimulant
Half-life: 4–6 hours
Clinically important, potentially hazardous interactions with: fluoxetine, fluvoxamine, MAO inhibitors, paroxetine, phenelzine, sertraline, tranylcypromine

Reactions

Skin
Diaphoresis (<1%)
Ecchymoses
Erythema (<1%)
Erythema multiforme
   (1997): Thaler D, Monona, WI (from internet) (observation)
Exanthems (<1%)
Flushing (<1%)
Pruritus (<1%)
Purpura (<1%)
Rash (sic)
Scleroderma
   (1991): Bourgeois P+, *Baillieres Clin Rheumatol* 5, 13
   (1990): Aeschlimann A+, *Scand J Rheumatol* 19, 87
Systemic sclerosis
   (1984): Tomlinson JW+, *J Rheumatol* 11, 254
Urticaria

Hair
Hair – alopecia (<1%)

Other
Dysgeusia
Gynecomastia
Headache
Myalgia (<1%)
Tremor
Xerostomia

DIETHYLSTILBESTROL

Synonyms: DES; stilbestrol
Trade names: Diethylstilbestrol; Stilphostrol
Other common trade names: *Diethyl Stilbestrol; Distilbene; Honvol; Stilboestrol*
Indications: Metastatic prostate carcinoma, progressive breast cancer
Category: Antineoplastic; Estrogen; Osteoporosis prophylactic
Half-life: 2–3 days

Reactions

Skin
Acanthosis nigricans
   (1974): Banuchi SR+, *Arch Dermatol* 109, 544
   (1971): Curth HO, *Birth Defects* 7, 31
Acne
Angioedema

(1942): Saphir WS+, *JAMA* 119, 557
Bullous eruption
    (1971): Kuchera LK, *JAMA* 218, 562
Chloasma (<1%)
Edema
Erythema multiforme
Erythema nodosum
Exanthems
    (1984): Lee M+, *J Urol* 131, 767
Exfoliative dermatitis
    (1942): Kasselberg LA, *JAMA* 120, 117
Flushing
    (1981): Ingle JN+, *N Engl J Med* 304, 16 (3%)
Hyperkeratosis of nipples
    (1980): Mold DE+, *Cutis* 26, 95
Lupus erythematosus
    (1989): Collins D, *J Rheumatol* 16, 408
Melasma (<1%)
Peripheral edema (>10%)
Pruritus
    (1971): Kuchera LK, *JAMA* 218, 562
Purpura
    (1984): Lee M+, *J Urol* 131, 767
Rash (sic) (<1%)
Urticaria
    (1989): Collins D, *J Rheumatol* 16, 408
    (1984): Lee M+, *J Urol* 131, 767

Hair

Hair – alopecia
Hair – hirsutism
    (1982): Peress MR+, *Am J Obstet Gynecol* 144, 135

Other

Gynecomastia (>10%)
Mastodynia (>10%)
Periarteritis nodosa
    (1967): Keyloun V+, *Vasc Dis* 4, 21
Porphyria cutanea tarda
    (1989): Coulson IH+, *Br J Urol* 63, 648
    (1978): Weimar VM+, *J Urol* 120, 643
    (1972): Reginster JP, *Arch Belg Dermatol Syphiligr* (French) 28, 179
    (1970): Domonkos AN, *Arch Dermatol* 102, 229
    (1970): Roenigk HH+, *Arch Dermatol* 102, 260
    (1969): Degos R+, *Ann Dermatol Syphiligr Paris* (French) 96, 5
    (1967): Thivolet J+, *Dermatologica* (French) 135, 455
    (1967): Vail JT, *JAMA* 201, 671
    (1966): Copeman PW+, *BMJ* 5485, 461
    (1966): Levere RD, *Blood* 28, 569
    (1965): Becker FT, *Arch Dermatol* 92, 252
    (1964): Theologides H+, *Metabolism* 13, 391
    (1963): Hurley HJ, *Arch Dermatol* 88, 233
    (1963): Walshe M, *Br J Dermatol* 75, 298
Vaginal candidiasis

DIFLUNISAL

Trade name: Dolobid (Merck)
Other common trade names: *Ansal; Apo-Diflunisal; Diflonid; Diflusal; Dolobis; Donobid; Fluniget; Flustar; Nu-Diflunisal*
Indications: Rheumatoid and osteoarthritis
Category: Nonsteroidal anti-inflammatory (NSAID) analgesic
Half-life: 8–12 hours
Clinically important, potentially hazardous interactions with: indomethacin

Reactions

Skin

Adverse effects (sic)
    (1985): Lee P+, *J Rheumatol* 12, 544
    (1983): McQueen EG, *N Z Med J* 96, 95
Angioedema (<1%)
Bullous eruption
    (1989): Street ML+, *J Am Acad Dermatol* 20, 850
Diaphoresis (<1%)
    (1986): Muncie HL+, *J Fam Pract* 23, 125
    (1979): Papatheodossiou N, *Curr Med Res Opinion* 6, 154
Edema (<1%)
Erythema multiforme (<1%)
    (1986): Grom JA+, *Hosp Formul Manage* 21, 353
    (1985): Bigby M+, *J Am Acad Dermatol* 12, 866 (5%)
    (1985): O'Brien WM+, *J Rheumatol* 12, 13
    (1982): Dubois A+, *Presse Med* (French) 11, 606
    (1978): Hunter JA+, *BMJ* 2, 1088
Erythroderma
    (1989): Street ML+, *J Am Acad Dermatol* 20, 850
    (1980): Chan LK+, *BMJ* 280, 84
Exanthems
    (1992): Breathnach SM+, *Adverse Drug Reactions and the Skin* Blackwell, Oxford, 180 (passim)
    (1988): Cook DJ+, *Can Med Assoc J* 138, 1029
    (1985): Bigby M+, *J Am Acad Dermatol* 12, 866 (5%)
    (1985): Bocanegra TS+, *Curr Res Med Opin* 9, 568 (1.7%)
Exfoliative dermatitis (<1%)
    (1985): Bigby M+, *J Am Acad Dermatol* 12, 866
Fixed eruption
    (1998): Mahboob A+, *Int J Dermatol* 37, 833
    (1991): Roetzheim RG+, *J Am Acad Dermatol* 24, 1021 (non-pigmenting)
Flushing (<1%)
Lichenoid eruption
    (1989): Street ML+, *J Am Acad Dermatol* 20, 850
Peripheral edema
Photosensitivity (<1%)
    (1989): Street ML+, *J Am Acad Dermatol* 20, 850
Pruritus (1–10%)
    (1992): Breathnach SM+, *Adverse Drug Reactions and the Skin* Blackwell, Oxford, 180 (passim)
    (1986): Hurme M+, *Int J Clin Pharmacol Res* 6, 53
    (1985): Bigby M+, *J Am Acad Dermatol* 12, 866 (5%)
Purpura
Rash (sic) (3–9%)
    (1987): Masden JJ+, *Curr Ther Res* 42, 319
    (1986): Bennett RM, *Clin Ther* 9, 27
    (1986): Turner RA+, *Clin Ther* 9, 37
Stevens–Johnson syndrome (<1%)
    (1992): Breathnach SM+, *Adverse Drug Reactions and the Skin* Blackwell, Oxford, 180 (passim)
    (1986): Grom JA+, *Hosp Formul Manage* 21, 353
    (1986): Szczeklik A, *Drugs* 32 (Suppl 4), 148

(1985): Bigby M+, *J Am Acad Dermatol* 12, 866
(1982): Dubois A+, *Presse Med* (French) 11, 606
(1979): *Curr Probl* 4, 2
(1978): Hunter JA+, *BMJ* 2, 1088
Toxic epidermal necrolysis (<1%)
(1990): Roujeau JC+, *Arch Dermatol* 126, 37
Urticaria (>1%)
(1995): Arias J+, *Ann Allergy Asthma Immunol* 74, 160
(1992): Breathnach SM+, *Adverse Drug Reactions and the Skin*
Blackwell, Oxford, 180 (passim)
(1987): Morse DR+, *Clin Ther* 9, 500
(1985): Bigby M+, *J Am Acad Dermatol* 12, 866 (5%)
(1983): Griffin JP, *Practitioner* 227, 1283 (passim)
(1980): Chan LK+, *BMJ* 280, 84
Vasculitis (<1%)

Hair

Hair – alopecia
(1978): Bresnihan B+, *Curr Med Res Opinion* 5, 556

Nails

Nails – onycholysis

Other

Anaphylactoid reactions (<1%)
Aphthous stomatitis
Headache
Hypersensitivity (<1%)
Oral lichen planus
(1983): Hamburger J+, *BMJ* 287, 1258
Oral ulceration
Paresthesias (<1%)
Pseudolymphoma
(2001): Werth V, *Dermatology Times* 18
Pseudoporphyria
(1987): Taylor BJ+, *N Z Med J* 100, 322
Stomatitis (<1%)
Tinnitus
Trembling (<1%)
Xerostomia
(1982): Ankri J+, *Clin Ther* 5, 85

DIGOXIN

Trade names: Lanoxicaps (GSK); Lanoxin (GSK)
Other common trade names: *Cardigox; Digacin; Digoxine; Eudigox; Lanicor; Lenoxin; Novo-Digoxin*
Indications: Congestive heart failure, atrial fibrillation
Category: Antiarrhythmic; Cardiac glycoside; Inotropic
Half-life: 36–48 hours
Clinically important, potentially hazardous interactions with: alprazolam, amiodarone, amphotericin B, arbutamine, bendroflumethiazide, benzthiazide, bumetanide, chlorothiazide, chlorthalidone, cholestyramine, clarithromycin, cyclosporine, cyclothiazide, demeclocycline, **devil's claw**, doxycycline, erythromycin, esomeprazole, ethacrynic acid, furosemide, hawthorn (fruit, leaf, flower extract), hydrochlorothiazide, hydroflumethiazide, indapamide, **licorice**, methyclothiazide, metolazone, minocycline, **mistletoe**, oxytetracycline, polythiazide, propafenone, propantheline, quinethazone, quinidine, rifampin, **sarsaparilla**, **senna**, **Siberian ginseng**, **St John's wort**, teriparatide, tetracycline, thiazide diuretics, trichlormethiazide, verapamil

Reactions

Skin

Angioedema
Bullous eruption
(1992): Breathnach SM+, *Adverse Drug Reactions and the Skin*
Blackwell, Oxford, 216 (passim)
Diaphoresis
(1980): Lofgren RP, *N Engl J Med* 302, 919
Exanthems (1.6%)
(1994): Martin SJ+, *JAMA* 271, 1905 (generalized)
(1994): Shelley WB+, *Cutis* 54, 76 (observation)
(1992): Breathnach SM+, *Adverse Drug Reactions and the Skin*
Blackwell, Oxford, 216 (passim)
Pruritus
(1994): Martin SJ+, *JAMA* 271, 1905 (generalized)
Psoriasis
(1981): David M+, *J Am Acad Dermatol* 5, 702
Purpura
(1992): Breathnach SM+, *Adverse Drug Reactions and the Skin*
Blackwell, Oxford, 216 (passim)
Rash (sic)
Urticaria
(1994): Shelley WB+, *Cutis* 54, 76 (observation)
(1992): Breathnach SM+, *Adverse Drug Reactions and the Skin*
Blackwell, Oxford, 216 (passim)
Vasculitis
(1972): Brauner GJ+, *Cutis* 10, 441

Hair

Hair – alopecia

Nails

Nails – loss (finger- and toenails)

Other

Dyschromatopsia (green vision)
(2002): Lawrenson JG+, *Br J Ophthalmol* 86(11), 1259
Gynecomastia
(2000): Hugues FC+, *Ann Med Interne (Paris)* (French) 151, 10
(passim)
Headache
Xanthopsia

DIHYDROERGOTAMINE

Trade names: D.H.E. 45 (Novartis); Migranal (Xcel)
Other common trade names: *Dergiflux; Dihydergot; Ergont; Ergovasan; Ikaran; Orstanorm; Seglor; Verladyn; Verteblan*
Indications: Prevention of vascular headaches
Category: Ergot alkaloid
Half-life: 1.3–3.9 hours
Clinically important, potentially hazardous interactions with: almotriptan, amprenavir, clarithromycin, delavirdine, efavirenz, erythromycin, indinavir, naratriptan, nelfinavir, ritonavir, rizatriptan, saquinavir, sibutramine, sumatriptan, troleandomycin, zolmitriptan

Reactions

Skin
Edema (>10%)
Pruritus

Other
Dysgeusia
Headache
Injection-site reactions (sic)
Myalgia
Paresthesias (>10%)
Xerostomia (>10%)

DIHYDROTACHYSTEROL

Trade names: DHT (Roxane); Hytakerol (Sanofi-Synthelabo)
Other common trade names: *AT 10; Dihydral; Dygratyl*
Indications: Hypocalcemia associated with hypoparathyroidism
Category: Fat-soluble vitamin
Half-life: N/A

Reactions

Skin
Calcification
 (1985): Michel B+, *Schweiz Med Wochenschr* (German) 115, 418
Exanthems
Livedo reticularis
 (1985): Michel B+, *Schweiz Med Wochenschr* (German) 115, 418
Pruritus (1–10%)

Other
Dysgeusia (metallic taste)
Myalgia
Ulcerative necrosis
 (1985): Michel B+, *Schweiz Med Wochenschr* (German) 115, 418
Xerostomia

DILTIAZEM

Trade names: Cardizem (Biovail); Cartia-XT; Dilacor XR (Watson); Diltia-XT; Teczem (Aventis); Tiazac (Forest)
Other common trade names: *Alti-Diltiazem; Britiazem; Calcicard; Deltazen; Dilrene; Diltahexal; Nu-Diltiaz; Presoken; Tiamate; Tilazem; Tildiem*
Indications: Angina, essential hypertension
Category: Antianginal; Antiarrhythmic; Calcium channel blocker
Half-life: 5–8 hours (for extended-release capsules)
Clinically important, potentially hazardous interactions with: amiodarone, aprepitant, carbamazepine, cyclosporine, epirubicin, **mistletoe**, simvastatin

Teczem is diltiazem and enalapril

Reactions

Skin
Acne
 (1989): Stern R+, *Arch Intern Med* 149, 829
Acute generalized exanthematous pustulosis (AGEP)
 (2002): Arroyo MP+, *J Drugs Dermatol* 1(1), 63
 (1998): Jan V+, *Dermatology* 197, 274
 (1998): Knowles S+, *J Am Acad Dermatol* 38, 201 (passim)
 (1997): Blodgett TP+, *Cutis* 60, 45
 (1997): Vincente-Calleja JM+, *Br J Dermatol* 137, 837
 (1996): Wolkenstein P+, *Contact Dermatitis* 35, 234
 (1995): Krasovec M+, *Schweiz Rundsch Med Prax* (German) 84, 814
 (1995): Moreau A+, *Int J Dermatol* 34, 263 (passim)
 (1995): Wakelin SH+, *Clin Exp Dermatol* 20, 341
 (1993): Janier M+, *Br J Dermatol* 129, 354
 (1992): Wittal RA+, *Australas J Dermatol* 33, 11
 (1988): Lambert DG+, *Br J Dermatol* 118, 308
Adverse effects (sic)
 (1993): Barbaud A+, *Therapie* (French) 48, 499
Angioedema
 (1998): Knowles S+, *J Am Acad Dermatol* 38, 201 (passim)
 (1989): Sadick NS+, *J Am Acad Dermatol* 21, 132
Ankle edema
 (1994): Litt JZ, Beachwood, OH (personal case) (observation)
Capillaritis (Schamberg's)
 (1999): Eastern JS, Belleville, NJ (from Internet) (observation)
Dermatitis (sic)
Diaphoresis
 (1988): Lambert DG+, *Br J Dermatol* 118, 308 (passim)
 (1985): Scolnick B+, *Ann Intern Med* 102, 558
Ecchymoses (<1%)
Edema (1–10%)
 (2001): Chugh SK+, *J Cardiovasc Pharmacol* 38(3), 356
 (1998): Knowles S+, *J Am Acad Dermatol* 38, 201 (passim)
 (1982): Hossack KF, *Am J Cardiol* 49, 567
 (1982): McGraw BF, *Drug Intell Clin Pharm* 16, 366
Erythema
 (1998): Knowles S+, *J Am Acad Dermatol* 38, 201 (passim)
 (1982): McGraw BF, *Drug Intell Clin Pharm* 16, 366
Erythema multiforme (<1%)
 (1998): Knowles S+, *J Am Acad Dermatol* 38, 201 (passim)
 (1995): Avila JR+, *Ann Pharmacother* 29, 317
 (1993): Kitamura K+, *J Dermatol* 20, 279 (psoriasiform) (31%)
 (1993): Sanders CJ+, *Lancet* 341, 967
 (1993): Sousa-Basto A+, *Contact Dermatitis* 29, 44
 (1992): Wittal RA+, *Australas J Dermatol* 33, 11
 (1989): Berbis P+, *Dermatologica* 179, 90
 (1989): Brown FH+, *Ann Dent* 48, 39
 (1989): Stern R+, *Arch Intern Med* 149, 829

Exanthems
  (2000): Heymann WR, *Cutis* 66, 129
  (1998): Knowles S+, *J Am Acad Dermatol* 38, 201 (passim)
  (1994): Baker BA+, *Ann Pharmacother* 28, 118
  (1993): Kitamura K+, *J Dermatol* 20, 279 (psoriasiform) (31%)
  (1993): Sousa-Basto A+, *Contact Dermatitis* 29, 44
  (1992): Romano A+, *Ann Allergy* 69, 31
  (1992): Wittal RA+, *Australas J Dermatol* 33, 11 (erythroderma)
  (1990): Wirebaugh SR+, *Drug Intell Clin Pharm* 24, 1046
  (1989): Jones SK+, *Clin Exp Dermatol* 14, 457
  (1989): Stern R+, *Arch Intern Med* 149, 829
  (1988): Hammentgen R+, *Dtsch Med Wochenschr* (German) 113, 1283
  (1988): Lambert DG+, *Br J Dermatol* 118, 308 (passim)
  (1988): Wakeel RA+, *BMJ* 296, 1071 (passim)
  (1986): Gibson RS+, *N Engl J Med* 315, 423 (0.7%)
  (1985): Chaffman M+, *Drugs* 29, 387 (1.3%)
  (1985): Scolnick B+, *Ann Intern Med* 102, 558
Exfoliative dermatitis (<1%)
  (1998): Knowles S+, *J Am Acad Dermatol* 38, 201 (passim)
  (1997): Odeh M, *J Toxicol Clin Toxicol* 35, 101
  (1993): Sousa-Basto A+, *Contact Dermatitis* 29, 44
  (1989): Stern R+, *Arch Intern Med* 149, 829
  (1988): Wakeel RA+, *BMJ* 296, 1071 (passim)
  (1986): Lavrijsen APM+, *Acta Derm Venereol* 66, 536 (in a patient with psoriasis)
Flushing (1–10%)
  (1992): Shelley WB+, *Advanced Dermatologic Diagnosis* WB Saunders, 583 (passim)
  (1988): Lambert DG+, *Br J Dermatol* 118, 308 (passim)
  (1985): Chaffman M+, *Drugs* 29, 387 (0.1–1%)
  (1983): Lewis JG, *Drugs* 25, 196
  (1982): McGraw BF, *Drug Intell Clin Pharm* 16, 366
Hyperkeratosis (feet)
  (1992): Ilia R+, *Int J Cardiol* 35, 115
Lichenoid eruption (photosensitive)
  (2001): Gladstone GC, *Dermatology Times* Worcester, MA (personal communication)
  (1988): Lambert DG+, *Br J Dermatol* 118, 308
Lupus erythematosus
  (1998): Callen JP, Academy '98 Meeting (4 patients)
  (1998): Knowles S+, *J Am Acad Dermatol* 38, 201 (passim)
  (1997): Crowson AN+, *Hum Pathol*
JC 28(1), 67
  (1995): Crowson AN+, *N Engl J Med* 333, 1429
  (1989): Stern R+, *Arch Intern Med* 149, 829
Palmar–plantar desquamation
  (1985): Scolnick B+, *Ann Intern Med* 102, 558
Periorbital edema
  (1993): Friedland S+, *Arch Ophthalmol* 111, 1027
Peripheral edema (5–8%)
  (2002): No Author, *Medscape Primary Care* 4
Petechiae (<1%)
Photosensitivity (<1%)
  (1998): Knowles S+, *J Am Acad Dermatol* 38, 201 (passim)
  (1997): O'Reilly FM+, American Academy of Dermatology Meeting, Poster #14
  (1996): Seggev JS+, *J Allergy Clin Immunol* 97, 852
  (1994): Shelley WB+, *Cutis* 53, 161 (observation)
  (1992): Wittal RA+, *Australas J Dermatol* 33, 11 (erythroderma)
  (1990): Young L+, *Clin Exp Dermatol* 15, 467
  (1989): Berbis P+, *Dermatologica* 179, 90
  (1988): Lambert DG+, *Br J Dermatol* 118, 308
  (1986): Lavrijsen APM+, *Acta Derm Venereol* 66, 536
  (1979): Hashimoto M+, *Acta Dermatol* (Kyoto) 74, 181
  (1976): Fujiwara N+, *Nippon Rinsho* (Japanese) 34, 3121
Pigmentation
  (2002): Chwala A+, *Arch Dermatol* 46, 468
  (2002): Schmutz JL+, *Ann Dermatol Venereol* 129(11), 1332

Pruritus (<1%)
  (2001): Gladstone GC, *Dermatology Times* (personal communication)
  (2000): Heymann WR, *Cutis* 66, 129
  (1998): Knowles S+, *J Am Acad Dermatol* 38, 201 (passim)
  (1994): Baker BA+, *Ann Pharmacother* 28, 118
  (1989): Stern R+, *Arch Intern Med* 149, 829
  (1986): Gibson RS+, *N Engl J Med* 315, 423 (0.7%)
  (1982): McGraw BF, *Drug Intell Clin Pharm* 16, 366
Psoriasis
  (2001): Smith KC, Niagara Falls, Ontario (from Internet) (observation)
  (1998): Knowles S+, *J Am Acad Dermatol* 38, 201 (passim)
  (1993): Kitamura K+, *J Dermatol* 20, 279 (psoriasiform) (31%)
Purpura (<1%)
  (2001): Inui S+, *J Dermatol* 28(2), 100 (lichenoid)
  (1998): Knowles S+, *J Am Acad Dermatol* 38, 201 (passim)
  (1992): Kuo M+, *Ann Pharmacother* 26, 1089
Pustular psoriasis
  (1989): Stern R+, *Arch Intern Med* 149, 829
Pustules
  (1993): Janier M+, *Br J Dermatol* 129, 354
  (1988): Lambert DG+, *Br J Dermatol* 118, 308
Rash (sic) (1.3%)
  (1998): Knowles S+, *J Am Acad Dermatol* 38, 201 (passim)
  (1989): Stern R+, *Arch Intern Med* 149, 829
  (1982): McGraw BF, *Drug Intell Clin Pharm* 16, 366
Side effects (sic)
  (1993): Kitamura K+, *J Dermatol* 20, 279 (psoriasiform) (31%)
  (1993): Sousa-Basto A+, *Contact Dermatitis* 29, 44
Stevens–Johnson syndrome
  (1998): Knowles S+, *J Am Acad Dermatol* 38, 201 (passim)
  (1993): Sanders CJ+, *Lancet* 341, 967
  (1990): Taylor J+, *Clin Pharmacy* 9, 948
  (1989): Stern R+, *Arch Intern Med* 149, 829
Subcorneal pustular dermatosis
  (2001): Reed B, Denver, CO (from Internet) (observation)
  (1992): Wittal RA+, *Australas J Dermatol* 33, 11
Thickening (sic)
  (1998): Knowles S+, *J Am Acad Dermatol* 38, 201 (passim)
  (1992): Ilia R+, *Int J Cardiol* 35, 115
Toxic dermatitis (sic)
  (1988): Wakeel RA+, *BMJ* 296, 1071
Toxic epidermal necrolysis
  (1998): Knowles S+, *J Am Acad Dermatol* 38, 201 (passim)
  (1991): No Author, *Lakartidningen* (Swedish) 88, 3489
  (1989): Stern R+, *Arch Intern Med* 149, 829
  (1988): Wakeel RA+, *BMJ* 296, 1071 (passim)
Toxic erythema
  (1998): Knowles S+, *J Am Acad Dermatol* 38, 201 (passim)
  (1988): Wakeel RA+, *BMJ* 296, 1071
Ulcerations of legs
  (1989): Jones SK+, *Clin Exp Dermatol* 14, 457
  (1988): Carmichael AJ+, *BMJ* 297, 562 (vasculitic)
Urticaria (<1%)
  (1998): Knowles S+, *J Am Acad Dermatol* 38, 201 (passim)
  (1989): Jones SK+, *Clin Exp Dermatol* 14, 457
  (1989): Sadick NS+, *J Am Acad Dermatol* 21, 132
  (1989): Stern R+, *Arch Intern Med* 149, 829
Vasculitis (<1%)
  (1998): Knowles S+, *J Am Acad Dermatol* 38, 201 (passim)
  (1992): Kuo M+, *Ann Pharmacother* 26, 1089
  (1992): Wittal RA+, *Australas J Dermatol* 33, 11
  (1989): Stern R+, *Arch Intern Med* 149, 829
  (1988): Sheehan-Dare RA+, *Br J Dermatol* 119, 134
  (1988): Sheehan-Dare RA+, *Postgrad Med J* 64, 467

Hair

Hair – alopecia (<1%)

(1998): Knowles S+, *J Am Acad Dermatol* 38, 201 (passim)
(1989): Stern R+, *Arch Intern Med* 149, 829
Hair – hirsutism
(1989): Stern R+, *Arch Intern Med* 149, 829

Nails
Nails – dystrophy
(1989): Stern R+, *Arch Intern Med* 149, 829

Other
Dysgeusia (<1%)
(2000): Zervakis J+, *Physiol Behav* 68, 405
Erythromelalgia
(1989): Stern R+, *Arch Intern Med* 149, 829
Fever
(2003): Jover-Saenz A+, *Med Clin* (Barc) 120(13), 517
Gingival hyperplasia (21%)
(1999): Ellis JS+, *J Periodontol* 70, 63 (74%)
(1998): Knowles S+, *J Am Acad Dermatol* 38, 201 (passim)
(1995): Moghadam BKH+, *Cutis* 56, 46 (passim)
(1993): King GN+, *J Clin Periodontol* 20, 286
(1990): Brown RS+, *Oral Surg* 70, 593
(1987): Giustiniani S+, *Int J Cardiol* 15, 247
Gynecomastia
(1994): Otto C+, *Arch Intern Med* 154, 351
Headache
Hypersensitivity
(1998): Knowles S+, *J Am Acad Dermatol* 38, 201 (passim)
Lymphadenopathy
(1985): Scolnick B+, *Ann Intern Med* 102, 558
Myoclonus
(2002): Jeret JS, *Neurology* 59(6), 962
Parageusia (<1%)
Paresthesias (<1%)
(1982): McGraw BF, *Drug Intell Clin Pharm* 16, 366
Parkinsonism
(2003): *Prescrire Int* 12(64), 62
(2001): Remblier C+, *Therapie* 56(1), 57
Pseudolymphoma
(1995): Magro CM+, *J Am Acad Dermatol* 32, 419
Rhabdomyolysis
(2002): Lewin JJ 3rd+, *Ann Pharmacother* 36(10), 1546
(2001): Kanathur N+, *Tenn Med* 94(9), 339 (with simvastatin)
(2001): Peces R+, *Nephron* 89(1), 117 (with simvastatin)
Tinnitus
Tremor (<1%)
Xerostomia (<1%)
(1983): Lewis JG, *Drugs* 25, 196
(1981): Pepine CJ+, *Am Heart J* 101, 719

DIMENHYDRINATE

Trade names: Calm-X; Dimetabs; Dramamine (Pharmacia); Marmine; Nico-Vert; Tega-Cert; Tega-Vert; Triptone; Vertab; Wehamine
Other common trade names: *Andrumin; Lomarin; Nauseatol; Nausicalm; Travel Tabs; Vomacur; Vomex A; Vomisen*
Indications: Motion sickness, dizziness, nausea, vomiting
Category: Antihistamine H$_1$-blocker
Half-life: N/A

Reactions

Skin
Angioedema (<1%)
Diaphoresis

Eczema (sic)
Edema (<1%)
Exanthems
Fixed eruption (<1%)
(2000): Ozkaya-Bayazit E+, *Eur J Dermatol* 10, 288
(2000): Saenz de San Pedro B+, *Allergy* 55, 297
(2000): Smith KC, Niagara Falls, Ontario (from Internet) (observation) (recurrent)
(1999): Gallagher W, *The Schoch Letter*, 49, #1, 2
(1998): Smola H+, *Br J Dermatol* 138, 920
(1997): Gonzalo-Garijo MA+, *Br J Dermatol* 135, 661
(1992): Hatzis J+, *Cutis* 50, 50
(1989): Hogan DJ+, *J Am Acad Dermatol* 20, 503
(1982): Schnyder UW+, *Dermatologica* 165, 292
(1960): Kirshbaum BA+, *Am J Med Sci* 240, 512
(1960): Stritzler C+, *J Invest Dermatol* 34, 319
Flushing
Photosensitivity (<1%)
(1976): Horio T, *Arch Dermatol* 112, 1125
Rash (sic) (<1%)
Systemic eczematous contact dermatitis
Urticaria

Other
Acute intermittent porphyria
Anaphylactoid reactions
Headache
Injection-site pain (<1%)
Myalgia (<1%)
Paresthesias (<1%)
Xerostomia (1–10%)

DIPHENHYDRAMINE

Trade names: Allermax; Benadryl (Parke-Davis); Benylin (Warner Lambert); Compoz; Sominex 2 (GSK); Valdrene
Other common trade names: *Allerdryl; Allermin; Banophen; Benahist; Dibrondrin; Dolestan; Genahist; Insomnal; Nytol; Resmin; Sediat*
Indications: Allergic rhinitis, urticaria
Category: Antidyskinetic; Antiemetic; Antihistamine; Sedative-hypnotic
Half-life: 2–8 hours
Clinically important, potentially hazardous interactions with: alcohol, anticholinergics, chloral hydrate, CNS depressants, glutethimide, MAO inhibitors

Reactions

Skin
Allergic reactions (sic)
(1970): Fidel VG, *Klin Med Mosk* (Russian) 48, 109
Angioedema (<1%)
(1988): Self F+, *J R Soc Med* 81, 544
Dermatitis
(1998): Yamada S+, *Contact Dermatitis* 38, 282
(1983): Coskey RJ, *J Am Acad Dermatol* 8, 204
(1976): Horio T, *Arch Dermatol* 112, 1124
(1972): Shelley WB+, *Acta Derm Venereol* (Stockh) 52, 376
Diaphoresis
Eczema (sic)
(1981): Lawrence CM+, *Contact Dermatitis* 7, 276
(1972): Shelley WB+, *Acta Derm Venereol* (Stockh) 52, 376
Edema (<1%)
Exanthems

(1965): Davenport PM+, *Arch Dermatol* 92, 577
Fixed eruption
  (1993): Dwyer CM+, *J Am Acad Dermatol* 29, 496
  (1973): Csonka GW, *Br J Vener Dis* 49, 316
  (1970): Savin JA, *Br J Dermatol* 83, 546
  (1961): Welsh AM, *Arch Dermatol* 84, 1004
Livedo reticularis
  (1996): Morell A+, *Dermatology* 193, 50
Photosensitivity (<1%)
  (2000): Danby FW, Manchester, NH (from Internet)
    (observation)
  (1976): Horio T, *Arch Dermatol* 112, 1124
  (1974): Emmett EA, *Arch Dermatol* 110, 249
  (1962): Schreiber M+, *Arch Dermatol* 86, 58
Pruritus
  (1998): Litt JZ, Beachwood, OH (personal case) (observation)
    (following varicella)
  (1972): Shelley WB+, *Acta Derm Venereol* (Stockh) 52, 376
  (1965): Davenport PM+, *Arch Dermatol* 92, 577
Purpura
  (1996): Morell A+, *Dermatology* 193, 50
Rash (sic) (<1%)
Toxic epidermal necrolysis
  (1991): Epishin AV+, *Klin Med Mosk* (Russian) 69, 92
  (1978): Soskin IaM+, *Akush Ginekol Kruglikova* (Russian)
    January, 67
  (1972): Timperman J+, *Z Rechtsmed* (German) 71, 139
Urticaria
Vasculitis
  (1965): Davenport PM+, *Arch Dermatol* 92, 577

Other
Anaphylactoid reactions
  (1998): Barranco P+, *Allergy* 53, 814
  (1995): Manhart AR+J, *Toxicol Clin Toxicol* 33, 189
  (1994): Watanabe T+, *J Toxicol Clin Toxicol* 32, 593
  (1980): Sandler BB, *Sov Med* (Russian) (9) 119
Death
  (2003): Baker AM+, *J Forensic Sci* 48(2), 425
Hypersensitivity
Injection-site gangrene
  (1989): Ramsdell WM, *J Am Acad Dermatol* 21, 1318
Injection-site necrosis
  (1989): Ramsdell WM, *J Am Acad Dermatol* 21, 1318
Myalgia (<1%)
Paresthesias (<1%)
Rhabdomyolysis
  (2003): Haas CE+, *Ann Pharmacother* 37(4), 538
  (2003): Stucka KR+, *Pediatr Emerg Care* 19(1), 25
  (1996): Emadian SM+, *Am J Emerg Med* 14(6), 574
Tinnitus
Tremor
Xerostomia (1–10%)

DIPHENOXYLATE

Trade names: Logen; Lomanate; Lomotil (Pharmacia); Lonox (Geneva)
Other common trade names: *Lamocot; Lofene; Low-Quel*
Indications: Diarrhea
Category: Antidiarrheal
Half-life: 2.5 hours

*Note: Diphenoxylate is almost always prescribed with atropine sulfate

Reactions

Skin
Angioedema
Diaphoresis (<1%)
Flushing
Pruritus (<1%)
Urticaria (<1%)

Other
Anaphylactoid reactions
Gingivitis
Headache
Paresthesias
Xerostomia (3%)

DIPHENYLHYDANTOIN

(See PHENYTOIN)

DIPYRIDAMOLE

Trade names: Aggrenox (Boehringer Ingelheim); Persantine (Boehringer Ingelheim)
Other common trade names: *Cardoxin; Cleridium; Coronarine; Coroxin; Curantyl N; Dipridacot; Lodimol; Novo-Dipiradol; Persantin*
Indications: Thromboembolic complications following cardiac valve replacement
Category: Platelet aggregation inhibitor
Half-life: 10–12 hours
Clinically important, potentially hazardous interactions with: adenosine, **dong quai**, fondaparinux, reteplase

Aggrenox is dipyridamole and aspirin

Reactions

Skin
Allergic reactions (sic) (<1%)
Angioedema
  (1971): Sullivan JM+, *N Engl J Med* 284, 1391
Diaphoresis (0.4%)
Edema (0.3%)
Erythema multiforme
Exanthems
  (1971): Sullivan JM+, *N Engl J Med* 284, 1391
Flushing (3.4%)
Pruritus
  (1971): Sullivan JM+, *N Engl J Med* 284, 1391
Psoriasis
  (1971): Sullivan JM+, *N Engl J Med* 284, 1391

Purpura (1.4%)
  (1993): Kaufman DW+, *Blood* 82, 2714
Rash (sic) (2.3%)
  (1971): Sullivan JM+, *N Engl J Med* 284, 1391
Stevens–Johnson syndrome
  (1971): Sullivan JM+, *N Engl J Med* 284, 1391
Toxic epidermal necrolysis
  (1993): Seoane-Leston JM+, *Rev Stomatol Chir Maxillofac*
    (French) 94, 281
Ulcerations (<1%)
Urticaria
  (1971): Sullivan JM+, *N Engl J Med* 284, 1391

Other
Anaphylactoid reactions
  (1994): Weinmann P+, *Am J Med* 97, 488
Dysgeusia (0.1%)
Gingivitis (<1%)
Headache
Hyperesthesia (0.5%)
Injection-site pain (0.1%)
Injection-site reactions (sic) (0.4%)
Mastodynia (0.03%)
Myalgia (0.9%)
Paresthesias (1.3%)
Pseudopolymyalgia rheumatica
  (1990): Chassagne P+, *BMJ* 301, 875
Tremor (<1%)

DIRITHROMYCIN

Trade name: Dynabac (Muro)
Indications: Various infections caused by susceptible organisms
Category: Macrolide antibiotic
Half-life: 8 hours
**Clinically important, potentially hazardous interactions
with:** pimozide, warfarin

Reactions

Skin
Allergic reactions (sic) (<1%)
Bullous eruption
Diaphoresis (<1%)
Edema (<1%)
Flu-like syndrome (sic) (<1%)
Peripheral edema (<1%)
Pruritus (1.2%)
Rash (sic) (1.4%)
Urticaria (1.2%)

Other
Anaphylactoid reactions
Dysgeusia (<1%)
Headache
Myalgia (<1%)
Oral ulceration (<1%)
Paresthesias (<1%)
Torsades de pointes
  (2002): Shaffer D+, *Clin Infect Dis* 35(2), 197
Tremor (<1%)
Vaginal candidiasis (<1%)
Vaginitis (<1%)
Xerostomia (<1%)

DISOPYRAMIDE

Trade name: Norpace (Pharmacia)
Other common trade names: *Dimodan; Dirythmin SA;
Disonorm; Durbis; Isorythm*
Indications: Ventricular arrhythmias
Category: Antiarrhythmic
Half-life: 4–10 hours
**Clinically important, potentially hazardous interactions
with:** arsenic, ciprofloxacin, clarithromycin, enoxacin,
erythromycin, gatifloxacin, lomefloxacin, moxifloxacin,
norfloxacin, ofloxacin, quinolones, sparfloxacin

Reactions

Skin
Angioedema
Dermatitis (sic)
Edema (1–3%)
Erythema nodosum
  (1985): Niv Y+, *Harefuah* (Hebrew) 108, 490
Exanthems (1–5%)
  (1987): Brogden RN+, *Drugs* 34, 151 (1–2%)
  (1973): 11, 3
Lupus erythematosus (<1%)
  (1985): Epstein A+, *Arthritis Rheum* 28, 158
  (1981): Wanner WR+, *Am Heart J* 101, 687
Photosensitivity
  (1987): Brogden RN+, *Drugs* 34, 151
Pruritus (1–3%)
Purpura
  (1987): Brogden RN+, *Drugs* 34, 151
Rash (sic) (generalized) (1–3%)
Urticaria
Xerosis

Hair
Hair – alopecia

Other
Gynecomastia (<1%)
Headache
Oral mucosal lesions (40%)
  (1987): Brogden RN+, *Drugs* 34, 151
Paresthesias (<1%)
Xerostomia (32%)
  (1987): Brogden RN+, *Drugs* 34, 151 (40%)

DISULFIRAM

Trade name: Antabuse (Odyssey)
Other common trade names: *Antabus; Busetal; Esperal; Nocbin; Refusal; Tetradin*
Indications: Alcoholism
Category: Deterrent to alcohol consumption
Half-life: N/A
Clinically important, potentially hazardous interactions with: alcohol, anisindione, anticoagulants, **capsicum**, cyclosporine, dicumarol, ethanolamine, ethotoin, fosphenytoin, mephenytoin, metronidazole, phenytoin, warfarin

Reactions

Skin
Acne
  (1967): Hitch JM, *JAMA* 200, 879
  (1964): Fegeler F, *Arch Klin Exp Dermatol* (German) 219, 335
  (1953): Barefoot SW, *JAMA* 147, 1653
Adverse effects (sic) (from beer-containing shampoo)
  (1980): Stoll D+, *JAMA* 244, 2045
Allergic reactions (sic)
Bullous eruption
  (1990): Larbre B+, *Ann Dermatol Venereol* (French) 117, 721
  (1979): Webb PK+, *JAMA* 241, 2061
Dermatitis (on exposure to rubber)
  (1996): Rebandel P+, *Contact Dermatitis* 35, 48
  (1995): Fisher AA, *Cutis* 56, 131
  (1994): Mathelier-Fusade P+, *Contact Dermatitis* 31, 121
  (1992): Baptista A+, *Contact Dermatitis* 26, 140
  (1989): Minet A+, *Ann Dermatol Venereol* (French) 116, 543
  (1988): Olfson M, *Am J Psychiatry* 145, 651
  (1984): van Hecke E+, *Contact Dermatitis* 10, 254
  (1982): Fisher AA, *Cutis* 30, 461 (passim)
  (1979): *Contact Dermatitis* 5, 199
  (1979): Webb PK+, *JAMA* 241, 2061
  (1976): Lachapelle JM+, *Nouv Presse Med* (French) 5, 1536
  (1975): Lachapelle JM, *Contact Dermatitis* 1, 218
  (1974): Kobayasi T+, *Arch Dermatol Forsch* (German) 249, 125
  (1970): Gunther WW, *Med J Aust* 1, 1177
  (1968): van Ketel WG, *Ned Tijdschr Geneeskd* (Dutch) 112, 406
Dermatitis recall (nickel)
  (1993): Gamboa P+, *Contact Dermatitis* 28, 255
  (1992): Klein LR+, *J Am Acad Dermatol* 26, 645
  (1987): Grondahl-Hansen V+, *Ugeskr Laeger* (Danish) 149, 2401
  (1987): Kaaber K+, *Derm Beruf Umwelt* (German) 35, 209
Diaphoresis (<1%) (with alcohol)
Eczema (sic)
  (1994): Mathelier-Fusade P+, *Contact Dermatitis* 31, 121
  (1981): Goitre M+, *Contact Dermatitis* 7, 272
Exanthems
  (1992): Breathnach SM+, *Adverse Drug Reactions and the Skin* Blackwell, Oxford, 204 (passim)
  (1989): Minet A+, *Ann Dermatol Venereol* (French) 116, 543
Fixed eruption (<1%)
  (2000): Sorkin M, Denver, CO (from Internet) (observation)
  (1961): Welsh AL+, *Arch Dermatol* 84, 1004
  (1950): Lewis HM+, *JAMA* 142, 1141
Flushing (<1%) (with alcohol)
  (1992): Breathnach SM+, *Adverse Drug Reactions and the Skin* Blackwell, Oxford, 204 (passim)
  (1992): Shelley WB+, *Advanced Dermatologic Diagnosis* WB Saunders, 582 (passim)
  (1982): Fisher AA, *Cutis* 30, 461 (passim)
  (1981): Wilkins JK, *Ann Intern Med* 95, 468
Purpura

  (1982): Thompson CC+, *J Am Dent Assoc* 105, 465
Pustules
  (1990): Larbre R+, *Ann Dermatol Venereol* (French) 117, 721
Rash (sic) (1–10%)
Systemic eczematous contact dermatitis (sic)
  (1966): Fisher AA, *Ann Allergy* 24, 406
Toxic epidermal necrolysis
  (1989): Stern RS+, *J Am Acad Dermatol* 21, 317
Urticaria
  (1992): Breathnach SM+, *Adverse Drug Reactions and the Skin* Blackwell, Oxford, 204 (passim)
  (1989): Minet A+, *Ann Dermatol Venereol* (French) 116, 543
  (1982): Fisher AA, *Cutis* 30, 461 (passim)
Vasculitis
  (1985): Sanchez NP+, *Arch Dermatol* 121, 220
Yellow palms
  (1997): Santonastaso M+, *Lancet* 350, 266

Other
Dysgeusia (metallic or garlic aftertaste) (1–10%)
Headache
Hypogeusia
Paresthesias
Periarteritis nodosa
  (1970): Zanini S+, *Fracastoro* (Italian) 63, 117
  (1975): Telerman-Toppet N+, *Acta Clin Belg* (French) 30, 101

DIVALPROEX

(See VALPROIC ACID)

DOBUTAMINE

Trade name: Dobutrex (Lilly)
Other common trade names: *Cardiject; Dobril; Dobuject; Dobutamin; Inotrex; Oxiken; Tobrex*
Indications: Cardiac surgery, heart failure
Category: Adrenergic agonist; Inotropic sympathomimetic; Vasopressor
Half-life: 2 minutes
Clinically important, potentially hazardous interactions with: furazolidone

Reactions

Skin
Cellulitis
  (1994): Cernek PK, *Ann Pharmacother* 28, 964
Erythema
  (1991): Wu CC+, *Chest* 99, 1547
Necrosis
  (1979): Hoff JV+, *N Engl J Med* 300, 1280
Pruritus
  (1991): Wu CC+, *Chest* 99, 1547
  (1986): McCauley CS+, *Ann Intern Med* 105, 966 (scalp)

Other
Headache
Hypersensitivity (sic)
  (1991): Wu CC+, *Chest* 99, 1547
Injection-site pain
Injection-site phlebitis
Paresthesias (1–10%)
Phlebitis

DOCETAXEL

Trade name: Taxotere (Aventis)
Indications: Metastatic breast cancer
Category: Antineoplastic
Half-life: 11–18 hours
Clinically important, potentially hazardous interactions with: aldesleukin, aprepitant

Reactions

Skin

Acral erythrodysesthesia syndrome
(2002): Eich D+, *Am J Clin Oncol* 25(6), 599 (2 cases)
(1995): Zimmerman GC+, *Arch Dermatol* 131, 202
(1994): Zimmerman GC+, *J Natl Cancer Inst* 86, 557
(1993): Vukelja SJ+, *J Natl Cancer Inst* 85, 1432
Allergic reactions (sic)
(2001): Talla M+, *Therapie* 56(5), 632
Angioedema
Ankle edema
(1995): Zimmerman GC+, *Arch Dermatol* 131, 202
Edema (1–20%)
(2002): Eich D+, *Am J Clin Oncol* 25(6), 599 (passim)
(1996): Edmonson JH+, *Am J Clin Oncon* 19, 574
(1993): Schrijvers D+, *Ann Oncol* 4, 610 (20%)
Edema of leg
(2002): Koukourakis MI+, *Anticancer Res* 22(4), 2491
Erythema (0.9%)
(2002): Hirai K+, *Gynecol Obstet Invest* 53(2), 118
(1995): Cortes JE+, *J Clin Oncol* 13, 2643
Exanthems
(1995): Cortes JE+, *J Clin Oncol* 13, 2643
(1995): Zimmerman GC+, *Arch Dermatol* 131, 202
Fixed eruption (erythematous plaque)
(2000): Chu CY+, *Br J Dermatol* 142, 808
Flushing
Infections
(2002): Bonneterre J+, *Br J Cancer* 87(11), 1210 (2%)
(2002): Koukourakis MI+, *Anticancer Res* 22(4), 2491
(2002): Souglakos J+, *Cancer* 95(6), 1326 (11.7%)
Peripheral edema (1–10%)
Photo-recall phenomenon
(1995): Zimmerman GC+, *Arch Dermatol* 131, 202
Photosensitivity
(2002): Eich D+, *Am J Clin Oncol* 25(6), 599 (passim)
(1995): Zimmerman GC+, *Arch Dermatol* 131, 202
Pruritus
(1995): Cortes JE+, *J Clin Oncol* 13, 2643
Radiation recall
(2002): Magne N+, *Cancer Radiother* 6(5), 281 (2 cases)
(2002): Morkas M+, *J Clin Oncol* 20(3), 867
(2002): Piroth MD+, *Onkologie* 25(5), 438
(2001): Giesel BU+, *Strahlenther Onkol* 177(9), 487
Rash (sic) (0.9%)
(1996): Edmonson JH+, *Am J Clin Oncon* 19, 574
Scleroderma
(2002): Eich D+, *Am J Clin Oncol* 25(6), 599 (passim)
(2001): Hassett G+, *Clin Exp Rheumatol* 19(2), 197
(1995): Battafarano DF+, *Cancer* 76,110
Seborrheic keratoses
(2001): Chu CY+, *Acta Derm Venereol* 81(4), 316
Squamous syringometaplasia
(2002): Karam A+, *Br J Dermatol* 146(3), 524
Toxic epidermal necrolysis
(2002): Dourakis SP+, *J Clin Oncol* 20(13), 3030

Urticaria
Xerosis
(1995): Cortes JE+, *J Clin Oncol* 13, 2643

Hair

Hair – alopecia (80%)
(2002): Eich D+, *Am J Clin Oncol* 25(6), 599 (passim)
(2002): Koukourakis MI+, *Anticancer Res* 22(4), 2491
(2002): Rein DT+, *Gynecol Oncol* 87(1), 98 (with carboplatin)
(1995): Lemenager M+, *Lancet* 346, 371

Nails

Nails – Beau's lines (transverse nail bands)
(2001): Camidge DR+, *Lancet Oncol* 2(6), 342
(1999): Correia O+, *Dermatology* 198, 288
Nails – changes (sic)
(2003): Kuroi K+, *Breast Cancer* 10(1), 10
(2002): Pavithran K+, *Br J Dermatol* 146(4), 709
(2001): Kuroi K+, *Gan To Kagaku Ryoho* (Japanese) 28(6), 797
(2001): Wasner G+, *Lancet* 357(9260), 910
Nails – hyponychial dermatitis
(2003): Chen GY+, *Br J Dermatol* 148, 1071 (with capecitabine)
Nails – loss
(2003): Maisano R+, *Anticancer Res* 23(2C), 1923
Nails – onycholysis
(2002): Eich D+, *Am J Clin Oncol* 25(6), 599 (passim)
(1999): Correia O+, *Dermatology* 198, 288
(1998): Obermair A+, *Ann Oncol* 9, 230
(1996): Dreyfuss AL+, *J Clin Oncol* 14, 1672
(1996): Trudeau ME, *Semin Oncol* 22, 17
(1995): Zimmerman GC+, *Arch Dermatol* 131, 202
Nails – paronychia
(1999): Correia O+, *Dermatology* 198, 288 (painful)
Nails – pigmentation
(2002): Eich D+, *Am J Clin Oncol* 25(6), 599 (passim)
(1999): Correia O+, *Dermatology* 198, 288 (orange discoloration)
(1998): Jacob CI+, *Arch Dermatol* 134, 1167 (nail bed dyschromia)
Nails – subungual abscess
(2000): Vanhooteghem O+, *Br J Dermatol* 143, 462
Nails – subungual hemorrhages
(1999): Correia O+, *Dermatology* 198, 288
Nails – subungual hyperkeratosis
(1999): Correia O+, *Dermatology* 198, 288
Nails – transverse superficial loss of nail plate
(1999): Correia O+, *Dermatology* 198, 288
(1997): Llombart-Cussac A+, *Arch Dermatol* 133, 1466

Other

Application-site fixed eruption
(1995): Zimmerman GC+, *Arch Dermatol* 131, 202
Asthenia
(2003): Kuroi K+, *Breast Cancer* 10(1), 10
Death
(2002): Morris MJ+, *Urology* 60(6), 1111
Dysesthesia (3.9%)
Dysgeusia
(2003): Maisano R+, *Anticancer Res* 23(2C), 1923
Dysphagia
(2002): Koukourakis MI+, *Anticancer Res* 22(4), 2491
Fatigue
(2003): Kuroi K+, *Breast Cancer* 10(1), 10
(2002): Paciucci PA+, *Anticancer Drugs* 13(8), 791
Fibrosis
(2000): Cleveland MG+, *Cancer* 88, 1078 (generalized)
Hypersensitivity (0.9%)
(2002): Denman JP+, *J Clin Oncol* 20(11), 2760 (previous hypersensitivity to paclitaxel)

(2002): Eich D+, *Am J Clin Oncol* 25(6), 599 (passim)
(1996): Hudis CA+, *J Clin Oncol* 14, 58
(1995): Bedikian AY+, *J Clin Oncol* 13, 2895
(1993): Schrijvers D+, *Ann Oncol* 4, 610 (28%)
Injection-site dermatitis
  (2002): Hirai K+, *Gynecol Obstet Invest* 53(2), 118
Injection-site erythema
  (2002): Hirai K+, *Gynecol Obstet Invest* 53(2), 118
  (1995): Zimmerman GC+, *Arch Dermatol* 131, 202
Injection-site exanthems
  (2002): Hirai K+, *Gynecol Obstet Invest* 53(2), 118
Injection-site extravasation
  (2000): Raley J+, *Gynecol Oncol* 78, 259
  (1995): Zimmerman GC+, *Arch Dermatol* 131, 202
Injection-site pigmentation
  (2000): Schrijvers D+, *Br J Dermatol* 142, 1069
  (1995): Zimmerman GC+, *Arch Dermatol* 131, 202
Injection-site reactions
  (2002): Eich D+, *Am J Clin Oncol* 25(6), 599 (passim)
Mucositis
  (2003): Suzuki M+, *Jpn J Clin Oncol* 33(6), 297
  (2002): Marx G+, *Br J Cancer* 87(8), 846 (with ifosfamide)
  (2002): Rein DT+, *Gynecol Oncol* 87(1), 98 (with carboplatin)
Myalgia (>10%)
Pain
  (2002): Paciucci PA+, *Anticancer Drugs* 13(8), 791
Paresthesias (3.9%)
  (2002): Eich D+, *Am J Clin Oncol* 25(6), 599 (passim)
Stomatitis (42.3%)
  (2002): Bonneterre J+, *Br J Cancer* 87(11), 1210 (5%)
  (2002): Eich D+, *Am J Clin Oncol* 25(6), 599 (passim)
  (1996): Edmonson JH+, *Am J Clin Oncon* 19, 574
Tearing
  (2003): Kuroi K+, *Breast Cancer* 10(1), 10
  (2003): Maisano R+, *Anticancer Res* 23(2C), 1923

DOCOSANOL

Synonyms: Behenyl Alcohol; n-Docosanol
Trade name: Abreva (GSK)
Indications: Herpes simplex (labialis)
Category: Antiviral (topical)
Half-life: N/A

Reactions

Skin
  Irritation (sic) (local)

DOCUSATE

Trade names: Colase (Purdue Frederick); Dialose; Diocto; Disonate; DOK; Doxinate; Peri-Colase (Purdue Frederick); Regutol; Sulfalax; Surfak (Pharmacia)
Other common trade names: *Coloxyl; Doxate-S; Hisof; Jamylene; Lambanol; Mollax; Regulex; Selax; SoFlax; Softon*
Indications: Constipation
Category: Laxative; Stool softener
Onset of action: 12–72 hours

Reactions

Skin
  Dermatitis
    (1998): Lee AY+, *Contact Dermatitis* 38, 355
  Diaphoresis
  Exanthems (1%)
  Rash (sic)

Other
  Dysgeusia

DOFETILIDE

Trade name: Tikosyn (Pfizer)
Indications: Conversion of atrial fibrillation and atrial flutter to normal sinus rhythm
Category: Class III antiarrhythmic
Half-life: 10 hours
Clinically important, potentially hazardous interactions with: atazanavir, chlorpromazine, cimetidine, co-trimoxazole, fluphenazine, ketoconazole, medroxyprogesterone, megestrol, mesoridazine, phenothiazines, prochlorperazine, progestins, promethazine, thioridazine, trifluoperazine, trimethoprim, verapamil

Reactions

Skin
  Angioedema (<2%)
  Diaphoresis (>2%)
  Edema
  Flu-like syndrome (sic) (4%)
  Peripheral edema (>2%)
  Rash (sic) (3%)

Other
  Headache
  Paresthesias (<2%)

DOLASETRON

Trade name: Anzemet (Aventis)
Indications: Prevention of nausea and vomiting
Category: Antiemetic
Half-life: 7.3 hours

Reactions

Skin
  Chills (>2%)

Diaphoresis
Edema
Facial edema
Flushing
Peripheral edema
Pruritus
Purpura
Rash (sic)
Urticaria

Other

Anaphylactoid reactions
Dysgeusia
Headache
Myalgia
Ocular pigmentation
Paresthesias
Thrombophlebitis
Twitching (sic)

DOMPERIDONE

Trade names: Evoxin; Motilium (Janssen)
Indications: Investigational antiemetic, gastroesophageal reflux disease (GERD), nausea and vomiting
Category: Peripherally-acting dopamine-2-receptor antagonist
Half-life: 7–8 hours

Note: Domperamol is domperidone & acetaminophen

Reactions

Skin

Diaphoresis
Edema
Edema of lip
Facial edema
Facial erythema
Lupus erythematosus
    (1986): Yasue T+, *J Dermatol* 13(4), 292
Neuroleptic malignant syndrome (<0.1%)
    (1992): Spirt MJ+, *Dig Dis Sci* 37(6), 946
Pruritus
Rash (sic)
    (1981): Nagler J+, *Am J Gastroenterol* 76(6), 495
Redness of face
Urticaria

Other

Anaphylactoid reactions
Breast changes (sic)
Death
    (1984): Giaccone G+, *Lancet* 2(8415):1336 (2 cases)
    (1982): Joss RA+, *Lancet* 1(8279):1019
Depression
    (1999): Patterson D+, *Am J Gastroenterol* 95(5), 1230
Dry mucous membranes
Galactorrhea
    (1992): Bozzolo M+, *Schweiz Rundsch Med Prax* 81:1511
    (1991): Nijhawan S+, *Indian J Gastroenterol* 10(3), 113
    (1986): Maddern GJ+, *J Clin Gastroenterol* 8(2), 135
    (1983): Cann PA+, *BMJ (Clin Res Ed)* 286(6375), 1395
    (1983): Maddern GJ, *Med J Aust* 2(11), 539
Gynecomastia
    (1991): Keating JP+, *Postgrad Med J* 67(786), 401
    (1982): van der Steen M+, *Lancet* 2(8303), 884 (in a male infant)

Hypersensitivity
Parkinsonism
    (1994): Llau ME+, *Rev Neurol* (Paris) (French) 150:757
Rhabdomyolysis
    (2002): Bourlon S+, *Therapie* 57(6), 597
Tremor

DONEPEZIL

Synonym: E2020
Trade name: Aricept (Roerig) (Endo)
Indications: Mild dementia of the Alzheimer's type
Category: Cholinergic; Reversible acetylcholinesterase inhibitor for Alzheimer's disease
Half-life: 50–70 hours
Clinically important, potentially hazardous interactions with: galantamine

Reactions

Skin

Dermatitis (sic) (<1%)
Diaphoresis (>1%)
Ecchymoses (4%)
Erythema (<1%)
Facial edema (<1%)
Flushing
    (1996): Rogers SL+, *Dementia* 7, 293 (3%)
Hyperkeratosis (sic) (<1%)
Neurodermatitis (sic) (<1%)
Neuroleptic malignant syndrome
    (2001): Ueki A+, *Nippon Ronen Igakkai Zasshi* 38(6), 822 (with bromperidol)
Periorbital edema (<1%)
Pigmentation (<1%)
Pruritus (>1%)
Purpura (1–10%)
    (1998): Bryant CA+, *BMJ* 317, 787
Striae (<1%)
Ulcerations (<1%)
Urticaria (>1%)

Hair

Hair – alopecia (<1%)
Hair – hirsutism (<1%)

Other

Anxiety
    (2002): Gauthier S+, *Int Psychogeriatr* 14(4), 389 (49%)
Depression
    (2002): Gauthier S+, *Int Psychogeriatr* 14(4), 389 (52%)
Dizziness
    (2002): Pratt RD+, *Int J Clin Pract* 56(9), 710
Dysgeusia (<1%)
Fatigue
    (2002): Pratt RD+, *Int J Clin Pract* 56(9), 710
Gingivitis (<1%)
Headache
    (2002): Pratt RD+, *Int J Clin Pract* 56(9), 710
Paresthesias (<1%)
Rhinitis
    (2002): Pratt RD+, *Int J Clin Pract* 56(9), 710
Tongue edema (<1%)
Vaginitis (<1%)
Xerostomia (<1%)

DONG QUAI

Scientific name: *Angelica sinensis (Angelica polymorpha sinensis)*
Family: Umbelliferae; Apioideae
Trade and other common names: Dang Gui; Dang Kwai; Danggui; Dong qua; Tan Kue; Tang Quai; Tank Kuei
Category: Immunostimulant; Phytoestrogen
Purported indications and other uses: Menopausal symptoms, PMS, menstrual disorders, anemia, constipation, insomnia, rheumatism, neuralgia, hypertension, hypopigmentation, psoriasis
Half-life: N/A
Clinically important, potentially hazardous interactions with: acetaminophen, dipyridamole, heparin, tamoxifen, ticlopidine, warfarin

Reactions

Skin
Photodermatitis
Phototoxicity

Other
Gynecomastia
  (2001): Goh SY+, *Singapore Med J* 42(3), 115
  (2001): Kiong HN, *Singapore Med J* 42(6), 286

Note: Some recent research has questioned the efficacy of Dong Quai, and also suggested that it may be a potential carcinogen

DOPAMINE

Trade names: Dopastat; Intropin
Other common trade names: *Cardiosteril; Dopamin; Dopamin AWD; Dynatra; Revimine*
Indications: Hemodynamic imbalances present in shock
Category: Adrenergic agonist; Inotropic sympathomimetic; Vasopressor
Half-life: 2 minutes
Clinically important, potentially hazardous interactions with: ethotoin, fosphenytoin, furazolidone, MAO inhibitors, mephenytoin, phenelzine, phenytoin, tranylcypromine

Reactions

Skin
Exanthems
Necrosis
  (2001): Subhani M+, *J Perinatol* 21(5), 324
Piloerection (goose bumps)
Pruritus
Raynaud's phenomenon (<1%)
Urticaria

Hair
Hair – alopecia

Other
Headache
Injection-site extravasation
  (1998): Chen JL+, *Ann Pharmacother* 32, 545
  (1989): Denkler KA+, *Plast Reconstr Surg* 84, 811
Injection-site gangrene
  (1977): Boltax RS+, *N Engl J Med* 296, 823
Injection-site necrosis (<1%)

  (1992): Breathnach SM+, *Adverse Drug Reactions and the Skin*
    Blackwell, Oxford, 233 (passim)
  (1982): Pillgram-Larsen J+, *Tidsskr Nor Laegeforen* (Norwegian)
    102, 1583
  (1976): Green SI+, *N Engl J Med* 294, 114
Injection-site piloerection and vasoconstriction (sic)
  (1991): Ross M, *Arch Dermatol* 127, 586
Peripheral ischemia
  (1983): Coakley J, *Lancet* 2, 633
Symmetric peripheral gangrene (sic)
  (1997): Weinberg JM+, *Arch Dermatol* 133, 249

DORZOLAMIDE

Trade names: Cosopt (Merck); Trusopt (Merck)
Indications: Glaucoma, ocular hypertension
Category: Carbonic anhydrase inhibitor (sulfonamide)
Half-life: about 4 months

Cosopt is dorzolamide and timolol

Reactions

Skin
Blepharoconjunctivitis
  (2001): Mancuso G+, *Contact Dermatitis* 45(4), 243
Burning
  (2003): Hommer A+, *Br J Ophthalmol* 87(5), 592
Dermatitis
  (2001): Shimada M+, *Contact Dermatitis* 45(1), 52
  (1998): Aalto-Korte K, *Contact Dermatitis* 39, 206
Eyelid edema
  (1998): Adamsons IA+, *J Glaucoma* 7, 395
Periorbital dermatitis
  (2002): Delaney YM+, *Br J Ophthalmol* 86(4), 378
Rash (sic) (<1%)
Stinging (ocular) (33%)
  (2000): Stewart WC+, *Am J Ophthalmol* 129, 723
  (1998): Adamsons IA+, *J Glaucoma* 7, 395

Other
Dysgeusia (25%)
  (2000): Sall K, *Surv Ophthalmol* 44, S155
  (2000): Sugrue MF, *Prog Retin Eye Res* 19(1), 87
Headache
Ocular burning (33%)
Ocular irritation
  (2001): Seong GJ+, *Ophthalmologica* 215(3), 188

*Note: Dorzolamide is a sulfonamide and can be absorbed systemically. Sulfonamides can produce severe, possibly fatal, reactions such as toxic epidermal necrolysis and Stevens–Johnson syndrome

DOXACURIUM

Trade name: Nuromax (GSK)
Indications: Neuromuscular blockade
Category: Neuromuscular blocker; Skeletal muscle relaxant
Half-life: 100–200 minutes
**Clinically important, potentially hazardous interactions
with:** amikacin, aminoglycosides, carbamazepine, cyclopropane,
enflurane, gentamicin, halothane, isoflurane, kanamycin,
methoxyflurane, neomycin, piperacillin, streptomycin, tobramycin

Reactions

Skin
  Rash (sic)
  Urticaria (<1%)

DOXAPRAM

Trade name: Dopram (Elkins-Sinn)
Indications: Chronic obstructive pulmonary disease, drug-
induced CNS depression
Category: CNS stimulant; Respiratory stimulant
Duration of action: 3.4 hours

Reactions

Skin
  Diaphoresis (<1%)
  Flushing
    (1972): *Drug Ther Bull* 10, 43
  Pruritus
    (1972): *Drug Ther Bull* 10, 43

Other
  Injection-site erythema
  Injection-site pain
  Injection-site phlebitis (<1%)
  Oral mucosal lesions
  Paresthesias

DOXAZOSIN

Trade name: Cardura (Pfizer)
Other common trade names: *Alfadil; Cardoxan; Cardular;
Dedralen; Diblocin; Supressin*
Indications: Hypertension
Category: Alpha-adrenoceptor blocker; Antihypertensive
Half-life: 19–22 hours

Reactions

Skin
  Bruising
    (1991): Anon, *Arch Intern Med* 151, 1413
  Diaphoresis (1.4%)
    (1988): Young JL+, *Drugs* 35, 525
  Eczema (sic) (<0.5%)
  Edema (4%)
  Exanthems (1.7%)
    (1988): Young JL+, *Drugs* 35, 525

Facial edema (1%)
Flu-like syndrome (sic) (1.1%)
Flushing (1%)
  (1991): Anon, *Arch Intern Med* 151, 1413
Hot flashes (<1%)
Lichen planus
  (2001): Madnani N, Mumbai, India (from Internet) (observation)
Lichenoid eruption
  (2002): Mittal A, Udaipur, India (from Internet) (observation)
Lupus erythematosus
  (1992): Feurle GE, *Dtsch Med Wochenschr* (German) 117, 157
Pallor (<1%)
Peripheral edema
Pruritus (1%)
Purpura (<0.5%)
Rash (sic) (1%)
  (1991): Anon, *Arch Intern Med* 151, 1413
Urticaria
  (1991): Anon, *Arch Intern Med* 151, 1413
Xerosis (<0.5%)

Hair
  Hair – alopecia (<0.5%)
    (1991): Anon, *Arch Intern Med* 151, 1413
  Hair – growth (sic)
    (1991): Anon, *Arch Intern Med* 151, 1413

Other
  Dysgeusia (<0.5%)
    (1991): Anon, *Arch Intern Med* 151, 1413
  Headache
  Hyperesthesia (<1%)
  Mastodynia (<1%)
  Myalgia (1%)
  Paresthesias
  Parosmia (<0.05%)
  Tinnitus
  Xerostomia (2%)
    (1991): Anon, *Arch Intern Med* 151, 1413

DOXEPIN

Trade names: Sinequan (Roerig); Zonalon (topical) (Bioglan)
Other common trade names: *Adapin; Alti-Doxepin; Anten;
Aponal; Doneurin; Gilex; Mareen; Novo-Doxepin; Sinquan; Triadapin*
Indications: Mental depression, anxiety
Category: Antipanic; Tricyclic antidepressant
Half-life: 6–8 hours
**Clinically important, potentially hazardous interactions
with: alcohol**, amprenavir, arbutamine, cholestyramine,
clonidine, CNS depressants, epinephrine, formoterol,
guanethidine, isocarboxazid, linezolid, MAO inhibitors,
phenelzine, QT interval prolonging agents, quinolones, selegiline,
sparfloxacin, sympathomimetics, tranylcypromine

Reactions

Skin
  Allergic reactions (sic)
  Ankle edema
    (1991): Dalack GW+, *Am J Psychiatry* 148, 1601
  Dermatitis (from topical)
    (2003): Bonnel RA+, *J Am Acad Dermatol* 48(2), 294
    (2003): Brancaccio RR+, *J Drugs Dermatol* 2(4), 409
    (1999): Wakelin SH+, *Contact Dermatitis* 40, 214

(1997): Koehn G, *The Schoch Letter* 47, 20 (observation)
(1996): Bilbao I+, *Contact Dermatitis* 35, 254
(1996): Rapaport MJ, *Arch Dermatol* 132, 1516
(1996): Shama S, *The Schoch Letter* 46, 36 (observation)
(1996): Shelley WB+, *J Am Acad Dermatol* 34, 143
(1996): Smith KC, Niagara Falls, Ontario (from Internet)
  (observation)
(1996): Taylor JS+, *Arch Dermatol* 132, 515
(1995): Goldblum O, *The Schoch Letter* 45, 26 (observation)
(1995): Greenberg JH, *Contact Dermatitis* 33, 281
(1995): Porres J, *The Schoch Letter* 45, 39 (observation)
Diaphoresis (1–10%)
Edema
Erythema
Erythroderma (sic)
(1991): Kastrup O+, *Dtsch Med Wochenschr* (German)
  116, 1748
Exanthems
(1970): Pöldinger P+, *Praxis* 59, 1006 (0.4%)
Flushing
(1998): Foster M+, *J Clin Dermatol* Winter, 7
Photosensitivity (<1%)
(1985): Walter-Ryan WG+, *JAMA* 254, 357
(1982): *Patient Care* June 15, 208 (list)
Pruritus
(1970): Pöldinger P+, *Praxis* 59, 1006
Purpura
(1972): Nixon DD, *JAMA* 220, 418
Rash (sic)
(1991): Roose SP+, *J Clin Psychiatry* 52, 338
Toxic dermatitis (sic)
(1995): Vo MY, *Arch Dermatol* 131, 1468
Urticaria
Vasculitis

Hair
Hair – alopecia (<1%)

Other
Aphthous stomatitis
(1980): Ives TJ+, *Am J Hosp Pharm* 37, 1551 (passim)
Application-site burning
Application-site edema
Dysgeusia (>10%)
Galactorrhea (<1%)
Glossalgia
(1980): Ives TJ+, *Am J Hosp Pharm* 37, 1551 (passim)
Glossitis
(1980): Ives TJ+, *Am J Hosp Pharm* 37, 1551
Gynecomastia (<1%)
Headache
Paresthesias
Parkinsonism
Pseudolymphoma
(1995): Magro CM+, *J Am Acad Dermatol* 32, 419
(1988): Kardaun SH+, *Br J Dermatol* 118(4), 545
Rhabdomyolysis
(1988): Hojgaard AD+, *Acta Med Scand* 223, 79 (with
  nitrazepam)
Stomatitis
(1981): Salem RB+, *Drug Intell Clin Pharm* 15, 992
Tinnitus
Tremor
Xerostomia (>10%)
(1998): Foster M+, *J Clin Dermatol* Winter, 7 (5%)
(1989): Assalian P+, *Drugs* 38(Suppl 1), 32
(1989): Lose G+, *J Urol* 142, 1024

DOXERCALCIFEROL

Trade name: Hectorol (Bone Care)
Indications: Secondary hyperparathyroidism
Category: Vitamin D analog (prohormone)
Half-life: 32–37 hours

Reactions

Skin
Edema (34.4%)
Pruritus (8.2%)

DOXORUBICIN

Trade names: Adriamycin (Pharmacia); Doxil (Ortho); Rubex
(Bristol-Myers Squibb)
Other common trade names: *Adiblastine; Adriablastine;
Adriacin; Adriblatina; Farmablastina*
Indications: Carcinomas, leukemias, sarcomas
Category: Antineoplastic; Cytotoxic antibiotic
Half-life: α phase: 0.6 hours; β phase: 16.7 hours
**Clinically important, potentially hazardous interactions
with:** aldesleukin

Reactions

Skin
Acral erythema
(1995): Komamura H+, *J Dermatol* 22(2), 116 (with vincristine,
  cyclophosphamide and GCSF)
Acral erythrodysesthesia syndrome (hand–foot syndrome)
(2002): Numico G+, *Lung Cancer* 35(1), 59
(2001): Goram AL+, *Pharmacotherapy* 21(6), 751
(2001): Verschraegen CF+, *Cancer* 92(9), 2327
(2000): Lotem M+, *Arch Dermatol* 136, 1475
(1995): Gordon KB+, *Cancer* 75, 2169
(1991): Baack BR+, *J Am Acad Dermatol* 24, 457
(1989): Jones AP+, *Br J Cancer* 59, 814
(1985): Levine LE+, *Arch Dermatol* 121, 102
(1985): Vogelzang NJ+, *Ann Intern Med* 103, 303
(1985): Walker IR+, *Arch Dermatol* 121, 1240
(1984): Lokich JJ+, *Ann Intern Med* 101, 798
(1982): Cordonnier C+, *Ann Intern Med* 97, 783
Actinic keratoses
(2001): Eisner J, Mt. Vernon, WA (from Internet) (observation)
(1987): Johnson TM+, *J Am Acad Dermatol* 17(2 pT 1), 192
Adverse effects (sic)
(2001): Verschraegen CF+, *Cancer* 92(9), 2327
Allergic reactions (sic) (<1%)
(2002): Cantu MG+, *J Clin Oncol* 20(5), 1232 (2%) (with
  cyclophosphamide and cisplatin)
(2002): McMenemin R+, *Invest New Drugs* 20(3), 331
(1979): Fallah-Sohy E+, *JAMA* 241, 1108
Angioedema
(1984): Collins JA, *Drug Intell Clin Pharm* 18, 402
(1983): Bronner AK+, *J Am Acad Dermatol* 9, 645
(1981): von Eyben FE+, *Cancer* 48, 1535 (passim)
(1981): Weiss RB+, *Ann Intern Med* 94, 66
(1979): Maldonado JE, *N Engl J Med* 301, 386
Cellulitis
Dermatitis
(1975): Reich SD+, *Cancer Chemother Rep* 59, 677
Dermatitis herpetiformis

(1986): Gottlieb D+, *Med J Aust* 145, 241

Exanthems
(1987): Lee M+, *J Urol* 138, 143
(1984): Collins JA, *Drug Intell Clin Pharm* 18, 402

Exfoliative dermatitis
(1975): Manalo FB+, *JAMA* 233, 56

Flushing (1–10%)
(1992): Curran CF, *Arch Dermatol* 128, 1408
(1987): Lee M+, *J Urol* 138, 143

Hand-foot syndrome
(2003): Skubitz KM, *Cancer Invest* 21(2), 167

Intertrigo
(2000): Lotem M+, *Arch Dermatol* 136, 1475

Keratoderma
(1975): Manalo FB+, *JAMA* 233, 56

Melanotic macules
(2000): Lotem M+, *Arch Dermatol* 136, 1475

Necrosis (local)
(1998): Bekerecioglu M+, *J Surg Res* 75, 61
(1982): Riegels-Nielsen P+, *Ugeskr-Laeger* (Danish) 144, 1313
(1981): von Eyben FE+, *Cancer* 48, 1535 (passim)
(1976): Rudolph R+, *Cancer* 38, 1087

Palmar–plantar dysesthesia
(2002): Fracasso PM+, *Cancer* 95(10), 2223 (with gemcitabine)
(2002): Hussein MA+, *Cancer* 95(10), 2160 (with vincristine and dexamethasone)

Palmar–plantar erythema (painful)
(1990): Pagliuca A+, *Postgrad Med J* 66, 242
(1989): Jones AP+, *Br J Cancer* 59, 814
(1989): Oksenhendler E+, *Eur J Cancer Clin Oncol* 25, 1181
(1988): Shall L+, *Br J Dermatol* 119, 249

Pigmentation
(1996): Schulte-Huermann P+, *Dermatology* 191, 65
(1992): Konohana A, *J Dermatol* 19, 250
(1990): Curran CF, *N Z Med J* 103, 517
(1990): Kumar L+, *N Z Med J* 103, 165
(1987): Loureiro C+, *J Clin Oncol* 5, 1705
(1983): Bronner AK+, *J Am Acad Dermatol* 9, 645 (palms and soles)
(1982): Alagaratnam TT+, *Aust N Z J Surg* 52, 531
(1981): Granstein RD+, *J Am Acad Dermatol* 5, 1 (brown-black)
(1980): Orr LE+, *Arch Dermatol* 116, 273
(1977): Kew MC+, *Lancet* 1, 811
(1976): Rubegni M+, *Nouv Presse Med* (French) 5, 798
(1974): Pratt CB+, *JAMA* 228, 460 (dermal creases)
(1974): Rothberg H+, *Cancer Chemother Rep* 58, 749

Postirradiation erythema

Pruritus
(1987): Lee M+, *J Urol* 138, 143
(1984): Solimando DA+, *Drug Intell Clin Pharm* 18, 808

Purpura
(1987): Lee M+, *J Urol* 138, 143
(1971): Wang JJ+, *Cancer* 28, 837

Pustular psoriasis
(2001): Kreuter A+, *Acta Derm Venereol* 81(3), 224

Radiation recall (<1%)
(2000): Lotem M+, *Arch Dermatol* 136, 1475
(1976): Greco FA+, *Ann Intern Med* 85, 294
(1975): Dreizen S+, *Postgrad Med* 58, 150
(1974): Etcubanas E+, *Cancer Chemother Rep* 58, 757

Rash (sic)
(2002): Fracasso PM+, *Cancer* 95(10), 2223 (with gemcitabine)
(2000): Israel VP+, *Gynecol Oncol* 78, 143
(1981): Karlin DA+, *Lancet* 2, 534

Raynaud's phenomenon
(1993): von Gunten CF+, *Cancer* 72, 2004

Scrotal skin toxicity (sic)
(2000): Toma S+, *Anticancer Res* 20, 485

Toxicity (sic)
(1981): von Eyben FE+, *Cancer* 48, 1535

Urticaria (<1%)
(1986): Wandt H, *Dtsch Med Wochenschr* (German) 111, 356
(1984): Collins JA, *Drug Intell Clin Pharm* 18, 402
(1984): Solimando DA+, *Drug Intell Clin Pharm* 18, 808
(1983): Bronner AK+, *J Am Acad Dermatol* 9, 645
(1981): Hatfield AK+, *Cancer Treat Rep* 65, 353
(1981): von Eyben FE+, *Cancer* 48, 1535 (passim)
(1981): Weiss RB+, *Ann Intern Med* 94, 66
(1978): Souhami J+, *JAMA* 240, 1624
(1974): Pratt CB+, *Am J Dis Child* 127, 534
(1974): Pratt CB+, *JAMA* 228, 460 (passim)

Hair

Hair – alopecia (>10%)
(2000): Lotem M+, *Arch Dermatol* 136, 1475 (passim)
(1995): Bonadonna G+, *JAMA* 273, 542 (96%)
(1994): Bogner JR+, *J Acquir Immune Defic Syndr* 7, 463
(1994): Rodrigeuz R+, *Ann Oncol* 5, 769
(1989): Henderson IC+, *J Clin Oncol* 7, 560 (>5%)
(1988): Giaccone G+, *Cancer Nurs* 11, 170
(1986): Martin-Jiminez M+, *N Engl J Med* 315, 894
(1986): Perez JE+, *Cancer Treat Rep* 70, 1213
(1984): Satterwhite B+, *Cancer* 54, 34
(1984): Wheelock JB+, *Cancer Treat Rep* 68, 1387
(1983): Howard N+, *Br J Radiol* 56, 963
(1983): Tigges FJ, *MMW Munch Med Wochenschr* (German) 125, 19
(1982): Gregory RP+, *Br Med J Clin Res Ed* 284, 1674
(1982): Hunt JM+, *Cancer Nurs* 5, 25
(1981): Anderson JE+, *Br Med J Clin Res* 282, 423
(1981): Cooke T+, *Br Med J Clin Res Ed* 282, 734
(1981): Hallett N, *Nurs Mirror* 152, 32
(1981): Tigges FJ, *MMW Munch Med Wochenschr* (German) 123, 737
(1980): Presser SE, *N Engl J Med* 302, 921
(1980): Timothy AR+, *Lancet* 1, 663
(1979): Dean JC+, *N Engl J Med* 301, 1427
(1979): Lovejoy NC, *Cancer Nurs* 2, 117
(1978): Soukop M+, *Cancer Treat Rep* 62, 489
(1977): Edelstyn GA+, *Lancet* 2, 253
(1975): Manalo FB+, *JAMA* 233, 56
(1974): Blum RH+, *Ann Intern Med* 80, 249 (85–100%)
(1974): Cortes EP+, *JAMA* 221, 1132 (100%)
(1974): Pratt CB+, *Am J Dis Child* 127, 534 (80%)
(1974): Pratt CB+, *JAMA* 228, 460 (passim)
(1971): Middleman E, *Cancer* 25, 844
(1971): Wang JJ+, *Cancer* 28, 837
(1969): Bonadonna G+, *BMJ* 3, 503 (60–100%)

Nails

Nails – Beau's lines (transverse nail bands)
(1994): Ben-Dayan D+, *Acta Haematol* 91, 89

Nails – onycholysis
(1990): Curran CF, *Arch Dermatol* 126, 1244
(1989): Jones AP+, *Br J Cancer* 59, 814
(1985): Kechijian P, *J Am Acad Dermatol* 12, 552
(1980): Runne U+, *Z Haut* (German) 55, 1590
(1975): Manalo FB+, *JAMA* 233, 56

Nails – pigmentation
(1999): Ghoshal UC+, *J Diarrhoeal Dis Res* 17, 43
(1983): Bronner AK+, *J Am Acad Dermatol* 9, 645
(1983): James WD+, *Arch Dermatol* 119, 334 (white lines)
(1983): Manigand G+, *Sem Hop* (French) 59, 1840
(1982): Sans-Ortiz J+, *Med Clin (Barc)* (Spanish) 79, 49
(1981): Giacobetti R+, *Am J Dis Child* 135, 317
(1980): Runne U+, *Z Haut* (German) 55, 1590
(1980): Sulis E+, *Eur J Cancer* 16, 1517
(1977): Kew MC+, *Lancet* 1, 811
(1977): Morris D+, *Cancer Chemother Rep* 61, 499

(1976): Nixon DW, *Arch Intern Med* 113, 1117
(1975): Priestman TJ+, *Lancet* 1, 3337
(1974): Pratt CB+, *JAMA* 228, 460 (21%)

Other

Anaphylactoid reactions (<1%)
  (1984): Collins JA, *Drug Intell Clin Pharm* 18, 402
  (1982): Dunagin WG, *Semin Oncol* 9, 14
Death
  (2002): Escudier B+, *J Urol* 168(3), 959 (with ifosfamide)
  (2002): McMenemin R+, *Invest New Drugs* 20(3), 331
Headache
Injection-site erythema
  (1984): Collins JA, *Drug Intell Clin Pharm* 18, 402
  (1983): Bronner AK+, *J Am Acad Dermatol* 9, 645
  (1982): Dunagin WG, *Semin Oncol* 9, 14
  (1981): von Eyben FE+, *Cancer* 48, 1535 (passim)
  (1981): Weiss RB+, *Ann Intern Med* 94, 66 (>5%)
  (1978): Souhami J+, *JAMA* 240, 1624
  (1974): Etcubanas E+, *Cancer Chemother Rep* 58, 757 (>5%)
Injection-site extravasation (>10%)
  (2000): Kassner E, *J Pediatr Oncon Nurs* 17, 135
  (2000): Lotem M+, *Arch Dermatol* 136, 1475
  (1999): Fleming A+, *J Hand Surg [Br]* 24, 390
  (1998): Emiroglu M+, *Ann Plast Surg* 41, 103
  (1989): Harwood KV+, *Oncol Nurs Forum* 16, 10
  (1984): Hankin FM+, *J Pediatr Orthop* 4, 96
  (1984): Sonneveld P+, *Cancer Treat Rep* 68, 895
  (1983): Cohen FJ+, *J Hand Surg Am* 8, 43
  (1983): Olver IN+, *Cancer Treat Rep* 67, 407
  (1983): Pitkanen J+, *J Surg Oncol* 23, 259
  (1980): Barden GA, *South Med J* 73, 1543
  (1978): Bowers DG+, *Plast Reconstr Surg* 61, 86
Injection-site necrosis (>10%)
  (1998): Bekerecioglu M+, *J Surg Res* 75, 61
  (1987): Dufresne RG, *Cutis* 39, 197
  (1983): Bronner AK+, *J Am Acad Dermatol* 9, 645
  (1978): Souhami J+, *JAMA* 240, 1624
  (1976): Rudolph R+, *Cancer* 38, 1087
Injection-site reactions
  (2001): Verschraegen CF+, *Cancer* 92(9), 2327
Injection-site ulceration (>10%)
  (1979): Petro JA+, *Surg Forum* 30, 535
  (1979): Zweig JI+, *Cancer Treat Rep* 63, 2101
  (1978): Mehta P+, *Clin Pediatr Phila* 17, 663
  (1977): Reilly JJ+, *Cancer* 40, 2053
Mucositis
  (2003): Skubitz KM, *Cancer Invest* 21(2), 167
  (2002): McMenemin R+, *Invest New Drugs* 20(3), 331
  (2001): Verschraegen CF+, *Cancer* 92(9), 2327
  (2000): Lotem M+, *Arch Dermatol* 136, 1475
Myalgia
  (2002): Cantu MG+, *J Clin Oncol* 20(5), 1232 (4%) (with
    cyclophosphamide and cisplatin)
Oral mucosal lesions
  (1975): Dreizen S+, *Postgrad Med* 58, 75 (71%)
  (1974): Blum RH+, *Ann Intern Med* 80, 249 (79%)
  (1974): Cortes EP+, *JAMA* 221, 1132 (61%)
  (1974): Pratt CB+, *Am J Dis Child* 127, 534 (37%)
  (1971): Middleman E, *Cancer* 25, 844
  (1971): Wang JJ+, *Cancer* 28, 837
  (1969): Bonadonna G+, *BMJ* 3, 503 (100%)
Oral mucosal pigmentation
  (1989): Kerker BJ+, *Semin Dermatol* 8, 173
Oral ulceration
  (1974): Pratt CB+, *JAMA* 228, 460 (passim)
Stomatitis (>10%)
  (2002): Fracasso PM+, *Cancer* 95(10), 2223 (with gemcitabine)
  (2002): Numico G+, *Lung Cancer* 35(1), 59

(2001): Goram AL+, *Pharmacotherapy* 21(6), 751
(2001): Verschraegen CF+, *Cancer* 92(9), 2327
(2000): Israel VP+, *Gynecol Oncol* 78, 143
(2000): Lotem M+, *Arch Dermatol* 136, 1475
(1994): Bogner JR+, *J Acquir Immune Defic Syndr* 7, 463
(1989): Henderson IC+, *J Clin Oncol* 7, 560 (8.4%)
(1981): von Eyben FE+, *Cancer* 48, 1535 (passim)
(1975): Dreizen S+, *Postgrad Med* 58, 75 (>5%)
(1975): Manalo FB+, *JAMA* 233, 56
(1969): Bonadonna G+, *BMJ* 3, 503 (60–100%)
Tongue pigmentation
  (1989): Kerker BJ+, *Semin Dermatol* 8, 173
  (1976): Rao SP+, *Cancer Treat Rep* 60, 1402

DOXYCYCLINE

Trade names: Adoxa (Bioglan); Doryx (Warner Chilcott);
Monodox (Oclassen); Vibra-Tabs (Pfizer); Vibramycin (Pfizer)
Other common trade names: *Apo-Dox; Apo-Doxy; Atridox;
Azudoxat; Bactidox; Doximed; Doxy-100; Doxylin; Doxytec;
Vibramycine; Vibravenos*
Indications: Various infections caused by susceptible organisms
Category: Tetracycline antibiotic
Half-life: 12–22 hours
**Clinically important, potentially hazardous interactions
with:** amoxicillin, ampicillin, antacids, bacampicillin, bismuth,
calcium, carbenicillin, cloxacillin, corticosteroids, digoxin, iron,
methoxyflurane, mezlocillin, nafcillin, oxacillin, penicillins,
piperacillin, retinoids, ticarcillin, zinc

Reactions

Skin

Actinic granuloma
  (2003): Lim DS+, *Australas J Dermatol* 44(1), 67
Acute generalized exanthematous pustulosis (AGEP)
  (1993): Trueb RM+, *Dermatology* 186, 75
Allergic reactions (sic) (0.47%)
  (1986): Bigby M+, *JAMA* 256, 3358
Angioedema
  (1997): Shapiro LE+, *Arch Dermatol* 133, 1224
Candidiasis
  (2002): Baxter BT+, *J Vasc Surg* 36(1), 1
Erythema multiforme
  (1988): Lewis-Jones MS+, *Clin Exp Dermatol* 13, 245
  (1987): Curley RK+, *Clin Exp Dermatol* 12, 124
  (1985): Albengres E+, *Therapie* (French) 38, 577
Erythroderma
  (2003): Batinac T+, *Tumori* 89(1), 91
Exanthems
  (1987): Bryant SG+, *Pharmacotherapy* 7, 125 (4.4%)
Exfoliative dermatitis
Fixed eruption (<1%)
  (2003): Drayton GE, Los Angeles, CA (from Internet)
    (observation)
  (2003): Gregg LJ, Tulsa, OK (from Internet) (observation) (3
    cases – all on glans penis)
  (2002): Walfish AE+, *Cutis* 69, 207 (Metronidazole, in the same
    patient, also produced a Fixed eruption)
  (1999): Correia O+, *Clin Exp Dermatol* 24, 137 (genital) (with
    minocycline)
  (1996): Marmelzat J, Los Angeles, CA (from Internet)
    (observation)
  (1989): Alanko K+, *Acta Derm Venereol* (Stockh) 69, 223
  (1988): Budde J+, *Aktuel Dermatol* (German) 14, 304
  (1987): Jolly HW+, *Arch Dermatol* 114, 1484
  (1984): Bargman H, *J Am Acad Dermatol* 11, 900

Lupus erythematosus

Maculopapular rash
  (2003): Batinac T+, *Tumori* 89(1), 91

Painful eruption of hands (sic)
  (1995): Levine N, *Geriatrics* 50, 23

Photosensitivity (<1%)
  (2002): Baxter BT+, *J Vasc Surg* 36(1), 1
  (2002): Litt JZ, Beachwood, OH (personal observation)
  (2002): Maffei K, Athens, GA (from Internet) (observation)
  (2002): Pages F+, *Trop Med Int Health* 7(11), 919
  (1997): O'Reilly FM+, American Academy of Dermatology Meeting, Poster #14
  (1997): Shapiro LE+, *Arch Dermatol* 133, 1224
  (1997): Tanaka N+, *Contact Dermatitis* 37, 93
  (1995): Nowakowski J+, *J Am Acad Dermatol* 32, 223
  (1992): Bennett MJ, *J R Army Med Corps* 138, 56
  (1987): Edwards R, *N Z Med J* 100, 640
  (1980): Möller H+, *Acta Derm Venereol* (Stockh) 60, 495
  (1977): Rey M+, *Nouv Presse Med* (French) 6, 3755
  (1973): Zuehlke RL, *Arch Dermatol* 108, 837
  (1968): Blank H+, *Arch Dermatol* 97, 1 (20%)

Phototoxicity
  (2002): Bohannon JS, Midlothian, VA (from Internet) (observation)
  (2002): Fishman CB, San Luis Obispo, CA (from Internet) (observation)
  (2002): Litt JZ, Beachwood, OH (personal case) (observation)
  (2002): Sorkin M, Denver, CO (from Internet) (observation)
  (2002): Thaler D, Monona, WI (from Internet) (observation)
  (1999): Litt JZ, Beachwood, OH (personal case) (observation)
  (1996): McCarty JR, Fort Worth, TX (from Internet) (observation)
  (1995): Smith EL+, *Br J Dermatol* 132, 316
  (1994): Bjellerup AM+, *Br J Dermatol* 130, 356
  (1993): Layton A+, *Clin Exp Dermatol* 18, 425
  (1993): Shea CR+, *J Invest Dermatol* 101, 329
  (1982): Rosen K+, *Acta Derm Venereol* 62, 246
  (1972): Frost P+, *Arch Dermatol* 105, 681

Pigmentation
  (2002): Bohm M+, *Am J Dermatopathol* 24(4), 345
  (1999): Westermann GW+, *J Intern Med* 246, 591
  (1980): Möller H+, *Acta Derm Venereol* (Stockh) 60, 495

Pruritus ani

Psoriasis
  (1988): Tsankov NK+, *Australas J Dermatol* 29, 111

Purpura

Rash (sic) (<1%)
  (1997): Shapiro LE+, *Arch Dermatol* 133, 1224

Seborrhea (sic)
  (1997): Rademaker M, New Zealand (from Internet) (observation)

Stevens–Johnson syndrome
  (1987): Curley RK+, *Clin Exp Dermatol* 12, 124

Toxic epidermal necrolysis
  (1999): Egan CA+, *J Am Acad Dermatol* 40, 458
  (1974): Aksnes K, *Tidsskr Nor Laegeforen* (Norwegian) 94, 1254

Urticaria
  (2002): Pages F+, *Trop Med Int Health* 7(11), 919
  (1997): Shapiro LE+, *Arch Dermatol* 133, 1224
  (1992): Deluze C+, *Allergol Immunopathol Madr* (Spanish) 20, 215
  (1989): Alanko K+, *Acta Derm Venereol* (Stockh) 69, 223

Vasculitis
  (1981): Rockl H, *Hautarzt* (German) 32, 467

Nails

Nails – discoloration (painful)
  (1993): Coffin SE+, *Pediatr Infect Dis J* 12, 702

Nails – onycholysis

Nails – photo-onycholysis
  (2000): Yong CK+, *Pediatrics* 106, E13
  (1995): Shapero H, *The Schoch Letter* 45 #6, 21 (observation)
  (1988): Quirce-Gancedo S+, *Med Clin* (Barc) (Spanish) 90, 636
  (1987): Baran R+, *J Am Acad Dermatol* 17, 1012
  (1985): Gventer M+, *J Am Podiatr Med Assoc* 75, 658
  (1982): Jeanmougin M+, *Ann Dermatol Venereol* (French) 109, 165
  (1981): Cavens TR, *Cutis* 27, 53
  (1972): Ramelli G+, *Cutis* 10, 155
  (1971): Frank SB+, *Arch Dermatol* 103, 520

Other

Anaphylactoid reactions

Anosmia
  (1990): Bleasel AF+, *Med J Aust* 152, 440

Dysgeusia
  (2001): Bunker C, United Kingdom (personal communication)

Fever
  (2003): Batinac T+, *Tumori* 89(1), 91

Glossitis

Headache

Hyperesthesia
  (2002): Sorkin M, Denver, CO (from Internet) (two observations)

Hypersensitivity

Injection-site phlebitis (<1%)

Mouth ulcers
  (2002): Pages F+, *Trop Med Int Health* 7(11), 919

Paresthesias
  (1995): Shapero H, *The Schoch Letter* 45, 21 (observation)
  (1994): Blanchard L, *The Schoch Letter* 44, #6 (observation)
  (1994): Liss W, *The Schoch Letter* 44, 16 (observation)
  (1993): Held J, *The Schoch Letter* 43, 27 (observation)

Phlebitis (<1%)

Pseudotumor cerebri

Serum sickness
  (1997): Shapiro LE+, *Arch Dermatol* 133, 1224

Tongue pigmentation

Tooth discoloration (>10%) (in children)
  (2002): Baxter BT+, *J Vasc Surg* 36(1), 1
  (1998): Lochary ME+, *Pediatr Infect Dis J* 17, 429 (staining of permanent teeth)

Tooth pigmentation
  (2002): Baxter BT+, *J Vasc Surg* 36(1), 1

Vaginitis
  (1995): Nowakowski J+, *J Am Acad Dermatol* 32, 223

DRONABINOL

Synonyms: tetrahydrocannabinol; THC
Trade name: Marinol (Solvay) (Unimed)
Indications: Chemotherapy-induced nausea
Category: Antiemetic; Appetite stimulant
Half-life: 19–24 hours

Reactions

Skin
  Diaphoresis (<1%)
  Flushing (<1%)

Other
  Myalgia (<1%)
  Paresthesias
  Tinnitus
  Xerostomia (1–10%)

DROPERIDOL

Trade names: Droperidol (AstraZeneca); Inapsine (Akorn)
Other common trade names: *Dehydrobenzperidol; Droleptan; Inapsin; Sintodian*
Indications: Tranquilizer and antiemetic in surgical procedures
Category: Antiemetic; Antipsychotic
Half-life: 2.3 hours

Reactions

Skin
Chills
Diaphoresis
Pruritus
  (2003): Culebras X+, *Anesth Analg* 97(3), 816 (6.1%)
Shivering (sic)

Other
Anxiety
  (2003): Silberstein SD+, *Neurology* 60(2), 315 (30%)
Death
  (2001): Glassman AH+, *Am J Psychiatry* 158(11), 1774
Seizures
  (2002): Chase PB+, *Acad Emerg Med* 9(12), 1402 (3 cases)

DROTRECOGIN ALFA

Trade name: Xigris (Lilly)
Indications: Severe sepsis
Category: Recombinant human activated protein C
Half-life: 1.6 hours

Reactions

Skin
Bleeding (severe)
Purpura (>10%)

DUTASTERIDE

Trade name: Avodart (GSK)
Indications: Benign prostatic hyperplasia, male pattern baldness (anecdotal)
Category: 5-alpha-reductase inhibitor
Half-life: 3–5 weeks

Reactions

Skin
None

Other
Gynecomastia (1%)
Mastodynia

ECHINACEA

Scientific names: *Echinacea angustifola; Echinacea pallida; Echinacea purpurea*
Family: Asteraceae; Compositae
Trade and other common names: Black Sampson; Black Susans; Comb Flower; Indian Head; Purple-Cone Flower; Snakeroot
Category: Antiseptic; Antiviral; Immunomodulator
Purported indications and other uses: Colds, upper respiratory infections, peripheral vasodilator, urinary tract infections, yeast infections, ulcers, psoriasis, herpes simplex, septicemia, boils, abscesses, rheumatism, migraine, dyspepsia, eczema, bee stings and hemorrhoids
Half-life: N/A
Clinically important, potentially hazardous interactions with: corticosteroids, cyclosporine

Reactions

Skin
Adverse effects (sic)
 (2002): Bielory L, *Ann Allergy Asthma Immunol* 88(1), 7
 (2002): Ernst E, *Ann Intern Med* 136(1), 42
 (2002): Haller CA+, *Adverse Drug React Toxicol Rev* 21(3), 143
 (2002): Mattsson K+, *Lakartidningen* 99(50), 5095
Allergic reactions (sic)
Angioedema
 (2000):
  www.aaaai.org/media/pressreleases/2000/03/000307.html
Erythema nodosum
 (2001): Crawford R, *J Am Acad Dermatol* 44, 298 (recurrent)
Rash (sic)
 (2002): Mullins RJ+, *Ann Allergy Asthma Immunol* 88(1), 42
Sensitization
 (2002): Paulsen E, *Contact Dermatitis* 47(4), 189
Urticaria
 (2002): Mullins RJ+, *Ann Allergy Asthma Immunol* 88(1), 42
 (2000):
  www.aaaai.org/media/pressreleases/2000/03/000307.html

Other
Anaphylactoid reactions
 (2002): Mullins RJ+, *Ann Allergy Asthma Immunol* 88(1), 42
 (2000):
  www.aaaai.org/media/pressreleases/2000/03/000307.html
 (1998): Mullins RJ, *Med J Aust* 168, 170
Dizziness
 (2003): Kligler B, *Am Fam Physician* 2003 Jan 67(1), 77
Hypersensitivity
 (2002): Mullins RJ+, *Ann Allergy Asthma Immunol* 88(1), 42
 (2000):
  www.aaaai.org/media/pressreleases/2000/03/000307.html (23 cases)
Paresthesias
Sialorrhea

Note: Individuals with atopy may be more likely to experience an allergic reaction when taking Echinacea

EDROPHONIUM

Trade names: Enlon (Baxter); Reversol (Organon); Tensilon (ICN)
Indications: Myasthenia gravis diagnosis
Category: Anticholinesterase; Antidote; Neuromuscular blocker
Half-life: 1.8 hours
Clinically important, potentially hazardous interactions with: corticosteroids, galantamine

Reactions

Skin
Diaphoresis (>10%)
Flushing
Rash (sic)
Urticaria

Other
Anaphylactoid reactions
Headache
Hypersensitivity (<1%)
Sialorrhea (>10%)
Thrombophlebitis (<1%)

EFAVIRENZ

Trade name: Sustiva (Bristol-Myers Squibb)
Indications: HIV infection
Category: Antiretroviral non-nucleoside reverse transcriptase inhibitor (NNRTI)
Half-life: 52–76 hours
Clinically important, potentially hazardous interactions with: alprazolam, benzodiazepines, chlordiazepoxide, clonazepam, clorazepate, diazepam, dihydroergotamine, ergot, flurazepam, lorazepam, methysergide, midazolam, oral contraceptives, oxazepam, quazepam, temazepam, triazolam

Reactions

Skin
Eczema (sic) (<2%)
Erythema
 (2003): Foti JL+, *AIDS Patient Care STDS* 17(1), 1
Exanthems (27%)
 (2001): Hartmann M+, *HIV Clin Trials* 2(5), 421
 (1998): Adkins JC+, *Drugs* 56, 1055
Exfoliation (sic) (<2%)
Flushing (<2%)
Folliculitis (<2%)
Hot flashes (<2%)
Peripheral edema (<2%)
Photosensitivity
 (2000): Newell A+, *Sex Transm Infect* 76, 221
Pruritus (<2%)
Rash (sic) (5–20%)
 (2002): Perez-Molina JA, *HIV Clin Trials* 3(4), 279 (5.8%)
Urticaria (<2%)
Vasculitis
 (2002): Domingo P+, *Arch Intern Med* 162(3), 355

Hair
Hair – alopecia (<2%)

Other
Depression
  (2002): Puzantian T, *Pharmacotherapy* 22(7), 930
Dysgeusia (<2%)
Fever
  (2003): Foti JL+, *AIDS Patient Care STDS* 17(1), 1
Gynecomastia
  (2002): Qazi NA+, *AIDS* 16(3), 506
  (2001): Arranz Caso JA+, *AIDS* 15(11), 1447
  (2001): Caso JA+, *AIDS* 15(11), 1447
  (2001): Mercie P+, *AIDS* 15(1), 126
Headache
Hyperesthesia (1–2%)
Hypersensitivity
  (2003): Foti JL+, *AIDS Patient Care STDS* 17(1), 1
  (2000): Bossi P+, *Clin Infect Dis* 30, 227
Myalgia (<2%)
Paresthesias (<2%)
Parosmia (<2%)
Thrombophlebitis (<2%)
Tremor (<2%)
Xerostomia (<2%)

EFLORNITHINE

Synonym: DFMO
Trade names: Ornidyl; Vaniqa (Women First)
Indications: Sleeping sickness, hypertrichosis
Category: Ornithine decarboxylase inhibitor
Half-life: IV: 3–3.5 hours; topical: 8 hours

Reactions

Skin
Acne (24.3%)
  (2001): Thaler D, Monona, WS (perioral) (from Internet)
    (observation))
Burning (4.3%)
Cheilitis (<1%)
Dermatitis (<1%)
Edema of lip (<1%)
Erythema (1.3%)
  (2001): Hickman JG+, *Curr Med Res Opin* 16, 235
Facial edema (0.3–3%)
Folliculitis (0.5%)
Herpes simplex (<1%)
Irritation (1%)
Pruritus (3.8%)
  (2001): Hickman JG+, *Curr Med Res Opin* 16, 235
Rash (sic) (2.8%)
Rosacea (<1%)
Stinging (7.9%)
Xerosis (1.8%)
  (2001): Hickman JG+, *Curr Med Res Opin* 16, 235

Hair
Hair – alopecia (1.5%)
  (2003): Burri C+, *Parasitol Res* 90(Suppl 1), S49 (5–10%)
Hair – ingrown (0.3–2%)
Hair – pseudofolliculitis barbae (5–15%)

Other
Paresthesias (3.6%)
Seizures
  (2003): Burri C+, *Parasitol Res* 90(Suppl 1), S49 (7%)

Thrombocytopenia
  (2003): Burri C+, *Parasitol Res* 90(Suppl 1), S49 (25%)

ELETRIPTAN

Trade name: Relpax (Pfizer)
Indications: Migraine headaches
Category: Serotonin agonist
Half-life: 4–5 hours

Reactions

Skin
Abscess (<1%)
Allergic reactions (sic) (<1%)
Candidiasis (<1%)
Chills (<1%)
Diaphoresis (<1%)
Edema (<1%)
Exanthems (<1%)
Exfoliative dermatitis (<1%)
Facial edema (<1%)
Peripheral edema (<1%)
Pigmentation (<1%)
Pruritus (<1%)
Psoriasis (<1%)
Rash (sic) (<1%)
Urticaria (<1%)
Xerosis (<1%)

Hair
Hair – alopecia

Other
Arthralgia (<1%)
Depression (<1%)
Dysgeusia (<1%)
Foetor ex ore (halitosis) (<1%)
Gingivitis (<1%)
Headache
Hyperesthesia (<1%)
Mastodynia (<1%)
Myalgia (<1%)
Myopathy (<1%)
Paresthesias (<1%)
Parosmia (<1%)
Sialorrhea (<1%)
Stomatitis (<1%)
Tinnitus (<1%)
Tongue disorder (<1%)
Tooth disorder (sic) (<1%)
Tremor (<1%)
Twitching (<1%)
Vaginitis (<1%)

ENALAPRIL

Trade names: Lexxel (AstraZeneca); Teczem (Aventis); Vasotec (Merck)
Other common trade names: Amprace; Apo-Enalapril; Enaladil; Enapren; Glioten; Innovace; Pres; Renitec; Reniten; Xanef
Indications: Hypertension
Category: Angiotensin-converting enzyme (ACE) inhibitor; Antihypertensive
Half-life: 11 hours
Clinically important, potentially hazardous interactions with: amiloride, spironolactone, triamterene

Lexxel is enalapril and felodipine; Teczem is enalapril and diltiazem; Vaseretic is enalapril and hydrochlorothiazide

Reactions

Skin

Acantholysis (sic)
  (1999): Lo Schiavo A+, Dermatology 198, 391
Angioedema (<1%)
  (2003): Olesen AL+, Ugeskr Laeger 165(10), 1041
  (2003): Regner KR+, Mayo Clin Proc 78(5), 655
  (2002): Abdi R+, Pharmacotherapy 22(9), 1173
  (2002): Kaur S+, J Dermatol 29(6), 336
  (2001): Cohen EG+, Ann Otol Rhinol Laryngol 110(8), 701 (64 cases)
  (2000): Babadzhan VD+, Lik Sprava (Russian) Apr-Jun, (3–4), 54
  (1998): Prescrire Int 7, 92
  (1998): Leuwer A+, HNO (German) 46, 56 (9 cases)
  (1997): Brown NJ+, JAMA 278, 232
  (1996): Kind B+, Schweiz Rundsch Med Prax (German) 85, 567
  (1996): Langauer-Messmer S+, Postgrad Med J 72, 383
  (1996): Mullins RJ+, Med J Aust 165, 319 (visceral)
  (1996): Pillans PI+, Eur J Clin Pharmacol 51, 123
  (1995): Forslund T+, J Intern Med 238, 179
  (1995): Juarez-Giminez JC+, Ann Pharmacother 29, 317
  (1995): Kozel MM+, Clin Exp Dermatol 20, 60
  (1995): Waldfahrer F+, HNO (German) 43, 35
  (1994): Dupasquier E, Arch Mal Coeur Vaiss (French) 87, 1371
  (1994): Dyer PD, J Allergy Clin Immunol 93, 947
  (1994): Farraye FA+, Am J Gastroenterol 89, 1117
  (1994): Lehmke J, Med Klin (German) 89, 508
  (1994): Nielsen EW+, Tidsskr Nor Laegeforen (Norwegian) 114, 804
  (1994): Varma JR+, J Am Board Fam Pract 7, 433
  (1993): Oike Y+, Intern Med 32, 308 (fatal)
  (1993): Thompson T+, Laryngoscope 103, 10
  (1992): Bielory L+, Allergy Proc 13, 85
  (1992): Diehl KL+, Dtsch Med Wochenschr (German) 117, 727
  (1992): Dobroschke R+, Anasthesiol Intensivmed Notfallmed Schmerzther (German) 27, 510
  (1992): Finley CJ+, Am J Emerg Med 10, 550
  (1992): Hedner T+, BMJ 304, 941
  (1992): Jain M+, Chest 102, 871
  (1992): Venable RJ, J Fam Pract 34, 201
  (1991): Abidin MR+, Arch Otolaryngol Head Neck Surg 117, 1059
  (1991): Candelaria LM+, J Oral Maxillofac Surg 49, 1237
  (1991): Lanting PJ+, Ned Tijdschr Geneeskd (Dutch) 135, 335
  (1991): Roberts JR+, Ann Emerg Med 20, 555
  (1990): Chin HL+, Ann Intern Med 112, 312
  (1990): DiNardo LJ+, Trans Pa Acad Ophthalmol Otolaryngol 42, 998
  (1990): Gannon TH+, Laryngoscope 100, 1156
  (1990): Gianos ME+, Am J Emerg Med 8, 124
  (1990): Gonnering RS+, Am J Ophthalmol 110, 566
  (1990): McAreavey D+, Drugs 40, 326 (0.2%)

  (1990): Orfan N+, JAMA 264, 1287
  (1990): Seidman MD+, Otolaryngol Head Neck Surg 102, 727
  (1990): Zech J+, HNO (German) 38, 143
  (1989): Barna JS+, Va Med 116, 147
  (1989): Giannoccaro PJ+, Can J. Cardiol 5, 335 (fatal)
  (1989): Huwyler T+, Schweiz Med Wochenschr (German) 119, 1253
  (1989): Smith ME+, Otolaryngol Head Neck Surg 101, 93
  (1989): Todd PA+, Drugs 37, 141 (<0.1%)
  (1989): Werber JL+, Otolaryngol Head Neck Surg 101, 96
  (1988): Inman WH+, BMJ 297, 826
  (1988): Schilling H+, Z Kardiol 77 (German) (Suppl 3), 47
  (1988): Slater EE+, JAMA 260, 967 (0.1%)
  (1988): Wernze H, Z Kardiol (German) 77, 61
  (1987): Ferner RE+, BMJ 294, 1119
  (1987): Inman WHW, BMJ 294, 578
  (1987): Vaillant L+, Therapie (French) 42, 411
  (1987): Wood SM+, BMJ 294, 91
  (1986): Marichal JF+, Therapie (French) 41, 517
Bullous pemphigoid
  (1994): Mullins PD+, BMJ 309, 1411
  (1993): Smith EP+, J Am Acad Dermatol 29, 879
Diaphoresis (<1%)
  (1994): Nachbar F+, Dtsch Med Wochenschr (German) 119, 321
Erythema
  (1993): Carrington PR+, Cutis 51, 121
Erythema multiforme (<1%)
Exanthems
  (1993): Carrington PR+, Cutis 51, 121
  (1990): McAreavey D+, Drugs 40, 326 (1.4%)
  (1990): Ruiz AM+, Drugs 39 (Suppl 2) 77 (0.9%)
  (1989): Todd PA+, Drugs 37, 141
  (1988): Warner NJ+, Drugs 35 (Suppl 5), 89 (1.4%)
  (1986): Gavras H, Clin Ther 9, 24
  (1986): Todd PA+, Drugs 31, 198 (0.5%)
  (1984): Kubo SH+, Ann Intern Med 100, 616
  (1983): Barnes JN+, Lancet 2, 41
Exfoliative dermatitis (<1%)
Flushing (<1%)
  (1989): Healey LA+, N Engl J Med 321, 763
  (1987): Ferner RE+, BMJ (Clin Res) 294, 1119
Herpes zoster (<1%)
Lichenoid eruption
  (1995): Roten SV+, J Am Acad Dermatol 32, 293
  (1993): Kanwar AJ+, Dermatology 187, 80 (photosensitive)
Lupus erythematosus
  (1990): Schwarz D+, Lancet 336, 187
Mycosis fungoides
  (1986): Furness PN+, J Clin Pathol 39, 902
Pemphigus
  (2001): Thami GP+, Dermatology 202(4), 341
  (1997): Brenner S+, J Am Acad Dermatol 36, 919
  (1996): Mitchell DF, Charleston, SC (from Internet) (observation)
  (1995): Frangogiannis NG+, Ann Intern Med 122, 803 (larynx and esophagus)
  (1994): Kuechle MK+, Mayo Clin Proc 69, 1166
  (1994): Wolf R+, Dermatology 189, 1
  (1993): Brenner S+, Clin Dermatol 11, 501
  (1992): Ruocco V+, Int J Dermatol 31, 33
Pemphigus foliaceus
  (2000): Ong CS+, Australas J Dermatol 41(4), 242
  (1991): Shelton RM, J Am Acad Dermatol 24, 503
Pemphigus vegetans
  (1994): Bastiaens MT+, Int J Dermatol 33, 168 (3 cases)
Photodermatitis
  (1993): Shelley WB+, Cutis 52, 81 (observation)
Photosensitivity (<1%)
  (1997): O'Reilly FM+, American Academy of Dermatology Meeting, Poster #14

(1993): Kanwar AJ+, *Dermatology* 187, 80
Pruritus (<1%)
  (1993): Litt JZ, Beachwood, OH (personal case) (observation)
  (1990): Heckerling PS, *Ann Intern Med* 112, 879 (vulvovaginal)
  (1987): Nugent LW+, *J Clin Pharmacol* 27, 461
  (1986): Gavras H, *Clin Ther* 9, 24 (0.75%)
Psoriasis
  (1993): Coulter DM+, *N Z Med J* 106, 392
  (1990): Wolf R+, *Dermatologica* 181, 51
Purpura
  (1989): Grosbois B+, *BMJ* 298, 189 (with quinidine)
Rash (sic) (1.4%)
  (2000): Babadzhan VD+, *Lik Sprava* (Russian) Apr–Jun, (3–4), 54
  (1986): DiBianco R, *Med Toxicol* 1, 122 (passim)
  (1986): Irvin JD+, *Am J Med* 81, 46
  (1984): Davies RO+, *Am J Med* 77, 23
  (1984): McFate Smith W+, *J Hypertens* Suppl 2, S113
Stevens–Johnson syndrome (<1%)
Toxic epidermal necrolysis (<1%)
Toxic pustuloderma
  (1996): Ferguson JE+, *Clin Exp Dermatol* 21, 54
Urticaria (<1%)
  (1996): Pillans PI+, *Eur J Clin Pharmacol* 51, 123
  (1993): Carrington PR+, *Cutis* 51, 121
  (1988): Inman WH+, *BMJ* 297, 826
  (1988): Slater EE+, *JAMA* 260, 967
  (1987): Wood SM+, *BMJ* 294, 91
Vasculitis (<1%)
  (1993): Carrington PR+, *Cutis* 51, 121
  (1991): Ayani I+, *Med Clin* (Barc) (Spanish) 95, 596

Hair

Hair – alopecia (<1%)
  (1991): Ahmad S, *Arch Intern Med* 151, 404

Nails

Nails – dystrophy
  (1986): Gupta S+, *BMJ* 293, 140

Other

Ageusia
  (1988): Rumboldt Z+, *Int J Clin Pharmacol Res* 8(3), 181
  (1984): Davies RO+, *Am J Med* 77, 23
  (1984): McFate Smith W+, *J Hypertens* Suppl 2, S113
Anaphylactoid reactions (<1%)
  (1989): Todd PA+, *Drugs* 37, 141
Anosmia (<1%)
Cough
  (2002): Coca A+, *Clin Ther* 24(1), 126
  (2002): Cuspidi C+, *J Hypertens* 20(11), 2293
  (2001): Adigun AQ+, *West Afr J Med* 20(1), 46
  (2001): Lee SC+, *Hypertension* 38(2), 166
  (2001): Rake EC+, *J Hum Hypertens* 15(12), 863 (23%)
  (2000): Babadzhan VD+, *Lik Sprava* (Russian) Apr–Jun, (3–4), 54
  (1988): Rumboldt Z+, *Int J Clin Pharmacol Res* 8(3), 181
Death
  (2001): Gonzalez de la Puente MA+, *Ann Pharmacother* 35(11), 1492
Dysesthesia (<1%)
Dysgeusia (1–10%)
  (2000): Zervakis J+, *Physiol Behav* 68, 405
  (1988): Schilling H+, *Z Kardiol* (German) 77 (Suppl 3), 47
  (1986): DiBianco R, *Med Toxicol* 1, 122
  (1986): Irvin JD+, *Am J Med* 81, 46
  (1984): Davies RO+, *Am J Med* 77, 23
Glossitis (<1%)
Glossopyrosis
  (1989): Drucker CR+, *Arch Dermatol* 125, 1437
Gynecomastia

(1994): Llop R+, *Ann Pharmacother* 28, 671
Headache
Myalgia (<1%)
Oral bleeding (sic)
  (1984): Kubo SH+, *Ann Intern Med* 100, 616
Oral mucosal lesions
  (1986): Gavras H, *Clin Ther* 9, 24 (0.37%)
  (1986): Todd PA+, *Drugs* 31, 198 (0.5%)
  (1985): Gomez HJ+, *Drugs* 30 (Suppl 1), 13
  (1984): Kubo SH+, *Ann Intern Med* 100, 616
Oral mucosal lichenoid eruption
  (1989): Firth NA+, *Oral Surg Oral Med Oral Pathol* 67, 41
Oral ulceration
  (2000): Madinier I+, *Ann Med Interne (Paris)* 151, 248
  (1982): Viraben R+, *Arch Dermatol* 118, 959
Paresthesias (<1%)
Pseudopolymyalgia
  (1989): Leloët X+, *BMJ* 298, 325
  (1986): Furness PN+, *J Clin Pathol* 39, 902
Scalded mouth (sic)
  (1982): Vlasses PH+, *BMJ* 284, 1672
Stomatitis (<1%)
Tinnitus
Tongue edema
  (1996): Litt JZ, Beachwood, OH (personal case) (observation)
  (1990): Zech J+, *HNO* (German) 38, 143
  (1986): Marichal JF+, *Therapie* (French) 41, 517
Xerostomia (<1%)

ENFLURANE

Trade name: Ethrane (Baxter)
Other common trade names: *Alyrane; Efrane; Etrane*
Indications: Maintenance of general anesthesia
Category: General anesthetic
Half-life: N/A
**Clinically important, potentially hazardous interactions
with:** cisatracurium, doxacurium, pancuronium, rapacuronium

Reactions

Skin

Shivering

Other

Rhabdomyolysis
  (1987): Lee SC+, *J Oral Maxillofac Surg* 45(9), 789 (with succinylcholine)

ENFUVIRTIDE

Trade name: Fuzeon (Roche)
Other common trade name: *T-20*
Indications: HIV-1 Infection (in combination with other antiretroviral agents)
Category: Antiviral; Fusion inhibitor
Half-life: 3.8 hours

Reactions

Skin

Chills
Ecchymoses (48%)

Edema
Exanthems
Flu-like syndrome (3.9%)
Herpes simplex (5%)
Papillomas (4.2%)
Pruritus (62%)
Rash (sic)

Other
Abdominal pain (3%)
Anxiety (5.7%)
Asthenia (5.7%)
Conjunctivitis (2.4%)
Cough (7.4%)
Depression (8.65)
Dizziness
Dysgeusia (2.4%)
Fatigue (16.1%)
Fever
Guillain–Barré syndrome (fatal)
Hypersensitivity (<1%)
Injection-site erythema (89%)
Injection-site induration (89%)
Injection-site nodules (76%)
Injection-site pain (95%)
Injection-site pruritus
Injection-site reactions (sic) (98%)
  (2003): Lalezari JP+, *AIDS* 17(5), 691
  (2003): Lalezari JP+, *N Engl J Med* 348(22), 2175 (98%)
  (2002): Chen RY+, *Expert Opin Investig Drugs* 11(12), 1837
  (2002): Kilby JM+, *AIDS Res Hum Retroviruses* 18(10), 685
Myalgia (5%)
Paresthesias
Pneumonia
  (2003): Lalezari JP+, *N Engl J Med* 348(22), 2175
Sinusitis (6.2%)

ENOXACIN

Trade name: Penetrex (Aventis)
Other common trade names: *Bactidan; Comprecin; Enoxacine; Enoxen; Enoxor; Gyramid*
Indications: Urinary tract infections
Category: Fluoroquinolone antibiotic
Half-life: 3–6 hours
Clinically important, potentially hazardous interactions with: amiodarone, arsenic, bepridil, bretylium, disopyramide, erythromycin, phenothiazines, procainamide, quinidine, sotalol, tricyclic antidepressants

Reactions

Skin
Chills (<1%)
Diaphoresis (<1%)
Edema (<1%)
Erythema multiforme (<1%)
Erythema nodosum
Exanthems
  (1988): Henwood JM+, *Drugs* 32, 32 (0.57%)
Exfoliative dermatitis (<1%)
Photosensitivity (<1%)
  (1993): Kang JS+, *Photodermatol Photoimmunol Photomed* 9, 159
  (1992): Izu R+, *Photodermatol Photoimmunol Photomed* 9, 86

  (1990): Schauder S, *Z Hautkr* (German) 65, 253
  (1989): Kawabe Y+, *Photodermatology* 6, 57
  (1988): Henwood JM+, *Drugs* 32, 32 (0.57%)
Phototoxicity
  (1998): Martinez LJ+, *Photochem Photobiol* 67, 399
  (1994): Fujita H+, *Photodermatol Photoimmunol Photomed* 10, 202
  (1990): Przybilla B+, *Dermatologica* 181, 98
  (1990): Schauder S, *Z Hautkr* (German) 65, 253
Pigmentation
Pruritus (<1%)
Purpura (<1%)
Rash (sic) (<1%)
Stevens–Johnson syndrome (<1%)
Toxic epidermal necrolysis (<1%)
Urticaria (<1%)
  (1988): Henwood JM+, *Drugs* 32, 32 (0.57%)

Other
Dysgeusia
Hypersensitivity
Injection-site phlebitis
Myalgia (<1%)
Paresthesias (<1%)
Stomatitis (<1%)
Tendon rupture (<1%)
Tinnitus
Tremor (<1%)
Vaginal candidiasis (<1%)
Vaginitis (<1%)
Xerostomia (<1%)

ENOXAPARIN

Trade name: Lovenox (Aventis)
Other common trade names: *Clexan; Clexane 40; Klexane*
Indications: Prevention of deep vein thrombosis
Category: Anticoagulant; Low-molecular weight heparin
Half-life: 4.5 hours
Clinically important, potentially hazardous interactions with: butabarbital, danaparoid

Reactions

Skin
Angioedema
  (1992): Odeh M+, *Lancet* 340, 972
Ecchymoses (2%)
Edema (3%)
Erythema (1–10%)
  (1993): Phillips JK+, *Br J Haematol* 85, 837
Exanthems
  (2002): MacLaughlin EJ+, *Pharmacotherapy* 22, 1511
  (2001): Kim K & Lynfield Y, New York, NY (personal communication)
Necrosis (<1%)
  (2002): Toll A+, *World Congress Dermatol* Poster, 0130
Peripheral edema (3%)
Pruritus
  (2002): MacLaughlin EJ+, *Pharmacotherapy* 22, 1511
  (2001): Kim K & Lynfield Y, New York, NY (personal communication)
Purpura (1–10%)
Side effects (sic) (0.2%)
  (2000): Enrique E+, *Contact Dermatitis* 42, 43

Urticaria
   (1997): Downham TF, Taylor, MI (from Internet) (observation)
   (1992): Odeh M+, *Lancet - 2985213R* 340, 972
Vesicular eruptions (<1%)

Other

Anaphylactoid reactions (<1%)
   (2002): MacLaughlin EJ+, *Pharmacotherapy* 22(11), 1511
Anxiety
   (2002): MacLaughlin EJ+, *Pharmacotherapy* 22(11), 1511
Cough
   (2002): MacLaughlin EJ+, *Pharmacotherapy* 22(11), 1511
Erythematous macular rash
   (2002): MacLaughlin EJ+, *Pharmacotherapy* 22(11), 1511
Fat necrosis
   (2001): Davies J+, *Postgrad Med* 77(903), 43112
Hypersensitivity
   (2000): Romero Ortega MR+, *Aten Primaria* (Spanish) 25, 521
   (1998): Cabanas R+, *J Investig Allergol Clin Immunol* 8, 383
   (1998): Mendez J+, *Allergy* 53, 999
   (1996): Koch P+, *Contact Dermatitis* 34, 156
   (1996): Mendez J+, *Allergy* 51, 853
Injection-site erythema
   (2001): Kim K & Lynfield Y, New York, NY (personal
      communication)
Injection-site exanthems
   (2000): Szolar-Platzer C+, *J Am Acad Dermatol* 43, 920
Injection-site hematoma
   (2002): Robb DM+, *Pharmacotherapy* 22(9), 1105
Injection-site infiltrated plaques
   (1998): Mendez J+, *Allergy* 53, 999
   (1998): Valdes F+, *Allergy* 53, 625
Injection-site necrosis
   (1997): Lefebvre I+, *Ann Dermatol Venereol* (French) 124, 397
   (1997): Tonn ME+, *Ann Pharmacother* 31, 323
   (1996): Fried M+, *Ann Intern Med* 125, 521
Injection-site pain
   (2002): Robb DM+, *Pharmacotherapy* 22(9), 1105
Injection-site pruritus
   (2000): Szolar-Platzer C+, *J Am Acad Dermatol* 43, 920

ENTACAPONE

Trade name: Comtan (Novartis)
Other common trade name: *Comtess*
Indications: Parkinsonism
Category: Antiparkinsonian; Reverse COMT inhibitor
Half-life: 2.4 hours
**Clinically important, potentially hazardous interactions
with:** MAO inhibitors, phenelzine, tranylcypromine

Reactions

Skin

Bacterial infections (sic) (1%)
Diaphoresis (2%)
Purpura (2%)

Other

Dizziness
   (2003): Larsen JP+, *Eur J Neurol* 10(2), 137 (20%)
Dysgeusia (1%)
Dyskinesia
   (2003): Fenelon G+, *J Neural Transm* 110(3), 239 (31%)
Headache
Parkinsonism

   (2003): Larsen JP+, *Eur J Neurol* 10(2), 137 (17%)
Xerostomia (3%)

EPHEDRA

Scientific names: *Ephedra equisetina; Ephedra intermedia;
Ephedra sinica; Ephedra vulgaris*
Family: Gnetaceae
Trade and other common names: Joint Fir; Ma Huang;
Popotillo; Sea Grape; Teamster's Tea; Yellow Astringent; Yellow
Horse
Category: Cardiovascular stimulant; CNS stimulant
Purported indications and other uses: Bronchospasm,
asthma, bronchitis, allergy, appetite suppressant, colds, flu, fever,
chills, edema, headache, anhidrosis, diuretic, joint and bone pain
Half-life: N/A
**Clinically important, potentially hazardous interactions
with:** acetazolamide, amitriptyline, **caffeine**, corticosteriods,
ephedrine, epinephrine, guanethidine, MAO inhibitors,
olmesartan, phenelzine, phenylpropanolamine, selegiline,
sibutramine, sodium bicarbonate

Reactions

Skin

Adverse effects (sic)
   (2003): Bent S+, *Ann Intern Med* 138(6), 468
   (2002): Arditti J+, *Acta Clin Belg* Suppl (1), 34 (slimming pills)
   (2002): Haller CA+, *Adverse Drug React Toxicol Rev* 21(3), 143
Flushing

Other

Death
   (2003): Charatan F, *BMJ* 326(7387), 464
   (2002): Arditti J+, *Acta Clin Belg* Suppl (1), 34 (slimming pills)
Eosinophilia–myalgia syndrome
   (1999): Zaacks SM+, *J Toxicol Clin Toxicol* 37, 485
Hypersensitivity
Myalgia
Myopathy
Seizures
   (2002): Arditti J+, *Acta Clin Belg* Suppl (1), 34
   (2002): van der Hooft CS+, *Ned Tijdschr Geneeskd*
      146(28), 1335
Side effects (sic)
   (2002): Lawrence ME+, *J Clin Gastroenterol* 35(4), 299
Tremor
Xerostomia
   (2002): Boozer CN+, *Int J Obes Relat Metab Disord* 26(5), 593
      (with ephedra)

EPHEDRINE

Trade names: Ectasule; Efedron; Ephedsol; Marax; Pretz-D; Rynatuss (Wallace); Vicks Vatronol (Procter & Gamble)
Indications: Nasal congestion, acute hypotensive states, asthma
Category: Adrenergic agonist; Sympathomimetic bronchodilator
Half-life: 3–6 hours
Clinically important, potentially hazardous interactions with: antihypertensives, **ephedra**, furazolidone, guanethidine, MAO inhibitors, methyldopa, phenelzine, phenylpropanolamine, selegiline, tranylcypromine, tricyclic antidepressants

Reactions

Skin
Bullous eruption
  (1944): Lewis G, *Arch Dermatol* 49, 379
Dermatitis (following topical application)
  (1945): Spencer GA, *Arch Dermatol* 51, 48
  (1944): Lewis G, *Arch Dermatol* 49, 379
  (1936): Hollander L, *JAMA* February 29, 706
Dermatitis (sic)
  (1993): Villas-Martinez F+, *Contact Dermatitis* 29, 215
  (1991): Audicana M+, *Contact Dermatitis* 24, 223
Diaphoresis (1–10%)
Edema
Exanthems
  (1933): Abramovitz EW+, *Br J Dermatol* XLV, 236
Exfoliative dermatitis
  (1981): Serup J, *Ugeskr Laeger* (Danish) 143, 1660
Fixed eruption
  (2000): Tanimoto K+, *Masui* 49(12), 1374
  (1997): Garcia Ortiz JC+, *Allergy* 52, 229
  (1994): Krivda SJ+, *J Am Acad Dermatol* 31, 291 (non-pigmenting)
  (1968): Brownstein MH, *Arch Dermatol* 97, 115
  (1960): Englehardt AW, *Hautarzt* (German) 11, 49
Pallor (1–10%)
Purpura
  (1933): Abramovitz EW+, *Br J Dermatol* XLV, 236
Toxic epidermal necrolysis
  (2002): Yung A+, *Australas J Dermatol* 43(1), 35
Urticaria
  (1978): Speer F+, *Ann Allergy* 40, 32
  (1933): Abramovitz EW+, *Br J Dermatol* XLV, 236
Vasculitis
  (1978): Speer F+, *Ann Allergy* 40, 32

Other
Death
  (2003): Kanstrup MH+, *Ugeskr Laeger* 165(3), 239 (with caffeine)
Headache
Myalgia
  (2002): Gonzalez Rodriguez JL+, *Rev Esp Anestesiol Reanim* 49(9), 501
Seizures
  (2002): van der Hooft CS+, *Ned Tijdschr Geneeskd* 146(28), 1335
Trembling (1–10%)
Tremor (1–10%)
  (2002): Gonzalez Rodriguez JL+, *Rev Esp Anestesiol Reanim* 49(9), 501
Xerostomia (1–10%)

EPINEPHRINE

Synonym: adrenaline
Trade names: Adrenalin (Monarch); AsthmaHaler; Bronitin; Bronkaid; Epifrin (Allergan); Epipen (DEY); MedihalerEpi; Primatene; Sus-Phrine (Forest)
Other common trade names: *Adrenaline; Ana-Guard; Epi E-Z Pen; Eppy; Eppystabil; Isopto-Epinal; Primatene Mist; S-2; Simplene*
Indications: Cardiac arrest, hay fever, asthma, anaphylaxis
Category: Adrenergic agonist; Sympathomimetic bronchodilator
Duration of action: 1–4 hours
Clinically important, potentially hazardous interactions with: albuterol, alpha-blockers, amitriptyline, amoxapine, atenolol, beta-blockers, carteolol, chlorpromazine, clomipramine, cocaine, desipramine, doxepin, **ephedra**, ergotamine, furazolidone, halothane, imipramine, MAO inhibitors, metoprolol, nadolol, nortriptyline, penbutolol, phenelzine, phenoxybenzamine, phenylephrine, pindolol, prazosin, propranolol, protriptyline, sympathomimetics, terbutaline, thioridazine, timolol, tranylcypromine, tricyclic antidepressants, trimipramine, vasopressors

Reactions

Skin
Dermatitis
  (1993): Gaspari AA, *Contact Dermatitis* 28, 35
  (1980): Romaguera C+, *Contact Dermatitis* 6, 364
  (1976): Alani SD+, *Contact Dermatitis* 2, 147
  (1970): Gibbs RC, *Arch Dermatol* 101, 92
Diaphoresis (1–10%)
Exanthems
Fixed eruption
Flushing (1–10%)
Necrosis
  (1984): Antrum RM+, *Br J Clin Pract* 38, 191
Pallor (<1%)
Pemphigus (cicatricial)
  (1981): Vadot E+, *Bull Soc Ophtalmol Fr* (French) 81, 693
  (1977): Norn MS, *Am J Ophthalmol* 83, 138
Urticaria

Hair
Hair – alopecia
  (1972): Kass MA+, *Arch Ophthalmol* 88, 429 (eyelashes)

Other
Headache
Injection-site necrosis
Injection-site pain
Injection-site urticaria
Trembling (1–10%)
Xerostomia (<1%)

EPIRUBICIN

Trade name: Ellence (Pharmacia)
Indications: Adjuvant therapy in primary breast cancer
Category: Antineoplastic
Half-life: 33 hours
**Clinically important, potentially hazardous interactions
with:** amlodipine, bepridil, cimetidine, diltiazem, felodipine,
isradipine, nicardipine, nifedipine, nimodipine, nisoldipine,
verapamil

Reactions

Skin
Allergic reactions (sic)
  (1999): Ormrod D+, *Drugs Aging* 15, 389
Erythema
Erythroderma (sic) (0.7–5%)
Exfoliative dermatitis
Facial flushing
Hot flashes (5–39%)
Photosensitivity
Pigmentation
Pruritus (9%)
Radiation recall
  (1999): Wilson J+, *Clin Oncol (R Coll Radiol)* 11, 424
Rash (sic) (1–9%)
Ulcerations
Urticaria

Hair
Hair – alopecia (69–95%) (reversible)
  (2002): Colozza M+, *Eur J Cancer* 38(17), 2279
  (1999): Ormrod D+, *Drugs Aging* 15, 389
  (1991): Carmo-Pereira J+, *Cancer Chemother Pharmacol* 27, 394
    (95%)
  (1991): Fountzilas G+, *Tumori* 77, 232 (81%)
  (1986): Kimura K+, *Gan To Kagaku Ryoho* (Japanese) 13, 2440
    (71.4%)
  (1986): Sakata Y+, *Gan To Kagaku Ryoho* (Japanese) 13, 1887
  (1986): Tominaga T+, *Gan To Kagaku Ryoho* (Japanese) 13, 2187
    (66.7%)
  (1985): Holdener EE+, *Invest New Drugs* 3, 63 (54%)
  (1984): Lopez M+, *Invest New Drugs* 2, 315
  (1984): Schutte J+, *J Cancer Res Clin Oncol* 107, 38 (88%)
  (1980): Bonfante V+, *Recent Results Cancer Res* 74, 192

Nails
Nails – pigmentation

Other
Anaphylactoid reactions
Hypersensitivity
Injection-site extravasation
  (1999): Fleming A+, *J Hand Surg [Br]* 24, 390
Injection-site inflammation
Injection-site necrosis
Injection-site reactions (sic) (3–20%)
Injection-site ulceration
Mucositis
  (1999): Ormrod D+, *Drugs Aging* 15, 389
Myalgia
  (1995): Fountzilas G+, *Med Pediatr Oncol* 24, 23 (55%)
Oral ulceration
Phlebitis
Stomatitis
  (1995): Fountzilas G+, *Med Pediatr Oncol* 24, 23

(1991): Carmo-Pereira J+, *Cancer Chemother Pharmacol* 27, 394
    (35%)
(1991): Fountzilas G+, *Tumori* 77, 232 (24%)
(1986): Kimura K+, *Gan To Kagaku Ruoho* (Japanese) 13, 2440
    (12.5%)
(1986): Sakata Y+, *Gan To Kagaku Ryoho* (Japanese) 13, 1887
(1980): Bonfante V+, *Recent Results Cancer Res* 74, 192

EPLERENONE

Trade name: Inspra (Pharmacia)
Indications: Hypertension
Category: Antihypertensive; Selective aldosterone blocker
Half-life: 4–6 hours
**Clinically important, potentially hazardous interactions
with:** ACE inhibitors, angiotensin II receptor antagonists,
erythromycin, fluconazole, **grapefruit juice**, itraconazole,
ketoconazole, saquinavir, **St John's wort**, verapamil

Reactions

Skin
Flu-like syndrome (2%)

Other
Cough (2%)
Dizziness (3%)
Fatigue (2%)
Gynecomastia (males <1%)
Headache
Mastodynia (males <1%)

EPOETIN ALFA

Synonyms: erythropoietin; EPO
Trade names: Epogen (Amgen); Procrit (Ortho)
Other common trade names: *Epoxitin; Eprex; Erypo*
Indications: Anemia
Category: Colony stimulating factor; Growth factor
Half-life: 4–13 hours (in patients with chronic renal failure)

Reactions

Skin
Acne
  (1989): Faulds D+, *Drugs* 38, 863
Angioedema (1–5%)
Dermatitis
  (1993): Hardwick N+, *Contact Dermatitis* 28, 123
Edema (17%)
Exanthems
  (1990): Schröder-Kolb B, *Derm Beruf Umwelt* (German) 38, 12
    (papular)
Lichenoid eruption
  (1997): Puritz E, Smithtown, NY (from Internet) (observation)
Photosensitivity
  (1992): Harvey E+, *J Pediatr* 121, 749
Pruritus
  (1990): Schröder-Kolb B, *Derm Beruf Umwelt* (German) 38, 12
    (papular)
  (1989): Faulds D+, *Drugs* 38, 863
Rash (sic) (1–10%)
Urticaria

Hair
Hair – alopecia
  (2001): Reddy V+, *Nephrol Dial Transplant* 16(7), 1525
Hair – alopecia totalis
  (2001): Reddy V+, *Nephrol Dial Transplant* 16(7), 1525
Hair – hypertrichosis
  (1991): Kleiner MJ+, *Am J Kidney Dis* 18, 689

Other
Anaphylactoid reactions
Headache
Hypersensitivity (<1%)
Injection-site pain
  (1998): Veys N+, *Clin Nephrol* 49, 41
Injection-site reactions (sic) (7%)
Injection-site thrombophlebitis
Injection-site ulceration
  (1997): Siegel DM, New York, NY (from Internet) (observation)
Myalgia
Paresthesias (11%)
Porphyria cutanea tarda
  (1992): Harvey E+, *J Pediatr* 121, 749

EPROSARTAN

Trade name: Teveten (Biovail)
Indications: Hypertension
Category: Angiotensin II receptor antagonist; Antihypertensive
Half-life: 5–9 hours

Reactions

Skin
Angioedema
Diaphoresis (<1%)
Eczema (sic) (<1%)
Exanthems (<1%)
Facial edema (<1%)
Furunculosis (<1%)
Herpes simplex (<1%)
Hot flashes (<1%)
Peripheral edema (<1%)
Pruritus (<1%)
Purpura (<1%)
Rash (sic) (<1%)

Other
Burning mouth syndrome
  (2002): Castells X+, *BMJ* 325(7375), 1277
Cough
  (2001): Rake EC+, *J Hum Hypertens* 15(12), 863 (5%)
Dysgeusia
  (2002): Castells X+, *BMJ* 325(7375), 1277
Gingivitis (<1%)
Myalgia
Paresthesias (<1%)
Tendinitis (<1%)
Tremor (<1%)
Xerostomia (<1%)

EPTIFIBATIDE

Trade name: Integrilin (Millennium) (Schering)
Indications: Acute coronary syndrome, unstable angina
Category: Antiplatelet; Platelet aggregation inhibitor
Half-life: 2.5 hours
Clinically important, potentially hazardous interactions with: fondaparinux

Reactions

Skin
None

Other
Anaphylactoid reactions (<1%)
Injection-site reactions (sic)

ERGOCALCIFEROL

Synonyms: viosterol; vitamin D_2
Trade names: Calciferol (Schwartz); Deltalin (Lilly); Drisdol (Sanofi-Synthelabo)
Other common trade names: *Kalciferol; Ostoforte; Radiostol Forte; Sterogyl-15; Vigantol; Vitaminol*
Indications: Rickets, hypoparathyroidism
Category: Antihypocalcemic; Fat-soluble nutritional supplement
Half-life: 19–48 hours

Reactions

Skin
Granulomas (perforating)
  (1982): Aliaga A+, *Dermatologica* 164, 62
Pruritus (1–10%)

Other
Dysgeusia (1–10%) (metallic taste)
Myalgia
Xerostomia

ERTAPENEM

Synonyms: L-749,345; MK-0826
Trade name: Invanz (Merck)
Indications: Severe resistant bacterial infections caused by susceptible organisms
Category: Carbapenem antibiotic
Half-life: 4 hours
Clinically important, potentially hazardous interactions with: probenecid

Reactions

Skin
Candidiasis (>1%)
Chills (>1%)
Dermatitis (sic) (>1%)
Desquamation (>1%)
Diaphoresis (>1%)
Edema (3%)
Erythema (1–2%)

Facial edema (>1%)
Flushing (>1%)
Hematomas (<1%)
Necrosis (<1%)
Pruritus (1–2%)
Rash (sic) (2–3%)
Urticaria (>1%)
Vaginal pruritus (>1%)
Vulvovaginitis (>1%)

Other
Anaphylactoid reactions (some fatal)
Cough (1–2%)
Death (2.5%)
Depression (>1%)
Dysgeusia (>1%)
Headache
Hiccups (<1%)
Hyperesthesia (>1%)
Hypersensitivity
Injection-site extravasation (0.7–2%)
Injection-site induration (>1%)
Injection-site pain (>1%)
Limb pain (0.4–1%)
Oral candidiasis (0.1%)
Oral ulceration (>1%)
Pain (>1%)
Paresthesias (>1%)
Phlebitis (1.5–2%)
Seizures (0.5%)
Stomatitis (>1%)
Thrombophlebitis (1.5–2%)
Tremor (>1%)
Vaginal candidiasis (>1%)
Vaginitis (1–3%)

ERYTHROMYCIN

Trade names: E.E.S (Abbott); E-Mycin; Eramycin; Ery-Ped (Abbott); Ery-Tab (Abbott); Eryc (Warner Chilcott); Erypar; Erythrocin; Eryzole*; Ilosone; Ilotycin; PCE (Abbott); Pediazole* (Ross); Robimycin; Wintrocin; Wyamicin S
Other common trade name: *Too numerous to list*
Indications: Various infections caused by susceptible organisms
Category: Bacteriostatic macrolide antibiotic
Half-life: 1.4–2 hours
Clinically important, potentially hazardous interactions with: alfentanil, aminophylline, amoxicillin, ampicillin, anticonvulsants, astemizole, atorvastatin, benzodiazepines, bromocriptine, carbamazepine, ciprofloxacin, cisapride, clindamycin, colchicine, cyclosporine, digoxin, dihydroergotamine, disopyramide, enoxacin, eplerenone, ergotamine, fluoxetine, fluvastatin, gatifloxacin, imatinib, lomefloxacin, lorazepam, lovastatin, methadone, methysergide, midazolam, moxifloxacin, norfloxacin, ofloxacin, paroxetine, pimozide, pravastatin, quinolones, sertraline, sildenafil, simvastatin, sparfloxacin, tacrolimus, terfenadine, theophylline, triazolam, vinblastine, warfarin

*Note: Eryzole and Pediazole are combinations of erythromycin and sulfisoxazole

Reactions

Skin
Acne
  (1969): Weary PE+, *Arch Dermatol* 100, 179
Acute generalized exanthematous pustulosis (AGEP)
  (1995): Moreau A+, *Int J Dermatol* 34, 263 (passim)
  (1991): Roujeau J-C+, *Arch Dermatol* 127, 1333
Allergic reactions (sic) (<1%)
  (1986): Bigby M+, *JAMA* 256, 3358 (2.04%)
  (1976): Arndt KA+, *JAMA* 235, 918 (2.3%)
  (1967): Nichols JT+, *Oral Surg Oral Med Oral Pathol* 24, 323
Baboon syndrome
  (1997): Goossens C+, *Dermatology* 194, 421
Dermatitis (systemic)
  (1996): Valsecchi R+, *Contact Dermatitis* 34, 428
  (1995): Martins C+, *Contact Dermatitis* 33, 360
  (1994): Fernandez Redondo V+, *Contact Dermatitis* 30, 311
  (1994): Fernandez Redondo V+, *Contact Dermatitis* 30, 43
Eczema (sic)
Erythema multiforme
  (1985): Ting HC+, *Int J Dermatol* 24, 587
Exanthems (1–5%)
  (1995): Litt JZ, Beachwood, OH (personal case) (observation)
  (1991): Igea JM+, *Ann Allergy* 66, 216
  (1989): Pendleton N+, *Br J Clin Prac* 43, 464
  (1979): Hartigan DA+, *Lancet* 2, 411
  (1973): Shapera RM+, *JAMA* 226, 531 (3.5%)
Fixed eruption
  (1998): Mahboob A+, *Int J Dermatol* 37, 833
  (1991): Florido-Lopez JF+, *Allergy* 46, 77
  (1991): Mutalik S, *Int J Dermatol* 30, 751
  (1986): Kanwar AJ+, *Dermatologica* 172, 315
  (1984): Pigatto PD, *Acta Derm Venereol* (Stockh) 64, 272
  (1976): Naik RPC+, *Dermatologica* 152, 177 (bullous)
Pruritus
Pustules
  (1993): Manu Shah R+, *Eur J Dermatol* 3, 576
Rash (sic) (<1%)
  (1992): Shirin H+, *Ann Pharmacother* 26, 1522

(1989): Pendleton N+, *Br J Clin Pract* 43, 464
(1983): Furniss LD, *Drug Intell Clin Pharm* 17, 631
Red neck syndrome
(1992): Estrada V+, *Rev Clin Esp* (Spanish) 190, 100
Stevens–Johnson syndrome
(1998): N Z Medicines Adverse Reactions Committee (from Internet) (observation)
(1995): Lestico MR+, *Am J Health Syst Pharm* 52, 1805
(1995): Pandha HS+, *N Z Med J* 108, 13
(1993): Leenutaphong V+, *Int J Dermatol* 32, 428
(1983): Fischer PR+, *Am J Dis Child* 137, 914
Toxic epidermal necrolysis
(1995): Kuper K+, *Ophthalmologe* (German) 92, 823
(1995): Raymond F+, *Arch Pediatr* (French) 2, 494
(1993): Leenutaphong V+, *Int J Dermatol* 32, 428
(1991): Porteous DM+, *Arch Dermatol* 127, 740 (in AIDS)
(1987): Guillaume JC+, *Arch Dermatol* 123, 1166
(1985): Lund-Kofoed ML+, *Contact Dermatitis* 13, 273
(1974): Czaplinska W+, *Pol Tyg Lek* (Polish) 29, 1263
Urticaria
(1998): Siegfried EC+, *J Am Acad Dermatol* 39, 797 (passim)
(1993): Lopez-Serrano C+, *Allergol Immunopathol Madr* (Spanish) 21, 225
(1976): van Ketel WG, *Contact Dermatitis* 2, 363
(1960): Prasard AS, *N Engl J Med* 262, 139
Vasculitis
(1985): Sanchez NP+, *Arch Dermatol* 121, 220

Other

Anaphylactoid reactions
(1998): Siegfried EC+, *J Am Acad Dermatol* 39, 797 (passim)
(1996): Jorro G+, *Ann Allergy Asthma Immunol* 77, 456
Enamel hypoplasia (teeth)
(1965): Adno J+, *SA Tydskrif vir Geneeskunde* (English), 1124
Gingival hyperplasia
(1992): Valsecchi R+, *Acta Derm Venereol* (Stockh) 72, 157
Glossodynia
Headache
Hypersensitivity (1–10%)
(1999): Gallardo MA+, *Cutis* 64, 129
(1998): Kruppa A+, *Dermatology* 196(3), 335
(1982): Lombardi P+, *Contact Dermatitis* 8, 416
Injection-site extravasation
(2001): Zimmerman T+, *Clin Drug Invest* 21, 527 (58%)
Injection-site irritation
(1983): Marlin GE+, *Hum Toxicol* 3, 593
Injection-site pain
(2001): Zimmerman T+, *Clin Drug Invest* 21, 527 (25%)
Injection-site phlebitis (1–10%)
(1987): David LM, *Am J Hosp Pharm* 44, 732
(1986): Holt RJ+, *Clin Pharm* 5, 787
Oral candidiasis (1–10%)
Oral ulceration
(1980): Evens RP+, *Drug Intell Clin Pharm* 14, 217
Phlebitis
(2001): de Dios Garcia-Diaz J+, *Med Clin* (Barc) 116(4), 133 (from intravenous administration)
Rhabdomyolysis
(1988): Tobert JA, *Am J Cardiol* 62, 28J (with Cyclosporine)
Stomatodynia
Thrombophlebitis
Tinnitus
Tooth discoloration
(1965): Adno J+, *SA Tydskrif vir Geneeskunde* (English), 1124
Torsades de pointes
(2002): Shaffer D+, *Clin Infect Dis* 35(2), 197

ESCITALOPRAM

Synonyms: Lu-26-054; S-Citalopram
Trade name: Lexapro (Forest)
Indications: Major depressive disorders, anxiety
Category: Antidepressant; Selective serotonin reuptake inhibitor (SSRI)
Half-life: 27–32 hours
Clinically important, potentially hazardous interactions with: alcohol, **kava**, MAO inhibitors, selegiline, **St John's wort**, sumatriptan, **valerian**

Reactions

Skin
Acne (<1%)
Allergic reactions (sic) (1–10%)
Ankle edema
Chills (<1%)
Dermatitis (sic)
Diaphoresis (5%)
Eczema (<1%)
Edema (<1%)
Facial edema
Flu-like syndrome (5%)
Flushing (<1%)
Folliculitis (<1%)
Furunculosis (<1%)
Hot flashes (1–10%)
Pruritus (<1%)
Purpura (<1%)
Rash (sic) (1–10%)
Shivering
Xerosis (<1%)

Hair
Hair – alopecia (<1%)

Other
Anaphylactoid reactions
Anxiety (<1%)
Arthralgia (1–10%)
Arthritis (<1%)
Bruxism (<1%)
Conjunctivitis (<1%)
Cough (1–10%)
Depression (<1%)
Dizziness (5%)
Dysgeusia (<1%)
Headache
Limb pain (<1%)
Lipoma
Mouth vesiculation (1–19%)
Myalgia (1–10%)
Paresthesias (1–10%)
Restless legs syndrome (<1%)
Tic disorder (<1%)
Tinnitus (1–10%)
Toothache (1–10%)
Tremor (1–10%)
Twitching (<1%)
Xerostomia (6%)

ESMOLOL

Trade name: Brevibloc (Baxter)
Indications: Tachyarrhythmias, tachycardia
Category: Antiarrhythmic class II; Antihypertensive; Beta-adrenoceptor blocker
Half-life: 9 minutes
Clinically important, potentially hazardous interactions with: clonidine, verapamil

Reactions

Skin

Acne (<1%)
Cold extremities (sic)
Diaphoresis (>10%)
Eczema (<1%)
Edema (<1%)
Erythema (<1%)
Exfoliative dermatitis (<1%)
Facial edema
Flushing (<1%)
Necrosis (<1%)
Pallor (<1%)
Pigmentation (<1%)
Psoriasis (<1%)
Purpura
Rash (sic)
Urticaria

Hair

Hair – alopecia

Other

Dysgeusia
Injection-site inflammation
  (1987): Benfield P+, *Drugs* 33, 392
Injection-site pain (8%)
Injection-site reactions (sic) (1–10%)
Paresthesias (<1%)
Thrombophlebitis (<1%)
Xerostomia (<1%)

ESOMEPRAZOLE

Synonyms: Perprazole; H 19918
Trade name: Nexium (AstraZeneca)
Indications: Gastroesophageal Reflux Disease (GERD)
Category: Proton pump inhibitor
Half-life: 1.5 hours
Clinically important, potentially hazardous interactions with: benzodiazepines, chlordiazepoxide, clonazepam, clorazepate, diazepam, digoxin, flurazepam, lorazepam, midazolam, oxazepam, quazepam, temazepam

Reactions

Skin

Acne (<1%)
Allergic reactions (sic) (<1%)
Angioedema (<1%)
Candidiasis (<1%)
Dermatitis (sic) (<1%)

Diaphoresis (<1%)
Edema (<1%)
Exanthems (<1%)
Facial flushing (<1%)
Flushing (<1%)
Fungal infections (sic) (<1%)
Peripheral edema (<1%)
Photosensitivity
  (2003): Zabawski E, Longwood, TX (from Internet)
    (observation)
Pruritus (<1%)
Pruritus ani (<1%)
Urticaria (<1%)

Other

Arthralgia (<1%)
Depression (<1%)
Dysgeusia (<1%)
Fibromyalgia (<1%)
Headache
  (2002): Johnson TJ+, *Am J Health Syst Pharm* 59(14), 1333
Hyperesthesia (<1%)
Paresthesias (<1%)
Parosmia (<1%)
Polymyalgia (<1%)
Respiratory infection
  (2002): Johnson TJ+, *Am J Health Syst Pharm* 59(14), 1333
Rhabdomyolysis
  (2003): Sipe BE+, *Ann Pharmacother* 37(6), 808 (with atorvastatin and clarithromycin)
Tinnitus (<1%)
Tongue edema (<1%)
Ulcerative stomatitis (<1%)
Vaginitis (<1%)
Xerostomia

ESTAZOLAM

Trade name: ProSom (Abbott)
Other common trade names: *Domnamid; Esilgan; Eurodin; Kainever; Nuctalon; Tasedan*
Indications: Insomnia
Category: Benzodiazepine sedative-hypnotic
Half-life: 10–24 hours
Clinically important, potentially hazardous interactions with: indinavir, ritonavir

Reactions

Skin

Acne (<1%)
Allergic reactions (sic) (<1%)
Chills (<1%)
Dermatitis (sic) (<1%)
Diaphoresis (1–10%)
Edema (<1%)
Eyelid edema (<1%)
Flushing (1–10%)
Photosensitivity
Pruritus (1–10%)
Purpura (<1%)
Rash (sic) (>10%)
Urticaria (1–10%)

Xerosis (<1%)

Other
Dysgeusia (1–10%)
Glossitis
Gynecomastia (<1%)
Myalgia (1–10%)
Oral ulceration (<1%)
Paresthesias (1–10%)
Sialopenia (>10%)
Sialorrhea (<1%)
Vaginal pruritus (1–10%)
Xerostomia (>10%)

ESTRAMUSTINE

Trade name: Emcyt (Pharmacia)
Other common trade name: *Cellmusin*
Indications: Prostate carcinoma
Category: Antineoplastic; Nitrogen mustard
Half-life: 20 hours
**Clinically important, potentially hazardous interactions
with:** aldesleukin

Reactions

Skin
Allergic reactions (sic)
  (2001): Zelek L+, *Ann Oncol* 12(9), 1265
Edema (>10%)
Exanthems
  (1971): Anderes A+, *Praxis* (German) 60, 1276
Flushing (1%)
Hot flashes (<1%)
Night sweats (<1%)
Pigmentary changes (sic) (<1%)
Pruritus (2%)
  (1976): Nagel R+, *Med Klin* (German) 71, 1724
Purpura (3%)
Rash (sic) (1%)
Urticaria
Xerosis (2%)

Hair
Hair – alopecia (<1%)

Other
Death
  (2001): Zelek L+, *Ann Oncol* 12(9), 1265
Gynecomastia (>10%)
Injection-site thrombophlebitis (1–10%)
  (1976): Nagel R+, *Med Klin* (German) 71, 1724
Mastodynia (66%)
Thrombophlebitis (3%)
Tinnitus

ESTROGENS

Generic:
  Chlorotrianisene
    Trade name: Tace
  Diethylstilbestrol
    Trade names: Cyren A; Destrol; Stilphostrol
  Estradiol
    Trade names: Estrace (Warner Chilcott); Estraderm (Novartis)
  Estrogens, conjugated
    Trade name: Premarin (Wyeth)
  Estrogens, esterified
    Trade names: Estratab (Solvay); Menest (Monarch)
  Estrone
    Trade names: Estroject; Estronol; Gynogen; Theelin, etc.
  Estropipate
    Trade name: Ogen (Pharmacia)
  Ethinyl estradiol
    Trade name: Estinyl
  Quinestrol
    Trade name: Estrovis
**Clinically important, potentially hazardous interactions
with: black cohosh**

Reactions

Skin
Acanthosis nigricans
  (1974): Banuchi SR+, *Arch Dermatol* 109, 544
Acne
Angioedema
  (2002): van der Klooster JM+, *Ned Tijdschr Geneeskd*
    146(34), 1599
  (2000): McGlinchey PG+, *Am J Med Sci* 320, 212
  (1942): Saphir WS+, *JAMA* 119, 557
Ankle edema
Bullous eruption
  (1971): Kuchera LK, *JAMA* 218, 562
Chloasma (<1%)
Dermatitis (sic)
  (1995): Shelley WB+, *J Am Acad Dermatol* 32, 25
  (1981): Ljunggren B, *Contact Dermatitis* 7(3), 141
Eczema (sic)
  (1995): Shelley WB+, *J Am Acad Dermatol* 32, 25
Edema (<1%)
Erythema multiforme
  (1998): Moghadam BK+, *Oral Surg Oral Med Oral Pathol Oral
    Radiol Endod* 85, 537
Erythema nodosum
  (1990): Bartelsmeyer JA+, *Clin Obstet Gynecol* 33, 777
  (1980): Salvatore MA+, *Arch Dermatol* 116, 557
Exanthems
  (1999): Coustou D+, *Ann Dermatol Venereol* 125, 484
  (1999): Kumar A+, *Australas J Dermatol* 40, 96
  (1997): Litt JZ, Beachwood, OH (personal case) (observation)
  (1984): Lee M+, *J Urol* 131, 767
Exfoliative dermatitis
  (1942): Kasselberg LA, *JAMA* 120, 117
Fixed eruption (<1%)
Flushing
  (1981): Ingle JN+, *N Engl J Med* 304, 16 (3%)
  (1973): Delius L, *Dtsch Med Wochenschr* (German) 98, 1512
Hot flashes
  (2001): Spetz AC+, *J Urol* 166(2), 517
Hyperkeratosis of nipples
  (1980): Mold DE+, *Cutis* 26, 95
Irritation (sic) (from transdermal system)

Livedo reticularis

Lupus erythematosus

(1989): Colins D, *J Rheumatol* 16, 408

(1986): Barrett C+, *Br J Rheumatol* 25, 300

(1973): Elias PM, *Arch Dermatol* 108, 716

(1971): Kay DR+, *Arthritis Rheum* 14, 239 (5%) (ANA only)

(1971): Laugier P+, *Bull Soc Fr Syphiligr* (French) 78, 623 (SLE-induced)

(1969): Bole CG+, *Lancet* 1, 323

(1968): Hadida E+, *Bull Soc Fr Syphiligr* (French) 75, 616

(1968): Schleicher EM, *Lancet* 1, 821

(1966): Pimstone BL, *S Afr J Obstet Gynecol* 3, 62

Melasma (<1%)

(1992): Breathnach SM+, *Adverse Drug Reactions and the Skin* Blackwell, Oxford, 274 (passim)

(1967): Resnic S, *JAMA* 199, 601

Mucha–Habermann disease

(1973): Hollander A+, *Arch Dermatol* 107, 465

Papulo-vesicular eruption

(1999): Coustou D+, *Ann Dermatol* 125, 484

(1998): Coustou D+, *Ann Dermatol Venereol* (French) 125, 505

Peripheral edema

Photosensitivity

(1970): Mathison IW+, *Obstet Gynecol Surv* 25, 389

(1968): Erickson LR+, *JAMA* 203, 980

(1965): Daniels F, *Med Clin North Am* 49, 565

Pigmentation

(1999): Oakley A, Auckland, New Zealand (from Internet) (observation) (from topical, over vulva)

(1972): Ippen H+, *Hautarzt* (German) 23, 21 (chloasma)

(1967): Resnic S, *JAMA* 199, 601

Pruritus

(2000): Siepmann M+, *Dtsch Med Wochenschr* (German) 125, 557

(1999): Coustou D+, *Ann Dermatol Venereol* 125, 484

(1999): Kumar A+, *Australas J Dermatol* 40, 96

(1998): Coustou D+, *Ann Dermatol Venereol* (French) 125, 505

(1995): Shelley WB+, *J Am Acad Dermatol* 32, 25

(1971): Kuchera LK, *JAMA* 218, 562

Purpura

(1984): Lee M+, *J Urol* 131, 767

Rash (sic) (<1%)

Raynaud's phenomenon

(1998): Fraenkel L+, *Ann Intern Med* 129, 208

Scleroderma

(2000): D'Cruz D, *Toxicol Lett* 112 and 421

Spider nevi

(1992): Breathnach SM+, *Adverse Drug Reactions and the Skin* Blackwell, Oxford, 274 (passim)

Striae

Telangiectasia

(1970): Aram H+, *Acta Derm Venereol* 50, 302

Urticaria

(1998): Moghadam BK+, *Oral Surg Oral Med Oral Pathol Oral Radiol Endod* 85, 537

(1995): Shelley WB+, *J Am Acad Dermatol* 32, 25

(1984): Lee M+, *J Urol* 131, 767

(1964): Beall GN, *Medicine* (Baltimore) 43, 131

Vasculitis (cutaneous polyarteritis nodosa)

(1998): Cvancara JL+, *J Am Acad Dermatol* 39, 643

Vesicular eruptions

(1999): Kumar A+, *Australas J Dermatol* 40, 96

Hair

Hair – alopecia

(1992): Breathnach SM+, *Adverse Drug Reactions and the Skin* Blackwell, Oxford, 233 (passim)

Hair – hirsutism

(1971): Fusi S+, *Folia Endocrinol* (Italian) 24, 412

Hair – straight

(1994): Litt JZ, Beachwood, OH (personal case) (observation)

Nails

Nails – onycholysis

(1976): Byrne JP+, *Post Grad Med J* 52, 535

Other

Acute intermittent porphyria

Dry eyes

(2001): Schaumberg DA+, *JAMA* 286(17), 2114

Galactorrhea

Gingival hyperplasia

Gynecomastia (>10%)

(2000): Felner EI+, *Pediatrics* 105, E55 (3 prepubertal boys from an estrogen cream)

(1987): Schmidt KU+, *Dtsch Med Wochenschr* (German) 112, 926

(1984): Gottswinter JM+, *Haarwasser Med Klin* (German) 79, 181

(1978): Gabilove JL+, *Arch Dermatol* 114, 1672

(1969): Degos R+, *Ann Dermatol Syphiligr Paris* (French) 96, 5

(1969): Goebel M, *Hautarzt* (German) 20, 521

(1968): Stewart WM+, *Bull Soc Fr Dermatol Syphiligr* (French) 75, 294

Headache

Injection-site pain (1–10%)

Mastodynia (>10%)

(2002): Arrenbrecht S+, *Osteoporos Int* 13(2), 176 (17%)

Oral mucosal eruption

(1998): Moghadam BK+, *Oral Surg Oral Med Oral Pathol Oral Radiol Endod* 85, 537

Oral mucosal pigmentation

(1991): Perusse R+, *Cutis* 48, 61

Osteoma cutis

(2002): Stockel S+, *Hautarzt* 53(1), 37

Porphyria

(1994): Siersema PD+, *Eur J Gastroenterol Hepatol* 6, 371

(1989): CoulsonDH+, *Br J Urol* 63, 648

Porphyria cutanea tarda

(1995): Nonaka S+, *Nippon Rinsho* (Japanese) 53, 1427

(1990): Roger D+, *Ann Dermatol Venereol* (French) 117, 127

(1982): Enriquez de Salamanca R+, *Arch Dermatol Res* 274, 179

(1979): Grossman ME+, *Am J Med* 67, 277

(1979): Sweeney GD+, *Can Med Assoc J* 120, 803

(1978): Benedetto AV+, *Cutis* 21, 483

(1976): Byrne JP+, *Post Grad Med J* 52, 535

(1975): Haberman HF+, *Can Med Assoc J* 113, 653

(1975): Malina L+, *Br J Dermatol* 92, 707

(1975): Wanscher B, *Ugeskr Laeger* (Danish) 137, 623

(1973): Gajdos A+, *Nouv Presse Med* (French) 2, 1131

(1973): Palma-Carlos AG+, *Nouv Presse Med* (French) 2, 1996

(1971): Barth J+, *Dermatol Monatsschr* (German) 157, 160

(1971): Stein KM+, *Obstet Gynecol* 38, 755

(1970): Roenigk HH+, *Arch Dermatol* 102, 260

(1969): Duverne+, *Lyon Med* (French) 221, 1097

(1966): Levere RD, *Blood* 28, 569

(1965): Becker FT, *Arch Dermatol* 92, 252

(1964): Theologides H+, *Metabolism* 13, 391

(1963): Hurley HJ, *Arch Dermatol* 88, 233

(1963): Walshe M, *Br J Dermatol* 75, 298

Pseudolymphoma

(1996): Magro CM+, *Hum Pathol* 27(2), 125

Vaginal candidiasis

ETANERCEPT

Trade name: Enbrel (Immunex) (Wyeth)
Indications: Rheumatoid arthritis
Category: Antiarthritic; Antirheumatic; Biologic response modifier
Half-life: 98–300 hours
Clinically important, potentially hazardous interactions with: anakinra

Reactions

Skin

Adverse effects (sic)
  (2002): Brocq O+, *Presse Med* 31(39), 1836
  (2001): Sandborn WJ+, *Gastroenterology* 121(5), 1088
Allergic reactions (sic) (<3%)
Cellulitis
  (2002): Gorman JD+, *N Engl J Med* 346, 1349
Erythema
Exanthems
  (2002): Conaghan P+, *Skin & Allergy News* June, 40
Herpes zoster
  (2001): Hogarty T, (from Internet) (observation) (generalized)
Infections (sic) (<3%)
  (2003): Kroesen S+, *Rheumatology (Oxford)* 42(5), 617
  (2002): Gorman JD+, *N Engl J Med* 346, 1349
  (2002): Phillips K+, *Arthritis Rheum* 47(1), 17
  (2002): Steensma DP+, *Blood* 99(6), 2252
  (2001): Baghai M+, *Mayo Clin Proc* 76(6), 653
Lupus erythematosus
  (2003): Carlson E+, *Arthritis Rheum* 48(4), 1165
  (2003): Debandt M+, *Clin Rheumatol* 22(1), 56
  (2003): Lepore L+, *Clin Exp Rheumatol* 21(2), 276
  (2002): Cairns AP+, *Ann Rheum Dis* 61(11), 1031
  (2002): Ferraccioli GF+, *Lancet* 360(9333), 645
  (2002): Mohan AK+, *Lancet* 360(9333), 646
  (2002): Shakoor N+, *Lancet* 359 (4 cases)
  (2002): Takeuchi T+, *Nippon Rinsho* 60(12), 2390
  (2001): Bleumink GS+, *Rheumatology* (Oxford) 40, 1317
  (2001): Werth V, *Dermatology Times* 18
  (1999): Brion PH+, *Ann Intern Med* 131, 634 (discoid)
Lymphoma
  (2002): Brown SL+, *Arthritis Rheum* 46(12), 3151 (18 cases)
Malignancies (sic) (<3%)
Nodules
  (2002): Cunnane G+, *Arthritis Rheum* 47(4), 445
Pruritus
Purpura
  (2002): Mitchell DF, Thomasville, MD (from Internet) (observation)
Rash (sic) (5%)
  (2000): *Nurses' Drug Alert* 24, 4
  (1999): Brion PH+, *Ann Int Med* 131, 634
Squamous cell carcinoma
  (2001): Smith KJ+, *J Am Acad Dermatol* 45(6), 953 (7 cases)
  (2000): Smith KJ+, Academy of Dermatology Meeting San Francisco Poster Exhibit
Ulcerations
Upper respiratory infection
  (2001): Alldred A, *Expert Opin Pharmacother* 2(7), 1137
Urticaria
  (2000): Skytta E+, *Clin Exp Rheumatol* 18, 533
Vasculitis
  (2002): Conaghan P+, *Skin & Allergy News* June, 40
  (2002): Cunnane G+, *Arthritis Rheum* 47(4), 445
  (2002): Livermore PA+, *Rheumatology (Oxford)* 41(12), 1450
  (2001): Werth V, *Dermatology Times* 18
  (2000): Galaria NA+, *J Rheumatol* 27, 2041 (leukocytoclastic)
  (1999): Brion PH+, *Ann Intern Med* 131, 634 (necrotizing)

Other

Death
  (2002): Phillips K+, *Arthritis Rheum* 47(1), 17
  (2001): Baghai M+, *Mayo Clin Proc* 76(6), 653
Headache
  (2003): Fleischmann RM+, *J Rheumatol* 30(4), 691
Injection-site reactions (sic) (20–40%)
  (2003): Arnold EL+, *Arthritis Rheum* 48(7), 2078
  (2003): Edwards KR+, *J Drugs Dermatol* 2(2), 184
  (2003): Fleischmann RM+, *J Rheumatol* 30(4), 691
  (2003): *Prescrire Int* 12(66), 127
  (2002): Gorman JD+, *N Engl J Med* 346, 1349
  (2002): Steensma DP+, *Blood* 99(6), 2252
  (2001): Alldred A, *Expert Opin Pharmacother* 2(7), 1137
  (2001): Girolomoni G+, *Arch Dermatol* 137, 784
  (2001): Sandborn WJ+, *Gastroenterology* 121(5), 1088
  (2001): Werth V, *Dermatology Times* 18
  (2001): Werth VP+, *Arch Dermatol* 137(7), 953
  (2001): Zeltser R+, *Arch Dermatol* 137, 893 (20%)
  (2000): Bathon JM+, *N Engl J Med* 343, 1586
  (2000): Lovell DJ+, *N Engl J Med* 342, 763
  (2000): Mease PJ, *Lancet* 356, 385
  (2000): Murphy FT+, *Arch Dermatol* 136, 556
  (1999): Jarvis B+, *Drugs* 57, 945
  (1999): Moreland LW+, *Ann Intern Med* 130, 478
  (1999): Moreland LW+, *Arthritis Rheum* 41, S364 (Suppl)
  (1999): Weinblatt ME+, *N Engl J Med* 340, 253
Lymphoproliferative disease
  (2002): Brown SL+, *Arthritis Rheum* 46(12), 3151 (18 cases)
Multiple sclerosis
  (2001): Sicotte NL+, *Neurology* 57(10), 1885
Rheumatoid nodules (sic)
  (2002): Kekow J+, *Arthritis Rheum* 46(3), 843
Rhinitis
  (2003): Fleischmann RM+, *J Rheumatol* 30(4), 691
Tinnitus
  (2002): Gorman JD+, *N Engl J Med* 346, 1349

ETHACRYNIC ACID

Trade name: Edecrin (Merck)
Other common trade names: *Edecril; Edecrina; Hydromedin; Reomax*
Indications: Edema
Category: Loop diuretic
Half-life: 2–4 hours
Clinically important, potentially hazardous interactions with: amikacin, aminoglycosides, digoxin, gentamicin, kanamycin, neomycin, streptomycin, tobramycin

Reactions

Skin

Allergic reactions (sic)
Chills (<1%)
Exanthems
  (1966): Sherlock S+, *Lancet* 1, 1049
Photosensitivity
Purpura (<1%)
Rash (sic) (<1%)
Urticaria

Vasculitis
  (1992): Breathnach SM+, *Adverse Drug Reactions and the Skin*
    Blackwell, Oxford, 229 (passim)
  (1967): Bar-on H+, *Isr J Med Sci* 3, 113

Other
Injection-site pain
Thrombophlebitis (<1%)
Tinnitus
Xerostomia

ETHAMBUTOL

Trade name: Myambutol (Elan)
Other common trade names: *Apo-Ethambutol; Dexambutol; EMB; Etapiam; Etibi; Stambutol*
Indications: Tuberculosis
Category: Antimycobacterial
Half-life: 3–4 hours

Reactions

Skin
Acne
Angioedema
  (1985): Holdiness MR, *Int J Dermatol* 24, 280
Bullous eruption
  (1985): Holdiness MR, *Int J Dermatol* 24, 280
  (1981): Frentz G+, *Acta Derm Venereol* (Stockh) 61, 89
Chills
Dermatitis (sic)
  (1986): Holdiness MR, *Contact Dermatitis* 15, 282
  (1986): Holdiness MR, *Contact Dermatitis* 15, 96
Diaphoresis
  (1985): Holdiness MR, *Int J Dermatol* 24, 280
Erythema multiforme
  (1985): Holdiness MR, *Int J Dermatol* 24, 280
  (1981): Frentz G+, *Acta Derm Venereol* (Stockh) 61, 89
Exanthems
  (1985): Holdiness MR, *Int J Dermatol* 24, 280
  (1981): Frentz G+, *Acta Derm Venereol* (Stockh) 61, 89 (1–5%)
  (1977): Pasricha JS+, *Arch Dermatol* 113, 1122
Exfoliative dermatitis
  (1985): Holdiness MR, *Int J Dermatol* 24, 280
Lichenoid eruption
  (1995): Grossman ME+, *J Am Acad Dermatol* 33, 675
  (1981): Frentz G+, *Acta Derm Venereol* (Stockh) 61, 89
Lupus erythematosus
  (1986): Layer P+, *Dtsch Med Wochenschr* (German) 111,1603
  (1977): Djawari D, *Z Hautkr* (German) 53, 180
Photosensitivity
  (1994): Berger TG+, *Arch Dermatol* 130, 609 (in HIV-infected)
Pruritus (<1%)
  (1985): Holdiness MR, *Int J Dermatol* 24, 280
  (1981): Frentz G+, *Acta Derm Venereol* (Stockh) 61, 89
  (1969): Council on Drugs, *JAMA* 208, 2463
Purpura
  (1972): Levantine A+, *Br J Dermatol* 86, 651
Rash (sic) (<1%)
  (1995): Chaisson RE, *Infections in Medicine* 12, 48
  (1995): Wong PC+, *Eur Respir J* 8, 866
Stevens–Johnson syndrome
  (1979): Surjapranata FJ+, *Paediatr Indones* 19, 195
Toxic epidermal necrolysis
  (1985): Heng MCY, *Br J Dermatol* 106, 107
  (1981): Pegram PS+, *Arch Intern Med* 141, 1677

Urticaria
  (1985): Holdiness MR, *Int J Dermatol* 24, 280
  (1981): Frentz G+, *Acta Derm Venereol* (Stockh) 61, 89

Hair
Hair – alopecia
  (1985): Holdiness MR, *Int J Dermatol* 24, 280

Other
Anaphylactoid reactions (<1%)
Dyschromatopsia
Headache
Hypersensitivity
  (1995): Dhamgaye T+, *Tuber Lung Dis* 76,181
Paresthesias

ETHANOLAMINE

Trade name: Ethamolin (Cypros)
Other common trade name: *Ethanolamine oleate*
Indications: Bleeding esophageal varices
Category: Sclerosing agent
Half-life: N/A
Clinically important, potentially hazardous interactions with: acitretin, amobarbital, aprobarbital, butabarbital, disulfiram, insulin, mephobarbital, pentobarbital, phenobarbital, primidone, secobarbital, thiopental

Reactions

Skin
Dermatitis
  (2002): Bowling JC+, *Contact Dermatitis* 47(2), 116
  (1995): Kock P, *Contact Dermatitis* 33, 273
  (1994): Aranzabal A+, *Contact Dermatitis* 31, 121
  (1994): Ortiz-Frutos FJ+, *Contact Dermatitis* 31, 193
  (1994): Schnuch A, *Contact Dermatitis* 30, 243

Other
Anaphylactoid reactions (<1%)
Injection-site necrosis

ETHCHLORVYNOL

Trade name: Placidyl (Abbott)
Other common trade names: *Arvynol; Nostel*
Indications: Insomnia
Category: Sedative-hypnotic
Half-life: 10–20 hours
Clinically important, potentially hazardous interactions with: antihistamines, brompheniramine, buclizine, chlorpheniramine, clemastine, dexchlorpheniramine, meclizine, tripelennamine

Reactions

Skin
Allergic reactions (sic)
Bullous eruption (from overdose)
  (1990): Yell RP, *Am J Emerg Med* 8, 246
  (1980): Brodin MD+, *J Cutan Pathol* 7, 326
Diaphoresis
Fixed eruption
  (1965): Auerbach R, *Arch Dermatol* 92, 184

Pruritus
Purpura
  (1972): Jakobson ES, *Ann Intern Med* 77, 73 (fatal)
Rash (sic) (1–10%)
Urticaria

Other

Acute intermittent porphyria
Death
Dysgeusia (>10%)
Facial numbness (sic)
Hypersensitivity
Paresthesias
Pressure necrosis
  (1990): Chamberlain JM+, *Am J Emerg Med* 8, 467

ETHIONAMIDE

Trade name: Trecator-SC (Wyeth)
Other common trade names: *Ethatyl; Etiocidan; Myobid-250;*
Tubermin
Indications: Tuberculosis
Category: Tuberculostatic
Half-life: 2–3 hours

Reactions

Skin

Acne
  (1992): Breathnach SM+, *Adverse Drug Reactions and the Skin*
    Blackwell, Oxford (passim)
  (1965): *Drug Ther Bull* 3, 61
  (1963): Lees AW, *Am Rev Respir Dis* 88, 347
Allergic reactions (sic)
  (1971): *Med Lett* 13, 55 (1%)
Butterfly eruptions on the face (sic)
  (1992): Breathnach SM+, *Adverse Drug Reactions and the Skin*
    Blackwell, Oxford (passim)
Eczema (sic) (chiefly involving the forehead)
  (1992): Breathnach SM+, *Adverse Drug Reactions and the Skin*
    Blackwell, Oxford, 159 (passim)
Edema of foot
  (1987): Schmutz JL+, *Ann Dermatol Venereol* (French) 114, 569
Exanthems
  (1969): Agrawal R, *BMJ* 4, 540
  (1965): Carey VCI, *Tubercle* 46, 287
Ichthyosis
  (1972): Levantine A+, *Br J Dermatol* 86, 651
Lupus erythematosus
  (1973): Desmons MF, *Bull Soc Fr Dermatol Syphiligr* (French)
    80, 168
Photosensitivity
  (1966): Baran R, *Hôpital* (French) 54, 445
  (1966): Friedmann ME, *Bull Soc Franc Dermatol Syphiligr* (French)
    73, 510
Purpura
  (1992): Breathnach SM+, *Adverse Drug Reactions and the Skin*
    Blackwell, Oxford (passim)
Rash (sic) (<1%)
Seborrheic dermatitis
  (1972): Levantine A+, *Br J Dermatol* 86, 651
Urticaria (1–5%)

Hair

Hair – alopecia (<1%)

  (1992): Breathnach SM+, *Adverse Drug Reactions and the Skin*
    Blackwell, Oxford, 159 (passim)
  (1966): Baran R, *Hôpital* (French) 54, 445

Other

Dysgeusia (1–10%) (metallic taste)
Gynecomastia (<1%)
Headache
Oral ulceration
Sialorrhea
Stomatitis (<1%)
  (1992): Breathnach SM+, *Adverse Drug Reactions and the Skin*
    Blackwell, Oxford (passim)
Stomatodynia
Xerostomia

ETHOSUXIMIDE

Trade name: Zarontin (Parke-Davis)
Other common trade names: *Emeside; Ethymal; Petnidan;*
Pyknolepsinum; Simatin; Zarondan
Indications: Absence (petit mal) seizures
Category: Succinimide anticonvulsant
Half-life: 50–60 hours

Reactions

Skin

Erythema multiforme (<1%)
  (1966): Coursin DB, *JAMA* 198, 113
Exanthems (1–5%)
  (1991): Pelekanos J+, *Epilepsia* 32, 554
  (1966): Weinstein AW+, *Am J Dis Child* 111, 63 (2.2%)
Exfoliative dermatitis (<1%)
Lupus erythematosus (>10%)
  (1996): Miyasaka N, *Intern Med* 35, 527
  (1996): Takeda S+, *Intern Med* 35, 587
  (1996): Wallace SJ, *Drug Saf* 15, 378
  (1994): Riviello JJ+, *J Epilepsy* 7, 23
  (1994): Yung RL+, *Rheum Dis Clin North Am* 20, 61
  (1993): Ansell BM, *Lupus* 2, 193
  (1993): Drory VE+, *Clin Neuropharmacol* 16, 19 (passim)
  (1985): Lovisetto P+, *Recenti Prog Med* (Italian) 76, 84
  (1984): Koike K+, *Rinsho Ketsueki* 25, 1635
  (1981): Grossman J+, *Arthritis Rheum* 24, 927
  (1980): Condemi JJ, *Geriatrics* 35(3), 81
  (1979): Tor J+, *Med Clin (Barc)* (Spanish) 73, 443
  (1976): Singsen BH+, *Pediatrics* 57, 529
  (1975): Teoh PC+, *Arch Dis Child* 50, 658 (morphea-like)
  (1973): Beernink DH+, *J Pediatr* 82, 113
  (1970): Alter BP, *J Pediatr* 77, 1093
  (1970): Dabbous IA+, *J Pediatr* 76, 617
  (1968): Livingston S+, *JAMA* 203, 731
  (1968): Monnet P+, *Lyon Med* (French) 220, 467
Periorbital edema
Pruritus
Purpura
  (1967): Kontsouliers E, *Lancet* 2, 310
Rash (sic) (<1%)
Raynaud's phenomenon
  (1990): Rose CD+, *Arthritis Rheum* 33 (Suppl) R23
  (1975): Taaffe A+, *Br Dent J* 138, 172
  (1966): Coursin DB, *JAMA* 198, 113
Side effects (sic) (3.4%)
  (1966): Weinstein AW+, *Am J Dis Child* 111, 63
Stevens–Johnson syndrome (>10%)

(1975): Taaffe A+, *Br Dent J* 138, 172
Urticaria (1–5%)
  (1966): Weinstein AW+, *Am J Dis Child* 111, 63 (1%)

Hair
Hair – alopecia
Hair – hirsutism

Other
Acute intermittent porphyria
Gingival hyperplasia
Headache
Oral ulceration
Tongue edema

ETHOTOIN

Trade name: Peganone (Abbott)
Other common trade name: *Accenon*
Indications: Tonic–clonic (grand mal) seizures
Category: Hydantoin anticonvulsant
Half-life: 3–9 hours
**Clinically important, potentially hazardous interactions
with:** chloramphenicol, cyclosporine, disulfiram, dopamine,
imatinib, itraconazole

Reactions

Skin
Bullous eruption
Fixed eruption
Lupus erythematosus
Purpura
  (1967): Coleman WP, *Med Clin North Am* 51, 1073
Rash (sic)

Other
Gingival hyperplasia
Pseudolymphoma
  (1958): Salzstein SL+, *JAMA* 167, 1618

ETIDRONATE

Trade name: Didronel (Procter & Gamble)
Other common trade names: *Didronate; Difosfen; Dinol;
Diphos; Osteum*
Indications: Paget's disease, osteoporosis
Category: Antihypercalcemic; Bone resorption inhibitor
Half-life: 6 hours

Reactions

Skin
Angioedema (<1%)
Exanthems
Pruritus
  (1985): Holzmann H+, *Hautarzt* (German) 36, 326
Rash (sic) (<1%)
Stevens–Johnson syndrome
Toxic epidermal necrolysis
  (1995): Coakley G+, *Br J Rheumatol* 34, 798
Urticaria

Hair
Hair – alopecia

Other
Ageusia
Conjunctivitis
  (2003): Frauenfelder FW+, *N Engl J Med* 348, 1187
Dysgeusia (<1%)
Glossitis
Hypersensitivity (<1%)
Paresthesias
Stomatitis

ETODOLAC

Trade name: Lodine (Wyeth)
Other common trade names: *Antilak; Ecridoxan; Edolan;
Elderin; Lonine; Tedolan; Utradol; Zedolac*
Indications: Pain
Category: Nonsteroidal anti-inflammatory (NSAID)
Half-life: 7 hours
**Clinically important, potentially hazardous interactions
with:** aspirin, methotrexate

Reactions

Skin
Angioedema (<1%)
  (1991): Astorga-Paulsen G+, *Curr Med Res Opin* 12, 401
Bullous eruption
Dermatitis (sic)
Diaphoresis
Ecchymoses
Edema
Erythema multiforme (<1%)
Exanthems
  (1998): Litt JZ, Beachwood, OH (personal case) (observation)
  (1997): Litt JZ, Beachwood, OH (personal case) (observation)
  (1990): Schattenkirchner M, *Eur J Rheumatol Inflamm* 10, 56
  (1986): Lynch S+, *Drugs* 31, 288 (3%)
Exfoliation (sic)
Exfoliative dermatitis
Facial edema
  (1991): Astorga-Paulsen G+, *Curr Res Med Opin* 12, 401
  (1990): Freitas GG, *Curr Med Res Opin* 12, 255
Fixed eruption
  (1997): Blumenthal HL, Beachwood, OH (personal case)
    (observation)
Flushing
  (1991): Astorga-Paulsen G+, *Curr Med Res Opin* 12, 401
Furunculosis
  (1987): Waltham-Weeks CD, *Curr Med Res Opin* 10, 540
Peripheral edema
  (1990): Freitas GG, *Curr Med Res Opin* 12, 255
Photosensitivity
  (1987): Waltham-Weeks CD, *Curr Med Res Opin* 10, 540
Pigmentation
Pruritus (1–10%)
  (1998): Litt JZ, Beachwood, OH (personal case) (observation)
  (1991): Astorga-Paulsen G+, *Curr Res Med Opin* 12, 401
  (1991): Balfour JA+, *Drugs* 42, 274
  (1991): Bianchi-Porro G+, *J Intern Med* 229, 5
  (1991): *Med Lett Drug Ther* 33, 79
  (1991): Karbowski A, *Curr Med Res Opin* 12, 309
  (1990): Schattenkirchner M, *Eur J Rheumatol Inflamm* 10, 56

(1989): Ciocci A, *Curr Med Res Opin* 11, 471
Purpura
Rash (sic) (>10%)
  (1991): Anon, *Med Lett Drug Ther* 33, 79
  (1991): Astorga-Paulsen G+, *Curr Med Res Opin* 12, 401
  (1991): Balfour JA+, *Drugs* 42, 274
  (1989): Ciocci A, *Curr Med Res Opin* 11, 471
  (1989): Williams PI+, *Curr Med Res Opin*
Stevens–Johnson syndrome (<1%)
Toxic epidermal necrolysis (<1%)
Urticaria (<1%)
  (2000): Mitchell D, Thomasville, GA (from Internet)
    (observation)
  (1996): Thaler D, Monona, WI (personal case) (pressure)
    (observation)
Vasculitis
  (1996): Lie JT+, *J Rheumatol* 23, 183 (hypersensitivity)
  (1989): Willemin B+, *Ann Méd Int* (French) 140, 529
Vesiculobullous eruption

Hair
Hair – alopecia

Other
Gingival ulceration
Glossitis
Gynecomastia
Parageusia
Paresthesias
Sialorrhea
Stomatitis
Tinnitus
Ulcerative stomatitis
Xerostomia

ETOPOSIDE

Synonyms: epipodophyllotoxin; VP-16; VP-16–213
Trade name: VePesid (Bristol-Myers Squibb)
Other common trade names: *Aside; Etopos; Etosid; Lastet; Serozide; Vepeside; VP-TEC*
Indications: Lymphomas, carcinomas
Category: Antineoplastic
Half-life: terminal: 4–15 hours
Clinically important, potentially hazardous interactions with: aldesleukin, cyclosporine, **St John's wort**

Reactions

Skin
Allergic reactions (sic) (1–2%)
Diaphoresis
Ecchymoses
Eccrine squamous syringometaplasia
  (1997): Valks R+, *Arch Dermatol* 133, 873
Erythema
  (1994): Portal I+, *Cancer Chemother Pharmacol* 34, 181 (acral)
  (1993): Dechaufour F+, *Ann Dermatol Venereol* (French) 120, 219 (acral)
  (1993): Vukelja SJ+, *Cutis* 52, 89 (acral)
Erythema multiforme
  (1987): Yokel BK+, *J Cutan Pathol* 14, 326
Exanthems
  (1992): Beyer J+, *Bone Marrow Transplant* 10, 491

(1992): Breathnach SM+, *Adverse Drug Reactions and the Skin* Blackwell, Oxford, 301 (passim)
  (1987): Yokel BK+, *J Cutan Pathol* 14, 326
  (1981): Weiss RB+, *Ann Intern Med* 94, 66
Facial edema
Flushing (<1%)
  (1990): Henwood JM+, *Drugs* 39, 438
  (1988): Ogle KM+, *Am J Clin Oncol* 11, 663
  (1985): Tucci E+, *Chemioterapia* 4, 460
Infections
  (2002): Evans SR+, *J Clin Oncol* 20(15), 3236
Pigmentation
  (2001): Mutafoglu-Uysal K+, *Turk J Pediatr* 43(2), 172
  (1991): Singal R+, *Pediatr Dermatol* 8, 231
Pruritus
Purpura
Radiation recall
  (1993): Williams BJ+, *Clin Exp Dermatol* 18, 452 (ultraviolet)
  (1992): Breathnach SM+, *Adverse Drug Reactions and the Skin* Blackwell, Oxford, 301 (passim)
  (1987): Yokel BK+, *J Cutan Pathol* 14, 326
Rash (sic)
Stevens–Johnson syndrome
  (1992): Breathnach SM+, *Adverse Drug Reactions and the Skin* Blackwell, Oxford, 301 (passim)
  (1987): Yokel BK+, *J Cutan Pathol* 14, 326
  (1983): Jameson CH+, *Cancer Treat Rep* 67, 1050
Urticaria

Hair
Hair – alopecia (8–66%)
  (1990): Henwood JM+, *Drugs* 39, 438 (100%, dose-dependent)
  (1989): Smit EF+, *Thorax* 44, 631
  (1989): Wander HE+, *Cancer Chemother Pharmacol* 24, 261
  (1989): Yoshino M+, *Jpn J Clin Oncol* 19, 120 (57%)

Nails
Nails – Beau's lines (transverse nail bands)
  (1994): Ben-Dayan D+, *Acta Haematol* 91, 89
Nails – onycholysis
  (1995): Obermair A+, *Gynecol Oncol* 57, 436

Other
Anaphylactoid reactions (<2%)
  (2003): Taguchi A+, *Gan To Kagaku Ryoho* 30(8), 1187
  (1989): Siddall SJ+, *Lancet* 1, 394
  (1989): Wander HE+, *Cancer Chemother Pharmacol* 24, 261
Dysgeusia
Hypersensitivity (<1%)
  (2002): Siderov J+, *Br J Cancer* 86(1), 12
  (2001): Mutafoglu-Uysal K+, *Turk J Pediatr* 43(2), 172
  (1993): Hudson MM+, *J Clin Oncol* 11, 1080
  (1992): Weiss RB, *Semin Oncol* 19, 458
  (1991): Kellie SJ+, *Cancer* 67, 1070
  (1988): Ogle KM+, *Am J Clin Oncol* 11, 663
  (1985): Tucci E+, *Chemioterapia* 4, 460
  (1984): O'Dwyer PJ+, *Cancer Treat Rep* 68, 959
Injection-site pain
Mucositis (>10%)
Oral mucosal lesions
  (1990): Henwood JM+, *Drugs* 39, 438 (1–5%)
Paresthesias
Stomatitis (1–10%)
Thrombophlebitis (<1%)
Tongue edema

EXEMESTANE

Trade name: Aromasin (Pharmacia)
Indications: advanced breast cancer
Category: Antineoplastic (steroidal aromatase inactivator)
Half-life: 24 hours

Reactions

Skin
Diaphoresis (6%)
  (2000): Clemett D+, *Drugs* 59, 1279
  (1997): Thurlimann B+, *Eur J Cancer* 33, 1767 (12%)
Edema (7%)
Flu-like syndrome
Hot flashes (13%)
  (2002): Tabei T+, *Gan To Kagaku Ryoho* 29(7), 1199
  (2000): Clemett D+, *Drugs* 59, 1279
  (1999): Jones S+, *J Clin Oncol* 17, 3418
  (1998): Paridaens R+, *Anticancer Drugs* 9, 675 (30%)
  (1997): Thurlimann B+, *Eur J Cancer* 33, 1767 (21%)
Infections (sic)
Peripheral edema
  (1997): Thurlimann B+, *Eur J Cancer* 33, 1767 (9%)
Pruritus (2–5%)
Rash (sic) (2–5%)

Hair
Hair – alopecia (2–5%)

Other
Headache
  (2002): Tabei T+, *Gan To Kagaku Ryocho* 29(7), 1199

Hyperesthesia
Lymphedema (2–5%)
Paresthesias (2–5%)
Tumor pain
  (1998): Paridaens R+, *Anticancer Drugs* 9, 675 (30%)

EZETIMIBE

Trade name: Zetia
Indications: Hypercholesterolemia
Category: Selective cholesterol-absorption inhibitor
Half-life: 22 hours
**Clinically important, potentially hazardous interactions
with:** cyclosporine, gemfibrozil, fenofibrate, HMG-CoA Inhibitors
(statins)

Reactions

Skin
Viral infections (2.2%)

Other
Abdominal pain (2.2%)
Arthralgia (3.8%)
Back pain (4.1%)
Cough (2.3%)
Myalgia (5%)

FAMCICLOVIR

Trade name: Famvir (Novartis)
Indications: Acute herpes zoster, recurrent genital herpes
Category: Antiviral
Half-life: 2–3 hours

Reactions

Skin
Dermatitis (sic)
  (1996): Sacks SL+, *JAMA* 276, 44
Pruritus (3.7%)

Other
Headache
Hypersensitivity
  (2001): Kawsar M+, *Sex Transm Infect* 77(3), 204
Paresthesias (2.6%)

FAMOTIDINE

Trade name: Pepcid (Merck)
Other common trade names: *Amfamox; Apo-Famotidine; Durater; Famodil; Famoxal; Ganor; Gastro; Motiax; Mylanta AR; Nu-Famotidine; Pepcidine; Pepdul; Sigafam*
Indications: Duodenal ulcer, Gastroesophageal Reflux Disease (GERD)
Category: Antihistamine H$_2$-blocker
Half-life: 2.5–3.5 hours
Clinically important, potentially hazardous interactions with: cefditoren, **devil's claw**

Reactions

Skin
Acne (<1%)
Acute generalized exanthematous pustulosis (AGEP)
  (2003): Scheinfeld N+, *Acta Derm Venereol* 83(1), 76
Allergic reactions (sic) (<1%)
Angioedema
  (1986): Campoli-Richards DM+, *Drugs* 32, 197 (0.05%)
Candidiasis
  (2003): Orenstein SR+, *Aliment Pharmacol Ther* 17(9), 1097 (1 case)
Dermatitis
  (1994): Guimaraens D+, *Contact Dermatitis* 31, 259
  (1990): Monteseirin J+, *Contact Dermatitis* 22, 290
Dermographism
  (1994): Warner DMc+, *J Am Acad Dermatol* 31, 677
Erythema multiforme
  (1999): Horiuchi Y+, *Ann Intern Med* 131, 795
Exanthems
Facial edema
Flushing
  (1986): Campoli-Richards DM+, *Drugs* 32, 197 (0.2%)
Periorbital edema
Pruritus (<1%)
  (1994): Warner DMc+, *J Am Acad Dermatol* 31, 677
  (1990): Edge DP, *N Z Med J* 103, 150
Purpura
  (1996): Kallal SM+, *West J Med* 164, 446
Rash (sic)
  (1989): McCullough AJ+, *Gastroenterology* 97, 860

(1989): Schunack W, *J Int Med Res* 17 (Suppl 1), 9A
Side effects (sic)
  (1986): Campoli-Richards DM+, *Drugs* 32, 197 (0.4%)
Toxic epidermal necrolysis
  (1995): Brunner M+, *Br J Dermatol* 133, 814
Urticaria (<1%)
  (1994): Warner DMc+, *J Am Acad Dermatol* 31, 677
  (1986): Campoli-Richards DM+, *Drugs* 32, 197 (0.1%)
Vasculitis
  (1993): Torralba M+, *An Med Interna* (Spanish) 10, 621
  (1990): Andreo JA+, *Med Clin<D (Barc)* (Spanish) 95, 234
Xerosis (<1%)

Hair
Hair – alopecia

Other
Dysgeusia
Gynecomastia
Headache
  (2003): Orenstein SR+, *Aliment Pharmacol Ther* 17(9), 1097 (2 cases)
Hiccups
  (2003): Orenstein SR+, *Aliment Pharmacol Ther* 17(9), 1097 (1 case)
Injection-site pain
Myalgia
Oral mucosal lesions
  (1986): Campoli-Richards DM+, *Drugs* 32, 197 (0.15%)
Paresthesias (<1%)
  (1997): Litt JZ, Beachwood, OH (personal case) (observation)
  (1997): Litt JZ, Beachwood, OH (personal case) (observation) (prickly sensation)
Seizures
  (2002): von Einsiedel RW+, *Pharmacopsychiatry* 35(4), 152
Tinnitus
Xerostomia
  (1986): Campoli-Richards DM+, *Drugs* 32, 197 (0.15%)

FELBAMATE

Trade name: Felbatol (Wallace)
Other common trade names: *Felbamyl; Taloxa*
Indications: Partial seizures
Category: Antiepileptic
Half-life: 13–23 hours

Reactions

Skin
Acne (3.4%)
Bullous eruption (<1%)
Diaphoresis
Edema
Facial edema (3.4%)
Flushing
Idiosyncratic drug reactions
  (2002): Dieckhaus CM+, *Chem Biol Interact* 142(1), 99
Lichen planus
Livedo reticularis
Lupus erythematosus
Photosensitivity (<0.01%)
Pruritus (>1%)
Purpura
Pustules

(1994): Shelley WB+, *Cutis* 53, 282 (observation)
Rash (sic) (3.5%)
Stevens–Johnson syndrome
  (1994): Jackel RA, *Epilepsia* 35, 98
Toxic epidermal necrolysis
  (1995): Travaglini MT+, *Pharmacotherapy* 15, 260
Urticaria (<1%)

Hair

Hair – alopecia

Other

Anaphylactoid reactions (<0.01%)
Dysgeusia (6.1%)
Foetor ex ore (halitosis)
Gingivitis
Glossitis
Headache
Myalgia (2.6%)
Oral mucosal edema (>1%)
Paresthesias (3.5%)
Thrombophlebitis
Xerostomia (2.6%)

FELODIPINE

Trade names: Lexxel (AstraZeneca); Plendil (AstraZeneca)
Other common trade names: *AGON SR; Hydac; Modip; Munobal; Penedil; Renedil; Splendil*
Indications: Hypertension
Category: Antihypertensive; Calcium channel blocker
Half-life: 11–16 hours
Clinically important, potentially hazardous interactions with: carbamazepine, epirubicin, imatinib

Lexxel is enalapril and felodipine

Reactions

Skin

Ankle edema
  (1992): Morgan TO+, *Am J Hypertens* 5, 238
  (1992): Morgan TO+, *Kidney Int* Suppl 36, S78
  (1991): Dimenas E+, *Eur J Clin Pharmacol* 40, 141
  (1991): Liedholm H+, *Drug Intell Clin Pharm* 25, 1007
Diaphoresis
  (1988): Saltiel E+, *Drugs* 36, 387
Edema
  (1991): *Med Lett Drugs Ther* 33, 115
Erythema (1.5%)
Exanthems
  (1993): Litt JZ, Beachwood, OH (personal case) (observation)
  (1985): Lorimer AR+, *Drugs* 29 (Suppl 2), 154
Facial edema (1.5%)
Flu-like syndrome (sic) (<1%)
Flushing
  (1992): Morgan TO+, *Am J Hypertens* 5, 238
  (1991): Dimenas E+, *Eur J Clin Pharmacol* 40, 141
  (1991): Frewin DB+, *Eur J Clin Pharmacol* 41, 393
  (1991): *Med Lett Drugs Ther* 33, 115
  (1991): Liedholm H+, *Drug Intell Clin Pharm* 25, 1007
  (1991): Yedinak KC+, *Drug Intell Clin Pharm* 25, 1193
  (1988): Saltiel E+, *Drugs* 36, 387 (5–30%; dose-related)
  (1987): Elmfeldt D+, *Drugs* 34 (Suppl 3), 132
  (1985): Aberg H+, *Drugs* 29 (Suppl 2), 117 (44%)
  (1985): Lorimer AR+, *Drugs* 29 (Suppl 2), 154 (25%)

Peripheral edema (22%)
  (1991): Frewin DB+, *Eur J Clin Pharmacol* 41, 393
Pruritus (<1%)
Purpura
  (1991): Capewell S+, *Eur J Clin Pharmacol* 41, 95
Rash (sic) (1.5%)
Telangiectasia
  (2001): Silvestre JF+, *J Am Acad Dermatol* 45, 323 (facial; photodistributed)
  (1998): Karonen T+, *Dermatology* 196, 272 (truncal)
Urticaria (1.5%)

Nails

Nails – brittle
  (1985): Aberg H+, *Drugs* 29 (Suppl 2), 117 (44%)

Other

Gingival hyperplasia (2–10%)
  (1998): Young PC+, *Cutis* 62, 41
Gynecomastia (<1%)
Headache
Myalgia (1.5%)
Paresthesias (2.5%)
Tinnitus
Xerostomia (<1%)
  (1991): Dimenas E+, *Eur J Clin Pharmacol* 40, 141

FENOFIBRATE

Synonyms: procetofene; proctofene
Trade name: Tricor (Abbott)
Other common trade name: *Apo-Fenofibrate*
Indications: Hyperlipidemia
Category: Fibric acid cholesterol-lowering agent
Half-life: 20 hours
Clinically important, potentially hazardous interactions with: dicumarol, ezetimibe, lovastatin, nicotinic acid, warfarin

Reactions

Skin

Adverse effects (sic) (1–10%)
  (1989): Goldberg AC+, *Clin Ther* 11, 69
Exanthems
  (1990): Balfour JA+, *Drugs* 40, 260
Photosensitivity
  (1997): Leroy D+, *Photodermatol Photoimmunol Photomed* 13, 93
  (1997): Machet L+, *J Am Acad Dermatol* 37, 808
  (1996): Diemer S+, *J Dermatol Sci* 13, 172
  (1996): Leenutaphong V+, *J Am Acad Dermatol* 35, 775
  (1994): Miranda MA+, *Photochem Photobiol* 59, 171
  (1993): Gardeazabal J+, *Photodermatol Photoimmunol Photomed* 9, 156
  (1993): Jeanmougin M+, *Ann Dermatol Venereol* (French) 120, 549
  (1992): Serrano G+, *J Am Acad Dermatol* 27, 204
  (1990): Leroy D+, *Photodermatol Photoimmunol Photomed* 7, 136
  (1989): Merino MV+, *Actas Dermo-Sif* (Spanish) 80, 703
Phototoxicity
  (1993): Vargas F+, *Photochem Photobiol* 58, 471
  (1990): Merino V+, *Contact Dermatitis* 23, 284
Pruritus (4%)
Rash (sic) (4–8%)
  (2002): Najib J, *Clin Ther* 24(12), 2022
  (1989): Blane GF, *Cardiology* 76, 1
  (1989): *Am J Med* 83, 26 (2%)

Toxic epidermal necrolysis
  (2002): Correia O+, *Arch Dermatol* 138, 29 (two cases)
Urticaria

Hair

Hair – alopecia
  (1990): Gollnick H+, *Z Hautkr* (German) 65, 1128

Other

Headache
Muscle tenderness
  (1989): *Am J Med* 83, 26 (1%)
Muscle toxicity (sic)
  (1989): Muller JP+, *Presse Med* (French) 18, 1033
  (1982): Giraud P+, *Rev Rhum Mal Osteartic* (French) 49, 162
Myalgia (<1%)
  (2001): Rabasa-Lhoret R+, *Diabetes Metab* 27(1), 66
Myopathy
  (1991): Solsona L+, *Med Clin (Barc)* (Spanish) 97, 677
Myositis
  (2002): Najib J, *Clin Ther* 24(12), 2022
Paresthesias
Polymyositis
  (1991): Sauvaget F+, *Rev Med Interne* (French) 12, 52
Rhabdomyolysis
  (2000): Duda-Krol W+, *Wiad Lek* 53(7), 454
  (1992): Raimondeau J+, *Presse Med* 21(14), 663 (with
    pravastatin)
Septic–toxic shock (sic)
  (2000): Duda-Krol W+, *Wiad Lek* 53(7), 454
Vaginitis

FENOPROFEN

Trade name: Nalfon (Dista)
Other common trade names: *Fenoprex; Fenopron; Fepron; Feprona; Nalgesic; Progesic*
Indications: Arthritis
Category: Nonsteroidal anti-inflammatory (NSAID)
Half-life: 2.5–3 hours
Clinically important, potentially hazardous interactions with: methotrexate

Reactions

Skin

Acne
  (1974): Wojtulewski JA+, *BMJ* 2, 475
Angioedema (<1%)
Bruising (<1%)
Bullous eruption
Diaphoresis (<0.5%)
Erythema multiforme (<1%)
  (1988): Stotts JS+, *J Am Acad Dermatol* 18, 755
Exanthems
  (1985): Bigby M+, *J Am Acad Dermatol* 12, 866
  (1977): Davis JD+, *Clin Pharmacol Ther* 21, 52
Exfoliative dermatitis (<1%)
Hot flashes (<1%)
Peripheral edema (<1%)
Pruritus (3–9%)
  (1992): Breathnach SM+, *Adverse Drug Reactions and the Skin*
    Blackwell, Oxford, 186 (passim)
  (1985): Bigby M+, *J Am Acad Dermatol* 12, 866
  (1977): Davis JD+, *Clin Pharmacol Ther* 21, 52

Purpura (<1%)
  (1992): Breathnach SM+, *Adverse Drug Reactions and the Skin*
    Blackwell, Oxford, 186 (passim)
  (1978): Simpson RE+, *N Engl J Med* 298, 629
Rash (sic) (>10%)
Stevens–Johnson syndrome (<1%)
Toxic epidermal necrolysis (<1%)
  (1988): Stotts JS+, *J Am Acad Dermatol* 18, 755
Urticaria (1–3%)
  (1992): Breathnach SM+, *Adverse Drug Reactions and the Skin*
    Blackwell, Oxford, 186 (passim)
  (1985): Bigby M+, *J Am Acad Dermatol* 12, 866
Vesiculobullous eruption
  (1992): Breathnach SM+, *Adverse Drug Reactions and the Skin*
    Blackwell, Oxford, 186 (passim)

Hair

Hair – alopecia (<1%)

Other

Anaphylactoid reactions
Aphthous stomatitis (<1%)
Dysgeusia (<1%) (metallic taste)
Glossopyrosis (<1%)
Headache
Mastodynia (<1%)
Oral ulceration
Stomatitis
Tinnitus
Xerostomia (>1%)

FENTANYL

Trade names: Actiq (Cephalon); Duragesic (Janssen)
Other common trade names: *Beatryl; Durogesic; Fentanest; Leptanal; Sublimaze*
Indications: Chronic pain
Category: Narcotic agonist analgesic
Half-life: 1.5–6 hours
Clinically important, potentially hazardous interactions with: amiodarone, amprenavir, atazanavir, cimetidine, indinavir, nelfinavir, ranitidine, ritonavir, saquinavir

Reactions

Skin

Cold, clammy skin (<1%)
Diaphoresis (>10%)
  (2001): Litt JZ, Beachwood, OH (personal case) (observation)
  (1992): Calis KA+, *Clin Pharm* 11, 22
  (1992): Friesen RH+, *Anesthesiology* 76, 46
Edema
  (1990): Ducker P+, *Z Hautkr* (German) 65, 734
Erythema (at application site) (<1%)
  (1992): Mosser KH, *Am Fam Physician* 45, 2289
  (1990): Ducker P+, *Z Hautkr* (German) 65, 734
Exanthems
Exfoliative dermatitis
Fixed eruption
  (2001): Vaughan K, Lakewood, WA (from Internet) (observation)
    (from patch)
Flushing (3–10%)
Papulo-nodular lesions (sic) (>1%)
Pruritus (3–44%)
  (2002): Gurkan Y+, *Anesth Analg* 95(6), 1763

(2002): Henry A+, *Reg Anesth Pain Med* 27(5), 538 (intrathecal)
(2002): Nelson KE+, *Anesthesiology* 96(5), 1070
(1999): Herman NL+, *Anesth Analg* 89, 378
(1996): Larijani GE+, *Pharmacotherapy* 16, 958
(1994): Gerwels JW+, *J Dermatol Surg Oncol* 20, 823
(1992): Badner NH+, *Can J Anaesth* 39, 330
(1992): Belzarena SD, *Anesth Analg* 74, 653
(1992): Calis KA+, *Clin Pharm* 11, 22
(1992): Friesen RH+, *Anesthesiology* 76, 46 (facial)
(1992): Mosser KH, *Am Fam Physician* 45, 2289
(1992): Mourisse J+, *Acta Anaesthesiol Scand* 36, 70
(1992): Paech MJ, *Anaesth Intensive Care* 20, 15
(1992): Sandler ES+, *Pediatrics* 89, 631
(1992): Varrassi G+, *Anaesthesia* 47, 558
(1992): White MJ+, *Can J Anaesth* 39, 594
(1989): Ackerman WE+, *Can J Anaesth* 36, 388
(1989): Jorrot JC+, *Ann Fr Anesth Réanim* (French) 8, 321 (22%)
(1988): Davies GG+, *Anesthesiology* 69, 763
(1988): Monk JP+, *Drugs* 36, 286 (40%)
(1986): Shipton EA+, *S Afr Med J* 70, 325 (13%)
Purpura
(2001): Tweed WA+, *Anesth Analg* 92, 1442
Pustules (sic) (<1%)
Rash (sic) (>1%)
(1992): Sandler ES+, *Pediatrics* 89, 631
(1992): Stoukides CA+, *Clin Pharm* 11, 222
Urticaria (<1%)

Other
Anaphylactoid reactions
(2001): Girgis Y, *Anaesthesia* 56(10), 1016
(2001): Konarzewski W+, *Anaesthesia* 56(5), 497 (with propofol) (fatal)
(2001): Lewis S+, *Anaesthesia* 56(11), 1128
(1990): Ducker P+, *Z Hautkr* (German) 65, 734
Confusion
(2002): *Prescrire Int* 11(60), 106
Cough
(2002): Tsou CH+, *Acta Anaesthesiol Sin* 40(4), 165
(2001): Tweed WA+, *Anesth Analg* 92(6), 1442
Death
(2002): Mertes PM+, *Anaesthesia* 57(8), 821 (with propofol)
(2002): Reeves MD+, *Med J Aust* 177(10), 552
(2001): Girgis Y, *Anaesthesia* 56(10), 1016
Dizziness
(2002): *Prescrire Int* 11(60), 106
Dysesthesia (<1%)
Dysgeusia (<1%)
Headache
Paresthesias (<1%)
Syndrome of inappropriate antidiuretic hormone secretion (SIADH)
(2002): Kokko H+, *Pharmacotherapy* 22(9), 1188
Xerostomia (>10%)
(2001): Litt JZ, Beachwood, OH (personal case) (observation)
(1992): Calis KA+, *Clin Pharm* 11, 22

FEVERFEW

Scientific names: *Chrysanthemum parthenium; Pyrethrum parthenium; Tanacetum parthenium*
Family: Asteraceae; Compositae
Trade and other common names: Atamisa; Featerfoiul; Featherfew; Featherfoil; MIG-99; Santa Maria
Category: Stimulant and tonic
Purported indications and other uses: Fever, headache, migraine, menstrual irregularities, arthritis, psoriasis, allergy, asthma, tinnitus, vertigo, nausea, cold, earache, orthopedic disorders, swollen feet, diarrhea, dyspepsia
Half-life: N/A
Clinically important, potentially hazardous interactions with: anticoagulants, NSAIDs, warfarin

Reactions

Skin
Adverse effects (mild)
(2000): Ernst E+, *Public Health Nutr* 3(4A), 509
Angioedema (lips)
(1998): Awang DVC, *Int Med* 1, 11
(1985): Johnson ES+, *BMJ (Clin Res Ed)* 291, 569
Dermatitis
(2002): Paulsen E+, *Contact Dermatitis* 47(1), 14
(1996): Lamminpaa A+, *Contact Dermatitis* 34, 330
Prurigo nodularis
(2000): Sharma VK+, *Contact Dermatitis* 42(4), 235

Other
Ageusia
(1998): Awang DVC, *Int Med* 1, 11
(1985): Johnson ES+, *BMJ (Clin Res Ed)* 291, 569
Bleeding
(2001): Fessenden JM+, *Am Surg* 67(1), 33
Oral ulceration
(1998): Awang DVC, *Int Med* 1, 11
(1985): Johnson ES+, *BMJ (Clin Res Ed)* 291, 569

FEXOFENADINE

Trade name: Allegra (Aventis)
Indications: Allergic rhinitis, pruritus, urticaria
Category: Antihistamine H$_1$-blocker (nonsedating)
Half-life: 14.4 hours

Reactions

Skin
Acne
(1998): Litt JZ, Beachwood, OH (personal case) (observation)
Viral infections (sic) (2.5%)

Other
Headache

FILGRASTIM

(See GRANULOCYTE COLONY-STIMULATING FACTOR (GCSF))

FINASTERIDE

Trade names: Propecia (Merck); Proscar (Merck)
Other common trade names: *Pro-Cure; Proscar 5*
Indications: Benign prostatic hypertrophy, male-pattern baldness
Category: Antiandrogen; Antineoplastic; Hair growth stimulant
Half-life: 4.8–6 hours

Reactions

Skin

Folliculitis
  (2000): Price VH+, *J Am Acad Dermatol* 43, 768
Rash (sic)
  (1999): Cather JC+, *Cutis* 64, 167
Urticaria

Hair

Hair – hypotrichosis (sic)
  (1998): Panagotacos PJ (from Internet) (observation) ("reversal of graying hair")
Hair – patchy hair, loss of beard (sic)
  (1999): Mitchell D, Thomasville, GA (from Internet) (observation)
  (1998): Drayton GE, Los Angeles, CA (from Internet) (observation)

Nails

Nails – onychomycosis
  (1999): Mitchell D, Thomasville, GA (from Internet) (observation)

Other

Depression
  (2002): Altomare G+, *J Dermatol* 29(10), 665 (19 cases)
Edema of lip
Gynecomastia
  (2002): Ferrando J+, *Arch Dermatol* 138, 543
  (2000): Wade MS+, *Australas J Dermatol* 41, 55 (painful and reversible)
  (2000): Zimmerman RL+, *Arch Pathol Lab Med* 124, 625
  (1999): Cather JC+, *Cutis* 64, 167 (passim)
  (1999): Miller JA+, *South Med J* 92, 615
  (1997): Carlin BI+, *J Urol* 158, 547
  (1997): Staiman VR+, *Urology* 50, 929
  (1996): Green L+, *New Engl J Med* 335, 823
  (1996): Wilton L+, *Br J Urol* 78, 379
  (1995): Volpi R+, *Am J Med Sci* 309, 322
Mastodynia (<1%)
Myopathy (severe)
  (1999): Cather JC+, *Cutis* 64, 167

FLAVOXATE

Trade name: Urispas (Ortho-McNeil)
Other common trade names: *Bladderon; Genurin; Harnin; Patricin; Spasuret; Urispadol; Uronid*
Indications: Dysuria, urgency, nocturia
Category: Urinary antispasmodic
Half-life: Onset of action: 55–60 minutes
Clinically important, potentially hazardous interactions with: anticholinergics, arbutamine

Reactions

Skin

Exanthems
Rash (sic) (<1%)
  (1999): Enomoto U+, *Contact Dermatitis* 40, 337
Urticaria

Other

Headache
Hypersensitivity
  (1986): Hirohata S+, *Arch Intern Med* 146, 2409
Oral ulceration
  (1972): Strouthidis TM+, *Lancet* 1, 72
Xerostomia (>10%)

FLECAINIDE

Trade name: Tambocor (3M)
Other common trade names: *Almarytm; Apocard; Corflene; Flecaine; Tabco*
Indications: Atrial fibrillation
Category: Antiarrhythmic
Half-life: 7–22 hours
Clinically important, potentially hazardous interactions with: ritonavir

Reactions

Skin

Diaphoresis (<3%)
Edema (3.5%)
Exanthems
  (2003): Litt JZ, Beachwood, OH (personal case) (observation)
  (1985): Holmes B+, *Drugs* 27, 301 (1.4%)
Exfoliative dermatitis (<1%)
Flushing (<3%)
Pruritus (<1%)
  (2003): Litt JZ, Beachwood, OH (personal case) (observation)
Psoriasis
  (1988): Mancuso G+, *G Ital Dermatol Venerol* (Italian) 123, 171
  (1985): Holmes B+, *Drugs* 27, 301
Rash (sic) (<3%)
Urticaria (<1%)

Hair

Hair – alopecia (<1%)

Other

Dysgeusia (<1%) (metallic taste)
Headache
Hyperesthesia (1–10%)
Myalgia (<1%)

Oral edema
Paresthesias (<1%)
Tinnitus
Tongue edema (<1%)
Tremor (5%)
Xerostomia (<1%)

FLOXURIDINE

Trade name: FUDR (Roche)
Indications: Gastrointestinal carcinoma, metastatic to the liver
Category: Antimetabolite; Antineoplastic; Pyramidine analog
Half-life: N/A
Clinically important, potentially hazardous interactions with: cimetidine

Reactions

Skin
Abscess
Acne
Allergic reactions (sic)
Bullous eruption
Chills
Dermatitis (sic)
Erythema
Exanthems
Fissures
Petechiae
Photosensitivity
Pigmentation
Pruritus
Purpura
Rash (sic)
Xerosis

Hair
Hair – alopecia
Hair – brittle

Nails
Nails – loss

Other
Anaphylactoid reactions
Blurred vision
Cough
Depression
Dizziness
Fever
Fibromyositis
Gingivitis
Glossitis
Hiccups
Lacrimation
Mucositis
Oral ulceration
Paresthesias
Seizures
Stomatitis
Stomatodynia
Thrombophlebitis
Tongue edema

FLUCONAZOLE

Trade name: Diflucan (Roerig)
Other common trade names: *Biozolene; Flucazol; Flukezol; Fluzone; Fungata; Triflucan*
Indications: Candidiasis
Category: Broad-spectrum bis-triazole antifungal
Half-life: 25–30 hours
Clinically important, potentially hazardous interactions with: alprazolam, amphotericin B, anisindione, anticoagulants, dicumarol, eplerenone, methadone, midazolam, phenobarbital, phenytoin, sulfonylureas, vinblastine, vincristine, warfarin

Reactions

Skin
Acne
  (1998): Drake L, *J Am Acad Dermatol* 38, S87
Acute generalized exanthematous pustulosis (AGEP)
  (2002): Alsadhan A+, *J Cutan Med Surg* 6(2), 122
  (2002): Di Lernia V (Italy) (personal communication) (from Internet) (observation)
Angioedema
  (1999): Errico MR, Buenos Aires, Argentina (from Internet) (observation)
  (1991): Abbott M+, *Lancet* 2, 633
Bullous eruption
  (1994): Gupta AK+, *J Am Acad Dermatol* 30, 911
Erythema multiforme
  (1994): Gupta AK+, *J Am Acad Dermatol* 30, 911
  (1991): Gussenhoven MJE+, *Lancet* 338, 120
Exanthems
  (2001): Altman EM, West Orange, NJ (from Internet) (observation)
  (1990): Grant SM+, *Drugs* 39, 877 (1.8%) (in AIDS patients)
Exfoliative dermatitis
  (1994): Gupta AK+, *J Am Acad Dermatol* 30, 911 (passim)
  (1990): Grant SM+, *Drugs* 39, 877
Fixed eruption
  (2003): Lane JE+, *Oral Surg Oral Med Oral Pathol Oral Radiol Endod* 95(2), 129
  (2002): Ghislain P-D, *J Am Acad Dermatol* 46, 47 (recurrence)
  (2001): Hudson TF, Conway AR (from Internet) (observation)
  (2000): Heikkilä H+, *J Am Acad Dermatol* 42, 883
  (1997): Danby B, Kingston, Ontario (from Internet) (observation)
  (1997): Jaffe P, Columbia, SC (from Internet) (observation)
  (1994): Morgan JM+, *BMJ* 308, 454
Hypertrophy (sic)
  (1998): Drake L+, *J Am Acad Dermatol* 38, S87
Pallor (<1%)
Petechiae
  (1995): Mercurio MG+, *J Am Acad Dermatol* 32, 525
Pruritus
  (1999): Errico MR, Buenos Aires, Argentina (from Internet) (observation)
  (1991): Neuhaus G+, *BMJ* 302, 1341
Purpura
  (1990): Agarwal A+, *Ann Intern Med* 113, 899
Rash (sic) (1.8%)
  (1998): Scher RK+, *J Am Acad Dermatol* 38, S77
  (1995): Powderly WG, *Infections in Medicine* 257 (passim)
  (1994): Gupta AK+, *J Am Acad Dermatol* 30, 911 (1.8%)
Stevens–Johnson syndrome
  (1995): Powderly WG, *Infections in Medicine* 257 (passim)
  (1991): Gussenhoven MJE+, *Lancet* 1, 120
  (1990): Sugar AM+, *Rev Infect Dis* 12, S338

Toxic epidermal necrolysis
  (1993): Azon-Masoliver A+, *Dermatology* 187, 268
  (1990): Grant SM+, *Drugs* 39, 877
Urticaria

Hair

Hair – alopecia
  (2001): Ondo A, *Las Cruces, NM* (from Internet) (observation)
  (1996): Goldsmith LA, *Ann Intern Med* 125, 153
  (1995): Pappas PG+, *Ann Intern Med* 123, 354
  (1993): Weinroth SE+, *Ann Intern Med* 119, 637

Nails

Nails – changes (sic)
  (1998): Drake L+, *J Am Acad Dermatol* 38, S87
  (1998): Ling MR+, *J Am Acad Dermatol* 38, S95
Nails – melanonychia (longitudinal)
  (1998): Kar HK, *Int J Dermatol* 37, 719

Other

Anaphylactoid reactions (in AIDS patients)
Dysgeusia
  (1998): Quart AM+, *Infect Med* 15, 379
  (1991): Neuhaus G+, *BMJ* 302, 1341
Headache
Hypersensitivity (1–4%)
  (1997): Craig TJ, *J Am Osteopath Assoc* 97, 584
Oral ulceration
  (1998): Ling MR+, *J Am Acad Dermatol* 38, S95
  (1991): Abbott M+, *Lancet* 2, 633
Paresthesias
  (1991): Neuhaus G+, *BMJ* 302, 1341
Torsades de pointes
  (2002): Khazan M+, *Pharmacotherapy* 22(12), 1632
Xerostomia
  (1998): Quart AM+, *Infect Med* 15, 379

FLUCYTOSINE

Trade name: Ancobon (ICN)
Other common trade names: *5-FC; Alcobon; Ancotil*
Indications: Candidal and cryptococcal infections
Category: Antifungal
Half-life: 3–8 hours

Reactions

Skin

Exanthems
  (1987): Thyss A+, *Ann Dermatol Venereol* (French) 114, 1131
  (1972): Editorial, *N Engl J Med* 286, 777
Photosensitivity (<1%)
  (1987): Thyss A+, *Ann Dermatol Venereol* (French) 114, 1131
  (1983): Shelley WB+, *J Am Acad Dermatol* 8, 229
Pruritus
Purpura
Rash (sic) (1–10%)
Urticaria

Other

Anaphylactoid reactions (<1%)
Headache
Paresthesias (<1%)
Parkinsonism (<1%)
Xerostomia

FLUDARABINE

Trade name: Fludara (Berlex)
Indications: Chronic lymphocytic leukemia (B-cell)
Category: Purine nucleoside antineoplastic
Half-life: 9 hours
Clinically important, potentially hazardous interactions with: aldesleukin

Reactions

Skin

Chills (>10%)
Edema (>10%)
Exanthems
Paraneoplastic pemphigus
  (2001): Gooptu C+, *Br J Dermatol* 144(6), 1255 (3 cases)
  (1995): Bazarbachi A+, *Ann Oncol* 6, 730
Petechiae
  (2001): Churn M+, *Clin Oncol* 13, 273
Rash (sic) (>10%)
Squamous cell carcinoma
  (1997): Davidovitz Y+, *Acta Haematol* 98, 44 (flare-up)

Hair

Hair – alopecia (1–10%)

Other

Death
  (2002): Klasa RJ+, *J Clin Oncol* 20(24), 4649 (3 patients)
Dysgeusia (<1%) (metallic taste)
Myalgia (>10%)
Paresthesias (>10%)
Pneumonia
  (2002): Trojan A+, *Ann Hematol* 81(9), 535
Stomatitis (>10%)

FLUMAZENIL

Trade name: Romazicon (Roche)
Other common trade names: *Anexate; Lanexat*
Indications: Benzodiazepine overdose
Category: Benzodiazepine antidote
Half-life: terminal: 41–79 minutes
Clinically important, potentially hazardous interactions with: alcohol, neuromuscular blockers

Reactions

Skin

Diaphoresis (3–9%)
Flushing (1–3%)
Hot flashes (1–10%)
Rash (sic)
Urticaria (<1%)

Other

Headache
Hyperesthesia
Injection-site pain (3–9%)
Injection-site reactions (sic)
Paresthesias (1–10%)
Thrombophlebitis
Tinnitus

Tongue disorder (sic) (<1%)
Tremor (1–10%)
Xerostomia (1–10%)

FLUOROURACIL

Trade names: Adrucil (Pharmacia); Carac (Dermik); Efudex (ICN); Fluoroplex (Allergan)
Other common trade names: *Efudix; Efurix*
Category: Antineoplastic antimetabolite
Half-life: 8–20 minutes
Clinically important, potentially hazardous interactions with: aldesleukin, cimetidine, metronidazole

Reactions

Skin

Acral erythema
  (1995): Esteve E+, *Ann Med Interne Paris* (French) 146, 192
  (1992): Doll DC+, *Semin Oncol* 19(5), 580
  (1989): Vukelja SJ+, *Ann Intern Med* 111, 688
Actinic keratoses (sic)
  (1999): Nabai H+, *Cutis* 64, 43
  (1987): Johnson TM+, *J Am Acad Dermatol* 17(2 Pt 1), 192
  (1969): Omura EF+, *JAMA* 208, 150
  (1962): Falkson G+, *Br J Dermatol* 74, 229
Angioedema
Bullous eruption
  (1970): Bart BJ+, *Arch Dermatol* 102, 457
Dermatitis (sic) (>10%)
  (1999): Sanchez-Perez J+, *Contact Dermatitis* 41, 106
  (1997): Anderson LL+, *J Am Acad Dermatol* 36, 478
  (1996): Nadal C+, *Contact Dermatitis* 35, 124 (systemic)
  (1977): Goette DK+, *Arch Dermatol* 113, 1058
Eczema (sic)
  (1977): Bernstein T, *New Engl J Med* 297, 337
Edema of foot
  (1992): Breathnach SM+, *Adverse Drug Reactions and the Skin*
    Blackwell, Oxford, 193 (passim)
Erythema
  (1980): Hrushesky WJ, *Cutis* 26, 181
  (1962): Falkson G+, *Br J Dermatol* 74, 229
Erythema multiforme
  (1980): Ueki H+, *Hautarzt* (German) 31, 207
Erythematous eruption, linear serpentine (sic)
  (1998): Pujol RM+, *J Am Acad Dermatol* 39, 839
Exanthems (1–10%)
  (1994): Leo S+, *J Chemother* 6, 423
  (1994): Sollitto RB+, *Arch Dermatol* 130, 1194 (sun-exposed
    areas)
Fissures
Folliculitis (forehead)
  (2001): Schmid-Wendtner M-H+, *Lancet* 358, 1575 (passim)
Hand-foot syndrome
  (2002): Cure H+, *J Clin Oncol* 20(5), 1175 (38%)
  (2001): Elasmar SA+, *Jpn J Clin Oncol* 31(4), 172 (passim)
  (1997): Chiara S+, *Eur J Cancer* 33, 967
  (1997): Iurio A+, *Acta Oncol* 36, 653
  (1997): Thaler D, Monona, WI (from internet) (observation)
  (1995): Banfield GK+, *J R Soc Med* 88, 356
  (1994): Leo S+, *J Chemother* 6, 423
  (1993): Beard JS+, *J Am Acad Dermatol* 29, 325
  (1991): Jorda E+, *Int J Dermatol* 30, 653
  (1989): Curran CF+, *Ann Intern Med* 111, 858
  (1989): Vukelja SJ+, *Ann Intern Med* 111, 688

  (1988): Guillaume J-C+, *Ann Dermatol Venereol* (French)
    115, 1167
  (1987): Molina R+, *Proc Am Soc Clin Oncol* 4, 92
  (1985): Atkins JN, *Ann Intern Med* 102, 419
  (1985): Feldman LD+, *JAMA* 254, 3479
  (1984): Lokich JJ+, *Ann Intern Med* 101, 798
Infections
  (2002): Bonneterre J+, *Br J Cancer* 87(11), 1210 (7%) (with
    vinorelbine)
Keratoderma (palms)
  (2001): Schmid-Wendtner M-H+, *Lancet* 358, 1575 (passim)
Keratoses
  (2001): Kurzman MA, Staten Island, NY (from Internet)
    (observation)
  (2001): Lamberts RJ, Grand Rapids, MI (from Internet)
    (observation) (inflammation)
Necrosis
  (1980): Yaffee HS+, *Cutis* 25, 649 ("ecdysis")
Palmar–plantar pigmentation
  (2001): Schmid-Wendtner M-H+, *Lancet* 358, 1575 (passim)
Photosensitivity (<1%)
  (1999): von Moos R+, *Schweiz Med Wochenschr* (German)
    129, 52
  (1992): Breathnach SM+, *Adverse Drug Reactions and the Skin*
    Blackwell, Oxford, 193 (passim)
  (1962): Falkson G+, *Br J Dermatol* 74, 229
Phototoxicity
Pigmentation (<1%)
  (1997): Miller BH+, *J Am Acad Dermatol* 36, 72
  (1995): Allen BJ+, *Int J Dermatol* 34, 219 (reticulate)
  (1994): Leo S+, *J Chemother* 6, 423
  (1991): Vukelja SJ+, *J Am Acad Dermatol* 25, 905 (serpentine)
  (1980): Hrushesky WJ, *Cutis* 26, 181 (sun-exposed areas)
  (1977): Goette DK+, *Arch Dermatol* 113, 1058
  (1962): Falkson G+, *Br J Dermatol* 74, 229
Pruritus
Psoriasis
  (2002): Wetzig T+, *Br J Dermatol* 147(4), 824
Radiation recall
  (1992): Breathnach SM+, *Adverse Drug Reactions and the Skin*
    Blackwell, Oxford, 193 (passim)
Reactivation phenomenon (sic)
  (1997): Anderson LL+, *J Am Acad Dermatol* 36, 478
  (1993): Prussick R+, *Arch Dermatol* 129, 644
Recall reaction
  (2003): Kirkup ME+, *Dermatology* 206(2), 175
Seborrheic dermatitis
  (1962): Falkson G+, *Br J Dermatol* 74, 229
Side effects (sic)
  (2002): Moazzam N+, *J Clin Oncol* 20(13), 3032
Systemic lupus erythematosus
  (2002): Moazzam N+, *J Clin Oncol* 20(13), 3032
Urticaria
Xerosis (1–10%)

Hair

Hair – alopecia (>10%)
  (2003): Saini A+, *Br J Cancer* 88(12), 1859
  (2002): Sloan JA+, *J Clin Oncol* 20(6), 1491
  (2001): Madnani N, Mumbai, India (from Internet) (observation)
  (1992): Breathnach SM+, *Adverse Drug Reactions and the Skin*
    Blackwell, Oxford, 193 (passim)
  (1962): Falkson G+, *Br J Dermatol* 74, 229

Nails

Nails – onycholysis
Nails – pigmentation (<1%)
  (2001): Schmid-Wendtner M-H+, *Lancet* 358, 1575 (passim)
  (1962): Falkson G+, *Br J Dermatol* 74, 229

Other

Anaphylactoid reactions
(1992): Breathnach SM+, *Adverse Drug Reactions and the Skin* Blackwell, Oxford, 193 (passim)
Death
(2003): van Kuilenburg AB+, *Ann Oncol* 14(2), 341
Dysgeusia
Ectropion
(1997): Lewis JE, *Int J Dermatol* 36, 79
(1994): Hecker D+, *Cutis* 53, 137
Injection-site burning
(1998): Kraus S+, *J Am Acad Dermatol* 38, 438
(1997): Miller BH+, *J Am Acad Dermatol* 36, 72
Injection-site desquamation
(1998): Kraus S+, *J Am Acad Dermatol* 38, 438
(1997): Miller BH+, *J Am Acad Dermatol* 36, 72
(1997): Swinehart JM+, *Arch Dermatol* 133, 67
(1992): Breathnach SM+, *Adverse Drug Reactions and the Skin* Blackwell, Oxford, 193 (passim)
Injection-site edema
(1997): Miller BH+, *J Am Acad Dermatol* 36, 72
(1997): Swinehart JM+, *Arch Dermatol* 133, 67
(1992): Breathnach SM+, *Adverse Drug Reactions and the Skin* Blackwell, Oxford, 193 (passim)
Injection-site erythema
(1998): Kraus S+, *J Am Acad Dermatol* 38, 438
(1997): Miller BH+, *J Am Acad Dermatol* 36, 72
(1997): Swinehart JM+, *Arch Dermatol* 133, 67
(1992): Breathnach SM+, *Adverse Drug Reactions and the Skin* Blackwell, Oxford, 193 (passim)
Injection-site necrosis
(1998): Kraus S+, *J Am Acad Dermatol* 38, 438
(1997): Swinehart JM+, *Arch Dermatol* 133, 67
Injection-site pain
(1998): Kraus S+, *J Am Acad Dermatol* 38, 438
(1997): Swinehart JM+, *Arch Dermatol* 133, 67
Injection-site pigmentation
(2001): Schmid-Wendtner M-H+, *Lancet* 358, 1575 (passim)
Injection-site ulceration
(1997): Miller BH+, *J Am Acad Dermatol* 36, 72
(1997): Swinehart JM+, *Arch Dermatol* 133, 67
Mucositis (1–10%)
(2003): Chen JY+, *Ai Zheng* 22(4), 418
(2003): Nottage M+, *Support Care Cancer* 11(1), 41 (79%)
(2002): Cure H+, *J Clin Oncol* 20(5), 1175 (26%)
(2001): Hejna M+, *Eur J Cancer* 37(16), 1994
Oral ulceration
(2002): Xu D+, *Zhonghua Zhong Liu Za Zhi* 24(1), 93 (with leucovorin)
Paresthesias (<1%)
Phlebitis
(2002): Xu D+, *Zhonghua Zhong Liu Za Zhi* 24(1), 93 (with leucovorin)
Stomatitis (>10%)
(2003): Rossi A+, *Oncology* 64(4), 353
(2003): Saini A+, *Br J Cancer* 88(12), 1859
(2003): Tebbutt NC+, *Br J Cancer* 88(10), 1510
(2002): Bonneterre J+, *Br J Cancer* 87(11), 1210 (40%) (with vinorelbine)
(2002): Ito A+, *Gan To Kagaku Ryoho* 29(4), 563
(2002): McCollum AD+, *J Natl Cancer Inst* 94(15), 1160
(2002): Sloan JA+, *J Clin Oncol* 20(6), 1491
(2002): Ueno H+, *Cancer Chemother Pharmacol* 49(2), 155
Tongue pigmentation
(2001): Schmid-Wendtner M-H+, *Lancet* 358, 1575 (passim)

FLUOXETINE

Trade names: Prozac (Dista) (Lilly); Sarafem (Dermik)
Other common trade names: Adofen; Apo-Fluoxetine; Dom-Fluoxetine; Fluctin; Fluctine; Fludac; Fluoxac; Fluoxeren; Fluxil; Fontex
Indications: Depression, obsessive-compulsive disorder
Category: Antidepressant; Selective serotonin reuptake inhibitor (SSRI)
Half-life: 2–3 days
Clinically important, potentially hazardous interactions with: alprazolam, amphetamines, clarithromycin, clozapine, desipramine, dextroamphetamine, diethylpropion, erythromycin, haloperidol, imipramine, isocarboxazid, linezolid, lithium, MAO inhibitors, mazindol, meperidine, methamphetamine, midazolam, moclobemide, nortriptyline, phendimetrazine, phenelzine, phentermine, phenylpropanolamine, phenytoin, pimozide, pseudoephedrine, selegiline, serotonin agonists, sibutramine, **St John's wort**, sumatriptan, sympathomimetics, tramadol, tranylcypromine, trazodone, tricyclic antidepressants, troleandomycin, **tryptophan**

Reactions

Skin

Acne (<1%)
Allergic reactions (sic)
(1998): Beauquier B+, *Encephale* (French) 24, 62
Angioedema
(1991): Olfson M+, *J Nerv Mental Dis* 179, 504
Bruising
(1996): Pai VB+, *Ann Pharmacother* 30, 786
Bullous eruption (<1%)
Candidiasis
Cellulitis
Dermatitis (<1%)
Diaphoresis (8.4%)
(1985): Wernicke JF, *J Clin Psychiatry* 46, 59
Eczema (sic) (<1%)
Erythema multiforme
(1985): Wernicke JF, *J Clin Psychiatry* 46, 59
Erythema nodosum (<1%)
Exanthems (4%)
(1993): Gupta MA+, *Cutis* 51, 386 (3%) (passim)
(1993): Gupta RK+, *Med J Aust* 158, 722
(1993): Litt JZ, Beachwood, OH (personal case) (observation)
(1991): Olfson M+, *J Nerv Mental Dis* 159, 504
(1989): Miller LG+, *Am J Psychiatry* 146, 1616
(1988): Cooper GL, *Br J Psychiatry* 153, 77
(1985): Wernicke JF, *J Clin Psychiatry* 46, 59
Exfoliative dermatitis
Facial edema (<1%)
Flushing (<2%)
Furunculosis (<1%)
Herpes simplex (reactivation)
(1991): Reed SM+, *Am J Psychiatry* 148, 949
Herpes zoster
Hot flashes
Lichenoid eruption
Lupus erythematosus (discoid)
Mycosis fungoides (exacerbation)
(1996): Vermeer MH+, *J Am Acad Dermatol* 35, 635
Nodules (sic)
Peripheral edema (<1%)

Petechiae (<1%)
Photosensitivity
(1998): Pazzagli L+, *Pharm World Sci* 20, 136 (with alprazolam)
Phototoxicity (<1%)
(1995): Gaufberg E+, *J Clin Psychiatry* 56, 486
(1995): O'Brien T, *Australas J Dermatology* 36, 103
Pigmentation (<1%)
Pruritus (2.4%)
(1993): Gupta RK+, *Med J Aust* 158, 722
(1991): Olfson M+, *J Nerv Mental Dis* 159, 504
(1985): Wernicke JF, *J Clin Psychiatry* 46, 59
Pseudo-mycosis fungoides (sic)
(1996): Gordon KB+, *J Am Acad Dermatol* 34, 304
Psoriasis (<1%)
(1992): Hemlock C+, *Ann Pharmacother* 26, 211
Purpura (<1%)
Pustules (<1%)
Rash (sic) (6%)
(1989): Miller LG+, *Am J Psychiatry* 146, 1616
(1987): Zerbe RL, *Int J Obes* 11 (Suppl 3), 191
(1985): Wernicke JF, *J Clin Psychiatry* 46, 59
Raynaud's phenomenon
(2000): De Broucker+, *Ann Med Interne (Paris)* 151(5), 424
Seborrhea (<1%)
Stevens–Johnson syndrome
(1998): N Z Medicines Adverse Reactions Committee (from
Internet) (observation)
(1992): Bodokh I+, *Therapie* (French) 47, 441
Toxic epidermal necrolysis
(1992): Bodokh I+, *Therapie* (French) 47, 441
(1991): Rosenthal E+, *Presse Med* (French) 20, 1459
Ulcerations (<1%)
Urticaria (4%)
(1994): Blumenthal HL, Beachwood, OH (personal case)
(observation)
(1993): Gupta RK+, *Med J Aust* 158, 722
(1992): Leznoff A+, *J Clin Psychopharmacol* 12, 355
(1991): Olfson M+, *J Nerv Mental Dis* 159, 504
(1989): Miller LG+, *Am J Psychiatry* 146, 1616
Vasculitis
(1999): Fisher A+, *Aust N Z J Med* 29, 375 (focal necrotizing)
(1995): Roger D+, *Dermatology* 191, 164
Xerosis

Hair

Hair – alopecia (<1%)
(2000): Murlidhar MD, Madras, India (from Internet)
(observation)
(1996): Bhatara VS+, *J Clin Psychiatry* 57, 227
(1995): Seifritz E+, *Can J Psychiatry* 40, 362
(1995): Shelley WB+, *Cutis* 55, 144 (observation)
(1994): Mareth TR, *J Clin Psychiatry* 55, 163
(1994): Shelley WB+, *Cutis* 53, 282 (observation)
(1993): Ogilvie AD, *Lancet* 342, 1423
(1991): Ananth J+, *J Psychiatry* 36, 621
(1991): Gupta S+, *Br J Psychiatry* 159, 737
(1991): Jenike MA, *Am J Psychiatry* 148, 392
Hair – hirsutism (<1%)

Other

Ageusia (<1%)
Anaphylactoid reactions (<1%)
Aphthous stomatitis (<1%)
Black tongue
(2000): Heymann WR, *Cutis* 66, 25
Dysgeusia (1.8%)
(2000): Heymann WR, *Cutis* 66, 25
Galactorrhea

(2001): Peterson MC, *Mayo Clin Proc* 76, 215
Gingivitis (<1%)
Glossitis (<1%)
Glossodynia
(1994): Shelley WB+, *Cutis* 53, 242 (observation)
Gynecomastia (<1%)
(2003): Boulenger A+, *J Eur Acad Dermatol Venereol* 17(1), 109
Headache
(2003): Calabrese JR+, *J Clin Psychiatry* 64(5), 562 (27%)
Hyperesthesia (<1%)
Hypersensitivity
(1994): Beer K+, *Arch Dermatol* 130, 803
Mastodynia (<1%)
Myalgia
Myopathy (<1%)
Oral ulceration (<1%)
(2000): Madinier I+, *Ann Med Interne (Paris)* (French) 151, 248
Paresthesias
(2001): Ribeiro L+, *Braz J Med Biol Res* 34(10), 1303
(1996): Bhatara VS+, *J Clin Psychiatry* 57, 227
Parosmia (<1%)
Priapism (<1%)
Pseudolymphoma
(1995): Crowson AN+, *Arch Dermatol* 131, 925
(1995): Magro CM+, *J Am Acad Dermatol* 32, 419
(1988): Kardaun SH+, *Br J Dermatol* 118(4), 545
Rhabdomyolysis
(1990): Lazarus A, *J Clin Psychopharmacol* 10 (overdose)
Serotonin syndrome
(2003): Birmes P+, *CMAJ* 168(11), 1439
(2002): Chechani V, *Crit Care Med* 30(2), 473
(2002): Lange-Asschenfeldt C+, *J Clin Psychopharmacol*
22(4), 440 (with tramadol)
(2000): Manos GH, *Ann Pharmacother* 34(7–8), 871 (with
buspirone)
Serum sickness
(1991): Vincent A+, *Am J Psychiatry* 148, 1602
(1989): Miller LG+, *Am J Psychiatry* 146, 1616
Sialorrhea (<1%)
Stomatitis (<1%)
Thrombophlebitis (<1%)
Tinnitus
Tongue edema (<1%)
Tongue pigmentation (<1%)
Tremor (2–10%)
Vaginal anesthesia
(1993): King VL+, *Am J Psychiatry* 150, 984
Xerostomia (12%)
(2002): Krymchantowski AV+, *Headache* 42(6), 510 (with
amitriptyline)
(2000): Heymann WR, *Cutis* 66, 25
(1993): Beasley CM+, *Ann Clin Psychiatry* 5, 199
(1985): Wernicke JF, *J Clin Psychiatry* 46, 59

FLUOXYMESTERONE

Trade names: Android-F; Halotensin (Pharmacia)
Other common trade names: *Stenox; Vewon*
Indications: Breast carcinoma, hypogonadism, anemia
Category: Androgen; Antianemic; Antineoplastic
Half-life: 9.2 hours
Clinically important, potentially hazardous interactions with: anticoagulants, cyclosporine, warfarin

Reactions

Skin
Acne (>10%)
  (1992): Fryand O+, *Acta Derm Venereol* 72, 148
  (1990): Fuchs E+, *J Am Acad Dermatol* 23, 125
  (1989): Fryand O+, *Tidsskr Nor Laegeforen* (Norwegian) 109, 239
  (1989): Hartmann AA+, *Monatsschr Kinderheilkd* (German) 137, 466
  (1989): Heydenreich G, *Arch Dermatol* 125, 571 (fulminans)
  (1989): Scott MJ+, *Cutis* 44, 30
  (1989): von Muhlendahl KE+, *Dtsch Med Wochenschr* (German) 114, 712
  (1988): Traupe H+, *Arch Dermatol* 124, 414 (fulminans)
  (1987): Kiraly CL+, *Am J Dermatopathol* 9, 515
  (1984): Lamb DR, *Am J Sports Med* 12, 31
  (1965): Kennedy BJ, *J Am Geriatr Soc* 13, 230
  (1965): Rook A, *Br J Dermatol* 77, 115
Dermatitis
  (1989): Holdiness MR, *Contact Dermatitis* 20, 3 (from patch)
Edema (>10%)
Exanthems
Flushing (1–5%)
  (1965): Kennedy BJ, *J Am Geriatr Soc* 13, 230
Furunculosis
  (1989): Scott MJ+, *Cutis* 44, 30
Lichenoid eruption
  (1989): Aihara M+, *J Dermatol* (Tokio) 16, 330
Lupus erythematosus
  (1978): Robinson HM, *Z Haut* (German) 53, 349
Pruritus
Psoriasis
  (1990): O'Driscoll JB+, *Clin Exp Dermatol* 15, 68
Purpura
Seborrhea (sic)
Seborrheic dermatitis
  (1989): Scott MJ+, *Cutis* 44, 30
Striae
  (1989): Scott MJ+, *Cutis* 44, 30
Urticaria

Hair
Hair – alopecia
  (1989): Scott MJ+, *Cutis* 44, 30
  (1965): Kennedy BJ, *J Am Geriatr Soc* 13, 230
Hair – hirsutism (1–10%)
  (1994): Castillo-Ceballos A+, *Med Clin (Barc)* (Spanish) 102, 78
  (1991): Bates GW+, *Clin Obstet Gynecol* 34, 848
  (1991): No Author, *Obstet Gynecol* 78, 474
  (1991): Parker LU+, *Cleve Clin J Med* 58, 43
  (1991): Urman B+, *Obstet Gynecol* 77, 595
  (1989): Scott MJ+, *Cutis* 44, 30
  (1974): Baron J, *Zentralbl Gynakol* (German) 96, 129
  (1971): Fusi S+, *Folia Endocrinol* (Italian) 24, 412
  (1965): Kennedy BJ, *J Am Geriatr Soc* 13, 230

Other
Anaphylactoid reactions
Gynecomastia (<1%)
Hypersensitivity (<1%)
Injection-site pain
Mastodynia (>10%)
Paresthesias
Priapism (>10%)
Stomatitis

FLUPHENAZINE

Trade names: Permitil (Schering); Prolixin (Geneva)
Other common trade names: *Anatensol; Apo-Fluphenazine; Dapatum D25; Dapotum D; Fludecate; Modecate; Moditen*
Indications: Psychoses
Category: Phenothiazine antipsychotic
Half-life: 84–96 hours
Clinically important, potentially hazardous interactions with: antihistamines, arsenic, chlorpheniramine, dofetilide, quinolones, sparfloxacin

Reactions

Skin
Angioedema (<1%)
Dermatitis (sic)
Diaphoresis
Eczema (sic)
Edema
Erythema
Exanthems
Exfoliative dermatitis
Hypohidrosis (>10%)
Lupus erythematosus
  (1975): Gallien M+, *Ann Med Psychol* (Paris) (French) 1, 237
Peripheral edema
Photosensitivity
Pigmentation (<1%) (blue-gray)
  (1987): Krebs A, *Schweiz Rundsch Med Prax* (German) 76, 1069
Pruritus (<1%)
Purpura
Rash (sic) (1–10%)
Seborrhea
Toxic epidermal necrolysis
  (1972): Carli-Basset C+, *Sem Hôp* (French) 48, 497
Urticaria
Vitiligo
  (1987): Krebs A, *Schweiz Rundsch Med Prax* (German) 76, 1069
  (1985): Rampertaap MP, *Mo Med* 82, 24
Xerosis

Other
Anaphylactoid reactions
Galactorrhea (1–10%)
Gynecomastia (1–10%)
Headache
Injection-site reactions
Mastodynia (1–10%)
Parkinsonism
Priapism (<1%)
  (1986): Fishbain DA, *Psychosomatics* 27, 538
  (1985): Fishbain DA, *Ann Emerg Med* 14, 600

Rhabdomyolysis
  (1978): Mann SC+, *Am J Psychiatry* 135, 1097
Sialorrhea
  (1973): Johnson DAW, *Br J Psychiatry* 123, 519
Trembling (sic) (fingers)
Xerostomia (<1%)

FLURAZEPAM

Trade name: Dalmane (ICN); Flurazepam (ICN)
Other common trade names: *Apo-Flurazepam; Benozil; Dalmadorm; Flunox; Nergart; Novoflupam; Som Pam; Somnol; Valdorm*
Indications: Insomnia
Category: Benzodiazepine sedative-hypnotic
Half-life: 40–114 hours
Clinically important, potentially hazardous interactions with: amprenavir, chlorpheniramine, clarithromycin, efavirenz, esomeprazole, imatinib, indinavir, nelfinavir, ritonavir

Reactions

Skin
Dermatitis (sic) (1–10%)
Diaphoresis (>10%)
Exanthems
  (1976): Arndt KA+, *JAMA* 235, 918 (0.05%)
Flushing
Pruritus
Purpura
Rash (sic) (>10%)
Urticaria

Other
Acute intermittent porphyria
Dysgeusia (3.4%) (metallic taste)
  (1984): Greenblatt DJ+, *J Clin Psychiatry* 45, 192 (3%)
Headache
Oral mucosal lesions
  (1984): Greenblatt DJ+, *J Clin Psychiatry* 45, 192 (3%)
Paresthesias
Sialopenia (>10%)
Sialorrhea (1–10%)
Xerostomia (>10%)

FLURBIPROFEN

Trade name: Ansaid (Pharmacia)
Other common trade names: *Apo-Flurbiprofen; Cebutid; Flurofen; Flurozin; Froben; Lapole; Nu-Flurprofen*
Indications: Arthritis
Category: Nonsteroidal anti-inflammatory (NSAID)
Half-life: 3–4 hours
Clinically important, potentially hazardous interactions with: methotrexate

Reactions

Skin
Angioedema (<1%)
  (1997): Romano A+, *J Intern Med* 241, 81
Burning (ophthalmic)
Dermatitis
  (2000): Kawada A+, *Contact Dermatitis* 42, 167
Dermatitis herpetiformis
  (1994): Tousignant J+, *Int J Dermatol* 33, 199
Diaphoresis
Discoloration (sic)
Eczema (sic) (3–9%)
Edema (3–9%)
Erythema multiforme (<1%)
Exanthems
  (1997): Romano A+, *J Intern Med* 241, 81
  (1977): Cardoe N, *Curr Med Res Opin* 5, 99
  (1974): Calin A+, *BMJ* 4, 496 (3%)
Exfoliative dermatitis (<1%)
Fixed eruption
  (1993): *Dermatology* 186, 164
Flushing
Furunculosis
Herpes simplex
Herpes zoster
Hot flashes (<1%)
Peripheral edema
Photosensitivity (<1%)
Pruritus (1–5%)
  (1977): Cardoe N, *Curr Med Res Opin* 5, 99
Pseudoreactions (sic)
  (1991): VanArsdel PP, *JAMA* 266, 3343
Purpura
Rash (sic) (1–3%)
Seborrhea
Side effects (sic) (6%)
  (1986): Buson M, *J Int Med Res* 14, 1
  (1977): Sheldrake FE+, *Curr Med Res Opin* 5, 106
Stevens–Johnson syndrome (<1%)
Stinging (ophthalmic)
Toxic epidermal necrolysis (<1%)
  (1987): Gillaume JC+, *Arch Dermatol* 123, 1166
Ulcerations
Urticaria (<1%)
Vasculitis
  (1990): Wei M, *Ann Intern Med* 112, 550
Vulvovaginitis
Xerosis

Hair
Hair – alopecia (<1%)

Nails
Nails – changes (sic) (<1%)
Nails – pigmentation

Other
Anaphylactoid reactions (<1%)
Aphthous stomatitis
Dysgeusia (<1%)
Headache
Hypersensitivity
  (1997): Romano A+, *J Intern Med* 241, 81
Oral lichenoid eruption
  (2000): Madinier I+, *Ann Med Interne (Paris)* (French) 151, 248
  (1983): Hamburger J+, *BMJ* 287, 1258
Paresthesias (<1%)
Parosmia (<1%)
Stomatitis
Tinnitus
Xerostomia (<1%)

FLUTAMIDE

Trade name: Eulexin (Schering)
Other common trade names: *Drogenil; Euflex; Eulexine; Flucinom; Fluken; Flulem; Fugerel; Novo-Flutamide*
Indications: Metastatic prostate carcinoma
Category: Antiandrogen; Antineoplastic (prostate carcinoma)
Half-life: 6 hours

Reactions

Skin
Bullous eruption
Diaphoresis
  (1992): Schmeller N, *Internist Berl* (German) 33, 284
Edema (4%)
Erythema
Exanthems
  (1999): Fisher BJ, Toronto, Ontario (from Internet) (observation)
    (generalized)
  (1989): Brogden RN+, *Drugs* 38, 185
Flu-like syndrome (sic) (<1%)
Hot flashes (61%)
Lupus erythematosus
  (1998): Reid MB+, *J Urol* 159, 2098
Photosensitivity
  (2003): Kaur C+, *Br J Dermatol* 148(3), 603
  (1999): Tsien C+, *J Urol* 162, 494
  (1998): Vilaplana J+, *Contact Dermatitis* 38, 68
  (1998): Yokote R+, *Eur J Dermatol* 8, 427
  (1996): Fujimoto M+, *Br J Dermatol* 135, 496
  (1991): Moraillon I+, *Photodermatol Photoimmunol Photomed*
    8, 264
Rash (sic) (3%)
Toxic epidermal necrolysis
Urticaria

Other
Gynecomastia (9%)
  (1997): Staiman VR+, *Urology* 50, 929
  (1993): Aso Y+, *Hinyokika Kiyo* (Japanese) 39, 391
Injection-site irritation (3%)
Paresthesias (1–10%)
Pseudoporphyria
  (1999): Mantoux F+, *Ann Dermatol Venereol* (French) 126, 150
  (1999): Schmutz JL+, *Ann Dermatol Venereol* (French) 126, 374
  (1998): Borroni G+, *Br J Dermatol* 138, 711

FLUVASTATIN

Trade name: Lescol (Novartis) (Reliant)
Other common trade names: *Cranoc; Locol*
Indications: Hypercholesterolemia
Category: Antihyperlipidemic; HMG-CoA reductase inhibitor
Half-life: 1.2 hours
Clinically important, potentially hazardous interactions with: azithromycin, bosentan, clarithromycin, cyclosporine, erythromycin, gemfibrozil, imatinib

Reactions

Skin
Allergic reactions (sic) (2.6%)
Angioedema

Discoloration (sic)
Erythema multiforme
Flu-like syndrome (sic)
Flushing
Lupus erythematosus
  (1998): Sridhar MK+, *Lancet* 352, 114 (fatal)
Photosensitivity
Pruritus
Purpura
Rash (sic) (2.7%)
  (1998): N Z Medicines Adverse Reactions Committee (from
    Internet) (observation) (2 patients)
Stevens–Johnson syndrome
Toxic epidermal necrolysis
Upper respiratory infection (16%)
Urticaria
Vasculitis
Xerosis

Hair
Hair – alopecia
  (2002): Litt JZ, Beachwood, OH (personal case) (observation)
Hair – changes (sic)

Nails
Nails – changes (sic)

Other
Anaphylactoid reactions
Death
Dysgeusia
Gynecomastia
Headache
Myalgia (5–6%)
  (1997): Australian Adverse Drug Reactions Bulletin
    16(1), February
Myopathy
  (1997): Australian Adverse Drug Reactions Bulletin
    61(1), February
  (1995): Garnett WR, *Am J Health Syst Pharm* 52(15), 1639
Myositis
  (2002): Lawrence JM+, *Expert Opin Pharmacother* 3(11), 1631
  (1997): Australian Adverse Drug Reactions Bulletin
    16(1), February
Paresthesias
Rhabdomyolysis
  (2002): Lawrence JM+, *Expert Opin Pharmacother* 3(11), 1631
  (2002): Modi JR+, *Ann Pharmacother* 36(12), 1870
  (2002): Sica DA+, *Am J Geriatr Cardiol* 11(1), 48
  (2002): Sica DA+, *Curr Opin Nephrol Hypertens* 11(2), 123
  (1999): Bottorff M, *Atherosclerosis* 147(Suppl 1), S23
  (1995): Farmer JA+, *Baillieres Clin Endocrinol Metab* 9(4), 825
  (1995): Garnett WR, *Am J Health Syst Pharm* 52(15), 1639

FLUVOXAMINE

Trade name: Luvox (Solvay)
Other common trade names: *Apo-Fluvoxamine; Dumirox; Dumyrox; Faverin; Favoxil; Fevarin; Maveral*
Indications: Obsessive-compulsive disorder, depression
Category: Antidepressant; Selective serotonin reuptake inhibitor (SSRI)
Half-life: 15 hours
Clinically important, potentially hazardous interactions with: alprazolam, amphetamines, dextroamphetamine, diethylpropion, isocarboxazid, linezolid, MAO inhibitors, mazindol, methamphetamine, phendimetrazine, phenelzine, phentermine, phenylpropanolamine, pseudoephedrine, selegiline, sibutramine, **St John's wort**, sumatriptan, sympathomimetics, tacrine, tramadol, tranylcypromine, trazodone, troleandomycin, **tryptophan**

Reactions

Skin
Acne (<1%)
Allergic reactions (sic) (<1%)
 (1998): Beauquier B+, *Encephale* (French) 24, 62
Angioedema
 (1993): No Author, *Lakartidningen* (Swedish) 90, 54
Bullous eruption
Dermatitis (sic) (<1%)
Diaphoresis (7%)
 (1986): Benfield P+, *Drugs* 32, 313 (5%)
Ecchymoses (<1%)
Edema (<1%)
Exanthems
Exfoliative dermatitis (<1%)
Furunculosis (<1%)
Photosensitivity (<1%)
 (1996): Gillet-Terver MN+, *Australas J Dermatol* 37, 62
 (1993): *Lakartidningen* (Swedish) 90, 54
Pigmentation (<1%)
Pruritus
Purpura (<1%)
Rash (sic)
Seborrhea (<1%)
Stevens–Johnson syndrome
Toxic epidermal necrolysis (<1%)
 (1993): Wolkenstein P+, *Lancet* 342, 304
Urticaria (<1%)
Xerosis (<1%)

Hair
Hair – alopecia (<1%)
Hair – alopecia areata
 (1996): Parameshwar E, *Am J Psychiatry* 153, 581

Other
Ageusia (<1%)
Anaphylactoid reactions
Dysgeusia (3%)
Fatigue
 (2003): Sugie Y+, *No To Hattatsu* 35(3), 233
Gingivitis (<1%)
Glossitis (<1%)
Headache
Hyperactivity
 (2003): Sugie Y+, *No To Hattatsu* 35(3), 233

Mastodynia (<1%)
Myalgia
Myopathy (<1%)
Oral mucosal lesions
 (1986): Benfield P+, *Drugs* 32, 313 (10%)
Paresthesias
Parosmia (<1%)
Priapism
Serotonin syndrome
 (2001): Demers JC+, *Ann Pharmacother* 35(10), 1217 (with mirtazapine)
 (2001): Isbister GK+, *Ann Pharmacother* 35(12), 1674 (with mirtazapine)
 (2001): Kaneda Y+, *Int J Neurosci* 109(3), 165
Sialorrhea
Stomatitis (<1%)
Vaginitis (<1%)
 (2003): Versea L+, *Clin J Oncol Nurs* 7(3), 307
Xerostomia (14%)
 (1986): Benfield P+, *Drugs* 32, 313 (10%)

FOLIC ACID

Synonyms: folacin; folate; vitamin B$_9$
Trade name: Folvite (Wyeth)
Other common trade names: *Acfol; Apo-Folic; Dalisol; Flodine; Folacin; Folina; Folinsyre; Folitab; Folsan; Lexpec*
Indications: Anemias
Category: Nutritional supplement; Water-soluble vitamin
Half-life: N/A

Reactions

Skin
Acne
 (1964): Fegeler F, *Arch Klin Exp Dermatol* (German) 219, 335
Allergic reactions (sic) (<1%)
Dermatitis (sic)
 (1966): Pedersen JT, *Ugeskr Laeger* (Danish) 128, 708
Erythema
 (1966): Pedersen JT, *Ugeskr Laeger* (Danish) 128, 708
Exanthems
 (1985): Sparling R+, *Clin Lab Haematol* 7, 184
 (1964): Fegeler F, *Arch Klin Exp Dermatol* (German) 219, 335
Flushing (<1%)
Pruritus (<1%)
 (1966): Mathur BP, *Indian J Med Sci* 20, 133
 (1966): Pedersen JT, *Ugeskr Laeger* (Danish) 128, 708
Rash (sic) (<1%)
Urticaria
 (1985): Sparling R+, *Clin Lab Haematol* 7, 184

Other
Anaphylactoid reactions
 (2000): Dykewicz MS+, *J Allergy Clin Immunol* 106, 386
 (1966): Woodliff HJ, *Med J Aust* 53, 351

FOMEPIZOLE

Synonyms: 4-Methylpyrazole; 4-MP
Trade name: Antizol (Orphan Medical)
Indications: Toxicity to methanol and ethylene glycol
Category: Antidote
Half-life: N/A (varies with dose)
Clinically important, potentially hazardous interactions with: alcohol

Reactions

Skin

Facial flushing (~3%)
Rash (sic) (~3%)
(2002): Dean P+, *Pharmacotherapy* 22(3), 365 (passim)
(1986): Baud FJ+, *J Toxicol Clin Toxicol* 24(6), 463

Other

Anxiety (1–10%)
Application-site reactions (1–10%)
Back pain (1–10%)
Dizziness (6%)
(2002): Dean P+, *Pharmacotherapy* 22(3), 365
(1988): Jacobsen D+, *Alcohol Clin Exp Res* 12(4), 516
Dysgeusia (6%)
Hiccups (1–10%)
Injection-site inflammation (1–10%)
Injection-site pain (1–10%)
Mouth vesiculation (~3%)
(1988): Jacobsen D+, *Alcohol Clin Exp Res* 12(4), 516
Parosmia (1–10%)
Pharyngitis (~3%)
Phlebitis (1–10%)
Seizures (~3%)
Shock (~3%)

FONDAPARINUX

Trade names: Arixtra (Sanofi-Synthelabo) (Organon)
Indications: Prophylaxis of deep vein thrombosis
Category: Factor Xa inhibitor
Half-life: 17–21 hours
Clinically important, potentially hazardous interactions with: abciximab, anagrelide, anticoagulants, cilostazol, clopidogrel, dipyridamole, eptifibatide, salicylates, ticlopidine, tirofiban. Many **herbals** that possess anticoagulant or antiplatelet activity

Reactions

Skin

Bullous eruption (3%)
Edema (9%)
Purpura (4%)
Rash (sic) (8%)

Other

Injection-site bleeding (1–10%)
Injection-site pruritus (1–10%)
Injection-site rash (sic) (1–10%)
Pain (2%)

FORMOTEROL

Synonym: Formoterol fumarate
Other common trade name: *Oxeze*
Indications: Asthma, bronchospasm
Category: Beta-2-adrenergic agonist
Half-life: 10–14 hours
Clinically important, potentially hazardous interactions with: clomipramine, desipramine, doxepin, imipramine, nortriptyline, protriptyline, trimipramine

Reactions

Skin

Angioedema
Erythema
Infections (sic) (3%)
Pruritus
Rash (sic) (1.1%)
Urticaria
Viral infections (17.2%)

Other

Anaphylactoid reactions (1%)
Cough
(1990): Schultze-Werninghaus G, *Lung* 168 (Suppl 83-9)
Headache
Hyperesthesia
(1995): van den Berg BT+, *Fundam Clin Pharmacol* 9(6), 593
Myalgia
Tremor (1.9%)
(1998): Bartow RA+, *Drugs* 55(2), 303
(1995): van den Berg BT+, *Fundam Clin Pharmacol* 9(6), 593
(1992): Lipworth BJ, *Drug Saf* 7(1), 54
(1991): Faulds D+, *Drugs* 42(1), 115
(1990): Schultze-Werninghaus G, *Lung* 168 (Suppl 83-9) (6%)
Xerostomia
(1990): Schultze-Werninghaus G, *Lung* 168 (Suppl 83-9) (1%)

FOSCARNET

Trade name: Foscavir (AstraZeneca)
Other common trade name: *Foscovir*
Indications: Cytomegalovirus retinitis in patients with AIDS
Category: Antiviral; Viral DNA and RNA polymerase inhibitor
Half-life: ~3 hours
Clinically important, potentially hazardous interactions with: adefovir, cyclosporine

Reactions

Skin

Acne
Dermatitis (sic) (<1%)
Diaphoresis (>5%)
Edema (<1%)
Edema of leg (<1%)
Eosinophilic pustular folliculitis
(2001): Roos TC+, *J Am Acad Dermatol* 44, 546
Exanthems (>5%)
(2001): Roos TC+, *J Am Acad Dermatol* 44, 546
(1990): Green ST, *J Infection* 21, 227
Facial edema (>5%)

Fixed eruption
  (1990): Connolly GM+, *Genitourin Med* 66, 97
Flushing (1–5%)
Herpes simplex (<1%)
Penile ulcers
  (1997): English JC+, *J Am Acad Dermatol* 37, 1
  (1996): Agcaoili DJ+, *Infect Med* 13, 35
  (1996): Papini M+, *Ann Dermatol Venereol* (French) 123, 679
  (1995): Fitzgerald E+, *Arch Dermatol* 131, 1447
  (1993): Bodian AB, *Int J Dermatol* 32, 526
  (1993): Brockmeyer NH+, *Int J Clin Pharmacol Ther Toxicol* 31, 204
  (1993): Gross AS+, *Clin Infect Dis* 17, 1076
  (1993): Moyle G+, *AIDS* 7, 140
  (1993): Schiff TA+, *Int J Dermatol* 32, 526
  (1992): Evans LM+, *J Am Acad Dermatol* 27, 124
  (1992): Katlama C+, *J Acquir Immune Defic Syndr* 5 (Suppl 1), S18
  (1991): Chrisp P+, *Drugs* 41, 104
  (1990): Fégueux S+, *Lancet* 335, 547
  (1990): Gilquin J+, *Lancet* 335, 287
  (1990): Lernestedt J-O+, *Lancet* 335, 548
  (1990): Moyle G+, *Lancet* 335, 547 (4.7%)
  (1990): Van Der Pijl JW+, *Lancet* 335, 286 (30%)
Periorbital edema
Peripheral edema (<1%)
Pigmentation (>5%)
Pruritus (>5%)
  (2001): Roos TC+, *J Am Acad Dermatol* 44, 546
Pruritus ani (<1%)
Psoriasis (<1%)
Rash (sic) (generalized) (>5%)
  (1991): Blanshard C, *J Infect* 23, 336
  (1990): Green ST+, *J Infect* 21, 227
Seborrhea (>5%)
Toxic epidermal necrolysis
  (1999): Wharton JR+, *Cutis* 63, 333
  (1997): Lauglin CL, Little Rock, Arkansas, American Academy of Dermatology Meeting, (SF) (gross and microscopic)
Ulcerations (>5%)
Urticaria (<1%)
  (2001): Roos TC+, *J Am Acad Dermatol* 44, 546
Vulvar ulceration
  (1993): Caumes E+, *J Am Acad Dermatol* 28, 799 (erosion)
  (1992): Lacey HB+, *Genitourin Med* 68, 182
Warts (<1%)
Xerosis (<1%)

Hair
Hair – alopecia (<1%)

Other
Dysgeusia (>5%)
Gynecomastia (<1%)
Headache
Hyperesthesia (<1%)
Injection-site pain (1–10%)
Injection-site thrombophlebitis
  (1991): Chrisp P+, *Drugs* 41, 104
Myalgia (>5%)
Oral leukoplakia
Oral ulceration
  (2000): Madinier I+, *Ann Med Interne (Paris)* (French) 151, 248
  (1990): Fégueux S+, *Lancet* 335, 547
  (1990): Gilquin J+, *Lancet* 335, 287
  (1990): Moyle G+, *Lancet* 335, 547
Paresthesias (1–10%)
  (1990): Safrin S+, *J Infect Dis* 161, 1078
Stomatitis (<1%)

Thrombophlebitis (<1%)
Tinnitus
Tongue ulceration (<1%)
Ulcerative stomatitis (>5%)
Xerostomia

FOSFOMYCIN

Trade name: Monurol (Forest)
Indications: Urinary tract infections
Category: Antibiotic (acute cystitis)
Half-life: 3–9 hours

Reactions

Skin
Angioedema
Exanthems (<1%)
Pruritus (<1%)
Rash (sic) (1.4%)

Other
Anaphylactoid reactions
  (1998): Rosales MJ+, *Allergy* 53, 905
Myalgia (<1%)
Paresthesias (<1%)
Vaginitis (7.6%)
Xerostomia (<1%)

FOSINOPRIL

Trade name: Monopril (Bristol-Myers Squibb)
Other common trade names: *Acenor-M; Dynacil; Fosinorm; Fozitec; Staril; Vasopril*
Indications: Hypertension
Category: Angiotensin-converting enzyme (ACE) inhibitor; Antihypertensive
Half-life: 11.5 hours
Clinically important, potentially hazardous interactions with: amiloride, spironolactone, triamterene

Reactions

Skin
Angioedema (<1%)
  (2001): Cohen EG+, *Ann Otol Rhinol Laryngol* 110(8), 701 (64 cases)
  (1997): Graumuller S+, *HNO* (German) 45, 1016
Bullous pemphigoid
Diaphoresis (<1%)
Edema (<1%)
Eosinophilic fasciitis
  (1997): Biasi D+, *J Rheumatol* 24(6), 1242
Eosinophilic vasculitis
Exfoliative dermatitis
Flu-like syndrome (sic) (<1%)
Flushing
Pemphigus
  (2002): Parodi A+, *Dermatology* 204, 139
Pemphigus foliaceus
  (2000): Ong CS+, *Australas J Dermatol* 41(4), 242
Photosensitivity (<1%)

Pruritus (<1%)
  (2001): Nunes AC+, *Eur J Gastroenterol Hepatol* 13, 279
Rash (sic) (<1%)
  (1990): Pool JL, *Clin Ther* 12, 520 (0.9%)
Scleroderma
  (1997): Biasi D+, *J Rheumatol* 24(6), 1242
Urticaria (<1%)
Vasculitis

Other
Ageusia (<1%)
Anaphylactoid reactions
Cough
  (2001): Adigun AQ+, *West Afr J Med* 20(1), 46–7
  (2001): Lee SC+, *Hypertension* 38(2), 166
Dysgeusia (<1%)
  (1992): Murdoch D+, *Drugs* 43, 123
Gynecomastia
Headache
Myalgia (<1%)
Paresthesias (<1%)
Tinnitus
Tremor (<1%)
Xerostomia (<1%)

FOSPHENYTOIN

Trade name: Cerebyx (Parke-Davis)
Indications: Seizure prophylaxis, status epilepticus
Category: Anticonvulsant
Half-life: 15 minutes
**Clinically important, potentially hazardous interactions
with:** chloramphenicol, cyclosporine, disulfiram, dopamine,
imatinib, itraconazole

Fosphenytoin is a prodrug of phenytoin

Reactions

Skin
Acne (<1%)
Bullous eruption
  (2001): Hebert AA+, *J Clin Psychiatry* 62(suppl 14), 22
Chills (sic)
Ecchymoses
Erythema multiforme (<1%)
  (2001): Hebert AA+, *J Clin Psychiatry* 62(suppl 14), 22
Exanthems
Exfoliative dermatitis (<1%)
  (2001): Hebert AA+, *J Clin Psychiatry* 62(suppl 14), 22
Facial edema
Lupus erythematosus
  (2001): Hebert AA+, *J Clin Psychiatry* 62(suppl 14), 22
Pruritus (48.9%)
  (2002): Coplin WM+, *Neurol Res* 24(8), 842
  (2001): Hebert AA+, *J Clin Psychiatry* 62(suppl 14), 22
  (1998): Knapp LE+, *J Child Neurol* 13, S15
  (1998): Luer MS, *Neurol Res* 20, 178
Rash (sic) (<1%)
Stevens–Johnson syndrome
Toxic epidermal necrolysis

Other
Dysgeusia (3.3%)
Gingival hyperplasia

  (2001): Hebert AA+, *J Clin Psychiatry* 62(suppl 14), 22
Headache
Hyperesthesia (2.2%)
Injection-site pain
  (2002): Coplin WM+, *Neurol Res* 24(8), 842
Paresthesias (4.4%)
  (2002): Coplin WM+, *Neurol Res* 24(8), 842
  (1998): Luer MS, *Neurol Res* 20, 178
Tongue disorder (sic)
Xerostomia (4.4%)

FROVATRIPTAN

Trade name: Frova (Elan)
Indications: Migraine headaches
Category: 5-HT1 (serotonin) receptor agonist; Antimigraine
Half-life: 26 hours

Reactions

Skin
Bullous eruption (<1%)
Cheilitis (<1%)
Diaphoresis (1%)
Flushing (4%)
Hot flashes (<1%)
Pruritus (<1%)
Purpura (<1%)
Rash (sic)

Other
Arthralgia (<1%)
Bone or joint pain (3%)
Conjunctivitis (<1%)
Depression (<1%)
Dysesthesia (1%)
Dysgeusia (<1%)
Headache
Hyperesthesia (<1%)
Myalgia (<1%)
Pain (1%)
Paresthesias (4%)
  (2001): Easthope SE+, *CNS Drugs* 15(12), 969
Sialopenia (3%)
Sialorrhea (<1%)
Stomatitis (<1%)
Tinnitus (1%)
Toothache (1%)
Tremor (<1%)
Xerostomia

FULVESTRANT

Synonyms: ICI 182; 780
Trade name: Faslodex (AstraZeneca)
Indications: Metastatic breast cancer
Category: Antineoplastic; Estrogen receptor antagonist
Half-life: ~40 days

Reactions

Skin
Diaphoresis (5%)
Edema (9%)
Flu-like syndrome (7.1%)
Hot flashes
  (2002): Lynn J, *Cancer Nurs* 25, 12S
Peripheral edema
Rash (sic) (7%)

Other
Arthritis (3%)
Back pain (14%)
Bone or joint pain (16%)
Cough (10%)
Depression (6%)
Headache
Injection-site reactions (11%)
  (2002): Lynn J, *Cancer Nurs* 25, 12S
Myalgia (<1%)
Pain (19%)
Paresthesias (6%)
Vaginitis
  (2003): Versea L+, *Clin J Oncol Nurs* 7(3), 307

FURAZOLIDONE

Trade name: Furoxone (Shire)
Other common trade names: *Furion; Furoxona; Fuxol*
Indications: Various infections caused by susceptible organisms
Category: Antidiarrheal; Antiprotozoal; Nitrofuran antibiotic
Half-life: N/A
**Clinically important, potentially hazardous interactions
with:** amphetamines, benzphetamine, chloroquine, dapsone,
dobutamine, dopamine, ephedrine, epinephrine, meperidine,
morphine, phenylephrine, phenylpropanolamine,
pseudoephedrine, sympathomimetics

Reactions

Skin
Dermatitis
  (1990): de Groot AC+, *Contact Dermatitis* 22, 202
  (1980): Goette DK+, *Cutis* 26, 406
  (1978): Novak M, *Cesk Dermatol* (Czech) 53, 128
  (1974): Bleumink E+, *Hautarzt* (German) 25, 403
Erythema multiforme
  (1986): Fisher AA, *Cutis* 37, 158
  (1980): Goette DK+, *Cutis* 26, 406
Exanthems (<1%)
Flushing (with alcohol) (<1%)
Photosensitivity
  (1980): Goette DK+, *Cutis* 26, 406
Pruritus

Pruritus ani
Rash (sic) (<1%)
Urticaria (<1%)
  (1969): Aaronson CM, *JAMA* 210, 557

Other
Disulfiram-like reaction (with alcohol) (<1%)*
Serum sickness
  (1978): Wolfe MS+, *Am J Trop Med Hyg* 27, 762

*Note: The disulfiram-like reaction consists of facial flushing,
diaphoresis, tachycardia, and pounding headache

FUROSEMIDE*

Trade name: Lasix (Aventis)
Other common trade names: *Apo-Furosemide; Discoid; Dryptal;
Edenol; Frusid; Furorese; Furoside; Fusid; Henexal; Lasilix; Novo-
Semide; Urex; Uritol*
Indications: Edema
Category: Antihypertensive; Sulfonamide loop diuretic
Half-life: 0.5–1 hour
**Clinically important, potentially hazardous interactions
with:** amikacin, amyl nitrite, digoxin, gentamicin, kanamycin,
neomycin, streptomycin, tobramycin

Reactions

Skin
Acute febrile neutrophilic dermatosis (Sweet's syndrome)
  (1989): Cobb MW, *J Am Acad Dermatol* 21, 339
Acute generalized exanthematous pustulosis (AGEP)
  (1995): Moreau A+, *Int J Dermatol* 34, 263 (passim)
Bullous eruption (<1%)
  (1995): Tamimi NA+, *Nephrol Dial Transplant* 10, 1943
  (1993): Landor M+, *Ann Allergy* 70, 196
  (1992): Van Olden RW+, *Am J Nephrol* 12, 351 (photosensitive)
  (1989): Sfar Z+, *Tunis Med* (French) 67, 805
  (1985): Anderson CD+, *Photodermatol* 2, 111
  (1982): Hallan H+, *Tidsskr Nor Laegeforen* (Norwegian) 102, 630
  (1980): Guin JD, *Cutis* 25, 534
  (1980): Rees RB+, *J Am Acad Dermatol* 2, 244
  (1977): Hertzenberg S, *Tidsskr Nor Laegeforen* (Norwegian)
    97, 792
  (1977): Heydenreich G+, *Acta Med Scand* 202, 61
  (1977): Heydenreich G+, *Ugeskr Laeger* (Danish) 139, 1847
  (1976): Burry JN+, *Ann Intern Med* 84, 493
  (1976): Coles GA+, *BMJ* 2, 525
  (1976): Gilchrist B+, *Ann Intern Med* 84, 494
  (1976): Keczkes K+, *BMJ* 2, 236
  (1975): Gilchrist B+, *Ann Intern Med* 83, 480
  (1969): Ebringer A+, *Med J Aust* 1, 768
Bullous pemphigoid
  (2003): Ng C, Jackson Beach, FL (from Internet) (observation)
  (2002): Thaler D, Monona, WI (from Internet) (observation)
  (1997): Panayiotou BN+, *Br J Clin Pract* 51, 49 (2 patients)
  (1996): Koch CA+, *Cutis* 58, 340
  (1995): Siddiqui MA+, *J Am Geriatr Soc* 43, 1183
  (1991): Shelley WB+, *Cutis* 48, 367 (passim)
  (1986): Ingber A+, *Z Hautarzt* (German)
  (1984): Halevy S+, *Harefuah* (Hebrew) 106, 125
  (1981): Castel T, *Clin Exp Dermatol* 6, 635
  (1980): Neufeld R+, *Cutis* 26, 290
  (1976): Fellner J+, *Arch Dermatol* 112, 75
Diaphoresis
Epidermolysis bullosa
  (1976): Kennedy AC+, *BMJ* 1, 1509

(1976): Kennedy AC, *Br J Dermatol* 94, 495

Erythema multiforme (<1%)
(1980): Zugerman C, *Arch Dermatol* 116, 518
(1970): Gibson TP+, *JAMA* 212, 1709
(1969): Ebringer A+, *Med J Aust* 1, 768

Erythema nodosum
(1975): Dargie HJ+, *Meyler's Side Effects of Drugs* Vol 8, Amsterdam, Excerpta Medica, 483

Exanthems
(1999): Litt JZ, Beachwood, OH (personal case) (observation)
(1988): Lin RY, *N Y State J Med* 88, 439
(1979): Lowe J+, *BMJ* 2, 360 (0.2%)
(1979): Naranjo CA+, *Clin Pharmacol Ther* 25, 154 (0.6%)
(1978): Bjoerndal N+, *Ugeskr Laeger* (Danish) 140, 1084
(1977): Greenblatt DJ+, *Am Heart J* 94, 6 (0.2%)
(1970): Gibson TP+, *JAMA* 212, 1709
(1966): Sherlock S+, *Lancet* 1, 1049 (12%)

Exfoliative dermatitis
(1992): Breathnach SM+, *Adverse Drug Reactions and the Skin* Blackwell, Oxford, 230 (passim)
(1978): Bjoerndal N+, *Ugeskr Laeger* (Danish) 140, 1084
(1975): Dargie HJ+, *Meyler's Side Effects of Drugs* Vol 8, Amsterdam, Excerpta Medica, 483

Flushing
(1977): Greenblatt DJ+, *Am Heart J* 94, 6

Grinspan's syndrome**
(1990): Lamey PJ+, *Oral Surg Oral Med Oral Path* 70, 184

Lichenoid eruption
(1990): West AJ+, *J Am Acad Dermatol* 23, 689
(1981): Ota J+, *Skin Res* (Japanese) 23, 639

Linear IgA bullous dermatosis
(1999): Cerottini J-P+, *J Am Acad Dermatol* 41, 103

Lupus erythematosus
(1988): Lin RY, *N Y State J Med* 88, 439

Periorbital edema
(1987): Hansbrough JR+, *J Allergy Clin Immunol* 80, 538

Photosensitivity (1–10%)
(1989): Cobb MW, *J Am Acad Dermatol* 21, 339
(1977): Heydenreich G+, *Acta Med Scand* 202, 61

Phototoxicity
(1998): Vargas F+, *J Photochem Photobiol B* 42, 219
(1976): Burry JN+, *Ann Intern Med* 84, 493
(1976): Burry JN, *Br J Dermatol* 94, 495

Porokeratosis (disseminated superficial)
(2000): Kroiss MM+, *Acta Derm Venereol* 80, 52

Pruritus (<1%)
(1993): Litt JZ, Beachwood, OH (personal case) (observation)
(1987): Hansbrough JR+, *J Allergy Clin Immunol* 80, 538
(1978): Sibbald RG+, *Can Med Assoc J* 118, 142

Purpura
(1989): Nishioka K+, *J Dermatol* 16, 220 (pigmented)
(1983): Michel M+, *Rev Geriat* (French) 8/10, 505
(1969): Ebringer A+, *Med J Aust* 1, 768

Pustules
(1990): Mothiron C+, *Presse Med* (French) 19, 1504
(1989): Cobb MW, *J Am Acad Dermatol* 21, 339

(1973): Macmillan AL, *Dermatologica* 146, 285

Rash (sic) (<1%)

Side effects (sic)
(1986): Bigby M+, *JAMA* 256, 3358 (0.05%)
(1976): Arndt KA+, *JAMA* 235, 918 (0.26%)

Stevens–Johnson syndrome
(1991): Chan JC+, *Drug Saf* 6, 230
(1978): Ward B+, *Am J Ophthalmol* 86, 133

Toxic epidermal necrolysis
(1999): Egan CA+, *J Am Acad Dermatol* 40, 458

Urticaria
(1987): Hansbrough JR+, *J Allergy Clin Immunol* 80, 538
(1967): Milla Santos J, *Summa Med* (Spanish) 10, 3
(1966): Atkins LL, *Geriatrics* 21, 143

Vasculitis
(1990): Bourgain C+, *Presse Med* (French) 19, 1504
(1989): Cobb MW, *J Am Acad Dermatol* 21, 339
(1988): Lin RY, *N Y State J Med* 88, 439
(1982): de la Chapelle C+, *LARC Med* (French) 2, 760
(1978): Sibbald RG+, *Can Med Assoc J* 118, 142
(1977): Hendricks WM+, *Arch Dermatol* 113, 375 (necrotizing)
(1971): Pathy MS, *Gerontol Clin* 13, 261

Other

Acute intermittent porphyria

Anaphylactoid reactions
(1987): Hansbrough JR+, *J Allergy Clin Immunol* 80, 538

Headache

Injection-site erythema (<1%)

Injection-site pain

Paresthesias

Porphyria
(1984): Harber LC+, *J Invest Dermatol* 82, 207

Porphyria cutanea tarda
(1992): Shelley WB+, *Advanced Dermatologic Diagnosis* WB Saunders, 414 (passim)
(1983): Goldsman CI+, *Cleve Clin Q* 50, 151
(1977): Rufli T+, *Schweiz Med Wochenschr* (German) 107, 1093

Pseudolymphoma
(1995): Magro CM+, *J Am Acad Dermatol* 32, 419

Pseudoporphyria cutanea tarda
(1998): Breier F+, *Dermatology* 197, 271

Thrombophlebitis

Tinnitus

Ulcerative stomatitis
(1988): Lin RY, *N Y State J Med* 88, 439

Xanthopsia

Xerostomia
(1967): Milla Santos J, *Summa Med* (Spanish) 10, 3

*Note: Furosemide is a sulfonamide and can be absorbed systemically. Sulfonamides can produce severe, possibly fatal, reactions such as toxic epidermal necrolysis and Stevens–Johnson syndrome

**Note: Grinspan's syndrome is the triad of oral lichen planus, diabetes mellitus, and hypertension

GABAPENTIN

Trade name: Neurontin (Parke-Davis)
Indications: Seizures
Category: Anticonvulsant
Half-life: 5–6 hours

Reactions

Skin
Acne (>1%)
Acute febrile neutrophilic dermatosis (Sweet's syndrome)
  (2001): Popescu C, Bucharest, Romania (from Internet)
    (observation)
  (1999): Smith W (from Internet) (observation)
Edema
  (2002): Gueguen A+, *Presse Med* 31(33), 1559
  (2002): *Prescrire Int* 11(60), 111
Exanthems
Facial edema (<1%)
Peripheral edema (1.7%)
  (2002): *Prescrire Int* 11(60), 111
  (1998): Rowbotham M+, *JAMA* 280, 1837
Pruritus (1.3%)
Purpura (<1%)
  (2003): Poon DY+, *Singapore Med J* 44(1), 42
Rash (sic) (>1%)
Stevens–Johnson syndrome
  (1998): Gonzalez-Sicilia L+, *Am J Med* 105, 455
Urticaria

Hair
Hair – alopecia
  (1997): Picard C+, *Ann Pharmacother* 31, 1260

Other
Dizziness
  (2002): *Prescrire Int* 11(60), 111
  (2002): Serpell MG, *Pain* 99(3), 557
  (2002): Wilton LV+, *Epilepsia* 43(9), 983
Foetor ex ore (halitosis)
  (1998): Backonja M+, *JAMA* 280, 1831
Gingivitis (<1%)
Glossitis
Gynecomastia
  (2000): Zylicz Z, *J Pain Symptom Manage* 20, 2
Myalgia (2%)
Paresthesias (<1%)
Priapism
  (2001): Matthews SC+, *Psychosomatics* 42(3), 280
Sialorrhea
Stomatitis
Tinnitus
Tooth discoloration
Tremor (1–10%)
  (2002): Viteri C, *Rev Neurol* 34(3), 292
Xerostomia (1.7%)

GALANTAMINE

Trade name: Reminyl (Janssen)
Indications: Alzheimer's disease
Category: Acetylcholinesterase inhibitor
Half-life: 6–8 hours
Clinically important, potentially hazardous interactions
with: bethanechol, cimetidine, donepezil, edrophonium,
physostigmine, pilocarpine, rivastigmine, succinylcholine, tacrine

Note: Derived from snowdrop (*Galanthus* sp) bulbs

Reactions

Skin
Acute generalized exanthematous pustulosis (AGEP)
  (2002): Gantcheva M+, *World Congress Dermatol* Poster, 1588
Edema
Peripheral edema (>2%)
Purpura (>2%)
Upper respiratory infection (>2%)

Other
Depression (5%)
Headache
Paresthesias
Sialorrhea
Tremor (1–10%)
Xerostomia

GANCICLOVIR

Trade name: Cytovene (Roche)
Other common trade names: *Cymevan; Cymeven; Cymevene;*
Vitrasert
Indications: Cytomegalovirus retinitis in immunocompromised
patients
Category: Antiviral
Half-life: 2.5–3.6 hours
Clinically important, potentially hazardous interactions
with: amphotericin B, dapsone, imipenem cilastatin, zidovudine

Reactions

Skin
Acne (<1%)
Bullous eruption (<1%)
Chills (<1%)
Diaphoresis
Edema (<1%)
Exanthems (<1%)
  (1987): Chachoua A+, *Ann Intern Med* 107, 133 (4.9%)
  (1979): Eyanson S+, *Arch Dermatol* 115, 54 (2%)
Exfoliative dermatitis
Facial edema (<1%)
Fixed eruption (<1%)
Photosensitivity (<1%)
Pigmentation (<1%)
Pruritus (5%)
Psoriasis
Purpura
Rash (sic) (>10%)
Stevens–Johnson syndrome

Urticaria (<1%)

Hair

Hair – alopecia (<1%)
(1990): Faulds D+, *Drugs* 39, 597

Other

Anaphylactoid reactions
Anosmia
Dysgeusia (<1%)
Gingival hypertrophy
Headache
Hyperesthesia (<1%)
Injection-site edema (<1%)
Injection-site inflammation (2%)
Injection-site pain
(1990): Faulds D+, *Drugs* 39, 597 (4%)
Mastodynia (<1%)
Myalgia (<1%)
Oral ulceration (<1%)
Paresthesias (6–10%)
Phlebitis (2%)
Tongue disorder (sic) (<1%)
Tremor (<1%)
Xerostomia (<1%)

GANIRELIX

Trade name: Antagon (Organon)
Indications: Infertility
Category: Antigonadotropic hormone
Half-life: 16.2 hours

Reactions

Skin

Hot flashes (4–5%)
Pruritus

Other

Injection-site reactions
(2001): Fluker M+, *Fertil Steril* 75(1), 38 (11.9%)
(2000): Gillies PS+, *Drugs* 59, 107
(2000): Oberye J+, *Hum Reprod* 15, 245

GARLIC

Scientific name: *Allium sativum*
Family: Liliaceae
Trade and other common names: Ail; Ajo; Camphor of the Poor; Nectar of the Gods; Poor Man's Treacle; Rust Treacle; Stinking Rose
Category: Antioxidant; Antiseptic; Immune stimulant
Purported indications and other uses: Hypertension, hypercholesterolemia, atherosclerosis, earache, menstrual disorders, allergy, 'flu, arthritis, diarrhea, bacterial and fungal infections, tinea corporis, tinea pedis, onychomycosis, vaginitis
Half-life: N/A
Clinically important, potentially hazardous interactions with: atazanavir, HIV medications, lisinopril, olmesartan, saquinavir, ticlopidine, warfarin

Reactions

Skin

Allergic reactions (sic)
(2002): Moneret-Vautrin DA+, *Allerg Immunol (Paris* (Paris) 34(4), 135
(2002): Pires G+, *Allergy* 57(10), 957
(2000): Sanchez-Hernandez MC+, *Allergy* 55(3), 297
Bullous eruption
(1993): Garty BZ, *Pediatrics* 91, 658
Burning
(2002): Groppo FC+, *Int Dent J* 52(6), 433
(2001): Baruchin AM+, *Burns* 27(7), 781
(2000): Hviid K+, *Ugeskr Laeger* 162(50), 6853
(2000): Rafaat M+, *Peditar Dermatol* 17(6), 475
(1997): Roberge RJ+, *Am J Emerg Med* 15(5), 548
(1987): Parish RA+, *Pediatr Emerg Care* 3(4), 258
Dermatitis
(2002): Hughes TM+, *Contact Dermatitis* 47(1), 48
(2001): McGovern TW+, *Cutis* 67, 193
(2000): Fernandez-Vozmediano JM+, *Contact Dermatitis* 42(2), 108
(1999): Eming SA+, *Br J Dermatol* 141(2), 391 (toxic)
(1999): Jappe U+, *Am J Contact Dermat* 10, 37
(1997): Bruynzeel DP, *Contact Dermatitis* 37, 70
(1996): Delaney TA+, *Australas J Dermatol* 37, 109
(1996): Kanerva L+, *Contact Dermatitis* 35(3), 157
(1993): Acciai MC+, *Contact Dermatitis* 29, 48
(1992): McFadden JP+, *Contact Dermatitis* 27(5), 333
(1991): Lee TY+, *Contact Dermatits* 24(3), 193
(1991): Lembo G+, *Contact Dermatitis* 25(5), 330
(1987): Cronin E, *Contact Dermatitis* 17, 265
(1985): Fernandez de Corres L+, *Allergol Immunopathol (Madr)* 13(4), 291
(1983): Papegeorgiou C+, *Arch Dermatol Res* 275(4), 229
(1981): Martinescu E, *Rev Med Chir Soc Med Nat Iasi* 85(3), 541
(1980): Mitchell JC, *Contact Dermatitis* 6(5), 356
(1978): van Ketel WF+, *Contact Dermatitis* 4(1), 53
(1977): Sinha SM+, *Arch Dermatol* 113(6), 776
Hemorrhage
(2002): Carden SM+, *Clin Experiment Ophthalmol* 30(4), 303
Pemphigus
(1996): Ruocco V+, *Dermatology* 192(4), 373
Rhinoconjunctivitis
(2002): Jimenez-Timon A+, *Allergol Immunopathol (Madr)* 30(5), 295
Urticaria
(2001): McGovern TW+, *Cutis* 67, 193 (passim)

Other
Anaphylactoid reactions
   (1999): Perez-Pimiento AJ+ 54(6), 626
Bleeding
   (2001): Ang-Lee MK+, *JAMA* 286(2), 208
   (2001): Fessenden JM+, *Am Surg* 67(1), 33
Foetor ex ore (halitosis)
Hypersensitivity
   (2001): McGovern TW+, *Cutis* 67, 193 (passim)
   (1982): Campolmi P+, *Contact Dermatitis* 8(5), 352
Sensitization
   (2002): Moneret-Vautrin DA+, *Allerg Immunol* (Paris) 34(4), 135
Stomatodynia

GATIFLOXACIN

Trade name: Tequin (Bristol-Myers Squibb)
Indications: Various infections caused by susceptible organisms
Category: Fluoroquinolone antibiotic
Half-life: 7–14 hours
Clinically important, potentially hazardous interactions
with: amiodarone, arsenic, bepridil, bretylium, disopyramide, erythromycin, phenothiazines, procainamide, quinidine, sotalol, tricyclic antidepressants

Reactions

Skin
Allergic reactions (sic) (0.1–3%)
   (2002): Medeiros EA, *Braz J Infect Dis* 6(4), 149 (0.18%)
Angioedema
Burning (sic)
Candidiasis
Cheilitis (<0.1%)
Chills (0.1–3%)
   (2002): Nicholson SC+, *Diagn Microbiol Infect Dis* 44(1), 117
Diaphoresis (0.1–3%)
Ecchymoses (<0.1%)
Edema (<0.1%)
Erythema
Exanthems (<0.1%)
Facial edema (<0.1%)
Fixed eruption
   (2000): Zabawski E, Longwood, TX (from Internet)
      (observation)
Peripheral edema (0.1–3%)
Photosensitivity
   (2000): Stein GE+, *Inf Med* 17, 564
Pruritus (<0.1%)
Rash (sic) (0.1–3%)
Stevens–Johnson syndrome
Toxic epidermal necrolysis
Urticaria
Vasculitis
Vesiculobullous eruption (<0.1%)

Other
Anaphylactoid reactions
Anxiety
   (2002): Medeiros EA, *Braz J Infect Dis* 6(4), 149
Dizziness
   (2002): Medeiros EA, *Braz J Infect Dis* 6(4), 149
   (2002): Sher LD+, *Otolaryngol Head Neck Surg* 127(3), 182
      (1.8%)

Dysgeusia (0.1–3%)
   (2002): Medeiros EA, *Braz J Infect Dis* 6(4), 149 (0.46%)
   (2000): Stein GE+, *Inf Med* 17, 564
Foetor ex ore (halitosis) (<1%)
Gingivitis (<0.1%)
Glossitis (0.1–3%)
Headache
   (2002): Medeiros EA, *Braz J Infect Dis* 6(4), 149 (0.42%)
Hyperesthesia (<0.1%)
Hypersensitivity
Injection-site reactions (sic) (5%)
   (2002): Perry CM+, *Drugs* 62(1), 169
   (2000): Gajjar DA+, *Pharmacotherapy* 20, 49S
Mastodynia (<0.1%)
Myalgia (<0.1%)
Oral candidiasis (0.1–3%)
Oral ulceration (0.1–3%)
Paresthesias (0.1–3%)
Parosmia (<0.1%)
Serum sickness
Stomatitis (0.1–3%)
Tendinitis
Tendon rupture
Tongue edema (<0.1%)
Tremor (0.1–3%)
Vaginitis (6%)
   (2000): Stein GE+, *Inf Med* 17, 564

GEFITINIB

Trade name: Iressa (AstraZeneca)
Other common trade name: *ZD1839*
Indications: Advanced non-small cell lung cancer
Category: Epidermal growth factor receptor (EGFR) inhibitor
Half-life: 12–51 hours

Reactions

Skin
Acne
   (2002): Herbst RS+, *J Clin Oncol* 20(18), 3815 (46%) (follicular)
   (2002): Van Doorn R+, *Br J Dermatol* 147(3), 598
Folliculitis
   (2002): Van Doorn R+, *Br J Dermatol* 147(3), 598
Pruritus
Rash (sic)
   (2000): Meric JB+, *Bull Cancer* 87(12), 873
Scaling (sic)
   (2002): Van Doorn R+, *Br J Dermatol* 147(3), 598

Hair
Hair – growth
   (2002): Van Doorn R+, *Br J Dermatol* 147(3), 598

Nails
Nails – paronychia
   (2003): Nakano J+, *J Dermatol* 30(3), 261
   (2002): Di Lernia V Reggio Emilia, Italy (from Internet)
      (observation)

Other
Death

GEMCITABINE

Trade name: Gemzar (Lilly)
Indications: Pancreatic carcinoma
Category: Antineoplastic nucleoside analog
Half-life: 42–94 minutes
Clinically important, potentially hazardous interactions with: aldesleukin

Reactions

Skin

Allergic reactions (sic) (4%)
Dermatitis (sic)
  (2001): Fogarty G+, *Lung Cancer* 33(2), 299
Diaphoresis
Edema (13%)
  (2000): Geffen DB+, *Isr Med Assoc J* 2, 552
  (1995): Tonato M+, *Anticancer Drugs* 6, 27
Erysipelas (sic)
  (2000): Brandes A+, *Anticancer Drugs* 11, 15 (confined to areas
    of lymphedema)
Exanthems
  (2001): Chu CY+, *Acta Derm Venereol* 81(6), 426
  (1996): Chen YM+, *J Clin Oncol* 14, 1743
Flu-like syndrome (sic) (>10%)
  (2002): Eckel F+, *Cancer Invest* 20(2), 180
Hand-foot syndrome
  (2003): Michaelson MD+, *Cancer* 97(1), 148
  (2003): Scheithauer W+, *Ann Oncol* 14(1), 97
  (2002): Dalbagni G+, *J Clin Oncol* 20(15), 3193
Infections (sic) (16%)
  (2002): Poggi MM+, *Int J Radiat Oncol Biol Phys* 54(3), 670
Lipodermatosclerosis
  (2001): Chia-Yu C+, *Acta Dermato-Venereol* 81(6), 426
Palmar–plantar dysesthesia
  (2002): Fracasso PM+, *Cancer* 95(10), 2223 (with doxorubicin)
Peripheral edema (20%)
  (2002): Voorburg AM+, *Lung Cancer* 36(2), 203 (with cisplatin)
  (1995): Tonato M+, *Anticancer Drugs* 6, 27
  (1994): Abratt RP+, *J Clin Oncol* 12, 1535
Petechiae (16%)
Pruritus (13%)
Pruritus ani
  (1999): Hejna M+, *N Engl J Med* 340, 655
Radiation recall
  (2002): Jeter MD+, *Int J Radiat Oncol Biol Phys* 53(2), 394
  (2001): Bar-Sela G+, *Tumori* 87(6), 428
  (2001): Fogarty G+, *Lung Cancer* 33(2–3), 299
  (2000): Burstein HJ, *J Clin Oncol* 18, 693
Rash (sic) (30%)
  (2003): Sumii T+, *Gan To Kagaku Ryoho* 30(7), 971
  (2002): Fracasso PM+, *Cancer* 95(10), 2223 (with doxorubicin)
Vasculitis
  (2002): Voorburg AM+, *Lung Cancer* 36(2), 203
  (2000): Banach MJ+, *Arch Ophthalmol* 118, 726 (necrotizing)

Hair

Hair – alopecia (15%)
  (2002): Brugnatelli S+, *Oncology* 62(1), 33
  (2001): Chu CY+, *Acta Derm Venereol* 81(6), 426 (passim)
  (1999): Akrivakis K+, *Anticancer Drugs* 1999 10, 525
  (1995): Tonato M+, *Anticancer Drugs* 6, 27
  (1994): Abratt RP+, *J Clin Oncol* 12, 1535

Other

Anaphylactoid reactions

Dysgeusia
  (2001): Johnson FM, *Cancer Nurs* 24(2), 149
Fatigue
  (2002): Poggi MM+, *Int J Radiat Oncol Biol Phys* 54(3), 670
Headache
Injection-site reactions (4%)
Lymphedema
  (2000): Brandes A+, *Anticancer Drugs* 11, 15 (confined to areas
    of erysipeloid rash)
Mucositis
  (2002): Eckel F+, *Cancer Invest* 20(2), 180
Myalgia (>10%)
  (2002): Voorburg AM+, *Lung Cancer* 36(2), 203 (with cisplatin)
Myositis
  (2001): Fogarty G+, *Lung Cancer* 33(2), 299
Paresthesias (10%)
Pseudolymphoma
  (2001): Marucci G+, *Br J Dermatol* 145(4), 650
Stomatitis (11%)
  (2003): Michaelson MD+, *Cancer* 97(1), 148
  (2002): Bass AJ+, *J Clin Oncol* 20(13), 2995
  (2002): Brugnatelli S+, *Oncology* 62(1), 33
  (2002): Fracasso PM+, *Cancer* 95(10), 2223 (with doxorubicin)

GEMFIBROZIL

Trade name: Lopid (Parke-Davis)
Other common trade names: *Bolutol; Decrelip; Fibrocit; Gemlipid; Gen-Fibro; Gevilon Uno; Jezil; Lipur; Nu-Gemfibrozil*
Indications: Hyperlipidemia
Category: Antihyperlipidemic
Half-life: 1.5 hours
Clinically important, potentially hazardous interactions with: atorvastatin, bexarotene, cyclosporine, dicumarol, fluvastatin, lovastatin, nicotinic acid, pravastatin, simvastatin, warfarin

Reactions

Skin

Abscess
Acanthosis nigricans
Angioedema
Basal cell carcinoma
Dermatitis (sic) (0.4%)
  (1988): Todd PA+, *Drugs* 36, 314
Dermatomyositis (<1%)
Eczema (sic) (1.9%)
Erythema multiforme
Exanthems
  (1990): Fusella J+, *J Rheumatol* 17, 572
  (1988): Todd PA+, *Drugs* 36, 314 (2.1%)
Exfoliative dermatitis (<1%)
Ichthyosis
Lichen planus
Lupus erythematosus
Melanoma
Petechiae
Pruritus (0.8%)
  (1988): Todd PA+, *Drugs* 36, 314
Psoriasis
  (1989): Frick MH, *Arch Dermatol* 125, 132
  (1988): Fisher DA+, *Arch Dermatol* 124, 854
Rash (sic) (1.7%)

Raynaud's phenomenon (<1%)
  (1993): Smith GW+, *Br J Rheumatol* 32, 84
Seborrhea
Thickening (sic)
Urticaria (0.1%)
  (1988): Todd PA+, *Drugs* 36, 314
Vasculitis (<1%)
  (1993): Smith GW+, *Br J Rheumatol* 32, 84
Xerosis

Hair
Hair – alopecia
Hair – hirsutism

Nails
Nails – discoloration
  (1990): Klein ME, *The Schoch Letter* 40 (#7), 29 (#120)
    (observation)
Nails – growth (sic)

Other
Anaphylactoid reactions
Death
  (2001): Federman DG+, *South Med J* 94(10), 1023
  (2000): Ozdemir O+, *Angiology* 51(8), 695 (with cerivastatin)
Dysgeusia (<1%)
Headache
Hyperesthesia (<1%)
Myalgia (<1%)
  (2002): Atmaca H+, *Ann Pharmacother* 36(11), 1719 (with
    colchicine)
  (2001): Litt JZ (personal case) (observation)
Myopathy
Myositis
Paresthesias (<1%)
Polymyositis
  (1990): Fusella J+, *J Rheumatol* 17, 572
Pseudolymphoma
  (1995): Magro CM+, *J Am Acad Dermatol* 32, 419
Rhabdomyolysis
  (2003): Yen TH+, *Ren Fail* 25(1), 139
  (2002): Atmaca H+, *Ann Pharmacother* 36(11), 1719 (with
    colchicine)
  (2002): Backman JT+, *Clin Pharmacol Ther* 72(6), 685 (with
    cerivastatin)
  (2002): Carretero MM+, *Br J Gen Pract* 52(476), 235 (with
    cerivastatin)
  (2002): Su M+, *Am J Forensic Med Pathol* 23(3), 305 (with
    cerivastatin)
  (2001): Bosch Rovira T+, *Rev Clin Esp* 201(12), 731 (with
    cerivastatin)
  (2001): Bruno-Joyce J+, *Ann Pharmacother* 35(9), 1016 (with
    cerivastatin)
  (2001): de Arriba Mendez JJ+, *Med Clin* (Barc) 117(7), 278 (with
    cerivastatin)
  (2001): Federman DG+, *South Med J* 94(10), 1023 (with
    simvastatin)
  (2001): Hendriks F+, *Nephrol Dial Transplant* 16(12), 2418 (with
    cerivastatin)
  (2001): Tomlinson B+, *Am J Med* 110(8), 669 (with cerivastatin)
  (2000): Oldemeyer JB+, *Cardiology* 94(2), 127 (with simvastatin)
  (2000): Ozdemir O+, *Angiology* 51(8), 695 (with cerivastatin)
  (1998): Torbet JA, *Am J Cardiol* 62, 28J (with cyclosporine)
  (1990): Pierce LR+, *JAMA* 264(1), 71 (with lovastatin)

GEMIFLOXACIN

Synonyms: DW286; LA 20304a; SB-265805
Trade name: Factive
Indications: Infections due to various microorganisms
Category: Fluoroquinolone antibiotic
Half-life: 4-12 hours

Reactions

Skin
Angioedema
Candidiasis (<1%)
Dermatitis (<1%)
Eczema (<1%)
Exanthems
Flushing (<0.1%)
Fungal infections (<1%)
Hot flashes (<0.1%)
Pharyngitis (<1%)
Photosensitivity (<1%)
  (2002): Lode H+, *Clin Ther* 24(11), 1915
  (2000): Lowe MN+, *Drugs* 59(5), 1137
Urticaria (<1%)

Other
Abdominal pain (1%)
  (2000): Lowe MN+, *Drugs* 59(5), 1137
Anaphylactoid reactions
Arthralgia (1%)
Asthenia (<1%)
Back pain (<1%)
Candidiasis (genital) (<1%)
Dizziness (1%)
Dysgeusia (<1%)
Fatigue (<1%)
Headache
Hypersensitivity
Myalgia (<1%)
Pharyngitis (<1%)
Seizures
Tremor (<1%)
Vaginitis (<1%)
  (2003): Wilson R+, *Respir Med* 97, 242
  (2002): Lode H+, *Clin Ther* 24, 1915
  (2001): Ball P+, *Int J Antimicrob Agents* 18, 19
  (2001): Hammerschlag MR+, *Antimicrob Chemother* 48, 735
Xerostomia (<1%)

Note: The incidence of rash increases significantly when duration of
therapy exceeds seven days, reaching 7.4% at 14 days

GEMTUZUMAB

Trade name: Mylotarg (Wyeth)
Indications: Acute myeloid leukemia
Category: Antineoplastic monoclonal antibody
Half-life: 45 hours (initial dose)

Reactions

Skin
Chills (66%)
  (2001): Larson RA, *Semin Hematol* 38(Suppl 6), 24

Ecchymoses (15%)
Herpes simplex (22%)
Infections (sic) (28%)
  (2001): Larson RA, *Semin Hematol* 38(Suppl 6), 24 (23%)
  (2001): Sievers EL+, *Curr Opin Oncol* 13(6), 522
  (2001): Sievers EL+, *J Clin Oncol* 19(13), 3244 (28%)
Peripheral edema (21%)
Petechiae (21%)
Rash (sic) (23%)

Other
Arthralgia (10%)
Headache
Infusion-related syndrome
  (2001): Larson RA, *Semin Hematol* 38(Suppl 6), 24
Injection-site reactions (sic) (25%)
Mucositis (25%)
  (2001): Larson RA, *Semin Hematol* 38(Suppl 6), 24 (4%)
  (2001): Sievers EL+, *Curr Opin Oncol* 13(6), 522
  (2001): Sievers EL+, *J Clin Oncol* 19(13), 3244 (4%)
Pain
  (2001): Larson RA, *Semin Hematol* 38(SUppl 6), 24
Stomatitis (32%)

GENTAMICIN

Trade names: Garamycin (Schering); Genoptic (Allergan); Gentacidin; Jenamicin; Ocumycin; Pred-G (Allergan)
Other common trade names: *Alcomicin; Cidomycin; Diogent; Garatec; Gentalline; Gentalol; I-Gent; Refobacin; Sedanazin*
Indications: Various infections caused by susceptible organisms
Category: Aminoglycoside antibiotic
Half-life: 2–4 hours
Clinically important, potentially hazardous interactions with: adefovir, aldesleukin, aminoglycosides, atracurium, bumetanide, carbenicillin, cephalexin, cephalothin, doxacurium, ethacrynic acid, furosemide, methoxyflurane, non-polarizing muscle relaxants, pancuronium, pipecuronium, polypeptide antibiotics, rocuronium, succinylcholine, torsemide, tubocurarine, vecuronium

Reactions

Skin
Dermatitis
  (2002): Paniagua MJ+, *Allergy* 57(11), 1086
  (2001): Sanchez-Perez J+, *Contact Dermatitis* 44(1), 54 (with kanamycin)
  (1996): Merlob P+, *Cutis* 57, 429 (neonatal orbital)
  (1996): Munoz-Bellido FJ+, *Allergy* 51, 758
  (1989): van Ketel WG+, *Contact Dermatitis* 20, 303
  (1988): Robinson PM, *J Laryngol Otol* 102, 577
  (1970): Lynfield YL, *N Y State J Med* 70, 2235
  (1969): Braun W+, *Hautarzt* (German) 20, 108
Eczema (sic)
  (1988): Ghadially R+, *J Am Acad Dermatol* 19, 428
Edema (1–10%)
Erythema (1–10%)
Exanthems
  (2002): Spigarelli MG+, *Pediatr Pulmonol* 33(4), 311
  (1990): Flax SH+, *Cutis* 46, 59
  (1974): Hewitt WL, *Postgrad Med* 50 (Suppl 7), 55 (0.3%)
  (1971): Tümmers H+, *Med Welt* (German) 22, 1404 (1%)
  (1969): Braun W+, *Hautarzt* (German) 20, 108
Exfoliative dermatitis

  (1989): Guin JD+, *Cutis* 43, 564
Photosensitivity (<1%)
  (1990): Flax SH+, *Cutis* 46, 59 (photo recall)
  (1966): Hough CE+, *Clin Med Surg* 73, 55
Pruritus (1–10%)
Purpura
  (1974): Hewitt WL, *Postgrad Med* 50 (Suppl 7), 55 (0.3%)
Rash (sic)
  (2002): Spigarelli MG+, *Pediatr Pulmonol* 33(4), 311
Toxic epidermal necrolysis
  (1984): Sluchenkova LD+, *Pediatriia* (Russian) July, 57
Urticaria
  (1974): Hewitt WL, *Postgrad Med* 50 (Suppl 7), 55 (0.14%)
Vasculitis
  (1980): Bonnetblanc JM+, *Ann Dermatol Vénéréol* (French) 107, 1089

Hair
Hair – alopecia
  (1973): Levantine A+, *Br J Dermatol* 89, 549
  (1970): Yoshioka H+, *JAMA* 211, 123

Other
Anaphylactoid reactions
  (1983): Fisher AA, *Cutis* 32, 510
Headache
Hypersensitivity
  (2002): Spigarelli MG+, *Pediatr Pulmonol* 33(4), 311
Injection-site erythema
  (1990): Shen K, *Lancet* 336, 689
Injection-site induration
Injection-site necrosis
  (1990): Grob JJ+, *Dermatologica* 180, 258
  (1985): Doutre MS+, *Therapie* (French) 40, 266
  (1985): Duterque M+, *Ann Dermatol Venereol* (French) 112, 707
  (1984): Penso D+, *Presse Méd* (French) 13, 1575
  (1984): Taillandier J+, *Presse Méd* (French) 13, 1574
Injection-site pain (<1%)
Paresthesias
Phlebitis
Pseudotumor cerebri (<1%)
Sialorrhea (<1%)
Stomatitis
Thrombophlebitis
Tinnitus
Tremor (<1%)

GINGER

Scientific name: *Zingiber officinale*
Family: Zingiberaceae
Trade and other common names: African Ginger; Cochin Ginger; Gingembre; Jamaica Ginger; Race Ginger
Category: Anti-infective; Anti-nausea
Purported indications and other uses: Colic, dyspepsia, flatulence, rheumatoid arthritis, loss of appetite, nausea, vomiting, upper respiratory infections, cough, bronchitis, burns, tinnitus, flavoring agent, fragrance component
Half-life: N/A
Clinically important, potentially hazardous interactions with: heparin, ticlopidine, warfarin

Reactions

Skin
Dermatitis (sic)
   (1996): Kanerva L+, *Contact Dermatitis* 35(3), 157

Other
Bleeding
   (2001): Fessenden JM+, *Am Surg* 67(1), 33

GINKGO BILOBA

Scientific name: *Ginkgo biloba*
Family: Ginkgoaceae
Trade and other common names: Fossil Tree; Japanese Silver Apricot; Maidenhair Tree; Salisburia; Tanakan; Tebonin
Category: Antidementia; Improved cognition
Purported indications and other uses: Dementia, memory loss, headache, tinnitus, dizziness, mood disturbances, hearing disorders, intermittent claudication, attention deficit hyperactivity disorder, premenstrual syndrome, heart disease
Half-life: N/A
Clinically important, potentially hazardous interactions with: anticoagulants, aspirin, diuretics, NSAIDs, phenytoin, platelet inhibitors, SSRIs, **St John's wort**, warfarin

Reactions

Skin
Adverse effects (sic)
   (2002): Ernst E, *Ann Intern Med* 136(1), 42
   (2002): Haller CA+, *Adverse Drug React Toxicol Rev* 21(3), 143
   (2002): Mattsson K+, *Lakartidningen* 99(50), 5095
Allergic reactions (sic)
Dermatitis
   (1989): Lepoittevin JP+, *Arch Dermatol* 281, 227
   (1988): Tomb RR+, *Contact Dermatitis* 19, 281
Eruptions
   (2002): Chiu AE+, *J Am Acad Dermatol* 46(1), 145
Erythema
Exanthems
   (2002): Chiu AE+, *J Am Acad Dermatol* 46(1), 145
Pruritus
Rash (sic)
Vasculitis
Vesicular eruptions

Other
Coma

   (2000): Galluzzi S+, *J Neurol Neurosurg Psychiatry* 68(5), 679
      (with trazodone)
Hyphema
   (2002): Schneider C+, *J Fr Ophtalmol* 25(7), 731
Phlebitis
Rectal burning (sic)
Seizures
   (2002): Kajiyama Y+, *Pediatrics* 109(2), 325 (overdose)
   (2001): Granger AS, *Age Ageing* 30(6), 523
   (2001): Gregory PJ, *Ann Intern Med* 134(4), 344
   (2001): Miwa H+, *Epilepsia* Feb 42(2), 280
Spontaneous bleeding
   (2002): Hauser D+, *Transpl Int* 15(7), 377
   (2002): Purroy Garcia F+, *Med Clin* (Barc) 119(15), 596
   (2002): Tesch BJ, *Dis Mon* Oct 48(10), 671
   (2001): Ang-Lee MK+, *JAMA* 286(2), 208
   (2001): Benjamin J+, *Postgrad Med J* 77(904), 112
   (2001): Boniel T+, *Harefuah* 140(8), 780
   (2001): Fessenden JM+, *Am Surg* 67(1), 33
   (1999): Cupp MJ, *Am Fam Physician* 59(5), 1239
   (1998): Matthews MK, *Neurology* 50, 1933
   (1997): Gilbert GJ, *Neurology* 48, 1137
   (1997): Rosenblatt M+, *N Engl J Med* 336, 1108
   (1996): Rowen J+, *Neurology* 46, 1775
Stomatitis

Note: *Ginkgo biloba* is the oldest living tree species in the world. Ginkgo is the most frequently prescribed herbal medicine in Germany

GINSENG

Scientific name: *Panax ginseng*
Family: Araliaceae
Trade and other common names: Asian Ginseng; Asiatic Ginseng; Chinese Ginseng; Japanese Ginseng; Jintsam; Korean Ginseng; Korean Red; Ninjin; Red Ginseng; Ren She; Sang; Seng
Category: Immune stimulant
Purported indications and other uses: General tonic, improving stamina, cognitive function, concentration, diuretic, antidepressant, gastritis, neurasthenia, impotence, fever, hangover, cancer, cardiovascular diseases
Half-life: N/A
Clinically important, potentially hazardous interactions with: alcohol, aspirin, **caffeine**, digoxin, olmesartan, phenelzine, tamoxifen, ticlopidine, warfarin

Reactions

Skin
Adverse effects (sic)
   (2002): Ellis JM+, *Ann Pharmacother* 36(3), 375
   (2002): Ernst E, *Ann Intern Med* 136(1), 42
   (2002): Haller CA+, *Adverse Drug React Toxicol Rev* 21(3), 143
Allergic reactions (sic)
Burning (sensation)
   (1999): Choi HK+, *Int J Impot Res* 11(5), 261
Edema
Pruritus
Stevens–Johnson syndrome
   (2001): Boniel T+, *Harefuah* 140(8), 780
   (1996): Dega H+, *Lancet* 313, 756

Other
Bleeding
   (2001): Ang-Lee MK+, *JAMA* 286(2), 208
   (2001): Boniel T+, *Harefuah* 140(8), 780

(2001): Fessenden JM+, *Am Surg* 67(1), 33
(2000): Nocerino E+, *Fitoterapia* 71, S1 (vaginal)
Gynecomastia
  (1999): Palop V+, *Med Clin* (Barc) 112(19), 758
Mania
  (2002): Vazquez I+, *Acta Psychiatr Scand* 105(1), 76
  (2001): Engelberg D+, *J Clin Psychopharmacol* 21(5), 535
Mastalgia
  (2001): Boniel T+, *Harefuah* 140(8), 780
  (2000): Nocerino E+, *Fitoterapia* 71, S1
Mastodynia
  (1978): Palmer BV+, *BMJ* 1, 1284
Penile pain
Side effects (sic)
  (2002): Tesch BJ, *Dis Mon* Oct 48(10), 671

Note: Ginseng has been used for medicinal purposes for more than 2000 years. Approximately 6,000,000 Americans use it regularly

GLATIRAMER*

Trade name: Copaxone (Teva)
Indications: Multiple sclerosis
Category: Immunosuppressive
Half-life: N/A

***Note:** Also known as Copolymer-1

Reactions

Skin

Acne (>2%)
Allergic reactions (sic)
Angioedema
Atrophy
Cellulitis
Chills (4%)
Cyst (2%)
Dermatitis
Diaphoresis (15%)
Ecchymoses (8%)
Eczema
Edema (3%)
Erythema (4%)
Erythema nodosum
Exanthems
Facial edema (6%)
Flu-like syndrome (19%)
  (2002): Flechter S+, *J Neurol Sci* 197(1), 51 (26%)
Flushing
  (2001): Ziemssen T+, *Drug Saf* 24(13), 979
Fungal infections
Furunculosis
Herpes simplex (4%)
Herpes zoster
Infections (50%)
Lupus erythematosus
Nodules (2%)
Peripheral edema (7%)
Photosensitivity
Pigmentation
Pruritus (185)
Psoriasis
Purpura
Pustules

Rash (sic) (18%)
Striae
Urticaria
Vesiculobullous eruption
Xanthomas
Xerosis

Hair

Hair – alopecia (>2%)

Nails

Nails – changes (>2%)

Other

Ageusia
Anaphylactoid reactions
Arthralgia (24%)
Arthritis
Bone or joint pain
Cough (>2%)
Depression (>2%)
Dizziness (>2%)
Dry eyes
Dysgeusia (>2%)
Facial numbness
Gingival hemorrhage
Glossodynia
Gynecomastia
Hallucinations
Headache
Hyperesthesia (>2%)
Injection-site abscess
Injection-site atrophy
Injection-site ecchymoses (>2%)
Injection-site edema
Injection-site erythema (66%)
  (2001): Ziemssen T+, *Drug Saf* 24(13), 979
Injection-site fibrosis
Injection-site hematoma
Injection-site hemorrhage (5%)
Injection-site hypersensitivity
Injection-site induration (13%)
  (2001): Ziemssen T+, *Drug Saf* 24(13), 979
Injection-site inflammation (49%)
  (2001): Ziemssen T+, *Drug Saf* 24(13), 979
Injection-site pain (73%)
Injection-site pigmentation
Injection-site pruritus (40%)
Injection-site reactions (6.5%)
  (2002): Flechter S+, *J Neurol Sci* 197(1), 51 (67%)
  (2002): Ziemssen T+, *Nervenarzt* 73(4), 321
Injection-site urticaria (5%)
Lipoatrophy
  (2001): Hwang L+, *Cutis* 68(4), 287
  (1999): Drago F+, *Arch Dermatol* 135(10), 1277 (localized)
Lipoma
Lymphedema
Mastodynia (>2%)
Moon face
Mouth vesiculation (6%)
Myalgia (>2%)
Myasthenia (>2%)
Myasthenia gravis
  (2000): Frese A+, *J Neurol* 247(9), 713
Myopathy
Oral candidiasis

Oral ulceration
Pain (28%)
Paresthesias (>2%)
Pharyngitis (>2%)
Priapism
Serum sickness
Sinusitis (>2%)
Stomatitis
Tenosynovitis
Tinnitus (>2%)
Tongue edema
Tongue pigmentation
Trembling
Tremor (7%)
Tumors
Ulcerative stomatitis
Vaginitis
Xerostomia (>2%)

GLIMEPIRIDE*

Trade name: Amaryl (Aventis)
Indications: Non-insulin dependent diabetes type II
Category: Second generation sulfonylurea antidiabetic
Half-life: 5–9 hours

Reactions

Skin
Allergic reactions (sic) (<1%)
Diaphoresis
Edema (<1%)
Erythema (<1%)
Exanthems (<1%)
Exfoliation (sic)
Photosensitivity (<1%)
Pruritus (<1%)
Psoriasis
   (1997): Leal G, Fortaleza, Brazil (from Internet) (observation)
Rash (sic) (<1%)
   (2001): Deerochanawong C+, J Med Assoc Thai 84(9), 1221
Urticaria (<1%)

Other
Headache
Porphyria cutanea tarda

*Note: Glimepiride is a sulfonamide and can be absorbed systemically. Sulfonamides can produce severe, possibly fatal, reactions such as toxic epidermal necrolysis and Stevens–Johnson syndrome

GLIPIZIDE*

Trade names: Glucotrol (Roerig); Metaglip (Bristol-Myers Squibb)
Other common trade names: *Glibenese; Glipid; Glyde; Melizide; Mindiab; Minidiab; Minodiab*
Indications: Non-insulin dependent diabetes type II
Category: Second generation sulfonylurea antidiabetic
Half-life: 2–4 hours

Reactions

Skin
Eczema (sic)
Edema (<1%)
Erythema (<1%)
Exanthems (<1%)
Exfoliation (sic)
Flushing (<1%)
Grinspan's syndrome**
   (1990): Lamey PJ+, Oral Surg Oral Med Oral Path 70, 184
Lichenoid eruption
Photosensitivity (1–10%)
Phototoxicity
   (2000): Vargas F+, In Vitr Mol Toxicol 13, 17
Pigmented purpuric dermatosis
   (1999): Adams BB+, J Am Acad Dermatol 41, 827
Pruritus (<3%)
Psoriasis (induced)
   (1994): Litt JZ, Beachwood, OH (2 personal cases) (observation)
Purpura
Rash (sic) (1–10%)
Urticaria (1–10%)

Other
Headache
Hyperesthesia (<3%)
Myalgia (<3%)
Oral lichen planus
   (1990): Lamey PJ+, Oral Surg Oral Med Oral Path 70, 184
Paresthesias (<3%)
Porphyria (coproporphyria-like)
   (1991): Moder KG+, Mayo Clin Proc 66, 312
Porphyria cutanea tarda

*Note: Glipizide is a sulfonamide and can be absorbed systemically. Sulfonamides can produce severe, possibly fatal, reactions such as toxic epidermal necrolysis and Stevens–Johnson syndrome

**Note: Grinspan's syndrome: the triad of oral lichen planus, diabetes mellitus, and hypertension

GLUCAGON

Trade name: Glucagon Emergency Kit (Lilly)
Indications: Hypoglycemic reactions
Category: Antidote; Antihypoglycemic; Antispasmodic
Half-life: 3–10 minutes
Clinically important, potentially hazardous interactions with: warfarin

Reactions

Skin

Acute febrile neutrophilic dermatosis (Sweet's syndrome)
(1996): Glass LF+, J Am Acad Dermatol 34, 455 (passim)
(1994): Fukutoku M+, Br J Haematol 86, 645
(1994): Johnson ML+, Arch Dermatol 130, 77
(1993): Paydas S+, Br J Haematol 85, 191
(1992): Karp DL, Ann Intern Med 117, 875
(1992): Park JW+, Ann Intern Med 116, 996
(1991): Cohen PR+, J Am Acad Dermatol 25, 734
Angioedema
(1985): Gelfand DW+, Am J Roentgenol 144, 405
Epidermolysis bullosa acquisita
(1992): Ward JC+, Br J Haematol 81, 27
Erythema multiforme
(1980): Edell SL, Am J Roentgenol 134, 385
Erythema necrolyticum migrans
(2002): Wald M+, Eur J Pediatr 161(11), 600
Erythema nodosum
(1994): Nomiyama J+, Am J Hematol 47, 333
Exanthems
(1996): Glass LF+, J Am Acad Dermatol 34, 455
(1995): Scott GA, Am J Dermatopathol 17, 107
(1994): Sasaki O+, Intern Med 33, 641
(1993): Peters MS+, J Cutan Pathol 20, 465
(1993): Yamashita N+, J Dermatol 20, 473
(1992): Mehregan DR+, Arch Dermatol 128, 1055
(1976): Barber SG+, Lancet 20, 1138
Folliculitis
(1996): Glass LF+, J Am Acad Dermatol 34, 455 (passim)
(1992): Ostlere LS+, Br J Dermatol 127, 193
Glucagonoma syndrome (necrolytic migratory erythema)
(1988): Benhamou PY+, Ann Dermatol Venereol (French) 115, 717
Pyoderma gangrenosum
(1996): Glass LF+, J Am Acad Dermatol 34, 455 (passim)
(1994): Johnson ML+, Arch Dermatol 130, 77
(1991): Ross HJ+, Cancer 68, 441 (bullous)
Rash (sic)
(1979): Barber SG+, Ann Intern Med 91, 213
(1976): Barber SG+, Lancet 2, 1138
Urticaria (1–10%)
(1985): Gelfand DW+, Am J Roentgenol 144, 405
(1975): Kitabchi AE+, J Clin Endocrinol Metab 41, 863
Vasculitis
(1996): Glass LF+, J Am Acad Dermatol 34, 455 (passim)
(1995): Couderc LJ+, Respir Med 89, 237
(1995): Vidarsson B+, Am J Med 98, 589
(1994): Jain KK, J Am Acad Dermatol 31, 213
(1994): Johnson ML+, Arch Dermatol 130, 77
(1994): van Kamp H+, Br J Haematol 86, 415
(1991): Wodzinski MA+, Br J Haematol 77, 249
(1990): Welte Z+, Blood 75, 1056
(1989): Dreicer R+, Ann Intern Med 111, 91

Other

Headache

Injection-site reactions (sic)
(1996): Glass LF+, J Am Acad Dermatol 34, 455 (passim)
(1993): Samlaska CP+, Arch Dermatol 129, 645
(1992): Mehregan DR+, Arch Dermatol 128, 1055

GLUCOSAMINE

Trade names: Arthro-Aid (NutraSense); Chitosamine; Glucosamine sulfate (Rottapharm); Mericon
Other common trade names: 2-amino-2-deoxyglucose hydrochloride;; 2-amino-deoxyglucose sulfate; N-acetyl-glucosamine (NAG)
Indications: Arthritis, osteoarthritis, cartilage repair and maintenance, strained joints, improving joint function and range of motion, alleviating joint pain
Category: chondroprotective agent; Dietary supplement; immunosuppressant; nutraceutical
Half-life: N/A

Reactions

Skin

Adverse effects (sic)
(1998): Barclay TS+, Ann Pharmacother 32(5), 574
(1998): Qiu GX+, Arzneimittelforschung 48(5), 469 (6%)
(1994): Muller-Fassbender H+, Osteoarthritis Cartilage 2(1), 61 (6%)
Allergic reactions (sic)
(2001): Reginster JY+, Lancet 357(9252) (4%)
Eczema
(2003): Maffei KR, Athens, GA (from Internet) (observations)

Other

Asthma
(2002): Tallia AF+, J Am Board Fam Pract 15(6), 481 (with chondroitin)
Depression
(2001): Reginster JY+, Lancet 357(9252) (6%)
Fatigue
(2001): Reginster JY+, Lancet 357(9252) (9%)
Hypersensitivity
(1999): Matheu V+, Allergy 54(6), 643
Mouth vesiculation
(2001): Reginster JY+, Lancet 357(9252) (7%)

GLYBURIDE

Synonyms: glibenclamide; glybenclamide
Trade names: Diabeta (Aventis); Glucovance (Bristol-Myers Squibb); Glynase (Pharmacia); Micronase (Pharmacia)
Other common trade names: *Albert (Glyburide); Daonil; Euglucan; Euglucon; Glimel; Glucal; Hemi-Daonil; Med-Glibe; Miglucan; Norboral*
Indications: Non-insulin dependent diabetes type II
Category: Second generation sulfonylurea antidiabetic
Half-life: 5–16 hours
Clinically important, potentially hazardous interactions with: bosentan

Glucovance is glyburide and metformin

Reactions

Skin
Allergic reactions (sic) (0.21%)
  (1986): Bigby M+, *JAMA* 256, 3358
Angioedema
Bullous eruption
  (1981): Wongpaitoon V+, *Postgrad Med J* 57, 244
Eczema (sic)
Edema of foot
  (1988): Berova N+, *Dermatol Monatsschr* (German) 174, 50
Erythema (1–5%)
  (1988): Chee Ching S, *Photodermatol* 5, 42
Exanthems (1–5%)
  (1971): Editorial, *BMJ* 2, 644
  (1970): O'Sullivan DJ+, *BMJ* 2, 572 (0.5–1%)
  (1969): Müller R+, *Horm Metab Res* 1, 88
Exfoliation (sic)
Eyelid edema
  (1985): Yitalo P+, *Arzneimittelforsch* (German) 35, 1596
Flushing
  (1971): Fairman MJ+, *BMJ* 4, 297
  (1971): Wardle EN+, *BMJ* 3, 309
Lichenoid eruption
Linear IgA bullous dermatosis
  (1983): Väätäinen N+, *Acta Derm Venereol* (Stockh) 63, 169
Pemphigus
  (1993): Paterson AJ+, *J Oral Pathol Med* 22, 92
Photosensitivity (1–10%)
  (1995): Fujii S+, *Am J Hematol* 50, 223
  (1994): Shelley WB+, *Cutis* 53, 287 (observation)
  (1994): Shelley WB+, *Cutis* 53, 77 (observation)
  (1988): Chee-Ching S, *Photodermatology* 5, 42
  (1988): Sun CC, *Photodermatol* 5, 42
  (1987): Henrietta G, *Nursing* 17, 56
  (1969): Müller R+, *Horm Metab Res* 1, 88
Pruritus (1–10%)
  (1988): Chee Ching S, *Photodermatol* 5, 42
  (1987): *Physicians Drug Alert* 7, 71
  (1970): O'Sullivan DJ+, *BMJ* 2, 572
Psoriasis
  (1988): Milner JE, *The Schoch Letter* 38(5), Item 64 (observation)
  (1987): Goh CL, *Australas J Dermatol* 28, 30
Purpura
  (1986): Dickey W+, *BMJ* 293, 823
  (1983): Väätäinen N+, *Acta Derm Venereol* (Stockh) 63, 169
Rash (sic) (1–10%)
Urticaria (1–5%)
  (1994): Shelley WB+, *Cutis* 53, 77 (observation)
  (1991): Chichmanian RM+, *Therapie* (French) 46, 163
  (1986): Jordan NS+, *Hosp Pharm* 21, 462

  (1986): Kure J, *NC Med J* 47, 149
  (1969): Müller R+, *Horm Metab Res* 1, 88
Vasculitis
  (2003): Bukhalo M+, *Cutis* 71(3), 235
  (1986): Dickey W+, *BMJ* 293, 823
  (1980): Ingelmo M+, *Med Clin* (Barc) (Spanish) 75, 306
  (1974): Clarke BF+, *Diabetes* 23, 739
  (1970): O'Sullivan DJ+, *BMJ* 2, 572
Vesiculobullous eruption
  (1993): Landor M+, *Ann Allergy* 70, 196

Other
Dysgeusia
Headache
Hypersensitivity (generalized)
  (1974): Clarke BF+, *Diabetes* 23, 739
Leukocytoclastic vasculitis
  (2003): Bukhalo M+, *Cutis* 71(3), 235
Myalgia
Paresthesias (<1%)
Porphyria cutanea tarda

*Note: Glyburide is a sulfonamide and can be absorbed systemically. Sulfonamides can produce severe, possibly fatal, reactions such as toxic epidermal necrolysis and Stevens–Johnson syndrome

GLYCOPYRROLATE

Trade name: Robinul (Baxter) (Elkins-Sinn)
Other common trade names: *Gastrodyn; Sroton; Strodin*
Indications: Duodenal ulcer, irritable bowel syndrome
Category: Anticholinergic; Antispasmodic
Half-life: N/A
Clinically important, potentially hazardous interactions with: anticholinergics, arbutamine

Reactions

Skin
Allergic reactions (sic)
Flushing
Hypohidrosis (>10%)
Photosensitivity (1–10%)
Rash (sic) (<1%)
Urticaria
Xerosis (>10%)

Other
Anhidrosis
Dysgeusia
Headache
Injection-site irritation (>10%)
Xerostomia (>10%)
  (2001): Patel PS+, *Spec Care Dentist* 21(5), 176

GOLD and GOLD COMPOUNDS

Generic names:
Auranofin
Trade name: Ridaura (Prometheus)
Aurothioglucose
Trade name: Solganal (Schering)
Gold sodium thiomalate (sodium aurothiomalate)
Trade name: Myochrysine (Merck)
Other common trade names: *Aureotan; Aurolate; Aurothio; Miocrin; Myocrisine; Shiosol; Tauredon*
Indications: Rheumatoid arthritis
Category: Antiarthritic
Half-life: 5 days

Reactions

Skin

Acne
(1982): Bailin PL+, *Clin Rheum Dis* 8, 493 (passim)
(1977): Hjortshoj A, *Acta Derm Venereol* (Stockh) 57, 165
Angioedema (<1%)
(1989): Herbst WM+, *Hautarzt* (German) 40, 568
Angiofibromatosis
(1989): Herbst WM+, *Hautarzt* (German) 40, 568
Bullous eruption
(1970): Almeyda J+, *Br J Dermatol* 83, 707
(1951): Jaeger H, *Dermatologica* 103, 280
(1940): Wile UJ+, *Arch Dermatol* 42, 1005 (passim)
Bullous pemphigoid
(1983): Wozel G+, *Dermatol Monatsschr* (German) 169, 125
Cheilitis
(1982): Bailin PL+, *Clin Rheum Dis* 8, 493 (passim)
(1974): Penneys NS+, *Arch Dermatol* 109, 372
Chrysiasis (blue-green pigmentation)
(2001): Werth V, *Dermatology Times* 18
Dermatitis (sic)
(2002): Ahlgren C+, *Acta Derm Venereol* 82(1), 41 (dental gold alloy)
(2001): Lee AY+, *Contact Dermatitis* 45(4), 214
(2000): ter Borg EJ+, *Arthritis Rheum* 43, 1420
(2000): Trattner A+, *Contact Dermatitis* 42, 301
(2000): Vamnes JS+, *Contact Dermatitis* 42, 128
(1999): Bruze M+, *Contact Dermatitis* 40, 295
(1999): Fowler JF, *Skin and Allergy News* September, 34 (9.5%)
(1999): Räsänen L+, *Br J Dermatol* 141, 683
(1998): Estlander T+, *Contact Dermatitis* 38, 40
(1998): Moller H+, *Am J Contact Dermat* 9, 15
(1998): Wiesner M+, *Contact Dermatitis* 38, 52
(1997): Armstrong DK+, *Br J Dermatol* 136, 776
(1997): Choy EH+, *Br J Rheumatol* 36, 1054
(1997): Fleming C+, *Contact Dermatitis* 37, 298 (lymphomatoid)
(1997): Hostynek JJ, *Food Chem Toxicol* 35, 839
(1997): Kilpikari I, *Contact Dermatitis* 37, 130
(1997): Moller H+, *Acta Derm Venereol* 77, 370
(1997): Silva R+, *Contact Dermatitis* 37, 78
(1996): Bonnetblanc JM, *Presse Med* (French) 25, 1555
(1996): Sabroe RA+, *Contact Dermatitis* 34, 345
(1996): Tan E+, *Australas J Dermatol* 37, 218
(1994): Björkner B+, *Contact Dermatitis* 30, 144
(1994): Bruze M+, *J Am Acad Dermatol* 31, 579
(1994): Collet E+, *Ann Dermatol Venereol* (French) 121, 21
(1994): Osawa J+, *Contact Dermatitis* 31, 89
(1994): Webster CG+, *Cutis* 54, 25
(1993): Aro T+, *Contact Dermatitis* 28, 276
(1993): Hisa T+, *Contact Dermatitis* 28, 174
(1993): Koga T+, *Br J Dermatol* 128, 227
(1993): Koga T+, *Contact Dermatitis* 28, 303

(1990): Miller RA+, *J Am Acad Dermatol* 23, 360
(1990): Wijnands MJ+, *Lancet* 335, 867
(1989): Camarasa JG+, *Med Cutan Ibero Lat Am* (Spanish) 17, 187
(1988): Fowler JF, *Arch Dermatol* 124, 181
(1988): Goh CL, *Contact Dermatitis* 18, 122
(1988): Wicks IP+, *Ann Rheum Dis* 47, 421
(1987): Fisher AA, *Cutis* 39, 473
(1987): Fisher AA, *J Am Acad Dermatol* 17, 853
(1986): Minghetti G+, *G Ital Dermatol Venereol* (Italian) 121, 425
(1985): Kalamkarian AA+, *Vestn Dermatol Venerol* (Russian) August, 4
(1985): Rapson WS, *Contact Dermatitis* 13, 56
(1985): Silvennoinen-Kassinen S+, *Contact Dermatitis* 11, 156
(1985): Tosi S+, *Int J Clin Pharmacol Res* 5, 265
(1983): Monti M+, *Contact Dermatitis* 9, 150
(1983): Sigler JW, *Am J Med* 75, 59
(1982): Iwatsuki K+, *Arch Dermatol* 118, 608
(1980): Raith L+, *Dermatol Monatsschr* (German) 166, 382
(1978): Budden MG+, *Contact Dermatitis* 4, 172
(1977): Dick D, *BMJ* 1, 51
(1977): Fisher AA, *Cutis* 19, 156
(1977): Rennie N, *BMJ* 1, 446
(1975): Klaschka F, *Contact Dermatitis* 1, 264
(1975): Roeleveld CG+, *Contact Dermatitis* 1, 333
(1973): Petros H+, *Br J Dermatol* 88, 505
(1971): Nava C+, *Med Lav* (Italian) 62, 572
(1971): Rytter M+, *Dermatologica* (German) 142, 209
(1971): Walzer R+, *Arch Dermatol* 104, 107
(1958): Smith RT+, *JAMA* 167, 1197
(1940): Wile UJ+, *Arch Dermatol* 42, 1005 (passim)
Eczema (sic)
(1994): Lizeaux-Parneix V+, *Ann Dermatol Venereol* (French) 121, 793
(1986): Hofmann C+, *Z Rheumatol* (German) 45, 100
(1976): Rennie JAN, *BMJ* 2, 1294
Eruptions (sic)
(1998): Pandya AG+, *Arch Dermatol* 134, 1104
Erythema annulare centrifugum
(1992): Tsuji T+, *J Am Acad Dermatol* 27, 284
Erythema multiforme
(1982): Bailin PL+, *Clin Rheum Dis* 8, 493 (passim)
(1966): Cameron AJ+, *BMJ* 2, 1125
Erythema nodosum
(1998): Pandya AG+, *Arch Dermatol* 134, 1104 (passim)
(1982): Bailin PL+, *Clin Rheum Dis* 8, 493 (passim)
(1974): Penneys NS+, *Arch Dermatol* 109, 372
(1973): Stone RL+, *Arch Dermatol* 107, 602
Exanthems (>5%)
(2003): Sperber BR+, *Contact Dermatitis* 48(4), 204
(1999): Räsänen L+, *Br J Dermatol* 141, 683
(1998): Pandya AG+, *Arch Dermatol* 134, 1104 (passim)
(1996): Bonnetblanc JM, *Presse Med* (French) 25, 1555
(1994): Shelley WB+, *Cutis* 52, 87 (observation)
(1977): Voigt K+, *Hautarzt* (German) 28, 421
(1974): Penneys NS+, *Arch Dermatol* 109, 372
(1972): Walzer RA+, *Arch Dermatol* 106, 231
(1940): Wile UJ+, *Arch Dermatol* 42, 1005 (passim)
Exfoliative dermatitis
(2000): Lancucki J+, *Wiad Lek* (Polish) 21, 1347 (erythroderma)
(1998): Pandya AG+, *Arch Dermatol* 134, 1104 (passim)
(1996): Sigurdsson V+, *J Am Acad Dermatol* 35, 53
(1991): Wilson CL+, *Int J Dermatol* 30, 148
(1989): Ranki A+, *Am J Dermatopathol* 11, 22
(1984): Adachi JD+, *J Rheumatol* 11, 355
(1982): Bailin PL+, *Clin Rheum Dis* 8, 493 (passim)
(1974): Penneys NS+, *Arch Dermatol* 109, 372
(1940): Wile UJ+, *Arch Dermatol* 42, 1005 (passim)
Fixed eruption
Graft-versus-host reaction

(1998): Jappe U+, *Hautarzt* (German) 49, 126 (passim)

Granuloma annulare
(1990): Martin N+, *Arch Dermatol* 126, 1370
(1980): Rothwell RS+, *Arch Dermatol* 116, 863

Herpes zoster
(1981): Fam AG+, *Ann Intern Med* 94, 712

Lichen planus
(1996): Russell MA+, *N Engl J Med* 334, 603
(1990): Torrelo A+, *Actas Dermo-Sif* (Spanish) 81, 743
(1986): Hofmann C+, *Z Rheumatol* (German) 45, 100
(1986): Ingber A+, *Z Hautkr* (German) 61, 315
(1982): Bailin PL+, *Clin Rheum Dis* 8, 493 (passim)
(1979): Krebs A, *Hautarzt* (German) 30, 281
(1977): Hjorthsoj A, *Acta Derm Venereol* (Stockh) 57, 165
(1974): Delaby MC, *Arch Belg Dermatol* 30, 111
(1974): Penneys NS+, *Arch Dermatol* 109, 372 (32%)
(1937): Hartfall SJ+, *Lancet* 2, 838

Lichen spinulosus
(1932): Throne B+, *Arch Dermatol* 25, 494

Lichenoid eruption
(2001): Werth V, *Dermatology Times* 18
(1999): Räsänen L+, *Br J Dermatol* 141, 683
(1998): Pandya AG+, *Arch Dermatol* 134, 1104 (passim)
(1997): Choy EH+, *Br J Rheumatol* 36, 1054
(1996): Bonnetblanc JM, *Presse Med* (French) 25, 1555
(1994): Alzieu PH+, *Ann Dermatol Venereol* (French) 121, 798
(1994): Lizeaux-Parneix V+, *Ann Dermatol Venereol* (French) 121, 793
(1971): Almeyda J+, *Br J Dermatol* 85, 604

Lupus erythematosus
(1988): Balsa A+, *Rev Clin Esp* (Spanish) 182, 505
(1969): Goerz G, *Dtsch Med Wochenschr* (German) 94, 2040
(1967): Kapp W+, *Praxis* (German) 56, 1594

Lymphocytoma cutis
(1992): Kobayashi Y+, *J Am Acad Dermatol* 27, 457

Lymphomatoid eosinophilic reaction (sic)
(1999): Park YM+, *Contact Dermatitis* 40, 216

Pemphigus
(1978): Miyamoto Y+, *Arch Dermatol* 114, 1855

Photosensitivity
(1973): Machtey I, *Harefuah* (Hebrew) 85, 517
(1970): Almeyda J+, *Br J Dermatol* 83, 707

Pigmentation (chrysiasis)
(1998): Pandya AG+, *Arch Dermatol* 134, 1104 (passim)
(1997): Miller ML+, *Cutis* 59, 256
(1996): Fleming CJ+, *J Am Acad Dermatol* 34, 349
(1992): Cremer B+, *Dtsch Med Wochenschr* (German) 117, 558
(1990): Bonet M+, *Clin Rheumatol* 9, 254
(1984): Fam AG+, *Arthritis Rheum* 27, 119
(1984): Larsen FS+, *Clin Exp Dermatol* 9, 174
(1984): Pelachyk IM+, *J Cutan Pathol* 11, 491
(1982): Bailin PL+, *Clin Rheum Dis* 8, 493 (passim)
(1982): Beckett VL+, *Mayo Clin Proc* 57, 773
(1981): Granstein RD+, *J Am Acad Dermatol* 5, 1 (blue-gray)
(1975): Altmeyer P+, *Hautarzt* (German) 26, 330
(1974): Gottlieb NL+, *Arthritis Rheum* 17, 56
(1973): Cox AJ+, *Arch Dermatol* 108, 655
(1973): Levantine A+, *Br J Dermatol* 89, 105
(1971): Franken E, *Dtsch Gesundheitsw* (German) 26, 653
(1965): Bianchi O+, *Arch Argent Dermatol* (Spanish) 15, 464
(1941): Schmidt OEL, *Arch Dermatol* 44, 446
(1928): Hansborg H, *Acta Tuberc Scand* 4, 124

Pityriasis rosea
(1999): Räsänen L+, *Br J Dermatol* 141, 683
(1998): Pandya AG+, *Arch Dermatol* 134, 1104 (passim)
(1994): Lizeaux-Parneix V+, *Ann Dermatol Venereol* (French) 121, 793
(1992): Tsuji T+, *J Am Acad Dermatol* 27, 284
(1986): Hofmann C+, *Z Rheumatol* (German) 45, 100

(1982): Bailin PL+, *Clin Rheum Dis* 8, 493 (passim)
(1977): Maize JC+, *Arch Dermatol* 113, 1457
(1974): Penneys NS+, *Arch Dermatol* 109, 372
(1940): Wile UJ+, *Arch Dermatol* 42, 1005

Pruritus
(2003): Sperber BR+, *Contact Dermatitis* 48(4), 204
(1998): Pandya AG+, *Arch Dermatol* 134, 1104
(1996): Bonnetblanc JM, *Presse Med* (French) 25, 1555
(1982): Bailin PL+, *Clin Rheum Dis* 8, 493 (passim)
(1975): Gordon MH+, *Ann Intern Med* 82, 47
(1974): Pennys NS+, *Arch Dermatol* 109, 372 (84%)
(1958): Smith RT+, *JAMA* 167, 1197
(1940): Wile UJ+, *Arch Dermatol* 42, 1005 (passim)

Psoriasis
(1991): Smith DL+, *Arch Dermatol* 127, 268

Purpura
(1984): Adachi JD+, *J Rheumatol* 11, 355
(1982): Bailin PL+, *Clin Rheum Dis* 8, 493 (passim)
(1966): Saphir JR+, *JAMA* 195, 782

Pyoderma gangrenosum

Radiation keratosis
(1996): Helm KF+, *Cutis* 57, 435

Rash (sic) (>10%)
(1990): Fremont-Smith P+, *Ann Rheum Dis* 49, 271
(1989): Caspi D+, *Ann Rheum Dis* 48, 730
(1984): Grindulis KA+, *Ann Rheum Dis* 43, 398
(1982): Smith PJ+, *Br Med J (Clin Res Ed)* 285, 595
(1979): Kean WF+, *Arthritis Rheum* 22, 495
(1961): Bayles TB, *Med Clin North Am* 5, 1229
(1956): Bayles TB+, *Ann Rheum Dis* 15, 394

Seborrheic dermatitis
(1982): Bailin PL+, *Clin Rheum Dis* 8, 493 (passim)
(1981): Kanwar AJ+, *Arch Dermatol* 117, 65 (passim)
(1951): Merliss RR+, *Ann Intern Med* 35, 352

Squamous cell carcinoma
(1990): Miller RA+, *J Am Acad Dermatol* 23, 360 (from radioactive gold)
(1973): Holubar K+, *Hautarzt* (German) 24, 489 (from radioactive gold)

Toxic dermatitis (sic)
(1958): Smith RT+, *JAMA* 167, 1197

Toxic epidermal necrolysis
(1998): Pandya AG+, *Arch Dermatol* 134, 1104 (passim)
(1982): Braun-Falco O+, *MMM Munch Med Wochenschr* (German) 124, 757 (with benoxaprofen)
(1982): Feldman C+, *Rheumatol Rehabil* 21, 222 (with benoxaprofen)
(1951): Jaeger H, *Dermatologica* 103, 280

Urticaria (1-10%)
(1998): Pandya AG+, *Arch Dermatol* 134, 1104 (passim)
(1994): Lizeaux-Parneix V+, *Ann Dermatol Venereol* (French) 121, 793
(1982): Bailin PL+, *Clin Rheum Dis* 8, 493 (passim)
(1974): Penneys NS+, *Arch Dermatol* 109, 372
(1970): Almeyda J+, *Br J Dermatol* 83, 707
(1940): Wile UJ+, *Arch Dermatol* 42, 1005 (passim)
(1936): Roche H, *BMJ* 1, 31

Vasculitis
(1984): Hauteville D+, *Rev Rhum Mal Osteoartic* (French) 51, 56
(1982): Bailin PL+, *Clin Rheum Dis* 8, 493 (passim)
(1974): Roenigk HR+, *Arch Dermatol* 109, 253
(1974): Steele DR, *Arch Dermatol* 110, 297

Vitiligo
(1933): Pillsbury DM+, *Arch Dermatol* 27, 36

Xerosis
(1984): Grindulis KA+, *Ann Rheum Dis* 43, 398

Hair

Hair – alopecia (1-10%)

(1998): Pandya AG+, *Arch Dermatol* 134, 1104 (passim)
(1984): Grindulis KA+, *Ann Rheum Dis* 43, 398
(1982): Bailin PL+, *Clin Rheum Dis* 8, 493 (passim)
(1975): Gordon MH+, *Ann Intern Med* 82, 47
(1972): Walzer RA+, *Arch Dermatol* 106, 231
Hair – pigmentation
(1974): Gottlieb NL+, *Arthritis Rheum* 17, 56

Nails

Nails – dystrophy
(1977): Voigt K+, *Hautarzt* (German) 28, 421
Nails – exfoliation
(1938): Boon TH, *BMJ* 1, 780
Nails – lichen planus
(1990): Torrelo A+, *Actas Dermo-Sif* (Spanish) 81, 743
Nails – loss
(2000): ter Borg EJ+, *Arthritis Rheum* 43, 1420
Nails – onycholysis
(1977): Voigt K+, *Hautarzt* (German) 28, 421
Nails – pigmentation
(1984): Fam AG+, *Arthritis Rheum* 27, 119 (gold nails)
(1974): Gottlieb NL+, *Arthritis Rheum* 17, 56
Nails – yellow
(2001): Roest MA+, *Br J Dermatol* 145, 186

Other

Acute intermittent porphyria
Anaphylactoid reactions
Aphthous stomatitis
(1989): Caspi D+, *Ann Rheum Dis* 48, 730
(1979): Kean WF+, *Arthritis Rheum* 22, 495
(1976): Kuffer R+, *Rev Stomatol Chir Maxillofac* (French) 77, 747
Burning mouth syndrome
(1994): Laeijendecker R+, *J Am Acad Dermatol* 30, 205
Dysgeusia
(1996): Bonnetblanc JM, *Presse Med* (French) 25, 1555
(1974): Pennys NS+, *Arch Dermatol* 109, 372 (metallic taste)
(1970): Almeyda J+, *Br J Dermatol* 83, 707
(1940): Wile UJ+, *Arch Dermatol* 42, 1005 (passim)
Gingivitis (>10%)
(1976): Adams D+, *J Rheumatol Rehabilitation* 15, 245
(1970): Almeyda J+, *Br J Dermatol* 83, 707
Gingivostomatitis
(1982): Izumi AK, *Arch Dermatol Res* 272, 387 (allergic contact)
Glossitis (>10%)
(1976): Adams D+, *J Rheumatol Rehabilitation* 15, 245
(1975): Gordon MH+, *Ann Intern Med* 82, 47
Headache
Hypersensitivity
(1972): Walzer RA+, *Arch Dermatol* 106, 231
Injection-site pain
(1984): Grindulis KA+, *Ann Rheum Dis* 43, 398
Mucocutaneous reactions
(1996): Cheatum DE, *J Rheumatol* 23, 944
(1995): Klinkhoff AV+, *J Rheumatol* 22, 1657
Oral lichen planus
(1994): Laeijendecker R+, *J Am Acad Dermatol* 30, 205
(1994): Lizeaux-Parneix V+, *Ann Dermatol Venereol* (French) 121, 793
(1993): Brown RS+, *Cutis* 51, 183
Oral lichenoid eruption
(1990): Vallejo-Irastorza G+, *Av Odontoestomatol* (Spanish) 6, 131
Oral mucosal eruption
(1968): Bardadin T+, *Reumatologia* (Polish) 6, 287
Oral mucosal pigmentation
(1990): Torrelo A+, *Actas Dermo-Sif* (Spanish) 81, 743
(1984): Sutak J+, *Prakt Zubn Lek* (Czech) 32, 166
Oral ulceration

(2000): Madinier I+, *Ann Med Interne (Paris)* (French) 151, 248
(1999): Räsänen L+, *Br J Dermatol* 141, 683
(1984): Glenert U, *Oral Surg* 58, 52
(1982): Bailin PL+, *Clin Rheum Dis* 8, 493 (passim)
(1979): Kean WF+, *Arthritis Rheum* 22, 495
(1976): Adams D+, *J Rheumatol Rehabilitation* 15, 245
Pseudolymphoma
(2002): Kim KJ+, *Br J Dermatol* 146, 882 (gold acupuncture)
(1996): Kalimo K+, *J Cutan Pathol* 23, 328
(1993): Kerl H+, *Dermatology in General Medicine* McGraw-Hill New York
Stomatitis (>10%)
(2001): Werth V, *Dermatology Times* 18
(1997): Tosti A+, *Semin Cutan Med Surg* 16, 314
(1996): Bonnetblanc JM, *Presse Med* (French) 25, 1555
(1994): Laeijendecker R+, *J Am Acad Dermatol* 30, 205
(1992): Svensson A+, *Ann Rheum Dis* 51, 326
(1989): Caspi D+, *Ann Rheum Dis* 48, 730
(1987): Tumiati B+, *J Rheumatol* 14, 177
(1984): Glenert U, *Oral Surg* 58, 52
(1983): Sigler JW, *Am J Med* 75, 59
(1982): Bailin PL+, *Clin Rheum Dis* 8, 493 (passim)
(1979): Belkahaia C+, *Tunis Med* (French) 57, 234
(1979): Fregert S+, *Contact Dermatitis* 5, 63
(1975): Gordon MH+, *Ann Intern Med* 82, 47
(1971): Myers AR, *Mod Treat* 8, 761
(1970): Almeyda J+, *Br J Dermatol* 83, 707
(1970): Schopf E+, *Hautarzt* (German) 21, 422
(1958): Smith RT+, *JAMA* 167, 1197
Vaginitis
(1978): Webster JC+, *Am J Obstet Gynecol* 131, 700

Note: Adverse reactions can occur months after therapy has been discontinued

GOSERELIN

Trade name: Zoladex (AstraZeneca)
Other common trade name: *Prozoladex*
Indications: Breast and prostate carcinoma, endometriosis
Category: Gonadotropin-releasing analog hormone
Half-life: 5 hours

Reactions

Skin

Chills
Diaphoresis (1–10%)
Edema (1–10%)
Hot flashes (>10%)
(2002): Gommersall LM+, *Expert Opin Pharmacother* 3(12), 1685
(1993): Bressler LR+, *Ann Pharmacother* 27, 182
Rash (sic) (1–10%)
Urticaria

Hair

Hair – alopecia
(2002): Jonat W+, *J Clin Oncol* 20(24), 4628

Other

Anaphylactoid reactions
(1996): Raj SG+, *Am J Med Sci* 312, 187
Gynecomastia (>10%)
Hypersensitivity
(1996): Raj SG+, *Am J Med Sci* 312, 187
Injection-site pain (1–10%)
Injection-site papules & nodules (sic)
(2002): Cunha AP+, *World Congress Dermatol* Poster, 0095

Mastodynia (1–10%)
  (2002): Gommersall LM+, *Expert Opin Pharmacother* 3(12), 1685
Relapsing polychondritis
  (1997): Labarthe MP+, *Dermatology* 195, 391

GRANISETRON

Trade name: Kytril (Roche)
Other common trade name: *Kevatril*
Indications: Chemotherapy-related emesis
Category: Antiemetic; Serotonin antagonist
Half-life: 3–4 hours; cancer patients: 10–12 hours

Reactions

Skin
Allergic reactions (sic)
  (2001): Kanny G+, *J Allergy Clin Immunol* 108(6), 1059
Exanthems
Hot flashes (<1%)
Rash (sic)
Urticaria

Hair
Hair – alopecia (3%)

Other
Anaphylactoid reactions
Dysgeusia (2%)
Headache
Hypersensitivity

GRANULOCYTE COLONY-STIMULATING FACTOR (GCSF)

Generic name:
  Filgrastim (rG-CSF)
    Trade name: Neupogen (Amgen)
  Sargramostin (rGM-CSF)
    Trade names: Leukine (Immunex) (Berlex); Prokine
Other common trade names: *Grasin; Leucogen; Neupogen 30*
Indications: Bone marrow allograft and autograft
Category: Hematopoietic growth factor; Neutrophil stimulator
Half-life: filgrastim: 3.5 hours; sargramostin: 2–3 hours

Reactions

Skin
Acne
  (1996): Lee PK+, *J Am Acad Dermatol* 34, 855
Acral erythema
  (1995): Komamura H+, *J Dermatol* 22(2), 116
Acute febrile neutrophilic dermatosis (Sweet's syndrome)
  (2002): Brazzelli V+, *World Congress Dermatol* Poster, 0089
  (2001): Matsumura T+, *Br J Haematol* 113(1), 1
  (2001): Prendiville J+, *Pediatr Dermatol* 18(5), 417 (2 cases)
  (2000): Malone JC+, *Arch Dermatol* 345 (passim)
  (1999): Arbetter KR+, *Am J Hematol* 61, 126
  (1999): Veres K+, *Orv Hetil* (Hungarian) 140, 1059
  (1998): Chao SC+, *J Formos Med Assoc* 96, 276
  (1998): Hasegawa M+, *Eur J Dermatol* 8, 503 (2 patients)
  (1998): Merkel PA, *Curr Opin Rheumatol* 10, 45
  (1996): Garty BZ+, *Pediatrics* 97, 401
  (1996): Jain KK, *Cutis* 57, 107

(1996): Petit T+, *Lancet* 347, 690
(1996): Prevost-Blank PL+, *J Am Acad Dermatol* 35, 995
(1996): Richard MA+, *J Am Acad Dermatol* 35, 629
(1996): Shimizu T+, *J Pediatr Hematol Oncol* 18, 282
(1995): Shiga Y+, *Rinsho Ketsueki* (Japanese) 36, 353
(1995): Suzuki Y+, *Br J Dermatol* 133, 483
(1994): Fukutoku M+, *Br J Haematol* 86, 645
(1994): Johnson ML+, *Arch Dermatol* 130, 77
(1994): Reuss-Borst MA+, *Leuk Lymphoma* 15, 261
(1994): van Kamp H+, *Br J Haematol* 86, 415
(1993): Paydas S+, *Br J Haematol* 85, 191
(1992): Karp DL, *Ann Intern Med* 117, 875
(1992): Park JW+, *Ann Intern Med* 116, 996
(1991): Ross HJ+, *Cancer* 68, 441
(1990): Morioka N+, *J Am Acad Dermatol* 23, 247
(1989): Groopman JE+, *N Engl J Med* 321, 1449
(1989): Kluin-Nelemans JC+, *Br J Haematol* 73, 419
Diaphoresis
  (2000): Khoury H+, *Bone Marrow Transplant* 25, 1197
Erythema
  (1990): Farmer KL+, *Arch Dermatol* 126, 1243
  (1989): Groopman JE+, *N Engl J Med* 321, 1449
Erythema nodosum
  (1994): Nomiyama J+, *Am J Hematol* 47, 333
Exanthems
  (1996): Glass LF+, *J Am Acad Dermatol* 34, 455
  (1995): McMullin MF+, *Clin Rheumatol* 14, 204
  (1995): Scott GA, *Am J Dermatopathol* 17, 107
  (1994): Sasaki O+, *Intern Med* 33, 641
  (1993): Samlaska CP+, *Arch Dermatol* 129, 645
  (1993): Yamashita N+, *J Dermatol* 20, 473
  (1991): Cohen PR+, *J Am Acad Dermatol* 25, 734
  (1991): Horn TD+, *Arch Dermatol* 127, 49 (>5%)
  (1990): Farmer KL+, *Arch Dermatol* 126, 1243
  (1990): Lazarus H+, *Proc Am Soc Clin Oncol* 9, 15
  (1988): Brandt SJ+, *N Engl J Med* 318, 869 (63%)
Exfoliative dermatitis
  (1988): Brandt SJ+, *N Engl J Med* 318, 869 (10%)
Flushing (>10%)
  (2000): Khoury H+, *Bone Marrow Transplant* 25, 1197
Folliculitis
  (1992): Ostlere LS+, *Br J Dermatol* 127, 193
Lichenoid eruption
  (2002): Brazzelli V+, *World Congress Dermatol* Poster, 0089
Linear IgA bullous dermatosis
  (1999): Kano Y+, *Eur J Dermatol* 9, 122
Neutrophilic eccrine hidradenitis
  (1998): Bachmeyer C+, *Br J Dermatol* 139, 354
Panniculitis, necrotizing
  (2000): Dereure O+, *Br J Dermatol* 142, 834
Peripheral edema (1–10%)
Pruritus
  (1990): Farmer KL+, *Arch Dermatol* 126, 1243
  (1990): Steward WP+, *Int J Cell Cloning* 8, 335
  (1989): Steward WP+, *Br J Cancer* 59, 142 (1–5%)
Psoriasis
  (2001): Yonei T+, *Nihon Kokyuki Gakkai Zasshi* 39(6), 438
  (1998): Cho SG+, *J Korean Med Sci* 13, 685
  (1996): Kavanaugh A, *Am J Med* 101, 567
Pyoderma gangrenosum
  (1998): Merkel PA, *Curr Opin Rheumatol* 10, 45
  (1991): Ross HJ+, *Cancer* 68, 441
Rash (sic)
Urticaria
Vasculitis
  (1999): Andavolu MV+, *Ann Hematol* 78, 79
  (1998): Merkel PA, *Curr Opin Rheumatol* 10, 45
  (1995): Couderc LJ+, *Respir Med* 89, 237
  (1995): Farhey YD+, *J Rheumatol* 22, 1179

(1995): Vidarsson B+, *Am J Med* 98, 589
(1994): Jain KK, *J Am Acad Dermatol* 31, 213
(1994): Johnson ML+, *Arch Dermatol* 130, 77
(1990): Farmer KL+, *Arch Dermatol* 126, 1243
(1989): Kluin-Nelemans JC+, *Br J Haematol* 73, 419

Hair
Hair – alopecia (>10%)
(1990): Lazarus H+, *Proc Am Soc Clin Oncol* 9, 15

Other
Anaphylactoid reactions (<1%)
(2000): Khoury H+, *Bone Marrow Transplant* 25, 1197
(1999): Dupre D+, *Ann Dermatol Venereol* (French) 126, 161
(1999): Keung YK+, *Bone Marrow Transplant* 23, 200
Arthralgia
(2002): Tsukadaira A+, *Ann Rheum Dis* 61(9), 849
Death
(2002): Kikuchi M+, *Nippon Ronen Igakkai Zasshi* 39(4), 433
Injection-site bullous eruption
(1990): Farmer KL+, *Arch Dermatol* 126, 1243
Injection-site erythema
(1995): Scott GA, *Am J Dermatopathol* 17, 107
Injection-site lichenoid reaction
(1999): Viallard AM+, *Dermatology* 198, 301
Injection-site nodules (sic)
(1990): Farmer KL+, *Arch Dermatol* 126, 1243
Injection-site pain (1–10%)
Injection-site pruritus
(1990): Farmer KL+, *Arch Dermatol* 126, 1243
Injection-site urticaria
(1995): Scott GA, *Am J Dermatopathol* 17, 107
Lymphoproliferative disease
(1994): De la Rubia J+, *Bone Marrow Transplantation* 14, 475
(1994): Kawach Y+, *Leukemia and Lymphoma* 13, 509
Mucositis
(1999): Crawford J+, *Cytokines Cell Mol Ther* 5, 187
Myalgia (>10%)
Oral mucosal lesions
(1990): Lazarus H+, *Proc Am Soc Clin Oncol* 9, 15
Stomatitis (>10%)

GREEN TEA

Scientific names: *Camellia sinensis; Camellia thea; Camellia theifera; Thea bohea; Thea sinensis; Thea viridis*
Family: Theaceae
Trade and other common names: Chinese tea
Category: Astringent; Improved cognition
Purported indications and other uses: Improving cognitive performance, stomach disorders, nausea, vomiting, diarrhea, anticancer, headaches, Crohn's disease. Topical: soothe sunburn, bleeding gums, reduce sweating
Half-life: N/A
Clinically important, potentially hazardous interactions with: warfarin

Reactions

Skin
None

Other
Confusion
(2003): Jatoi A+, *Cancer* 97(6), 1442

Note: Tea is consumed as a beverage

GREPAFLOXACIN*

Indications: Various infections caused by susceptible organisms
Category: Fluoroquinolone antibiotic
Half-life: 5–12 hours

Reactions

Skin
Acne (<1%)
Balanitis (<1%)
Cheilitis (<1%)
Diaphoresis (<1%)
Edema (<1%)
Exanthems (<1%)
Exfoliative dermatitis (<1%)
Facial edema (<1%)
Fungal dermatitis (sic) (<1%)
Herpes simplex (<1%)
Peripheral edema (<1%)
Photosensitivity
(1997): Ferguson J+, *J Antimicrob Chemother* 40, 93
(1997): Stahlmann R+, *J Antimicrob Chemother* 40, 83
Phototoxicity (2%)
(2000): Traynor NJ+, *Toxicol Vitr* 14, 275
(1998): Lode H, *Infect Med* 15 (Suppl 1), 28
Pruritus (<1%)
Rash (sic) (1.9%)
(1998): Lode H, *Infect Med* 15 (Suppl 1), 28
(1997): Stahlmann R+, *J Antimicrob Chemother* 40, 83
Toxic epidermal necrolysis (<1%)
Urticaria (<1%)
Vesiculobullous eruption (<1%)
Xerosis (<1%)

Hair
Hair – alopecia (<1%)

Other
Ageusia (<1%)
Bromhidrosis (<1%)
Dysgeusia (17%) (metallic taste)
(1998): Chodosh S+, *Antimicrob Agents Chemother* 42, 114
(1998): Lode H, *Infect Med* 15 (Suppl 1), 28
(1997): Stahlmann R+, *J Antimicrob Chemother* 40, 83
Gingivitis (<1%)
Glossitis (<1%)
Hyperesthesia (<1%)
Hypersensitivity
Myalgia (<1%)
Oral candidiasis (<1%)
Oral ulceration (<1%)
Paresthesias (<1%)
Parosmia (<1%)
Stomatitis (<1%)
Tendinitis
Tendon rupture
Tongue disorder (sic) (<1%)
Tongue edema (<1%)
Tongue pigmentation (<1%)
Vaginitis (3.3%)
Xerostomia (1.1%)

*Note: Grepafloxacin has been withdrawn in the USA

GRISEOFULVIN

Trade names: Fulvicin (Schering); Grifulvin V (Ortho); Gris-PEG (Allergan)
Other common trade names: *Fulcin; Fulvina P/G; Grisefuline; Griseostatin; Grisovin; Likudin M; Polygris*
Indications: Fungal infections of the skin, hair and nails
Category: Antifungal
Half-life: 9–24 hours
Clinically important, potentially hazardous interactions with: alcohol, midazolam

Reactions

Skin
Allergic reactions (sic) (1–5%)
  (1971): *Med Lett* 13, 55
Angioedema (<1%)
  (1994): Gupta AK+, *J Am Acad Dermatol* 30, 677 (passim)
  (1989): Rustin MHA+, *Br J Dermatol* 120, 455
  (1961): Goldblatt S, *Arch Dermatol* 83, 936
Angular stomatitis
  (1994): Gupta AK+, *J Am Acad Dermatol* 30, 677 (passim)
Bullous eruption (<1%)
  (1995): Meffert JJ+, *Cutis* 56, 279
  (1960): O'Farrell NM, *Arch Dermatol* 82, 424
Candidiasis
  (1972): Bessiere L, *Bull Soc Fr Dermatol Syphiligr* (French) 79, 560
Cold urticaria
  (1989): Rustin MHA+, *Br J Dermatol* 120, 455
  (1965): Chang T, *JAMA* 193, 848
Erythema multiforme (<1%)
  (1994): Gupta AK+, *J Am Acad Dermatol* 30, 677 (passim)
  (1990): Almeida L+, *J Am Acad Dermatol* 23, 855
  (1989): Rustin MHA+, *Br J Dermatol* 120, 455
  (1981): Walinga H+, *Ned Tijdschr Geneeskd* (Dutch) 125, 729
  (1961): Sternberg TH+, *Med Clin North Am* 45, 781
Exanthems
  (1997): Litt JZ, Beachwood, OH (personal case) (observation in a 10–year–old boy)
  (1994): Gupta AK+, *J Am Acad Dermatol* 30, 677 (passim)
  (1993): Gaudin JL+, *Gastroenterol Clin Biol* 17, 145
  (1992): Breathnach SM+, *Adverse Drug Reactions and the Skin* Blackwell, Oxford, 169 (passim)
  (1989): Miyagawa S+, *Am J Med* 87, 100
  (1972): Von Pohler M+, *Dermatol Monatsschr* (German) 158, 383
Exfoliative dermatitis
  (1989): Rustin MHA+, *Br J Dermatol* 120, 455
  (1964): Reaves LE, *J Am Geriatr Soc* 12, 889
Fixed eruption (<1%)
  (1998): Mahboob A+, *Int J Dermatol* 37, 833
  (1994): Gupta AK+, *J Am Acad Dermatol* 30, 677 (passim)
  (1989): Boudghene-Stambouli O+, *Dermatologica* 179, 92
  (1989): Rustin MHA+, *Br J Dermatol* 120, 455
  (1984): Feinstein A+, *J Am Acad Dermatol* 10, 915
  (1981): Thyagarajan K+, *Mykosen* (German) 24, 482
  (1977): Savage J, *Br J Dermatol* 97, 107
Flushing
  (1992): Shelley WB+, *Advanced Dermatologic Diagnosis* WB Saunders, 582 (passim)
Hemorrhage (sic)
  (1992): Breathnach SM+, *Adverse Drug Reactions and the Skin* Blackwell, Oxford, 169 (passim)
Herpes zoster
  (1969): Chistiakov AM, *Vestn Dermatol Venerol* (Russian) 43, 76
Hypohidrosis

  (1986): Duvanel T, *Ann Dermatol Venereol* (French) 113, 471
Jarisch–Herxheimer reaction
  (1993): Amita DB+, *Clin Exp Dermatol* 18, 389
Leprosy (exacerbation)
  (1982): Shulman DG+, *Arch Dermatol* 118, 909
Lichenoid eruption
  (1994): Gupta AK+, *J Am Acad Dermatol* 30, 677 (passim)
  (1961): Sternberg TH+, *Med Clin North Am* 45, 781
Lupus erythematosus
  (1995): Bonilla-Felix M+, *Pediatr Nephrol* 9, 478
  (1994): Gupta AK+, *J Am Acad Dermatol* 30, 677 (passim)
  (1994): Yung RL+, *Rheum Dis Clin North Am* 20, 61
  (1990): Okazaki H+, *Ryumachi* (Japanese) 30, 418
  (1989): Miyagawa S+, *Am J Med* 87, 100
  (1989): Miyagawa S+, *J Am Acad Dermatol* 21, 343
  (1985): Madhok R+, *BMJ* 291, 249 (fatal)
  (1980): Condemi JJ, *Geriatrics* 35(3), 81
  (1976): Watsky MS+, *Cutis* 17, 361
  (1968): Shinskii GE+, *Sov Med* (Russian) 31, 92
  (1966): Anderson W+, *J Med Soc N J* 63, 161
  (1966): Lee SL+, *Arch Intern Med* 117, 620
  (1963): Steagall RW, *Arch Dermatol* 88, 218
  (1962): Alexander S, *Br J Dermatol* 74, 72
Mucocutaneous lymph node syndrome (Kawasaki syndrome)
Petechiae
  (1994): Gupta AK+, *J Am Acad Dermatol* 30, 677 (passim)
  (1960): Smith NG, *Arch Dermatol* 81, 981
Photosensitivity (1–10%)
  (1994): Gupta AK+, *J Am Acad Dermatol* 30, 677 (passim)
  (1989): Kojima K+, *J Dermatol* (Tokio) 15, 76
  (1989): Miyagawa S+, *Am J Med* 87, 100
  (1989): Rustin MHA+, *Br J Dermatol* 120, 455
  (1988): Kawabe Y+, *Photodermatol* 5, 272
  (1988): Kojima T+, *J Dermatol* 15, 76
  (1986): Ljunggren B+, *Photodermatol* 3, 26
  (1983): Hawk JLM, *Clin Exp Dermatol* 9, 300
  (1977): Martins JE+, *Rev Hosp Clin Fac Med Sao Paulo* (Portuguese) 32, 1
  (1976): Jarratt M, *Int J Dermatol* 15, 317
  (1972): Gotz H, *Arch Dermatol Forsch* (German) 244, 391
  (1969): Kalivas J, *JAMA* 209, 1706
  (1967): Tarsitani F+, *Policlinico Prat* (Italian) 74, 329
  (1966): Kobori T+, *J Asthma Res* 3, 213
  (1965): Chang T, *JAMA* 193, 848
  (1961): Lamb JH+, *Arch Dermatol* 83, 568
  (1961): Sternberg TH+, *Med Clin North Am* 45, 781
  (1960): Quero R, *J Invest Dermatol* 34, 283
Pigmentation
  (1968): Vollum DI, *Trans St Johns Hosp Dermatol Soc* 54, 204
  (1964): Durand P+, *Minerva Med* (Italian) 55, 2422
Pityriasis rosea
Pruritus (<1%)
  (1994): Gupta AK+, *J Am Acad Dermatol* 30, 677 (passim)
  (1989): Rustin MHA+, *Br J Dermatol* 120, 455
  (1960): Quero R, *J Invest Dermatol* 34, 283
  (1960): Smith NG, *Arch Dermatol* 81, 981
Purpura
  (1967): Lockey SD, *Med Sci* 18, 43
Rash (sic) (>10%)
Seborrheic dermatitis
  (1962): Brodthagen H, *Acta Derm Venereol* (Stockh) 42, 345
Stevens–Johnson syndrome
  (1989): Rustin MHA+, *Br J Dermatol* 120, 455
  (1981): Walinga H+, *Ned Tijdschr Geneeskd* (Dutch) 125, 729
  (1973): Belkin BG+, *Vestn Dermatol Venerol* (Russian) 47, 61
Toxic epidermal necrolysis
  (1991): Correia O+, *Ann Fr Anesth Reanim* (French) 10, 493
  (1990): Mion G+, *Ann Fr Anesth Reanim* (French) 9, 305 (fatal)
  (1989): Mion G+, *Lancet* 2, 1331 (fatal)

(1988): Taylor B+, *J Am Acad Dermatol* 19, 565
Urticaria (>10%)
  (1989): Rustin MHA+, *Br J Dermatol* 120, 455
  (1984): Feinstein A+, *J Am Acad Dermatol* 10, 915
  (1963): Driscoll BJO, *BMJ* 2, 503
  (1963): Fisher AA, *Arch Dermatol* 87, 660
  (1961): Goldblatt S, *Arch Dermatol* 83, 936
Vasculitis
  (1994): Gupta AK+, *J Am Acad Dermatol* 30, 677 (passim)
  (1970): Livingood CS+, *Cutis* 6, 1346

Nails

Nails – subungual hemorrhages
Nails – yellow
  (1986): Duvanel T, *Ann Dermatol Venereol* (French) 113, 471

Other

Acute intermittent porphyria
  (1965): Berman A+, *JAMA* 192, 1005
Anaphylactoid reactions
  (1977): Fel'ker Ala+, *Vestn Dermatol Venerol* (Russian)
    February, 78
Black tongue
  (1994): Gupta AK+, *J Am Acad Dermatol* 30, 677 (passim)
Death
Dysgeusia
  (1995): Hofmann H+, *Arch Dermatol* 131, 919
  (1994): Gupta AK+, *J Am Acad Dermatol* 30, 677 (passim)
  (1971): Fogan L, *Ann Intern Med* 74, 795
Glossodynia
  (1994): Gupta AK+, *J Am Acad Dermatol* 30, 677 (passim)
Gynecomastia
  (1994): Gupta AK+, *J Am Acad Dermatol* 30, 677 (passim)
  (1968): Vollum DI, *Trans St Johns Hosp Dermatol Soc* 54, 204
Headache
Hypogeusia
  (1971): Fogan L, *Ann Intern Med* 74, 795
Oral candidiasis (1–10%)
  (1994): Gupta AK+, *J Am Acad Dermatol* 30, 677 (passim)
Paresthesias
  (1994): Gupta AK+, *J Am Acad Dermatol* 30, 677 (passim)
Porphyria
  (1980): Smith AG+, *Clin Haematol* 9, 399
  (1969): Kalivas J, *JAMA* 209, 1706
  (1968): Watson CJ+, *Arch Dermatol* 98, 451
  (1967): Lochhead AC+, *Br J Dermatol* 79, 96
  (1966): Ziprowski L+, *Arch Dermatol* 93, 21
  (1965): Berman A+, *JAMA* 192, 1005
  (1964): Redeker AG+, *JAMA* 188, 466
  (1963): Editorial, *Lancet* 1, 870
  (1963): Rimington C+, *Lancet* 2, 318
Porphyria cutanea tarda
  (1970): Thiers H+, *Arch Belg Dermatol Syphiligr* (French) 26, 463
Protoporphyria
  (1990): Gederaas OA+, *Photodermatol Photoimmunol Photomed* 7, 82
  (1983): Poh-Fitzpatrick MB+, *J Clin Invest* 72, 1449
  (1970): Perrot H+, *Experientia* (French) 26, 256
Serum sickness
  (1994): Gupta AK+, *J Am Acad Dermatol* 30, 677 (passim)
  (1989): Rustin MHA+, *Br J Dermatol* 120, 455
Stomatodynia
Xerostomia
  (1994): Gupta AK+, *J Am Acad Dermatol* 30, 677 (passim)

GUANABENZ

Trade name: Wytensin (Wyeth)
Other common trade names: *Rexitene; Wytens*
Category: Alpha-2-adrenoceptor blocker; Antihypertensive
Half-life: 7–10 hours

Reactions

Skin
Edema (<3%)
Hyperhidrosis
Pruritus (<3%)
Rash (sic) (<3%)

Other
Dysgeusia (<3%)
Gynecomastia (<3%)
Headache
Sialorrhea
Xerostomia (28%)
  (1988): Bork K, *Cutaneous Side Effects of Drugs* WB Saunders, 307

GUANADREL

Trade name: Hylorel (Medeva)
Indications: Hypertension
Category: Adrenergic agonist; Antihypertensive
Half-life: 5–45 hours (terminal)

Reactions

Skin
Peripheral edema (28.6%)

Other
Glossitis (8.4%)
Headache
Paresthesias (25.1%)
Xerostomia (1.7%)

GUANETHIDINE

Trade name: Ismelin (Novartis)
Other common trade names: *Apo-Guanethidine; Ismeline*
Indications: Hypertension
Category: Alpha-2-adrenoceptor blocker; Antihypertensive
Half-life: 5–10 days
Clinically important, potentially hazardous interactions with: amitriptyline, amoxapine, benzphetamine, chlorpromazine, clomipramine, desipramine, doxepin, **ephedra**, ephedrine, imipramine, insulin, insulin glargine, minoxidil, nortriptyline, protriptyline, tricyclic antidepressants, trimipramine

Reactions

Skin
Dermatitis (sic)
Exanthems
Fixed eruption
  (1966): Rastogi SK, *J Indian Med Assoc* 47, 31

Lupus erythematosus
Peripheral edema (>10%)
Purpura
Urticaria
Vasculitis
  (1964): Dewar HA+, *BMJ* 2, 609 (polyarteritis nodosa?)

Hair
Hair – alopecia

Other
Glossitis (5%)
Headache
Myalgia
Paresthesias (16%)
Priapism
Sialorrhea
Xerostomia (1–10%)

GUANFACINE

Trade name: Tenex (Wyeth)
Other common trade names: *Entulic; Estulic*
Indications: Hypertension
Category: Alpha-2-adrenoceptor blocker; Antihypertensive
Half-life: 10–30 hours

Reactions

Skin
Dermatitis (sic) (<3%)

Diaphoresis (<3%)
  (1991): Wilson MF+, *J Clin Pharmacol* 31, 318
  (1990): Mosqueda-Garcia R, *Am J Med Sci* 299, 73
  (1986): Sorkin EM+, *Drugs* 31, 301 (3%)
Edema
Exanthems
Exfoliative dermatitis
Peripheral edema
  (1991): Oster JR+, *Arch Intern Med* 151, 1638
Pruritus (<3%)
  (1991): Wilson MF+, *J Clin Pharmacol* 31, 318
Purpura (<3%)
Rash (sic)
  (1990): Lewin A+, *J Clin Pharmacol* 30, 1081
Urticaria

Hair
Hair – alopecia

Other
Dysgeusia (<3%)
  (1988): Cornish LA, *Clin Pharm* 7, 187
Headache
Paresthesias (<3%)
Sialorrhea
Tinnitus
Xerostomia (47%)
  (1991): Wilson MF+, *J Clin Pharmacol* 31, 318
  (1990): Lewin A+, *J Clin Pharmacol* 30, 1081
  (1990): Mosqueda-Garcia R, *Am J Med Sci* 299, 73
  (1988): Board AW+, *Clin Ther* 10, 761
  (1988): Cornish LA, *Clin Pharm* 7, 187
  (1988): Van Zweiten PA, *Am J Cardiol* 61, 6D

HALOPERIDOL

Trade name: Haldol (Ortho-McNeil)
Other common trade names: *Dozic; Duraperidol; Haloper; Peridol; Seranace; Serenace*
Indications: Psychoses, Tourette's disorder
Category: Phenothiazine antipsychotic; Sedative
Half-life: 20 hours
Clinically important, potentially hazardous interactions with: fluoxetine, lithium, methotrexate, propranolol

Reactions

Skin
Acne
Cellulitis
  (1982): Sacks HS, *Hosp Pract Off Ed* 17, 179
Dermatitis (<1%)
Diaphoresis
  (2001): Kane JM+, *Arch Gen Psychiatry* 58(10), 965
Exanthems
Exfoliative dermatitis
Flushing
  (1972): Meyler L+, *Side Effects of Drugs Annual* 7 Excerpta Medica, Amsterdam
Neuroleptic malignant syndrome
  (2003): Spivak M+, *Can J Psychiatry* 48(1), 66 (with clozapine)
  (2002): Bhan S+, *Asian Cardiovasc Thorac Ann* 10(4), 365
  (2002): Neu P+, *Pharmacopsychiatry* 35(1), 26
  (2001): Reeves RR+, *Ann Pharmacother* 35(6), 698 (with risperidone and mirtazapine)
  (2001): Russell CS+, *Obstet Gynecol* 98(5), 906
  (2001): Wang HC+, *Mov Disord* 16(4), 765
Pemphigus foliaceus
  (2003): Perez Espana+, *Med Clin* (Barc) 120(3), 117
Photo-recall phenomenon
  (2002): Thami GP+, *Postgrad Med J* 78(916), 116
Photosensitivity (<1%)
  (2002): Thami GP+, *Postgrad Med* 78(916), 116 (pellagra-like)
  (1970): *Med Lett* 12, 104
  (1964): Gerle B, *Acta Psychiatr Scand* 40, 65
Pigmentation (<1%)
Pruritus (<1%)
Purpura
Rash (sic) (<1%)
Seborrheic dermatitis
  (1984): Binder RL+, *J Clin Psychiatry* 45, 125
  (1983): Binder RL+, *Arch Dermatol* 119, 473
Urticaria

Hair
Hair – alopecia (<1%)
  (2000): Mercke Y+, *Ann Clin Psychiatry* 12, 35
Hair – alopecia areata
  (1994): Kubota T+, *Jpn J Psychiatry Neurol* 48, 579
  (1993): Kubota T+, *Acta Neurol Napoli* 15, 200 (3 cases)
Hair – depigmentation
  (1964): Simpson GM+, *Clin Pharmacol Ther* 5, 310 (graying and fading)

Other
Death
  (2002): Remijnse PL+, *Ned Tijdschr Geneeskd* 146(16), 768
  (2002): Veltkamp R, *Ned Tijdschr Geneeskd* 146(27), 1301
  (2002): Vorel-Havelkova E+, *Ned Tijdschr Geneeskd* 146(27), 1301
  (2001): Glassman AH+, *Am J Psychiatry* 158(11), 1774
Galactorrhea (<1%)

Gynecomastia (<1%)
Headache
Injection-site hypersensitivity
  (1992): Hay J, *J Clin Psychiatry* 53, 256
Injection-site pain
  (1990): Hamann GL+, *J Clin Psychiatry* 51, 502
Injection-site reactions (sic)
  (1995): Maharaj K+, *J Clin Psychiatry* 56, 172
  (1992): Reinke M+, *J Clin Psychiatry* 53, 415
  (1990): Hamann GL+, *J Clin Psychiatry* 51, 502
Mastodynia
Parkinsonism (pseudo)
Priapism (<1%)
Rhabdomyolysis
  (1996): Meltzer HY+, *Neuropsychopharmacology* 15(4), 395
  (1984): Cavanaugh JJ+, *J Clin Psychiatry* 45, 356
Sialorrhea
  (2001): Kane JM+, *Arch Gen Psychiatry* 58(10), 965
Tardive dyskinesia
  (1990): Miller LG+, *South Med J* 83(5), 525 (37%)
Torsades de pointes
  (2003): Hassaballa HA+, *Am J Ther* 10(1), 58
Tremor
  (2001): Russell CS+, *Obstet Gynecol* 98(5), 906
Xerostomia (<1%)
  (2001): Kane JM+, *Arch Gen Psychiatry* 58(10), 965

HALOTHANE

Trade name: Fluothane (Wyeth)
Other common trade names: *Halothan; Trothane*
Indications: Induction and maintenance of general anesthesia
Category: Anesthetic
Half-life: N/A
Clinically important, potentially hazardous interactions with: aminophylline, atracurium, cisatracurium, doxacurium, epinephrine, non-depolarizing muscle relaxants, pancuronium, rapacuronium, rifampin, theophylline, vecuronium, xanthines

Reactions

Skin
Acne
  (1987): Guldager H, *Lancet* 1, 1211
  (1973): Gomez SW, *Anesth Analg* 52, 861
  (1973): Soper LE+, *Anesth Analg* 52, 125
Angioedema
  (1988): Slegers-Karsmakers S+, *Anesthesia* 43, 506
Exanthems
  (1988): Slegers-Karsmakers S+, *Anesthesia* 43, 506
Sensitivity (sic)
  (1979): Bodman R, *Br J Anaesth* 51, 1092 (to vapors)
Urticaria
  (1964): Cole WHJ, *Med J Aust* 2, 925

Hair
Hair – alopecia
  (1990): Gollnick H+, *Z Haut* (German) 65, 1128

Other
Rhabdomyolysis
  (1987): Rubiano R+, *Anesthesiology* 67(5), 856
  (1985): Sodano R+, *Minerva Anestesiol* 51(3), 109
  (1979): Bomholt A, *Ugeskr Laeger* 141, 925
  (1976): Moore WE+, *Anesth Analg* 55(5), 680 (with succinylcholine)

HAWTHORN (FRUIT, LEAF, FLOWER EXTRACT)

Scientific names: *Crataegus laevigata; Crataegus monogyna; Crataegus oxyacantha; Crataegus pentagyna*
Family: Rosaceae
Trade and other common names: Arterio-K; Aubepine; Basticrat; Born; Cardiplant; Cordapur; Coronal; Cratamed; Harthorne; Haw; HeartCare (Nature's Way); Hedgethorne; Maythorn; Nan Shanzha; Naranocor; Regulacor; Shanzha; Thorn Plum; Whitethorn
Trade names: Arterio-K, Basticrat, Born, Cardiplant, Cordapur, Coronal, Cratamed, HeartCare (Natures Way), Naranocor, Regulacor
Category: Improves cardiac function
Purported indications and other uses: Amenorrhea, arrhythmias, atherosclerosis, diuretic, hyperlipidemia, hypertension, hypotension, sedative, appetite stimulant, arthritis, enteritis, indigestion, sore throats. Topical: boils, sores and ulcers
Half-life: N/A
Clinically important, potentially hazardous interactions with: digoxin, vasodilators

Note: The American Herbal Products Association (AHPA) gives hawthorn a class 1 safety rating, indicating that it is very safe. However, hawthorn should be used with caution in patients with heart disease

Reactions

Skin
Allergic reactions (sic)
Diaphoresis
  (2002): Rigelsky JM+, *Am J Health Syst Pharm* 59(5), 417
Rash (sic) (hands)
  (2002): Rigelsky JM+, *Am J Health Syst Pharm* 59(5), 417
  (1996): Newall CA+, *A Guide For Healthcare Professionals* (London UK, Pharmaceutical Press)
Toxiderma
  (1984): Rogov VD, *Vestn Dermatol Venerol* 7, 46

Other
Dizziness
  (2003): Pittler MH+, *Am J Med* 114(8), 665
  (2002): Rigelsky JM+, *Am J Health Syst Pharm* 59(5), 417
Hypersensitivity
  (1984): Steinman HK+, *Contact Dermatitis* 11(5), 321

HENNA*

Scientific names: *Lawsonia alba; Lawsonia inermis*
Family: Lythraceae
Trade and other common names: Alcanna; Egyptian Privet; Hinai; Hinna; Inai; Jamaica Kina; Lawsone (2-hydroxy-1:4naphthaquione); Mehandi; Mehndi
Category: Anti-inflammatory
Purported indications and other uses: Analgesic, antipyretic, seborrheic dermatitis, fungal infections, gastrointestinal ulcers, sunscreen, dandruff, scabies, headache, jaundice, decorative tattoos, Used in cosmetics, body paint, hair dyes, hair care products
Half-life: N/A

Note: Black Henna is Henna plus paraphenylenediamine (PPD). PPD is added to henna to make it stain black. PPD is a transdermal toxin and may be used alone as hair dye or to stain skin black. Other products called 'black henna' may have indigo or food dyes added, and are generally not harmful to the skin. The (+PPD) following the references, below, indicates that this is Black Henna

Reactions

Skin
Adverse effects (sic)
  (2003): De Souza B+, *Plast Reconstr Surg* 111(7), 2487
  (2003): Wolf R+, *Dermatol Online J* 9(1), 3
Allergic reactions (sic)
  (2000): US Food and Drug Administration, Office of Cosmetics and Colors Fact Sheet
  (1970): Blohm SG+, *Acta Derm Venereol* 50, 49
  (1970): Rajka G+, *Acta Derm Venereol* 50, 51
Bullous eruption
Burning
Dermatitis
  (2003): Leggiadro RJ+, *J Pediatr* 142(5), 586
  (2003): Wolf R+, *Dermatol Online J* 9(1), 3
  (2002): Marcoux D+, *Pediatr Dermatol* 19(6), 498
  (2002): Neri I+, *Pediatr Dermatol* 19(6), 503
  (2002): Pegas JR+, *J Investig Allergol Clin Immunol* 12(1), 62
  (2002): Temesvari E+, *Contact Dermatitis* 47(4), 240
  (2002): van Zuuren+, *Ned Tijdschr Geneeskd* 146(28), 1332
  (2001): Di Lando A+, *Am J Contact Dermat* 12(3), 186
  (2001): Kulkarni PD+, *Cutis* 68(3):187, 229 (+PPD)
  (2001): Lauchl S+, *Swiss Med Wkly* 131, 199 (+PPD)
  (2001): Onder M+, *Int J Dermatol* 40(9), 577 (+PPD)
  (2001): Oztass MO+, *J Eur Acad Dermatol Venereol* 15(1), 91
  (2001): Thami GP+, *Allergy* 56(10), 1013
  (2000): Le Coz CJ+, *Arch Dermatol* 136(12), 1515 (+PPD)
  (2000): Lyon MJ+, *Arch Dermatol* 136(1), 124
  (2000): Nikkels AF+, *J Eur Acad Dermatol Venereol* 15(2), 140 (+PPD)
  (2000): Raison-Peyron N+, *Ann Dermatol Venereol* 127(12), 1083 (+PPD)
  (2000): Sidbury R+, *Am J Contact Dermat* 11(3), 182 (+PPD)
  (2000): Tosti A+, *Contact Dermatitis* 42(6), 356
  (1999): Gallo R+, *Contact Dermatitis* 40(1), 57
  (1999): Lestringant GG+, *Br J Dermatol* 141(3), 598
  (1999): Lewin PK, *CMAJ* 160(3), 310
  (1998): Nigam PK+, *Contact Dermatitis* 18(1), 55
  (1998): Wakelin SH+, *Contact Dermatitis* 39(2), 92 (+PPD)
  (1997): Downs AMR+, *Br Med J* 315, 1772 (+PPD)
  (1997): Etienne A+, *Contact Dermatitis* 37(4), 183
  (1997): Garcia Ortiz JC+, *Int Arch Allergy Immunol* 114(3), 298
  (1996): al-Sheik OA+, *Int J Dermatol* 35(7), 493
  (1992): Wantke F+, *Contact Dermatitis* 27(5), 346 (from Azo dyes)
  (1986): Gupta BN+, *Contact Dermatitis* 15(5), 303
  (1980): Pasricha JS+, *Contact Dermatitis* 6(4), 288
Eczema
  (2002): Suarez Fernandez R+, *Allergol Immunopathol (Madr)* 30(5), 292
Edema
  (2002): Marcoux D+, *Pediatr Dermatol* 19(6), 498
  (2001): Lauchl S+, *Swiss Med Wkly* 131, 199 (+PPD)
  (2001): Wohrl S+, *Eur Acad Dermatol Venereol* 15(5), 470 (+PPD)
Erythema
  (2002): Marcoux D+, *Pediatr Dermatol* 19(6), 498
  (2002): Schultz E+, *Int J Dermatol* 41(5), 301
  (2001): Lauchl S+, *Swiss Med Wkly* 131, 199 (+PPD)
Erythema multiforme
  (2001): Jappe U+, *Contact Dermatitis* 45(4), 249 (+PPD)
Keloid

(1999): Lewkin PK, *CMAJ* 160(3), 310
Lichenoid dermatitis
  (2002): Ferrer P+, *Cosmetic Dermatology* 15, 11
Lichenoid eruption
  (2002): Chung WH+, *Arch Dermatol* 138(1), 88 (+PPD)
  (2002): Schultz E+, *Int J Dermatol* 41(5), 301
  (2000): Rubegni P+, *Contact Dermatitis* 42(2), 117
Photosensitivity
Pigmentation
  (2002): Marcoux D+, *Pediatr Dermatol* 19(6), 498
  (2002): van Zuuren+, *Ned Tijdschr Geneeskd* 146(28), 1332
  (2001): Wohrl S+, *J Eur Acad Dermatol Venereol* 15(5), 470
    (+PPD)
Pruritus
  (2002): Suarez Fernandez+, *Allergol Immunopathol* (Madr)
    30(5), 292
  (2001): Lauchl S+, *Swiss Med Wkly* 131, 199 (+PPD)
  (2000): Sidbury R+, *Am J Contact Dermat* 11(3), 182 (+PPD)
Psoriasis
  (1991): El-Gammal SY, *Bull Indian Inst Hist Med Hyderabad*
    121(2), 125
Rash (sic)
Urticaria
  (1997): Downs AMR+, *Br Med J* 315, 1722
  (1996): Majoie IM+, *Am J Contact Dermat* 7(1), 38

Other
Death
  (2001): Devecioglu C+, *Turk J Pediatr* 43(1), 65
  (2001): Raupp P+, *Arch Dis Child* 85(5), 411
  (1992): Sir Hashim M+, *Ann Trop Paediatr* 12(1), 3 (+PDD)
Hypersensitivity
  (2001): Bolhaar ST+, *Allergy* 56(3), 248
  (2001): Kulkarni PD+, *Cutis* 68(3), 187 (+PPD)
  (2000): Lyon MJ+, *Arch Dermatol* 136(1), 124
  (2000): Nikkels AF+, *J Eur Acad Dermatol Venereol* 15(2), 140
    (+PPD)
  (1996): Abdulla KA+, *Lancet* 348(9028), 658 (+PPD)
  (1996): Majoie IM+, *Am J Contact Dermat* 7(1), 38
  (1996): Ozsoylu S, *Lancet* 348(9035), 1173
  (1982): Starr JC+, *Ann Allergy* 48(2), 98
  (1979): Cronin E, *Contact Dermatitis* 5(3), 198
  (1976): Pepys J+, *Clin Allergy* 6(4), 399
Side effects (sic)
  (2000): Ernst E, *Br J Dermatol* 143(5), 923

*Note: Adverse side effects to pure henna are rare; those reported above may be due to additives. Henna tattoos were popularized by Madonna. Her black patterns, however, were created with body paint, not henna

HEPARIN

Trade names: Hep-Flush (Wyeth); Hep-Lock (Elkins-Sinn); Liquaemin (Organon)
Other common trade names: *Calcilean; Calciparin; Caprin; Hepalean; Heparin-Leo; Heparine; Liquemin; Uniparin*
Indications: Venous thrombosis, pulmonary embolism
Category: Anticoagulant
Half-life: 1.5 hours
Clinically important, potentially hazardous interactions with: aspirin, bivalirudin, butabarbital, **capsicum**, danaparoid, **dong quai**, **ginger**, **horse chestnut (bark, flower, leaf, seed)**, **red clover**, salicylates, tirofiban

Reactions

Skin
Allergic reactions (sic) (1–10%)
  (1997): Hermes B+, *Acta Derm Venereol* 77, 35
  (1972): Lebeaupin R+, *Anesth Analg* (Paris) (French) 29, 487
Angioedema (<1%)
Baboon syndrome
  (1993): Herfs H+, *Hautarzt* (German) 44, 466
Burning (sic) (soles)
  (1992): Breathnach SM+, *Adverse Drug Reactions and the Skin*
    Blackwell,Oxford, 249 (passim)
Chills
Dermatitis
  (1996): Boehncke WH+, *Contact Dermatitis* 35, 73
  (1996): Koch P+, *Contact Dermatitis* 34, 1256
  (1995): Krasovec M+, *Contact Dermatitis* 32, 135
  (1992): Valsecchi R+, *Contact Dermatitis* 26, 129
  (1988): Young E, *Contact Dermatitis* 19, 152
Ecchymoses
  (1985): Tuneu A+, *J Am Acad Dermatol* 12, 1072
  (1979): Stavorovsky M+, *Dermatologica* 158, 451
Erythema
Erythematous plaques (sic)
Exanthems
  (1996): Warkentin TE, *Br J Haematol* 92, 494
  (1994): Greiner D+, *Hautarzt* (German) 45, 569
Fixed eruption
  (1995): Mohammed KN, *Dermatology* 190, 91
Hemorrhage
  (1992): Breathnach SM+, *Adverse Drug Reactions and the Skin*
    Blackwell, Oxford, 249 (passim)
  (1986): Levine M+, *Semin Thromb Hemost* 12, 39
Lesions (sic)
  (1996): Warkentin TE, *Br J Haematology* 92, 494
Livedo reticularis
  (1993): Gross AS+, *Int J Dermatol* 32, 276
Necrosis
  (2003): Takwale A+, *Br J Dermatol* 148(6), 1292
  (2002): Denoel C+, *Rev Med Liege* 57(8), 502
  (2002): Wong G+, *World Congress Dermatol* Poster, 0133
  (2001): Andolfatto S+, *Ann Biol Clin* (Paris) 59(5), 651 (2 cases)
  (2001): Denton MD+, *Am J Nephrol* 21(4), 289
  (1997): Carter RL, *N Engl J Med* 336, 589
  (1997): Kumar PD, *N Engl J Med* 336, 588
  (1997): Libow LF+, *Cutis* 59, 242
  (1997): McCloskey RV, *N Engl J Med* 336, 588
  (1997): Schechter FG, *N Engl J Med* 336, 589
  (1996): Christiaens GC+, *N Engl J Med* 335, 715
  (1996): Whitmore SE+, *Arch Dermatol* 132, 341
  (1995): Balestra B, *Schweiz Med Wochenschr* (German) 125, 361
  (1994): Griffin JP, *Adverse Drug React Toxicol Rev* 13, 157

(1994): Leblanc M+, *Nephron* 68, 133
(1994): Peluso AM+, *Eur J Dermatol* 4, 127
(1994): Yoon TY+, *Ann Dermatol* 6, 74
(1993): Humphries JE, *Acta Haematol* 90, 52
(1993): Warkentin TE+, *Am J Med* 95, 662
(1993): Yates P+, *Clin Exp Dermatol* 18, 138
(1992): Calzavara-Pinton PG+, *EJD* 2, 171
(1992): Soundararajan R+, *Am J Med* 93, 467
(1992): Thomas D+, *Chest* 102, 1578
(1991): Humphries JE+, *Am J Kidney Dis* 17, 233
(1991): Ritchie AJ+, *Ulster Med J* 60, 248
(1990): Adcock DM+, *Semin Thromb Hemost* 16, 283
(1990): Bircher AJ+, *Br J Dermatol* 123, 507 (passim)
(1990): Fowlie J+, *Postgrad Med J* 66, 573
(1989): Armengol R+, *Med Clin (Barc)* (Spanish) 93, 699
(1989): Diem E, *Hautarzt* (German) 40, 239
(1989): Rongioletti F+, *Dermatologica* 178, 47
(1989): Vinti H+, *Presse Med* (French) 18, 128
(1988): Cohen GR+, *Obstet Gynecol* 73, 498
(1988): Hartman AR+, *J Vasc Surg* 7, 781
(1987): Alegre A+, *Med Clin (Barc)* (Spanish) 88, 170
(1987): Jones BF+, *Australas J Dermatol* 28, 117
(1986): Lim KB+, *Singapore Med J* 27, 356
(1985): Barthelemy H+, *Ann Dermatol Venereol* (French) 112, 245
(1985): Tuneu A+, *J Am Acad Dermatol* 12, 1072
(1984): Hasegawa GR, *Drug Intell Clin Pharm* 18, 313
(1984): Mathieu A+, *Ann Dermatol Venereol* (French) 111, 733
(1984): Monreal M+, *Lancet* 2, 820
(1984): Nodel'son SE+, *Ter Arkh* (Russian) 56, 118
(1984): Ulrick PJ+, *Med J Aust* 140, 287
(1983): Jehn U+, *Dtsch Med Wochenschr* (German) 108, 1148
(1983): Levine LE+, *Arch Dermatol* 119, 400
(1982): Isaacs P+, *Br Med J Clin Res Ed* 284, 201
(1982): No Author, *Am J Hosp Pharm* 39, 412
(1982): Shelley WB+, *J Am Acad Dermatol* 7, 674
(1981): Berkessy S+, *Orv Hetil* (Hungarian) 122, 3075
(1981): Jackson AM+, *Br Med J Clin Res Ed* 283, 1087
(1981): Kelly RA+, *JAMA* 246, 1582
(1980): Hall JC+, *JAMA* 244, 1831
(1979): White PW+, *Ann Surg* 190, 595

Peripheral edema
(1993): Phillips JK+, *Br J Haematol* 84, 349

Petechiae
(1979): Stavorovsky M+, *Dermatologica* 158, 451

Pruritus (<1%)

Purpura (>10%)

Rash (sic)

Scleroderma
(1985): Barthelemy H+, *Ann Dermatol Venereol* (French) 112, 245

Toxic dermatitis (sic)
(1996): Gallais V+, *Presse Med* (French) 25, 1040

Toxic epidermal necrolysis
(1991): Lemziakov TG+, *Vrach Delo* (Ukrainian) November, 113
(1985): Leung A, *JAMA* 253, 201

Ulcerations
(2001): Denton MD+, *Am J Nephrol* 21(4), 289

Urticaria (<1%)
(1992): Breathnach SM+, *Adverse Drug Reactions and the Skin* Blackwell, Oxford, 249 (passim)
(1990): Bircher AJ+, *Br J Dermatol* 123, 507 (passim)
(1975): Hancock BW+, *BMJ* 3, 746
(1964): Zinn WJ, *Am J Cardiol* 14, 36
(1962): Rajka G+, *Acta Derm Venereol* (Stockh) 42, 27

Vasculitis
(1989): Guillet G+, *J Am Acad Dermatol* 20, 1130
(1989): Korstanje MJ+, *Contact Dermatitis* 20, 283
(1982): Kearsley JH+, *Aust N Z J Med* 12, 288

(1979): Ranft K+, *Med Welt* (German) 30, 1489
(1979): Stavorovsky M+, *Dermatologica* 158, 451

Hair
Hair – alopecia
(1980): Jaques LB, *Pharmacol Rev* 31, 99
(1969): Baker H+, *Br J Dermatol* 81, 236

Nails
Nails – discoloration

Other
Anaphylactoid reactions
(1992): Breathnach SM+, *Adverse Drug Reactions and the Skin* Blackwell, Oxford, 249 (passim)
(1990): Bircher AJ+, *Br J Dermatol* 123, 507 (passim)

Gingivitis (>10%)

Headache

Hypersensitivity
(2002): Mora A+, *Contact Dermatitis* 47(3), 177
(2002): Nicolie B+, *Allerg Immunol (Paris* (Paris) 34(2), 47
(2000): Koch P+, *J Am Acad Dermatol* 42, 612
(1995): Sanders MN+, *Int J Dermatol* 34, 443
(1994): Patriarca G+, *Allergy* 49, 292
(1993): Dupin N+, *Ann Dermatol Venereol* (French) 120, 845
(1993): O'Donnell BF+, *Br J Dermatol* 129, 634
(1992): de Kort WJ+, *Ned Tijdschr Geneeskd* (Dutch) 136, 2379
(1992): Manoharan A, *Eur J Haematol* 48, 234
(1991): Rivers JK+, *Aust N Z J Surg* 61, 865
(1989): Korstanje MJ+, *Contact Dermatitis* 20, 383
(1989): Patrizi A+, *Contact Dermatitis* 20, 309
(1973): Curry N+, *Arch Intern Med* 132, 744

Injection-site eczematous patches (<1%)
(2000): Koch P+, *J Am Acad Dermatol* 42, 612
(1995): Mathelier-Fusade P+, *Presse Med* (French) 24, 323
(1993): Phillips JK+, *Br J Haematol* 84, 349 (erythema)
(1990): Bircher AJ+, *Br J Dermatol* 123, 507

Injection-site hematoma

Injection-site induration
(1993): Phillips JK+, *Br J Haematol* 84, 349
(1989): Guillet G+, *J Am Acad Dermatol* 20, 1130
(1989): Klein GF+, *J Am Acad Dermatol* 21, 703
(1987): Mayou SC+, *Br J Dermatol* 117, 664

Injection-site necrosis (<1%)
(1995): Mar AW+, *Australas J Dermatol* 36, 201
(1988): Cohen GR+, *Obstet and Gyn* 72, 498
(1984): Hasegawa GR, *Drug Intell Clin Pharm* 18, 313
(1980): Hall JC+, *JAMA* 244, 1831

Injection-site nodules
(2002): Funt SA+, *J Comput Assist Tomogr* 26(4), 520

Injection-site pain
(2001): Chan H, *J Adv Nurs* 35(6), 882

Injection-site plaques
(2000): Koch P+, *J Am Acad Dermatol* 42, 612
(1990): Bircher AJ+, *Br J Dermatol* 123, 507

Injection-site purpura
(2001): Chan H, *J Adv Nurs* 35(6), 882

Injection-site urticaria
(1995): Mathelier-Fusade P+, *Presse Med* (French) 24, 323

Priapism
(2001): Bauduer F+, *Presse Med* 30(8), 376
(2001): Bschleipfer TH+, *Int J Impot rES* 13(6), 357

HEPATITIS B VACCINE

Trade names: Comvax (Merck); Engerix B (GSK); Pediatrix (GSK); Recombivax HB (Merck); Twinrix (GSK)
Other common trade name: *Heptavax-B*
Indications: For immunization of infection caused by all known subtypes of hepatitis B virus
Category: Vaccine
Half-life: N/A

Reactions

Skin

Anetoderma
  (1997): Daoud MS+, *J Am Acad Dermatol* 36 (5 Pt 1), 779
Angioedema
  (1998): Barbaud A+, *Br J Dermatol* 139(5), 925
Bullous pemphigoid
  (2002): Erbagci Z, *J Dermatol* 29(12), 781
  (2002): Erbagci Z, *World Congress Dermatol* Poster 0315
Chills
Dermatomyositis
  (1998): Fernandez-Funez A+, *Med Clin* (Barc) 111(17), 675
Diaphoresis
Eczema (sic)
  (1999): Mc Kenna KE, *Contact Dermatitis* 40(3), 158
Erythema
Erythema multiforme
  (2000): Loche F+, *Clin Exp Dermatol* 25(2), 167
  (1994): Di Lernia+, *Pediatr Dermatol* 11(4), 363
Erythema nodosum
  (1993): Castresana-Isla CJ+, *J Rheumatol* 20(8), 1417
  (1990): Rogerson SJ+, *BMJ* 301, 345
  (1989): Goolsby PL, *N Engl J Med* 321, 1198
Erythromelalgia
  (1999): Rabaud C+, *J Rheumatol* 26(1), 233
Flushing
Gianotti–Crosti syndrome
  (2001): Tay YK, *Pediatr Dermatol* 18(3), 262
Granuloma annulare
  (1998): Wolf F+, *Eur J Dermatol* 8(6), 435 (generalized)
Granulomas (necrobiotic)
  (1998): Ajithkumar K+, *Clin Exp Dermatol* 23(5), 222
Granulomatous dermatitis (Churg–Strauss syndrome)
  (1998): Vanoli M+, *Ann Rheum Dis* 57(4), 256
Herpes zoster
Lichen planus
  (2002): Calista D+, *World Congress Dermatol* Poster, 0090
  (2001): Al-Khenaizan S, *J Am Acad Dermatol* 45(4), 614
  (2001): Aron-Moar A+, *Lupus* 10(3), 237
  (2000): Agrawal S+, *J Dermatol* 27(9), 618
  (1999): Rebora A+, *Dermatology* 198(1), 1
  (1999): Schupp P+, *Int J Dermatol* 38(10), 799
  (1998): Ferrando MN+, *Br J Dermatol* 139(2), 350
  (1998): Merigou D+, *Ann Dermatol Venereol* 125(6-7), 399
  (1997): Gisserot O+, *Presse Med* 26(16), 760
  (1995): Lefort A+, *Ann Dermatol Venereol* 122(10), 701
  (1994): Aubin F+, *Arch Dermatol* 130(10), 1329
  (1993): Trevisan G+, *Acta Derm Venereol* 73(1), 73
  (1990): Ciaccio M+, *Br J Dermatol* 122, 424
Lichen planus
  (2002): Schuh T+, *Hautarzt* 53(10), 650
Lichenoid eruption
  (2001): Usman A+, *Pediatr Dermatol* 18(2), 123
  (1997): Saywell CA+, *Australas J Dermatol* 38(3), 152
Lupus erythematosus

  (2000): Maillefert JF+, *Arthritis Rheum* 43(2), 468
  (1999): Senecal JL+, *Arthritis Rheum* 42(6), 1307
  (1998): Grotto I+, *Vaccine* 16(4), 329
  (1996): Grezard P+, *Ann Dermatol Venereol* 123(10), 657
  (1996): Guiserix J, *Nephron* 74(2), 441
  (1994): Mamoux V+, *Arch Pediatr* 1(3), 307
  (1992): Tudela P+, *Nephron* 62(2), 236
Morphea
  (2000): Schmutz JL+, *Presse Med* 29(19), 1046
Petechiae
Purpura
  (2002): Chave TA+, *World Congress Dermatol* Poster, 0093
  (2001): Conesa V+, *Haematologica* 86(3), E09
  (1999): Lliminana C+, *Med Clin* (Barc) 113(1), 39
  (1999): Muller A+, *Eur J Pediatr* 158 Suppl 3, S209
  (1998): Ronchi F+, *Arch Dis Child* 78(3), 273 (3 cases)
  (1994): Poullin P+, *Lancet* 344(8932), 1293
Rash (sic)
Raynaud's phenomenon
  (1990): Cockwell P+, *BMJ* 301, 1281
Reiter's syndrome
  (1994): Fraser PA+, *BMJ* 309(6967), 1513
  (1994): Hassan W+, *BMJ* 309(6947), 94
Sjøgren's syndrome
  (2000): Toussirot E+, *Arthritis Rheum* 43(9), 2139
Stevens–Johnson syndrome
Urticaria
  (2000): Barbaud A+, *Ann Dermatol Venereol* 127(6-7), 662
  (1998): Barbaud A+, *Br J Dermatol* 139(5), 925
  (1998): Grotto I+, *Vaccine* 16(4), 329
Vasculitis
  (2001): Saadoun D+, *Rev Med Interne* 22(2), 172
  (1999): Le Hello C, *Pathol Biol* (Paris) 47(3), 252
  (1999): Le Hello+, *J Rheumatol* 26(1), 191 (3 cases)
  (1998): Bui-Quang D+, *Presse Med* 27(26), 1321
  (1998): Grotto I+, *Vaccine* 16(4), 329
  (1998): Masse I+, *Presse Med* 27(20), 965
  (1997): Kerleau JM+, *Rev Interne Med* 18(6), 491 (necrotizing)
  (1993): Allen MB+, *Thorax* 48(5), 580
  (1990): Cockwell P+, *BMJ* 301, 1281

Hair

Hair – alopecia
  (1997): Wise RP+, *JAMA* 278(14), 1176 (46 cases)

Other

Anaphylactoid reactions
  (2000): *Prescrire Int* 9(46), 59
  (1998): Grotto I+, *Vaccine* 16(4), 329
  (1996): *MMWR Morb Mortal Wkly Rep* 45(RR-12), 1
  (1994): Stratton KR+, *JAMA* 271(20), 1602
Aphthous stomatitis
  (1996): Grezard P+, *Ann Dermatol Venereol* 123(10), 657
Arthralgia
Arthus reaction
  (2001): Froelich H+, *Clin Infect Dis* 33(6), 906 (with skin necrosis)
Death
  (1999): Niu MT+, *Pediatr Adolesc Med* 153(12), 1279
Guillain–Barré syndrome
  (2000): Sinsawaiwong S+, *J Med Assoc Thai* 83(9), 1124
  (1997): Kakar A+, *Indian J Pediatr* 64(5), 710
Headache
Hyperesthesia
Hypersensitivity
Injection-site ecchymoses
Injection-site edema
Injection-site erythema
Injection-site induration

Injection-site nodules (sic)
Injection-site pain (22%)
Injection-site pruritus
Myalgia
Oral lichenoid eruption
  (2000): Pemberton MN+, *Oral Surg Oral Med Oral Pathol Oral Radiol Endod* 89(6), 717
Paresthesias
Periarteritis nodosa
  (2003): Bourgeais AM+, *Ann Dermatol Venereol* 130(2), 205
  (2001): Saadoun D+, *Rev Med Interne* 22(2), 172
  (1988): Le Goff P+, *Presse Med* 17, 1763
Polymyalgia rheumatica
  (2001): Saadoun D+, *Rev Med Interne* 22(2), 172
Sclerotic plaques (sic)
  (1998): Gout O+, *Rev Neurol* (Paris) 154(3), 205
Serum sickness
  (2002): Arkachaisri T, *J Med Assoc Thai* 85, S607
Still's disease
  (1998): Grasland A+, *Rev Med Interne* 19(2), 134
Tinnitus
White dot syndrome (retinal)
  (1996): Baglivo E+, *Am J Ophthalmol* 122(3), 431

HEROIN

Trade name: Heroin
Indications: Recreational drug
Category: Diacetylmorphine; Semisynthetic narcotic; Substance abuse drug
Half-life: N/A

Reactions

Skin

Abscess
  (1990): Rasokat H, *Z Haut* (German) 65, 351
  (1987): Muller F+, *Infection* 15, 201
  (1987): Podzamczer D+, *J Am Acad Dermatol* 16, 386
  (1984): O'Sullivan M+, *Ir Med J* 77, 68
  (1980): Espiritu MB+, *Laryngoscope* 90, 1111 (neck)
  (1979): Webb D+, *West J Med* 130, 200
  (1971): Young AW+, *Arch Dermatol* 104, 80
Acanthosis nigricans
  (1973): Young AW+, *Am Fam Physician* 7, 79
  (1971): Young AW+, *Arch Dermatol* 104, 80
Acne
  (1973): Young AW+, *Am Fam Physician* 7, 79
Angioedema
  (1973): Young AW, *N Y State J Med* 73, 1681
Blistering (arms)
  (1995): Mielke-Ibrahim R+, *Dtsch Med Wochenschr* (German) 120, 55
Bullous impetigo
  (1973): Young AW, *N Y State J Med* 73, 1681
Burning
  (2002): Warner-Smith M+, *Addiction* 97(8), 963 (24%)
Candidiasis
  (1987): Bielsa I+, *Int J Dermatol* 26, 314 (systemic)
  (1987): Puig L+, *Int J Dermatol* 26, 257
  (1985): Calandra T+, *Eur J Clin Microbiol* 4, 340 (disseminated)
Cellulitis
  (1988): O'Rourke MG+, *Med J Aust* 148, 54
  (1984): Alguire PC, *Cutis* 34, 93 (necrotizing of the scrotum)
  (1975): Lewis RJ+, *JAMA* 232, 54

Dermatitis
  (1973): Young AW+, *Am Fam Physician* 7, 79
Ecthyma
  (1990): Rasokat H, *Z Haut* (German) 65, 351
Ecthyma gangrenosum
  (1977): Mandell IN+, *Arch Dermatol* 113, 199
Edema
  (1990): Rasokat H, *Z Haut* (German) 65, 351
  (1973): McCabe WP+, *Plast Reconstr Surg* 52, 538
  (1973): Young AW+, *Am Fam Physician* 7, 79
  (1973): Young AW, *N Y State J Med* 73, 1681 (eyelids)
  (1971): Weidman AJ+, *N Y State J Med* 71, 2643 (eyelids)
  (1971): Young AW+, *Arch Dermatol* 104, 80
Exanthems
  (1973): Young AW, *N Y State J Med* 73, 1681
  (1970): Vollum DI, *BMJ* 2, 647
Excoriations
  (1990): Rasokat H, *Z Haut* (German) 65, 351
Fixed eruption
  (1983): Westerhof W+, *Br J Dermatol* 109, 605 (tongue)
  (1973): Young AW, *N Y State J Med* 73, 1681
Folliculitis (candidal)
  (1987): Cristobal-Rodriguez P+, *Med Cutan Ibero Lat Am* (Spanish) 15, 411
  (1986): Darcis JM+, *Am J Dermatopathol* 8, 501 (with septicemia)
  (1986): Leclerc G+, *Int J Dermatol* 25, 100
  (1985): Calandra T+, *Eur J Clin Microbiol* 4, 340
Glucagonoma syndrome (necrolytic migratory erythema)
  (1994): Bencini PL+, *Dermatology* 189, 72
Infections
  (2002): Warner-Smith M+, *Addiction - 9304118* 97(8), 963 (13%)
Kaposi's sarcoma
  (1986): Schofer H+, *Hautarzt* (German) 37, 159
Necrosis
  (2002): Oehler U+, *Pathologe* 23(4), 318
  (1990): Rasokat H, *Z Haut* (German) 65, 351
  (1972): Dunne JH+, *Arch Dermatol* 105, 544
Necrotizing fasciitis
  (1990): Rasokat H, *Z Haut* (German) 65, 351
Pemphigus
  (1989): Civatte J, *Dermatol Monatsschr* (German) 175, 1
Pemphigus erythematosus
  (1978): Fellner MJ+, *Int J Dermatol* 17, 308
Pemphigus vegetans
  (1998): Downie JB+, *J Am Acad Dermatol* 39, 872
Perforating collagenosis
  (1989): Bank DE+, *J Am Acad Dermatol* 21, 371
Photosensitivity
  (1973): Young AW, *N Y State J Med* 73, 1681
  (1971): Young AW+, *Arch Dermatol* 104, 80
Pigmentation
  (1990): Rasokat H, *Z Haut* (German) 65, 351
  (1973): Young AW+, *Am Fam Physician* 7, 79
  (1973): Young AW, *N Y State J Med* 73, 1681 (photolocalized)
  (1971): Young AW+, *Arch Dermatol* 104, 80 (photolocalized)
Pruritus
  (1990): Rasokat H, *Z Haut* (German) 65, 351
  (1973): Young AW+, *Am Fam Physician* 7, 79
  (1973): Young AW, *N Y State J Med* 73, 1681
  (1971): Young AW+, *Arch Dermatol* 104, 80
  (1970): Vollum DI, *BMJ* 2, 647
  (1967): Minkin W+, *N Engl J Med* 277, 473
Purpura
  (1973): Young AW+, *Am Fam Physician* 7, 79
Pustules
  (1993): Badillet G+, *Ann Dermatol Venereol* (French) 110, 691 (candidal)

(1992): Gallais V+, *Presse Med* (French) 21, 677 (candidal)
(1990): Altes J+, *Enferm Infecc Microbiol Clin* (Spanish) 8, 464
(1985): Cabre L+, *Med Clin (Barc)* (Spanish) 84, 542 (candidal)
(1984): Pinilla-Moraza J+, *Med Clin (Barc)* (Spanish) 83, 557
Side effects (sic) (85%)
Toxic epidermal necrolysis
(1990): Llibre LM+, *Med Clin (Barc)* (Spanish) 94, 799
(1974): Lewis RJ, *JAMA* 230, 375
Ulcerations
(1990): Abidin MR+, *Ann Plast Surg* 24, 268
(1990): Rasokat H, *Z Haut* (German) 65, 351
(1973): McCabe WP+, *Plast Reconstr Surg* 52, 538
(1971): Young AW+, *Arch Dermatol* 104, 80
Urticaria
(1990): Shaikh WA, *Allergy* 45, 555
(1973): Young AW+, *Am Fam Physician* 7, 79
(1973): Young AW, *N Y State J Med* 73, 1681
Vasculitis
(1984): Rosman JB+, *Neth J Med* 27, 50
(1979): Redmond WJ, *Arch Dermatol* 115, 111

Other
Death
(2003): Sheedy DL+, *Am J Addict* 12(1), 52
(2002): Darke S+, *Addiction* 97(8), 977
(2002): Davidson PJ+, *Addiction* 97(12), 1511
(1996): Amoiridis G+, *Nervenarzt* 67(12), 1023
Dental decay
(1999): Fazzi M+, *Minerva Stomatol* (Italian) 48, 485
Hypersensitivity
(1990): Rasokat H, *Z Haut* (German) 65, 351
Injection-site scarring
(1990): Rasokat H, *Z Haut* (German) 65, 351
Injection-site ulceration
(1995): Hatton MQ+, *Clin Oncol R Coll Radiol* 7, 268
(1982): White WB+, *Cutis* 29, 63 (penis)
(1973): Bennett RG+, *Arch Dermatol* 107, 121
Myopathy
(1990): Shoji S, *Nippon* (Rinsho) (Japanese) 48, 1517
Necrotizing vasculitis (tongue)
(1995): Jurgensen O+, *Schweiz Monatsschr Zahnmed* (German, French) 105, 54
Oral mucosal ulceration (tongue)
(1983): Westerhof W+, *Br J Dermatol* 109, 605
Polyarteritis nodosa
(1982): Ojeda E+, *Rev Clin Esp* (Spanish) 167, 275
Rhabdomyolysis
(2002): Oehler U+, *Pathologe* 23(4), 318
(2000): Richards JR, *J Emerg Med* 19(1), 51
(1996): Amoiridis G+, *Nervenarzt* 67(12), 1023 (fatal)
(1992): Zele I+, *Minerva Med* 83(12), 847 (30%)
(1991): Nolte KB+, *Am J Forensic Med Pathol* 12(3), 273
(1990): Larpin R+, *Presse Med* 19(30), 1403
(1988): Hecker E+, *Schweiz Med Wochenschr* 118(52), 1982 (5 cases)
(1988): Uzan M+, *Nephrologie* 9(5), 217 (13 cases)
(1981): Palmucci L+, *Ital J Neurol Sci* 2(3), 275
Seizures
(2002): Warner-Smith M+, *Addiction - 9304118* 97(8), 963 (2%)
Serum sickness
(1971): Weidman AJ+, *NY State J Med* 71, 2643
Sweat gland necrosis
(1986): Rocamora A+, *J Dermatol* 13, 49
Tongue pigmentation (fixed eruption)
(1983): Westerhof W+, *Br J Dermatol* 109, 605

HORSE CHESTNUT (BARK, FLOWER, LEAF, SEED)

Scientific name: *Aesculus hippocastanum*
Family: Hippocastanaceae
Trade and other common names: Buckeye; Hippocastani; Marron Europeen; Venostat; Venostatin Retard
Category: Diuretic
Purported indications and other uses: Oral: malaria, dysentery, tinnitus, pancreatitis, cough, arthritis, rheumatism, chronic venous insufficiency. Topical: lupus, skin ulcers eczema, phlebitis, varicose veins, hemorrhoids, rectal problems
Half-life: N/A
Clinically important, potentially hazardous interactions with: heparin, NSAIDs, ticlopidine, warfarin

Reactions

Skin
Adverse effects (sic) (mild)
(2002): Pittler MH+, *Cochrane Database Syst Rev* (1), CD003230
Dermatitis (flower)
(1980): Comaish JS+, *Contact Dermatitis* 6(2), 150
Purpura
(1998): Brinker F, *Herb Contraindications & Interactions* Eclectic Medical Publications (2nd Ed)

Other
Anaphylactoid reactions (seed)
(1998): Gruenwald J+, *PDR for Herbal Medicines*. 1st ed Montvale, NJ: Medical Economics Company, Inc
Depression (seed)
Twitching (seed)

*Note: The active ingredient is a toxic glycoside, escin

HYDRALAZINE

Trade names: Apresazide (Novartis); Apresoline (Novartis); Ser-Ap-Es (Novartis)
Other common trade names: *Alphapress; Apdormin; Apresolin; Novo-Hylazin; Nu-Hydral; Solesorin; Stable*
Indications: Hypertension
Category: Antihypertensive; Vasodilator
Half-life: 3–7 hours

Apresazide is hydralazine and hydrochlorothiazide; Ser-Ap-Es is hydralazine, reserpine and hydrochlorothiazide

Reactions

Skin
Acute febrile neutrophilic dermatosis (Sweet's syndrome)
(1995): Gilmour E+, *Br J Dermatol* 133, 490
(1991): Juanola X+, *J Rheumatol* 18, 948
(1990): Ramsay-Goldman R+, *J Rheumatol* 17, 682
(1987): Servitje O+, *Arch Dermatol* 123, 1436
(1986): Sequeira W+, *Am J Med* 81, 558
Allergic reactions (sic)
(1986): Bigby M+, *JAMA* 236, 3358
Angioedema (<1%)
Bullous eruption
(1988): Dodd HJ+, *Br J Dermatol* 119 (Suppl 33), 27
Chills

Diaphoresis

Edema (<1%)

Erythema nodosum
(1984): Peterson LL, *J Am Acad Dermatol* 10, 379

Exanthems
(1984): Peterson LL, *J Am Acad Dermatol* 10, 379
(1984): Schapel GJ, *Med J Aust* 141, 765
(1981): Finlay AY+, *BMJ* 282, 1703
(1967): Alarcon-Segovia D+, *Medicine* (Baltimore) 46, 1

Fixed eruption (<1%)
(1986): Sehgal VN+, *Int J Dermatol* 25, 394

Flushing (>10%)
(1967): Alarcon-Segovia D+, *Medicine* (Baltimore) 46, 1

Lupus
(2002): Pape L+, *Pediatr Transplant* 6(4), 337

Lupus erythematosus
(1998): Hari CK+, *J Laryngol Otol* 112, 875
(1997): Yung R+, *Arthritis Rheum* 40, 1436
(1996): Miyasaka N, *Intern Med* 35, 587
(1996): Pirmohamed M, *Hum Exp Toxicol* 15, 361
(1995): Price EJ+, *Drug Saf* 12(4), 283
(1994): Cohen MG, *J Rheumatol* 21, 578
(1994): Hofstra AH, *Drug Metab Rev* 26, 485
(1994): Nassberger L+, *Scand J Rheumatol* 23, 206
(1994): Yung RL+, *Rheum Dis Clin North Am* 20, 61
(1992): Rubin RL, *Clin Biochem* 25, 223
(1992): Skaer TL, *Clin Ther* 14, 496
(1992): Yonga GO, *East Afr Med J* 69, 649
(1991): Alarcon-Segovia D+, *Baillieres Clin Rheumatol* 5, 1
(1991): Hess EV, *Curr Opin Rheumatol* 3, 809
(1991): Juanola X+, *J Rheumatol* 18, 948
(1990): Mulder H, *Eur J Clin Pharmacol* 38, 303
(1990): Nassberger L+, *Clin Exp Immunol* 81, 380
(1990): Ramsay-Goldman R+, *J Rheumatol* 17, 682
(1990): Richards FM+, *Am J Med* 88, 56N
(1989): Fleming MG+, *Int J Dermatol* 28, 321 (bullous)
(1989): Mitchell JA+, *Clin Exp Immunol* 78, 354
(1989): Palsson L+, *Clin Pharmacol Ther* 46, 177
(1989): Sim E, *Complement Inflamm* 6, 119
(1989): Speirs C+, *Lancet* 1, 922
(1989): Yemini M+, *Eur J Obstet Gynecol Reprod Biol* 30, 193
(1988): Chong WK+, *BMJ* 297, 660
(1988): Dodd HJ+, *Br J Dermatol* 119 (Suppl 33), 27
(1988): Jiang M, *Chung Kuo I Hsueh Yuan Hsueh Pao* (Chinese) 10, 379
(1988): Sturman SG+, *Lancet* 2, 1304 (fatal)
(1988): Uetrecht JP, *Chem Res Toxicol* 1, 133
(1987): Andersson OK, *Eur J Clin Pharmacol* 31, 741
(1987): Craft JE+, *Arthritis Rheum* 30, 689
(1987): Hobbs RN+, *Ann Rheum Dis* 46, 408
(1987): Martinez-Vea A+, *Am J Nephrol* 7, 71
(1987): Servitje O+, *Arch Dermatol* 123, 1436
(1986): Asherson RA+, *Ann Rheum Dis* 45, 771
(1986): Innes A+, *Br J Rheumatol* 25, 225
(1986): Sequeira W+, *Am J Med* 81, 558
(1985): Cush JJ+, *Am J Med Sci* 290, 36
(1985): Doherty M+, *Br Med J Clin Res Ed* 290, 675
(1985): Epstein A+, *Arthritis Rheum* 28, 158
(1985): Kale SA, *Postgrad Med* 77, 231
(1985): Lovisetto P+, *Recenti Prog Med* (Italian) 76, 110
(1985): Stratton MA, *Clin Pharm* 4, 657
(1985): Totoritis MC+, *Postgrad Med* 78, 149
(1984): Brand C+, *Lancet* 1, 462
(1984): Cameron HA+, *BMJ* 289, 410 (6.7%)
(1984): Christophidis N, *Lancet* 2, 868
(1984): French WJ, *Ala J Med Sci* 21, 427
(1984): Naparstek Y+, *Arthritis Rheum* 27, 822
(1984): No Author, *Lancet* 2, 441
(1984): Peterson LL, *J Am Acad Dermatol* 10, 379
(1984): Ramsay LE+, *Br Med J Clin Res Ed* 289, 1310

(1984): Shapiro KS+, *Am J Kidney Dis* 3, 270
(1984): Sim E+, *Lancet* 2, 422
(1984): Timbrell JA+, *Eur J Clin Pharmacol* 27, 555
(1984): Weiser GA+, *Arch Intern Med* 144, 2271
(1984): Wollina U, *Z Gesamte Inn Med* (German) 39, 69
(1983): Macleod WN, *Scott Med J* 28, 181
(1983): Shoenfeld Y+, *Br Med J Clin Res Ed* 286, 224
(1982): Aylward PE+, *Aust N Z J Med* 12, 546
(1982): Freestone S+, *Br Med J Clin Res Ed* 285, 1536
(1982): Harmon CE+, *Clin Rheum Dis* 8, 121
(1982): Hess EV, *Arthritis Rheum* 25, 857
(1982): Mansilla-Tinoco R+, *BMJ* 284, 936
(1982): Ohe A+, *Osaka City Med J* 28, 149
(1982): Portanova JP+, *Clin Immunol Immunopathol* 25(1), 67
(1982): Ramsay LE+, *Br Med J Clin Res Ed* 284, 1711
(1981): Chisholm JC, *J Natl Med Assoc* 73, 278
(1981): Dubroff LM+, *Arthritis Rheum* 24, 1082
(1981): Grossman J+, *Arthritis Rheum* 24, 927
(1981): Neville E+, *Postgrad Med* 57, 378
(1981): Perry HM, *Arthritis Rheum* 24, 1093
(1981): Reidenberg MM, *Arthritis Rheum* 24, 1004
(1981): Sinclair AJ+, *Hum Toxicol* 1, 65
(1980): Batchelor JR+, *Lancet* 1, 1107
(1980): Condemi JJ, *Geriatrics* 35(3), 81
(1980): Harland SJ+, *BMJ* 281, 273
(1980): Weinstein A, *Prog Clin Immunol* 4, 1
(1979): Kissin MW+, *BMJ* 2, 1330
(1979): Ryan PF+, *Lancet* 2, 1248
(1978): Anderson B+, *JAMA* 239, 1392
(1978): Jones WN+, *Ariz Med* 35, 16
(1978): Weinstein J, *Am J Med* 65, 553
(1976): Berkowitz HS, *S Afr Med J* 50, 797
(1976): Demay-Wechsler P, *Rev Stomatol Chir Maxillofac* (French) 77, 727
(1976): Hess EV+, *Arthritis Rheum* 19, 122
(1975): Irias JJ, *Am J Dis Child* 129, 862
(1975): Johansson M+, *Lakartidningen* (Swedish) 72, 153
(1975): Lee SL+, *Semin Arthritis Rheum* 5, 83
(1974): Blumenkrantz N+, *Acta Med Scand* 195, 443
(1973): Almeyda J+, *Br J Dermatol* 88, 313 (13%)
(1973): Perry HM, *Am J Med* 54, 58 (12%)
(1971): Alkalay I+, *Ann Allergy* 29, 35
(1967): Alarcon-Segovia D+, *Medicine* (Baltimore) 46, 1
(1966): White AB, *J Am Geriatr Soc* 14, 361
(1963): Shulman LE+, *Arthritis Rheum* 6, 558 (1–3%)

Photosensitivity
(1967): Alarcon-Segovia D+, *Medicine* (Baltimore) 46, 1

Pruritus
(1984): Peterson LL, *J Am Acad Dermatol* 10, 379

Purpura
(1984): Peterson LL, *J Am Acad Dermatol* 10, 379
(1980): Petty R+, *BMJ* 280, 482
(1967): Alarcon-Segovia D+, *Medicine* (Baltimore) 46, 1

Pyoderma gangrenosum
(1984): Peterson LL, *J Am Acad Dermatol* 10, 379

Rash (sic) (<1%)

Sjøgren's syndrome
(1988): Darwaza A+, *Int J Oral Maxillopfac* 17, 92

Systemic eczematous contact dermatitis
(1964): van Ketel WG, *Acta Derm Venereol* (Stockh) 44, 49

Ulcerations
(1980): Brooks AP+, *BMJ* 280, 482
(1980): Petty R+, *BMJ* 280, 482

Urticaria

Vasculitis
(2003): Norris JH+, *Ren Fail* 25(2), 311
(1998): Merkel PA, *Curr Opin Rheumatol* 10, 45
(1993): Reynolds NJ+, *Br J Dermatol* 129, 82
(1982): Kincaid-Smith P+, *Lancet* 2, 348

(1981): Finlay AY+, *Br Med J Clin Res Ed* 282, 1703
(1981): Peacock A+, *BMJ* 282, 1121
(1980): Bernstein RM+, *BMJ* 280, 156
(1980): Brooks AP+, *BMJ* 280, 482

Other
Arthralgia
    (2002): Pape L+, *Pediatr Transplant* 6(4), 337
Death
Headache
Hypersensitivity
Myalgia
    (2002): Pape L+, *Pediatr Transplant* 6(4), 337
Oral ulceration
    (1984): Peterson LL, *J Am Acad Dermatol* 10, 379
    (1980): Brooks AP+, *BMJ* 280, 482
Orogenital ulceration
    (1984): Peterson LL, *J Am Acad Dermatol* 10, 379
    (1981): Neville E+, *Postgrad Med* 57, 378
Paresthesias
Relapsing polychondritis
    (1983): Dahlqvist A+, *Acta Otolaryngol Stockh* 96, 355
Tremor

HYDROCHLOROTHIAZIDE

Trade names: Accuretic (Parke-Davis); Aldactazide (Pharmacia); Aldoril (Merck); Atacand HCT (AstraZeneca); Avalide (Bristol-Myers Squibb); Capozide (Par); Diovan (Novartis); Dyazide (GSK); Hydrodiuril (Merck); Hyzaar (Merck); Inderide (Wyeth); Lopressor (Novartis); Lotensin (Novartis); Maxzide (Bertek); Micardis (Boehringer Ingelheim); Microzide (Watson); Moduretic (Merck); Prinizide (Merck); Teveten HCT (Biovail); Timolide (Merck); Uniretic (Schwarz Pharma); Vaseretic (Biovail); Zestoretic (AstraZeneca); Ziac (Wyeth)
Other common trade names: *Apo-Hydro; Clothia; Dichlotride; Diu-Melsin; Diuchlor H; Esidrex; Hydrosaluric; Urozide*
Indications: Edema
Category: Antihypertensive; Thiazide diuretic
Half-life: 5.6–14.8 hours
Clinically important, potentially hazardous interactions with: digoxin, lithium

Aldactazide is spironolactone and hydrochlorothiazide; Aldoril is methyldopa and hydrochlorothiazide; Avalide is irbesartan and hydrochlorothiazide; Capozide is captopril and hydrochlorothiazide; Dyazide is triamterene and hydrochlorothiazide; Maxzide is triamterene and hydrochlorothiazide; Moduretic is amiloride and hydrochlorothiazide; Prinizide is lisinopril and hydrochlorothiazide; Ser-Ap-Es is reserpine, hydralazine and hydrochlorothiazide

Reactions

Skin
Actinic reticuloid
    (1985): Robinson HN+, *Arch Dermatol* 121, 522
Acute generalized exanthematous pustulosis (AGEP)
    (2001): Petavy-Catala C+, *Acta Derm Venereol* 81(3), 209
Bullous eruption (<1%)
Dermatitis (sic)
    (1984): Fisher RS+, *J Am Acad Dermatol* 11, 146
    (1960): Smirk H+, *BMJ* 1, 515
Diaphoresis
    (1979): Fan WJ+, *Pediatrics* 64, 698
Erythema annulare centrifugum
    (1988): Goette DK+, *Int J Dermatol* 27, 129

(1973): Rekant SI+, *Arch Dermatol* 107, 424
Erythema multiforme (<1%)
    (1985): Ting HC+, *Int J Dermatol* 24, 587
Exanthems
    (1960): Smirk H+, *BMJ* 1, 515
Exfoliative dermatitis
Fixed eruption
    (1985): Kauppinen K+, *Br J Dermatol* 112, 575
Lichenoid eruption
    (1986): Halevy S+, *Ann Allergy* 56, 402
    (1971): Almeyda J+, *Br J Dermatol* 85, 604
    (1959): Harber LC+, *J Invest Dermatol* 33, 83
    (1959): Harber LC+, *N Engl J Med* 261, 1378
Lupus erythematosus
    (2002): Boye T+, *World Congress Dermatol* Poster, 0088
    (1998): Callen JP, Academy '98 Meeting (5 patients)
    (1996): Litt JZ, Beachwood, OH (personal case) (observation)
    (1995): Brown CW+, *Clin Toxicol* 33, 729
    (1995): Rich MW+, *J Rheumatol* 22, 1001
    (1993): Goodrich AL+, *J Am Acad Dermatol* 28, 1001
    (1991): Wollenberg A+, *Hautarzt* (German) 42, 709
    (1989): Alanko K+, *Acta Derm Venereol* (Stockh) 69, 223
    (1989): Fine RM, *Int J Dermatol* 28, 375 (Comment)
    (1989): Parodi A+, *Photodermatology* 6, 100
    (1988): Darken M+, *J Am Acad Dermatol* 18, 38
    (1986): Berbis Ph, *Ann Dermatol Venereol* 113, 1245 (thiazides)
    (1985): Reed BR+, *Ann Intern Med* 103, 49
    (1977): Weiss RB, *W V Med J* 73, 101
Photosensitivity (<1%)
    (2002): Johnston GA, *Clin Exp Dermatol* 27(8), 670
    (2000): Wagner SN+, *Contact Dermatitis* 43, 245 (with ramipril)
    (1994): Bielan B, *Dermatol Nurs* 6, 30
    (1994): Shelley WB+, *Cutis* 53, 77 (observation)
    (1987): Addo HA+, *Br J Dermatol* 116, 749
    (1985): Reed BR+, *Ann Intern Med* 103, 49
    (1985): Robinson HN+, *Arch Dermatol* 121, 522
    (1984): Ophir O+, *Harefuah* (Hebrew) 107, 14
    (1983): White IR, *Contact Dermatitis* 9, 237
    (1982): No Author, *Ugeskr Laeger* (Danish) 144, 1101
    (1981): Journet M, *Union Med Can* 110, 356
    (1980): Okrasinski H, *Lakartidningen* (Swedish) 77, 2718
    (1980): Torinuki W, *J Dermatol* (Tokio) 7, 293
    (1969): Kalivas J, *JAMA* 209, 1706
    (1965): Fellner MJ+, *Med Clin North Am* 49, 709
    (1965): Jung EG+, *Int Arch Allergy Appl Immunol* 27, 313
    (1959): Harber LC+, *J Invest Dermatol* 33, 83
    (1959): Harber LC+, *N Engl J Med* 261, 1378
    (1959): Norins AL, *Arch Dermatol* 79, 592
Phototoxicity
    (1989): Diffey BL, *Arch Dermatol* 125, 1355
    (1987): Addo HA+, *Br J Dermatol* 116, 749
    (1982): Rosen K+, *Acta Derm Venereol* (Stockh) 62, 246
Porokeratosis (Mibelli)
    (1984): Inamoto N+, *J Am Acad Dermatol* 11, 359
Pruritus (<1%)
    (1992): Shelley WB+, *Cutis* 49, 391 (observation)
    (1969): Kalivas J, *JAMA* 209, 1706
Purpura
    (1980): Miescher PA+, *Clin Haematol* 9, 505
    (1971): Eisner EW+, *JAMA* 215, 480
    (1966): Smith JW+, *Ann Intern Med* 65, 629
    (1963): Bettman JW, *Arch Intern Med* 112, 840
    (1960): Ball P, *JAMA* 173, 663
    (1960): Gesink MH+, *JAMA* 172, 556
Rash (sic)
    (1976): Weisburst M+, *South Med J* 69, 126
Stevens–Johnson syndrome
    (1978): Assaad D+, *Can Med Assoc* 118, 154
Systemic eczematous contact dermatitis

Toxic epidermal necrolysis
(1978): Assaad D+, Can Med Assoc J 118, 154
(1973): Björnberg A, Acta Derm Venereol (Stockh) 53, 149
Urticaria
(1960): Smirk H+, BMJ 1, 515
Vasculitis
(1989): Grunwald MH+, Isr J Med Sci 25, 572
(1965): Björnberg A+, Lancet 2, 982

Other
Dysgeusia
(2000): Zervakis J+, Physiol Behav 68, 405
Headache
Oral lichenoid eruption (erosive)
(1990): Espana A+, Med Clin (Barc) (Spanish) 94, 559
Paresthesias
Pseudoporphyria
(1990): Motley RJ, BMJ 300, 1468
Xanthopsia
Xerostomia

*Note: Hydrochlorothiazide is a sulfonamide and can be absorbed systemically. Sulfonamides can produce severe, possibly fatal, reactions such as toxic epidermal necrolysis and Stevens–Johnson syndrome

HYDROCODONE*

Trade names: Bacomine; Ban-Tuss HC; Codamine; Duratuss (UCB Pharma); Entex HC (Andrx); Hycotuss (Endo); Lortab (UCB Pharma); Maxidone (Watson); Morcomine; Norco (Watson); Prolex-DH (Blansett); Propachem; Ru-Tuss; Tussgen; Tussionex (Celltech); Tussogest; Vicodin (Abbott); Vicoprofen (Abbott); Zydone (Endo)
Indications: Acute pain, coughing
Category: Narcotic analgesic antitussive
Half-life: 3.8 hours

Reactions

Skin
Diaphoresis
Edema
Erythema multiforme
Exanthems
(2000): Litt JZ, Beachwood, OH (personal case) (observation)
Flushing
Hot flashes
Pruritus (1–10%)
(2000): Litt JZ, Beachwood, OH (personal case) (observation)
(1999): Litt JZ, Beachwood, OH (personal case) (observation)
(1999): Sorkin MJ, Denver, CO (from Internet) (observation)
Rash (sic) (>10%)
Stevens–Johnson syndrome
Toxic epidermal necrolysis
Urticaria (>10%)

Other
Headache
Xerostomia

*Note: Hydrocodone is included in many combination drugs. Other medications that can be included in these preparations include: phenylpropanolamine, phenylephrine, pyrilamine, pseudoephedrine, acetaminophen, ibuprofen, and others

HYDROFLUMETHIAZIDE*

Trade name: Diucardin (Wyeth)
Other common trade names: Diademil; Hydravern; Hydrenox; Leodrine; Rivosil; Rontyl
Indications: Hypertension, edema
Category: Antihypertensive; Thiazide diuretic
Duration of action: 12–24 hours
Clinically important, potentially hazardous interactions with: digoxin, lithium

Reactions

Skin
Photosensitivity (<1%)
Purpura
Rash (sic) (<1%)
Urticaria
Vasculitis

Other
Dysgeusia
Paresthesias (<1%)
Xanthopsia

*Note: Hydroflumethiazide is a sulfonamide and can be absorbed systemically. Sulfonamides can produce severe, possibly fatal, reactions such as toxic epidermal necrolysis and Stevens–Johnson syndrome

HYDROMORPHONE

Trade name: Dilaudid (Abbott)
Other common trade names: Dilaudid HP; HydroStat IR; Palladone
Indications: Pain
Category: Narcotic analgesic antitussive
Half-life: 1–3 hours
Clinically important, potentially hazardous interactions with: cimetidine

Reactions

Skin
Diaphoresis
Exanthems
(1992): de Cuyper C+, Contact Dermatitis 27, 220 (generalized)
Flushing (1–10%)
Pruritus (<1%)
(1992): Chaplan SR+, Anesthesiology 77, 1090 (11.5%)
Rash (sic) (<1%)
Urticaria (<1%)

Hair
Hair – alopecia

Other
Dizziness
(2003): Coda BA+, Anesth Analg 97(1), 117
Dysgeusia
Injection-site reactions (sic)
Paresthesias
Xerostomia (1–10%)

HYDROXYCHLOROQUINE

Trade name: Plaquenil (Sanofi-Synthelabo)
Other common trade names: *Ercoquin; Oxiklorin; Plaquinol; Quensyl; Toremonil; Yuma*
Indications: Malaria, lupus erythematosus, rheumatoid arthritis
Category: Antimalarial; Antirheumatic
Half-life: elimination in blood: 50 days
Clinically important, potentially hazardous interactions with: chloroquine, cholestyramine, dapsone, penicillamine

Reactions

Skin

Acute generalized exanthematous pustulosis (AGEP)
  (1996): Assier-Bonnet H+, *Dermatology* 193, 70
  (1995): Bonnetblanc JM+, *Ann Dermatol Venereol* (French) 122, 604
  (1995): Moreau A+, *Int J Dermatol* 34, 263 (passim)
  (1993): Assier H+, *Ann Dermatol Venereol* (French) 120, 848
Angioedema (<1%)
Atrophy
  (2001): Vassallo C+, *Clin Exp Dermatol* 26(2), 141
Bullous eruption
  (2001): Klein AD, Statesboro, GA (from Internet) (observation)
  (1995): Kutz DC+, *Arthritis Rheum* 38, 440 Statesboro, GA (from Internet) (observation)
Dermatitis
  (1999): Meier H+, *Hautarzt* (German) 50, 665
Dermatomyositis
  (1994): Bloom BJ+, *J Rheumatology* 21, 2171
Erythema annulare centrifugum
  (1985): Hudson LD, *J Am Acad Dermatol* 36, 129
  (1982): Koralewski F, *Dermatosen* (German) 30, 125
  (1967): Ashurst PJ, *Arch Dermatol* 95, 37
Erythema multiforme (<1%)
  (1997): Rudolph R, Wyomissing, PA (from Internet) (observation)
Erythema nodosum
  (1996): Jarrett P+, *Br J Dermatol* 134, 373 (chronic)
Erythroderma
  (1990): Simoneaux PW, *Curr Concept Skin Dis* Winter, 15
  (1985): Slagel GA+, *J Am Acad Dermatol* 12, 857
Exanthems (1–5%)
  (2001): Werth V, *Dermatology Times* 18
  (1995): Blumenthal HL, Beachwood, OH (personal case) (observation)
  (1991): Ochsendorf FR+, *Hautarzt* (German) 42, 140
  (1990): Simoneaux PW, *Curr Concept Skin Dis* Winter, 15
Exfoliative dermatitis
  (1995): Blumenthal HL, Beachwood, OH (personal case) (observation)
  (1986): Lavrijsen APM+, *Acta Derm Venereol* (Stockh) 66, 536
  (1985): Slagel GA+, *J Am Acad Dermatol* 12, 857
  (1980): Koranda FC, *J Am Acad Dermatol* 4, 650 (passim)
Fixed eruption (<1%)
Lichenoid eruption
  (1990): Simoneaux PW, *Curr Concept Skin Dis* Winter, 15
  (1980): Koranda FC, *J Am Acad Dermatol* 4, 650 (passim)
  (1958): Savage J, *Br J Dermatol* 70, 181
  (1948): Alving AS+, *J Clin Invest* 27, 56
Photosensitivity
  (2002): Litt JZ, Beachwood, OH (personal observation)
  (2001): Metayer I+, *Ann Dermatol Venereol* 128(6), 729 (4 cases)
  (2000): Ainsworth GE, Salina, KS (from Internet) (observation)
  (1991): Ochsendorf FR+, *Hautarzt* (German) 42, 140
  (1982): van Weelden H, *Arch Dermatol* 118, 290
  (1981): Journet M, *Union Med Can* (French) 110, 356

Phototoxicity
  (2001): Metayer I+, *Ann Dermatol Venereol* 128(6), 729 (4 cases)
Pigmentation (1–10%)
  (1991): Ochsendorf FR+, *Hautarzt* (German), 42, 140
  (1982): Levy H, *S Afr Med J* 2, 735
  (1980): Koranda FC, *J Am Acad Dermatol* 4, 650 (passim)
  (1963): Tuffanelli D+, *Arch Dermatol* 88, 419
  (1959): Dall JLC+, *BMJ* 1, 1387
Polymorphous light eruption
  (1968): Reed WB+, *Arch Dermatol* 98, 327
Pruritus (>10%)
  (2002): Litt JZ, Beachwood, OH (personal observation)
  (2001): Silver B, Deerfield, IL (from Internet) (observation)
  (1999): Holme SA+, *Acta Derm Venereol* (Stockh) 79, 333
  (1995): Blumenthal HL, Beachwood, OH (personal case) (observation)
  (1994): Fain O+, *Rev Med Interne* (French) 15, 433
  (1991): Mnyika KS+, *J Trop Med Hyg* 94, 27 (47% incidence)
  (1990): Abdulkadir SA+, *Trans Roy Soc Trop Med Hyg* 84, 898
  (1990): Simoneaux PW, *Curr Concept Skin Dis* Winter, 15
  (1984): Osifo NG, *Arch Dermatol* 120, 80
  (1982): Spencer HC+, *BMJ* 285, 1703
  (1969): Olatunde IA, *J Nigerian Med Assoc* 6, 23
  (1964): Ekpechi OL+, *Arch Dermatol* 120, 80
Psoriasis (exacerbation)
  (2001): Spencer L, Crawfordsville, IN (from Internet) (2 observations)
  (2001): Thaler D, Monona, WI (from Internet) (exacerbation) (observation)
  (1993): Potter B, *Cutis* 52, 229 (passim)
  (1988): Nicolas J-F+, *Ann Dermatol Venereol* (French) 115, 289
  (1985): Gray RG, *J Rheumatol* 12, 391
  (1982): Abel EA+, *J Am Acad Dermatol* 15, 2007
  (1982): Luzar MJ, *J Rheumatol* 9, 462
  (1981): Olsen TG, *Ann Intern Med* 94, 546
  (1966): Baker H, *Br J Dermatol* 78, 161
  (1957): Cornbleet T+, *Arch Dermatol* 75, 286
Purpura
Pustular psoriasis
  (2003): Welsch MJ, *J Drugs Dermatol* 2, 193
  (1996): Vine JE+, *J Dermatol* 23, 357
  (1987): Friedman SJ, *J Am Acad Dermatol* 16, 1256
Pustules
  (1990): Lotem M+, *Acta Derm Venereol* (Stockh) 70, 250
Rash (sic) (1–10%)
Stevens–Johnson syndrome
  (2002): Leckie MJ+, *Rheumatology* (Oxford) 41(4), 473
Telangiectasia
  (2001): Vassallo C+, *Clin Exp Dermatol* 26(2), 141
Toxic epidermal necrolysis
  (2002): Chavez JS, (Santiago) (Chile) March AAD Poster
  (2001): Murphy M+, *Clin Exp Dermatol* 26(5), 457 (fatal)
Urticaria
  (2002): Litt JZ, Beachwood, OH (personal case) (observation)
  (1990): Simoneaux PW, *Curr Concept Skin Dis* Winter, 15
  (1980): Koranda FC, *J Am Acad Dermatol* 4, 650 (passim)
Vasculitis

Hair

Hair – alopecia
Hair – pigmentation (bleaching) (1–10%)
  (1999): Lecocq P+, *Presse Med* (French) 28, 741
  (1991): Ochsendorf FR+, *Hautarzt* (German) 42, 140
  (1985): Dupré A+, *Arch Dermatol* 121, 1164
  (1980): Koranda FC, *J Am Acad Dermatol* 4, 650 (passim)
  (1978): Dubois EL, *Semin Arthritis Rheum* 8, 33
  (1976): Sams WM, *Int J Dermatol* 15, 99
  (1965): Rook A, *Br J Dermatol* 77, 115

Nails

Nails – discoloration
(1991): Zic JA+, Arch Dermatol 127, 1037
Nails – pigmentation
(2001): Vassallo C+, Clin Exp Dermatol 26(2), 141
(1980): Koranda FC, J Am Acad Dermatol 4, 650 (passim)
(1963): Tuffanelli D+, Arch Dermatol 88, 419

Other

Death
(2001): Murphy M+, Clin Exp Dermatol 26(5), 457
Dysgeusia
(1996): Weber JC+, Presse Med (French) 25, 213
Gingival pigmentation
(1992): Veraldi S+, Cutis 49, 281
Headache
Leukocytoclastic vasculitis
(2003): Welsch MJ, J Drugs Dermatol 2(2), 193
Lymphoproliferative disease
(1980): Schechter SL+, Arthritis Rheum 23, 256
Mucosal atrophy
(2001): Vassallo C+, Clin Exp Dermatol 26(2), 141
Myopathy
(1998): Richards AJ, J Rheumatol 25, 1642
(1969): Chapman RS+, Br J Dermatol 81, 217
Oral mucosal pigmentation
(1992): Veraldi S+, Cutis 49, 281
(1991): Zic JA+, Arch Dermatol 127, 1037
(1980): Koranda FC, J Am Acad Dermatol 4, 650 (passim)
(1971): Giansanti JS+, Oral Surg 31, 66
Oral mucosal ulceration
Oral pigmentation
(2001): Vassallo C+, Clin Exp Dermatol 26(2), 141
Porphyria
(1993): Potter B, Cutis 52, 229 (passim)
(1976): Baler GR, Cutis 17, 96
(1974): Kordac V+, Br J Dermatol 90, 95
(1962): Cripps DL+, Arch Dermatol 86, 575
(1959): Marsden CW, Br J Dermatol 71, 219
(1957): Davis MJ+, Arch Dermatol 75, 796
(1954): Linden IH+, Calif Med 81, 235
Stomatitis
(2001): Vassallo C+, Clin Exp Dermatol 26(2), 141
Stomatopyrosis
Tinnitus

HYDROXYUREA

Trade names: Droxia (Bristol-Myers Squibb); Hydrea (Bristol-Myers Squibb); Mylocel
Other common trade names: Litalir; Onco-Carbide
Indications: Leukemia, malignant tumors
Category: Antineoplastic
Half-life: 3–4 hours
Clinically important, potentially hazardous interactions with: adefovir, aldesleukin

Reactions

Skin

Acral erythema
(1993): Brincker H+, Cancer Chemother Pharmacol 32, 496 (edema and soreness)
(1992): Parodi A+, G Ital Dermatol Venereol (Italian) 127, 361 (fingers and toes)
(1991): Baack BR+, J Am Acad Dermatol 24, 457

(1989): Kampmann KK+, Cancer 63, 2482 (passim)
(1984): Sigal M+, Ann Dermatol Venereol (French) 111, 895 (band-like)
(1983): Silver FS+, Ann Intern Med 98, 675
Acral ulcers
(2001): Vassallo C+, Clin Exp Dermatol 26(2), 141
Acrodermatitis perstans
(2001): Eming SA+, J Am Acad Dermatol 45, 321
Acute febrile neutrophilic dermatosis (Sweet's syndrome)
(2002): Guennoc B+, World Congress Dermatol Poster 0102
Atrophy
(1997): Ena P+, J Geriatr Dermatol 5, 310
Baboon syndrome
(1999): Chowdhury MM+, Clin Exp Dermatol 24, 336
Band-like erythema
(1984): Sigal M+, Ann Dermatol Venereol (French) 111, 895 (fingers and toes)
Collodion-like skin
(1996): Gauthier O+, Ann Dermatol Venereol (French) 123, 727
Dermatitis (sic) (dry, scaly)
(1984): Sigal M+, Ann Dermatol Venereol (French) 111, 895
(1975): Kennedy BJ+, Arch Dermatol 111, 183
Dermatomyositis
(2002): Dacey MJ+, Louisville, KY, March AAD Poster
(2002): Oskay T+, Eur J Dermatol 12(6), 586
(2001): Vassallo C+, Clin Exp Dermatol 26(2), 141
(2000): Kirby B+, Clin Exp Dermatol 25, 256
(1998): Suehiro M+, Br J Dermatol 139, 748
(1998): Velez A+, Clin Exp Dermatol 23, 94
(1997): Ena P+, J Geriatr Dermatol 5, 310
(1996): Bahadoran P+, Br J Dermatol 134, 1161
(1995): Senet P+, Br J Dermatol 133, 455
(1995): Weber L+, Hautarzt 46, 717
(1994): Kelly RI+, Australas J Dermatol 35, 61
(1994): Perrot JL+, Ann Dermatol Venereol (French) 121, 499
(1989): Richard M+, J Am Acad Dermatol 21, 797
(1984): Sigal M+, Ann Dermatol Venereol (French) 111, 895
Edema of leg
(2002): Kumar B+, Clin Exp Dermatol 27(1), 8
Erythema multiforme (<1%)
Exanthems (1–10%)
(1992): Breathnach SM+, Adverse Drug Reactions and the Skin Blackwell, Oxford, 303 (passim)
Facial erythema (<1%)
(1975): Kennedy BJ+, Arch Dermatol 111, 183
Fixed eruption (<1%)
(1991): Boyd AS+, J Am Acad Dermatol 25, 518
(1976): Moschella SL, Int J Dermatol 15, 373
(1972): Hunter GA+, Aust J Dermatol 13, 93
(1969): Moschella SL+, Arch Dermatol 107, 363
Ichthyosis
(2002): Kumar B+, Clin Exp Dermatol 27(1), 8
(1997): Ena P+, J Geriatr Dermatol 5, 310
Keratoacanthoma
(2001): Vassallo C+, Clin Exp Dermatol 26(2), 141 (sun-exposed areas)
Keratoses
(1998): Salmon-Her V+, Dermatology 196, 274
(1995): Grange F+, Ann Dermatol Venereol (French) 122, 16
Lichen planus
(1998): Bohn J+, J Eur Acad Dermatol Venereol 10, 187 (ulcerative)
(1991): Renfro L+, J Am Acad Dermatol 24, 143 (ulcerative)
(1975): Kennedy BJ+, Arch Dermatol 111, 183 (atrophic)
Lichenoid acrodermatitis
(2001): Eming SA+, J Am Acad Dermatol 45(2), 321
Lichenoid eruption
(1997): Daoud MS+, J Am Acad Dermatol 36, 178

(1997): Ena P+, *J Geriatr Dermatol* 5, 310

Lupus erythematosus
  (1994): Layton AM+, *Br J Dermatol* 130, 687
  (1994): Layton AM+, *Br J Dermatol* 131, 581

Palmar–plantar keratoderma
  (2001): Chaine B+, *Arch Dermatol* 137, 467 (2 cases)
  (1997): Ena P+, *J Geriatr Dermatol* 5, 310 (plantar)
  (1992): Breathnach SM+, *Adverse Drug Reactions and the Skin*
    Blackwell, Oxford, 303 (passim)
  (1992): Parodi A+, *G Ital Dermatol Venereol* (Italian) 127, 361
  (1989): Richard M+, *J Am Acad Dermatol* 21, 797 (passim)
  (1984): Sigal M+, *Ann Dermatol Venereol* (French) 111, 895

Peripheral edema
  (2002): Kumar B+, *Clin Exp Dermatol* 27(1), 8

Photosensitivity
  (1992): Breathnach SM+, *Adverse Drug Reactions and the Skin*
    Blackwell, Oxford, 303 (passim)

Pigmentation (1–10%)
  (2002): Kumar B+, *Clin Exp Dermatol* 27(1), 8 (58.6%)
  (2001): Chaine B+, *Arch Dermatol* 137, 467 (29%)
  (2001): O'Branski EE+, *J Am Acad Dermatol* 44, 859 (palmar
    creases) (2 patients; both had sickle cell anemia)
  (1995): Weber L+, *Hautarzt* (German) 46, 717
  (1993): Brincker H+, *Cancer Chemother Pharmacol* 32, 496
  (1993): Gropper CA+, *Int J Dermatol* 32, 731
  (1990): Majumdar G+, *BMJ* 300, 1468
  (1989): Layton AM+, *Br J Dermatol* 121, 647
  (1989): Richard M+, *J Am Acad Dermatol* 21, 797 (passim)
  (1984): Sigal M+, *Ann Dermatol Venereol* (French) 111, 895
    (band-like)
  (1982): Jeanmougin M+, *Ann Dermatol Venereol* (French)
    109, 169
  (1975): Kennedy BJ+, *Arch Dermatol* 111, 183
  (1972): Dahl MH+, *BMJ* 4, 585 (yellow-gray-brown)
  (1966): Kennedy BJ+, *JAMA* 195, 162

Poikiloderma
  (1997): Daoud MS+, *J Am Acad Dermatol* 36, 178

Pruritus (<1%)
  (1995): Weber L+, *Hautarzt* 46, 717
  (1992): Vosburgh E, *Am J Hematol* 41, 70
  (1975): Kennedy BJ+, *Arch Dermatol* 111, 183

Psoriasis
  (2002): Kumar B+, *Clin Exp Dermatol* 27(1), 8

Purpura
  (1973): Moschella SL+, *Arch Dermatol* 107, 363
  (1973): Roe LD+, *Arch Dermatol* 108, 426

Radiation recall (sic)
  (1974): Levantine A+, *Br J Dermatol* 90, 239
  (1964): Sears ME, *Cancer Chemother Rep* 40, 31

Rash (sic)

Side effects (sic)
  (1998): Radaelli F+, *Am J Hematol* 58, 82
  (1975): Kennedy BJ+, *Arch Dermatol* 111, 183 (35%)
  (1973): Moschella SL+, *Arch Dermatol* 107, 363 (7%)

Squamous cell carcinoma
  (2001): Vassallo C+, *Clin Exp Dermatol* 26(2), 141 (sun-exposed
    areas)
  (2000): Bateman B, *Skin and Allergy News* August, 3 (observation)

Telangiectasia
  (1997): Daoud MS+, *J Am Acad Dermatol* 36, 178
  (1995): Weber L+, *Hautarzt* (German) 46, 717

Ulceration of foot
  (2003): Aragane Y+, *Br J Dermatol* 148(3), 599

Ulcerations
  (2001): Chaine B+, *Arch Dermatol* 137, 467 (29%) (leg)
  (2001): Olesen LH+, *Ugeskr Laeger* 163(49), 6908 (5 cases)
  (2001): Vassallo C+, *Clin Exp Dermatol* 26(2), 141
  (2001): Young HS+, *Clin Exp Dermatol* 26(8), 664 (fatal)
  (2000): Tarumoto T+, *Jpn J Clin Oncol* 30, 159 (heels)

(1999): Kato N+, *J Dermatol* 26, 56
(1999): Sirieix M-E+, *Arch Dermatol* 135, 818
(1999): Stagno F+, *Blood* 94, 1479
(1998): Best PJ+, *Ann Intern Med* 128, 29 (leg)
(1998): Disla E+, *Ann Intern Med* 129, 252
(1998): Kennedy BJ, *Ann Intern Med* 129, 252
(1998): Kido M+, *Br J Dermatol* 139, 1124
(1998): Liebschutz S+, *Rev Med Interne* (French) 19, 360
  (malleolar)
(1998): Radaelli F+, *Am J Hematol* 58, 82 (hands)
(1998): Reichenberger F, *Schweiz Rundsch Med Praxis* (German)
  87, 1370
(1998): Ruiz-Arguelles GL+, *Mayo Clin Proc* 73, 1125
(1998): Suehiro M+, *Br J Dermatol* 139, 748 (large leg ulcer)
(1998): Weinlich G+, *J Am Acad Dermatol* 39, 372 (painful) (legs)
  (2 cases)
(1997): Best PJ+, *Ann Int Med* 128, 29
(1997): Cox C+, *Ann Plastic Surg* 39, 546 (ankle)
(1997): Ena P+, *J Geriatr Dermatol* 5, 310 (malleolar squamous
  cell)
(1997): Glazier DB+, *Wounds* 9, 169
(1996): Callot-Mellot C+, *Arch Dermatol* 132, 1395
(1996): Esteve E+, *Ann Dermatol Venereol* (French) 123, 271
(1996): Iwama H+, *Gan To Kagaku Ryoho* (Japanese) 23, 937
(1995): Masuoka H+, *Rinsho Ketsueki* (Japanese) 36, 156
(1993): Nguyen TV+, *Cutis* 52, 217 (painful legs ulcers)
(1986): Montefusco E+, *Tumori* (Italian) 72, 317 (legs) (17 cases)
(1985): Stahl RL+, *Am J Med* 78, 869
(1984): Sigal M+, *Ann Dermatol Venereol* (French) 111, 895

Ulcerations of legs
  (2003): Sastre JL+, *Haematologica* 88(2), EIM01
  (2002): Demircay Z+, *Int J Dermatol* 41(12), 872

Urticaria

Vasculitis
  (2001): Young HS+, *Clin Exp Dermatol* 26(8), 664
  (1997): Reed BR, Denver, CO (from Internet) (observation)
  (1992): Breathnach SM+, *Adverse Drug Reactions and the Skin*
    Blackwell, Oxford, 303 (passim)
  (1989): Richard M+, *J Am Acad Dermatol* 21, 797 (passim)
  (1976): Moschella SL+, *Int J Dermatol* 15, 373
  (1973): Moschella SL+, *Arch Dermatol* 107, 363
  (1973): Roe LD+, *Arch Dermatol* 108, 426

Xerosis (1–10%)
  (2002): Kumar B+, *Clin Exp Dermatol* 27(1), 8
  (2001): Chaine B+, *Arch Dermatol* 137, 467 (6 cases)
  (1995): Weber L+, *Hautarzt* (German) 46, 717
  (1989): Richard M+, *J Am Acad Dermatol* 21, 797 (passim)
  (1984): Sigal M+, *Ann Dermatol Venereol* (French) 111, 895
  (1975): Kennedy BJ+, *Arch Dermatol* 111, 183

Hair

Hair – alopecia (1–10%)
  (2002): Kumar B+, *Clin Exp Dermatol* 27(1), 8 (diffuse)
  (1992): Breathnach SM+, *Adverse Drug Reactions and the Skin*
    Blackwell, Oxford, 303 (passim)
  (1989): Layton AM+, *Br J Dermatol* 121, 647
  (1989): Richard M+, *J Am Acad Dermatol* 21, 797 (passim)
  (1976): Bergstresser PR+, *Arch Dermatol* 112, 977
  (1975): Kennedy BJ+, *Arch Dermatol* 111, 183

Nails

Nails – atrophic
  (1984): Daniel CR+, *J Am Acad Dermatol* 10, 250
  (1984): Sigal M+, *Ann Dermatol Venereol* (French) 111, 895
  (1975): Kennedy BJ+, *Arch Dermatol* 111, 183

Nails – dystrophy
  (1992): Breathnach SM+, *Adverse Drug Reactions and the Skin*
    Blackwell, Oxford, 303 (passim)
  (1989): Richard M+, *J Am Acad Dermatol* 21, 797 (passim)

Nails – onycholysis

(1992): Breathnach SM+, *Adverse Drug Reactions and the Skin* Blackwell, Oxford, 303 (passim)
(1989): Richard M+, *J Am Acad Dermatol* 21, 797 (passim)

Nails – pigmentation
(2002): Aste N+, *J Am Acad Dermatol* 47(1), 146 (9 cases)
(2002): Kumar B+, *Clin Exp Dermatol* 27(1), 8
(2001): Chaine B+, *Arch Dermatol* 137, 467 (9%)
(2001): O'Branski EE+, *J Am Acad Dermatol* 44, 859 (longitudinal bands) (patient had sickle cell anemia)
(1999): Hernández-Martin A+, *J Am Acad Dermatol* 40, 333
(1997): Cakir B+, *Int J Dermatol* 36, 234
(1997): Ena P+, *J Geriatr Dermatol* 5, 310
(1996): Kwong YL, *J Am Acad Dermatol* 35, 275
(1995): Delmas-Marsalet B+, *Nouv Rev Fr Hematol* (French) 37, 205
(1994): Pirard C+, *Ann Dermatol Venereol* (French) 121, 106 (longitudinal)
(1993): Gropper CA+, *Int J Dermatol* 32, 731
(1992): Kelsey PR, *Clin Lab Haematol* 14, 337
(1991): Vomvouras S+, *J Am Acad Dermatol* 24, 1016
(1989): Baran R+, *J Am Acad Dermatol* 21, 1165
(1984): Sigal M+, *Ann Dermatol Venereol* (French) 111, 895
(1982): Jeanmougin M+, *Ann Dermatol Venereol* 109, 169

Other

Death
(2001): Young HS+, *Clin Exp Dermatol* 26(8), 664
Gangrene (toes)
(2002): Leo E+, *Ann Hematol* 81(8), 467
Glossitis
(2001): Vassallo C+, *Clin Exp Dermatol* 26(2), 141
Leg ulcers
(2002): Demircay Z+, *Int J Dermatol* 41(12), 872 (3 cases)
Mucocutaneous eruption
(2002): Kumar B+, *Clin Exp Dermatol* 27(1), 8
Myositis
(1998): Ikeda K+, *Rinsho Ketsueki* (Japanese) 39, 676
Oral mucosal lesions
(1976): Bergstresser PR+, *Arch Dermatol* 112, 977
(1975): Kennedy BJ+, *Arch Dermatol* 111, 183
Oral mucosal pigmentation
(2002): Kumar B+, *Clin Exp Dermatol* 27(1), 8
Oral mucosal ulceration
(2001): Vassallo C+, *Clin Exp Dermatol* 26(2), 141
Oral pigmentation
(2002): Kumar B+, *Clin Exp Dermatol* 27(1), 8
(2001): Chaine B+, *Arch Dermatol* 137, 467 (29%)
Oral squamous cell carcinoma
(2001): Esteve E+, *Ann Dermatol Venereol* 128(8), 919
Oral ulceration
(2002): Kumar B+, *Clin Exp Dermatol* 27(1), 8
(1997): Norhaya MR+, *Singapore Med J* 38, 283
(1989): Richard M+, *J Am Acad Dermatol* 21, 797 (passim)
Porphyria cutanea tarda
(2002): Zweegman S+, *Ned Tijdschr Geneeskd* 146(49), 2353
Scleral pigmentation
(2002): Kumar B+, *Clin Exp Dermatol* 27(1), 8
Stomatitis (>10%)
(1993): Brincker H+, *Cancer Chemother Pharmacol* 32, 496
(1992): Breathnach SM+, *Adverse Drug Reactions and the Skin* Blackwell, Oxford, 303 (passim)
(1989): Richard M+, *J Am Acad Dermatol* 21, 797 (passim)
Tongue pigmentation
(2001): Chaine B+, *Arch Dermatol* 137, 467 (29%)
(1997): Ena P+, *J Geriatr Dermatol* 5, 310
(1993): Gropper CA+, *Int J Dermatol* 32, 731
Tumors
(1998): Best PJ+, *Mayo Clin Proc* 73, 961 (multiple malignant)

(1998): De Simone C+, *Eur J Dermatol* 8, 114 (multiple squamous cell)
(1998): Salmon-Her V+, *Dermatology* 196, 274
(1993): Papi M+, *J Am Acad Dermatol* 28, 485 (on light-exposed areas)
(1992): Stasi R+, *Eur J Haematol* 48, 121

HYDROXYZINE

Trade names: Atarax (Roerig); Marax; Vistaril (Pfizer)
Other common trade names: *AH3 N; Anaxanil; Bobsule; Iremofar; Masmoran; Multipax; Otarex; Paxistil; Quiess; Rezine; Vamate*
Indications: Anxiety and tension, pruritus
Category: Antihistamine; Anxiolytic
Half-life: 3–7 hours
Clinically important, potentially hazardous interactions with: alcohol, barbiturates, CNS depressants, narcotics, non-narcotic analgesics

Reactions

Skin

Angioedema (<1%)
(1971): *Drug Ther Bull* 9, 84
(1964): Welsh AL, *Med Clin North Am* 48, 459
(1958): Cohen AE+, *J Allergy* 29, 542
Dermatitis
(1997): Menne T, *Am J Contact Dermat* 8, 1
Diaphoresis
Edema (<1%)
Erythema multiforme (<1%)
(1959): Wright W, *JAMA* 171, 1642
Exanthems
(1964): Welsh AL, *Med Clin North Am* 48, 459
(1959): Wright W, *JAMA* 171, 1642
(1958): Cohen AE+, *J Allergy* 29, 542
Fixed eruption
(2002): Assouere MN+, *Ann Dermatol Venereol* 129(11), 1295
(1997): Cohen HA+, *Ann Pharmacother* 31, 327 (penis)
(1996): Cohen HA+, *Cutis* 57, 431 (scrotum)
Flushing
(1998): Foster M+, *J Clin Dermatol* Winter, 7
Photosensitivity (<1%)
Purpura
Rash (sic) (<1%)
Urticaria
(1964): Welsh AL, *Med Clin North Am* 48, 459
(1959): Wright W, *JAMA* 171, 1642

Other

Hypersensitivity
(1978): Massoud N, *J Pediatr* 93, 308
Injection-site necrosis
(1995): Tokodi G+, *J Am Osteopath Assoc* 95, 609
Myalgia (<1%)
Priapism
(1994): Thavundayil JX+, *Neuropsychobiology* 30, 4
Xerostomia (10%)
(1998): Foster M+, *J Clin Dermatol* Winter, 7 (12.5%)
(1990): Kalivas J+, *J Allergy Clin Immunol* 86, 1014

HYOSCYAMINE

Synonyms: Hyoscyamine sulfate; hyoscyamine sulfate

Trade names: Anaspaz (Ascher); Cytospaz (PolyMedica); Donnamar; ED-SPAZ; Gastrosed; Hyco; Hycosol Sl; Hyospaz; IB-Stat (InKline); Levbid (Schwartz); Levsin (Schwartz); Levsin/SL (Schwartz); Levsinex (Schwartz); Medispaz; Nulev (Schwartz); Pasmex; Setamine; Urised (PolyMedica)

Other common trade names: *Duboisine; Egacene Durettes; Egazil; Peptard*

Indications: Treatment of gastrointestinal tract disorders caused by spasm, Adjunctive therapy for peptic ulcers, cystitis, parkinsonism, biliary & renal colic

Category: Anticholinergic

Duration of action: 13–38 min

Clinically important, potentially hazardous interactions with: anticholinergics, arbutamine

Reactions

Skin

Allergic reactions (sic)
Flushing
Hypohidrosis (>10%)
Photosensitivity (1–10%)
Rash (sic) (<1%)
Urticaria
Xerosis (>10%)

Other

Ageusia
Anaphylactoid reactions
Dysgeusia
Headache
Injection-site inflammation (>10%)
Xerostomia (>10%)

IBRITUMOMAB

Synonyms: In-111 Zevalin; Y-90 Zevalin
Trade name: Zevalin (IDEC)
Indications: Non-Hodgkin's lymphoma
Category: Antineoplastic monoclonal antibody;
Radiopharmaceutical
Half-life: 30 hours

Reactions

Skin
Allergic reactions (sic) (2%)
Angioedema (5%)
Chills (24%)
Diaphoresis (4%)
Ecchymoses (7%)
Flushing (6%)
Infections (sic) (29%)
Peripheral edema (8%)
Petechiae (3%)
Pruritus (9%)
Purpura (7%)
Rash (sic) (8%)
Urticaria (4%)

Other
Anaphylactoid reactions
Arthralgia (7%)
Arthritis (<1%)
Back pain (8%)
Cough (10%)
Death
Hypersensitivity
Injection-site reactions (sic) (fatal)
Myalgia (7%)
Pain (13%)

IBUPROFEN

Trade names: Advil (Wyeth); Genpril; Haltran; Medipren; Midol 220; Motrin (McNeil); Nuprin; Pamprin; Profen; Rufen; Trendar; Vicoprofen
Other common trade names: Act-3; Actiprofen; Anco; Apsifen; Brufen; Ebufac; Lidifen; Proflex; Tabalom; Urem
Indications: Arthritis, pain
Category: Antipyretic; Nonsteroidal anti-inflammatory (NSAID)
Half-life: 2–4 hours
Clinically important, potentially hazardous interactions with: aspirin, diuretics, methotrexate, NSAIDs, salicylates, tacrolimus, urokinase

Reactions

Skin
Angioedema (<1%)
  (1994): Halpern SM, *Arch Dermatol* 130, 259 (passim)
  (1987): Shelley ED+, *J Am Acad Dermatol* 17, 1057
  (1985): Bigby M+, *J Am Acad Dermatol* 12, 866
  (1984): Stern RS+, *JAMA* 252, 1433
  (1982): Bailin PL+, *Clinics in Rheumatic Diseases* WB Saunders 8, 493 (passim)
Bullous eruption (<1%)

  (1994): Halpern SM, *Arch Dermatol* 130, 259 (passim)
  (1988): Laing VB+, *J Am Acad Dermatol* 19, 91
  (1984): Stern R+, *JAMA* 252, 1433
Bullous pemphigoid
  (1993): Fellner MJ, *Clin Dermatol* 11, 515
  (1981): Pompeova L, *Cesk Dermatol* (Czech) 56, 256
Dermatitis (<1%)
  (1993): Ophaswongse S+, *Contact Dermatitis* 29, 57
  (1986): Veronesi S+, *Contact Dermatitis* 15, 103
  (1985): Valsecchi R+, *Contact Dermatitis* 12, 286
Dermatitis herpetiformis
  (1994): Tousignant J+, *Int J Dermatol* 33, 199
Diaphoresis
  (1974): Regalado RG+, *J Int Med Res* 2, 115
Eczema (sic)
  (1986): Veronesi S+, *Contact Dermatitis* 15, 103
Edema (<1%)
Erythema multiforme (<1%)
  (1995): Lesko SM+, *JAMA* 273, 929
  (1994): Halpern SM, *Arch Dermatol* 130, 259 (passim)
  (1992): Breathnach SM+, *Adverse Drug Reactions and the Skin* Blackwell, Oxford, 186 (passim)
  (1985): Bigby M+, *J Am Acad Dermatol* 12, 866
  (1985): O'Brien WM+, *J Rheumatol* 12, 13
  (1984): Stern R+, *JAMA* 252, 1433
  (1978): Sternlieb P+, *N Y State J Med* 78, 1239
Erythema nodosum
  (1994): Halpern SM, *Arch Dermatol* 130, 259 (passim)
Exanthems
  (1994): Halpern SM, *Arch Dermatol* 130, 259 (passim)
  (1994): Litt JZ, Beachwood, OH (personal case) (observation)
  (1985): Bigby M+, *J Am Acad Dermatol* 12, 866
  (1980): Shoenfeld Y+, *JAMA* 244, 547
  (1979): Finch WR+, *JAMA* 241, 2616
  (1978): Sonnenblick M+, *BMJ* 1, 619
  (1975): Blechman WJ+, *JAMA* 233, 336 (3.4%)
  (1974): Regalado RG+, *J Int Med Res* 2, 115 (0.86%)
  (1973): Mills SB+, *BMJ* 4, 82 (>5%)
Fixed eruption (<1%)
  (2003): Litt JZ, Beachwood, OH (glans penis) (personal case) (pbservation)
  (2003): Litt JZ, Beachwood, OH (personal case) (observation)
  (2001): Diaz Jara M+, *Pediatr Dermatol* 18, 66
  (2000): Zabawski E, Longview, TX (from Internet) (observation)
  (1998): Mahboob A+, *Int J Dermatol* 37, 833
  (1996): Eichwald M, Redding, CA (from Internet) (observation)
  (1994): Shelley WB+, *Cutis* 53, 282 (observation)
  (1992): Breathnach SM+, *Adverse Drug Reactions and the Skin* Blackwell, Oxford, 186 (passim)
  (1991): Kuligowski ME+, *Contact Dermatitis* 25, 259
  (1990): Bharija SC+, *Dermatologica* 181, 237
  (1985): Bigby M+, *J Am Acad Dermatol* 12, 866
  (1984): Kanwar AJ+, *J Dermatol* 11, 383
  (1984): Stern R+, *JAMA* 252, 1433
Flushing
Hot flashes (<1%)
Linear IgA bullous dermatosis
  (2002): Au S+, (Vancouver) (Canada) March AAD Poster
Livedo reticularis
  (1979): Finch WR+, *JAMA* 241, 2616
Lupus erythematosus
  (1996): Vigouroux C+, *Rev Med Interne* (French) 14, 856
  (1985): O'Brien WM+, *J Rheumatol* 12, 13
  (1980): Bar-Sela S+, *J Rheumatol* 7, 379
  (1978): Pereyo-Torrellas N, *Arch Dermatol* 114, 1097
  (1978): Sonnenblick M+, *BMJ* 1, 619 (exacerbation)
Pemphigus
  (1988): Laing VB+, *J Am Acad Dermatol* 19, 91
Periorbital edema

(1979): Finch WR+, *JAMA* 241, 2616
Photosensitivity
  (1994): Berger TG+, *Arch Dermatol* 130, 609 (in HIV-infected)
    (5 cases)
  (1994): Halpern SM, *Arch Dermatol* 130, 259 (passim)
  (1992): Bergner T+, *J Am Acad Dermatol* 26, 114
  (1990): Bergner T+, *J Allergy Clin Immunol* 85, 177
  (1985): Bigby M+, *J Am Acad Dermatol* 12, 866
  (1982): Bailin PL+, *Clinics in Rheumatic Diseases* WB Saunders 8,
    493
Pruritus (1–5%)
  (1994): Halpern SM, *Arch Dermatol* 130, 259 (passim)
  (1992): Breathnach SM+, *Adverse Drug Reactions and the Skin*
    Blackwell, Oxford, 186 (passim)
  (1985): Bigby M+, *J Am Acad Dermatol* 12, 866 (1–5%)
  (1979): Finch WR+, *JAMA* 241, 2616
  (1975): Blechman WJ+, *JAMA* 233, 336 (1.8%)
Psoriasis (palms)
  (1986): Ben-Chetrit E+, *Cutis* 38, 45 (exacerbation)
  (1985): Bigby M+, *J Am Acad Dermatol* 12, 866
Purpura
  (1969): Ward T, *BMJ* 4, 430
Rash (sic) (>10%)
  (1974): Regalado RG+, *J Int Med Res* 2, 115
Stevens–Johnson syndrome (<1%)
  (1994): Halpern SM, *Arch Dermatol* 130, 259 (passim)
  (1978): Sternlieb P+, *N Y State J Med* 78, 1239
Toxic epidermal necrolysis (<1%)
  (1994): Halpern SM, *Arch Dermatol* 130, 259 (passim)
  (1980): Sternlieb P+, *Ann Intern Med* 92, 570
Urticaria (>10%)
  (2001): Diaz Jara M+, *Pediatr Dermatol* 18, 66
  (1994): Halpern SM, *Arch Dermatol* 130, 259 (passim)
  (1993): Litt JZ, Beachwood, OH (personal case) (observation)
  (1987): Shelley ED+, *J Am Acad Dermatol* 17, 1057
  (1985): Bigby M+, *J Am Acad Dermatol* 12, 866
  (1984): Stern RS+, *JAMA* 252, 1433
  (1982): Bailin PL+, *Clinics in Rheumatic Diseases* WB Saunders 8,
    493 (passim)
  (1975): Blechman WJ+, *JAMA* 233, 336 (0.2%)
Vasculitis
  (2001): Davidson KA+, *Cutis* 67, 303 (bullous leukocytoclastic)
  (1996): Peters F+, *J Rheumatol* 23, 2008
  (1994): Halpern SM, *Arch Dermatol* 130, 259 (passim)
  (1992): Breathnach SM+, *Adverse Drug Reactions and the Skin*
    Blackwell, Oxford, 186 (passim)
  (1985): Bigby M+, *J Am Acad Dermatol* 12, 866
  (1984): Stern R+, *JAMA* 252, 1433
  (1982): Labbe A+, *Ann Dermatol Venereol* (French) 109, 995
  (1978): Pereyo-Torrellas N, *Arch Dermatol* 114, 1097
Vesiculobullous eruption
  (1992): Breathnach SM+, *Adverse Drug Reactions and the Skin*
    Blackwell, Oxford, 186 (passim)
  (1988): Laing VB+, *J Am Acad Dermatol* 19, 91 (passim)

Hair

Hair – alopecia (<1%)
  (1985): O'Brien WM+, *J Rheumatol* 12, 13
  (1979): Meyer HC, *JAMA* 242, 142
Hair – disorders (sic)
  (1994): Halpern SM, *Arch Dermatol* 130, 259 (passim)

Nails

Nails – changes (sic)
  (1994): Halpern SM, *Arch Dermatol* 130, 259 (passim)
Nails – onycholysis
  (1982): Bailin PL+, *Clinics In Rheumatic Diseases* WB Saunders 8,
    493

Other

Anaphylactoid reactions (<1%)
  (2001): Verma S, Baroda, India (from Internet) (observation)
    (with acetaminophen)
  (2000): Takahama H+, *J Dermatol* 27, 337
  (1998): Menendez R+, *Ann Allergy Asthma Immunol* 80, 225
  (1985): O'Brien WM+, *J Rheumatol* 12, 13
  (1979): Finch WR+, *JAMA* 241, 2616
Aphthous stomatitis
Death
  (2001): Stevenson R+, *Scott Med J* 46(3), 84
DRESS syndrome
  (2001): Descamps V+, *Arch Dermatol* 137, 301
Embolia cutis medicamentosa (Nicolau syndrome)
  (2003): Reding EL+, *J Am Acad Dermatol* 48(3), 472 (passim)
Gingival ulceration (<1%)
Gynecomastia (<1%)
Headache
Hypersensitivity
  (2001): McMahon AD+, *J Clin Epidemiol* 54(12), 1271
  (1981): Ruppert GB+, *South Med J* 74, 241
Impaired wound healing
  (1988): Proper SA+, *J Am Acad Dermatol* 18, 1173
Myopathy
  (1987): Ross NS+, *JAMA* 257, 62
Oral lichenoid eruption
  (1983): Hamburger J+, *BMJ* 287, 1258
Oral mucosal lesions
  (1974): Regalado RG+, *J Int Med Res* 2, 115
Oral ulceration
  (1974): Regalado RG+, *J Int Med Res* 2, 115
Paresthesias
Pseudolymphoma
  (2001): Werth V, *Dermatology Times* 18
Pseudoporphyria
  (2000): De Silva B+, *Pediatr Dermatol* 17, 480
  (1992): Petersen CS+, *Ugeskr Laeger* (Danish) 154, 1713
Rhabdomyolysis
  (1989): Menzies DG+, *Med Toxicol Adverse* 4(6), 468
Serum sickness
  (1995): Lesko SM+, *JAMA* 273, 929
Stomatitis
Tinnitus
Xerostomia (<1%)

IBUTILIDE

Trade name: Corvert (Pharmacia)
Indications: Atrial fibrillation and flutter
Category: Antiarrhythmic class III
Half-life: 2–12 hours

Reactions

Skin

Bullous eruption
Dermatitis
  (1998): Dodds ES+, *Pharmacotherapy* 18, 880 (bullous)

Other

Headache
Torsades de pointes
  (2002): Gowda RM+, *Am J Ther* 9(6), 527

IDARUBICIN

Synonyms: 4-demethoxydaunorubicin; 4-DMDR
Trade name: Idamycin (Pharmacia)
Other common trade name: *Zavedos*
Indications: Acute myeloid leukemia
Category: Antineoplastic antibiotic
Half-life: 14–35 hours (oral)
Clinically important, potentially hazardous interactions with: aldesleukin

Reactions

Skin

Acral erythema
  (1993): Cohen PR, *Cutis* 51, 175
Bullous eruption (palms and soles)
Erythematous streaking (sic) (>10%)
Exanthems (<1%)
Radiation recall
  (1995): Gabel C+, *Gynecol Oncol* 57, 266
Rash (sic) (>10%)
  (1998): Stuart NS+, *Cancer Chemother Pharmacol* 21, 351
  (1997): Maloney DG+, *J Clin Oncol* 15, 3266
Urticaria (>10%)
  (1997): Maloney DG+, *J Clin Oncol* 15, 3266

Hair

Hair – alopecia (77%)
  (2000): No author, *Prescrire Int* 9, 103
  (1993): Ogawa M+, *Gan To Kaguku Ryoho* (Japanese) 20, 897
  (1993): Ogawa M+, *Gan To Kaguku Ryoho* (Japanese) 20, 907
  (1991): Hollingshead LM+, *Drugs* 42, 690
  (1988): Gillies H+, *Cancer Chemother Pharmacol* 21, 261
  (1986): Dodion P+, *Invest New Drugs* 4, 31
  (1986): Lopez M+, *Invest New Drugs* 4, 39

Nails

Nails – pigmentation
  (1997): Borecky Derrick J+, *Cutis* 59, 203

Other

Extravasation-site necrosis (>10%)
Injection-site urticaria
Mucositis (50%)
  (2000): Creutzig U+, *Klin Padiatr* 212, 163
  (1986): Dodion P+, *Invest New Drugs* 4, 31
Stomatitis (>10%)

IFOSFAMIDE

Trade name: Ifex (Bristol-Myers Squibb)
Other common trade names: *Holoxan; Ifoxan; Mitoxana; Tronoxal*
Indications: Cancers, sarcomas, leukemias, lymphomas
Category: Antineoplastic; Nitrogen mustard
Half-life: 4–15 hours
Clinically important, potentially hazardous interactions with: aldesleukin, aprepitant

Reactions

Skin

Allergic reactions (sic) (1–10%)
Dermatitis (sic) (1–10%)

Pigmentation (1–10%)
  (1994): Yule SM+, *Cancer* 73, 240
  (1993): Teresi ME+, *Cancer* 71, 2873

Hair

Hair – alopecia (50–83%)
  (1988): Negretti E+, *Tumori* (Italian) 74, 163 (100%)
  (1971): Kunz W+, *Schweiz Med Wochenschr* (German) 101, 1151

Nails

Nails – ridging (1–10%)
  (1994): Ben Dayan D+, *Acta Haematol* 91, 89

Other

Anaphylactoid reactions
Death
  (2002): Escudier B+, *J Urol* 168(3), 959 (with doxorubicin)
Oral mucosal lesions
Phlebitis (2%)
Sialorrhea (<1%)
Stomatitis (<1%)

IMATINIB

Synonyms: CGP57148; ST1571; STi571
Trade name: Gleevec (Novartis)
Other common trade name: *Glivec*
Indications: Chronic myeloid leukemia
Category: Antineoplastic; Signal transduction inhibitor; Tyrosine kinase inhibitor
Half-life: 18 hours
Clinically important, potentially hazardous interactions with: amlodipine, anisindione, anticoagulants, aprepitant, atorvastatin, barbiturates, benzodiazepines, butabarbital, carbamazepine, chlordiazepoxide, clarithromycin, clonazepam, clorazepate, corticosteroids, cyclosporine, diazepam, dicumarol, erythromycin, ethotoin, felodipine, flurazepam, fluvastatin, fosphenytoin, isradipine, itraconazole, ketoconazole, lorazepam, lovastatin, mephenytoin, mephobarbital, midazolam, nicardipine, nifedipine, nimodipine, nisoldipine, oxazepam, pentobarbital, phenobarbital, phenytoin, pimozide, pravastatin, primidone, quazepam, rifampin, secobarbital, simvastatin, **St John's wort**, temazepam, warfarin

Reactions

Skin

Acute generalized exanthematous pustulosis (AGEP)
  (2002): Schwarz M+, *Eur J Haematol* 69(4), 254 (2 cases)
Edema (1–5%)
  (2003): *Prescrire Int* 12(64), 49 (%)
  (2003): Shimazaki C+, *Leukemia* 17(4), 804
  (2003): Valeyrie L+, *J Am Acad Dermatol* 48(2), 201 (35 cases)
  (2002): Demetri GD+, *N Engl J Med* 347(7), 472
  (2002): Pindolia VK+, *Pharmacotherapy* 22(10), 1249
  (2002): Tefferi A+, *Blood* 99(10), 3854
  (2001): van Oosterom AT+, *Lancet* 358(9291), 1421
Necrolysis
  (2003): Schaich M+, *Ann Hematol* 82(5), 303
Night sweats (8–10%)
Periorbital edema
  (2003): Ramar K+, *J Clin Oncol* 21(1), 172
  (2002): Esmaeli B+, *Cancer* 95(4), 881
Peripheral edema
Petechiae (1–10%)
Photosensitivity

(2003): Rousselot P+, *Br J Haematol* 120(6), 1091
Pruritus (6–10%)
    (2003): Valeyrie L+, *J Am Acad Dermatol* 48(2), 201 (22 cases)
Rash (sic) (32–39%)
    (2003): Valeyrie L+, *J Am Acad Dermatol* 48(2), 201 (36 cases)
    (2001): van Oosterom+, *Lancet* 358(9291), 1421
Squamous cell carcinoma
    (2003): Baskaynak G+, *Eur J Haematol* 70(4), 231
Stevens–Johnson syndrome
    (2002): Vidal D+, *Br J Haematol* 119(1), 274

Other
Arthralgia (21–26%)
Fatigue
    (2002): Demetri GD+, *N Engl J Med* 347(7), 472
Gynecomastia (male)
    (2003): Gambacorti-Passerini C+, *Lancet* 361(9373), 1954
Headache
Joint pains
    (2003): *Prescrire Int* 12(64), 49 (%)
Myalgia (7–18%)
    (2002): Tefferi A+, *Blood* 99(10), 3854
Myositis
    (2002): Tefferi A+, *Blood* 99(10), 3854
Porphyria cutanea tarda
    (2003): Ho AY+, *Br J Haematol* 121(2), 375

IMIPENEM/CILASTATIN

Synonym: imipemide
Trade name: Primaxin (Merck)
Other common trade names: *Tenacid; Tienam; Tienam 500; Zienam*
Indications: Various infections caused by susceptible organisms
Category: Carbapenem antibiotic
Half-life: 1 hour
Clinically important, potentially hazardous interactions with: cyclosporine, ganciclovir

Reactions

Skin
Acute generalized exanthematous pustulosis (AGEP)
    (1989): Escallier F+, *Ann Dermatol Venereol* (French) 116, 407
Allergic reactions (sic) (1–3%)
    (1994): Pleasants RA+, *Chest* 106, 1124 (in patients with cystic fibrosis)
Angioedema (0.2%)
    (1987): Clissold SP+, *Drugs* 33, 183
Candidiasis (0.2%)
Diaphoresis (0.2%)
Erythema multiforme (0.2%)
    (1987): Clissold SP+, *Drugs* 33, 183
Exanthems (<1%)
    (1989): Escallier F+, *Ann Dermatol Venereol* (French) 116, 407
    (1987): Clissold SP+, *Drugs* 33, 183
    (1985): Calandra GB+, *Am J Med* 78, 73 (1–5%)
Flushing (0.2%)
Pruritus (0.3%)
    (1991): Machado ARL+, *J Allergy Clin Immunol* 87, 754
    (1989): Escallier F+, *Ann Dermatol Venereol* (French) 116, 407
    (1987): Clissold SP+, *Drugs* 33, 183
Pruritus vulvae (0.2%)
Pustules
    (1994): Spencer JM+, *Br J Dermatol* 130, 514

Rash (sic) (4%)
    (1994): Grayson ML+, *Clin Infect Dis* 18, 683
Toxic epidermal necrolysis (0.2%)
Urticaria (0.2%)
    (1991): Hantson P+, *BMJ* 302, 294
    (1989): Escallier F+, *Ann Dermatol Venereol* (French) 116, 407
    (1987): Clissold SP+, *Drugs* 33, 183
Vasculitis
    (1997): Reiner MR+, *J Am Podiatr Med Assoc* 87, 245

Other
Dysgeusia (0.2%)
Glossitis (0.2%)
Hypersensitivity
    (1988): Donowitz GR+, *N Engl J Med* 318, 490
Injection-site erythema (0.4%)
Injection-site pain
    (1991): *Drug Ther Bull* 29, 43
    (1985): Calandra GB+, *Am J Med* 78, 73 (0.7%)
Injection-site phlebitis
    (1991): *Drug Ther Bull* 29, 43
    (1988): Gould IM+, *Drugs Exp Clin Res* 14, 555
    (1987): Clissold SP+, *Drugs* 33, 183 (2%)
    (1985): Calandra GB+, *Am J Med* 78, 73 (3.8%)
Oral mucosal lesions
Paresthesias (0.2%)
Phlebitis (3%)
Sialorrhea (0.2%)
Thrombophlebitis (3.1%)
Tinnitus

IMIPRAMINE

Trade name: Tofranil (Mallinckrodt) (Novartis)
Other common trade names: *Apo-Imipramine; Imidol; Imipramin; Impril; Novo-Pramine; Primonil; Pryleugan*
Indications: Depression
Category: Tricyclic antidepressant
Half-life: 6–18 hours
Clinically important, potentially hazardous interactions with: amprenavir, arbutamine, clonidine, epinephrine, fluoxetine, formoterol, guanethidine, isocarboxazid, linezolid, MAO inhibitors, phenelzine, quinolones, sparfloxacin, tranylcypromine

Reactions

Skin
Acne
Allergic reactions (sic)
Angioedema (<1%)
    (1971): Almeyda J, *Br J Dermatol* 84, 298
Ankle edema
Bullous eruption
    (1977): Varma AJ+, *Arch Intern Med* 137, 1207 (passim)
Diaphoresis (1–25%)
    (2002): Mavissakalian M+, *J Clin Psychopharmacol* 22(2), 155
    (1990): Leeman CP, *J Clin Psychiatry* 51, 258
    (1989): Butt MM, *J Clin Psychiatry* 50, 146
    (1971): Almeyda J, *Br J Dermatol* 84, 298
    (1962): Busfield BL+, *J Nerv Ment Dis* 134, 339 (25%)
    (1961): Kiloh LG+, *BMJ* 1, 168
    (1959): Mann AM+, *Can Psychiatr Assoc J* 4, 38
Edema
    (1961): Kiloh LG+, *BMJ* 1, 168
Erythema

Exanthems (1–6%)
  (1992): Breathnach SM+, *Adverse Drug Reactions and the Skin*
    Blackwell, Oxford, 197 (passim)
  (1988): Warnock JK+, *Am J Psychiatry* 145, 425 (6%)
  (1985): Walter-Ryan WG+, *JAMA* 254, 357
  (1971): Almeyda J, *Br J Dermatol* 84, 298
  (1968): Powell WJ+, *JAMA* 206, 642
  (1959): Mann AM+, *Can Psychiatr Assoc J* 4, 38
Exfoliative dermatitis
  (1992): Breathnach SM+, *Adverse Drug Reactions and the Skin*
    Blackwell, Oxford, 197 (passim)
  (1971): Almeyda J, *Br J Dermatol* 84, 298
  (1968): Powell WJ+, *JAMA* 206, 642
  (1959): Mann AM+, *Can Psychiatr Assoc J* 4, 38
Fixed eruption (<1%)
  (1978): Sehgal VN+, *Int J Dermatol* 17, 78
Flushing
  (1961): Kiloh LG+, *BMJ* 1, 168
Lichen planus
  (1971): Almeyda J, *Br J Dermatol* 84, 298
Lupus erythematosus
  (1971): Almeyda J, *Br J Dermatol* 84, 298
Petechiae
Photosensitivity (<1%)
  (1985): Walter-Ryan WG+, *JAMA* 354, 357
  (1971): Almeyda J, *Br J Dermatol* 84, 298
  (1960): Gesensway D+, *Am J Psychiatry* 116, 1027
Pigmentation
  (2003): Dean CE+, *Ann Pharmacother* 37(6), 825
  (2002): Angel TA+, *Int J Dermatol* 41(6), 327 (slate gray)
    (photodistributed)
  (1999): Ming ME+, *J Am Acad Dermatol* 40, 159 (4 cases)
  (1999): Sicari MC+, *J Am Acad Dermatol* 40(2), 290 (slate gray)
    (2 cases)
  (1991): Hashimoto K+, *J Am Acad Dermatol* 25, 357 (slate-gray)
  (1990): Goldberg NC, *Dermatology Perspectives* 6, 8
  (1989): Hashimoto K+, *Am Soc Dermatopath* San Francisco, CA
    (abstract)
  (1988): Warnock JK+, *Am J Psychiatry* 145, 425
  (1970): Hare PJ, *Br J Dermatol* 83, 420 ("visage mauve")
Pruritus
  (1988): Warnock JK+, *Am J Psychiatry* 145, 425 (3%)
  (1987): Pohl R+, *Am J Psychiatry* 144, 237
  (1971): Almeyda J, *Br J Dermatol* 84, 298
  (1968): Powell WJ+, *JAMA* 206, 642
  (1961): Kiloh LG+, *BMJ* 1, 168
  (1959): Mann AM+, *Can Psychiatr Assoc J* 4, 38
Purpura
  (1988): Warnock JK+, *Am J Psychiatry* 145, 425
  (1971): Almeyda J, *Br J Dermatol* 84, 298
  (1971): Kosakova M, *Cesk Dermatol* (Czech) 46, 158
Rash (sic)
Urticaria
  (1992): Breathnach SM+, *Adverse Drug Reactions and the Skin*
    Blackwell, Oxford, 197 (passim)
  (1987): Pohl R+, *Am J Psychiatry* 144, 237
  (1985): Burnett GB+, *South Med J* 78, 71
  (1971): Almeyda J, *Br J Dermatol* 84, 298
  (1961): Kiloh LG+, *BMJ* 1, 168
  (1959): Mann AM+, *Can Psychiatr Assoc J* 4, 38
Vasculitis
  (1992): Breathnach SM+, *Adverse Drug Reactions and the Skin*
    Blackwell, Oxford, 197 (passim)
Xerosis

Hair

Hair – alopecia (<1%)
  (1994): Friedman M, *J Fam Pract* 39, 114
  (1991): Warnock JK+, *J Nerv Ment Dis* 179, 441

Hair – alopecia areata
  (1987): Baral J+, *Int J Dermatol* 26, 198

Nails

Nails – parrot-beak
  (1971): Kandil E, *J Med Liban* (French) 24, 433

Other

Black tongue
Dysgeusia (>10%) (metallic taste)
  (1961): Kiloh LG+, *BMJ* 1, 168
Galactorrhea (<1%)
  (1964): Klein JJ+, *N Engl J Med* 271, 510
Glossitis
  (1992): Breathnach SM+, *Adverse Drug Reactions and the Skin*
    Blackwell, Oxford, 197 (passim)
  (1959): Delay J+, *Can Psychiatr Assoc J* 4, 100
Glossodynia
Gynecomastia (<1%)
  (1964): Klein JJ+, *N Engl J Med* 271, 510
Hypogeusia
Mucous membrane desquamation
  (1968): Powell WJ+, *JAMA* 206, 642
Oral mucosal lesions
  (1971): Almeyda J, *Br J Dermatol* 84, 298
  (1964): Pollack B+, *Am J Psychiatry* 121, 384
  (1962): Busfield BL+, *J Nerv Ment Dis* 134, 339 (21%)
Oral ulceration
Paresthesias
Parkinsonism (1–10%)
Stomatitis
  (1992): Breathnach SM+, *Adverse Drug Reactions and the Skin*
    Blackwell, Oxford, 197 (passim)
  (1964): Pollack B+, *Am J Psychiatry* 121, 384
Tremor
Vaginitis
Xerostomia (>10%)
  (2002): Mavissakalian M+, *J Clin Psychopharmacol* 22(2), 155
  (1971): Almeyda J, *Br J Dermatol* 84, 298
  (1962): Busfield BL+, *J Nerv Ment Dis* 134, 339 (21%)
  (1961): Kiloh LG+, *BMJ* 1, 168
  (1959): Mann AM+, *Can Psychiatr Assoc J* 4, 38

IMIQUIMOD

Trade name: Aldara (3M)
Indications: External genital and perianal warts
Category: Immune response modifier (interferon inducer)
Half-life: N/A

Reactions

Skin

Bullous eruption
  (2002): Chen TM+, *Dermatol Surg* 28, 344 (for BCCs)
Burning (9–31%)
  (2001): Gollnick H+, *Int J STD AIDS* 12(1), 22
  (1999): Perry CM+, *Drugs* 58(2), 375
  (1998): Beutner KR+, *J Am Acad Dermatol* 38(2), 230 (31.3%)
Edema (12–17%)
Erosions (10–32%)
  (1999): Perry CM+, *Drugs* 58(2), 375
  (1998): Beutner KR+, *J Am Acad Dermatol* 38(2), 230 (10.4%)
Erythema (33–67%)
  (2002): Chen TM+, *Dermatol Surg* 28, 344 (for BCCs)
  (2001): Fife KH+, *Sex Transm Dis* 28(4), 226

(2001): Garland SM+, *Int J STD AIDS* 12(11), 722 (67%)
(2001): Gollnick H+, *Int J STD AIDS* 12(1), 22
(1999): Gilson RJ+, *AIDS* 13(17), 2397 (41.9%)
(1999): Perry CM+, *Drugs* 58(2), 375 (67%)
(1998): Beutner KR+, *J Am Acad Dermatol* 38(2), 230 (33.3%)
(1998): Edwards L+, *Arch Dermatol* 134(1), 25
Excoriations (18–25%)
(2001): Fife KH+, *Sex Transm Dis* 28(4), 226
(1999): Perry CM+, *Drugs* 58(2), 375
Flaking (18–25%)
(1999): Perry CM+, *Drugs* 58(2), 375 (67%)
Flu-like syndrome (1–3%)
Fungal infections (2–11%)
Irritation (sic)
(1998): Beutner KR+, *J Am Acad Dermatol* 38(2), 230 (16.7%)
Pigmentation
(2000): Geisse JK, *Dermatol Surg* 26, 579
Pruritus (22–67%)
(2001): Gollnick H+, *Int J STD AIDS* 12(1), 22
(1999): Perry CM+, *Drugs* 58(2), 375 (67%)
(1998): Beutner KR+, *J Am Acad Dermatol* 38(2), 230 (54.2%)
Scabbing (4%)
Tenderness (local)
(2002): Schroeder TL+, *J Am Acad Dermatol* 46(4), 545
(1998): Beutner KR+, *J Am Acad Dermatol* 38(2), 230 (12.5%)
Ulcerations (5–10%)
(2002): Chen TM+, *Dermatol Surg* 28, 344 (for BCCs) (focal)
(2002): Emmet S, Solana Beach, CA (from Internet)
(observation) (topical on lips)
(2001): Fife KH+, *Sex Transm Dis* 28(4), 226
(1998): Beutner KR+, *J Am Acad Dermatol* 38(2), 230 (10.4%)
Vesiculation (2–3%)
(2001): Fife KH+, *Sex Transm Dis* 28(4), 226

Hair

Hair – pigmentation (of white hair)
(2002): Kirschenbaum MB, Chicago, IL (from Internet)
(observation)

Other

Aphthous stomatitis
(2002): Goldblum O, Pittsburgh, PA (from Internet)
(observation) (topical on face and lips)
(2002): Kaufmann MD, New York, NY (from Internet)
(observation) (topical on face)
Application-site reactions (sic)
(2001): Barba AR+, *Dermatol Online J* 7(1), 20
(2001): Gollnick H+, *Int J STD AIDS* 12, 22
(2000): Kagy MK+, *Dermatol Surg* 26(6), 577 (for BCCs)
Depression
(1998): Goldstein D+, *J Infect Dis* 178(3), 858 (oral intake)
Headache
Induration (5%)
Myalgia (1%)
(2002): Sorkin MJ, Denver, CO (from Internet) (observation)
(topical)
Pain (2–8%)
(2001): Gollnick H+, *Int J STD AIDS* 12(1), 22
(1998): Beutner KR+, *J Am Acad Dermatol* 38(2), 230

INAMRINONE

Trade name: Inocor (Sanofi-Synthelabo)
Other common trade names: *Amcoral; Cartonic; Vestistol*
Indications: Congestive heart failure
Category: Positive inotropic agent
Half-life: 4.6 hours

Reactions

Skin
None

Other
Hypersensitivity
Injection-site burning (0.2%)

INDAPAMIDE*

Trade name: Lozol (Aventis)
Other common trade names: *Dapa-tabs; Fludex; Ipamix; Lozide; Naplin; Natrilix; Pamid*
Indications: Edema
Category: Antihypertensive sulfonamide diuretic
Half-life: 14–18 hours
Clinically important, potentially hazardous interactions with: digoxin, lithium

Reactions

Skin
Angioedema
(1994): Gales BJ+, *Am J Hosp Pharm* 51, 118
(1992): Spinler SA+, *Cutis* 50, 200
(1987): Stricker BHC+, *Br Med J Clin Res Ed* 295, 1313
Bullous eruption
Diaphoresis
Erythema multiforme
(1994): Gales BJ+, *Am J Hosp Pharm* 51, 118
(1987): Stricker BHC+, *Br Med J Clin Res Ed* 295, 1313
Exanthems
(1987): Stricker BHC+, *Br Med J Clin Res Ed* 295, 1313
Fixed eruption
(1998): De Barrio M+, *J Investig Allergol Clin Immunol* 8, 253
Flushing (<5%)
(1985): Chaignon M+, *Arch Mal Coeur Vaiss* (French) 78, 67
Necrotizing angiitis
Pemphigus foliaceus
(2002): Schmutz JL+, *Ann Dermatol Venereol* 129(8-9), 1085
Peripheral edema (<5%)
Photosensitivity (<1%)
Pigmentation
(2002): Roy-Peaud F+, *Rev Med Interne* 23(7), 674
Pruritus (<5%)
(1985): Kirsten R+, *Z Kardiol* (German) 74, 66
(1982): Brennan L+, *Clin Ther* 5, 121
Purpura
Rash (sic) (<5%)
(1988): Kandela D+, *BMJ* 296, 573
(1985): Kirsten R+, *Z Kardiol* (German) 74, 66
(1983): Slotkoff L, *Am Heart J* 106, 233
(1982): Brennan L+, *Clin Ther* 5, 121
Stevens–Johnson syndrome
(1992): Spinler SA+, *Cutis* 50, 200

Toxic epidermal necrolysis
  (1993): Partanen J+, *Arch Dermatol* 129, 793
  (1990): Black RJ+, *Br Med J Clin Res Ed* 301, 1280
  (1987): Stricker BHC+, *Br Med J Clin Res Ed* 295, 1313
Urticaria (<5%)
  (1987): Stricker BHC+, *Br Med J Clin Res Ed* 295, 1313
Vasculitis (<5%)

Other
Anaphylactoid reactions
Headache
Paresthesias (<5%)
Xanthopsia
Xerostomia (<5%)
  (1985): Kirsten R+, *Z Kardiol* (German) 74, 66
  (1982): Brennan L+, *Clin Ther* 5, 121

*Note: Indapamide is a sulfonamide and can be absorbed systemically. Sulfonamides can produce severe, possibly fatal, reactions such as toxic epidermal necrolysis and Stevens–Johnson syndrome

INDINAVIR

Trade name: Crixivan (Merck)
Indications: HIV infection
Category: Antiretroviral; Protease inhibitor
Half-life: ~1.8 hours
Clinically important, potentially hazardous interactions with: alprazolam, atazanavir, chlordiazepoxide, clonazepam, clorazepate, delavirdine, diazepam, dihydroergotamine, ergot alkaloids, estazolam, fentanyl, flurazepam, halazepam, methysergide, midazolam, phenytoin, pimozide, quazepam, sildenafil, **St John's wort**, triazolam

Reactions

Skin
Allergic reactions (sic)
  (1998): Rijnders B+, *Clin Infect Dis* 26, 523
Cheilitis
  (2001): Scully C+, *Oral Dis* 7, 205 (passim)
  (2000): Bonfanti P+, *J Acquir Immune Defic Syndr* 23(3), 236
  (2000): Calista D+, *Eur J Dermatol* 10, 292 (51.7%)
  (2000): Fox PA+, *Sex Transm Infect* 76, 323
Dermatitis (sic) (<2%)
Diaphoresis (<2%)
Erythema multiforme
Exanthems
  (1999): Fung HB+, *Pharmacotherapy* 19, 1328
Eyelid edema (<2%)
Flushing (<2%)
Folliculitis (<2%)
Herpes simplex (<2%)
Herpes zoster (<2%)
Pigmentation
Pruritus
  (2000): Calista D+, *Eur J Dermatol* 10, 292 (11.9%)
  (1999): Gajewski LK+, *Ann Pharmacother* 33, 17 (86%)
Pyogenic granuloma
  (1998): Bouscarat F+, *N Engl J Med* 338, 1776 (great toes)
Rash (sic)
  (2002): Albrecht D+, *AIDS* 16(15), 2098
  (1999): Gajewski LK+, *Ann Pharmacother* 33, 17 (67%)
Seborrhea (<2%)

Stevens–Johnson syndrome
  (1998): Teira R+, *Scand J Infect Dis* 30, 634
Striae
  (1999): Darvay A+, *J Am Acad Dermatol* 41, 467
Urticaria (<2%)
Vasculitis
  (2001): Rachline A+, *Br J Dermatol* 143, 1112
Xerosis
  (2000): Bonfanti P+, *J Acquir Immune Defic Syndr* 23(3), 236
  (2000): Calista D+, *Eur J Dermatol* 10, 292 (11.9%)

Hair
Hair – alopecia
  (2002): Ginarte M+, *AIDS* 16(12), 1695 (with ritonavir)
  (2000): Bonfanti P+, *J Acquir Immune Defic Syndr* 23(3), 236
  (2000): Calista D+, *Eur J Dermatol* 10, 292 (11.9%)
  (1999): Bouscarat F+, *N Engl J Med* 341, 618
  (1998): d'Arminio Monforte A+, *AIDS* 12, 328
Hair – loss
  (2002): Ginarte M+, *AIDS* 16(12), 1695

Nails
Nails – ingrown
  (2001): James CW+, *Ann Pharmacother* 35(7), 881 (with ritonavir)
  (2000): Heim M+, *Haemophilia* 6, 191
  (2000): Miot HA, Sao Paulo, Brazil (from internet) (observation)
Nails – paronychia
  (2001): Colson AE+, *Clin Infect Dis* 32, 140
  (2001): Garcia Garcia+, *Rev Clin Esp* 201(8), 455
  (2000): Dauden E+, *Br J Dermatol* 142, 1063 (toes and finger)
  (2000): Sass JO+, *Dermatology* 200(1), 40
  (1998): Bouscarat F+, *N Engl J Med* 338, 1776 (great toes)
Nails – pyogenic granulomas
  (2000): Calista D+, *Eur J Dermatol* 10, 292 (5.9%)
  (2000): Sass JO+, *Dermatology* 200(1), 40

Other
Aphthous stomatitis (<2%)
Bromhidrosis (<2%)
Bruxism (<2%)
Buffalo hump
  (2000): Calista D+, *Eur J Dermatol* 10, 292
Buffalo neck
  (1999): Milpied-Homsi B+, *Ann Dermatol Venereol* (French) 126, 254
Dysesthesia (<2%)
Dysgeusia (2.6%)
Foetor ex ore (halitosis) (<2%)
Gingivitis (<2%)
Gynecomastia
  (2001): Manfredi R+, *Ann Pharmacother* 35, 438
  (1998): Caeiro JP+, *Clin Infect Dis* 27, 1539
  (1998): Lui A+, *Clin Infect Dis* 26, 1482
  (1998): Toma E+, *AIDS* 12, 681
Headache
Hyperesthesia (<2%)
Lipoatrophy
  (2001): Lichtenstein KA+, *AIDS* 15(11), 1389
Lipodystrophy
  (2002): Reid S, *Can Adv Drug Reaction Newsletter* 12, 5
  (2000): Calista D+, *Eur J Dermatol* 10, 292 (14.3%)
  (2000): Hartmann M+, *Hautarzt* (German) 51, 159
  (1999): Hermieu JF+, *Prog Urol* (French) 9, 537
  (1999): Krautheim A, *Schweiz Rundsch Med Prax* (German) 88, 285
  (1998): Miller KD+, *Lancet* 351, 871
  (1998): Viraben R+, *AIDS* 12, F37
  (1997): Herry I+, *Clin Infect Dis* 25, 937 (breast hypertrophy)

Lipomatosis
  (2000): Calista D+, *Eur J Dermatol* 10, 292
  (1997): Hengel RL+, *Lancet* 350, 1596 (benign symmetric)
Myalgia (<2%)
Paresthesias (<2%)
  (2001): McMahon D+, *Antivir Ther* 6(2), 105
Porphyria (acute)
  (2001): Schmutz JL+, *Ann Dermatol Venereol* 128(2), 184
  (1999): Fox PA+, *AIDS* 16, 322
Tendinitis
  (2002): Florence E+, *Ann Rheum Dis* 61(1), 82
Tuberculosis
  (2003): Taylor JC+, *Rheumatology* (Oxford) 42(7), 901
Xerostomia (0.5%)

*Note: Protease inhibitors cause dyslipidemia which includes elevated triglycerides and cholesterol and redistribution of body fat centrally to produce the so-called "protease paunch," breast enlargement, facial atrophy, and "buffalo hump"

INDOMETHACIN

Synonym: indometacin
Trade name: Indocin (Merck)
Other common trade names: *Amuno; Apo-Indomethacin; Durametacin; Imbrilon; Indochron; Indolar SR; Indotec; Nu-Indo; Rhodacine; Vonum*
Indications: Arthritis
Category: Antipyretic; Nonsteroidal anti-inflammatory (NSAID)
Half-life: 4.5 hours
Clinically important, potentially hazardous interactions with: aldesleukin, aspirin, diflunisal, diuretics, methotrexate, NSAIDs, sermorelin, triamterene, urokinase

Reactions

Skin
Angioedema (<1%)
  (1981): Juhlin L, *Br J Dermatol* 104, 369
  (1966): Rothermich ND, *JAMA* 195, 531 (0.5%)
Bullous eruption (<1%)
  (1986): Harrington CI+, *Br J Dermatol* 114, 265
  (1969): Duperrat B+, *Bull Soc Franc Dermatol Syphiligr* (French) 76, 26
Dermatitis
  (1999): Pulido Z+, *Contact Dermatitis* 41, 112
  (1998): Ueda K+, *Contact Dermatitis* 39, 323
  (1993): Goday-Bujan JJ+, *Contact Dermatitis* 28, 111
  (1993): Ophaswongse S+, *Contact Dermatitis* 29, 57
  (1987): Beller U+, *Contact Dermatitis* 17, 121
Dermatitis herpetiformis (exacerbation)
  (1986): Harrington CI+, *Br J Dermatol* 114, 265
  (1985): Griffiths CEM+, *Br J Dermatol* 112, 443
Diaphoresis (<1%)
Ecchymoses (<1%)
Eczema (sic)
  (1987): Beller U+, *Contact Dermatitis* 17, 121
Edema (3–9%)
  (1978): Castles JJ+, *Arch Intern Med* 138, 362 (5.6%)
Erythema multiforme (<1%)
  (1985): Ting HC+, *Int J Dermatol* 24, 58
Erythema nodosum (<1%)
  (1982): Elizaga FV, *Ann Intern Med* 96, 383
Exanthems
  (1978): Castles JJ+, *Arch Intern Med* 138, 362 (5.6%)
  (1976): Arndt KA+, *JAMA* 235, 918 (0.4%)

  (1975): Pasquariello G+, *Curr Med Res Opin* 3, 109 (1.8%)
  (1973): Thorne N, *Practitioner* 211, 606
  (1970): Almeyda J+, *Br J Dermatol* 83, 707
  (1967): Boardman PL+, *Ann Rheum Dis* 26, 127 (1.7%)
  (1967): *Clin Pharmacol Ther* 8, 11 (11%)
Exfoliative dermatitis (<1%)
  (1983): O'Sullivan M+, *Br J Rheumatol* 22, 47
Fixed eruption
  (1998): Mahboob A+, *Int J Dermatol* 37, 833
  (1976): Mackie BS, *Arch Dermatol* 112, 122
Flushing (>1%)
Generalized eruption (sic)
  (1966): Kern AB, *Arch Dermatol* 93, 239
Granulomas (plasma cell)
  (1975): Shelley WB+, *Acta Derm Venereol* (Stockh) 55, 489
Hot flashes (<1%)
Lichen planus
  (1983): Hamburger J+, *BMJ* 287, 1258
Pemphigus
Periorbital edema
  (1970): Almeyda J+, *Br J Dermatol* 83, 707
  (1966): Rothermich NO, *JAMA* 195, 531
Peripheral edema
Petechiae (>1%)
Photosensitivity
  (1984): Stern RS+, *JAMA* 252, 1433
Pruritus (1–10%)
  (1973): Thorne N, *Practitioner* 211, 606
  (1970): Almeyda J+, *Br J Dermatol* 83, 707
  (1967): *Clin Pharmacol Ther* 8, 11 (5%)
Psoriasis
  (1993): Shelley WB+, *Cutis* 51, 415 (observation)
  (1989): Lazarova AZ+, *Clin Exp Dermatol* 14, 260 (from topical application)
  (1987): Powles AV+, *Br J Dermatol* 117, 799
  (1987): Sendagorta E+, *Dermatologica* 175, 300
  (1986): Abel EA+, *J Am Acad Dermatol* 15, 1007
  (1981): Katayama H+, *J Dermatol* (Tokio) 8, 323
  (1980): Katayama H+, *Nippon Hifuka Gakkai Zasshi* (Japanese) 90, 1027
Purpura (<1%)
  (1984): Camba L+, *Acta Hematol* 71, 350
  (1974): Cuthbert MF, *Curr Med Res Opin* 2, 600
  (1973): Thorne N, *Practitioner* 211, 606
  (1970): Almeyda J+, *Br J Dermatol* 83, 707
  (1968): Bartoletti L+, *Riv Crit Clin Med* (Italian) 68, 279
Pustular psoriasis
  (1987): Sendagorta E+, *Dermatologica* 175, 300
Rash (sic) (>10%)
  (1967): Boardman PL+, *Ann Rheum Dis* 26, 127
Reiter's syndrome (exacerbation)
  (1989): Allegue F+, *Med Cutan Ibero Lat Am* (Spanish) 17, 113
Side effects (sic)
  (1986): Bigby M+, *JAMA* 256, 3358 (0.21%)
Stevens–Johnson syndrome (<1%)
Toxic epidermal necrolysis (<1%)
  (1996): Lear JT+, *Postgrad Med J* 72, 186
  (1990): Roujeau JC+, *Arch Dermatol* 126, 37
  (1989): Roth DE+, *Med Clin North Am* 73, 1275
  (1986): Johnson VB+, *La Pharm* 45, 4
  (1985): Heng MCY, *Br J Dermatol* 113, 597
  (1983): O'Sullivan M+, *Br J Rheumatol* 22, 47
Urticaria
  (1995): Gebhardt M+, *Z Rheumatol* (German) 54, 405
  (1992): Shelley WB+, *Cutis* 50, 87 (observation)
  (1985): O'Brien WM+, *J Rheumatol* 12, 13
  (1981): Juhlin L, *Br J Dermatol* 104, 369
  (1974): Mathews JI+, *Ann Intern Med* 80, 771

(1973): Thorne N, *Practitioner* 211, 606
(1970): Almeyda J+, *Br J Dermatol* 83, 707
Urticaria pigmentosa
(1968): Vissian L+, *Bull Soc Franc Dermatol Syphiligr* (French) 75, 591
Vasculitis (<1%)
(1988): Gamboa PM+, *Allergol Immunopathol Madr* (Spanish) 16, 53
(1985): Bigby M, *J Am Acad Dermatol* 12, 866
(1985): O'Brien WM+, *J Rheumatol* 12, 13
(1971): Marsh FP+, *Ann Rheum Dis* 30, 501
(1970): Almeyda J+, *Br J Dermatol* 83, 707

Hair

Hair – alopecia (<1%)

Nails

Nails – onycholysis

Other

Ageusia
(1967): Boardman PL+, *Ann Rheum Dis* 26, 127
Anaphylactoid reactions (<1%)
Aphthous stomatitis
Gynecomastia (<1%)
Headache
Hypersensitivity (<1%)
Oral lichenoid eruption
(1983): Hamburger J+, *BMJ* 287, 1258
Oral mucosal lesions
(1967): Boardman PL+, *Ann Rheum Dis* 26, 127 (0.5%)
(1967): *Clin Pharmacol Ther* 8, 11 (7%)
Oral ulceration
(2000): Madinier I+, *Ann Med Interne (Paris)* (French) 151, 248
(1983): Hamburger J+, *BMJ* 287, 1258
(1975): Guggenheimer J+, *J Am Dent Assoc* 90, 632
(1967): Boardman PL+, *Ann Rheum Dis* 26, 127
Paresthesias (<1%)
Pseudolymphoma
(2000): Werth V, *Dermatology Times* 18
Pseudoporphyria
(2000): De Silva B+, *Pediatr Dermatol* 17, 480
Serum sickness
(1985): Ferraccioli G+, *Acta Haematol* 73, 45
Temporal arteritis
(1985): O'Brien WM+, *J Rheumatol* 12, 13
(1967): Easterbrook WM+, *Can Med Assoc J* 97, 296
Tinnitus
Tongue edema
(1967): Boardman PL+, *Ann Rheum Dis* 26, 127
Ulcerative stomatitis (<1%)
(1982): Bailin PL+, *Clin Rheum Dis* 8, 493 (passim)
Xerostomia

INFLIXIMAB

Trade name: Remicade (Centocor)
Indications: Crohn's disease
Category: Monoclonal antibody; Tumor necrosis factor alpha blocker
Half-life: 9.5 days

Reactions

Skin

Acute febrile neutrophilic dermatosis (Sweet's syndrome)

(2003): Matzkies FG+, *Ann Rheum Dis* 62(1), 81
Adverse effects (sic)
(2001): Serrano MS+, *Ann Pharmacother* 35(7), 823
Allergic reactions (sic)
(2002): Brocq O+, *Presse Med* 31(39), 1836
Bullous eruption
(2002): Kent PD+, *Arthritis Rheum* 46(8), 2257
Candidiasis (5%)
Chills (5–9%)
Edema
(1999): Lichenstein GR+, *Biologics in Clinical Practice Symposium*, Orlando, FL, May 19 (from Internet) (observation)
Eruptions
(2002): Bartolucci P+, *Rheumatology (Oxford)* 41(10), 1126 (2 cases)
Herpes simplex
(2001): Voigtländer C+, *Arch Dermatol* 137, 1571
Herpes zoster
(2002): Baumgart DC+, *Ann Rheum Dis* 61(7), 661
Infections (sic) (21%)
(2003): Kroesen S+, *Rheumatology (Oxford)* 42(5), 617
(2003): Mikuls TR+, *Drug Saf* 26(1), 23
(2002): Brocq O+, *Presse Med* 31(39), 1836
(2001): Ouraghi A+, *Gastroenterol Clin Biol* 25(11), 949
(2001): Serrano MS+, *Ann Pharmacother* 35(7), 823
Lupus erythematosus
(2003): Debandt M+, *Clin Rheumatol* 22(1), 56
(2003): Klapman JB+, *Inflamm Bowel Dis* 9(3), 176
(2003): Mikuls TR+, *Drug Saf* 26(1), 23
(2002): Ali Y+, *Ann Intern Med* 137(7), 625
(2000): Charles PJ+, *Arthritis Rheum* 43(11), 2383
Lymphoma
(2002): Brown SL+, *Arthritis Rheum* 46(12), 3151 (8 cases)
(2001): Aithal GP+, *Aliment Pharmacol Ther* 15(8), 1101
(1992): Greenstein AJ+, *Cancer* 69, 1119
Molluscum contagiosum (eyelids)
(2002): Cursiefen C+, *Am J Ophthalmol* 134(2), 270
Necrotizing fasciitis
(2002): Chan AT+, *Postgrad Med J* 78(915), 47
Photosensitivity
(2002): Smith JG, Mobile, AL (from Internet) (observation) (2 cases)
Pruritus (5%)
(2001): Finkelstein RP, Stratford, NJ (from Internet) (observation)
(1999): Lichenstein GR+, *Biologics in Clinical Practice Symposium*, Orlando, FL, May 19
Psoriasis
(2002): Smith SZ, Louisville, KY (from Internet) (observation)
(2001): Finkelstein RP, Stratford, NJ (from Internet) (observation)
Pustules
(2002): Chan AT+, *Postgrad Med J* 78(915), 47
(2001): Finkelstein RP, Stratford, NJ (from Internet) (observation)
Rash (sic) (6%)
(2002): Ljung T+, *Scand J Gastroenterol* 37(9), 1108
(2001): Serrano MS+, *Ann Pharmacother* 35(7), 823
(2000): Hyams JS+, *J Pediatr* 137(2), 192
(1999): Baert S+, *Int J Colorectal Dis* 14, 47
(1999): Lichenstein GR+, *Biologics in Clinical Practice Symposium* Orlando, FL, May 19
Red man syndrome
(2003): Lobel EZ+, *J Clin Gastroenterol* 36(2), 186
Ulcerations (foot)
(2002): Conaghan P+, *Skin & Allergy News* June, 40
Urticaria
(1999): Lichenstein GR+, *Biologics in Clinical Practice Symposium*, Orlando, FL, May 19
(1997): Van Deventer SJH, *Clin Nutr* 16, 271
Vasculitis

(2003): McIlwain L+, *J Clin Gastroenterol* 36(5), 411

Other

Anaphylactoid reactions
  (2002): Diamanti A+, *J Pediatr* 140(5), 636
  (2002): O'Connor M+, *Dig Dis Sci* 47(6), 1323
  (2002): Sample C+, *Can J Gastroenterol* 16(3), 165
  (2000): Soykan I+, *Am J Gastroenterol* 95(9), 2395
Arthralgia
  (2002): Kugathasan S+, *Am J Gastroenterol* 97(6), 1408
  (2002): Riegert-Johnson DL+, *Inflamm Bowel Dis* 8(3), 186
  (2001): Serrano MS+, *Ann Pharmacother* 35(7), 823
Death
  (2002): de' Clari F+, *Circulation* 105(21), E183
  (2002): Su C+, *Am J Gastroenterol* 97(10), 2577
  (2001): Lankarani KB, *J Clin Gastroenterol* 33(3), 255
  (2001): Srinivasan R, *Am J Gastroenterol* 96, 2274 (neonatal)
Headache
Hypersensitivity
  (2002): Riegert-Johnson DL+, *Inflamm Bowel Dis* 8(3), 186
  (1999): Lichenstein GR+, *Biologics in Clinical Practice Symposium* Orlando, FL, May 19
  (1997): Van Deventer SJH, *Clin Nutr* 16, 271
Injection-site reactions (sic) (16%)
  (2003): Cheifetz A+, *Am J Gastroenterol* 98(6), 1315 (6.1%)
  (2003): Crandall WV+, *Aliment Pharmacol Ther* 17(1), 75 (35 cases)
  (2002): Kugathasan S+, *Am J Gastroenterol* 97(6), 1408
  (2002): Steinfeld SD+, *Arthritis Rheum* 46(12), 3301
  (1989): Morrison SL, *Hosp Prac* 24, 65
Lymphoproliferative disease
  (2002): Brown SL+, *Arthritis Rheum* 46(12), 3151 (8 cases)
Myalgia (5%)
  (2002): Kugathasan S+, *Am J Gastroenterol* 97(6), 1408
  (2002): Riegert-Johnson DL+, *Inflamm Bowel Dis* 8(3), 186
  (1999): Baert S+, *Int J Colorectal Dis* 14, 47
  (1999): Lichenstein GR+, *Biologics in Clinical Practice Symposium* Orlando, FL, May 19
Oral mucosal reaction
  (2002): Kugathasan S+, *Am J Gastroenterol* 97(6), 1408
Paresthesias (1–4%)
  (2002): Conaghan P+, *Skin & Allergy News* June, 40
Parkinsonism
  (2003): Hrycaj P+, *Rheumatology* (Oxford) 42(5), 702
Pneumonia
  (2002): Ljung T+, *Scand J Gastroenterol* 37(9), 1108
Polychondritis
  (2003): Matzkies FG+, *Ann Rheum Dis* 62(1), 81
Tuberculosis
  (2003): Arend SM+, *Neth J Med* 61(4), 111
  (2003): Long R+, *CMAJ* 168(9), 1153
  (2002): Liberopoulos EN+, *Am J Med* 113(7), 615
  (2002): Ramos Gonzalez A+, *Med Clin* (Barc) 119(16), 636
  (2001): Keane J+, *N Engl J Med* 345(15), 1098 (70 cases)

INH

(See ISONIAZID)

INSULIN

Trade names: Humulin (Lilly); Iletin Lente (Lilly); Novolin R (Novo Nordisk); NPH (Lilly); Velosulin (Novo Nordisk)
Other common trade names: *Humalog; Huminsulin; Insuman; Monotard; Velosuline Humaine*
Indications: Diabetes
Category: Hypoglycemic
Duration of action: 5–28 hours
Clinically important, potentially hazardous interactions with: alcohol, ethanolamine, guanethidine, pegvisomant, propranolol, sermorelin, vidarabine

Note: About 25% of patients with insulin allergy have a concomitant history of penicillin allergy

Reactions

Skin

Allergic reactions (sic) (local)
  (2002): Lee AY+, *Acta Derm Venereol* 82(2), 114
  (1989): Zinman B, *N Engl J Med* 321, 363
  (1988): Plantin P+, *Ann Dermatol Venereol* (French) 115, 813 (>5%)
  (1985): Bruni B+, *Diabetes Care* 8, 201
  (1984): Grammer LC+, *JAMA* 251, 1459
  (1982): Carveth-Johnson AO+, *Lancet* 2, 1287
  (1982): Patterson R+, *JAMA* 248, 2637 (passim)
  (1981): Hasche H+, *Dtsch Med Wochenschr* (German) 106, 1451
  (1981): Kahn CB, *Handbook of Diabetes Mellitus* Garland STPM, 75
  (1980): Jegasothy BV, *Int J Dermatol* 19, 139 (immediate and delayed) (10–56%)
  (1979): Borsey DQ+, *Postgrad Med J* 55, 199
  (1969): Aubert J+, *Rev Fr Allergol* (French) 9, 40
  (1961): Hanauer L+, *Diabetes* 10, 105
  (1939): Kern RA+, *JAMA* 113, 198
Angioedema
  (1983): Grammer LC+, *J Allergy Clin Immunol* 71, 250
  (1981): Kahn CB, *Handbook of Diabetes Mellitus* Garland STPM, 75
  (1979): Lynfield Y+, *Arch Dermatol* 115, 591 (passim)
  (1978): Galloway JA+, *Med Clin North Am* 62, 663
  (1976): Lamkin N+, *J Allergy Clin Immunol* 58, 213
  (1952): Dolger H, *Med Clin North Am* 36, 783
Bullous eruption
  (1974): Haroon TS, *Scott Med J* 19, 257
Dermatitis
  (1994): Goldfine AB+, *Curr Ther Endocrinol Metab* 5, 461
  (1989): Geldof BA+, *Contact Dermatitis* 20, 384
Diaphoresis (1–10%)
Edema (1–10%)
  (1981): Galloway JA+, *Diabetes Mellitus* Bowie 5, 117
  (1979): Lawrence JR+, *BMJ* 2, 445
Exanthems
  (1978): Galloway JA+, *Med Clin North Am* 62, 663
Flushing
  (1961): Hanauer L+, *Diabetes* 10, 105
Granulomas (zinc)
  (1989): Jordaan HF+, *Clin Exp Dermatol* 14, 227
Hematomas
  (2003): Camata DG, *Rev Lat Am Enfermagem* 11(1), 119
Hyperkeratotic verrucous papules
  (1989): Jordaan HF+, *Clin Exp Dermatol* 14, 277
  (1986): Fleming MG+, *Arch Dermatol* 122, 1054 (resembling acanthosis nigricans)
  (1969): Erickson L+, *JAMA* 209, 934

Keloid
  (1970): Jelinek JE, *Year Book of Dermatology* Chicago 5–35
Necrosis
  (1974): Rohan P+, *Arch Dermatol Forsch* 250, (German) 121
Pallor (1–10%)
Pigmentation
  (1970): Jelinek JE, *Year Book of Dermatology* Chicago 5–35
Pigskin appearance (sic)
  (1925): Lawrence RD, *Lancet* 1, 1125
Pruritus (1–10%)
  (2002): Lee AY+, *Acta Derm Venereol* 82(2), 114
  (1981): Knick B, *Munch Med Wochenschr* (German) 123, 1197
  (1925): Lawrence RD, *Lancet* 1, 1125
  (1922): Banting FG+, *J Metab Res* 2, 547
Purpura
  (1976): Lamkin N+, *J Allergy Clin Immunol* 58, 213
  (1956): Constam GR, *Diabetes* 5, 121
Urticaria (1–10%)
  (1996): Rowland-Payne CM+, *Br J Dermatol* 134, 184
  (1995): Chng HH+, *Allergy* 50, 984
  (1988): Plantin P+, *Ann Dermatol Venereol* (French) 115, 813
  (1983): Grammer LC+, *J Allergy Clin Immunol* 71, 250
  (1982): Mirouze J+, *Nouv Presse Med* (French) 11, 3121
  (1982): Patterson R+, *JAMA* 248, 2637 (passim)
  (1981): Kahn CB, *Handbook of Diabetes Mellitus* Garland
    STPM, 75
  (1979): Levy WJ+, *Cleve Clin Q* 46, 155
  (1979): Lynfield Y+, *Arch Dermatol* 115, 591 (passim)
  (1978): Galloway JA+, *Med Clin North Am* 62, 663
  (1978): Reisner C+, *BMJ* 2, 56
  (1976): Lamkin N+, *J Allergy Clin Immunol* 58, 213
  (1962): Arkins JA+, *J Allergy* 33, 69
  (1952): Dolger H, *Med Clin North Am* 36, 783
  (1925): Lawrence RD, *Lancet* 1, 1125
  (1922): Banting FG+, *J Metab Res* 2, 547
Vasculitis
  (2002): Mandrup-Poulsen T+, *Diabetes Care* 25(1), 242
  (1983): Grammer LC+, *J Allergy Clin Immunol* 71, 250
Xanthomatosis
  (1975): Vermeer BJ+, *Dermatologica* 151, 43

Other

Amyloidosis (localized)
  (2002): Swift B, *Diabet Med* 19(10), 881
Anaphylactoid reactions (1–10%)
  (1983): Grammer LC+, *J Allergy Clin Immunol* 71, 250
  (1982): Patterson R+, *JAMA* 248, 2637 (passim)
  (1981): Kahn CB, *Handbook of Diabetes Mellitus* Garland
    STPM, 75
  (1979): Lynfield Y+, *Arch Dermatol* 115, 591 (passim)
  (1978): Galloway JA+, *Med Clin North Am* 62, 663
  (1976): Lamkin N+, *J Allergy Clin Immunol* 58, 213
  (1952): Dolger H, *Med Clin North Am* 36, 783
  (1925): Lawrence RD, *Lancet* 1, 1125
Atrophy
  (1978): Oakley WG+, *Diabetes and its Management* Blackwell,
    103
Headache
Hypersensitivity
  (2003): Wittrup M+, *Ugeskr Laeger* 165(21), 2207
  (1983): Berman BA+, *Cutis* 32, 320
  (1982): deShazo RD+, *J Allergy Clin Immunol* 69, 229
  (1974): Federlin K, *Dtsch Med Wochenschr* (German) 99, 535
Hypertrophic lipodystrophy
  (1983): Johnson DA+, *Cutis* 32, 273
Injection-site calcification
  (1995): Ullman HR+, *J Comput Assist Tomogr* 19, 657
Injection-site cancer (sic)
  (1976): Sampson WI, *JAMA* 235, 374

Injection-site induration
  (1983): White WB+, *Am J Med* 74, 909
  (1981): Galloway JA+, *Diabetes Mellitus* Bowie 5, 117
  (1979): Feinglos MN+, *Lancet* 1, 122 (due to zinc)
  (1979): Lynfield Y+, *Arch Dermatol* 115, 591 (with erythema)
  (1978): Galloway JA+, *Med Clin North Am* 62, 663
Injection-site pruritus
  (1988): Plantin P+, *Ann Dermatol Venereol* (French) 115, 813
  (1979): Lynfield Y+, *Arch Dermatol* 115, 591
Injection-site reactions (sic)
  (2003): HOE 901/2004, *Diabet Med* 20(7), 545 (1 case)
Lipoatrophy (1–10%)
  (2003): Ampudia-Blasco FJ+, *Diabetes Care* 26(3), 953
  (2003): Chowdhury TA+, *BMJ* 327(7411), 383
  (2003): Felner EI, *J Pediatr* 142(4), 448
  (1998): Murao S+, *Intern Med* 37, 1031
  (1996): Logwin S+, *Diabetes Care* 19, 255
  (1993): Chantelau E+, *Exp Clin Endocrinol* 101, 194
  (1992): Igea JM+, *Allergol Immunopathol Madr* (Spanish) 20, 173
  (1989): Gyimesi A+, *Orv Hetil* (Hungarian) 130, 2751
  (1989): Zinman B, *N Engl J Med* 321, 363
  (1988): McNally PG+, *Postgrad Med J* 64, 850
  (1988): Perrot H, *Ann Dermatol Venereol* (French) 115, 523
  (1983): Blickle JF+, *Presse Med* (French) 12, 2534
  (1982): Levandoski LA+, *Diabetes Care* 5, 6
  (1981): Jones GR+, *BMJ* 282, 190
  (1981): Kahn CB, *Handbook of Diabetes Mellitus* Garland
    STPM, 75
  (1980): Reeves WG+, *BMJ* 280, 1500
  (1979): Asherov J+, *Diabete Metab* 5, 1
  (1978): Aw TC+, *Singapore Med J* 19, 227
  (1978): Galloway JA+, *Med Clin North Am* 62, 663
  (1978): Oakley WG+, *Diabetes and its Management* Blackwell,
    103
  (1978): Talantov VV, *Sov Med* (Russian) June, 104
  (1977): Kumar O+, *Diabetes* 26, 296
  (1976): Maaz E, *Z Gesamte Inn Med* (German) 31, 941
  (1976): Whitley TH+, *JAMA* 235, 839
  (1975): Jablonska S+, *Acta Derm Venereol* 55, 135
  (1974): Talantov VV, *Sov Med* (Russian) 37, 80
  (1974): Teuscher A, *Diabetologia* 10, 211
  (1972): Bloom A, *BMJ* 4, 366
Lipodystrophy
  (1990): Kohli V+, *Indian Pediatr* 27, 1120
  (1988): Field LM, *J Am Acad Dermatol* 19, 570
  (1988): Verbenko EV+, *Sov Med* (Russian) 3, 104
  (1987): Goldman JM+, *Am J Med* 83, 195
  (1985): Valenta LJ+, *Ann Intern Med* 102, 790
  (1984): Campbell IW+, *Postgrad Med J* 60, 439
  (1984): De Mattia G+, *Clin Ter* (Italian) 111, 169
  (1984): Tebuev AM, *Pediatriia* (Russian) December 59
  (1982): Levandoski LA+, *Diabetes Care* 5, 6
  (1981): Libman E+, *Med Pregl* (Serbo-Croatian-Roman) 34, 49
  (1981): Pisarskaia IV+, *Med Sestra* (Russian) 40, 54
  (1979): Welk DS, *Nursing* 9, 42
  (1978): da Cruz-Borges RC+, *Rev Bras Enferm* (Portuguese)
    31, 252
  (1974): Mehnert H, *Dtsch Med Wochenschr* (German) 99, 1274
  (1973): Watson D+, *Med J Aust* 1, 248
  (1972): Mehnert H, *Med Klin* (German) 67, 1384
  (1971): Sapelkina LV+, *Pediatriia* (Russian) 50, 18
  (1969): Todorovic M, *Med Pregl* (Serbo-Croatian-Cyrillic) 22, 177
  (1968): Gleize J+, *Diabete* (French) 16, 281
  (1968): Thosteson GC, *Mich Med* 67, 609
  (1967): Hintz R, *Pol Tyg Lek* (Polish) 22, 828
  (1967): Hintz R, *Pol Tyg Lek* (Polish) 22, 902
  (1967): Jablonska S+, *Pol Tyg Lek* (Polish) 22, 977
  (1965): Aubertin E+, *J Med Bord* (French) 142, 605
Lipohypertrophy (1–10%)
  (1996): Hauner H+, *Exp Clin Endocrinol Diabetes* 104, 106

(1990): Schiazza L+, *J Am Acad Dermatol* 22, 148
(1989): Zinman B, *N Engl J Med* 321, 363
(1988): McNally PG+, *Postgrad Med J* 64, 850
(1987): Samadaei A+, *J Am Acad Dermatol* 17, 506
(1984): Young RJ+, *Diabetes Care* 7, 479
(1983): Johnson DA+, *Cutis* 32, 273
(1982): Mier A+, *BMJ* 285, 1539
(1969): Erickson L+, *JAMA* 209, 934
Panniculitis
(1988): Verbenko EV+, *Vestn Dermatol Venerol* (Russian) 1, 63
Paresthesias (1–10%)
Tremor (1–10%)
Tumors (nodules)
(1981): Galloway JA+, *Diabetes Mellitus* Bowie 5, 117
(1978): Oakley WG+, *Diabetes and its Management* Blackwell, 103
(1960): Oakley WG, *Br Med Bull* 16, 247

INSULIN GLARGINE

Trade name: Lantus (Aventis)
Indications: Type 1 & type 2 diabetes
Category: Long-acting recombinant human insulin analog
Half-life: N/A
Clinically important, potentially hazardous interactions with: alcohol, guanethidine, propranolol

Reactions

Skin
Allergic reactions (sic)
Edema
Pruritus
Rash (sic)

Other
Injection-site pain (2.7%)
Lipodystrophy

INTERFERON BETA 1-A

Synonym: rIFN-b
Trade name: Avonex (Biogen)
Other common trade name: *Rebif*
Indications: Multiple sclerosis
Category: Immunomodulator; Interferon
Half-life: 10 hours

Reactions

Skin
Basal cell carcinoma (<1%)
Bullae
Cellulitis
Chills (21%)
(1998): Mohr DC+, *Mult Scler* 4(6), 487
Cold, clammy skin
Dermatitis
Diaphoresis
Ecchymoses
Erythema
(2000): Beghi E+, *Neurology* 54(2), 469 (local)
Exanthems

(2002): Beaudet LD, Trois-Rivieres, Quebec (from Internet) (observation)
Facial edema
Flu-like syndrome (61%)
(2002): Clanet M+, *Neurology* 59(10), 1507
(2000): Beghi E+, *Neurology* 54(2), 469
(2000): Gottberg K+, *Mult Scler* 6(5), 349
(1998): *Prescrire Int* 7(37), 142
(1998): Mohr DC+, *Mult Scler* 4(6), 487
Furunculosis
Genital pruritus
Herpes simplex (2–3%)
Herpes zoster (3)
Infections (sic) (11%)
Lupus erythematosus
(2000): Schmutz J+, *Ann Dermatol Venereol* 127(2), 237
(1998): Nousari HC+, *Lancet* 352(9143), 1825 (Subacute cutaneous)
Nevi (3%)
Petechiae
Photosensitivity (<1%)
Pigmentation
Pruritus
(2002): Beaudet LD, Trois-Rivieres, Quebec (from Internet) (observation)
Raynaud's phenomenon
(2000): De Broucker+, *Ann Med Interne* (Paris) 151(5), 424
Seborrhea
Spider angiomas
Telangiectasia
Ulcerations
Upper respiratory infection (31%)
Urticaria (5%)
(2003): Mazzeo L+, *Br J Dermatol* 148(1), 172

Hair
Hair – alopecia (4%)

Other
Anaphylactoid reactions
(1999): Corona T+, *Neurology* 52(2), 425
Arthralgia (9%)
Arthritis
(2002): Altintas A+, *Mult Scler* 8(6), 534
Death
(2000): Beghi E+, *Neurology* 54(2), 469
Depression
(2003): Goeb JL+, *Clin Neuropharmacol* 26(1), 5
(2002): Lana-Peixoto MA+, *Arq Neuropsiquiatr* 60(3-B), 721
(1999): Mohr DC+, *Arch Neurol* 56(10), 1263
(1998): Mohr DC+, *Mult Scler* 4(6), 487
Gingivitis
Headache
Hiccups
Hyperesthesia
Hypersensitivity (3%)
Injection-site atrophy
Injection-site burning
Injection-site ecchymoses (2%)
Injection-site edema
Injection-site hypersensitivity
Injection-site inflammation (3%)
Injection-site necrosis
(1999): Radziwill AJ+, *J Neurol Neurosurg Psychiatry* 67(1), 115
Injection-site purpura (2%)
Injection-site reactions (sic) (4%)
(2002): Panitch H+, *Neurology* 59(10), 1496

Joint pains
Lipoma
Lymphadenopathy
Mastodynia (7%)
Myalgia (34%)
Pain (24%)
Paresthesias
  (1998): Mohr DC+, *Mult Scler* 4(6), 487
Peyronie's disease
Rhabdomyolysis
  (2002): Lunemann JD+, *J Neurol Neurosurg Psychiatry* 72(2), 274
Seizures
  (2002): Dubisar BM+, *Pharmacotherapy* 22(11), 1504
Tongue disorder (sic)
Toothache
Vaginitis (4%)
Xerostomia

INTERFERON BETA-1B

Synonyms: IFNB-1b; IFN-beta1b
Trade names: Betaseron (Berlex); Rebif (Serono)
Indications: Relapsing multiple sclerosis, cancers
Category: Immunomodulatory agent; Recombinant human interferon beta(ser), rHuIFN-beta(ser)
Half-life: N/A

Reactions

Skin

Abscess
Acral cyanosis
  (1987): Grunberg SM+, *Cancer Res* 47(4), 1174
Adverse effects (sic)
  (1999): Rice GP+, *Neurology* 52(9), 1893
  (1998): Rio J+, *Neurologia* 13(9), 422
Allergic reactions (sic)
  (1998): Cohen BA+, *Allergy Asthma Proc* 19(2), 85
  (1997): Elgart GW+, *J Am Acad Dermatol* 37(4), 553
  (1996): Neilley LK+, *Neurology* 46(2), 552
Balanitis
Cellulitis
Cheilitis
Chills (46%)
  (1998): Williams GJ+, *J Interferon Cytokine Res* 18(11), 967
  (1997): Munschauer FE+, *Clin Ther* 19(5), 883
  (1994): Connelly JF, *Ann Pharmacother* 28(5), 610
  (1991): Allen J+, *J Clin Oncol* 9(5), 783
  (1990): Fetell MR+, *Cancer* 65(1), 78
  (1990): Von Hoff+, *J Interferon Res* 10(5), 531
  (1990): Yung WK+, *J Neurooncol* 9(1), 29
  (1987): Grunberg SM+, *Cancer Res* 47(4), 1174
Cyst (4%)
Dermatitis
Diaphoresis (23%)
Edema (generalized) (8%)
Erythema
  (1999): Fortuno Y+, *Med Clin* (Barc) 113(12), 447 (9 cases)
  (1997): Elgart GW+, *J Am Acad Dermatol* 37(4), 553
  (1989): Glaspy JA+, *Cancer* 64(2), 409
Erythema nodosum
Exanthems
Exfoliative dermatitis
Flu-like syndrome (76%)

  (2002): Exton MS+, *Neuropsychobiology* 45(4), 199
  (2002): Flechter S+, *J Neurol Sci* 197(1-2), 51 (35%)
  (2002): Yang CH+, *Chang Gung Med J* 25(11), 774
  (2000): Bayas A+, *Drug Saf* 22(2), 149
  (2000): Gottberg K+, *Mult Scler* 6(5), 349
  (2000): *Prescrire Int* 9(48), 110
  (1999): Rice GP+, *Neurology* 52(9), 1893
  (1998): Rio J+, *Neurologia* 13(9), 422 (90%)
  (1997): Munschauer FE+, *Clin Ther* 19(5), 883
  (1996): Huber S+, *Schweiz Med Wochenschr* 126(35), 1475 (50%)
  (1996): Lublin FD+, *Neurology* 46(1), 12
  (1996): Mohr DC+, *Mult Scler* 2(5), 222
  (1996): Neilley LK+, *Neurology* 46(2), 552
  (1995): Logan-Clubb L+, *J Neurosci Nurs* 27(6), 344
  (1994): Connelly JF, *Ann Pharmacother* 28(5), 610
  (1989): Glaspy JA+, *Cancer* 64(2), 409
  (1987): Lillis PK+, *Cancer Treat Rep* 71(10), 965
Furunculosis
Granulomatous dermatitis
  (1998): Mehta CL+, *J Am Acad Dermatol* 39(6), 1024
Hyperhidrosis
  (1997): Schwid SR+, *Arch Neurol* 54(9), 1169
  (1994): Connelly JF, *Ann Pharmacother* 28(5), 610
Infections (sic)
Leucoderma
Lichenoid dermatitis
Necrosis
  (2002): Yang CH+, *Chang Gung Med J* 25(11), 774
  (1999): Sasseville D+, *J Cutan Med Surg* 3(6), 320
  (1998): Weinberg JM, *J Am Acad Dermatol* 39(5 Pt 1), 807
  (1997): Albani C+, *Minerva Med* 88(6), 271
  (1997): Fruland JE+, *J Am Acad Dermatol* 37(3 Pt 1), 488
  (1997): Weinberg JM+, *Acta Derm Venereol* 77(2), 146
  (1995): Sheremata WA+, *N Engl J Med* 332(23), 1584
  (1995): Shinohara K, *N Engl J Med* 333(18), 1222
Photosensitivity
Psoriasis
Pustular psoriasis
  (1996): Webster GF+, *J Am Acad Dermatol* 34(2 Pt 2), 365
Scleroderma
  (1999): Fortuno Y+, *Med Clin* (Barc) 113(12), 447 (9 cases)
  (1997): Elgart GW+, *J Am Acad Dermatol* 37(4), 553
Seborrhea
Squamous cell carcinoma
  (1997): Fruland JE+, *J Am Acad Dermatol* 37(3), 488
Ulcerations
  (1999): Fortuno Y+, *Med Clin* (Barc) 113(12), 447 (9 cases)
Urticaria
  (2001): Brown DL+, *Neurology* 56(10), 1416
Vasculitis
  (1998): Cohen BA+, *Allergy Asthma Proc* 19(2), 85
Vesiculobullous eruption

Hair

Hair – alopecia
  (1997): Schwid SR+, *Arch Neurol* 54(9), 1169
Hair – hirsutism

Other

Ageusia
Anaphylactoid reactions
  (1999): Clear D, *J Neurol Neurosurg Psychiatry* 66(5), 690
Anxiety
  (2002): Exton MS+, *Neuropsychobiology* 45(4), 199
Aphthous stomatitis
Arthralgia
  (1997): Munschauer FE+, *Clin Ther* 19(5), 883
Arthritis

(2002): Altintas A+, *Mult Scler* 8(6), 534

Death

(1991): Yung WK+, *J Clin Oncol* 9(11), 1945 (2 cases)

Depression

(2002): Feinstein A+, *J Neurol* 249(7), 815
(2000): Arnoldus JH+, *Mult Scler* 6(5), 338
(1998): Rio J+, *Neurologia* 13(9), 422
(1997): *Rev Neurol* 25(148), 1876
(1997): Schwid SR+, *Arch Neurol* 54(9), 1169
(1996): Mohr DC+, *Mult Scler* 2(5), 222
(1996): Neilley LK+, *Neurology* 46(2), 552

Dizziness (35%)

Dysgeusia

Fatigue

(2002): Exton MS+, *Neuropsychobiology* 45(4), 199
(2002): Yang CH+, *Chang Gung Med J* 25(11), 774
(2000): Gottberg K+, *Mult Scler* 6(5), 349
(1998): Wadler S+, *Cancer J Sci Am* 4(5), 331
(1997): Schwid SR+, *Arch Neurol* 54(9), 1169
(1996): Huber S+, *Schweiz Med Wochenschr* 126(35), 1475
   (31%)
(1996): Neilley LK+, *Neurology* 46(2), 552
(1991): Allen J+, *J Clin Oncol* 9(5), 783
(1988): Schiller JH+, *J Interferon Res* 8(5), 581
(1987): Grunberg SM+, *Cancer Res* 47(4), 1174
(1987): Schiller JH+, *Cancer Treat Rep* 71(10), 945

Fever

(2002): Yang CH+, *Chang Gung Med J* 25(11), 774
(1999): Garcia-Moreno JM+, *Neurologia* 14(4), 154
(1998): Williams GJ+, *J Interferon Cytokine* 18(11), 967
(1997): Munschauer FE+, *Clin Ther* 19(5), 883
(1994): Connelly JF, *Ann Pharmacother* 28(5), 610
(1991): Allen J+, *J Clin Oncol* 9(5), 783
(1990): Fetell MR+, *Cancer - 0374236* 65(1), 78
(1990): Von Hoff+, *J Interferon Res* 10(5), 531
(1990): Yung WK+, *J Neurooncol* 9(1), 29
(1987): Grunberg SM+, *Cancer Res* 47(4), 1174
(1987): Lillis PK+, *Cancer Treat Rep* 71(10), 965
(1986): Rinehart J+, *Cancer Res* 46(10), 5364
(1986): Sarna G+, *Cancer Treat Rep* 70(12), 1365

Fibrosis

(1997): Elgart GW+, *J Am Acad Dermatol* 37(4), 553

Gingivitis

Glossitis

Graves' disease

(2000): Rotondi M+, *J Endocrinol Invest* 23(5), 321
(1997): Schwid SR+, *Arch Neurol* 54(9), 1169

Headache

Hiccups

Hyperesthesia

Induration

(2001): Durieu C+, *Ann Dermatol Venereol* 128(12), 1336
(1989): Glaspy JA+, *Cancer* 64(2), 409

Injection-site erythema

(1987): Grunberg SM+, *Cancer Res* 47(4), 1174

Injection-site necrosis

(1998): Gaines AR+, *Mult Scler* 4(2), 70

Injection-site pain

(2000): Gottberg K+, *Mult Scler* 6(5), 349
(1996): Mohr DC+, *Mult Scler* 2(5), 222

Injection-site panniculitis

(2002): Heinzerling L+, *Eur J Dermatol* 12(2), 194

Injection-site reactions

(2002): Flechter S+, *J Neurol Sci* 197(1), 51
(2000): Bayas A+, *Drug Saf* 22(2), 149
(2000): *Prescrire Int* 9(48), 110
(1999): Rice GP+, *Neurology* 52(9), 1893
(1998): Gaines AR+, *Mult Scler* 4(2), 70

(1997): Munschauer FE+, *Clin Ther* 19(5), 883
(1996): Huber S+, *Schweiz Med Wochenschr* 126(35), 1475
   (63%)
(1996): Lublin FD+, *Neurology* 46(1), 12
(1996): Webster GF+, *J Am Acad Dermatol* 34(2 Pt 2), 365
(1995): Logan-Clubb L+, *J Neurosci Nurs* 27(6), 344
(1994): Connelly JF, *Ann Pharmacother* 28(5), 610
(1990): Miles SA+, *Ann Intern Med* 112(8), 582
(1989): Glaspy JA+, *Cancer* 64(2), 409 (56%)

Injection-site ulceration

(2002): Yang CH+, *Chang Gung Med J* 25(11), 774
(1997): Elgart GW+, *J Am Acad Dermatol* 37(4), 553
(1997): Weinberg JM+, *Acta Derm Venereol* 77(2), 146

Mastodynia (7%)

Mucosal bleeding

(1988): Sperber SJ+, *J Infect Dis* 158(1), 166 (12.5–38%)

Myalgia (44%)

(2002): Yang CH+, *Chang Gung Med J* 25(11), 774
(1998): Williams GJ+, *J Interferon Cytokine Res* 18(11), 967
(1997): Munschauer FE+, *Clin Ther* 19(5), 883
(1994): Connelly JF, *Ann Pharmacother* 28(5), 610
(1988): Schiller JH+, *J Interferon Res* 8(5), 581
(1987): Grunberg SM+, *Cancer Res* 47(4), 1174

Myasthenia gravis

(1997): Blake G+, *Neurology* 49(6), 1747

Myopathy

Myositis

Oral candidiasis

Oral mucosal bleeding

(1988): Sperber SJ+, *J Infect Dis* 158(1), 166 (12.5–38%)

Pain (52%)

(2002): Heinzerling L+, *Eur J Dermatol* 12(2), 194 (52%)

Panniculitis

(2002): Heinzerling L+, *Eur J Dermatol* 12(2), 194

Paresthesias

(1987): Grunberg SM+, *Cancer Res* 47(4), 1174

Parosmia

Seizures (2%)

Sialorrhea

Thrombophlebitis

(1999): Fortuno Y+, *Med Clin* (Barc) 113(12), 447 (2 cases)
(1997): Elgart GW+, *J Am Acad Dermatol* 37(4), 553

Tremor

Vaginal bleeding

(1997): Pakulski LA+, *Ann Pharmacother* 31(1), 50

Xerostomia

INTERFERONS, ALFA-2

Synonyms: IFLrA; IFN; rLFN-A; INF; INF-alpha-2
Trade names: Alferon N; Infergen (Intermune); Intron A
(Schering); Rebetron (Schering); Roferon-A (Roche)
Other common trade names: *Green-Alpha; Introna; Introne;
Laroferon; Roceron-A*
Indications: Chronic hepatitis C virus infection
Category: Biologic response modulator
Half-life: 2 hours

Note: Many of the adverse reactions depend on the nature of the
disease being treated. Either hairy cell leukemia [L] or AIDS-related
Kaposi's sarcoma [K]

Reactions

Skin
Acne (1%)

Acral sclerosis
  (2002): Saydam G+, *Acta Haematol* 107(1), 43
Acrocyanosis
  (1998): Campo-Voegeli A+, *Dermatology* 196, 361
Allergic reactions (sic)
  (1996): Azagury M+, *Eur J Cancer* 32A, 1821 (severe)
Angioedema
  (2001): Ohmoto K, *Am J Gastroenterol* 96, 1311
Atrophie blanche
  (2002): Bugatti L+, *Dermatology* 204(2), 154
Behçet's disease
  (1995): Segawa F+, *J Rheumatol* 22, 1183
Bullous eruption
  (2002): Pouthier D+, *Nephrol Dial Transplant* 17(1), 174
  (1995): Chang LW+, *Cutis* 56, 144
  (1993): Andry P+, *Ann Dermatol Venereol* (French) 120, 843
  (1993): Parodi A+, *Dermatology* 186, 155
Candidiasis (1%)
Chills
  (2002): Alpsoy E+, *Arch Dermatol* 138, 467
  (2000): Cornejo P+, *Arch Dermatol* 136, 429
  (2000): Shenefelt PD+, *Arch Dermatol* 136, 837
Dermatitis
  (1995): Chang LW+, *Cutis* 56, 144
Dermatitis herpetiformis
  (1995): Dmochowski M+, *Postepy Dermatol* 12, 7
Diaphoresis (22%) [L]; (7%) [K]
  (1999): Angulo MP+, *Pediatr Cardiol* 20, 293 [L]
Discoloration (sic) (<1%)
Ecchymoses ([L])
Eczema (sic)
  (2002): Dereure O+, *Br J Dermatol* 147(6), 1142 (with ribavirin)
  (1999): Sookoian S+, *Arch Dermatol* 135, 999 ([K]) (with ribavirin)
  (1989): Detmar U+, *Contact Dermatitis* 20, 149
Edema (11%) [L]
  (2002): Goldberg JS+, *Cancer* 95(6), 1220 (1 case)
Erythema
  (1999): Sookoian S+, *Arch Dermatol* 135, 999 (with ribavirin) (malar) ([K])
Erythema nodosum
  (2001): Leveque L+, *Rev Med Interne* 22(12), 1248 (with ribavirin)
Exanthems
  (2002): Farady KK, Austin, TX (with ribavirin) (from Internet) (observation)
  (1994): Sollitto RB+, *Arch Dermatol* 130, 1194
  (1994): Toyofuku K+, *J Dermatol* 21, 732
  (1986): Quesada JR+, *Lancet* 1, 1466
Flu-like syndrome (sic) (>10%)
  (2002): Alpsoy E+, *Arch Dermatol* 138, 467
  (2002): Giuliani M+, *Arch Dermatol* 138, 535
Fungal infections (sic) (<1%)
Herpes simplex (1%)
  (1995): Chang LW+, *Cutis* 56, 144
  (1992): Breathnach SM+, *Adverse Drug Reactions and the Skin* Blackwell, Oxford, 322 (passim)
Hot flashes (sic) (1%)
Infections
  (2002): Goldberg JS+, *Cancer* 95(6), 1220 (1 case)
Kaposi's sarcoma
  (2002): Giuliani M+, *Arch Dermatol* 138(4), 535
  (1993): Ariad S+, *South Afr Med J* 83, 430
Keratoses
  (1994): Sollitto RB+, *Arch Dermatol* 130, 1194
Lichen myxedematosus
  (1998): Rongioletti F+, *J Am Acad Dermatol* 38, 760
Lichen planus

  (1999): Herstoff JK, Newport, RI (from Internet) (observation)
  (1999): Sookoian S+, *Arch Dermatol* 135, 999 ([K]) (with ribavirin)
  (1998): Dalekos GN+, *Eur J Gastroenterol Hepatol* 10, 933
  (1995): Chang LW+, *Cutis* 56, 144
  (1995): Fornaciari G+, *J Clin Gastroenterol* 20, 346
  (1995): Hyrailles V+, *Gastroenterol Clin Biol* (French) 19, 833
  (1993): Boccia S+, *Gastroenterology* 105, 1921
  (1993): Heintges T+, *J Hepatol* 18, 129
  (1993): Protzer U+, *Gastroenterology* 104, 903
Lichenoid eruption
  (2002): Bohannon JS, Midlothian, VA (from Internet) (observation)
Linear IgA bullous dermatosis
  (1993): Parodi A+, *Dermatology* 187, 155
  (1990): Guillaume JC+, *Ann Dermatol Venereol* (French) 117, 899
Lupus erythematosus
  (2001): Werth V, *Dermatology Times* 18
  (1998): Garcia-Porrua C+, *Clin Exp Rheumatol* 16, 107
  (1994): Flores A+, *Br J Rheumatol* 33, 787
  (1994): Fritzler MJ, *Lupus* 3, 455
  (1994): Sanchez Roman J+, *Med Clin (Barc)* (Spanish) 102, 198
  (1992): Mehta ND+, *Am J Hematol* 41, 141
  (1992): Tolaymat A+, *J Pediatr* 120, 429
  (1991): Hess EV, *Curr Opin Rheumatol* 3, 809
  (1991): Schilling JP+, *Cancer* 68, 1536
Lupus syndrome
  (2002): Pouthier D+, *Nephrol Dial Transplant* 17(1), 174
Malignancies (sic)
  (1991): Wagner RF+, *Arch Dermatol* 127, 272
Melanoma
  (1988): Bork K+, *Dermatologica* 177, 249 (exacerbation)
Necrosis
  (1998): Sickler JB+, *Am J Gastroenterol* 93, 463
  (1997): de Ledinghen V+, *Gastroenterol Clin Biol* 21, 523
  (1995): Chang LW+, *Cutis* 56, 144
  (1995): Trautinger F+, *N Engl J Med* 333, 1222
  (1991): Cnudde F+, *Int J Dermatol* 30, 147
  (1989): Rasokat H+, *Dtsch Med Wochenschr* (German) 114, 458
Nodules (sic) (painful)
  (1995): Chang LW+, *Cutis* 56, 144
Pemphigus
  (1995): Kirsner RS+, *Br J Dermatol* 132, 474
  (1994): Niizeki H+, *Dermatology* 189 (Suppl), 129
Photosensitivity (<1%)
  (2002): Dereure O+, *Br J Dermatol* 147(6), 1142 (with ribavirin)
  (1994): Sollitto RB+, *Arch Dermatol* 130, 1194
Pigmentation
  (2003): Willems M+, *Br J Dermatol* 149(2), 390
Pigmented purpuric dermatosis (capillaritis)
  (2000): Gupta G+, *J Am Acad Dermatol* 43, 937
Pruritus (13%) [L]; (5%) [K]
  (2002): Bohannon JS, Midlothian VA (from Internet) (observation)
  (2001): Beaudet LD (from Internet) (observation)
  (1994): Czarnetzki BM+, *J Am Acad Dermatol* 30, 500
  (1992): Breathnach SM+, *Adverse Drug Reactions and the Skin* Blackwell, Oxford, 322 (passim)
Psoriasis
  (2002): Oliveira-Soares+, *World Congress Dermatol* Poster, 0123 (aggravation in 3 cases)
  (2001): Werth V, *Dermatology Times* 18
  (2000): Taylor C+, *Postgrad Med J* 76, 365
  (1996): Wolfer LU+, *Hautarzt* (German) 47, 124
  (1995): Chang LW+, *Cutis* 56, 144
  (1995): Wolfe JT+, *J Am Acad Dermatol* 32, 887
  (1994): Matsuoka H+, *Rinsho Ketsueki* (Japanese) 35, 309
  (1993): Cleveland MG+, *J Am Acad Dermatol* 29, 788
  (1993): Garcia-Lora E+, *Dermatology* 187, 280

(1993): Georgetson MJ+, *Am J Gastroenterol* 88, 756
(1993): Pauluzzi P+, *Acta Derm Venereol* 73, 395
(1991): Funk J+, *Br J Dermatol* 125, 463
(1990): Fierlbeck G+, *Arch Dermatol* 126, 351 (at injection site)
(1990): Jucgla A+, *Arch Dermatol* 127, 910 (exacerbation)
(1990): Kowalzick L+, *Arch Dermatol* 126, 1515 (at injection site)
(1990): Kusec R+, *Dermatologica* 181, 170
(1989): Harrison P, *J Invest Dermatol* 93, 555
(1989): Hartmann F+, *Dtsch Med Wochenschr* (German) 114, 96 (exacerbation)
(1986): Quesada JR+, *Lancet* 1, 1466 (exacerbation)

Purpura
(2001): Toubai T+, *Nippon Naika Gakkai Zasshi* 90(7), 1330

Radiation recall
(2002): Thomas R+, *J Clin Oncol* 20(1), 355

Rash (sic) (44%) [L]; (11%) [K]
(1999): Sookoian S+, *Arch Dermatol* 135, 999 (with ribavirin) ([K])

Raynaud's phenomenon
(1996): Creutzig A+, *Ann Intern Med* 125, 423
(1994): Arslan M+, *J Intern Med* 235, 503

Reiter's syndrome (incomplete)
(1993): Cleveland MG+, *J Am Acad Dermatol* 29, 788

Sarcoidosis
(2002): Cogrel O+, *Br J Dermatol* 146(2), 320 (with ribavirin)
(2002): Gitlin N, *Eur J Gastroenterol Hepatol* 14(8), 883
(2002): Li SD+, *J Gastroenterol* 37(1), 50
(2002): Wendling J+, *Arch Dermatol* 138, 546 (2 cases) (with ribavirin)
(2001): Leveque L+, *Rev Med Interne* 22(12), 1248 (with ribavirin)
(2001): Neglia V+, *J Cutan Med Surg* 5(5), 406
(2001): Ravenel JG+, *Am J Roentgenol* 177(1), 199
(1999): Pietropaoli A+, *Chest* 116, 569
(1993): Blum L+, *Rev Med Interne* (Paris) (French) 14, 1161

Seborrheic dermatitis
(1986): Quesada JR+, *Lancet* 1, 1466

Sjøgren's syndrome
(1994): Lunel F, *Gastroenterol Clin Biol* (French) 19, 442

Systemic sclerosis
(2002): Beretta L+, *Br J Dermatol* 147(2), 385

Telangiectasia
(1989): Dreno B+, *Ann Intern Med* 111, 95

Toxicity (sic)
(1993): Miglino M+, *Haematologica* 78(6), 411
(1989): Dreno B+, *Ann Intern Med* 111, 95

Ulcerations
(1992): Orlow SJ+, *Arch Dermatol* 128, 566

Urticaria (<3%) [K]
(1994): Czarnetzki BM+, *J Am Acad Dermatol* 30, 500
(1992): Breathnach SM+, *Adverse Drug Reactions and the Skin* Blackwell, Oxford, 322 (passim)

Vasculitis
(2001): Toubai T+, *Nippon Naika Gakkai Zasshi* 90(7), 1330
(2001): Werth V, *Dermatology Times* 18
(1998): Gordon AC+, *J Infect* 36, 229
(1996): Pateron D+, *Clin Exp Rheumatol* 14, 79
(1995): Chang LW+, *Cutis* 56, 144
(1992): Liet JM+, *Rev Med Interne* (French) 13, 169
(1983): Sangster G+, *Eur J Cancer Clin Oncol* 19, 1647

Vitiligo
(1997): Nouri K+, *Cutis* 60, 289
(1996): Le Gal F-A+, *J Am Acad Dermatol* 35, 650
(1996): Simsek H+, *Dermatology* 193, 65
(1995): Bernstein D+, *Am J Gastroenterol* 90, 1176
(1994): Scheibenbogen C+, *Eur J Cancer* 30A, 1209

Xerosis (17%) [L]; (22%) [K]

Hair

Hair – alopecia (1–10%)
(2002): Alpsoy E+, *Arch Dermatol* 138, 467
(2001): Zucker DM+, *Gastroenterol Nurs* 24(4), 192 (with ribavirin)
(1997): Brehler R+, *J Am Acad Dermatol* 36, 983 (passim)
(1995): Chang LW+, *Cutis* 56, 144
(1994): Czarnetzki BM+, *J Am Acad Dermatol* 30, 500
(1992): Tosti A+, *Dermatology* 184, 124
(1989): Olsen EA+, *J Am Acad Dermatol* 20, 395
(1987): Werter MJBP, *Ned Tijdschr Geneeskd* (Dutch) 131, 2081

Hair – alopecia areata
(1999): Kernland KH+, *Dermatology* 198, 418

Hair – hypertrichosis
(1996): Ariyoshi K+, *Am J Hematol* 53, 50 (eyebrows)
(1990): Berglund EF+, *South Med J* 83, 363
(1984): Foon KA+, *N Engl J Med* 19, 1259 (eyelashes)

Hair – pigmentation
(1996): Fleming CJ+, *Br J Dermatol* 135, 337
(1995): Bernstein D+, *Am J Gastroenterol* 90, 1176 (canities)

Hair – straight
(2002): Bessis D+, *Br J Dermatol* 147(2), 392

Other

Ageusia
(2001): Manzano Alonso ML+, *Gastroenterol Hepatol* 24(8), 412

Anosmia
(2001): Manzano Alonso ML+, *Gastroenterol Hepatol* 24(8), 412
(1998): Maruyama S+, *Am J Gastroenterol* 93, 122

Aphthous stomatitis
(1998): Dalekos GN+, *Eur J Gastroenterol Hepatol* 10, 933

Arthralgia
(2001): Karim A+, *Am J Med Sci* 322(4), 233
(2001): Leveque L+, *Rev Med Interne* 22(12), 1248 (with ribavirin)
(2001): Zucker DM+, *Gastroenterol Nurs* 24(4), 192 (with ribavirin)

Depression
(2002): Bonaccorso S+, *J Clin Psychopharmacol* 22(1), 86
(2002): Castera L+, *Hepatology* 35(4), 978
(2002): Farah A, *J Clin Psychiatry* 63(2), 166
(2002): Herrine SK, *Ann Intern Med* 136(10), 747
(2001): Bonaccorso S+, *Psychiatry Res* 105(1), 45
(2001): Debien C+, *Encephale* 27(4), 308 (5–15%)
(2001): Kraus MR+, *N Engl J Med* 345(5), 375
(2001): Maes M+, *Mol Psychiatry* 6(4), 475
(2001): Malik UR+, *Cancer* 92(6), 1664

Dysgeusia (25%) (metallic taste) [K]
(1995): Chang LW+, *Cutis* 56, 144

Embolia cutis medicamentosa (Nicolau syndrome)
(2003): Reding EL+, *J Am Acad Dermatol* 48(3), 472 (passim)

Fatigue
(2002): Goldberg JS+, *Cancer* 95(6), 1220 (2 cases)

Fever
(2002): Goldberg JS+, *Cancer* 95(6), 1220 (2 cases)

Halo dermatitis
(1999): Krischer J+, *J Am Acad Dermatol* 40, 105

Headache
(2002): Goldberg JS+, *Cancer* 95(6), 1220 (1 case)

Hyperesthesia

Hypersensitivity
(2001): Beckman DB+, *Allergy* 56(8), 806

Injection-site alopecia
(1999): Lang AM+, *Arch Dermatol* 135, 1127

Injection-site erythema
(1995): Chang LW+, *Cutis* 56, 144

Injection-site induration
(1997): Siegel M, New York, NY (from Internet) (observation)

(1995): Chang LW+, *Cutis* 56, 144
Injection-site necrosis
  (1998): Krainick U+, *J Interferon Cytokine Res* 18, 823
  (1997): Weinberg JM+, *Acta Derm Venereol* (Stockh) 77, 146
  (1996): Konohana A+, *J Am Acad Dermatol* 35, 788
  (1996): Kontochristopoulos G+, *J Hepatol* 25, 271
  (1995): Shinohara K, *N Engl J Med* 333, 1222
  (1994): Akiyama Y+, *Jpn J Dermatol* (Japanese) 104, 436
  (1994): Tone T+, *Jpn J Dermatol* 104, 1047
  (1993): Christian B+, *Presse Med* (French) 22, 783
  (1993): Mihara K+, *Miyazakiikaishi* (Japanese) 17, 40
  (1993): Nagai A+, *Int J Hematol* 58, 129
  (1993): Oeda E+, *Am J Hematol* 44, 213
  (1992): Orlow SJ+, *Arch Dermatol* 128, 566
  (1991): Cnudde F+, *Int J Dermatol* 30, 147
  (1989): Rasokat H+, *Dtsch Med Wochenschr* (German) 114, 158
Injection-site pruritus
  (1989): Detmar U+, *Contact Dermatitis* 20, 149
Injection-site vasculitis
  (1997): Christian MM+, *J Am Acad Dermatol* 37, 118
Malignant lymphoma
  (1994): Arico M+, *Blood* 83, 869
Myalgia (71%) [L]; (69%) [K]
  (2002): Alpsoy E+, *Arch Dermatol* 138, 467
  (2002): Herrine SK, *Ann Intern Med* 136(10), 747
  (2001): Karim A+, *Am J Med Sci* 322(4), 233
  (2000): Shenefelt PD+, *Arch Dermatol* 136, 837
  (1999): Spieth K+, *Arch Dermatol* 135, 1035
  (1997): Brehler R+, *J Am Acad Dermatol* 36, 983 (passim)
  (1984): Foon KA+, *N Engl J Med* 19, 1259 (passim)
Myasthenia gravis
  (2001): Weegink CJ+, *J Gastroenterol* 36(10), 723 (with ribavirin)
Myopathy
  (1998): Dippel E, *Arch Dermatol* 134, 880 (4 patients)
Oral lichen planus
  (1997): Kutting B+, *Br J Dermatol* 137, 836
  (1997): Schlesinger TE+, *J Am Acad Dermatol* 36, 1023 (erosive)
  (1995): Chang LW+, *Cutis* 56, 144
  (1994): Papini M+, *Int J Dermatol* 33, 221
  (1994): Perreard M+, *Gastroenterol Clin Biol* (French) 18, 1051
  (1993): Sassigneux P+, *Gastroenterol Clin Biol* (French) 17, 764
Oral pemphigus
  (2001): Marinho RT+, *Eur J Gastroenterol Hepatol* 13(7), 869
Oropharyngeal pemphigus
  (2001): Marinho RT+, *Eur J Gastroenterol Hepatol* 13(7), 869
Paresthesias (12%) [L]; (8%) [K]
Parkinsonism
  (2002): Sarasombath P+, *Hawaii Med J* 61(3), 48
Polyarteritis nodosa
  (2001): *Drug & Ther Perspect* 17, 15
Polymyositis
  (2002): Lee SW+, *J Korean Med Sci* 17(1), 141
Rhabdomyolysis
  (2001): van Londen GJ+, *J Clin Oncol* 19(17), 3794
  (1995): Anderlini P+, *Cancer* 76, 678
Sialopenia
Stomatitis (1–10%)
Tinnitus
Xerostomia (>10%)

INTERLEUKIN-2

(See ALDESLEUKIN)

IPODATE

Trade names: Bilivist (Berlex); Oragrafin (Bristol-Myers Squibb)
Indications: Cholecystography
Category: Cholecystographic contrast medium
Half-life: N/A

Reactions

Skin
Allergic reactions (sic)
  (1986): Bigby M+, *JAMA* 256, 3358 (2.78%)
Exanthems
Pruritus
Purpura
  (1966): Stacher A, *Wien Klin Wochenschr* (German) 75, 820
Rash (sic)
Urticaria

Other
Anaphylactoid reactions
Hypersensitivity
Serum sickness

IPRATROPIUM

Trade names: Atrovent (Boehringer Ingelheim); Combivent (Boehringer Ingelheim); Duoneb (DEY)
Other common trade names: *Alti-Ipratropium; Novo-Ipramide*
Indications: Bronchospasm
Category: Anticholinergic; Antimuscarinic bronchodilator
Half-life: 2 hours

Combivent is albuterol and ipratropium

Reactions

Skin
Dermatitis
  (1988): Eedy DJ+, *Postgrad Med J* 64, 306
Exanthems
Flushing (<1%)
Miliaria profunda
  (1990): Saurat JH+, *Pediatr Dermatol* 7, 325
Pruritus (<1%)
Rash (sic) (1.2%)
Urticaria (<1%)

Hair
Hair – alopecia (<1%)

Other
Anaphylactoid reactions
  (1993): Bone WD+, *Chest* 103, 981
Death
  (2003): Ringbaek T+, *Respir Med* 97(3), 264 (in patients with asthma and COPD)
Dysgeusia (1%) (metallic taste)
  (2002): Cuvelier A+, *Respir Care* 47(2), 159
  (1980): Pakes GE+, *Drugs* 20, 237
Headache
Oral mucosal lesions (1–5%)
  (1980): Pakes GE+, *Drugs* 20, 237
Oral mucosal ulceration (<1%)
  (1987): High AS, *BMJ* 294, 375

(1986): Spencer PA, *BMJ* 292, 380
Paresthesias (<1%)
Stomatitis (<1%)
Trembling (1–10%)
Xerostomia (3.2%)
  (1980): Pakes GE+, *Drugs* 20, 237

IRBESARTAN

Trade names: Avalide (Bristol-Myers Squibb); Avapro (Bristol-Myers Squibb) (Sanofi-Synthelabo)
Indications: Hypertension
Category: Angiotensin II receptor antagonist; Antihypertensive
Half-life: 11–15 hours

Avalide is irbesartan and hydrochlorothiazide (a sulfonamide)*

Reactions

Skin
Angioedema
  (2002): Touraud JP+, *Ann Dermatol Venereol* 129(8), 1033
Chills (<1%)
Dermatitis (sic) (<1%)
Ecchymoses (<1%)
Eczema
  (2002): Touraud JP+, *Ann Dermatol Venereol* 129(8), 1033 (2 cases)
Edema (1–10%)
Erythema (<1%)
Eyelid edema
  (2002): Cohen PR, *J Drugs Dermatol* 1(3), 329
Facial edema (<1%)
Flushing (<1%)
Pemphigus herpetiformis (sic)
  (2002): Viseux V+, *World Congress Dermatol* Poster, 0360
Pruritus (<1%)
Rash (sic) (1–10%)
Urticaria (<1%)

Other
Cough
  (2002): Coca A+, *Clin Ther* 24(1), 126
  (2002): Touraud JP+, *Ann Dermatol Venereol* 129(8), 1033
Headache
Oral lesions (<1%)
Paresthesias (<1%)
Tremor (<1%)

*Note: Avalide contains a sulfonamide which can be absorbed systemically. Sulfonamides can produce severe, possibly fatal, reactions such as toxic epidermal necrolysis and Stevens–Johnson syndrome

IRINOTECAN

Synonyms: Camptothecin-11; CPT-11
Trade name: Camptosar (Pharmacia)
Indications: Metastatic colorectal carcinoma
Category: Antineoplastic
Half-life: 6–10 hours
Clinically important, potentially hazardous interactions with: aprepitant, atazanavir, **St John's wort**

Reactions

Skin
Allergic reactions (sic)
  (1997): Verschraegen CF+, *J Clin Oncol* 15, 625 (9%)
Chills (13.8%)
Diaphoresis (16%)
Edema (10.2%)
Exanthems
  (2002): Liu CY, *Ann Pharmacother* 36(12), 1897
Flushing (11%)
Hand-foot syndrome
  (2003): Gerbrecht BM, *Cancer Nurs* 26(2), 161
  (2002): Lin E+, *Oncology* (Huntingt) 16(12 Suppl 14), 31
Infections (sic)
  (2001): Ulrich-Pur H+, *Ann Oncol* 12(9), 1269 (3%)
Photodermatitis
  (2002): Willey A+, *J Am Acad Dermatol* 47(3), 453
Pigmentation
  (2002): Pui JC+, *J Drugs Dermatol* 1(2), 202
Pruritus
  (2002): Liu CY, *Ann Pharmacother* 36(12), 1897
Pyogenic granuloma
  (2002): Piguet V+, *Br J Dermatol* 147(6), 1270
Rash (sic) (12.8%)
  (1997): Verschraegen CF+, *J Clin Oncol* 15, 625 (21%)

Hair
Hair – alopecia (60.5%)
  (2002): Kollmannsberger C+, *Br J Cancer* 87(7), 729 (2 cases)
  (2001): Ulrich-Pur H+, *Ann Oncol* 12(9), 1269 (13%)
  (1999): Takahashi Y+, *Gan To Kagaku Ryoho* (Japanese) 26, 1193
  (1998): Berg D, *Oncol Nurs Forum* 25, 535
  (1997): Verschraegen CF+, *J Clin Oncol* 15, 625 (48%)
  (1996): Rougier P+, *Semin Oncol* 23, 34
  (1995): Abigerges D+, *J Clin Oncol* 13, 210 (53%)
  (1995): Catimel G+, *Ann Oncol* 6, 133
  (1994): de Forni M+, *Cancer Res* 54, 4347
  (1994): Sakata Y+, *Gan To Kagaku Ryoho* (Japanese) 21, 1039 (40%)
  (1994): Taguchi T+, *Gan To Kagaku Ryoho* (Japanese) 21, 1017 (30%)
  (1994): Taguchi T+, *Gan To Kagaku Ryoho* (Japanese) 21, 83 (61%)
  (1992): Fukuoka M+, *J Clin Oncol* 10, 16 (4%)
  (1991): Negoro S+, *Gan To Kagaku Ryoho* (Japanese) 18, 1013
  (1991): Takeuchi S+, *Gan To Kagaku Ryoho* (Japanese) 18, 1681 (33%)
  (1991): Takeuchi S+, *Gan To Kagaku Ryoho* (Japanese) 18, 579 (33%)
  (1990): Taguchi T+, *Gan To Kagaku Ryoho* (Japanese) 17, 115

Nails
Nails – onycholysis
  (2003): Munoz A+, *J Natl Cancer Inst* 95(16), 1252 (with capecitabine)

Other
Death
  (2003): Buckner JC+, *Cancer* 97(9 Suppl), 2352
Dizziness
  (2002): Liu CY, *Ann Pharmacother* 36(12), 1897
Dysgeusia (metallic taste)
Fatigue
  (2002): Vaishampayan UN+, *Int J Radiat Oncol Biol Phys*
    53(3), 675
Fever
  (2002): Kollmannsberger C+, *Br J Cancer* 87(7), 729 (1 case)
Headache
Mucositis (2%)
Oral ulceration
Sialorrhea
Stomatitis (12%)
  (2002): Bass AJ+, *J Clin Oncol* 20(13), 2995
  (2000): Adjei AA+, *J Clin Oncol* 18, 1116
  (1997): Verschraegen CF+, *J Clin Oncol* 15, 625 (14%)
Thrombophlebitis (1–10%)

ISOCARBOXAZID

Trade name: Marplan (Roche)
Other common trade name: *Enerzer*
Indications: Depression
Category: Antidepressant; Monoamine oxidase (MAO) inhibitor
Half-life: N/A
**Clinically important, potentially hazardous interactions
with:** amitriptyline, amoxapine, bupropion, citalopram,
clomipramine, desipramine, doxepin, fluoxetine, fluvoxamine,
imipramine, meperidine, nefazodone, nortriptyline, paroxetine,
protriptyline, rizatriptan, sertraline, sibutramine, sumatriptan,
trimipramine, **tryptophan**, venlafaxine, zolmitriptan

Reactions

Skin
Diaphoresis
  (1962): Busfield BL+, *J Nerv Ment Dis* 134, 339 (30%)
Exanthems (7%)
  (1962): Busfield BL+, *J Nerv Ment Dis* 134, 339
Peripheral edema (1–10%)
Photosensitivity (4%)
  (1962): Busfield BL+, *J Nerv Ment Dis* 134, 339
Pruritus (4%)
  (1962): Busfield BL+, *J Nerv Ment Dis* 134, 339
Rash (sic)
Telangiectasia

Other
Black tongue
Xerostomia (1–10%)
  (1962): Busfield BL+, *J Nerv Ment Dis* 134, 339 (11%)

ISOETHARINE

Trade names: Arm-a-Med; Beta-2; Bronkomed; Bronkometer
(Sanofi-Synthelabo); Bronkosol (Sanofi-Synthelabo); Dey-Lute
Other common trade names: *Asthmalitan; Numotac*
Indications: Bronchial asthma
Category: Adrenergic agonist; Bronchodilator;
Sympathomimetic
Half-life: N/A

Reactions

Skin
None

Other
Anaphylactoid reactions
  (1982): Twarog FJ+, *JAMA* 248, 2030
Trembling (1–10%)
Tremor
Xerostomia (1–10%)

ISOFLURANE

Trade names: Forane (Abbott); Forane (Abbott)
Other common trade names: *Aerrane; Floran; Forene; Forthane;
Isofluran; Isoflurano; Isofor; Isorane; Lisorane; Sofloran; Tensocold*
Indications: Maintenance of general anesthesia
Category: General Inhalation anesthetic
Onset of action: 7-10 minutes
**Clinically important, potentially hazardous interactions
with:** cisatracurium, doxacurium, muscle relaxants, pancuronium,
rapacuronium

Reactions

Skin
Shivering (post-operative)

ISONIAZID

Synonym: INH
Trade names: Rifamate (Aventis); Rifater (Aventis)
Other common trade names: *Cemidon; Diazid; Isotamine;
Isozid; Nicotibine; Nicozid; PMS-Isoniazid; Tibinide*
Indications: Tuberculosis
Category: Tuberculostatic
Half-life: 1–4 hours
**Clinically important, potentially hazardous interactions
with:** phenytoin, rifampin

Reactions

Skin
Acne
  (1988): Oliwiecki S+, *Clin Exp Dermatol* 13, 283
  (1988): Yamanaka M+, *Kekkaku* (Japanese) 63, 11
  (1982): Rosin MA+, *Southern Med J* 75, 81 (passim)
  (1974): Cohen LK+, *Arch Dermatol* 109, 377
  (1969): Lantis SH, *J Am Med Wom Assoc* 24, 305
  (1959): Bereston ES, *J Invest Dermatol* 33, 427
Acute generalized exanthematous pustulosis (AGEP)

Angioedema (<1%)
 (1989): Yagi S+, *Kekkaku* (Japanese) 64, 407
 (1959): Bereston ES, *J Invest Dermatol* 33, 427
Bullous eruption
 (1999): Scheid P+, *Allergy* 54, 294
Cutis laxa
 (1985): Koch SE+, *Pediatr Dermatol* 2, 282
Dermatitis
 (1993): Meseguer J+, *Contact Dermatitis* 28, 110 (systemic)
 (1986): Holdiness MR, *Contact Dermatitis* 15, 282
 (1978): Ippen H, *Derm Beruf Umwelt* (German) 26, 57
Dermatomyositis
 (1975): Fayolle J+, *Lyon Med* (French) 233, 135
Edema of foot
 (1999): Muratake T+, *Am J Psychiatry* 156, 660
 (1987): Schmutz JL+, *Ann Derm Venereol* (French) 114, 569
 (1983): Jorgensen J, *Int J Dermatol* 22, 44
 (1981): Meyrick Thomas RH+, *BMJ* 283, 287
 (1977): Comaish JS+, *Arch Dermatol* 113, 986
 (1977): Harrington CI, *Practitioner* 218, 716
 (1976): Comaish JS+, *Arch Dermatol* 112, 70
 (1974): Cohen LK+, *Arch Dermatol* 109, 377
 (1974): Forstrom L+, *Arch Dermatol* 110, 635
 (1974): Schlenzka K+, *Dermatol Monatsschr* (German) 160, 848
 (1972): Bjornstad RT, *Tidsskr Nor Laegeforen* (Norwegian) 92, 640
 (1972): Harber LC+, *J Invest Dermatol* 58, 327
 (1972): Jansen CT+, *Duodecim* 88, 928
 (1969): Polano MK+, *Arch Belg Dermatol Syphiligr* (Dutch) 25, 345
 (1967): Di Lorenzo PA, *Acta Derm Venereol* (Stockh) 47, 318
 (1964): Aspinall DL, *BMJ* 2, 1177
 (1959): Bereston ES, *J Invest Dermatol* 33, 427
 (1958): Haynes WS, *East Afr Med J* 35, 171
 (1956): Harrison RJ+, *BMJ* 2, 853
 (1955): Wood MM, *Br J Tuberc Dis Chest* 49, 20
 (1952): McConnell RB+, *Lancet* 2, 959
Erythema multiforme (<1%)
 (1988): Hira SK+, *J Am Acad Dermatol* 19, 451 (in AIDS patients)
 (1976): Bomb BS+, *Tubercle* 57, 229
Exanthems
 (1982): Rosin MA+, *Southern Med J* 75, 81 (passim)
 (1979): Byrd RB+, *JAMA* 241, 1239 (0.9%)
 (1963): Honeycutt WM+, *Arch Dermatol* 88, 190
 (1959): Bereston ES, *J Invest Dermatol* 33, 427
Exfoliative dermatitis
 (1985): Holdiness MR, *Int J Dermatol* 24, 280
 (1982): Rosin MA+, *Southern Med J* 75, 81
 (1969): Agrawal R, *BMJ* 4, 540
 (1963): Abrahams I+, *Arch Dermatol* 87, 96
 (1963): Honeycutt WM+, *Arch Dermatol* 88, 190
Flushing
 (1953): Witbind E+, *Dis Chest* 23, 16 (>5%)
Herpes zoster
 (1959): Bereston ES, *J Invest Dermatol* 33, 427
Keratoacanthoma
 (1966): Randazzo SD, *G Ital Dermatol Minerva Dermatol* (Italian) 107, 1195
Lichenoid eruption
 (2001): Sharma PK+, *J Dermatol* 28(12), 737
 (1974): Haldar B, *Indian J Dermatol* 19(3), 71
Lupus erythematosus
 (1994): Yung RL+, *Rheum Dis Clin North Am* 20, 61
 (1992): Hofstra AH+, *Drug Metab Dispos* 20, 205
 (1992): Rubin RL+, *J Clin Invest* 90, 165
 (1992): Salazar-Pama M+, *Ann Rheum Dis* 51, 1085
 (1992): Skaer TL, *Clin Ther* 14, 496
 (1991): Gatenby PA, *Autoimmunity* 11, 61

(1995): Moreau A+, *Int J Dermatol* 34, 263 (passim)

 (1990): Guleria R+, *Indian J Chest Dis Allied Sci* 32, 55
 (1989): Ueda Y+, *Kekkaku* (Japanese) 64, 613
 (1988): Jiang M, *Chung Kuo I Hsueh Ko Hsueh Yuan Hseuh Pao* (Chinese) 10, 379
 (1988): Umeki S, *Kekkaku* (Japanese) 63, 713
 (1986): Layer P+, *Dtsch Med Wochenschr* (German) 111, 1603
 (1985): Cush JJ+, *Am J Med Sci* 290, 36
 (1985): Holdiness MR, *Int J Dermatol* 24, 280
 (1985): Kale SA, *Postgrad Med* 77, 231
 (1985): Lovisetto P+, *Recenti Prog Med* (Ital) 76, 110
 (1985): Stratton MA, *Clin Pharm* 4, 657
 (1984): No Author, *Lancet* 2, 441
 (1984): Sim E+, *Lancet* 2, 422
 (1983): Escolar-Castellon F+, *Rev Clin Esp* (Spanish) 169, 209
 (1982): Grunwald M+, *Dermatologica* 165, 172
 (1982): Harmon CE+, *Clin Rheum Dis* 8, 121
 (1981): Reidenberg MM, *Arthritis Rheum* 24, 1004
 (1980): Agarwal MB+, *J Postgrad Med* 26, 263
 (1980): Condemi JJ, *Geriatrics* 35(3), 81
 (1980): Weinstein A, *Prog Clin Immunol* 4, 1
 (1977): Dandavino R+, *Ann Med Interne Paris* (French) 128, 39
 (1977): Seedat YK+, *S Afr Med J* 51, 335
 (1976): Cohmen G, *Med Klin* (German) 71, 789
 (1976): Dutt AK+, *Indian J Chest Dis Allied Sci* 18, 146
 (1975): Laroche C+, *Sem Hop* (French) 51, 2515
 (1974): Harpey JP, *Ann Allergy* 33, 256
 (1974): *Med Lett Drugs Ther* 16, 34
 (1974): McEwen J, *Lancet* 2, 1570
 (1974): No Author, *Va Med Mon* 101, 299 (passim)
 (1973): Alarcon-Segovia D, *Chest* 63, 299
 (1973): Bar-On H, *Harefuah* (Hebrew) 84, 25
 (1973): Blomgren SE, *Semin Hematol* 10, 345
 (1973): Durand JP+, *Cah Med* (French) 14, 9
 (1973): Godeau P+, *Ann Med Interne Paris* (French) 124, 181
 (1972): Dorfmann H+, *Nouv Presse Med* (French) 1, 2907
 (1972): Gaultier CI+, *Ann Pédiatr Paris* (French) 19, 459
 (1972): Goldman AL+, *Chest* 62, 71
 (1972): Greenberg JH+, *JAMA* 222, 191
 (1971): Delepierre F+, *Rev Tuberc Pneumol Paris* (French) 35, 397
 (1970): No Author, *BMJ* 2, 192
 (1970): Trad J+, *Sem Hop* (French) 46, 3013
 (1969): Alarcon-Segovia D, *Mayo Clin Proc* 44, 664
 (1967): Auquier L+, *Bull Mem Soc Med Hop Paris* (French) 118, 372
 (1967): Hothersall TE+, *Scott Med J* 13, 245
 (1967): Masel MA, *Med J Aust* 54, 738
 (1967): Siegel M+, *Arthritis Rheum* 10, 407
 (1963): Zingale SB+, *Arch Intern Med* 112, 63
Photosensitivity
 (1998): Lee AY+, *Photodermatol Photoimmunol Photomed* 14, 77 (lichenoid) (2 patients)
 (1987): Schmutz JL+, *Ann Dermatol Venereol* (French) 114, 569
 (1972): Kauppinen K, *Acta Derm Venereol* (Stock) 52, 68
 (1969): Kalivas J, *JAMA* 209, 1706
Pruritus
 (1953): Witbind E+, *Dis Chest* 23, 16 (>5%)
Purpura
 (1992): Breathnach SM+, *Adverse Drug Reactions and the Skin* Blackwell, Oxford, 159 (passim)
 (1982): Rosin MA+, *Southern Med J* 75, 81 (passim)
 (1980): Miescher PA+, *Clin Haematol* 9, 505
 (1979): Byrd RB+, *JAMA* 241, 1239
 (1965): Horowitz HI+, *Semin Hematol* 2, 287
 (1964): Duncan JT, *Am Rev Respir Dis* 89, 103
 (1959): Bereston ES, *J Invest Dermatol* 33, 427
Pustules
 (1993): Webster GF, *Clin Dermatol* 11, 541
 (1985): Yamasaki R+, *Br J Dermatol* 112, 504 (subcorneal)
Rash (sic) (<1%)
 (2000): Gordin F+, *JAMA* 283, 1445

Side effects (sic)
  (1985): Holdiness MR, *Int J Dermatol* 24, 280 (2%)
Stevens–Johnson syndrome
  (1976): Bomb BS+, *Tubercle* 57, 229
  (1965): Ingle VN+, *Indian Pediatr* 2, 305
Striae
  (1967): Hofer W, *Z Haut Geschlechtskr* (German) 42, 603
Systemic eczematous contact dermatitis
  (1993): Meseguer J+, *Contact Dermatitis* 28, 110
Toxic epidermal necrolysis (<1%)
  (1990): Nanda A+, *Arch Dermatol* 126, 125
  (1983): Katoch K+, *Lepr India* 55, 133
  (1976): Mital OP+, *Indian J Tuberc* 23, 32
  (1974): Faye I+, *Bull Soc Med Afr Noire Lang Fr* (French) 19, 185
    (fatal)
  (1973): Sehgal VN+, *Indian J Chest Dis* 15, 57
  (1967): Lowney ED+, *Arch Dermatol* 95, 359
Urticaria (1–5%)
  (1992): Breathnach SM+, *Adverse Drug Reactions and the Skin*
    Blackwell, Oxford, 159 (passim)
  (1982): Rosin MA+, *Southern Med J* 75, 81 (passim)
  (1959): Bereston ES, *J Invest Dermatol* 33, 427
  (1953): Cormia FE+, *Arch Dermatol* 68, 536 (4%)
Vasculitis
  (1982): Rosin MA+, *Southern Med J* 75, 81 (passim)
  (1963): Honeycutt WM+, *Arch Dermatol* 88, 190

Hair
Hair – alopecia
  (2001): Sharma PK+, *J Dermatol* 28(12), 737
  (1996): FitzGerald JM+, *Lancet* 347, 472
  (1978): Krivokhizh VN+, *Vestn Dermatol Venerol* (Russian) 3, 63

Nails
Nails – onycholysis

Other
Acute intermittent porphyria
Anaphylactoid reactions
  (2003): Crook MJ, *J Clin Pharmacol* 43(5), 545
Death
Gynecomastia
Hypersensitivity
  (2001): Rebollo S+, *Contact Dermatitis* 45(5), 306
  (1992): Dukes CS+, *Trop Geogr Med* 44, 308
  (1969): Rykowska Z, *Gruzlica* (Polish) 37, 777
Injection-site irritation
Myopathy
  (1989): Cronkright PJ+, *Ann Intern Med* 110, 945
Oral mucosal lesions
  (1973): Parish LC+, *Int J Dermatol* 12, 324
  (1971): *Med Lett* 13, 55 (1–5%)
Oral mucosal ulceration
Paresthesias
  (1982): Porter IH, *Handbook of Clinical Neurology* 44, 648
Rhabdomyolysis
  (2001): Panganiban LR+, *J Toxicol Clin Toxicol* 39(2), 143 (3%)
  (1995): Blowey DL+, *Am J Emerg Med* 13(5), 543
Serum sickness
  (1981): Simelaro J+, *J Am Osteopath Assoc* 80, 348
Side effects (sic)
  (2003): Yee D+, *Am J Respir Crit Care Med* 167(11), 1472
Tinnitus
Xerostomia

ISOPROTERENOL

Trade names: Aerolone; Isuprel (Sanofi-Synthelabo); Medihaler-ISO (3M); Norisodrine (Abbott)
Other common trade names: *Isopro; Isuprel Mistometer; Isuprel Nebulimetro; Saventrine; Vapo-Iso*
Indications: Bronchospasm, ventricular arrhythmias
Category: Adrenergic bronchodilator; Sympathomimetic
Half-life: 2.5–5 minutes

Reactions

Skin
Diaphoresis (1–10%)
Edema
Flushing (1–10%)
Pruritus
Rash (sic)
Urticaria

Other
Headache
Oral mucosal lesions
  (1969): Warth J+, *JAMA* 209, 417
Saliva discoloration (sic) (pinkish-red) (>10%)
Trembling
Tremor
Xerostomia (>10%)

ISOSORBIDE

Trade name: Ismotic
Indications: Acute angle-closure glaucoma
Category: Osmotic diuretic
Half-life: 5–9.5 hours

Reactions

Skin
Rash (sic) (<1%)
Other
Tinnitus

ISOSORBIDE DINITRATE

Synonyms: ISD; ISDN
Trade names: Dilatrate-SR (Schwartz); Isordil (Wyeth); Sorbitrate (AstraZeneca)
Other common trade names: *Apo-ISDN; Cedocard; Coradur*
Indications: Angina pectoris
Category: Antianginal; Vasodilator
Half-life: 4 hours (oral)
Clinically important, potentially hazardous interactions with: sildenafil

Reactions

Skin
Ankle edema
  (1981): Rodger JC, *BMJ* 283, 1365
Diaphoresis

Edema (<1%)
  (2002): Aquilina S+, *Clin Exp Dermatol* 27(8), 700
Flushing (>10%)
  (1981): Rodger JC, *BMJ* 283, 1365 (passim)
Maculopapular rash
  (2002): Aquilina S+, *Clin Exp Dermatol* 27(8), 700
Pallor
Peripheral edema

Other
  Headache
  Xerostomia

ISOSORBIDE MONONITRATE

Synonym: ISMN
Trade names: Imdur (Schering); Ismo (ESP Pharma); Monoket (Schwartz)
Indications: Angina pectoris
Half-life: ~4 hours
Clinically important, potentially hazardous interactions with: sildenafil

Reactions

Skin
  Ankle edema
    (1981): Rodger JC, *BMJ* 283, 1365
  Diaphoresis
  Edema (<1%)
  Flushing (>10%)
    (1981): Rodger JC, *BMJ* 283, 1365 (passim)
  Pruritus (<1%)
  Rash (sic) (<1%)

Other
  Headache
  Hyperesthesia (<1%)
  Tooth disorder (sic) (<1%)

ISOTRETINOIN

Synonym: 13-*cis*-retinoic acid
Trade names: Accutane (Roche); Amnesteem (Bertek)
Other common trade names: *Isotrex; Roaccutan; Roaccutane; Roacutan; Roacuttan*
Indications: Cystic acne
Category: Retinoid; Sebaceous gland function inhibitor
Half-life: 10–20 hours
Clinically important, potentially hazardous interactions with: acitretin, antacids, bexarotene, cholestyramine, co-trimoxazole, corticosteroids, **fish oil supplements**, minocycline, retinoids, tetracycline, vitamin A

Reactions

Skin
  Acne (fulminans)
    (2002): Moroz B+, *World Congress Dermatol* Poster, 0119
    (1997): Tan BB+, *Clin Exp Dermatol* 22, 26
    (1996): Faverge B+, *Arch Pediatr* (French) 3, 188
    (1993): Bottomley WW+, *Acta Derm Venereol* (Stockh) 73, 74
    (1993): Lepagney ML+, *Ann Dermatol Venereol* (French) 120, 917

  (1992): Choi EH+, *J Dermatol* 19, 378
  (1992): Hagler J+, *Int J Dermatol* 31, 199
  (1992): Jenkinson HA, *Br J Dermatol* 127, 62
  (1991): Elias LM+, *J Dermatol* 18, 366
  (1991): Joly P+, *Ann Dermatol Venereol* (French) 118, 369
  (1989): Rotoli M+, *G Ital Dermatol Venereol* (Italian) 124, 120
  (1988): Blanc D+, *Dermatologica* 177, 16
  (1985): Kellett JK+, *BMJ* 290, 820
  (1984): Darley CR+, *J R Soc Med* 77, 328
Acute febrile neutrophilic dermatosis (Sweet's syndrome)
  (2003): Gyorfy A+, *Med Pediatr Oncol* 40(2), 135
Bruising (sic)
  (1993): Green C, *Br J Dermatol* 128, 465
Cellulitis (1–10%)
Cheilitis (>90%)
  (2001): Önder M+, *J Dermatol Treat* 12, 115
  (1999): Graham BS+, *Arch Dermatol* 349
  (1997): Berger R, *The Schoch Letter* 47, 5
  (1997): Goulden V+, *Br J Dermatol* 137, 106
  (1988): Shalita AR+, *Cutis* 42, 10
  (1976): Peck GL+, *Lancet* 2, 1172
Desquamation (palms and soles) (5%)
  (1988): Shalita AR+, *Cutis* 42, 10
Diaphoresis
  (2000): Popescu C, Bucharest, Romania (from Internet) (observation)
  (1988): Rees JL+, *Br J Dermatol* 119, 79
  (1987): Kiistala R+, *Acta Derm Venereol* 67, 331 (increased number of active sweat glands)
Edema (subcutaneous, recurrent)
  (1999): Choquet-Kastylevsky G+, *Therapie* (French) 54, 263
  (1999): Graham BS+, *Arch Dermatol* 135, 349
Eruptive xanthoma
  (1983): Shalita AR+, *J Am Acad Dermatol* 9, 629
  (1980): Dicken CH+, *Arch Dermatol* 116, 951
Erythema multiforme
  (1988): Bigby M+, *J Am Acad Dermatol* 18, 543
Erythema nodosum
  (1997): Tan BB+, *Clin Exp Dermatol* 22, 26
  (1988): Bigby M+, *J Am Acad Dermatol* 18, 543
  (1985): Kellett JK+, *BMJ* 290, 820
Exanthems
  (1993): Litt JZ, Beachwood, OH (non-pruritic) (personal case) (observation)
  (1988): Bigby M+, *J Am Acad Dermatol* 18, 543
Exfoliation (1–10%)
Facial cellulitis
  (1994): Boffa MJ+, *J Am Acad Dermatol* 31, 800
Facial edema (1–10%)
Facial scarring
  (1994): Katz BE+, *J Am Acad Dermatol* 30, 852
Fixed eruption
  (1988): Bigby M+, *J Am Acad Dermatol* 18, 543
Flushing
  (1998): Frederickson K (from Internet) (observation)
  (1998): Gass M (from Internet) (2 observations)
Folliculitis
  (1990): Hughes BR+, *Br J Dermatol* 122, 683
Fragility
  (2000): *Prescrire Int* 7, 178 (from wax epilation)
  (1997): Litt JZ, Beachwood, OH (lips from wax epilation) (2 personal cases) (observations)
  (1997): Woollons A+, *Br J Dermatol* 137, 389
  (1995): Holmes SC+, *Br J Dermatol* 132, 165
Granulation tissue
  (1991): Rodland O+, *Tidsskr Nor Laegeforen* (Norwegian) 111, 2630
  (1985): Miller RA+, *J Am Acad Dermatol* 5, 888

(1984): Robertson DB+, *Br J Dermatol* 111, 689
Herpes (sic)
(1990): Joly P+, *Ann Dermatol Venereol* (French) 117, 860
Keloid
(1999): Ginarte M+, *Int J Dermatol* 38, 228
(1997): Bernestein LJ+, *Arch Dermatol* 133, 111
(1994): Katz BE+, *J Am Acad Dermatol* 30, 852
(1988): Zachariae H, *Br J Dermatol* 118, 703
Keratolysis exfoliativa
Leucoderma
(1988): Bigby M+, *J Am Acad Dermatol* 18, 543
Lichenoid eruption
(2001): Boyd AS+, *Cutis* 68, 301
Melasma
(1998): Thaler D, Monona, WI (from internet) (observation)
(1997): Verros CD, Tripolis, Greece (from Internet) (observation)
Miliaria
(1986): Gupta AK+, *Cutis* 38, 275
Mycosis fungoides
(1985): Molin L+, *Acta Derm Venereol* 65, 69
Nummular eczema
(1987): Bettoli V+, *J Am Acad Dermatol* 16, 617
Pallor (1–10%)
Pemphigus
(1995): Georgala S+, *Acta Derm Venereol* 75, 413
Photosensitivity (>10%)
(2002): Carlin CS+, *J Cutan Med Surg* 6(2), 125
(1991): Auffret N+, *J Am Acad Dermatol* 23, 321
(1986): Ferguson J+, *Br J Dermatol* 115, 275
(1986): Wong RC+, *J Am Acad Dermatol* 14, 1095
(1985): Diffey BL+, *J Am Acad Dermatol* 12, 119
(1983): McCormack LS+, *J Am Acad Dermatol* 9, 273
Pigmentation
(2002): Carlin CS+, *J Cutan Med Surg* 6(2), 125
(1988): Bigby M+, *J Am Acad Dermatol* 18, 543
Pityriasis rosea
(1984): Helfman RJ+, *Cutis* 33, 297
Pruritus (1–5%)
(1994): Yee KC+, *Dermatology* 189, 117
(1988): Shalita AR+, *Cutis* 42, 10
(1976): Peck GL+, *Lancet* 2, 1172
Pyoderma gangrenosum
(2002): Moroz B+, *World Congress Dermatol* Poster
(1997): Gangaram HP+, *Br J Dermatol* 136, 636
Pyogenic granuloma
(1992): Hagler J+, *Int J Dermatol* 31, 199 (fatal)
(1988): Blanc D+, *Dermatologica* 177, 16
(1984): Robertson DB+, *Br J Dermatol* 111, 689
(1983): Campbell JP+, *J Am Acad Dermatol* 9, 708
(1983): Exner JH+, *Arch Dermatol* 119, 808
(1983): Spear KL+, *Mayo Clin Proc* 58, 509
(1983): Valentic JP+, *Arch Dermatol* 119, 871
Rash (sic)
Sebaceous casts (sic)
(2000): Agarwal S+, *Br J Dermatol* 143, 228 (nasolabial follicular)
Telangiectasia
(1994): Thompson D, *The Schoch Letter* 44, 47 (#186) (observation)
Toxic epidermal necrolysis
(1994): Rosen T, *Arch Dermatol* 130, 260
Urticaria
(2000): Madnani N, Mumbai, India (from Internet) (observation)
(1988): Bigby M+, *J Am Acad Dermatol* 18, 543
Varicosities
(1994): Thompson D, *The Schoch Letter* 44, 47 (#186) (observation)
Vasculitis

(1990): Aractingi S+, *Lancet* 335, 362
(1989): Dwyer JM+, *Lancet* 2, 494
(1989): Reynolds P+, *Lancet* 2, 1216
(1987): Epstein EH, *Arch Dermatol* 123, 1124
Xerosis (>10%)
(1997): Berger R, *The Schoch Letter* 47, 5
(1988): Shalita AR+, *Cutis* 42, 10
(1976): Peck GL+, *Lancet* 2, 1172

Hair
Hair – alopecia (16%)
(2002): Hirsch R, Boston, MA (from Internet) (observation)
(2000): Dintiman BJ, Fairfax, VA (from Internet) (4 observations)
(2000): Frederickson KS, Novalo, CA (from Internet) (observation)
(2000): Rehbein HM, Jacksonville, FL (from Internet) (2 observations)
(1998): Litt JZ, Beachwood, OH (personal case) (observation)
(1998): Thaler D, Monona, WI (from Internet) (observation)
(1997): Berger R, *The Schoch Letter* 47, 5 (diffuse)
(1997): Thaler D, Monona, WI (from Internet) (observation)
(1994): Shelley WB+, *Cutis* 53, 237 (observation)
Hair – hirsutism
Hair – pili torti (curly hair)
(2002): Spencer L, Crawforsville, IN (from Internet) (observation)
(1996): van der Pijl JW+, *Lancet* 348, 622
(1990): Bunker CB+, *Clin Exp Dermatol* 15, 143
(1985): Hays SB+, *Cutis* 25, 466
Hair – trichotillomania
(1990): Mahr G, *Psychosomatics* 31, 235

Nails
Nails – brittle
(2001): Önder M+, *J Dermatol Treat* 12, 115
Nails – growth
(1994): Litt JZ, Beachwood, OH (personal case) (observation)
Nails – herpetic whitlow
(2003): Stetson CL+, *Int J Dermatol* 42(6), 496
Nails – median canaliform dystrophy
(1997): Dharmagunawardena B+, *Br J Dermatol*
(1992): Bottomley WW+, *Br J Dermatol* 127, 447
(1988): Bigby M+, *J Am Acad Dermatol* 18, 543
Nails – onycholysis
(2001): Önder M+, *J Dermatol Treat* 12, 115
(1988): Bigby M+, *J Am Acad Dermatol* 18, 543
Nails – paronychia
(1998): Lepine EM, Rock Hill, SC (from Internet) (observation)
(1988): Bigby M+, *J Am Acad Dermatol* 18, 543
(1986): DeRaeve L+, *Dermatologica* 172, 278
(1984): Blumental G, *J Am Acad Dermatol* 10, 677
Nails – periungual hemorrhage
(1997): Leal G, Fortaleza, Brazil (from Internet) (observation)

Other
Ageusia
(1996): Halpern SM+, *Br J Dermatol* 134(2), 378
Death
Depression
(2002): Robusto O, *Acta Med Port* 15(4), 325
Dysgeusia
(1990): Heise E+, *Eur Arch Otorhinolaryngol* 247, 382
Galactorrhea
(1985): Larsen GK, *Arch Dermatol* 121, 450
Gynecomastia
(1994): Shelley WB+, *Cutis* 54, 149 (passim)
(1992): Fluckiger R, *Schweiz Rundsch Med Prax* (German) 81, 1370
Headache

Mucosal denudation of lips
  (1999): Graham BS+, *Arch Dermatol* 349
Myalgia (>10%)
  (1998): Heudes AM+, *Ann Dermatol Venereol* 125(2), 94
Myopathy
  (1996): Fiallo P+, *Arch Dermatol* 132, 1521
  (1986): Hodak E, *BMJ* 293, 425
Parosmia
  (1990): Heise E+, *Eur Arch Otorhinolaryngol* 247, 382
Pseudoporphyria
  (1993): Riordan CA+, *Clin Exp Dermatol* 18, 69
Pseudotumor cerebri
  (1998): Sorkin MJ, Denver, CO (from Internet) (observation of 4
    cases)
  (1995): Lee AG, *Cutis* 55, 165
  (1988): Roytman M+, *Cutis* 42, 399
Rhabdomyolysis
  (2001): Trauner MA+, *Dermatology Online Journal* 5, 2
  (2001): Zabawski E, Longwood, TX (from Internet)
    (observation)
  (1998): Heudes AM+, *Ann Dermatol Venereol* 125(2), 94
Stiff-person syndrome
  (2002): Chroni E+, *Neuromuscul Disord* 12(9), 886
Tinnitus
Xerostomia (>10%)
  (1992): Breathnach SM+, *Adverse Drug Reactions and the Skin*
    Blackwell, Oxford, 259 (passim)

ISOXSUPRINE

Trade names: Vasodilan (Bristol-Myers Squibb); Voxsuprine
Other common trade names: *Duvadilan; Isoxine; Sincen;
Vasolan; Vasosuprina; Xuprin*
Indications: Peripheral vascular disease, Raynaud's phenomenon
Category: Peripheral vasodilator
Half-life: N/A

Reactions

Skin
Dermatitis (sic)
  (1978): Horowitz JJ+, *Am J Obstet Gynecol* 131, 225

ISRADIPINE

Trade name: DynaCirc (Reliant)
Other common trade names: *Dynacirc SRO; Lomir; Lomir SRO;
Prescal; Vascal*
Indications: Hypertension
Category: Antihypertensive; Calcium channel blocker
Half-life: 8 hours
**Clinically important, potentially hazardous interactions
with:** epirubicin, imatinib

Reactions

Skin
Diaphoresis (<1%)
Edema (7.2%)
  (1992): Lopez LM+, *Ann Pharmacother* 26, 789
  (1992): Madias NE+, *Am J Hypertens* 5, 141
  (1991): Eisner GM+, *Am J Hypertens* 4, 154S
  (1991): Galloe AM+, *J Intern Med* 229, 447

  (1991): Schachter M, *J Clin Pharm Ther* 16, 79
  (1990): Vidt DG, *Cleve Clin J Med* 57, 677
Exanthems
  (1993): Blumenthal HL, Beachwood, OH (personal case)
    (observation)
  (1990): Fitton A+, *Drugs* 40, 31 (1.5%)
Flushing (2.6%)
  (2002): Flynn JT+, *Pediatr Nephrol* 17(9), 748 (9.5%)
  (1992): Lopez LM+, *Ann Pharmacother* 26, 789
  (1991): Galloe AM+, *J Intern Med* 229, 447
  (1991): Schachter M, *J Clin Pharm Ther* 16, 79
  (1990): Fitton A+, *Drugs* 40, 31 (10–15%)
  (1990): Vidt DG, *Cleve Clin J Med* 57, 677
  (1990): Welzel D+, *Drugs* 40 (Suppl 2), 60
  (1990): Zubair M+, *Drugs* 40 (Suppl 2), 26 (7.8%)
Peripheral edema
Pruritus (<1%)
  (1990): Zubair M+, *Drugs* 40 (Suppl 2), 26 (5.9%)
Rash (sic) (1.5%)
Urticaria (<1%)

Other
Dizziness
  (2002): Flynn JT+, *Pediatr Nephrol* 17(9), 748 (9.5%)
Gingival hyperplasia (<1%)
Headache
  (2002): Flynn JT+, *Pediatr Nephrol* 17(9), 748 (9.5%)
Oral mucosal lesions
  (1990): Zubair M+, *Drugs* 40 (Suppl 2), 26 (5.9%)
Paresthesias (<1%)
Xerostomia (<1%)

ITRACONAZOLE

Trade name: Sporanox (Janssen) (Ortho)
Other common trade names: *Isox; Itranax; Sopronox; Sporacid;
Sporal; Sporanox 15 D*
Indications: Onychomycosis, deep mycoses
Category: Antifungal
Half-life: 21 hours
**Clinically important, potentially hazardous interactions
with:** alprazolam, amphotericin B, anisindione, antacids,
aprepitant, atorvastatin, bosentan, cimetidine, clorazepate,
dicumarol, didanosine, eplerenone, ethotoin, fosphenytoin,
grapefruit juice, HMG-CoA reductase inhibitors, imatinib,
lovastatin, mephenytoin, midazolam, phenytoin, pimozide,
quinidine, rifampin, sildenafil, simvastatin, triazolam, vinblastine,
vincristine, warfarin

Reactions

Skin
Acute generalized exanthematous pustulosis (AGEP)
  (1997): Park YM+, *J Am Acad Dermatol* 36, 794
  (1995): Heymann WR+, *J Am Acad Dermatol* 33, 130
Angioedema
  (1996): Foong H, Malaysia (from Internet) (observation)
Edema (3.5%)
  (1998): N Z Medicines Adverse Reactions Committee,
    (peripheral) (from Internet) (observation)
  (1996): Tailor SA+, *Arch Dermatol* 132, 350 (peripheral) (with
    nifedipine)
  (1994): Gupta AK+, *J Am Acad Dermatol* 30, 911
  (1994): Rosen T, *Arch Dermatol* 130, 260
  (1992): *Med Lett Drugs Ther* 34, 14
  (1991): Diaz M+, *Chest* 100, 682

(1991): Sharkey PK+, *Antimicrob Agents Chemother* 35, 707
(1990): Denning DW+, *J Am Acad Dermatol* 23, 602 (2%)
(1990): Sharkey PK+, *J Am Acad Dermatol* 23, 577
(1990): Tucker RM+, *J Antimicrob Chemother* 26, 561

Eruptions (sic)
(2000): Goto Y+, *Acta Derm Venereol* 80, 72
(1992): Cleary JD+, *Ann Pharmacother* 26(4), 502

Erythema multiforme
(1998): Rademaker M+, *New Zealand Adverse Drug Reactions Committee*, April, 1998 (from Internet)

Exanthems
(1999): Burrow WH, Jackson, MS, (from Internet) (2 cases) (observation)
(1999): Valentine MC, Everett, WA (from Internet) (2 cases) observation)
(1998): Litt JZ, Beachwood, OH (personal case) (observation)
(1997): Blumenthal HL, Beachwood, OH (personal case) (observation)
(1997): Danby FW, Kingston, Ontario (2 cases) (from Internet) (observation)
(1996): Degreef H, *Cutis* 58, 90
(1994): Litt JZ, Beachwood, OH (2 personal cases) (observation)
(1991): Smith DE+, *AIDS* 5, 1367
(1990): Roseeuw D+, *Clin Exp Dermatol* 15, 101 (2.6%)
(1990): Tucker RM+, *J Am Acad Dermatol* 23, 593 (3%)

Facial dermatitis (papular, id-like)
(1996): Thaler D, Monona, WI (2 cases) (from internet) (observation)

Fixed eruption
(1997): Perry S, *The Schoch Letter* 47, 19
(1994): Litt JZ, Beachwood, OH (personal case) (observation)

Flu-like syndrome
(2002): Faergemann J+, *Arch Dermatol* 138, 69

Peripheral edema (4%)

Photosensitivity
(1996): Moreland A, *The Schoch Letter* 46, 19 (observation)

Phototoxicity
(1999): Gass M, Davis, CA (from Internet) (observation)
(1995): Epstein E Jr, *The Schoch Letter* 45, 28 (observation)
(1994): Milstein H, *The Schoch Letter* 44, 5 (observation)

Pruritus (2.5%)
(2002): Faergemann J+, *Arch Dermatol* 138, 69
(1997): Gupta AK+, *J Am Acad Dermatol* 36, 789
(1994): Gupta AK+, *J Am Acad Dermatol* 30, 911 (0.7%)
(1992): Cleary JD+, *Ann Pharmacother* 26, 502
(1992): Lavrijsen AP+, *Lancet* 340, 251
(1991): De Beule K+, *Curr Ther Res* 49, 814
(1990): Tucker RM+, *J Antimicrob Chemother* 26, 561
(1989): Grant SM+, *Drugs* 39, 877 (0.6%)

Purpura
(1997): Kramer KE+, *J Am Acad Dermatol* 37, 994

Rash (sic) (8.6%)
(2003): Gallin JI+, *N Engl J Med* 348(24), 2416
(1996): Odom R+, *J Am Acad Dermatol* 35, 110 (severe)
(1994): Gupta AK+, *J Am Acad Dermatol* 30, 911 (1.1%)
(1990): Sharkey PK+, *J Am Acad Dermatol* 23, 577
(1990): Tucker RM+, *J Am Acad Dermatol* 23, 593
(1990): Tucker RM+, *J Antimicrob Chemother* 26, 561

Side effects (sic)
(1999): Gupta AK+, *Dermatology* 199, 248
(1997): Gupta AK+, *J Am Acad Dermatol* 36, 789

Stevens–Johnson syndrome

Urticaria
(2002): Faergemann J+, *Arch Dermatol* 138, 69
(1999): Valentine MC, Everett, WA (from Internet) (observation)
(1997): Billon S, *The Schoch Letter* 47, 32 (observation)
(1996): Thaler D, Monona, WI (from internet) (observation)
(1994): Litt JZ, Beachwood, OH (personal case) (observation)
(1993): Litt JZ, Beachwood, OH (personal case) (observation)

(1992): Piepponen T+, *J Antimicrob Chemother* 29, 195
Vasculitis
(1996): Odom R+, *J Am Acad Dermatol* 35, 110

Hair

Hair – alopecia
(1995): Litt JZ, Beachwood, OH (personal case) (observation)
(1992): de Gans J+, *AIDS* 6, 185
(1986): Moller Heilesen A, *BMJ* 293, 823

Nails

Nails – beading
(1994): Donker PD+, *Clin Exp Dermatol* 19, 404
Nails – onychocryptosis
(1995): Arenas R+, *Int J Dermatol* 34, 138

Other

Anaphylactoid reactions
Death
(2002): Legras A+, *Am J Med* 113(4), 352 (with leflunomide)
Gynecomastia (<1%)
(1994): Gupta AK+, *J Am Acad Dermatol* 30, 911
Headache
Myalgia (1%)
Rhabdomyolysis
(2002): Vlahakos DV+, *Transplantation* 73(12), 1962
Serum sickness
(1998): Park H+, *Ann Pharmacother* 32, 1249
Tinnitus
Xerostomia
(1990): Tucker RM+, *J Am Acad Dermatol* 23, 593
(1990): Tucker RM+, *J Antimicrob Chemother* 26, 561

IVERMECTIN

Trade name: Stromectol (Merck)
Indications: Various infections caused by susceptible helmintic organisms
Category: Antihelmintic antibiotic
Half-life: 16–35 hours
Clinically important, potentially hazardous interactions with: alprazolam, barbiturates, benzodiazepines, diazepam, midazolam, valproic acid

Reactions

Skin

Bullous eruption
(1993): Burnham GM, *Trans R Soc Trop Med Hyg* 87, 313
Bullous pemphigoid
(2001): Trindade P, Natal, Brazil (personal communication)
Burning
(1999): Editorial, *Arch Dermatol* 135, 705
Dermatitis (sic)
(1999): Editorial, *Arch Dermatol* 135, 705
Edema
(1998): Jaramillo-Ayerbe F+, *Arch Dermatol* 134, 143
(1995): Darge K+, *Trop Med Parasitol* 46, 206 (arms and legs) (10%)
(1993): Burnham GM, *Trans R Soc Trop Med Hyg* 87, 313
(1992): Chijioke CP+, *Trans R Soc Trop Med Hyg* 86, 284
(1992): Collins RC+, *Am J Trop Med Hyg* 47, 156 (facial) (31.8%)
(1992): Zea-Flores R+, *Trans R Soc Trop Med Hyg* 86, 663 (53%)
(1991): Bryan RT+, *Lancet* 337, 304
(1991): Guderian RH+, *Lancet* 337, 188 (leg)
Exanthems

(1993): Burnham GM, *Trans R Soc Trop Med Hyg* 87, 313
(1991): Whitworth JAG+, *Lancet* 337, 625 (1–5%)
(1990): Ette EI+, *Drug Intell Clin Pharm* 24, 426 (34%)
Facial edema (1.2%)
(1998): Jaramillo-Ayerbe F+, *Arch Dermatol* 134, 143
(1993): Burnham GM, *Trans R Soc Trop Med Hyg* 87, 313
Peripheral edema
Pruritus (2.8%–27.5%)
(1998): Jaramillo-Ayerbe F+, *Arch Dermatol* 134, 143
(1995): Darge K+, *Trop Med Parasitol* 46, 206
(1993): Burnham GM, *Trans R Soc Trop Med Hyg* 87, 313
(1993): Kar SK+, *Acta Trop* 55, 21
(1992): Chijioke CP+, *Trans R Soc Trop Med Hyg* 86, 284 (71.2%)
(1992): Collins RC+, *Am J Trop Med Hyg* 47, 156 (34%)
(1991): Bryan RT+, *Lancet* 337, 304
(1991): Whitworth JAG+, *Lancet* 337, 625 (8%)
(1990): Ette EI+, *Drug Intell Clin Pharm* 24, 426 (9.6%)
(1989): Guderian RH+, *Eur J Epidemiol* 5, 294 (4%)
Pustules
Rash (sic) (0.9%)
(1998): Jaramillo-Ayerbe F+, *Arch Dermatol* 134, 143
(1993): Kar SK+, *Acta Trop* 55, 21
(1991): Bryan RT+, *Lancet* 337, 304 (93%)
(1991): Guderian RH+, *Lancet* 337, 188
(1991): Whitworth JAG+, *Lancet* 337, 625 (8%)
(1989): Guderian RH+, *Eur J Epidemiol* 5, 294 (4%)
Urticaria (0.9–22.7%)

Other

Myalgia
(1995): Darge K+, *Trop Med Parasitol* 46, 206 (20%)
(1993): Kar SK+, *Acta Trop* 55, 21
Tremor

JUNIPER

Scientific names: *Juniperus communis; Juniperus oxycedrus; Juniperus phoenicea; Juniperus virginiana*
Family: Cupressaceae
Trade and other common names: Baccae Juniperi; Cade Oil; Enebro; Gemeiner Wachholder; Genevrier; Ginepro; Juniper Tar Oil; Zimbro
Category: Anti-inflammatory; Antirheumatic; Carminative; Diuretic; Stomachic; Urinary antiseptic; Uterine stimulant
Purported indications and other uses: Cystitis, urethritis, urinary tract infections, flatulent colic, rheumatism, arthritis, gout, leucorrhea, blenorrhea, scrofula. Topical: joint pain, muscle pain, neuralgia, chronic eczema. Inhalant:: bronchitis, lung infections. Condiment, flavor component (gin, Chartreuse, bitters), perfume
Half-life: N/A
Clinically important, potentially hazardous interactions with: loop diuretics, spironolactone, thiazide diuretics, triamterene

Reactions

Skin
Allergic reactions (sic)
  (1973): Rothe A+, *Berufsdermatosen* 21(1), 11
Dermatitis
  (1996): Meding B+, *Contact Dermatitis* 34(3), 185
Edema
Erythema
Sensitivity (sic)
  (2001): *Int J Toxicol* 20, 41
Vesicular eruptions

KANAMYCIN

Trade name: Kantrex (Geneva)
Other common trade names: *Kanamicina; Kanamycine; Kanamytrex; Kanescin; Kannasyn; Randikan*
Indications: Various infections caused by susceptible organisms
Category: Aminoglycoside antibiotic
Half-life: 2–4 hours
Clinically important, potentially hazardous interactions with: aldesleukin, atracurium, bumetanide, doxacurium, ethacrynic acid, furosemide, methoxyflurane, non-depolarizing muscle relaxants, pancuronium, polypeptide antibiotics, rocuronium, succinylcholine, torsemide, vecuronium

Reactions

Skin
Burning
Edema (>10%)
Erythema (<1%)
Exanthems
Photosensitivity (<1%)
Pruritus (1–10%)
Rash (sic) (1–10%)
Systemic eczematous contact dermatitis
  (1986): Holdiness MR, *Contact Dermatitis* 15, 282
Urticaria

Other
Hypersensitivity
Injection-site irritation
Injection-site pain (<1%)
Paresthesias
Phlebitis
Pseudotumor cerebri
Sialorrhea (<1%)
Tremor

KAVA

Scientific name: *Piper methysticum*
Family: Piperaceae
Trade and other common names: Ava; Awa; Intoxicating Pepper; Kavosporal; Kew; Sakau; Tonga
Category: Anxiolytic; Sedative
Purported indications and other uses: Psychosis, depression, headache, migraines, colds, rheumatism, cystitis, vaginal prolapse, otitis, abscesses, antistress, analgesic, local anesthetic, anticonvulsant
Half-life: N/A
Clinically important, potentially hazardous interactions with: alcohol, alprazolam, benzodiazepines, escitalopram, levodopa

'Products containing herbal extracts of kava have been implicated in cases of severe liver toxicity in Germany and Switzerland' says the FDA letter. 'Approximately 25 reports of [liver] toxicity associated with the use of products containing kava extracts have been reported in these countries. Serious adverse effects include hepatitis, cirrhosis and liver failure. At least one patient required a liver transplant.' In both Switzerland and Germany, regulatory agencies have prohibited the sale of kava extract-containing products. The FDA is investigating whether the use of kava-containing dietary supplements poses a similar health hazard in the U.S., according to the letter. The agency has received several reports of serious injury allegedly associated with the use of kava-containing dietary supplements

Note: Products containing kava have been implicated in cases of severe liver toxicity. Serious adverse effects include hepatitis, cirrhosis and liver failure. At least one patient required a liver transplant. Kava has now been banned in many countries

Reactions

Skin
Adverse effects (sic)
  (2003): Bent S+, *Ann Intern Med* 138(6), 468
  (2002): Denham A+, *J Altern Complement Med* 8(3), 237
  (2002): Ernst E, *Ann Intern Med* 136(1), 42
  (2002): Haller CA+, *Adverse Drug React Toxicol Rev* 21(3), 143
  (2002): Stevinson C+, *Drug Saf* 25(4), 251
  (2000): Ernst E, *Br J Dermatol* 143(5), 923
Dermopathy (pellagra-like syndrome)
  (2003): Cairney S+, *Neuropsychopharmacology* 28(2), 389
  (2003): Clough A, *Drug Alcohol Rev* 22(1), 43
  (2002): Singh YN+, *CNS Drugs* 16(11), 731
Lymphocytic inflammation of the dermis (sic)
Photosensitivity
Pigmentation (yellow)
Pruritus
Rash (sic)
Scaly rash (sic)
Seborrheic dermatitis
  (2000): Caro I, *Skin & Aging* 80
Xerosis

Hair
Hair – pigmentation

Nails
Nails – pigmentation

Other
Death
  (2003): Gow PJ+, *Med J Aust* 178(9), 442
Dizziness
  (2001): Wheatley D, *Phytother Res* 15(6), 549
Hypersensitivity
  (2000): Schmidt P+, *Contact Dermatitis* 42(6), 363
Mouth numbness (sic)
Parkinsonism
  (2002): Meseguer E+, *Mov Disord* 17(1), 195
Seizures
  (2003): Cairney S+, *Neuropsychopharmacology* 28(2), 389
Side effects (sic)
  (2001): Kava R, *Pac Health Dialog* 8(1), 115
  (2000): Ernst E, *Br J Dermatol* 143(5), 923
  (1999): Tinsley JA, *Minn Med* 82(5), 29

Note: Kava was discovered by Captain Cook, who named the plant 'intoxicating pepper.' In the South Pacific, kava is a popular social drink, similar to alcohol in Western societies

KETAMINE

Trade name: Ketalar (Monarch)
Other common trade names: *Calypsol; Ketalin; Ketanest; Ketolar; Petar*
Indications: Induction of anesthesia
Category: Anesthetic; Sedative-hypnotic
Half-life: 2–3 hours

Reactions

Skin
Erythema
Exanthems
Pruritus
 (2001): Burstal R+, *Anaesth Intensive Care* 29(3), 246
 (2001): Subramaniam K+, *J Clin Anesth* 13(5), 339 (with morphine)
Rash (sic) (1–10%)

Other
Injection-site erythema
Injection-site pain (1–10%)
Sialorrhea (<1%)
 (2001): Green SM+, *Pediatr Emerg Care* 17(4), 244
Tremor (>10%)

KETOCONAZOLE

Trade name: Nizoral (Janssen) (McNeil)
Other common trade names: *Aquarius; Fungarest; Fungoral; Ketoderm; Ketoisidin; Nazoltec*
Indications: Fungal infections
Category: Imidazole antifungal
Half-life: initial: 2 hours; terminal: 8 hours
Clinically important, potentially hazardous interactions with: alcohol, almotriptan, alprazolam, amphotericin B, anisindione, anticoagulants, aprepitant, aripiprazole, benzodiazepines, bosentan, chlordiazepoxide, cimetidine, clorazepate, cyclosporine, dicumarol, didanosine, dofetilide, eplerenone, gastric alkanizers, HMG-CoA reductase inhibitors, imatinib, midazolam, nevirapine, non-sedating antihistamines, pimozide, proton pump inhibitors, rifampin, ritonavir, saquinavir, sildenafil, sucralfate, tacrolimus, triazolam, vinblastine, vincristine, warfarin

Reactions

Skin
Allergic reactions (sic)
 (1983): van Ketel WG, *Contact Dermatitis* 9, 313
Angioedema
 (1994): Gonzalez-Delgado P+, *Ann Allergy* 73, 326
 (1994): Gupta AK+, *J Am Acad Dermatol* 30, 677 (passim)
 (1983): van Dijke CPH+, *BMJ* 287, 1673
Chills (1–3%)
Dermatitis
 (1993): Lodi A+, *Contact Dermatitis* 29, 97
 (1993): Valsecchi R+, *Contact Dermatitis* 29, 162
 (1992): Santucci B+, *Contact Dermatitis* 27, 274
Dry skin
 (2002): Harris KA+, *J Urol* 168(2), 542
Eczema (generalized)
 (1989): Garcia-Bravo B+, *Contact Dermatitis* 21, 346

Exanthems
 (1985): Bradsher RW+, *Ann Intern Med* 103, 872 (2%)
 (1985): Study Group, *Ann Intern Med* 103, 861 (9.7%)
 (1984): Ford GP+, *Br J Dermatol* 111, 603 (5%)
 (1984): Kahana M+, *Arch Dermatol* 120, 837
 (1983): Dismukes WE+, *Ann Intern Med* 98, 13 (4%)
 (1983): Rand R+, *Arch Dermatol* 119, 97
 (1982): Heel RC+, *Drugs* 23, 1 (0.7%)
Exfoliative dermatitis
 (1984): Parent D+, *Ann Dermatol Venereol* (French) 111,339
 (1983): Rand R+, *Arch Dermatol* 119, 97
Fixed eruption
 (1994): Gupta AK+, *J Am Acad Dermatol* 30, 677 (passim)
 (1988): Bharija SC+, *Int J Dermatol* 27, 278
Jarisch–Herxheimer reaction
Photosensitivity
 (1988): Mohamed KN, *Clin Exp Dermatol* 13, 54
Pigmentation
 (1992): Gallais V+, *Ann Dermatol Venereol* (French) 119, 471
 (1990): Poizot-Martin I+, *Int Conf AIDS* 6, 357
 (1985): Tucker WS+, *JAMA* 253, 2413
Pruritus (1.5%)
 (1994): Gupta AK+, *J Am Acad Dermatol* 30, 677 (passim)
 (1988): Mohamed KN, *Clin Exp Dermatol* 13, 54 (passim)
 (1985): Study Group, *Ann Intern Med* 103, 861 (9.7%)
 (1983): Rand R+, *Arch Dermatol* 119, 97 (1.5%)
 (1982): Heel RC+, *Drugs* 23, 1 (1.7%)
Purpura
 (1994): Gupta AK+, *J Am Acad Dermatol* 30, 677 (passim)
 (1982): Heel RC+, *Drugs* 23, 1
Rash (sic) (1–3%)
 (1994): Gupta AK+, *J Am Acad Dermatol* 30, 677 (passim)
Urticaria (1–3%)
 (1994): Gupta AK+, *J Am Acad Dermatol* 30, 677 (passim)
 (1985): Bradsher RW+, *Ann Intern Med* 103, 872 (2%)
Vasculitis
 (1982): Heel RC+, *Drugs* 23, 1
Xerosis
 (1994): Gupta AK+, *J Am Acad Dermatol* 30, 677 (passim)
 (1985): Study Group, *Ann Intern Med* 103, 861

Hair
Hair – alopecia
 (1994): Gupta AK+, *J Am Acad Dermatol* 30, 677 (passim)
 (1990): Venturoli S+, *J Clin Endocrinol Metab* 71, 335
 (1985): Study Group, *Ann Intern Med* 103, 861 (3.7%)
 (1982): Heel RC+, *Drugs* 23, 1 (0.2%)
Hair – trichoptilosis
 (1993): Aljabre SH, *Int J Dermatol* 32, 150

Nails
Nails – pigmentation
 (1985): Dreessen K, *Z Hautkr* (German) 60, 679 (black longitudinal bands)

Other
Anaphylactoid reactions
 (1994): Gupta AK+, *J Am Acad Dermatol* 30, 677 (passim)
 (1983): van Dijke CPH+, *BMJ* 287, 1673
Death
 (2001): Duman D+, *Am J Med* 111(9), 737
Depression
 (2002): Harris KA+, *J Urol* 168(2), 542
Fatigue
 (2002): Harris KA+, *J Urol* 168(2), 542
Gingival hyperplasia
 (1988): Veraldi S+, *Int J Dermatol* 27, 730
Gingivitis
 (1994): Gupta AK+, *J Am Acad Dermatol* 30, 677 (passim)

(1983): Dismukes WE+, *Ann Intern Med* 98, 13
Gynecomastia (1–3%)
  (1994): Gupta AK+, *J Am Acad Dermatol* 30, 677 (passim)
  (1993): Thompson DF+, *Pharmacotherapy* 13, 37
  (1982): Moncada B, *J Am Acad Dermatol* 7, 557
  (1981): DeFelice R+, *Antimicrob Agents Chemo* 19, 1073
Headache
Hypersensitivity
  (1994): Gonzalez-Delgado P+, *Ann Allergy* 73, 326
  (1992): Verschueren GL+, *Contact Dermatitis* 26, 47
  (1989): Garcia-Bravo B+, *Contact Dermatitis* 21, 346
Myopathy
  (1991): Garty BZ+, *Am J Dis Child* 145, 970
Oral lichenoid eruption
  (1993): Ficarra G+, *Oral Surg Oral Med Oral Pathol* 76, 460
  (1986): Markitziu A+, *Mykosen* (German) 29, 317
Oral mucosal lesions
  (1994): Gupta AK+, *J Am Acad Dermatol* 30, 677 (passim)
  (1985): Study Group, *Ann Intern Med* 103, 861 (1–5%)
  (1983): Dismukes WE+, *Ann Intern Med* 98, 13 (2%)
Oral pigmentation
  (1991): Poizot-Martin I+, *Presse Med* (French) 20, 632
  (1989): Langford A+, *Oral Surg Oral Med Oral Pathol* 67, 301 (in HIV-infected patients)
Paresthesias
  (1994): Gupta AK+, *J Am Acad Dermatol* 30, 677 (passim)
Tongue pigmentation
  (1982): Heel RC+, *Drugs* 23, 1

KETOPROFEN

Trade names: Orudis (Wyeth); Oruvail (Wyeth)
Other common trade names: *Alrheumat; Alrheumun; Aneol; Bi-Profenid; Gabrilen Retard; Keduril; Novo-Keto; Rhodis; Rhovail*
Indications: Arthritis
Category: Nonsteroidal anti-inflammatory (NSAID) analgesic
Half-life: 1.5–4 hours
Clinically important, potentially hazardous interactions with: aspirin, methotrexate, probenecid

Reactions

Skin
Allergic reactions (sic) (<1%)
Angioedema (<1%)
  (1978): Frith P+, *Lancet* 2, 847
Bullous eruption (<1%)
Dermatitis
  (2001): Preisz K+, *Orv Hetil* 142(51), 2841
  (1998): Baudot S+, *Therapie* (French) 53, 137
  (1997): *Lakartidningen* (Swedish) 94, 2664
  (1996): Jeanmougin M+, *Ann Dermatol Venereol* (French) 123, 251
  (1996): Pigatto P+, *Am J Contact Dermat* 7, 220
  (1995): Gebhardt M+, *Z Rheumatol* (German) 54, 405
  (1995): Navarro LA+, *Contact Dermatitis* 32, 181
  (1994): Mastrolonardo M+, *Contact Dermatitis* 30, 110
  (1994): Oh VM, *BMJ* 309, 512
  (1993): Ophaswongse S+, *Contact Dermatitis* 29, 57
  (1990): Mozzanica N+, *Contact Dermatitis* 23, 336
  (1990): Tosti A+, *Contact Dermatitis* 23, 112
  (1990): Valsecchi R+, *Contact Dermatitis* 21, 345
  (1989): Lanzarini M+, *Contact Dermatitis* 21, 51
  (1989): Romaguera C+, *Contact Dermatitis* 20, 310

  (1987): Mozzanica N, *Contact Dermatitis* 17, 325
  (1985): Camarasa JG, *Contact Dermatitis* 12, 121
  (1983): Angelini G+, *Contact Dermatitis* 9, 234
  (1983): Valsecchi R+, *Contact Dermatitis* 9, 163
Diaphoresis (<1%)
  (1989): Roth DE+, *Med Clin North Am* 73, 1275
Eczema (sic) (<1%)
  (1990): Tosti A+, *Contact Dermatitis* 23, 112
  (1987): Mozzanica N, *Contact Dermatitis* 17, 325
Erythema multiforme (<1%)
Exanthems
  (1975): Hingorani K+, *Curr Med Res Opin* 3, 407
Exfoliative dermatitis (<1%)
Facial edema (<1%)
Hot flashes (<1%)
Pemphigus (localized)
  (2001): Kanitakis J+, *Acta Derm Venereol* 81(4), 304
Peripheral edema (1–3%)
Photoallergic reaction
  (2002): Vigan M+, *Ann Dermatol Venereol* 129(10 Pt 1), 1125 (11%)
Photodermatitis
  (2002): Valenzuela N+, *Contact Dermatitis* 47(4), 237
  (2002): Vigan M+, *Ann Dermatol Venereol* 129(10), 1125
  (2001): Milpied-Homsi B, *Presse Med* 30(12), 605 (from gel)
  (2001): Sugiyama M+, *Am J Contact Dermat* 12(3), 180
  (2000): Matsushita T+, *Photodermatol Photoimmunol Photomed* 17(1), 26 (from gel) (5 cases)
  (1998): Baudot S+, *Therapie* (French) 53, 137
  (1998): Le Coz CJ+, *Contact Dermatitis* 38, 245
  (1997): Bastien M+, *Ann Dermatol Venereol* (French) 124, 523 (5 cases)
  (1997): Leroy D+, *Photodermatol Photoimmunol Photomed* 13, 93
  (1997): Mirande-Romero A+, *Contact Dermatitis* 37, 242 (connubial)
  (1996): Jeanmougin M+, *Ann Dermatol Venereol* (French) 123, 251
  (1995): Nabeya R+, *Contact Dermatitis* 32, 52
  (1993): Ophaswongse S+, *Contact Dermatitis* 29, 57 (phototoxic and photoallergic)
  (1992): Serrano G+, *J Am Acad Dermatol* 27, 204 (passim)
  (1990): Black AK+, *Br J Dermatol* 123, 277
  (1990): Mozzanica N+, *Contact Dermatitis* 23, 336
  (1989): Roth DE+, *Med Clin North Am* 73, 1275
  (1987): Cusano F+, *Contact Dermatitis* 17, 108
  (1987): Cusano F+, *Contact Dermatitis* 27, 50
  (1985): Alomar A, *Contact Dermatitis* 12, 112
Photosensitivity (<1%)
  (2001): Kawada A+, *Contact Dermatitis* 44(6), 370
Pigmentation (<1%)
Pruritus (1–10%)
  (1975): Hingorani K+, *Curr Med Res Opin* 3, 407
Psoriasis
  (1992): Shelley WB+, *Cutis* 51, 23 (observation)
Purpura (<1%)
  (1989): Roth DE+, *Med Clin North Am* 73, 1275
Rash (sic) (>10%)
Side effects (sic)
  (1989): Le-Loet X, *Scand J Rheumatol* Suppl 83, 21 (0.7%)
Stevens–Johnson syndrome (<1%)
Toxic epidermal necrolysis (<1%)
  (1995): Tijhuis GJ+, *Dermatology* 190, 176
Urticaria (<1%)
  (1978): Frith P+, *Lancet* 2, 847

Hair

Hair – alopecia (<1%)
(1989): Roth DE+, *Med Clin North Am* 73, 1275

Nails

Nails – onycholysis (<1%)
(1989): Roth DE+, *Med Clin North Am* 73, 1275

Other

Acute intermittent porphyria
Anaphylactoid reactions (<1%)
(1985): O'Brien WM+, *J Rheumatol* 12, 13
(1978): Frith P+, *Lancet* 2, 847
Aphthous stomatitis
Dysgeusia (<1%)
Gynecomastia (<1%)
Headache
Myalgia (<1%)
Oral mucosal lesions
(1975): Hingorani K+, *Curr Med Res Opin* 3, 407
Oral mucosal numbness
(2001): Passali D+, *Clin Ther* 23(9), 1508
Oral mucosal paresthesias
(2001): Passali D+, *Clin Ther* 23(9), 1508
Paresthesias (<1%)
Pseudolymphoma
(2001): Werth V, *Dermatology Times* 18
Pseudoporphyria
(1992): Breathnach SM+, *Adverse Drug Reactions and the Skin*
Blackwell, Oxford (passim)
(1987): Taylor BJ+, *N Z Med J* 100, 322
Sialorrhea (<1%)
Stomatitis (<1%)
Tinnitus
Xerostomia (<1%)
(2001): Passali D+, *Clin Ther* 23(9), 1508

KETOROLAC

Trade names: Acular (Allergan); Toradol (Roche)
Other common trade names: *Dolac; Kelac; Ketonic; Nodine; Topadol; Torolac; Torvin*
Indications: Pain
Category: Nonsteroidal anti-inflammatory (NSAID)
Half-life: 2–8 hours
Clinically important, potentially hazardous interactions with: aspirin, methotrexate, probenecid, salicylates

Reactions

Skin

Allergic reactions (sic)
(2000): Reinhart DI, *Drug Saf* 22, 487
Angioedema
(1994): Shapiro N, *J Oral Maxillofac Surg* 52, 626
Dermatitis (sic) (3–9%)
Diaphoresis (1–10%)
(1990): Buckley MMT+, *Drugs* 39, 86
Edema (3–9%)
Exanthems (3–9%)

(1990): Buckley MMT+, *Drugs* 39, 86
Excoriations
(1994): Shelley WB+, *Cutis* 53, 235 (observation)
Exfoliative dermatitis (<1%)
Flushing (<1%)
Pruritus (3–9%)
Purpura (>1%)
(1994): Shelley WB+, *Cutis* 54, 149 (palpable) (observation)
Rash (sic) (>1%)
Side effects (sic) (0.7%)
(1990): Buckley MMT+, *Drugs* 39, 86
Stevens–Johnson syndrome (<1%)
Stinging (from topical)
(2000): Shiuey Y+, *Ophthalmology* 107, 1512
Toxic epidermal necrolysis (<1%)
Urticaria
(1990): Buckley MMT+, *Drugs* 39, 86

Other

Anaphylactoid reactions (<1%)
Aphthous stomatitis (<1%)
(1990): Buckley MMT+, *Drugs* 39, 86
Dysgeusia
Headache
Hypersensitivity
(2000): Reinhart DI, *Drug Saf* 22, 487
Injection-site pain (1–10%)
Myalgia
Paresthesias
Stomatitis (>1%)
Tinnitus
Tongue edema (<1%)
Xerostomia
(1990): Buckley MMT+, *Drugs* 39, 86

KETOTIFEN

Trade name: Zaditor (Novartis)
Indications: Allergic conjunctivitis
Category: Ophthalmic antihistamine H$_1$-blocker
Half-life: 22 hours

Reactions

Skin

Allergic reactions (sic) (1–10%)
Burning (1–10%)
(2003): Ganz M+, *Adv Ther* 20(2), 79
Photosensitivity
Pityriasis rosea
(1985): Wolf R+, *Dermatologica* 171, 355
Pruritus (1–10%)
(2003): Sowunmi A, *Ann Trop Med Parasitol* 97(2), 103
Rash (sic) (1–10%)
Stinging (1–10%)

Other

Headache
(2003): Ganz M+, *Adv Ther* 20(2), 79
Xerophthalmia (1–10%)

L-CARNITINE

Trade names: Aplegin; L-Carnipure
Other common trade names: B(t)Factor; Carnitine; Carnitor; Levocarnitine; Vitacarn; Vitamin B(t)
Other Trade names: Acetyl-L-carnitine, propionyl-L-carnitine
Indications: Improves lipid metabolism, red blood cell count, and antioxidant status, chronic fatigue syndrome, dementia, angina, post-MI cardioprotection, congestive heart failure, valproate toxicity, anorexia
Category: Dietary supplement

Note: Mixed D, L-carnitine has been associated with myasthenic syndrome.

LABETALOL

Trade names: Normodyne (Schering); Normozide; Trandate (Prometheus)
Other common trade names: Abetol; Amipress; Hybloc; Ipolab; Labrocol; Presolol; Salmagne
Indications: Hypertension
Category: Antihypertensive; Beta-adrenoceptor blocker
Half-life: 3–8 hours

Normozide is labetalol and hydrochlorothiazide

Note: Cutaneous side effects of beta-receptor blockaders are clinically polymorphous. They apparently appear after several months of continuous therapy. Atypical psoriasiform, lichen planus-like, and eczematous chronic rashes are mainly observed. (1983): Hödl St, *Z Hautkr* (German) 1:58, 17

Reactions

Skin

Angioedema
  (1986): Ferree CE, *Ann Intern Med* 104, 729
Dermatitis
  (1990): Bause GS+, *Contact Dermatitis* 23, 51
Diaphoresis (<1%)
Eczema (sic)
Edema (<2%)
Exanthems
  (1989): Goa KL+, *Drugs* 37, 583
  (1984): Prichard BNC, *Drugs* 28 (Suppl 2), 51 (1–5%)
  (1978): Branford WA+, *Practitioner* 221, 765
  (1978): Finlay AY+, *BMJ* 1, 987
Exfoliative dermatitis
Facial edema
Flushing
  (1978): Harris C, *Curr Med Res Opin* 5, 618 (19%)
Lichen planus (bullous)
  (1978): Gange RW+, *BMJ* 1, 816
Lichenoid eruption
  (1982): Bertani E+, *G Ital Dermatol Venereol* (Italian) 117, 229
  (1980): Staughton R+, *Lancet* 2, 581
  (1978): Branford WA+, *Practitioner* 221, 765
  (1978): Finlay AY+, *BMJ* 1, 987
  (1978): Savage RL+, *BMJ* 1, 987
Lupus erythematosus
  (1984): Prichard BNC, *Drugs* 28 (Suppl 2), 51
  (1981): Brown RC+, *Postgrad Med J* 57, 189
  (1979): Griffiths ID+, *BMJ* 2, 496
Peripheral edema

Pigmentation (slate-gray)
  (1978): Branford WA+, *Practitioner* 221, 765
Pityriasis rubra pilaris
  (1978): Branford WA+, *Practitioner* 221, 765
  (1978): Finlay AY+, *BMJ* 1, 987
Pruritus (1–10%)
  (1984): Prichard BNC, *Drugs* 28 (Suppl 2), 51 (1–5%)
  (1978): Finlay AY+, *BMJ* 1, 987
  (1978): Harris C, *Curr Med Res Opin* 5, 618 (7.5%)
Psoriasis (exacerbation)
  (1987): Savola J+, *BMJ* 295, 637 (induction)
  (1986): Czernielewski J+, *Lancet* 1, 808
  (1984): Arntzen N+, *Acta Derm Venereol* (Stockh) 64, 346
Purpura
  (1978): Harris C, *Curr Med Res Opin* 5, 618
Rash (sic) (<1%)
Raynaud's phenomenon (<1%)
Side effects (sic) (5.5%)
  (1982): Waal-Manning HJ+, *Br J Clin Pharmacol* 13 (Suppl 1), 65S
  (1978): No Author, *BMJ* 1, 987
Urticaria
  (1986): Ferree CE, *Ann Intern Med* 104, 729
Xerosis

Hair

Hair – alopecia (reversible)
  (1978): Finlay AY+, *BMJ* 1, 987

Other

Anaphylactoid reactions
  (1990): Bause GS+, *Contact Dermatitis* 23, 51
  (1986): Ferree CE, *Ann Intern Med* 104, 729
Dysgeusia (1–10%)
  (2000): Zervakis J+, *Physiol Behav* 68, 405
Headache
Hyperesthesia (1%)
Hypersensitivity
Myopathy
  (1989): Willis J+, *Ann Neurology* 26, 456
  (1981): Teicher A+, *BMJ* 282, 1824
  (1977): Bolli P+, *N Z Med J* 86, 557
  (1976): Andersson O+, *Br J Clin Pharmacol* 3, 757
Paresthesias (7%)
  (1984): Prichard BNC, *Drugs* 28 (Suppl 2), 51 (scalp) (6%)
  (1977): Bailey RR, *Lancet* 2, 720 (tingling of scalp)
Peyronie's disease
  (1979): Kristensen BO, *Acta Med Scand* 206, 511
Priapism
Scalp tingling
  (1979): Coulter DM, *N Z Med J* 90, 397
  (1977): Bailey RR, *Lancet* 2, 720
  (1977): Hua AS+, *Lancet* 2, 295
Xerostomia

LAMIVUDINE

Synonym: 3TC
Trade names: Combivir (GSK); Epivir (GSK); Trizivir (GSK)
Indications: HIV progression
Category: Antiretroviral; Nucleoside reverse transcriptase inhibitor (NRTI)
Half-life: 5–7 hours

Combivir is lamivudine and zidovudine

Reactions

Skin
Angioedema
  (1996): Kainer MA+, *Lancet* 348, 1519
Chills (1–10%)
Dermatitis
  (2000): Smith KJ+, *Cutis* 65, 227
Exanthems
Pruritus
  (2000): Smith KJ+, *Cutis* 65, 227
Rash (sic) (9%)
Urticaria
  (1996): Kainer MA+, *Lancet* 348, 1519

Hair
Hair – alopecia
  (1994): Fong IW, *Lancet* 344, 1702

Nails
Nails – ingrown
  (2001): James CW+, *Ann Pharmacother* 35(7), 881 (with ritonavir)
Nails – paronychia
  (1998): Zerboni R+, *Lancet* 351, 1256

Other
Anaphylactoid reactions
  (1996): Kainer MA+, *Lancet* 348(9040), 1519
Buffalo hump
  (2000): Carr A+, *AIDS* 14, F25
Gynecomastia
  (2001): Manfredi R+, *Ann Pharmacother* 35(4), 438 (with savudine) (3 cases)
Headache
Hypersensitivity
  (2002): Winston A+, *Int J STD AIDS* 13(3), 213
Myalgia (8%)
Paresthesias (>10%)
Rhabdomyolysis
  (1997): Mendila M+, *Dtsch Med Wochenschr* 122(33), 1003

LAMOTRIGINE

Synonyms: BW-430C; LTG
Trade name: Lamictal (GSK)
Indications: Epilepsy
Category: Anticonvulsant
Half-life: 24 hours

Reactions

Skin
Acne (1.3%)

Acute generalized exanthematous pustulosis (AGEP)
  (2001): Wensween CA+, *Ned Tijdschr Geneeskd* 145(31), 1525
Adverse effects (sic)
  (2002): Hurley SC, *Ann Pharmacother* 36(5), 860
Angioedema (1–10%)
  (2001): Hebert AA+, *J Clin Psychiatry* 62(suppl 14), 22 (~1%)
Bullous eruption
  (1997): Australian Adverse Drug Reactions Bulletin 16(1), February
Diaphoresis (<1%)
Ecchymoses (<1%)
Eczema (sic) (<1%)
Erythema (<1%)
  (2001): Hebert AA+, *J Clin Psychiatry* 62(suppl 14), 22 (~10%)
Erythema multiforme
  (1997): Australian Adverse Drug Reactions Bulletin 16(1), February
Exanthems (1–10%)
  (2001): Hebert AA+, *J Clin Psychiatry* 62(suppl 14), 22 (~10%)
  (1997): Australian Adverse Drug Reactions Bulletin 16(1), February
  (1997): Hyson C+, *Can J Neurol Sci* 24, 245
  (1996): Dooley J+, *Neurology* 46, 240 (7%)
  (1996): Li LM+, *Arq Neuropsiquiatr* 54, 47
  (1995): Brodie MJ, *Can J Neurol Sci* 23, S6 (<5%)
  (1995): Fitton A+, *Drugs* 50, 691
  (1995): Makin AJ+, *BMJ* 311, 292
  (1995): Tavernor SJ+, *Seizure* 4, 67
  (1994): Tavernor SJ+, *Epilepsia* 35, 72
Facial edema (<1%)
Fixed eruption
  (2001): Hsiao C-J+, *Br J Dermatol* 144, 1289
Flu-like syndrome (sic) (7%)
Flushing (<1%)
Hot flashes (1–10%)
Lupus erythematosus
  (1997): Mackay FJ+, *Epilepsia* 38, 881
Petechiae (<1%)
Photosensitivity
  (1999): Borowitz SM, *Pediatric Pharmacotherapy* 5, 3
  (1999): Bozikas V+, *Am J Psychiatry* 156, 2015
Pruritus (3.1%)
  (2001): Hebert AA+, *J Clin Psychiatry* 62(suppl 14), 22 (~1%)
Rash (sic) (10%)
  (2003): Choi H+, *Expert Opin Pharmacother* 4(2), 243
  (2002): Anderson GD, *Epilepsia* 43(Suppl 3), 53 (10–20%)
  (2002): Hurley SC, *Ann Pharmacother* 36(5), 860
  (2002): Labiner DM, *J Clin Psychiatry* 63(11), 1010
  (2001): Eisenberg E+, *Neurology* 57, 505
  (2000): Besag FM+, *Seizure* 9, 282
  (2000): Husain AM+, *South Med J* 93, 335
  (2000): Jurynczyk J+, *Neurol Neurochir Pol* (Polish) 34, 43
  (2000): Messenheimer JA+, *Drug Saf* 22, 303
  (2000): Messenheimer JA+, *Epilepsia* 41, 488
  (2000): Parmeggiani L+, *J Child Neurol* 15, 15
  (1999): Faught E+, *Epilepsia* 40, 1135
  (1999): Gericke CA+, *Epileptic Disord* 1, 159
  (1999): Guberman AH+, *Epilepsia* 40, 985
  (1999): Matsuo F, *Epilepsia* 40, S30
  (1998): Buzan RD+, *J Clin Psychiatry* 59, 87 (re-challenged)
  (1998): Messenheimer JA, *Can J Neurol Sci* 25, S14
  (1997): Mackay FJ+, *Epilepsia* 38, 881
Stevens–Johnson syndrome (1–10%)
  (2001): Hebert AA+, *J Clin Psychiatry* 62(suppl 14), 22 (~10%)
  (2000): Popescu C, Bucharest, Romania (from Internet) (observation)
  (2000): Yalcin B+, *J Am Acad Dermatol* 43, 898 (with valproic acid)

(1999): Bocquet H+, *Ann Dermatol Venereol* (French) 126, 46
(1999): Borowitz SM, *Pediatric Pharmacotherapy* 5, 3
(1999): Guberman AH+, *Epilepsia* 40, 985
(1999): Rzany B+, *Lancet* 353, 2190
(1998): *Drugs and Therapy Perspectives* 11, 11
(1998): Schlienger RG+, *Epilepsia* 39, S22
(1998): Zachariae CO+, *Ugeskr Laeger* (Danish) 160, 6656
(1997): Australian Adverse Drug Reactions Bulletin 16(1), February
(1997): Mackay FJ+, *Epilepsia* 38, 881
(1997): Sachs B+, *Dermatology* 195, 60
(1996): Dooley J+, *Neurology* 46, 240 (7%)
(1995): Campistol J+, *Rev Neurol* (Spanish) 23, 1236
(1995): Duval X+, *Lancet* 345, 1301
Toxic epidermal necrolysis
(2002): Wirtzer A, Sherman Oaks, CA (from Internet) (observation)
(2001): Hebert AA+, *J Clin Psychiatry* 62(suppl 14), 22 (~1%)
(2001): Wensween CA+, *Ned Tijdschr Geneeskd* 145(31), 1525
(2000): Bhushan M+, *Clin Exp Dermatol* 25, 349
(2000): Fernandez-Calvo C+, *Rev Neurol* 31(12), 1162
(1999): Bocquet H+, *Ann Dermatol Venereol* (French) 126, 46
(1999): Borowitz SM, *Pediatric Pharmacotherapy* 5, 3
(1999): *Actas Dermosifiliogr* (Spanish) 90, 612
(1999): Rzany B+, *Lancet* 353, 2190
(1998): *Drugs and Therapy Perspectives* 11, 11
(1998): Page RL+, *Pharmacotherapy* 18, 392 (fatal)
(1998): Schlienger RG+, *Epilepsia* 39, S22
(1998): Zachariae CO+, *Ugeskr Laeger* (Danish) 160, 6656
(1997): Australian Adverse Drug Reactions Bulletin 16(1), February
(1997): Chaffin JJ+, *Ann Pharmacother* 31, 720 (suspected)
(1997): Fogh K+, *Seizure* 6, 63
(1997): Vukelic D+, *Dermatology* 195, 307
(1996): Sachs B+, *Lancet* 348, 1597
(1996): Sullivan JR+, *Australas J Dermatol* 37, 208
(1996): Wadelius M+, *Lancet* 348, 1041
(1995): Duval X+, *Lancet* 345, 1301
(1995): Sterker M+, *Int J Clin Pharmacol Ther* 33, 595
Urticaria (<1%)
Xerosis (<1%)

Hair

Hair – alopecia (1.3%)
Hair – hirsutism (<1%)

Other

Anaphylactoid reactions
(1999): Borowitz SM, *Pediatric Pharmacotherapy* 5, 3
Anticonvulsant hypersensitivity syndrome
(2003): Bin-Nakhi HA+, *Med Princ Pract* 12(3), 197
(2002): Metin A+, *World Congress Dermatol* Poster, 0116
Death
Dysgeusia (<1%)
(2001): Avoni P+, *Neurology* 57(8), 1521 (3 cases)
Foetor ex ore (halitosis) (<1%)
Gingival hyperplasia (<1%)
Gingivitis (<1%)
Headache
Hyperesthesia (<1%)
Hypersensitivity (1–10%)
(2001): Hebert AA+, *J Clin Psychiatry* 62(suppl 14), 22
(2001): Lalanza J+, *Aten Primaria* 28(3), 213
(2000): Schaub N+, *Allergy* 55, 191
(1999): Borowitz SM, *Pediatric Pharmacotherapy* 5, 3
(1999): Brown TS+, *Pediatr Dermatology* 16, 46
(1999): Guberman AH+, *Epilepsia* 40, 985
(1999): Knowles SR+, *Drug Safety* 21, 489
(1999): Mylonakis E+, *Ann Pharmacol* 33, 557
(1998): Chapman MS+, *Br J Dermatol* 138, 710

(1998): Iannetti P+, *Epilepsia* 39, 502
(1998): Tugendhaft P+, *J Am Acad Dermatol* 38, 785 (phenytoin-like)
(1997): Jones D+, *J Am Acad Dermatol* 36, 1016 (phenytoin-like)
Myalgia (>1%)
Oral ulceration (<1%)
Paresthesias (>1%)
Porphyria
(1996): Gregersen H+, *Ugeskr Laeger* (Danish) 158, 4091
Pseudolymphoma
(1998): Pathak P+, *Neurology* 50, 1509
Sialorrhea (<1%)
Stomatitis (<1%)
Tic disorder
(2000): Sotero de Menezes MA+, *Epilepsia* 41, 862
Tremor
(2002): Robillard M+, *Can J Psychiatry* 47(8), 767
(2000): Messenheimer JA+, *Drug Saf* 22, 303
Vaginal candidiasis (<1%)
Vaginitis (4.1%)
Xerostomia (1%)

LANSOPRAZOLE

Trade name: Prevacid (TAP)
Indications: Active duodenal ulcer
Category: Gastric acid secretion (proton pump) inhibitor
Half-life: 2 hours
Clinically important, potentially hazardous interactions with: sucralfate

Reactions

Skin

Acne (<1%)
Acute generalized exanthematous pustulosis (AGEP)
(1997): Dewerdt S+, *Acta Derm Venereol* (Stockh) 77, 250
Candidiasis (<1%)
Dermatitis
(2001): Vilaplana J+, *Contact Dermatitis* 44, 47 (with omeprazole)
Diaphoresis
(2000): Natsch S+, *Ann Pharmacother* 34, 474
Edema (<1%)
Erythroderma
(1999): Cockayne SE+, *Br J Dermatol* 141, 173
Exanthems
(1996): Blumenthal HL, Beachwood, OH (personal case) (observation)
(1996): Litt JZ, Beachwood, OH (personal case) (observation)
Facial edema
(2000): Natsch S+, *Ann Pharmacother* 34, 474
Lichenoid eruption
(2000): Bong JL+, *BMJ* 320, 283
Peripheral edema
(2001): Brunner G+, *Dig Dis Sci* 46(5), 993
Pruritus (3–10%)
(2000): Natsch S+, *Ann Pharmacother* 34, 474
Rash (sic) (3–10%)
Urticaria (<1%)
(2000): Gerson LB+, *Aliment Pharmacol* 14, 397 (1%)
(2000): Natsch S+, *Ann Pharmacother* 34, 474

Hair

Hair – alopecia (<1%)
(2000): Litt JZ, Beachwood, OH (personal case) (observation)

Other

Anaphylactoid reactions
(2000): Natsch S+, *Ann Pharmacother* 34, 474
Black tongue
(1997): Greco S+, *Ann Pharmacother* 31, 1548
Dysgeusia (<1%)
Foetor ex ore (halitosis) (<1%)
Glossitis
(1997): Greco S+, *Ann Pharmacother* 31, 1548
Gynecomastia (<1%)
(2000): Comas A+, *Med Clin (Barc)* (Spanish) 114, 397
Headache
Hypersensitivity
(1999): Baudot S, *Therapie* (French) 54, 491
Mastodynia (<1%)
Myalgia (<1%)
(1998): Smith JD+, *Ann Pharmacother* 32, 196 (with eosinophilia)
Paresthesias (<1%)
Stomatitis (<1%)
(1997): Greco S+, *Ann Pharmacother* 31, 1548
Xerostomia (<1%)

LATANOPROST

Trade name: Xalatan (Pharmacia)
Indications: Glaucoma
Category: Antiglaucoma; Prostaglandin ophthalmic
Half-life: 17 minutes

Reactions

Skin

Allergic reactions (sic) (1.1%)
Blepharitis (0.4%)
Ecchymoses (0.2%)
Eczema (sic) (0.7%)
Eyelid burning (1.1%)
Eyelid edema (1–4%)
(2001): Stewart WC+, *Am J Ophthalmol* 131(5), 631
Eyelid erythema (1–4%)
Eyelid pigmentation
(2003): Herndon LW+, *Am J Ophthalmol* 135(5), 713
(2001): Wand M+, *Arch Ophthalmol* 119(4), 614
(2000): Kook MS+, *Am J Ophthalmol* 129, 804
Eyelid pruritus (1.7%)
Eyelid stinging (0.4%)
Facial rash
(1997): Rowe JA+, *Am J Ophthalmol* 124, 683
Herpes simplex (ocular)
(2001): Morales J+, *Am J Ophthalmol* 132(1), 114 (2 cases)
Local irritation
(1999): Hejkal TW+, *Semin Ophthalmol* 14, 114
Ocular erythema
Pruritus (0.2%)
(1997): Crowe MA, Puyallup, WA (from Internet) (observation)
Rash (sic) (1–10%)

Hair

Eyelashes – change in color
(2002): Johnstone MA+, *Surv Ophthalmol* 47(Suppl 1), S185
Eyelashes – growth
(2003): Noecker RS+, *Am J Ophthalmol* 135(1), 55
(2002): Eisenberg DL+, *Surv Ophthalmol* 47(Suppl 1), S105
(2002): Johnstone MA+, *Surv Ophthalmol* 47(Suppl 1), S185
Eyelashes – hyperpigmentation

(1999): Hejkal TW+, *Semin Ophthalmol* 14, 114
(1998): Reynolds A+, *Eye* 12, 741
(1997): Johnstone MA, *Am J Ophthalmol* 124, 544
(1997): Wand M, *Arch Ophthalmol* 115, 1206
Eyelashes – lengthening
(2003): Herndon LW+, *Am J Ophthalmol* 135(5), 713
(2002): Johnstone MA+, *Surv Ophthalmol* 47(Suppl 1), S185
(2002): Sugimoto M+, *Can J Ophthalmol* 37(6), 342
Hair – hypertrichosis
(2001): Demitsu T+, *J Am Acad Dermatol* 44, 721 (eyelashes) (77%)
(2001): Strober BE+, *Cutis* 67, 109 (eyelashes)
(1997): Johnstone MA, *Am J Ophthalmol* 124, 544

Other

Conjuctival hyperemia
(2001): DuBiner H+, *Surv Opthalmol* 45(Suppl 4), S353–60
(2001): Gandolfi S+, *Adv Ther* 18(3), 110
Eyelid pain (0.4%)
Gynecomastia (0.2%)
Myalgia (1–10%)
Ocular irritation
Ocular pigmentation
(2002): Novack GD+, *J Am Geriatr Soc* 50(5), 956
(2002): Stjernschantz JW+, *Surv Ophthalmol* 47(Suppl 1), S162
(2001): Aung T+, *Am J Ophthalmol* 131(5), 636
(2001): Netland PA+, *Am J Ophthalmol* 132(4), 472 (5.2%)
(2001): Stewart WC+, *Am J Ophthalmol* 131(5), 631
(2000): Alm A+, *Acta Ophthalmol Scand* 78, 71
(2000): Camras CB+, *J Glaucoma* 9, 95
(1999): Hejkal TW+, *Semin Ophthalmol* 14, 114
(1997): Bito LAZ, *Surv Ophthalmol* 41(Suppl 2), S1
(1997): Wistrand JP+, *Surv Ophthalmol* 41(Suppl 2), S129

LAVENDER

Scientific names: *Lavandula angustifolia; Lavandula dentata; Lavandula spica; Lavandula vera*
Family: Lamiaceae
Trade and other common names: Alhucema; English Lavender; French Lavender; Spanish Lavender; Spike Lavender
Category: Sedative
Purported indications and other uses: Restlessness, insomnia, loss of appetite, flatulence, colic, giddiness, nervous headache, migraine, toothache, sprains, neuralgia, rheumatism, acne, pimples, nausea, vomiting. Flavoring, fragrance, insect repellent
Half-life: N/A

Reactions

Skin

Dermatitis
(2002): Schempp CM+, *Hautarzt* 53(2), 93
(1999): Coulson IH+, *Contact Dermatitis* 41(2), 111

LEFLUNOMIDE

Trade name: Arava (Aventis)
Indications: Rheumatoid arthritis
Category: Antimetabolite; Immunosuppressant
Half-life: 14–15 days

Reactions

Skin

Acne (1–10%)
Allergic reactions (sic) (2%)
  (2000): Smolen JS+, *Rheumatology* (Oxford) 39 (Suppl 1), 48
  (1999): Goldenberg MM, *Clin Ther* 21, 1837
  (1997): Silva Junior HT+, *Am J Med Sci* 313, 289
  (1995): Mladenovic V+, *Arthritis Rheum* 38, 1595
Bullous eruption
  (2000): Lepine G, Rock Hill, SC, (from Internet) (observation)
    (occurred 6 months after starting drug)
Dermatitis (sic) (1–10%)
Diaphoresis (1–10%)
Eczema (sic) (2%)
Herpes (sic) (1–10%)
Infections (sic) (4%)
  (2001): Cohen S+, *Arthritis Rheum* 44(9), 1984
Nodules (sic) (1–10%)
Peripheral edema (1–10%)
Pigmentation (1–10%)
Pruritus (4%)
Purpura (1–10%)
Rash (sic) (10%)
  (2002): Hirohata S, *Nippon Rinsho* 60(12), 2357
  (2002): Sanders S+, *Am J Med Sci* 323(4), 190
  (2001): Cohen S+, *Arthritis Rheum* 44(9), 1984
  (2000): Emery P+, *Rheumatology* (Oxford) 39, 655
  (2000): Nousari HC+, *Arch Dermatol* 136, 1204
  (1999): Goldenberg MM, *Clin Ther* 21, 1837
  (1999): Smolen JS+, *Lancet* 353, 259
  (1997): Silva Junior HT+, *Am J Med Sci* 313, 289
  (1995): Mladenovic V+, *Arthritis Rheum* 38, 1595
Squamous cell carcinoma
  (2002): Shelly J (from Internet) (observation)
Stevens–Johnson syndrome
Toxic epidermal necrolysis
Ulcerations (1–10%)
Urticaria (<1%)
Vasculitis (1–10%)
  (2003): Chan AT+, *Rheumatology* (Oxford) 42(3), 492
Xerosis (2%)

Hair

Hair – alopecia (10%)
  (2002): Gottenberg JE+, *J Rheumatol* 29(8), 1806
  (2002): Hirohata S, *Nippon Rinsho* 60(12), 2357
  (2002): Sanders S+, *Am J Med Sci* 323(4), 190
  (2001): Cohen S+, *Arthritis Rheum* 44(9), 1984
  (2000): Emery P+, *Rheumatology* (Oxford) 39, 655
  (2000): Nousari HC+, *Arch Dermatol* 136, 1204
  (2000): Smolen JS+, *Rheumatology* (Oxford) 39 (Suppl 1), 48
  (1999): Goldenberg MM, *Clin Ther* 21, 1837
  (1999): Smolen JS+, *Lancet* 353, 259 (8%)
  (1997): Silva Junior HT+, *Am J Med Sci* 313, 289
  (1995): Mladenovic V+, *Arthritis Rheum* 38, 1595
Hair – alopecia areata
  (2002): Gottenberg JE+, *J Rheumatol* 29(8), 1806
Hair – pigmentation (1–10%)

Nails

Nails – changes (sic) (1–10%)

Other

Anaphylactoid reactions (<1%)
Death
  (2002): Legras A+, *Am J Med* 113(4), 352 (also taking
    itraconazole)
Dysgeusia (1–10%)
Gingivitis (1–10%)
Headache
Myalgia (1–10%)
Oral candidiasis (3%)
Oral ulceration (3%)
Paresthesias (2%)
Stomatitis (3%)
Tendon rupture (1–10%)
Tooth disorder (sic) (1–10%)
Vaginal candidiasis (1–10%)
Xerostomia (1–10%)

LETROZOLE

Trade name: Femara (Novartis)
Indications: Breast cancer
Category: Antineoplastic; Nonsteroidal aromatase inhibitor
Half-life: ~2 days

Reactions

Skin

Diaphoresis (<5%)
Exanthems (5%)
Hot flashes (6%)
Pruritus (2%)
Psoriasis (5%)
Rash (sic) (1–10%)
Vesicular eruptions (5%)

Hair

Hair – alopecia (<5%)

Other

Headache

LEUCOVORIN

Synonyms: citrovorum factor; folinic acid
Trade name: Leucovorin
Other common trade names: *Antrex; Citrec; Lederfolin;
Refolinin; Rescufolin; Rescuvolin*
Indications: Overdose of methotrexate
Category: Antidote; Methotrexate toxicity prophylactic agent
Half-life: 15 minutes

Reactions

Skin

Erythema (<1%)
Pruritus (<1%)
Rash (sic) (<1%)
Urticaria (<1%)

Hair

Hair – alopecia
  (2001): Madnani N, Mumbai, India (from Internet) (observation)

Other

Anaphylactoid reactions (<1%)
Hypersensitivity
Oral ulceration
  (2002): Xu D+, *Zhonghua Zhong Liu Za Zhi* 24(1), 93 (with
    fluorouracil)
Phlebitis
  (2002): Xu D+, *Zhonghua Zhong Liu Za Zhi* 24(1), 93 (with
    fluorouracil)

LEUPROLIDE

Synonym: leuprorelin acetate
Trade names: Eligard (Sanofi-Synthelabo); Lupron (TAP); Viadur
(Bayer)
Other common trade names: *Carcinil; Enantone; Lucrin;*
Procren Depot; Procrin; Tapros
Indications: Prostate carcinoma, endometriosis
Category: Gonadotropin-releasing hormone
Half-life: 3–4 hours

Reactions

Skin

Acne
Dermatitis (sic) (5%)
Diaphoresis
Ecchymoses (<5%)
Edema (1–10%)
Exanthems
Flushing
  (1989): Crawford ED+, *N Engl J Med* 321, 419 (61%)
Hot flashes
  (2002): Chu FM+, *J Urol* 168(3), 1199 (12–57%)
  (2002): Perez-Marreno R+, *Clin Ther* 24(11), 1902 (56.7%)
  (1993): Bressler LR+, *Ann Pharmacother* 27, 182
Lupus erythematosus
  (1994): Fritzler MJ, *Lupus* 3, 455
Nodules
  (2003): Saxby M, *BJU Int* 91(1), 125
Peripheral edema (12%)
  (1989): Crawford ED+, *N Engl J Med* 321, 419 (4%)
Photosensitivity
Pigmentation (<5%)
Pruritus (<5%)
Purpura (<1%)
Rash (sic) (1–10%)
Stickiness
  (2001): Sander HM, Austin, TX (from Internet) (observation)
Urticaria
Xerosis (<5%)

Hair

Hair – alopecia (<5%)
Hair – growth (sic) (<1%)

Other

Depression
  (2003): Freeman MP+, *J Clin Psychiatry* 64(3), 341
Dysgeusia (<5%)
Gynecomastia (7%)

Headache
Injection-site granuloma
  (2003): Saxby M, *BJU Int* 91(1), 125
  (2002): Whitaker IS+, *BJU Int* 90(3), 350
Injection-site inflammation
  (1989): Crawford ED+, *N Engl J Med* 321, 419 (2.1%)
Injection-site pruritus
  (1989): Crawford ED+, *N Engl J Med* 321, 419 (2.1%)
Injection-site reactions
  (2001): Fluker M+, *Fertil Steril* 75(1), 38 (24.4%)
Mastodynia (7%)
Myalgia (3%)
Myopathy
  (2002): Van Gerpen JA+, *J Am Geriatr Soc* 50(10), 1746
Paresthesias (<5%)
Thrombophlebitis (2%)
Vaginitis

LEVALBUTEROL

Synonym: R-albuterol
Trade name: Xopenex (Sepracor)
Indications: Bronchospasm
Category: Beta-2-agonist
Half-life: 3.3–4.0 hours

Reactions

Skin

Chills (<2%)
Diaphoresis (<2%)
Flu-like syndrome (1–4%)
Ocular pruritus (<2%)
Viral infections (7–12%)

Other

Cough (1–4%)
Headache
Hyperesthesia (<2%)
Hypersensitivity
Leg cramps (~3%)
Myalgia (<2%)
Pain (1–3%)
Paresthesias (<2%)
Tremor (~7%)

LEVAMISOLE

Trade name: Ergamisol (Janssen)
Other common trade names: *Ascaridil; Decaris; Detrax 40;*
Ketrax; Solaskil; Termizole
Indications: Susceptible helmintic organism infections, colorectal
carcinoma
Category: Antineoplastic; Immunomodulator
Half-life: 2–6 hours
**Clinically important, potentially hazardous interactions
with: alcohol**, aldesleukin

Reactions

Skin

Angioedema (<1%)

(1978): Multiple Authors, *Lancet* 2, 1007
Dermatitis (sic) (1–10%)
Edema (1–10%)
Erythema annulare
  (1989): Lioté F+, *Rev Rhum Mal Ostéoartic* (French) 56, 11
Erythema multiforme
  (1979): Hodinka L+, *Int Arch Allergy Appl Immunol* 58, 362
Exanthems
  (1989): Lioté F+, *Rev Rhum Mal Ostéoartic* (French) 56, 11
  (1980): Miller B+, *Arthritis Rheum* 23, 172 (>10%)
  (1978): Multiple Authors, *J Rheumatol* 5 (Suppl 4), 5
  (1978): Pinals RS, *J Rheumatol* 5 (Suppl 4), 71 (>5%)
  (1978): Secher L+, *Acta Derm Venereol* 58, 372
  (1978): Symoens J+, *Cancer Treat Rep* 62, 1721 (2.6%)
  (1976): Rosenthal M+, *N Engl J Med* 295, 1204
Exfoliative dermatitis
Fixed eruption
  (1994): Clavère P+, *Ann Dermatol Venereol* (French) 121, 238
    (pigmented)
  (1991): Thankappen TP+, *Int J Dermatol* 30, 867 (0.88%)
Hemorrhage (sic)
  (1982): Papageorgiou P+, *J Clin Lab Immunol* 8, 121
Infections (sic) (1–10%)
Lichen planus
  (1980): Kirby JD+, *J R Soc Med* 73, 208 (passim)
Lichenoid eruption
  (1980): Kirby JD+, *J R Soc Med* 73, 208
  (1978): Multiple Authors, *Lancet* 2, 1007
  (1978): Pinals RS, *J Rheumatol* 5 (Suppl 4), 71
Necrosis
  (2002): Kumar B+, *Clin Exp Dermatol* 27(1), 8
  (2002): Powell J+, *Clin Exp Dermatol* 27(1), 32
Pemphigus
  (1980): Mashkilleison NA, *Vestn Dermatol Venerol* (Russian)
    October 46
Pruritus (<1%)
  (1992): Breathnach SM+, *Adverse Drug Reactions and the Skin*
    Blackwell, Oxford, 178 (passim)
  (1989): Lioté F+, *Rev Rhum Mal Ostéoartic* (French) 56, 11
  (1980): Kirby JD+, *J R Soc Med* 73, 208
  (1978): Pinals RS, *J Rheumatol* 5 (Suppl 4), 71
  (1978): Secher L+, *Acta Derm Venereol* 58, 372
Psoriasis
  (1980): Kirby JD+, *J R Soc Med* 73, 208 (passim)
Purpura
  (1999): Rongioletti F+, *Br J Dermatol* 140(5), 948
Rash (sic)
  (1980): Husain Z+, *J Rheumatol* 7, 825
  (1980): Kinsella PL+, *J Rheumatol* 7, 288
  (1980): Miller B+, *Arthritis Rheum* 23, 172
  (1979): Scherak O+, *Wien Klin Wochenschr* (German) 91, 758
  (1978): Pinals RS, *J Rheumatol* 5 (Suppl 4), 71
  (1978): Secher L+, *Acta Derm Venereol* 58, 372
  (1978): Symoens J+, *Cancer Treat Rep* 62, 1721
  (1977): Parkinson DR+, *Lancet* 2, 1129
Side effects (sic)
  (1978): Multiple Authors, *Lancet* 2, 1007 (20%)
Stevens–Johnson syndrome (<1%)
Urticaria (<1%)
  (1992): Breathnach SM+, *Adverse Drug Reactions and the Skin*
    Blackwell, Oxford, 178 (passim)
  (1989): Lioté F+, *Rev Rhum Mal Ostéoartic* (French) 56, 11
  (1979): Hodinka L+, *Int Arch Allergy Appl Immunol* 58, 362
  (1978): Pinals RS, *J Rheumatol* 5 (Suppl 4), 71
Vasculitis
  (1999): Rongioletti F+, *Br J Dermatol* 140(5), 948
  (1989): Lioté F+, *Rev Rhum Mal Ostéoartic* (French) 56, 11
  (1983): Ferlazzo B+, *Boll Ist Sieroter Milan* (Italian) 62, 107

(1980): Huskisson EC, *Agents Actions* Suppl 7, 55
(1978): MacFarlane DG+, *BMJ* 1, 407
(1978): Multiple Authors, *Lancet* 2, 1007
(1978): Scheinberg MA+, *BMJ* 1, 408
Xerosis
  (1980): Kirby JD+, *J R Soc Med* 73, 208

Hair

Hair – alopecia (1–10%)
  (1980): Kirby JD+, *J R Soc Med* 73, 208

Other

Anaphylactoid reactions
Dysgeusia (1–10%) (metallic taste)
  (1977): Runge LA+, *Arthritis Rheum* 20, 1445
  (1977): Veys EM+Willoughby DA+, *Perspectives in Inflammation*
    Lancaster, England, MTP Press, W3 FU966 v3
Myalgia (1–10%)
Oral mucosal lesions
  (1989): Lioté F+, *Rev Rhum Mal Ostéoartic* (French) 56, 11
    (2.1%)
  (1980): Miller B+, *Arthritis Rheum* 23, 172 (>10%)
  (1978): Multiple Authors, *J Rheumatol* 5 (Suppl 4), 5 (2.3%)
  (1978): Multiple Authors, *Lancet* 2, 1007 (5.9%)
  (1978): Symoens J+, *Cancer Treat Rep* 62, 1721 (0.3%)
Oral ulceration
  (1978): Symoens J+, *Cancer Treat Rep* 62, 1721
Paresthesias (1–10%)
Parosmia (<1%)
Stomatitis (1–10%)
  (1980): Kinsella PL+, *J Rheumatol* 7, 288
  (1978): Multiple Authors, *Lancet* 2, 1007 (6%)

LEVETIRACETAM

Trade name: Keppra (UCB Pharma)
Indications: Partial onset seizures
Category: Anticonvulsant
Half-life: 7 hours

Reactions

Skin

Ecchymoses (<1%)
Flu-like syndrome (sic)
  (2000): Cereghino JJ+, *Neurology* 55, 236
Fungal infections (>1%)
Infections (sic) (13%)
  (2002): Boon P+, *Epilepsy Res* 48(1), 77
  (2002): Glauser TA+, *Epilepsia* 43(5), 518
  (2001): Nash EM+, *Am J Health Syst Pharm* 58(13), 1195
  (2000): Cereghino JJ+, *Neurology* 55, 236
Rash (sic) (>1%)

Other

Gingivitis (>1%)
Headache
Pain
  (2002): Boon P+, *Epilepsy Res* 48(1), 77
Paresthesias (2%)

LEVOBETAXOLOL

Trade name: Betaxon (Alcon)
Other common trade name: *L-betaxolol*
Indications: Chronic open-angle glaucoma, ocular hypertension
Category: Antiglaucoma; Beta-adrenoceptor blocker (ophthalmic)
Half-life: 20 hours

Reactions

Skin
Dermatitis (sic) (<2%)
Infections (sic) (<2%)
Psoriasis (<2%)
Rash (sic)
Xerosis

Hair
Hair – alopecia (<2%)

Other
Breast abscess (<2%)
Dysgeusia (<2%)
Ocular transient discomfort (sic) (11%)
Tendinitis (<2%)
Tinnitus (<2%)

LEVOBUNOLOL

Trade name: Betagan (Allergan)
Other common trade names: *Bunolgan; Gotensin; Vistagan; Vistagen*
Indications: Glaucoma, ocular hypertension
Category: Beta-adrenoceptor blocker (ophthalmic)
Half-life: N/A

Reactions

Skin
Burning eyes
Dermatitis
  (2001): Holdiness MR, *Am J Contact Dermat* 12(4), 217
  (1999): Erdmann S+, *Contact Dermatitis* 41, 44
  (1995): di Lernia V+, *Contact Dermatitis* 33, 57
  (1995): Koch P, *Contact Dermatitis* 33, 140
  (1995): Zucchelli V+, *Contact Dermatitis* 33, 66
  (1993): van der Meeren HL+, *Contact Dermatitis* 28, 41
  (1989): Schultheiss E, *Derm Beruf Umwelt* (German) 37, 185
Erythema
Lichen planus
  (1995): Beckman KA+, *Am J Ophthalmol* 120, 530
Pruritus (<1%)
Rash (sic) (<1%)
Stinging eyes
Urticaria

Hair
Hair – alopecia (1–10%)

Other
Headache
Hypersensitivity

*****Note:** Peak effect: 1–7 days

LEVOBUPIVACAINE

Trade name: Chirocaine (Purdue)
Indications: Regional anesthesia for surgery, postoperative pain management
Category: Local anesthetic
Half-life: 1.3 hours

Reactions

Skin
Angioedema
Chills
Diaphoresis (<1%)
Edema (<1%)
Erythema
Pigmentation (<1%)
Pruritus (3.7%)
Purpura (1.4%)
Rash (sic)
  (2003): Taylor R+, *Paediatr Anaesth* 13(2), 114
Shivering
  (2002): Cheng CR+, *Acta Anaesthesiol Sin* 40(1), 13
Urticaria

Other
Anaphylactoid reactions
Back pain (6%)
Cough (1%)
Hyperesthesia (3%)
Mastodynia (1%)
Pain (7–18%)
Paresthesias (2%)
Seizures
  (2003): Breslin DS+, *Reg Anesth Pain Med* 28(2), 144
  (2003): Crews JC+, *Anesth Analg* 96(4), 1188
  (2003): Cumming C+, *Anaesthesia* 58(6), 610
  (2003): Dhileepan S+, *Anaesthesia* 58(6), 611
  (2002): Pirotta D+, *Anaesthesia* 57(12), 1187
Tinnitus
Tremor (<1%)

LEVODOPA

Synonym: L-dopa
Trade names: Sinemet (Bristol-Myers Squibb)
Other common trade names: *Brocadopa; Dopaflex; Doparl; Eldopal; Levodopa-Woelm*
Indications: Parkinsonism
Category: Antidyskinetic; Antiparkinsonian
Half-life: 1–3 hours
Clinically important, potentially hazardous interactions with: kava, MAO inhibitors, phenelzine, pyridoxine, selegiline, tranylcypromine

Sinemet is carbidopa and levodopa

Reactions

Skin
Diaphoresis
  (1995): Sage JI+, *Ann Neurol* 37, 120
Exanthems
  (1976): Arndt KA+, *JAMA* 235, 918

(1970): Schwarz GA+, *Med Clin North Am* 54, 773
Flushing
Hot flashes
Hypomelanosis guttata
  (2001): Mocci A, Panama City, Panama (from Internet)
    (observation)
Leukoplakia
Lupus erythematosus
  (1985): Stratton MA, *Clin Pharm* 4, 657
  (1979): Massarotti G+, *BMJ* 2, 553
Melanoma
  (1997): Pfützner W+, *J Am Acad Dermatol* 37, 332
  (1996): Kleinhans M+, *Hautarzt* (German) 47, 432
  (1993): Weiner WJ+, *Neurology* 43, 674
  (1992): Haider SA+, *Br J Ophthalmol* 76, 246
  (1992): Sandyk R, *Int J Neurosci* 63, 137
  (1989): Kande'l EI, *Zh Nevropatol Psikhiatr* (Russian) 89, 126
  (1987): Morpurgo G+, *Eur J Cancer Clin Oncol* 23, 1213
  (1985): Kochar AS, *Am J Med* 79, 119
  (1985): Przybilla B+, *Acta Derm Venereol* (Stockh) 65, 556
  (1985): Rampen FHJ, *J Neurol Neurosurg Psychiatry* 48, 585
  (1984): Abramson DH+, *JAMA* 252, 1011
  (1984): Rosin MA+, *Cutis* 33, 572
  (1982): Van Rens GH+, *Ophthalmology* 89, 1464
  (1980): Bernstein JE+, *Arch Dermatol* 116, 1041
  (1980): Warner TF+, *J Cutan Pathol* 7, 50
  (1979): Botteri A+, *Lakartidningen* (Swedish) 76, 316
  (1979): Fermaglich J+, *JAMA* 241, 883
  (1978): Fermaglich J, *Neurology* 28, 404
  (1978): Sober AJ+, *JAMA* 240, 554
  (1977): Fermaglich J+, *J Neurology* 215, 221
  (1975): Pelfrene AF, *Nouv Presse Med* (French) 4, 1365
  (1974): Happle R, *Fortschr* (German) 92, 1065
  (1974): Liebermann AN+, *Neurology* 24, 340
  (1973): Robinson E+, *Arch Pathol* 95, 213
  (1972): Skibba JL+, *Arch Pathol* 93, 556
Neuroleptic malignant syndrome
  (2003): Serrano-Duenas M, *Parkinsonism Relat Disord* 9(3), 175
    (drug withdrawal)
Pemphigus
  (1986): Pisani M+, *G Ital Dermatol Venereol* (Italian) 121, 39
Purpura
  (1976): Wanamaker WM+, *JAMA* 235, 2217
Rash (sic)
  (1984): Goetz CG, *Clin Neuropharmacol* 7, 107
  (1983): Goetz CG, *N Engl J Med* 309, 1387
Urticaria
Vitiligo
  (1999): Sabate M+, *Ann Pharmacother* 33, 1228 (with tolcapone)

Hair

Hair – alopecia
  (1971): Marshall A+, *BMJ* 1, 407
Hair – repigmentation
  (1989): Reynolds NJ+, *Clin Exp Dermatol* 14, 317
  (1973): Grainger KM, *Lancet* 1, 97

Nails

Nails – growth
  (1984): Danial CR+, *J Am Acad Dermatol* 10, 250
  (1973): Miller E, *N Engl J Med* 288, 916

Other

Ageusia
Black cartilage
  (1986): Connolly CE+, *Lancet* 1, 690
Bruxism
Chromhidrosis (1–10%)
Dysgeusia

Dyskinesia
  (2003): Keijsers NL+, *Hum Mov Sci* 22(1), 67
  (2003): Keijsers NL+, *Mov Disord* 18(1), 70
  (2002): Arabia G+, *Neurol Sci* 23(Suppl 2), S53
  (2002): Lucetti C+, *Neurol Sci* 23(Suppl 2), S83
  (2002): Zegers de Beyl D, *Acta Neurol Belg* 102(4), 163
Glossopyrosis
Headache
Paresthesias
Phlebitis
Priapism
Sialorrhea
Xerostomia (1–10%)

LEVOFLOXACIN

Trade names: Levaquin (Ortho-McNeil); Quixin (Santen)
Indications: Various infections caused by susceptible organisms
Category: Fluoroquinolone antibiotic
Half-life: 6–8 hours

Reactions

Skin

Candidiasis (0.3%)
Diaphoresis (0.1%)
Edema (0.1%)
Erythema
  (1992): Kanzaki H+, *Jpn J Antibiot* (Japanese) 45, 576
Erythema multiforme
Erythema nodosum (<3%)
Exanthems
  (2000): Paily R, *J Dermatol* 27, 405
Exfoliative dermatitis
  (2001): Sienkiewicz G, Johnson City, NY (from Internet)
    (observation)
Photosensitivity (<0.1%)
  (2000): Boccumini LE+, *Ann Pharmacol* 34, 453
Phototoxicity
  (2001): Carbon C, *Therapie* 56(1), 35
Pruritus (1.6%)
Purpura (<0.5%)
Rash (sic) (1.7%)
Side effects
  (2002): Papastavros T+, *CMAJ* 167(2), 131 (with pyrazinamide)
    (14 cases)
Stevens–Johnson syndrome
Toxic epidermal necrolysis
Urticaria (<0.5%)
  (2001): Eisner J (from Internet) (personal reaction)
Vasculitis
  (2003): Welsch MJ, *J Drugs Dermatol* 2, 193
  (2002): Drayton G, Los Angeles, CA (from Internet)
    (observation)

Other

Anaphylactoid reactions
  (2001): *Drug & Ther Perspect* 17, 15
Death
  (2001): Spahr L+, *J Hepatol* 35(2), 308
Dysgeusia (0.2%)
Headache
Injection-site reactions (sic)
Myalgia (<0.5%)
  (2003): Litt JZ, Beachwood, OH (personal case) (observation)

(2002): Papastavros T+, *CMAJ* 167(2), 131 (with pyrazinamide)
(14 cases)
Paresthesias
Seizures
(2001): Kushner JM+, *Ann Pharmacother* 35(10), 1194
Tendinitis
(2003): Bernacer L+, *Med Clin* (Barc) 120(2), 78
(2003): Cebrian P+, *Foot Ankle Int* 24(2), 122
(2003): *Prescrire Int* 12(63), 20
(2003): Litt JZ, Beachwood, OH (personal case) (observation)
(2003): Tomas ME+, *Gastroenterol Hepatol* 26(1), 53
(2002): Aros C+, *Rev Med Chil* 130(11), 1277 (4 cases)
(2002): Greene BL, *Phys Ther* 82(12), 1224
(2001): Carbon C, *Therapie* 56(1), 35
(2001): Emmet S, Solana Beach, CA (from Internet)
(observation) (Achilles; long-lasting)
(2000): Casado Burgos E+, *Med Clin (Barc)* (Spanish) 114, 319
(1999): Lewis JR+, *Ann Pharmacother* 33(7), 792 (Achilles, bilateral)
Tendon rupture
(2003): Bernacer L+, *Med Clin* (Barc) 120(2), 78
(2003): Cebrian P+, *Foot Ankle Int* 24(2), 122
(2003): Mathis AS+, *Ann Pharmacother* 37(7), 1014
(2003): Tomas ME+, *Gastroenterol Hepatol* 26(1), 53
(2001): Nuno Mateo FJ+, *Rev Clin Esp* 201(9), 539
Tremor
Vaginitis (1.8%)
Xerostomia (<1%)

LEVOTHYROXINE

Synonyms: L-thyroxine sodium; T_4
Trade names: Eltroxin; Levo-T; Levothyroid (Forest); Levoxyl (Jones); Synthroid (Abbott); Unithroid (Watson)
Other common trade names: *Berlthyrox; Droxine; Eferox; Levo-T; Levothyrox; Thevier*
Indications: Hypothyroidism
Category: Synthetic thyroid hormone
Half-life: 6–7 days
Clinically important, potentially hazardous interactions with: dicumarol, oral anticoagulants, warfarin

Reactions

Skin
Acne
Allergic reactions (sic)
Angioedema
(1991): Levesque H+, *Lancet* 338, 393
(1990): Pandya AG+, *Arch Dermatol* 126, 1238
Dermatitis herpetiformis
(1974): From E+, *Br J Dermatol* 91, 221
Diaphoresis (<1%)
Flushing
Nevi
(1976): Tofahrn J+, *Z Hautkr* (German) 51, 617 (eruption)
Pruritus
(1990): Pandya AG+, *Arch Dermatol* 126, 1238
Rash (sic)
Urticaria
(2000): Drayton GE, Los Angeles, CA (from Internet)
(observation)
(1994): Magner J+, *Thyroid* 4, 341 (from the blue dye)
(1990): Pandya AG+, *Arch Dermatol* 126, 1238
(1966): Romanski B+, *Pol Med Sci Hist* 9, 92

Xerosis
Hair
Hair – alopecia (<1%)
Other
Headache
Hypersensitivity
Myalgia (<1%)
Pseudotumor cerebri (in infants)
Tremor

LICORICE

Scientific names: *Glycyrrhiza glabra; Glycyrrhiza uralensis*
Family: Fabaceae; Leguminosae
Trade and other common names: Alcazuz; Gan Cao; Gan Zao; Orozuz; Reglisse; Subholz; Sweet Root
Category: Anti-inflammatory
Purported indications and other uses: Upper respiratory tract infection, gastric and duodenal ulcers, bronchitis, colic, dry cough, arthritis, lupus, sore throat, malaria, sores, abscesses, contact dermatitis. Flavoring in foods, beverages and tobacco
Half-life: N/A
Clinically important, potentially hazardous interactions with: cascara, digoxin, hydrocortisone, oral contraceptives, prednisolone

Reactions

Skin
Dermatitis
(1999): Nishioka K+, *Contact Dermatitis* 40(1), 56
Edema
(2000): Negro A+, *Ann Ital Med Int* 15(4), 296
(2000): Olukoga A+, *J R Soc Health* 120(2), 83

Other
Hypertension
(2001): Brouwers AJ+, *Ned Tijdschr Geneeskd* 145(15), 744
Myopathy
Rhabdomyolysis
(2002): Firenzuoli F+, *Recenti Prog Med* 93(9), 482
(2002): Sardi A+, *Ann Ital Med Int* 17(2), 126
(1997): Barrella M+, *Ital J Neurol Sci* 18(4), 217
(1995): Berlango Jimenez A+, *An Med Interna* 12(1), 33
(1992): Caradonna P+, *Ultrastruct Pathol* 16(5), 529
(1989): Achar KN+, *Aust N Z J Med* 19(4), 365
(1988): Maresca MC+, *Minerva Med* 79(1), 55 (3 cases)
(1983): Corsi FM+, *Ital J Neurol Sci* 4(4), 493
(1983): Heidemann HT+, *Klin Wochenschr* 61(6), 303
(1980): Cumming AM+, *Postgrad Med J* 56(657), 526
(1979): Mourad G+, *J Urol Nephrol* (Paris) 85(4), 315
(1970): Nielsen H, *Nord Med* 84(31), 999
(1970): Nielsen H+, *Ugeskr Laeger* 132(38), 1778
(1970): Tourtellotte CR+, *Calif Med* 113(4), 51
(1966): Geerling J, *Ned Tijdschr Geneeskd* 110(43), 1919
(1966): Gross EG+, *N Engl J Med* 274(11), 602

LIDOCAINE

Synonym: lignocaine
Trade names: Anamantle HC (Doak); Anestacon (PolyMedica); ELA-Max (Ferndale); EMLA (AstraZeneca); Lidoderm (Endo); Xylocaine (AstraZeneca)
Other common trade names: *Dentipatch; DermaFlex; Dilocaine; Lidodan; Lidoject-2; Octocaine; Xylocard*
Indications: Ventricular arrhythmias, topical anesthesia
Category: Anesthetic; Antiarrhythmic
Half-life: terminal: 1.5–2 hours
Clinically important, potentially hazardous interactions with: amprenavir, antiarrhythmics, cimetidine

Reactions

Skin

Allergic reactions (sic)
 (2002): Helfman M, *N Y State Dent J* 68(10), 24
Angioedema
 (1987): Bricker SR+, *Anaesthesia* 42, 323
 (1961): Noble DS+, *Lancet* 2, 1436
 (1961): Rajka G, *Allergie Asthma* (German) 7, 237
Bullous eruption
Dermatitis
 (2003): Gammaitoni AR+, *J Clin Pharmacol* 43(2), 111
 (2002): Kaufmann JM+, *J Drugs Dermatol* 1(2), 192
 (2001): Breit S+, *Contact Dermatitis* 45(5), 296
 (1999): Lodi A+, *Contact Dermatitis* 41(4), 221
 (1998): Downs AM+, *Contact Dermatitis* 39, 33
 (1997): Kawada A+, *Contact Dermatitis* 37(1), 45
 (1996): Bassett IB+, *Australas J Dermatol* 37, 155
 (1996): Bircher AJ+, *Contact Dermatitis* 34, 387
 (1996): Whalen JD+, *Arch Dermatol* 132, 1256
 (1995): Thakur BK+, *J Allergy Clin Immunol* 95, 776
 (1994): Hardwick N+, *Contact Dermatitis* 30, 245
 (1993): Duggan M+, *Contact Dermatitis* 28, 190
 (1993): Handfield-Jones SE+, *Clin Exp Dermatol* 18, 342
 (1990): Black RJ+, *Contact Dermatitis* 23, 117
 (1989): Budde J+, *Derm Beruf Umwelt* (German) 37, 181
 (1986): Curley KR, *Arch Dermatol* 122, 924
 (1985): Fernandes-de-Corres L+, *Contact Dermatitis* 12, 114
 (1983): Nurse DS+, *Contact Dermatitis* 9, 513
 (1983): van Ketel WG+, *Contact Dermatitis* 9(6), 512
 (1980): Chin TM+, *Int J Dermatol* 19, 147
 (1979): Fregert S+, *Contact Dermatitis* 5, 185
 (1979): Kernekamp AS+, *Contact Dermatitis* 5, 403
 (1977): Turner TW, *Contact Dermatitis* 3, 210
 (1976): Roed-Petersen J, *Contact Dermatitis* 2(4), 235
 (1963): Calnan CD+, *Trans St Johns Hosp Dermatol Soc* 49, 9
Eczema (sic)
 (1990): Huwyler T+, *Schweiz Monatsschr Zahnmed* (German) 100, 751
 (1986): Curley KR, *Arch Dermatol* 122, 924
 (1961): Rajka G, *Allergie Asthma* (German) 7, 237
Edema (<1%)
 (2001): Breit S+, *Contact Dermatitis* 45(5), 296
Erythema
 (2001): Breit S+, *Contact Dermatitis* 45(5), 296
Erythema multiforme
 (1987): Arrowsmith JB+, *Ann Intern Med* 107, 693
Exanthems
 (2003): Gammaitoni AR+, *J Clin Pharmacol* 43(2), 111
Exfoliative dermatitis
 (1987): Arrowsmith JB+, *Ann Intern Med* 107, 693
 (1975): Hoffmann H+, *Arch Dermatol* 111, 266
Fixed eruption

 (1997): Garcia JC+, *J Investig Allergol Clin Immunol* 7, 127
 (1996): Kawada A+, *Contact Dermatitis* 35, 375
Lupus erythematosus
 (1988): Oliphant LD+, *Chest* 94, 427
Pigmentation
 (1987): Curley RK+, *Br Dent J* 162, 113
Pruritus (<1%)
 (2001): Breit S+, *Contact Dermatitis* 45(5), 296
 (1961): Rajka G, *Allergie Asthma* (German) 7, 237
Purpura
Rash (sic) (<1%)
Shivering (1–10%)
Stevens–Johnson syndrome
 (1987): Arrowsmith JB+, *Ann Intern Med* 107, 693
Urticaria
 (1980): Chin TM+, *Int J Dermatol* 19, 147
 (1969): Aldrete JA+, *JAMA* 207, 356
 (1961): Rajka G, *Allergie Asthma* (German) 7, 237

Other

Acute intermittent porphyria
Anaphylactoid reactions
 (2001): Browne IM+, *Am J Obstet Gynecol* 185(5), 1253
 (1999): Bircher AJ+, *Aust Dent J* 44, 64
 (1984): Metzner HH+, *Dermatol Monatsschr* (German) 170, 648
 (1980): Agathos M, *Contact Dermatitis* 6, 236
 (1975): Tannenbaum H+, *J Allergy Clin Immunol* 56, 226
Application-site edema
 (2001): Wahlgren CF+, *Plast Reconstr Surg* 107(3), 750
Application-site erythema
 (2001): Wahlgren CF+, *Plast Reconstr Surg* 107(3), 750
Application-site pallor
 (2001): Wahlgren CF+, *Plast Reconstr Surg* 107(3), 750
Death
 (2002): Nisse P+, *Acta Clin Belg* Suppl 1, 51
Embolia cutis medicamentosa (Nicolau syndrome)
 (1990): Wand A+, *Aktuel Dermatol* (German) 16, 128
Headache
Hypersensitivity
 (2003): Mackley CL+, *Arch Dermatol* 139(3), 343
 (1998): Marks JG+, *J Am Acad Dermatol* 38(6), 911
 (1996): Bircher AJ+, *Contact Dermatitis* 34, 387
 (1996): Whalen JD+, *Arch Dermatol* 132, 1256
 (1991): Klein CE+, *Contact Dermatitis* 25(1), 45
 (1975): Ravindranathan N, *Br Dent J* 138, 101
Injection-site pain
Injection-site phlebitis
Paresthesias (<1%)
 (2003): Dower JS Jr, *Dent Today* 22(2), 64
Seizures
 (2002): DeToledo JC+, *Anesthesiology* 97(3), 737
 (2002): Yamashita S+, *J Pain Symptom Manage* 24(5), 543
Stomatitis
 (1987): Arrowsmith JB+, *Ann Intern Med* 107, 693
Tinnitus
Tremor

LINCOMYCIN

Trade name: Lincocin (Pharmacia)
Other common trade names: *Albiotic; Cillimicina; Cillimycin; Lincocine; Princol; Zumalin*
Indications: Various infections caused by susceptible organisms
Category: Macrolide antibiotic
Half-life: 2–11.5 hours

Reactions

Skin

Allergic reactions (sic)
  (1971): *Med Lett* 13, 55 (1–5%)
Angioedema
Dermatitis
  (1991): Vilaplana J+, *Contact Dermatitis* 24, 225
  (1985): Conde-Salazar L+, *Contact Dermatitis* 12, 59 (erythema multiforme-like)
Erythema multiforme
Exanthems
Exfoliative dermatitis
Photosensitivity
Pruritus
  (1965): Kanee B, *Can Med Assoc J* 93, 220
Pruritus ani (<1%)
Purpura
  (1973): Raff M, *Ann Intern Med* 78, 779
Rash (sic) (<1%)
Stevens–Johnson syndrome (<1%)
  (1973): Pickering LK+, *JAMA* 223, 1392
Urticaria (<1%)
Vesiculobullous eruption

Other

Anaphylactoid reactions
Glossitis (<1%)
Injection-site erythema
  (1990): Shen K, *Lancet* 336, 689
Oral mucosal lesions
Serum sickness
Stomatitis (<1%)
Tinnitus
Vaginitis (<1%)

LINDANE

Synonyms: Hexachlorocyclohexane; Gamma Benzene Hexachloride
Trade names: Aphtiria; G-Well (Goldline); Hexicid; Kwell; Lorexane; Scabex
Other common trade names: *Benhex Cream; Bicide; Bio-Well; Davesol; Delice; Elentol; GAB; Gamabenceno; Gambex; Gamene; Gammalin; GBH; Herklin; Hexit; Jacutin; Kildane; Kwildane; Lencid; Locion-V; PMS-Lindane; Quellada; Sacbexyl; Sarconyl; Scabecid; Scabene; Scabi; Scabisan; Thinex; Varsan*
Indications: Scabies, pediculosis capitis, pediculosis pubis
Category: Pediculicide; Topical scabicide
Half-life: 17–22 hours
Clinically important, potentially hazardous interactions with: oil-based hair dressings

Reactions

Skin

Adverse effects (sic)
  (2000): Hernandez Contreras N+, *Rev Cubana Med Trop* 52(3), 228 (2.54%)
  (1999): Hall RC+, *Psychosomatics* 40(6), 513
  (1995): Brown S+, *Clin Infect Dis* 20 (Suppl 1), S104
  (1981): Rasmussen JE, *J Am Acad Dermatol* 5(5), 507
Bullous dermatosis
  (1994): Bouree P+, *Bull Soc Fr Parasitol* 12, 75
Dermatitis
  (1990): Andersen KE, *Occupational Skin Disease* 2nd ed, 73–88
  (1983): Farkas J, *Derm Beruf Umwelt* (German) 31(6), 189
  (1983): Fiumara NJ+, *Am Fam Physician* 28(1), 137
  (1983): *AMA Drug Evaluations* 5th ed, 1850
Ecchymoses
Eczema
Erythema
  (1987): Bowerman JG+, *Pediatr Infect Dis* 6(3), 252 (2.6%)
  (1980): Smith DE+, *Cutis* 26(6), 618
Irritation (sic)
Lymphoma (non-Hodgkins)
  (1998): Blair A+, *Am J Ind Med* 33(1), 82
Papulo-nodular lesions
  (2000): Hashimoto K+, *J Dermatol* 27(3), 181
Pruritus
  (2000): Hashimoto K+, *J Dermatol* 27(3), 181
  (1999): Revenga Arranz F+, *Rev Clin Esp* 199(2), 101
  (1998): Bowie C+, *Public Health* 112(4), 249
  (1990): Schultz MW+, *Arch Dermatol* 126(2), 167
  (1987): Bowerman JG+, *Pediatr Infect Dis* 6(3), 252 (2.6%)
Purpura
  (1981): Fagan JE, *Pediatrics* 67, 310
Toxicity (sic)
  (1999): Hall RC+, *Psychosomatics* 40(6), 513
Urticaria (0.16%)
  (1996): Shuster J, *Hosp. Pharm* 31, 370
  (1994): Fischer TF, *Ann Emerg Med* 24(5), 972

Other

Death
  (2003): Katsumata K+, *Intern Med* 42(4), 367
  (2000): Walker GJ+, *Cochrane Database Syst Rev* 3, CD00
  (1996): Lewis RJ, *Sax's Dangerous Properties of Industrial Materials* 9th ed, 338
  (1995): Aks SE+, *Ann Emerg Med* 26(5), 647
  (1995): Surber C+, *Hautarzt* (German) 46(8), 528
  (1994): Fischer TF, *Ann Emerg Med* 24(5), 972
  (1989): Vercel M+, *Cah Anesthesiol* 37(7), 543

(1988): Sunder Ram Rao CV+, *Vet Hum Toxicol* 30(2), 132
(1985): *American Hospital Formulary Service-Drug Information* 85, 1601
(1984): Gosselin RE+, *Clinical Toxicology of Commercial Products* 5th ed, III–239
(1983): Davies JE+, *Arch Dermatol* 119(2), 142
(1982): Telch J+, *Can Med Assoc* 126(6), 662
(1982): Telch J+, *Can Med Assoc* 127(9), 821
(1980): Powell GM, *Cent Afr J Med* 26(7), 170
(1980): Rasmussen JE, *Arch Dermatol* 116(11), 1226
(1979): IARC, *Monographs on the Evaluation of the Carcinogenic Risk of Chemicals to Man* 20, 220
(1977): Wheeler M, *West J Med* 127, 518
(1970): Macnamara BG, *Br Med J* 3(722), 585
(1966): Sovljanski R+, *Med Pregl* 19(6), 349
Paresthesias
Pseudotumor cerebri
(1991): Verderber L+, *J Neurol Neurosurg Psychiatry* 54(12), 1123
(1976): Heuser M+, *Acta Univ Carol Med Monogr* 75, 133
Rhabdomyolysis
(1988): Sunder Ram Rao CV+, *Vet Hum Toxicol* 30(2), 132
(1984): Jaeger U+, *Vet Hum Toxicol* 26(1), 11
(1977): Munk ZM+, *Can Med Assoc* 117(9), 1050
Seizures
(2002): Simpson WM Jr+, *Am Fam Physician* 65(8), 1599
(2000): Cox R+, *J Miss Med Assoc* 41(8), 690
(2000): Nordt SP+, *J Emerg Med* 18(1), 51
(1995): Solomon BA+, *J Fam Pract* 40(3), 291
(1994): Fischer TF, *Ann Emerg Med* 24(5), 972
(1991): Ramchander V+, *West Indian Med J* 40(1), 41
(1991): Tenenbein M, *J Am Geriatr Soc* 39(4), 394
(1987): Friedman SJ, *Arch Dermatol* 123(8), 1056
(1984): Jaeger U+, *Vet Hum Toxicol* 26(1), 11
(1979): Pramanik AK+, *Arch Dermatol* 115(10), 1224
(1977): Munk ZM+, *Can Med Assoc J* 117(9), 1050

LINEZOLID

Trade name: Zyvox (Pharmacia)
Indications: Various infections caused by susceptible organisms
Category: Oxazolidinone antibiotic
Half-life: 4–5 hours
Clinically important, potentially hazardous interactions with: amitriptyline, amoxapine, clomipramine, desipramine, dextromethorphan, doxepin, fluoxetine, fluvoxamine, imipramine, meperidine, nortriptyline, paroxetine, protriptyline, sertraline, sibutramine, trazodone, tricyclic antidepressants, trimipramine, venlafaxine

Reactions

Skin
Adverse effects (sic)
(2003): Birmingham MC+, *Clin Infect Dis* 36(2), 159 (4%)
Allergic reactions (sic)
(2003): Birmingham MC+, *Clin Infect Dis* 36(2), 159 (4%)
Fungal infections (0.1–2%)
Pruritus
Rash (sic) (2%)

Other
Candidal vaginitis (1–2%)
Dysgeusia (1–2%)
Headache
Oral candidiasis (<1%)
Serotonin syndrome

(2003): Bernard L+, *Clin Infect Dis* 36(9), 1197
(2002): Wigen CL+, *Clin Infect Dis* 34(12), 1651
(2001): Lavery S+, *Psychosomatics* 42(5), 432
Tongue pigmentation (<1%)
Tooth discoloration
(2003): Matson KL+, *Pharmacotherapy* 23(5), 682

LINSEED

Scientific name: *Linum usitatissimum*
Family: Linaceae
Trade and other common names: alpha-linolenic acid; Flaxseed; flaxseed oil; L-310; Igroco; Lini Semen; linseed oil; lint bells; Salinum; winterlien
Category: Anodyne; Anti-inflammatory; Antiseptic; Antitussive; Demulcent; Emollient; Expectorant; Laxative; Phytoestrogen
Purported indications and other uses: Dry mouth, menopause, osteoporosis, heart disease, catarrh, bronchitis, furunculosis, pleuritic pains, constipation, high cholesterol, benign prostatic hyperplasia, bladder inflammation, gastritis, enteritis, irritable bowel syndrome. Topical: poultice for skin inflammation. Ophthalmologic: oil used for removal of foreign bodies from the eye.
Half-life: N/A

Reactions

Skin
Allergic reactions (sic)
Erythema
Eyelid edema
Irritation

Other
Anaphylactoid reactions
(2003): Leon F+, *Allergol Immunopathol* (Madr) 31(1), 47 (seed)
(1996): Alonso L+, *J Allergy Clin Immunol* 98(2), 469 (seed)
Fever

Note: Linum is cultivated for both its stem fibers (the source of linen and some paper) and its seeds (oil used in cooking and in margarine). The oil is used in paints and varnishes and the seed residues are used in cattle cake

LIOTHYRONINE

Synonym: T$_3$ sodium
Trade names: Cytomel (Jones); Triostat (Jones)
Other common trade names: *Cynomel; T3; Tertroxin; Thyronine; Trijodthyronin BC N*
Indications: Hypothyroidism
Category: Synthetic thyroid hormone
Half-life: 16–49 hours
Clinically important, potentially hazardous interactions with: anticoagulants, dicumarol, warfarin

Reactions

Skin
Allergic reactions (sic)
Diaphoresis (<1%)
Rash (sic)
Urticaria

(1994): Magner J+, *Thyroid* 4, 341 (from the blue dye)
(1990): Pandya AG+, *Arch Dermatol* 126, 1238
(1966): Romanski B+, *Pol Med Sci Hist* 9, 92
Xerosis

Hair

Hair – alopecia (<1%)

Other

Headache
Hypersensitivity
Myalgia (<1%)
Phlebitis (1%)
Pseudotumor cerebri
Tremor

LISINOPRIL

Trade names: Prinivil (Merck); Prinizide (Merck); Zestoretic (AstraZeneca); Zestril (AstraZeneca)
Other common trade names: *Acerbon; Alapril; Apo-Lisinopril; Carace; Coric; Prinil; Tensopril; Vivatec*
Indications: Hypertension
Category: Angiotensin-converting enzyme (ACE) inhibitor; Antihypertensive
Half-life: 12 hours
Clinically important, potentially hazardous interactions with: amiloride, **garlic**, spironolactone, triamterene

Prinizide is lisinopril and hydrochlorothiazide; Zestoretic is lisinopril and hydrochlorothiazide

Reactions

Skin

Angioedema
(2001): Cohen EG+, *Ann Otol Rhinol Laryngol* 110(8), 701 (64 cases)
(1999): Guo X+, *J Okla State Med Assoc* 92, 71
(1999): Maestre ML+, *Rev Esp Anestesiol Reanim* (Spanish) 46, 88
(1999): Neutel JM+, *Am J Ther* 6, 161
(1997): Brown NJ+, *JAMA* 278, 232
(1997): Pavletic AJ, *J Am Board Fam Pract* 10, 370
(1996): Pillans PI+, *Eur J Clin Pharmacol* 51, 123
(1995): Bauwens LJ+, *Ned Tijdschr Geneeskd* (Dutch) 139, 674
(1995): Frontera Y+, *J Am Dent Assoc* 126, 217
(1995): Kuo DC+, *J Emerg Med* 13, 327 (uvular)
(1994): Krikorian RK+, *Chest* 106, 1922
(1993): Soo Hoo GW+, *West J Med* 158, 412
(1992): McElligott S+, *Ann Intern Med* 116, 426
(1992): Shelley WB+, *Cutis* 49, 391 (tongue) (observation)
(1990): Laher MS, *Drugs* 39 (Suppl 2), 55
(1990): McAreavey D+, *Drugs* 40, 326 (0.4%)
(1990): Orfan N+, *JAMA* 264, 1287
(1988): Lancaster SG+, *Drugs* 35, 646 (0.6%)
(1987): Rush JE+, *J Cardiovasc Pharmacol* 9, s99
Bullous eruption
(1988): Barlow RJ+, *Clin Exp Dermatol* 13, 117
Diaphoresis (<1%)
Edema (1%)
Erythema (1%)
Exanthems
(1990): Laher MS, *Drugs* 39 (Suppl 2), 55
(1990): McAreavey D+, *Drugs* 40, 326 (3.2%)
(1988): Barlow RJ+, *Clin Exp Dermatol* 13, 117
(1988): Lancaster SG+, *Drugs* 35, 646 (3.2%)
Facial edema (<1%)

Flushing (<1%)
(1997): Litt JZ, Beachwood, OH (personal case) (observation)
(1990): Laher MS, *Drugs* 39 (Suppl 2), 55
(1989): Healy LA+, *N Engl J Med* 321, 763
Lichenoid eruption
(1992): Shelley WB+, *Cutis* 50, 182 (observation)
Lupus erythematosus
Pemphigus
Pemphigus foliaceus
(2000): Ong CS+, *Australas J Dermatol* 41(4), 242
Peripheral edema (<1%)
(1988): Uretsky BF+, *Am Heart J* 116, 480
Photosensitivity (<1%)
Pruritus (1.2%)
(2000): Kalikhman ZM, (from Internet) (observation)
Purpura
(1993): Sztern B+, *Presse Med* (French) 22, 967
(1988): Barlow RJ+, *Clin Exp Dermatol* 13, 117
Rash (sic) (1.5%)
(1999): Horiuchi Y+, *J Dermatol* 26, 128
(1989): Giles TD+, *J Am Coll Cardiol* 13, 1240
(1988): Uretsky BF+, *Am Heart J* 116, 480
(1987): Bolzano K+, *J Cardiovasc Pharmacol* 9, s43
(1987): Rush JE+, *J Cardiovasc Pharmacol* 9, s99
Rosacea
(1999): Oakley A, Hamilton, New Zealand (from Internet) (observation)
Stevens–Johnson syndrome
Telangiectasia
(1999): Oakley A, Hamilton, New Zealand (from Internet) (observation)
Toxic epidermal necrolysis
Ulcerations (sic) (ischemic skin ulcer)
(1987): Rush JE+, *J Cardiovasc Pharmacol* 9, s99
Urticaria (<1%)
(1996): Pillans PI+, *Eur J Clin Pharmacol* 51, 123
(1989): Cameron HA+, *J Human Hypertension* 3, 177
Vasculitis (<1%)
(1988): Barlow RJ+, *Clin Exp Dermatol* 13, 117

Hair

Hair – alopecia (<1%)

Other

Anaphylactoid reactions (<1%)
Cough
(2001): Adigun AQ+, *West Afr J Med* 20(1), 46–7
(2001): Lee SC+, *Hypertension* 38(2), 166
Dysesthesia (<1%)
Dysgeusia
(1988): Uretsky BF+, *Am Heart J* 116, 480
Headache
Mastodynia (<1%)
Myalgia (0.5%)
Paresthesias (0.8%)
Tinnitus
Tremor
Xerostomia (<1%)

LITHIUM

Trade names: Eskalith (GSK); Lithobid (Solvay); Lithonate; Lithotabs
Other common trade names: *Carbolith; Duralith; Hynorex Retard; Lithicarb; Lithizine; Priadel; Teralithe*
Indications: Manic-depressive states
Category: Antidepressant; Antipsychotic
Half-life: 18–24 hours
Clinically important, potentially hazardous interactions with: acetazolamide, acitretin, bendroflumethiazide, benzthiazide, chlorothiazide, chlorthalidone, fluoxetine, haloperidol, hydrochlorothiazide, hydroflumethiazide, indapamide, meperidine, methotrexate, methyclothiazide, metolazone, olmesartan, pegfilgrastim, polythiazide, quinethazone, rofecoxib, sibutramine, thiazides, trichlormethiazide, valdecoxib

Note: An excellent review of the cutaneous conditions associated with lithium can be found in (1983): Sarantidis D+, *Br J Psychiatry* 143, 42

Reactions

Skin

Acanthosis nigricans
  (1979): Arnold HL+, *J Am Acad Dermatol* 1, 93
Acne
  (2001): Oztas P+, *Ann Pharmacother* 35(7), 961
  (1991): Srebrnik A+, *Cutis* 48, 65
  (1986): Remmer HI+, *J Clin Psychiatry* 47, 48
  (1985): Albrecht G, *Hautarzt* (German) 36, 77 (passim)
  (1984): Lambert D+, *Ann Med Interne Paris* (French) 135, 637
  (1983): Sarantidis D+, *Br J Psychiatry* 143, 42 (11%)
  (1982): Deandrea D+, *J Clin Psychopharmacol* 2, 199
  (1982): Heng MCY, *Arch Dermatol* 118, 246
  (1982): Heng MCY, *Br J Dermatol* 106, 107
  (1982): Lambert D+, *Ann Dermatol Venereol* (French) 109, 19
  (1980): Vestergaard P+, *Acta Psychiatrica Scand* 62, 193
  (1978): Oei TT+, *Ned Tijdschr Geneeskd* (Dutch) 122, 1302
  (1977): Okrasinski H, *Dermatologica* 154, 251
  (1977): Reiffers J+, *Dermatologica* 155, 155
  (1975): Yoder FW, *Arch Dermatol* 111, 396
  (1971): Kusumi Y, *Dis Nerv Syst* 32, 853
Angioedema
  (1985): Berova N+, *Dermatol Venerol* (Sofia) (Bulgarian) 24, 23
  (1982): Lambert D+, *Ann Dermatol Venereol* (French) 109, 19
Angular cheilitis
  (1983): Sarantidis D+, *Br J Psychiatry* 143, 42 (1%)
Atopic dermatitis
  (1983): Sarantidis D+, *Br J Psychiatry* 143, 42 (3%)
Bullous eruption
  (1987): McWhirter JD+, *Arch Dermatol* 123, 1122
Darier's disease
  (1995): Rubin MB, *J Am Acad Dermatol* 32, 674
  (1990): Milton GP, *J Am Acad Dermatol* 23, 926 (exacerbation)
  (1986): Clark RD Jr+, *Psychosomatics* 27, 800 (exacerbation)
Dermatitis (sic)
  (1980): Aldoroty N+, *Am J Psychiatry* 137, 870
  (1973): Kurtin SB, *JAMA* 223, 802
  (1973): Ruiz-Maldonado R+, *JAMA* 224, 1534
  (1972): Posey RE, *JAMA* 221, 1517
Dermatitis herpetiformis
  (1985): Albrecht G, *Hautarzt* (German) 36, 77 (passim)
  (1983): Sarantidis D+, *Br J Psychiatry* 143, 42
  (1982): Heng MCY, *Arch Dermatol* 118, 246
Discoloration of fingers and toes (sic) (<1%)

Eczema (sic)
  (1980): Vestergaard P+, *Acta Psychiatrica Scand* 62, 193
Edema
  (1984): Lambert D+, *Ann Med Interne Paris* (French) 135, 637
  (1975): Baldessarini RJ+, *Ann Intern Med* 83, 527
  (1970): Demers R+, *JAMA* 214, 1845 (pretibial)
Erythema
  (1996): Wakelin SH+, *Clin Exp Dermatol* 21, 296
Erythema multiforme
  (1991): Balldin J+, *J Am Acad Dermatol* 24, 1015
Exanthems
  (1985): Albrecht G, *Hautarzt* (German) 36, 77 (passim)
  (1983): Sarantidis D+, *Br J Psychiatry* 143, 42
  (1982): Deandrea D+, *J Clin Psychopharmacol* 2, 199
  (1982): Lambert D+, *Ann Dermatol Venereol* (French) 109, 19
  (1980): Meinhold JM+, *J Clin Psychiatry* 41, 395
  (1975): Baldessarini RJ+, *Ann Intern Med* 83, 527
  (1970): No Author, *Ann Intern Med* 73, 291
  (1968): Callaway CL+, *Am J Psychiatry* 124, 1124
Exfoliative dermatitis
  (1985): Albrecht G, *Hautarzt* (German) 36, 77 (passim)
  (1983): Sarantidis D+, *Br J Psychiatry* 143, 42 (1%)
  (1979): Kuhnley EJ+, *Am J Psychiatry* 136, 1340
Follicular keratosis (sic)
  (1996): Wakelin SH+, *Clin Exp Dermatol* 21, 296
  (1982): Lambert D+, *Ann Dermatol Venereol* (French) 109, 19
  (1977): Reiffers J+, *Dermatologica* 155, 155
Folliculitis
  (1985): Hogan DJ+, *J Am Acad Dermatol* 13, 245 (passim)
  (1983): Sarantidis D+, *Br J Psychiatry* 143, 42
  (1973): Kurtin SB, *JAMA* 223, 803
  (1973): Rifkin A+, *Am J Psychiatry* 130, 1018
Hidradenitis suppurativa
  (1997): Marinella MA, *Acta Derm Venereol* 77, 483
  (1996): Blumenthal HL, Beachwood, OH (personal case) (observation)
  (1995): Gupta AK+, *J Amer Acad Dermatol* 32, 382
  (1981): Stamm T+, *Psychiatr Prax* (German) 8, 152
Hyperplasia (verrucous)
  (1984): Frenk E, *Z Hautkr* (German) 2, 97
Ichthyosis
  (1983): Sarantidis D+, *Br J Psychiatry* 143, 42 (1%)
  (1977): Reiffers J+, *Dermatologica* 155, 155
Keratoderma
  (1991): Labelle A+, *J Clin Psychopharmacol* 11, 149
Keratosis pilaris
  (1985): Albrecht G, *Hautarzt* (German) 36, 77 (passim)
  (1973): Rifkin A+, *Am J Psychiatry* 130, 1018
Lichen planus
  (1994): Thompson DF+, *Pharmacotherapy* 14, 561
Lichen simplex chronicus
  (1984): Shukla S+, *Am J Psychiatry* 141, 909
Linear IgA bullous dermatosis
  (2002): Cohen LM+, *J Am Acad Dermatol* 46, S32 (passim)
  (1996): Tranvan A+, *J Am Acad Dermatol* 35, 865
  (1987): McWhirter JD+, *Arch Dermatol* 123, 1122
Lupus erythematosus
  (1994): Yung RL+, *Rheum Dis Clin North Am* 20, 61
  (1985): Stratton MA, *Clin Pharm* 4, 657
  (1982): Shukla VR+, *JAMA* 248, 921
  (1981): Hess EV, *Arthritis Rheum* 24, 6
Morphea
  (1982): Lambert D+, *Ann Dermatol Venereol* (French) 109, 19
Mycosis fungoides
  (2001): Francis GJ+, *J Am Acad Dermatol* 44, 308
Myxedema
  (1981): Kvetny J+, *Ugeskr Laeger* (Danish) 143, 1323
  (1979): Medley ES+, *J Fam Pract* 8, 855

(1978): Perrild H+, *BMJ* 1, 1108
(1973): Pousset G+, *Ann Endocrinol Paris* (French) 34, 454
(1973): Pousset G+, *Ann Endocrinol Paris* (French) 34, 549
(1972): Brandrup FO, *Ugeskr Laeger* (Danish) 134, 2710
(1972): Vestergaard PA+, *Lancet* 2, 427
(1972): Vestergaard PA+, *Ugeskr Laeger* (Danish) 134, 1282
(1972): Wiener JD, *JAMA* 220, 587
(1971): Luby ED+, *JAMA* 218, 1298

Papulo-nodular lesions (elbows)
(1973): Kurtin SB, *JAMA* 223, 802
(1972): Posey RE, *JAMA* 221, 1517

Port-wine stain
(1987): Leung AK, *J Natl Med Assoc* 79, 877

Prurigo nodularis
(1983): Sarantidis D+, *Br J Psychiatry* 143, 42 (1%)

Pruritus (<1%)
(1985): Berova N+, *Dermatol Venerol* (Sofia) (Bulgarian) 24, 23
   (1–5%)
(1984): Lambert D+, *Ann Med Interne Paris* (French) 135, 637
(1983): Sarantidis D+, *Br J Psychiatry* 143, 42
(1982): Lambert D+, *Ann Dermatol Venereol* (French) 109, 19
(1980): Vestergaard P+, *Acta Psychiatrica Scand* 62, 193
(1977): Reiffers J+, *Dermatologica* 155, 155
(1970): No Author, *Ann Intern Med* 73, 291
(1968): Callaway CL+, *Am J Psychiatry* 124, 1124

Psoriasis
(2003): Akkerhuis GW+, *Am J Psychiatry* 160(7), 1355
(1996): Ockenfels HM+, *Arch Dermatol Res* 288, 173
(1994): Dorevitch A, *Harefuah* (Hebrew) 127, 228
(1993): Hermle L+, *Nervenarzt* (German) 64, 208
(1992): Abel EA, *Semin Dermatol* 11, 269
(1992): Hemlock C+, *Ann Pharmacother* 26, 211
(1992): Rudolph RI, *J Am Acad Dermatol* 26, 135
(1989): Sasaki T+, *J Dermatol* (Tokio) 16, 59 (exacerbation)
(1988): Koo E+, *Orv Hetil* (Hungarian) 129, 1699
(1988): Zirilli G+, *Minerva Psichiatr* (Italian) 29, 43
(1987): Gupta MA+, *Gen Hosp Psychiatry* 9, 157
(1986): Abel EA+, *J Am Acad Dermatol* 15, 1007 (exacerbation)
(1986): Ghadirian AM+, *J Clin Psychiatry* 47, 212
(1986): Holy B+, *Acta Univ Carol Med Praha* (Czech) 32, 217
(1986): Pande AC+, *J Clin Psychiatry* 47, 330 (exacerbation)
(1986): Segui-Montesinos J+, *Med Clin (Barc)* (Spanish) 86, 261
(1985): Albrecht G, *Hautarzt* (German) 36, 77 (passim)
(1984): Alvarez WA+, *Int J Psychosom* 31, 21
(1984): Farber EM+, *J Am Acad Dermatol* 10, 511
(1984): Fox BJ+, *J Assoc Military Dermatol* 10, 35 (exacerbation)
(1984): Lambert D+, *Ann Med Interne Paris* (French) 135, 637
(1984): Lin HN+, *Taiwan I Hsueh Hui Tsa Chih* (Chinese)
   83, 1064
(1983): Hollander A, *Hautarzt* (German) 34, 487
(1983): Sarantidis D+, *Br J Psychiatry* 143, 42 (2%)
(1982): Deandrea D+, *J Clin Psychopharmacol* 2, 199
(1982): Heng MCY, *Arch Dermatol* 118, 246 (exacerbation)
(1982): Heng MCY, *Br J Dermatol* 106, 107 (exacerbation)
(1982): Lambert D+, *Ann Dermatol Venereol* (French) 109, 19
   (exacerbation)
(1982): Pincelli C+, *G Ital Dermatol Venereol* (Italian) 117, 113
(1981): No Author, *Drug Ther Bull* 19, 68
(1980): Bakris GL+, *Int J Psychiatry Med* 10, 327
(1980): Thiers B, *J Am Acad Dermatol* 3, 101
(1979): Evans DL+, *Am J Psychiatry* 136, 1326
(1979): Lazarus GS+, *Arch Dermatol* 115, 1183
(1979): Skoven I+, *Arch Dermatol* 115, 1185 (exacerbation)
(1979): Umbert P+, *Actas Dermosifiliogr* (Spanish) 70, 623
(1978): Mobacken H+, *Br J Dermatol* 98, 597
(1978): Robak OH, *Tidsskr Nor Laegeforen* (Norwegian) 98, 566
(1978): Thormann J, *Ugeskr Laeger* (Danish) 140, 721
(1977): No Author, *Lakartidningen* (Swedish) 74, 2109
(1977): Reiffers J+, *Dermatologica* 155, 155 (exacerbation)
(1977): Skott AH+, *Br J Dermatol* 96, 445 (exacerbation)

(1977): Skott AH+, *Br J Psychiatry* 131, 223
(1976): Bakker JB+, *Psychosomatics* 17, 143 (exacerbation)
(1972): Carter TN, *Psychosomatics* 13, 325

Purpura
(1984): Lambert D+, *Ann Med Interne Paris* (French) 135, 637
(1982): Lambert D+, *Ann Dermatol Venereol* (French) 109, 19

Pustular psoriasis
(1979): Evans DL+, *Am J Psychiatry* 136, 10
(1979): Skoven I+, *Arch Dermatol* 115, 1185
(1978): Lowe NJ+, *Arch Dermatol* 114, 1788

Pustules
(1993): Webster GF, *Clin Dermatol* 11, 541
(1982): White SW, *J Am Acad Dermatol* 7, 660 (palms and soles)

Rash (sic) (1–10%)
(1980): Bone S+, *Am J Psychiatry* 137:1, 103

Seborrheic dermatitis
(1984): Lambert D+, *Ann Med Interne Paris* (French) 135, 637
(1983): Sarantidis D+, *Br J Psychiatry* 143, 42
(1982): Lambert D+, *Ann Dermatol Venereol* (French) 109, 19

Side effects (sic)
(1985): Berova N+, *Dermatol Venerol* (Sofia) (Bulgarian) 24, 23
   (23%)
(1983): Sarantidis D+, *Br J Psychiatry* 143, 42 (up to one-third)
(1982): Lambert D+, *Ann Dermatol Venereol* (French) 109, 19

Subcorneal pustular dermatosis (Sneddon–Wilkinson)
(1988): Sterling GB+, *Cutis* 41, 165

Telangiectasia
(1983): Brinkmann W+, *Z Hautkr* (German) 9, 681

Tinea versicolor
(1997): Fearfield LA+, *Clin Exp Dermatol* 22, 57

Toxicoderma
(1985): Lambert D, *Dermatologica* (French) 171, 209

Ulcerations (lower extremities)
(1984): Lambert D+, *Ann Med Interne Paris* (French) 135, 637
(1975): Baldessarini RJ+, *Ann Intern Med* 83, 527
(1971): Kusumi Y, *Dis Nerv Syst* 32, 853
(1970): No Author, *Ann Intern Med* 73, 291
(1968): Callaway CL+, *Am J Psychiatry* 124, 1124

Urticaria
(1985): Berova N+, *Dermatol Venerol* (Sofia) (Bulgarian) 24, 23
(1984): Lambert D+, *Ann Med Interne Paris* (French) 135, 637
(1982): Lambert D+, *Ann Dermatol Venereol* (French) 109, 19

Vasculitis
(1994): Blumenthal HL, Beachwood, OH (personal case)
   (observation)
(1984): Lambert D+, *Ann Med Interne Paris* (French) 135, 637
(1982): Lambert D+, *Ann Dermatol Venereol* (French) 109, 19
(1970): *Ann Intern Med* 73, 291

Verrucous lesions (sic)
(1984): Frenk E, *Z Hautkr* (German) 59, 97

Warts
(1982): White SW, *Int J Dermatol* 21, 107

Xerosis
(1975): Hoxtell E+, *Arch Dermatol* 111, 1073

Hair

Hair – alopecia
(2001): Francis GJ+, *J Am Acad Dermatol* 44, 308
(2000): Mercke Y+, *Ann Clin Psychiatry* 12, 35 (12–19%)
(1999): van dem Bent PM+, *Ned Tijdschr Geneeskd* (Dutch)
   143, 990
(1998): Litt JZ, Beachwood, OH (personal case) (observation)
(1996): McKinney PA+, *Ann Clin Psychiatry* 8, 183 (10%)
(1991): Wagner KD+, *Psychosomatics* 32, 355
(1986): Ghadirian AM+, *J Clin Psychiatry* 47, 212
(1985): Albrecht G, *Hautarzt* (German) 36, 77 (passim)
(1984): Lambert D+, *Ann Med Interne Paris* (French) 135, 637
(1984): Mortimer PS+, *Int J Dermatol* 23, 603
(1983): Orwin A, *Br J Dermatol* 108, 503 (12%)

(1983): Shader RI, *J Clin Psychopharmacol* 3, 122
(1983): Yassa R+, *Can J Psychiatry* 28, 132
(1982): Dawber R+, *Br J Dermatol* 107, 125
(1982): Lambert D+, *Ann Dermatol Venereol* (French) 109, 19
(1982): Muniz CE+, *Psychosomatics* 23, 312
(1982): No Author, *Psychosomatics* 23, 563
Hair – alopecia areata
  (1988): Silvestri A+, *Gen Hosp Psychiatry* 10, 46
  (1983): Sarantidis D+, *Br J Psychiatry* 143, 42 (2%)
  (1980): Vestergaard P+, *Acta Psychiatr Scand* 62, 193
Hair – brittle
  (1970): No Author, *Ann Intern Med* 73, 291
Hair – changes in texture
  (1985): McCreadle RG+, *Acta Psychiatr Scand* 72, 387

Nails

Nails – Beau's lines (transverse nail bands)
  (1988): Don PC+, *Cutis* 41, 20
Nails – dystrophy
  (1988): Don PC+, *Cutis* 41, 20
  (1982): Lambert D+, *Ann Dermatol Venereol* (French) 109, 19
Nails – onychomadesis
  (1988): Don PC+, *Cutis* 41, 20
Nails – psoriasis
  (1992): Rudolph RI, *J Am Acad Dermatol* 26, 135

Other

Dysgeusia (>10%)
Geographic tongue
  (1992): Patki AH, *Int J Dermatol* 31, 386
Gingival hyperplasia
  (1968): Callaway CL+, *Am J Psychiatry* 124, 1124
Glossodynia
Headache
Lichenoid stomatitis
  (1995): Menni S+, *Ann Dermatol Venereol* (French) 122, 91
  (1991): Srebrnik A+, *Cutis* 48, 65
  (1985): Hogan DJ+, *J Am Acad Dermatol* 13, 245
Oral ulceration
  (2000): Madinier I+, *Ann Med Interne (Paris)* (French) 151, 248
  (1985): Bar Nathan EA+, *Am J Psychiatry* 142, 1126
  (1985): Hogan DJ+, *J Am Acad Dermatol* 13, 245
Parkinsonism
  (2000): Muthane UB+, *J Neurol Sci* 176, 78
Pseudolymphoma
  (1995): Magro CM+, *J Am Acad Dermatol* 32, 419
Pseudotumor cerebri (<1%)
Rhabdomyolysis
  (1991): Bateman AM+, *Nephrol Dial Transplant* 6(3), 203
  (1982): Unger J+, *Acta Clin Belg* 39, 216 (overdose)
Sialorrhea
Stomatitis
  (1985): Bar Nathan EA+, *Am J Psychiatry* 142, 1126
  (1978): Muniz CE+, *JAMA* 239, 2759
Stomatodynia
  (1985): Bar Nathan EA+, *Am J Psychiatry* 142, 1126
Stutter
  (2001): Netski AL+, *Ann Pharmacother* 35(7), 961
Tinnitus
Tremor
Vaginal ulceration
  (1991): Srebrnik A+, *Cutis* 48, 65
Xerostomia (<1%)
  (1980): Bone S+, *Am J Psychiatry* 137:1, 103

LOMEFLOXACIN

Trade name: Maxaquin (Elan)
Other common trade names: *Logiflox; Ontop*
Indications: Various infections caused by susceptible organisms
Category: Broad-spectrum fluoroquinolone antibacterial
Half-life: 4–6 hours
**Clinically important, potentially hazardous interactions
with:** amiodarone, antacids, arsenic, bepridil, bismuth, bretylium, didanosine, disopyramide, erythromycin, NSAIDs, phenothiazines, procainamide, quinidine, sotalol, sucralfate, tricyclic antidepressants, zinc salts

Reactions

Skin

Allergic reactions (sic) (<1%)
Ankle edema
Chills (<1%)
Diaphoresis (<1%)
  (1992): Crome P+, *Am J Med* 92 (Suppl 4A), 126S
  (1992): Iravani A, *Am J Med* 92, 75S
Eczema (sic)
Edema (<1%)
Exanthems
Exfoliation (sic) (<1%)
Facial edema (<1%)
Flu-like syndrome (sic) (<1%)
Flushing (<1%)
Genital pruritus (sic)
  (1992): Iravani A, *Am J Med* 92, 75S
Photosensitivity (2.4%)
  (2000): Ferguson J+, *J Antimicrob Chemother* 45, 503
  (1998): Arata J+, *Antimicrob Agents Chemother* 42, 3141
  (1998): Kimura M+, *Contact Dermatitis* 38, 180
  (1996): Young AR+, *J Photochem Photobiol B* 32, 165
  (1994): Cohen JB+, *Arch Dermatol* 130, 805 (following tanning bed)
  (1994): Correia O+, *Arch Dermatol* 130, 808 (bullous)
  (1994): Lowe NJ+, *Clin Pharmacol Ther* 56, 587
  (1994): Poh-Fitzpatrick MB, *Arch Dermatol* 130, 261
  (1993): Tozawa K+, *Hinyokika Kiyo* (Japanese) 39, 801
  (1992): Crome P+, *Am J Med* 92 (Suppl 4A), 126S
  (1992): Iravani A, *Am J Med* 92, 75S
  (1992): Kurumaji Y+, *Contact Dermatitis* 26, 5
  (1992): Rizk E, *Am J Med* 92, 130S (2.4%)
  (1990): LeBel M+, *Antimicrob Agents Chemother* 34, 1254
Phototoxicity
  (2000): Traynor NJ+, *Toxicol Vitr* 14, 275
  (1998): Martinez LJ+, *Photochem Photobiol* 67, 399
Pruritus (<1%)
  (1992): Cox CE, *Am J Med* 92, 82S
  (1992): Gotfried MH+, *Am J Med* 92, 108S
  (1992): Kemper P+, *Am J Med* 92, 98S
  (1992): Klimberg IW+, *Am J Med* 92, 121S
  (1992): Mouton Y+, *Am J Med* 92, 87S
  (1991): Wadworth AN+, *Drugs* 42, 1018
Purpura (<1%)
Pustules
  (1992): Mouton Y+, *Am J Med* 92, 87S
Rash (sic) (<1%)
  (1992): Crome P+, *Am J Med* 92 (Suppl 4A), 126S
  (1992): Gotfried MH+, *Am J Med* 92, 108S
  (1992): Iravani A, *Am J Med* 92, 75S
  (1992): Mouton Y+, *Am J Med* 92, 87S
  (1991): Wadworth AN+, *Drugs* 42, 1018

Stevens–Johnson syndrome
Toxicoderma (sic)
  (1991): Wadworth AN+, *Drugs* 42, 1018
Urticaria (<1%)
  (1991): Wadworth AN+, *Drugs* 42, 1018
Vasculitis

Other
Dysgeusia (<1%)
Headache
Hypersensitivity
  (1991): Wadworth AN+, *Drugs* 42, 1018
Myalgia (<1%)
Paresthesias (<1%)
  (1992): Crome P+, *Am J Med* 92 (Suppl 4A), 126S
Tendon rupture (many reports)
Tinnitus
Tongue pigmentation (<1%)
Tremor
Vaginal candidiasis
Vaginitis (<1%)
Xerostomia (<1%)
  (1992): Mant TG, *Am J Med* 92, 26S

LOMUSTINE

Synonym: CCNU
Trade name: CeeNU (Bristol-Myers Squibb)
Other common trade names: *Belustine; Cecenu; Lomeblastin; Lucostine; Lundbeck*
Indications: Brain tumors, lymphomas, melanoma
Category: Nitrosurea alkylating antineoplastic
Half-life: 16–72 hours
Clinically important, potentially hazardous interactions with: aldesleukin

Reactions

Skin
Acral erythema
  (1989): Oksenhendler E+, *Eur J Cancer Clin Oncol* 25, 1181
Flushing
  (1992): Breathnach SM+, *Adverse Drug Reactions and the Skin* Blackwell, Oxford, 290
Neutrophilic eccrine hidradenitis
  (1996): Shear NH+, *J Am Acad Dermatol* 35, 819
Rash (sic) (1–10%)

Hair
Hair – alopecia (<1%)

Other
Stomatitis (1–10%)

LOPERAMIDE

Trade names: Imodium (McNeil); Maalox (Novartis)
Other common trade names: *Brek; Diar-Aid; Diarr-Eze; Diarstop-L; Imossel; Lop-Dia; Loperhoe; Maalox Anti-Diarrheal; Stopit; Vancotil*
Indications: Diarrhea
Category: Antidiarrheal
Half-life: 9–14 hours
Clinically important, potentially hazardous interactions with: St John's wort

Reactions

Skin
Erythema nodosum
Exanthems
Pruritus
Rash (sic)
Urticaria

Hair
Hair – alopecia
  (1993): Litt JZ, Beachwood, OH (personal case) (observation)

Other
Gingivitis
  (1990): DuPont HL+, *Am J Med* 88, 20S
Hypersensitivity
Oral mucosal lesions (1.1%)
  (1990): DuPont HL+, *Am J Med* 88, 20S
Xerostomia
  (1990): DuPont HL+, *Am J Med* 88, 20S

LORACARBEF

Trade name: Lorabid (Monarch)
Other common trade name: *Carbac*
Indications: Various infections caused by susceptible organisms
Category: Beta-lactam antibiotic (carbacephem)
Half-life: 60 minutes

Reactions

Skin
Candidiasis
Erythema multiforme (<1%)
Pruritus (<1%)
Rash (sic) (1.2%)
Stevens–Johnson syndrome (<1%)
Urticaria (<1%)

Other
Candidal vaginitis (1.3%)
Headache
Serum sickness (<1%)

LORATADINE

Trade names: Alavert (Wyeth); Claritin (Schering); Claritin-D (Schering)
Other common trade names: *Civeran; Claratyne; Claritine; Lisino; Lorastine; Velodan; Zeos*
Indications: Allergic rhinitis, urticaria
Category: Antihistamine H₁-blocker
Half-life: 3–20 hours

Reactions

Skin

Angioedema (>2%)
  (1989): Clissold SP+, *Drugs* 37, 42
Dermatitis (sic) (>2%)
Diaphoresis (>2%)
Erythema multiforme (>2%)
Exanthems
Fixed eruption
  (2002): Ruiz-Genao DP+, *Br J Dermatol* 146(3), 528
Flushing (>2%)
Peripheral edema (>2%)
Photosensitivity (>2%)
Pruritus (>2%)
  (1989): Barenholtz HA+, *Drug Intell Clin Pharm* 23, 445
Purpura (>2%)
Rash (sic) (>2%)
Urticaria (>2%)
  (1992): Boner AL+, *Allergy* 47, 98
  (1989): Clissold SP+, *Drugs* 37, 42
Xerosis (>2%)

Hair

Hair – alopecia (>2%)
Hair – dry (sic) (>2%)

Other

Anaphylactoid reactions (>2%)
Dysgeusia (>2%)
Gynecomastia (>2%)
Headache
Hyperesthesia (>2%)
Mastodynia (1–10%)
Myalgia (>2%)
Paresthesias (>2%)
Sialorrhea (>2%)
Stomatitis (>2%)
Tinnitus
Torsades de pointes
  (2003): Atar S+, *Pacing Clin Electrophysiol* 26(3), 785 (with amiodarone)
Vaginitis (>2%)
Xerostomia (>10%)
  (1992): Monroe EW+, *Arzneimittelforschung* (German) 42, 1119
  (1992): Olson OT+, *Arzneimittelforschung* (German) 42, 1227
  (1990): Del Carpio J+, *J Allergy Clin Immunology* 84, 741
  (1990): Irander K+, *Allergy* 45, 86
  (1990): Simons FE, *Clin Exp Allergy* 20, 19
  (1989): Barenholtz HA+, *Drug Intell Clin Pharm* 23, 445
  (1989): Bruttman G+, *J Allergy Clin Immunology* 83, 411
  (1988): Gutkowski A+, *J Allergy Clin Immunology* 81, 902

LORAZEPAM

Trade name: Ativan (Wyeth) (Baxter)
Other common trade names: *Apo-Lorazepam; Durazolam; Laubeel; Merlit; Nu-Loraz; Punktyl; Tavor; Temesta; Titus*
Indications: Anxiety, depression
Category: Anticonvulsant; Antiemetic; Benzodiazepine anxiolytic
Half-life: 10–20 hours
Clinically important, potentially hazardous interactions with: alcohol, amprenavir, barbiturates, chlorpheniramine, clarithromycin, CNS depressants, efavirenz, erythromycin, esomeprazole, imatinib, MAO inhibitors, narcotics, nelfinavir, phenothiazines, valproate

Reactions

Skin

Dermatitis (sic) (1–10%)
Diaphoresis (>10%)
Erythema multiforme
  (1991): Porteous DM+, *Arch Dermatol* 127, 741
Exanthems
Fixed eruption
  (1988): Jafferany M+, *Dermatologica* 177, 386
Pruritus
Purpura
Rash (sic) (>10%)
Stevens–Johnson syndrome
  (1991): Porteous DM+, *Arch Dermatol* 127, 741
Urticaria

Hair

Hair – alopecia
Hair – hirsutism

Other

Gingival lichenoid reaction
  (1986): Colvard MD+, *Periodont Case Rep* 8, 69
Headache
Injection-site pain (>10%)
  (1981): Ameer B+, *Drugs* 21, 161 (7–52%)
Injection-site phlebitis (>10%)
  (1981): Clarke RSJ, *Drugs* 22, 26 (15%)
Paresthesias
Pseudolymphoma
  (1995): Magro CM+, *J Am Acad Dermatol* 32, 419
  (1988): Kardaun SH+, *Br J Dermatol* 118(4), 545
Rhabdomyolysis
  (1983): Cauana RJ+, *N C Med J* 44, 18 (with amitriptyline and perphenazine)
Sialopenia (>10%)
Sialorrhea (<1%)
  (1978): Dodson ME+, *Br J Anaesth* 50, 1059
Tremor (1–10%)
Xerostomia (>10%)

LOSARTAN

Synonyms: DuP 753; MK 594
Trade names: Cozaar (Merck); Hyzaar (Merck)
Indications: Hypertension
Category: Angiotensin II receptor antagonist; Antihypertensive
Half-life: 2 hours

Hyzaar is losartan and hydrochlorothiazide

Reactions

Skin
Angioedema (<1%)
  (2002): Abdi R+, *Pharmacotherapy* 22(9), 1173
  (2001): Chiu AG+, *Laryngoscope* 111(10), 1729 (3 cases)
  (1999): Rivera JO, *Ann Pharmacother* 33, 933
  (1999): Rupprecht R+, *Allergy* 54, 81
  (1998): van Rijnsoever EW+, *Arch Intern Med* 158, 2063
  (1996): Boxer M, *J Allergy Clin Immunol* 98, 471
  (1996): *Med Sci Bull* 18, 6
  (1995): Acker CG+, *N Engl J Med* 333, 1572
Dermatitis (sic) (<1%)
Diaphoresis (<1%)
Ecchymoses (<1%)
Edema (<1%)
Erythema (<1%)
Exanthems
Facial edema (<1%)
Flushing (<1%)
  (1995): Ahmad S, *JAMA* 274, 1266
Photosensitivity (<1%)
Pruritus (<1%)
Purpura
  (2001): Brouard M+, *Br J Dermatol* 145(2), 362
  (1998): Bosch X, *Arch Intern Med* 158, 191
Rash (sic) (<1%)
Urticaria (<1%)
Xerosis (<1%)

Hair
Hair – alopecia (<1%)

Other
Ageusia
  (2002): Ohkoshi N+, *Eur J Neurol* 9(3), 315
  (1996): Schlienger RG+, *Lancet* 347, 471
Anaphylactoid reactions (<1%)
Aphthous stomatitis
  (1998): Goffin E+, *Clin Nephrol* 50, 197
Dysgeusia (<1%)
  (1998): Heeringa M+, *Ann Intern Med* 129, 72
Fetal death
  (2001): Saji H+, *Lancet* 357(9253), 363
Headache
Hyperesthesia (<1%)
Myalgia (1%)
Oral ulceration
  (2000): Madinier I+, *Ann Med Interne (Paris)* (French) 151, 248
Paresthesias (<1%)
  (1995): Ahmad S, *JAMA* 274, 1266
Pseudolymphoma
  (1999): Goldstein E, Toronto, ON (from Internet) (observation)
  (1997): Viraben R+, *Lancet* 350, 1366
Tremor (<1%)
Xerostomia (<1%)

LOVASTATIN

Trade names: Advicor (Kos); Altocor (Andryx); Mevacor (Merck)
Other common trade names: *Apo-Lovastatin; Lovalip; Mevinacor; Mevinolin; Nergadan; Rovacor; Taucor*
Indications: Hypercholesterolemia
Category: Antihyperlipidemic; HMG-CoA reductase inhibitor
Half-life: 1–2 hours
Clinically important, potentially hazardous interactions with: atazanavir, azithromycin, bosentan, cholestyramine, clarithromycin, cyclosporine, erythromycin, fenofibrate, gemfibrozil, **grapefruit juice**, imatinib, itraconazole, tacrolimus, verapamil

Reactions

Skin
Erythema
Erythema multiforme
Exanthems
  (1988): Henwood JM+, *Drugs* 36, 429 (5%)
  (1988): Tobert JA+, *Am J Cardiol* 62 (Suppl), 28J (0.3%)
  (1987): Havel RJ+, *Ann Intern Med* 107, 609 (1%)
Flushing
  (2002): Kashyap ML+, *Am J Cardiol* 89(6), 672 (with niacin) (10%)
Lupus erythematosus
  (1994): Yung RL+, *Rheum Dis Clin North Am* 20, 61
  (1993): Ahmad S, *Heart Dis Stroke* 2, 262
  (1991): Ahmad S, *Arch Intern Med* 151, 1667
Pruritus (5.2%)
  (2002): Kashyap ML+, *Am J Cardiol* 89(6), 672 (with niacin)
  (1988): Tobert JA+, *Am J Cardiol* 62 (Suppl), 28J
Purpura
  (1999): Stein EA+, *JAMA* 281, 137
Rash (sic) (5.2%)
  (2002): Kashyap ML+, *Am J Cardiol* 89(6), 672 (with niacin)
  (1993): Krasovec M+, *Dermatology* 186, 248
  (1993): Merck Laboratories, *The Lovastatin Study Groups I through IV* 153, 1079
Stevens–Johnson syndrome
  (1998): Downs JR+, *JAMA* 279, 1615
Toxic epidermal necrolysis
Urticaria
Vasculitis

Hair
Hair – alopecia (>1%)

Other
Dysgeusia (0.8%)
Gynecomastia (1–10%)
  (1999): Stein EA+, *JAMA* 281, 137
Headache
  (2002): Kashyap ML+, *Am J Cardiol* 89(6), 672 (with niacin)
Hypersensitivity
Hyposmia
  (1992): Weber R+, *Laryngorhinootologie* (German) 71, 483
Myalgia (2.4%)
Myopathy (1–10%)
  (1995): Garnett WR, *Am J Health Syst Pharm* 52(15), 1639
  (1990): Kogan AD+, *Postgrad Med J* 66, 294
  (1989): Vaher VMG+, *Lancet* 2, 1098
Paresthesias (>1%)
Pseudolymphoma

(1996): Magro CM+, *Hum Pathol* 27(2), 125
Rhabdomyolysis
  (2000): Davidson MH, *Curr Atheroscler Rep* 2(1), 14
  (1999): Bottorff M, *Atherosclerosis* 147(Suppl 1), S23
  (1999): Corsini A+, *Pharmacol Ther* 84, 413 (with either
    cyclosporine, mibefradil or nefazodone)
  (1998): Reaven P+, *Ann Intern Med* 109, 597 (with nicotinic acid)
  (1998): Tobert JA+, *Am J Cardiol* 62, 28J (with gemfibrozil)
  (1998): Wong PW+, *South Med J* 91(2), 202 (with erythromycin)
  (1997): Chu PH+, *Jpn Heart J* 38(4), 541
  (1997): Grunden JW+, *Ann Pharmacother* 31(7), 859 (with
    azithromycin and clarithromycin)
  (1997): Hermida Lazcano I+, *An Med Interne* 14, 488
  (1997): Olbricht C+, *Clin Pharmacol Ther* 62(3), 311 (with
    cyclosporine)
  (1996): Ballantyne CM+, *Am J Cardiol* 78(5), 532
  (1995): Farmer JA+, *Baillieres Clin Endocrinol Metab* 9(4), 825
  (1995): Garnett WR, *Am J Health Syst Pharm* 52(15), 1639 (with
    either cyclosporine, gemfibrozil or niacin)
  (1994): Dallaire M+, *CMAJ* 150(12), 1991 (with danazol)
  (1992): Hume AL, *Ann Pharmacother* 26(10), 1303
  (1992): Wallace CS+, *Ann Pharmacother* 26(2), 190
  (1990): Pierce LR+, *JAMA* 264(1), 71 (with gemfibrozil)
  (1990): Tobert JA+, *Am J Cardiol* 65(Suppl), 23F
  (1988): Tobert JA+, *Am J Cardiol* 62, 28J (with cyclosporine)
Stomatitis
Xerostomia (>1%)

LOXAPINE

Trade name: Loxitane (Watson)
Other common trade names: *Desconex; Loxapac*
Indications: Psychoses
Category: Anxiolytic; Tricyclic antipsychotic
Half-life: 12–19 hours (terminal)

Reactions

Skin
  Dermatitis (sic)

(1992): Breathnach SM+, *Adverse Drug Reactions and the Skin*
    Blackwell, Oxford, 203 (passim)
Diaphoresis
Exanthems
Facial edema
Neuroleptic malignant syndrome
  (2002): Tajima Y, *Rinsho Byori* 50(2), 133 (with pravastatin)
Photosensitivity (<1%)
  (1991): Anon, *Drug Ther Bull* 29, 41
Pigmentation (<1%)
Pruritus (<1%)
  (1992): Breathnach SM+, *Adverse Drug Reactions and the Skin*
    Blackwell, Oxford, 203 (passim)
Purpura
Rash (sic) (1–10%)
Seborrhea
  (1992): Breathnach SM+, *Adverse Drug Reactions and the Skin*
    Blackwell, Oxford, 203 (passim)
Side effects (sic)
Urticaria

Hair
  Hair – alopecia

Other
  Galactorrhea (<1%)
  Gynecomastia (1–10%)
  Headache
  Myopathy
    (1984): Thase ME+, *J Clin Psychopharmacol* 4, 46
  Paresthesias
  Parkinsonism
  Priapism (<1%)
  Rhabdomyolysis
    (1996): Meltzer HY+, *Neuropsychopharmacology* 15(4), 395
  Xerostomia (>10%)

MAFENIDE*

Trade name: Sulfamylon (Bertek)
Indications: Second and Third degree burns
Category: Antibiotic (topical)
Half-life: N/A

*****Note:** Mafenide is a sulfonamide and can be absorbed systemically.
Sulfonamides can produce severe, possibly fatal, reactions such as
toxic epidermal necrolysis and Stevens-Johnson syndrome

Reactions

Skin

Allergic reactions (sic)
  (1995): McKenna SR+, *Burns* 21(4), 310
Bullous eruption
Burning
Dermatitis
  (1993): Sanz de Galdeano C+, *Contact Dermatitis* 28(4), 249
  (1992): Fernandez JC+, *Contact Dermatitis* 27(4), 262
Edema
Erythema
Excoriations
Facial edema
Pruritus (2.8%)
  (1993): Kucan JO+, *J Burn Care Rehabil* 14(2 Pt 1), 158
Rash (sic) (4.6%)
  (1993): Kucan JO+, *J Burn Care Rehabil* 14(2 Pt 1), 158

Other

Anaphylactoid reactions
Application-site burning
Chondritis
  (2002): Pickus EJ+, *Ann Plast Surg* 48(2), 202
  (1987): Kroll SS+, *Plast Reconstr Surg* 80(2), 298
Death
Diarrhea
Hypersensitivity
  (1988): Perry AW+, *J Burn Care Rehabil* 9(2), 145
Pain
  (1993): Kucan JO+, *J Burn Care Rehabil* 14(2 Pt 1), 158
  (1975): Harrison HN+, *Arch Surg* 110(12), 1446
Porphyria
Pseudochondritis (erythema, edema, pruritus)
  (1988): Perry AW+, *J Burn Care Rehabil* 9(2), 145

MAPROTILINE

Trade name: Ludiomil (Novartis)
Other common trade names: *Delgian; Maprostad; Melodil;
Mirpan; Nono-Maprotiline; Psymion; Retinyl*
Indications: Depression, anxiety
Category: Tetracyclic antidepressant
Half-life: 27–58 hours

Reactions

Skin

Acne
  (1988): Warnock JK+, *Am J Psychiatry* 145, 425
  (1985): Oakley AM+, *Aust N Z J Med* 15, 256
  (1982): Ponte CD, *Am J Psychiatry* 139, 141
Diaphoresis
  (1977): Pinder RM+, *Drugs* 13, 321 (3–8%)

Edema
Erythema
Erythema multiforme
  (1990): Zukervar P+, *J Toxicol Clin Exp* 10, 169
Exanthems (1–5%)
  (1988): Warnock JK+, *Am J Psychiatry* 145, 425
  (1977): Pinder RM+, *Drugs* 13, 321 (3–9%)
  (1976): Johnson NM+, *Lancet* 2, 1357 (4%)
Flushing
Ichthyosis
  (1991): Niederauer HH+, *Hautarzt* (German) 42, 455
Petechiae
Photosensitivity
  (1989): Koch P+, *Derm Beruf Umwelt* (German) 37, 203
  (1988): Warnock JK+, *Am J Psychiatry* 145, 425
Pruritus
Purpura
  (1988): Warnock JK+, *Am J Psychiatry* 145, 425
Rash (sic) (>10%)
Stevens–Johnson syndrome
  (1990): Zukervar P+, *J Toxicol Clin Exp* 10, 169
Urticaria
  (1988): Warnock JK+, *Am J Psychiatry* 145, 425
  (1976): Johnson NM+, *Lancet* 2, 1357 (4%)
Vasculitis
  (1985): Oakley AM+, *Aust N Z J Med* 15, 256

Hair

Hair – alopecia
  (2000): Mercke Y+, *Ann Clin Psychiatry* 12, 35
  (1991): Niederauer HH+, *Hautarzt* (German) 42, 455

Other

Black tongue
Dysgeusia
Galactorrhea
Gynecomastia (<1%)
Headache
Parkinsonism
Sialorrhea
Stomatitis
Tinnitus
Tremor
Xerostomia (22%)
  (1977): Pinder RM+, *Drugs* 13, 321 (30–40%)

MARIHUANA

Trade name: Marihuana
Indications: Nausea and vomiting, substance abuse drug
Category: Hallucinogen
Half-life: N/A
**Clinically important, potentially hazardous interactions
with:** atazanavir

Note: Marihuana is the popular name for the dried flowering leaves
of the hemp plant, *Cannabis sativa*. It contains tetrahydrocannabinols.
It is also known as 'pot,' 'grass,' 'hashish,' etc

Reactions

Skin

Allergic reactions (sic)
  (2000): Perez JA, *J Emerg Med* 18, 260
Exanthems
Pruritus

Squamous metaplasia
(2000): Holdcroft A, *Br J Anaesth* 84(3), 419
Urticaria

Other
Anaphylactoid reactions
(1971): Liskow B+, *Ann Intern Med* 75, 571

MAZINDOL

Trade names: Mazanor (Wyeth); Sanorex (Novartis)
Other common trade names: *Diestet; Liofindol; Solucaps; Teronac*
Indications: Obesity
Category: Anorexiant
Half-life: 10 hours
Clinically important, potentially hazardous interactions with: fluoxetine, fluvoxamine, MAO inhibitors, paroxetine, phenelzine, sertraline, tranylcypromine

Reactions

Skin
Diaphoresis
Edema
Exanthems
Rash (sic)
Urticaria

Other
Dysgeusia
Paresthesias
Xerostomia

MDMA*

Trade name: Ecstacy*
Indications: N/A
Category: Hallucinogenic 'designer drug'; Psychotherapeutic; Recreational drug
Half-life: N/A

Reactions

Skin
Acne
(1998): Wollina U+, *Dermatology* 197(2), 171 (2 cases)
Chills
Diaphoresis
(1999): Rochester JA+, *J Am Board Fam Pract* 12(2), 137
(1998): Weinmann W+, *Forensic Sci Int* 91(2), 91
(1988): Buchanan JF+, *Med Toxicol Adverse Drug Exp* 3(1), 1
Flushing
(1999): Rochester JA+, *J Am Board Fam Pract* 12(2), 137
Rash (sic)

Other
Bruxism
(2001): Murray JB, *Psychol Rep* 88(3 Pt 1), 895
(1999): Milosevic A+, *Community Dent Oral Epidemiol* 27(4), 283
Death
(2001): Braback L+, *Lakartidningen* 98(8), 817 (after one pill)
(2001): Doyon S, *Curr Opin Pediatr* 13(2), 170
(2001): Murray JB, *Psychol Rep* 88(3 Pt 1), 895

(2001): Nielsen S+, *Ugeskr Laeger* 163(16), 2253
(2001): Vickrey V, *Mich Med* 100(6), 53
(2000): Carter N+, *Int J Legal Med* 113(3), 168
(2000): Weir E, *CMAJ* 162(13), 1843
(1999): de la Torre R+, *Lancet* 353(9152), 593
(1999): Fineschi V+, *Forensic Sci Int* 104(1), 65
(1999): Hedetoft C+, *Ugeskr Laeger* 161(50), 6907
(1999): Lind J+, *Lancet* 354(9196), 2167
(1999): Ramsey JD+, *Lancet* 354(9196), 2166
(1999): Schwab M+, *Lancet* 352(9142), 1751
(1999): Walubo A+, *Hum Exp Toxicol* 18(2), 119
(1998): Byard RW+, *Am J Forensic Med Pathol* 19(3), 261 (5 cases)
(1998): Henry JA+, *Lancet* 352(9142), 1751
(1998): Mueller PD+, *Ann Emerg Med* 32(3 Pt 1), 377
(1998): Weinmann W+, *Forensic Sci Int* 91(2), 91
(1997): Parr MJ+, *Med J Aust* 166(3), 136
(1997): Thomasius R+, *Fortschr Neurol Psychiatr* 65(2), 49
(1996): Burnat P+, *Presse Med* 25(26), 1208
(1996): Dowsett RP, *Med J Aust* 164(11), 700
(1996): Fineschi V+, *Int J Legal Med* 108(5), 272
(1996): McCauley JC, *Med J Aust* 164(1), 56
(1996): Milroy CM+, *J Clin Pathol* 49, 149
(1995): Nielsen JC+, *Ugeskr Laeger* 157(6), 724
(1995): Squier MV+, *J Neurol Neurosurg Psychiatry* 58(6), 756
(1994): Szukaj M, *Nervenarzt* 65(11), 802
(1993): Cregg MT+, *Ir Med J* 86(4), 118
(1992): Henry JA, *BMJ* 305, 5
(1992): Henry JA+, *Lancet* 340, 284
(1988): Buchanan JF+, *Med Toxicol Adverse Drug Exp* 3(1), 1
(1988): Suarez RV+, *Am J Forensic Med Pathol* 9(4), 339
(1987): Dowling GP+, *JAMA* 257(12), 1615 (5 cases)
Depression
(2000): Morgan ML, *Psychopharmacol (Berl)* 152(3), 230
(2000): Shannon M, *Pediatr Emerg Care* 16(5), 377
(1999): Rochester JA+, *J Am Board Fam Pract* 12(2), 137
(1998): Liberg JP+, *Tidsskr Nor Laegeforen* 118(28), 4384
(1998): Pennings EJ+, *Ned Tijdschr Geneeskd* 142(35), 1942
(1997): Williamson S+, *Drug Alcohol Depend* 44(2-3), 87
(1993): Cregg MT+, *Ir Med J* 86(4), 118
Jaw clenching
(2001): Murray JB, *Psychol Rep* 88(3 Pt 1), 895
(1999): Milosevic A+, *Community Dent Oral Epidemiol* 27(4), 283
Myalgia
Paresthesias
(2000): Yates KM+, *N Z Med J* 113(1114), 315
Parkinsonism
(1999): Mintzer S+, *N Engl J Med* (340(18) 1443
Priapism
(2000): Dubin N+, *Urology* 56(6), 1057
Rhabdomyolysis
(2002): Smith KM+, *Am J Health Syst Pharm* 59(11), 1067
(2001): Halachanova V+, *Mayo Clin Proc* 76(1), 112
(2001): Kalant H, *CMAJ* 165(7), 917
(2001): Teter CJ+, *Pharmacotherapy* 21(12), 1486
(1999): Fineschi V+, *Forensic Sci Int* 104(1), 65
(1999): Hedetoft C+, *Ugeskr Laeger* 161(50), 6907
(1999): Rochester JA+, *J Am Board Fam Pract* 12(2), 137
(1998): Liberg JP+, *Tidsskr Nor Laegeforen* 118(28), 4384
(1998): Ramcharan S+, *J Toxicol Clin Toxicol* 36(7), 727
(1997): Cunningham M, *Intensive Crit Care Nurs* 13(4), 216
(1997): Trkulja V+, *Lijec Vjesn* 119(5-6), 158
(1997): Tsatsakis AM+, *Vet Hum Toxicol* 39(4), 241
(1996): Ellis AJ+, *Gut* 38(3), 454 (8 cases)
(1996): Fineschi V+, *Int J Legal Med* 108(5), 272
(1996): Gouzoulis-Mayfrank E+, *Nervenarzt* 67(5), 369
(1996): Roebroek RM+, *Ned Tijdschr Geneeskd* 140(4), 205
(1995): Lehmann ED+, *Postgrad Med J* 71(833), 186
(1995): Nielsen JC+, *Ugeskr Laeger* 157(6), 724

(1995): Steidle B+, *Rofo Fortschr Geb Roentgenstr Neuen Bildgeb Verfahr* 163(4), 353
(1994): Forrest AR+, *Forensic Sci Int* 64(1), 57 (fatal)
(1992): Henry JA+, *Lancet* 340(8816), 384 (7 fatal)
(1992): Screaton GR+, *Lancet* 339(8794), 677
(1992): Singarajah C+, *Anaesthesia* 47(8), 686
Serotonin syndrome
(1997): Dinse H, *Anaesthetist* 46(8), 697
(1997): Huether G+, *J Neural Transm* 104(8-9), 771
Tremor
Xerostomia
(1999): Milosevic A+, *Community Dent Oral Epidemiol* 27(4), 283

*Note: 3,4-Methylenedioxymethamphetamine

MEADOWSWEET

Scientific names: *Filipendula ulmaria; Spiraea ulmaria*
Family: Rosaceae
Trade and other common names: Bridewort; Dolloff; Dropwort; Meadow Queen; Meadow-Wart
Category: Anti-inflammatory; Diuretic
Purported indications and other uses: Colds, fevers, cough, bronchitis, dyspepsia, heartburn, peptic ulcer, gout, rheumatic disorders
Half-life: N/A
Clinically important, potentially hazardous interactions with: salicylates

Reactions

Skin
  Rash (sic)

Other
  Hypersensitivity

MEBENDAZOLE

Trade name: Vermox (McNeil)
Other common trade names: *Amycil; Bantenol; Helminzole; Lomper; Mebensole; Mindol; Nemasol; Pantelmin; Revapole; Toloxim; Vermicol*
Indications: Parasitic worm infestations
Category: Anthelmintic
Half-life: 1–12 hours

Reactions

Skin
  Allergic reactions (sic)
    (1979): Kern P+, *Tropenmed Parasitol* 30, 65 (2 in 7 patients)
  Angioedema (<1%)
  Exanthems
  Pruritus (<1%)
  Rash (sic) (<1%)
  Stevens–Johnson syndrome
    (2000): Ajonuma LC+, *Trop Doc* 30, 57
  Urticaria

Hair
  Hair – alopecia
    (1992): Breathnach SM+, *Adverse Drug Reactions and the Skin* Blackwell, Oxford, 177 (passim)

Other
  Xerostomia

MECAMYLAMINE

Trade name: Inversine (Layton Biosciences)
Other common trade name: *Mevasine*
Indications: Hypertension
Category: Antihypertensive; Peripherally acting antiadrenergic ganglion blocker
Half-life: N/A
Clinically important, potentially hazardous interactions with: alcohol, antibiotics, sulfonamides

Reactions

Skin
  Angioedema

Other
  Abdominal pain
  Depression
  Dizziness
  Glossitis
  Paresthesias
  Seizures
  Trembling
  Tremor
  Xerostomia

MECHLORETHAMINE

Synonyms: mustine; nitrogen mustard
Trade name: Mustargen (Merck)
Other common trade names: *Mustine; Mustine Hydrochloride Boots*
Indications: Hodgkin's disease, mycosis fungoides
Category: Antineoplastic
Half-life: <1 minute
Clinically important, potentially hazardous interactions with: aldesleukin, **vaccines**

Reactions

Skin
  Acanthosis nigricans
    (1988): Schweitzer WJ+, *J Am Acad Dermatol* 19, 951
  Angioedema
    (1981): Wilson KS+, *Ann Intern Med* 94, 823
  Bullous eruption
    (1990): Goday JJ+, *Contact Dermatitis* 22, 306
    (1981): Weiss RB+, *Ann Intern Med* 94, 66
  Cellulitis
    (1981): Wilson KS+, *Ann Intern Med* 94, 823
  Cyst
    (1991): Smith SP+, *J Am Acad Dermatol* 25, 940
  Dermatitis (sic)
    (1999): Estève E+, *Arch Dermatol* 135, 1349
    (1991): Sheehan MP+, *J Pediatr* 119, 317
    (1988): Ramsay DL+, *J Am Acad Dermatol* 19, 684
    (1986): Mauduit G+, *Br J Dermatol* 115, 82
    (1985): Arrazola JM+, *Int J Dermatol* 24, 608

(1985): Zachariae H, *Int J Clin Pharmacol Res* 5, 193
(1984): Ramsay DL+, *Arch Dermatol* 120, 1585
(1984): Vonderheid EC, *Int J Dermatol* 23, 180
(1983): Bronner AK+, *J Am Acad Dermatol* 9, 645
(1983): Nusbaum BP+, *Arch Dermatol* 119, 117
(1983): Price NM+, *Cancer* 52, 2214
(1982): Price NM+, *Arch Dermatol* 118, 234
(1981): Halprin KM+, *Br J Dermatol* 105, 71
(1981): Shelley WB, *Acta Derm Venereol* 61, 161
(1979): Handler RM+, *Int J Dermatol* 18, 758
(1978): du Vivier A+, *BMJ* 2, 1300
(1978): Volden G+, *BMJ* 2, 865
(1977): Price NM+, *Br J Dermatol* 97, 547
(1977): Sanchez-Yus E+, *Actas Dermosifiliogr* (Spanish) 68, 39
(1977): Volden G+, *Tidsskr Nor Laegeforen* (Norwegian) 97, 1671
(1976): Grunnet E, *Br J Dermatol* 94, 101
(1976): Pariser DM+, *Arch Dermatol* 112, 1113
(1975): Constantine VS+, *Arch Dermatol* 111, 484
(1975): Mitchell JC+, *Contact Dermatitis* 1, 363
(1971): Mandy S+, *Arch Dermatol* 103, 272
(1970): Van Scott EJ+, *Arch Dermatol* 102, 507
Erythema multiforme (<1%)
(1967): Brauer MJ+, *Arch Intern Med* 120, 499
Exanthems (<1%)
Fungal infections (sic)
(1981): Shelley WB, *Acta Derm Venereol* 61, 164
Herpes zoster (>10%)
Pigmentation
(1984): Vonderheid EC, *Int J Dermatol* 23, 180
(1983): Bronner AK+, *J Am Acad Dermatol* 9, 645
(1982): Price NM+, *Arch Dermatol* 118, 234
(1977): Price NM, *Arch Dermatol* 113, 1387
(1975): O'Doherty CS, *Lancet* 2, 365
(1973): Flaxman BA+, *J Invest Dermatol* 60, 321
(1970): Epstein E Jr+, *Arch Dermatol* 102, 504
(1970): Van Scott EJ+, *Arch Dermatol* 102, 507
Pruritus
(1981): Weiss RB+, *Ann Intern Med* 94, 66
(1981): Wilson KS+, *Ann Intern Med* 94, 823
Purpura
(1981): Weiss RB+, *Ann Intern Med* 94, 66
Rash (sic) (<1%)
Squamous cell carcinoma
(1991): Smith SP+, *J Am Acad Dermatol* 25, 940
(1982): Lee LA+, *J Am Acad Dermatol* 7, 590
(1978): du Vivier A+, *Br J Dermatol* 99, 61
Stevens–Johnson syndrome
(1997): Newman JM+, *J Am Acad Dermatol* 36, 112
Urticaria
(1981): Weiss RB+, *Ann Intern Med* 94, 66
(1981): Wilson KS+, *Ann Intern Med* 94, 823
(1973): Daughters D+, *Arch Dermatol* 107, 429
Xerosis
(1984): Vonderheid EC, *Int J Dermatol* 23, 180

Hair

Hair – alopecia (1–10%)

Other

Anaphylactoid reactions (1–10%)
(1983): Bronner AK+, *J Am Acad Dermatol* 9, 645
(1977): Sanchez-Yus E+, *Actas Dermosifiliogr* (Spanish) 68, 39
(1976): Grunnet E, *Br J Dermatol* 94, 101
(1973): Daughters D+, *Arch Dermatol* 107, 429
Dysgeusia (1–10%) (metallic taste)
Headache
Hypersensitivity (1–10%)
(1972): Zackheim HS+, *Arch Dermatol* 105, 702
Injection-site extravasation (1–10%)

(2000): Kassner E., *J Pediatr Oncol Nurs* 17, 135
Injection-site thrombophlebitis (1–10%)
(1989): Kerker BJ+, *Semin Dermatol* 8, 173
(1981): Wilson KS+, *Ann Intern Med* 94, 823
Tinnitus

MECLIZINE

Trade name: Antivert (Roerig)
Other common trade names: *Antrizine; Bonamine; Bonine; Dizmiss; Dramamine II; Dramine; Meni-D; Nico-Vert; Peremesin; Postadoxin; Postafen; Suprimal; Vergon*
Indications: Motion sickness
Category: Antiemetic; Antihistamine H$_1$-blocker
Half-life: 6 hours
Clinically important, potentially hazardous interactions with: alcohol, barbiturates, chloral hydrate, ethchlorvynol, paraldehyde, phenothiazines, zolpidem

Reactions

Skin

Angioedema (<1%)
Exanthems
  (2001): Litt JZ, Beachwood, OH (personal case) (observation)
Photosensitivity (<1%)
Rash (sic) (<1%)
Urticaria

Other

Myalgia (<1%)
Paresthesias (<1%)
Tremor
Xerostomia (1–10%)

MECLOFENAMATE

Trade name: Meclofenamate
Other common trade names: *Kyroxan; Melvon; Movens*
Indications: Arthritis
Category: Nonsteroidal anti-inflammatory (NSAID)
Half-life: 2 hours
Clinically important, potentially hazardous interactions with: methotrexate

Reactions

Skin

Angioedema (<1%)
(1984): Stern RS+, *JAMA* 252, 1433
Bullous eruption
Edema (>1%)
Erythema multiforme (<1%)
(1985): Bigby M+, *J Am Acad Dermatol* 12, 866
(1984): Stern RS+, *JAMA* 252, 1433
(1983): Harrington T, *J Rheumatol* 10, 169
Erythema nodosum (<1%)
Erythroderma
(1985): Bigby M+, *J Am Acad Dermatol* 12, 866
Exanthems (1–5%)
(1992): Breathnach SM+, *Adverse Drug Reactions and the Skin* Blackwell, Oxford, 190 (passim)
(1985): Bigby M+, *J Am Acad Dermatol* 12, 866 (3–9%)

(1984): Stern RS+, *JAMA* 252, 1433
(1978): Dresner AJ, *Curr Ther Res* 23, 107
Exfoliative dermatitis (<1%)
 (1992): Breathnach SM+, *Adverse Drug Reactions and the Skin*
  Blackwell, Oxford, 190 (passim)
 (1984): Stern RS+, *JAMA* 252, 1433
Fixed eruption (<1%)
 (1992): Breathnach SM+, *Adverse Drug Reactions and the Skin*
  Blackwell, Oxford, 190 (passim)
 (1985): Bigby M+, *J Am Acad Dermatol* 12, 866
 (1984): Stern RS+, *JAMA* 252, 1433
Hot flashes (<1%)
Lupus erythematosus
Peripheral edema
Photosensitivity
 (1985): Bigby M+, *J Am Acad Dermatol* 12, 866
 (1984): Stern RS+, *JAMA* 252, 1433
Pruritus (1–10%)
 (1992): Breathnach SM+, *Adverse Drug Reactions and the Skin*
  Blackwell, Oxford, 190 (passim)
 (1985): Bigby M+, *J Am Acad Dermatol* 12, 866
 (1984): Stern RS+, *JAMA* 252, 1433
Psoriasis (exacerbation)
 (1983): Meyerhoff JO, *N Engl J Med* 309, 496
Purpura (>1%)
 (1992): Breathnach SM+, *Adverse Drug Reactions and the Skin*
  Blackwell, Oxford, 190 (passim)
 (1985): Bigby M+, *J Am Acad Dermatol* 12, 866
 (1984): Stern RS+, *JAMA* 252, 1433
 (1981): Rodriguez J, *Drug Intell Clin Pharm* 15, 999
Rash (sic) (3–9%)
 (1984): Stern RS+, *JAMA* 252, 1433
Stevens–Johnson syndrome (<1%)
Toxic epidermal necrolysis (<1%)
Urticaria (>1%)
 (1985): Bigby M+, *J Am Acad Dermatol* 12, 866
 (1984): Stern RS+, *JAMA* 252, 1433
Vasculitis
 (1992): Breathnach SM+, *Adverse Drug Reactions and the Skin*
  Blackwell, Oxford, 190 (passim)
 (1985): Bigby M+, *J Am Acad Dermatol* 12, 866
 (1984): Stern RS+, *JAMA* 252, 1433
Vesiculobullous eruption
 (1992): Breathnach SM+, *Adverse Drug Reactions and the Skin*
  Blackwell, Oxford, 190 (passim)
 (1984): Stern RS+, *JAMA* 252, 1433

Hair

Hair – alopecia (<1%)

Other

Aphthous stomatitis
 (1996): Fetterman M, Hialeah, FL (from Internet) (observation)
Dysgeusia (<1%)
Headache
Hypersensitivity
 (1993): Fernandez-Rivas M+, *Ann Allergy* 71, 515
Oral ulceration
Paresthesias (<1%)
Porphyria
Serum sickness
Stomatitis (1–3%)
Tinnitus
Xerostomia

MEDROXYPROGESTERONE

Trade names: Amen (Carnrick); Cycrin (Wyeth); Depo-Provera (Pharmacia); Lunelle (Pharmacia); Premphase (Wyeth); Prempro (Wyeth); Provera (Pharmacia)
Other common trade names: *Alti-MPA; Aragest 5; Clinofem; Gestapuran; Novo-Medrone; Perlutex; Progevera; Ralovera*
Indications: Secondary amenorrhea, renal or endometrial carcinoma
Category: Antineoplastic; Contraceptive; Progestin
Half-life: 30 days
Clinically important, potentially hazardous interactions with: acitretin, dofetilide

Reactions

Skin

Acne (1–5%)
 (1974): Pochi PE, *Arch Dermatol* 109, 556
Allergic reactions (sic) (<1%)
Angioedema
Ankle edema
Chloasma (1–10%)
Diaphoresis (<1%)
 (1990): Willemse PHB+, *Eur J Cancer* 26, 337 (31%)
Edema (>10%)
Erythema nodosum
 (1974): Berant N, *Harefuah* (Hebrew) 87, 19
Exanthems
Flushing
 (1990): Willemse PHB+, *Eur J Cancer* 26, 337 (12%)
Hemorrhage (sic)
Hot flashes
Melasma (1–10%)
Mucha–Habermann disease
 (1973): Hollander A+, *Arch Dermatol* 107, 465
Photosensitivity
Pigmented purpuric eruption
 (2000): Tsao H+, *J Am Acad Dermatol* 43, 308
Pruritus (1–10%)
Rash (sic) (1–5%)
Scleroderma (<1%)
Striae
 (2000): Gupta M, *Br J Fam Plann* 26, 104
Urticaria
Xerosis (<1%)

Hair

Hair – alopecia (1–5%)
Hair – hirsutism (<1%)
 (1984): Delanoe D+, *Lancet* 1, 276

Other

Anaphylactoid reactions (<1%)
Bromhidrosis (<1%)
Galactorrhea (<1%)
 (1998): Cromwell P+, *J Adolesc Health* 23, 61
Gynecomastia (<1%)
Headache
Injection-site necrosis
 (2000): Clark SM+, *Br J Dermatol* 143, 1356
Injection-site pain (>10%)
Mastodynia (1–5%)
Paresthesias (<1%)
Thrombophlebitis (1–10%)
Vaginitis (1–5%)

MEFENAMIC ACID

Trade name: Ponstel (First Horizon)
Other common trade names: *Dysman; Lysalgo; Mefac; Mefic; Parkemed; Ponstan; Ponstyl*
Indications: Pain, dysmenorrhea
Category: Nonsteroidal anti-inflammatory (NSAID)
Half-life: 3.5 hours
Clinically important, potentially hazardous interactions with: methotrexate

Reactions

Skin
Angioedema (<1%)
Bullous pemphigoid
  (1986): Shepherd AN+, *Postgrad Med J* 62, 67
Diaphoresis
Edema
Erythema multiforme (<1%)
  (1990): Sowden JM+, *Clin Exp Dermatol* 15, 387
  (1985): Ting HC+, *Int J Dermatol* 24, 587
Exanthems
  (1992): Breathnach SM+, *Adverse Drug Reactions and the Skin*
    Blackwell, Oxford, 190 (passim)
Exfoliative dermatitis
  (1992): Breathnach SM+, *Adverse Drug Reactions and the Skin*
    Blackwell, Oxford, 190 (passim)
Facial edema
Fixed eruption
  (1998): Mahboob A+, *Int J Dermatol* 37, 833
  (1992): Long CC+, *Br J Dermatol* 126, 409
  (1991): Mohamed KN, *Aust N Z J Med* 21, 291
  (1990): Sowden JM+, *Clin Exp Dermatol* 15, 387
  (1986): Watson A+, *Australas J Dermatol* 27, 6
  (1986): Wilson CL+, *BMJ* 293, 1243
Hot flashes (<1%)
Photosensitivity
  (1997): O'Reilly FM+, American Academy of Dermatology
    Meeting, Poster #14
Pruritus (1–10%)
Purpura
Rash (sic) (>10%)
Stevens–Johnson syndrome (<1%)
  (1991): Chan JC+, *Drug Safety* 6, 230
Toxic epidermal necrolysis (<1%)
  (1991): Sakellariou G+, *Int J Artif Organs* 14, 634
  (1990): Black AK+, *Br J Dermatol* 123, 277
Urticaria (<1%)
  (1992): Breathnach SM+, *Adverse Drug Reactions and the Skin*
    Blackwell, Oxford, 190 (passim)
Vasculitis
  (1980): Malik S+, *Lancet* 2, 746

Other
Anaphylactoid reactions
  (1985): O'Brien WM+, *J Rheumatol* 12, 13
Glossitis
Headache
Oral ulceration
Pseudoporphyria
  (1998): O'Hagan AH+, *Br J Dermatol* 139, 1131
Sialorrhea
Xerostomia

MEFLOQUINE

Trade name: Lariam (Roche)
Other common trade names: *Laricam; Mephaquin; Mephaquine*
Indications: Malaria
Category: Antimalarial
Half-life: 21–22 days

Reactions

Skin
Erythema
  (1992): Breathnach SM+, *Adverse Drug Reactions and the Skin*
    Blackwell, Oxford, 176 (passim)
Erythema multiforme
Exanthems
  (1999): Smith HR+, *Clin Exp Dermatol* 24, 249 (30%)
Exfoliative dermatitis
  (1993): Martin GJ+, *Clin Infect Dis* 16, 341
Facial dermatitis
  (1991): Shlim DR, *JAMA* 266, 2560
Pruritus
  (1999): Smith HR+, *Clin Exp Dermatol* 24, 249 (4–10%)
  (1989): Sowunmi A+, *Lancet* 2, 313; 397
Psoriasis
  (1998): Potasman I+, *J Travel Med* 5, 156
Rash (sic) (1–10%)
Stevens–Johnson syndrome
  (1999): Smith HR+, *Clin Exp Dermatol* 24, 249
  (1991): Van den Enden E+, *Lancet* 337, 683
Toxic epidermal necrolysis
  (1999): Smith HR+, *Clin Exp Dermatol* 24, 249 (fatal)
  (1997): McBride SR+, *Lancet* 349, 101
Urticaria
  (1999): Smith HR+, *Clin Exp Dermatol* 24, 249
Vasculitis
  (1999): Smith HR+, *Clin Exp Dermatol* 24, 249
  (1995): White AC+, *Ann Intern Med* 123, 894
  (1993): Scerri L+, *Int J Dermatol* 32, 517

Hair
Hair – alopecia (<1%)

Other
Death
Depression
  (2002): van Riemsdijk MM+, *Clin Pharmacol Ther* 72(3), 294
Headache
Myalgia (1–10%)
Tinnitus

MELATONIN

Scientific name: *N-acetyl-5-methoxytryptamine*
Family: None
Trade and other common names: MEL; MLT
Category: Chemoprotectant; Circadian rhythm regulator
Purported indications and other uses: Jet lag, sleep disorders, Alzheimer's disease, free radical scavenger, chemotherapy adjunct, tinnitus, depression, migraine, cluster headache, hypertension, hyperpigmentation, osteoporosis, antioxidant. Skin protectant against sunburn
Half-life: N/A
Clinically important, potentially hazardous interactions with: acetaminophen, NSAIDs, warfarin, zoloft

Reactions

Skin
Fixed eruption
  (2001): Morera AL+, *Actas Esp Psiquiatr* 29(5), 334 (2 cases)
  (1998): Bardazzi F+, *Acta Derm Venereol* 78(1), 69
Photosensitivity
  (1999): Haga HJ+, *Lupus* 8(4), 269

Other
Confusion
  (2001): Morera AL+, *Actas Esp Psiquiatr* 29(5), 334 (overdose)
Crohn's disease
  (2002): Calvo JR+, *J Pineal Res* 32(4), 277
Seizures
  (2001): Morera AL+, *Actas Esp Psiquiatr* 29(5), 334 (4 cases)

MELOXICAM

Trade name: Mobic (Boehringer Ingelheim)
Indications: Osteoarthritis
Category: Nonsteroidal anti-inflammatory (NSAID)
Half-life: 15–20 hours

Reactions

Skin
Adverse effects (sic)
  (1996): Huskisson EC+, *Br J Rheumatol* 35, 29 (18%)
Allergic reactions (sic) (<2%)
Angioedema (<2%)
  (2000): Quaratino D+, *Ann Allergy Asthma Immunol* 84, 613
Bullous eruption (<2%)
Edema (2–5%)
Erythema multiforme (<2%)
  (1999): Nikas SN+, *Am J Med* 107, 532
Exanthems (<2%)
  (2000): Quaratino D+, *Ann Allergy Asthma Immunol* 84, 613
Facial edema
  (2000): Quaratino D+, *Ann Allergy Asthma Immunol* 84, 613
Hot flashes (<2%)
Photosensitivity (<2%)
Pruritus (<2%)
  (2001): Bunyaratavej N+, *J Med Assoc Thai* 84(Suppl 2), S542 (2%)
Purpura (<2%)
Rash (sic) (1–3%)
  (2001): Bunyaratavej N+, *J Med Assoc Thai* 84, S542 (2%)
Stevens–Johnson syndrome (<2%)

Toxic epidermal necrolysis (<2%)
  (2002): Eastern J, North Caldwell, NJ (from Internet) (observation)
Urticaria (<2%)
  (2000): Quaratino D+, *Ann Allergy Asthma Immunol* 84, 613
Vasculitis (<2%)

Other
Anaphylactoid reactions (<2%)
Dysgeusia (<2%)
Headache
Hypersensitivity
  (2001): Nettis E+, *Allergy* 56(8), 803
Paresthesias (<2%)
Tremor (<2%)
Ulcerative stomatitis (<2%)
Xerostomia (<2%)

MELPHALAN

Trade name: Alkeran (GSK)
Indications: Multiple myeloma, carcinomas
Category: Antineoplastic; Nitrogen mustard
Half-life: 90 minutes
Clinically important, potentially hazardous interactions with: aldesleukin, PEG-interferon alfa-2b

Reactions

Skin
Angioedema
  (1983): Bronner AK+, *J Am Acad Dermatol* 9, 645
  (1981): Weiss RB+, *Ann Intern Med* 94, 66
Eccrine squamous syringometaplasia
  (1997): Valks R+, *Arch Dermatol* 133, 873
Edema
Exanthems
  (1981): Harvey HA+, *Ann Intern Med* 94, 542
  (1981): Weiss RB+, *Ann Intern Med* 94, 66
  (1978): Levine N+, *Cancer Treat Rev* 5, 67
  (1969): Hoogstraten B+, *JAMA* 209, 251 (4%)
Petechiae
Pruritus (1–10%)
  (1983): Bronner AK+, *J Am Acad Dermatol* 9, 645
Purpura
Rash (sic) (1–10%)
Scleroderma (localized)
  (1998): Landau M+, *J Am Acad Dermatol* 39, 1011 (2 cases)
Urticaria
  (1983): Bronner AK+, *J Am Acad Dermatol* 9, 645
  (1981): Harvey HA+, *Ann Intern Med* 94, 542
  (1981): Weiss RB+, *Ann Intern Med* 94, 66
Vasculitis (1–10%)
  (1986): Hannedouche T+, *Ann Med Intern* (Paris) (French) 137, 57
Vesiculation (1–10%)

Hair
Hair – alopecia (1–10%)
  (1992): Zaun H+, *Hautarzt* (German) 43, 215
  (1978): Levine N+, *Cancer Treat Rev* 5, 67

Nails
Nails – Beau's lines (transverse nail bands)
  (1992): Zaun H+, *Hautarzt* (German) 43, 215
  (1983): James WD+, *Arch Dermatol* 119, 334

(1982): Jeanmougin M+, *Ann Dermatol Venereol* (French) 109, 169
(1977): Malacarne P+, *Arch Dermatol Res* 25, 81

Other

Anaphylactoid reactions
(1983): Bronner AK+, *J Am Acad Dermatol* 9, 645
(1982): Dunagin WG, *Semin Oncol* 9, 14
Death
(2001): Sanchorawala V+, *Bone Marrow Transplant* 28(7), 637 (14%)
Gynecomastia
(2000): Cohen JD+, *Presse Med* 29(35), 1936
Hypersensitivity (1–10%)
(1992): Weiss RB, *Semin Oncol* 19, 458
Injection-site edema
(1995): Vrouenraets BC+, *Melanoma Res* 5, 425
Mucositis
(2002): Moreau P+, *Blood* 99(3), 731
Oral mucosal lesions
Oral mucositis
(2000): Wardley AM+, *Br J Haematol* 110, 292
Oral ulceration
Perfusion edema
(1995): Vrouenraets BC+, *Melanoma Res* 5, 425
Stomatitis (1–10%)

MEPACRINE

(See QUINACRINE)

MEPERIDINE

Trade names: Demerol (Sanofi-Synthelabo); Mepergan (Wyeth)
Other common trade names: *Dolantin; Dolestine; Dolosal; Opistan; Pethidine; Petidin*
Indications: Pain
Category: Narcotic agonist analgesic
Half-life: 3–4 hours
Clinically important, potentially hazardous interactions with: acyclovir, **alcohol**, amphetamines, barbiturates, CNS depressants, fluoxetine, furazolidone, general anesthetics, isocarboxazid, linezolid, lithium, MAO inhibitors, moclobemide, phenelzine, phenobarbital, phenothiazines, phenytoin, ritonavir, selegiline, sibutramine, SSRIs, tranquilizers, tranylcypromine, tricyclic antidepressants, valacyclovir

Reactions

Skin

Angioedema
(1960): Schoenfeld MR, *N Y State J Med* 60, 2591
Diaphoresis
Flushing
Herpes (sic)
(1986): Acalovschi I, *Anaesthesia* 41, 1271
Necrotizing angiitis
(1971): Halpern M+, *Am J Roentgenol Radium Ther Nucl Med* 111, 663
Pruritus
(1993): Riley RH, *Anaesth Intensive Care* 21, 474
(1984): Saissy JM, *Ann Fr Anesth Reanim* (French) 3, 402
(1960): Schoenfeld MR, *N Y State J Med* 60, 2591
Rash (sic) (<1%)

Toxic epidermal necrolysis
(1967): Caldwell IW+, *Br J Dermatol* 79, 287
Urticaria (<1%)
(2000): Anibarro B+, *Allergy* 55, 305

Other

Cold microabscesses
(1978): Waisbren BA, *JAMA* 239, 1395
Embolia cutis medicamentosa (Nicolau syndrome)
(1995): Faucher L+, *Pediatr Dermatol* 12, 187
Injection-site erythema
(1993): Kundrotas L+, *Gastrointest Endosc* 39, 109
(1960): Schoenfeld MR, *N Y State J Med* 60, 2591
Injection-site pain (1–10%)
Injection-site scarring
(1994): Danielsen AG+, *Ugeskr Laeger* (Danish) 156, 162
Injection-site ulceration
(1994): Danielsen AG+, *Ugeskr Laeger* (Danish) 156, 162
Myopathy
(1968): Aberfeld DC+, *Arch Neurol* 19, 384
Tremor
Xerostomia (1–10%)

MEPHENYTOIN

Trade name: Mesantoin (Novartis)
Other common trade names: *Epilan-Gerot; Epilanex*
Indications: Partial seizures
Category: Hydantoin anticonvulsant
Half-life: 7 hours (for the active metabolite: 95–144 hours)
Clinically important, potentially hazardous interactions with: chloramphenicol, cyclosporine, disulfiram, dopamine, imatinib, itraconazole

Reactions

Skin

Acne
(1951): Frankel AZ+, *Ohio State Med J* 47, 1013
Angioedema
(1951): Frankel AZ+, *Ohio State Med J* 47, 1013
Bullous eruption
(1948): Ruskin DB, *JAMA* 137, 1031
Dermatomyositis
(1977): Zangemeister WH+, *Fortschr Neurol Psychiatr Grenzgeb* (German) 45, 501
Edema
Erythema multiforme
(1979): Pollack MA+, *Ann Neurol* 5, 262
(1951): Frankel AZ+, *Ohio State Med J* 47, 1013
(1951): Lindermayr W, *Hautarzt* (German) 2, 313
Exanthems
(1972): Levantine A+, *Br J Dermatol* 87, 646 (8–10%)
(1954): Dreyer R, *Dtsch Med Wochenschr* (German) 79, 1215
(1952): McArthur P, *Lancet* 1, 592 (5%)
(1951): Frankel AZ+, *Ohio State Med J* 47, 1013 (8.85%)
(1951): Lindermayr W, *Hautarzt* (German) 2, 313
Exfoliative dermatitis
(1951): Frankel AZ+, *Ohio State Med J* 47, 1013
Lupus erythematosus
(1989): Vivino FB+, *Arthritis Rheum* 32, 560
(1980): Condemi JJ, *Geriatrics* 35(3), 81
(1977): Zangemeister WH+, *Fortschr Neurol Psychiatr Grenzgeb* (German) 45, 501
(1976): Singsen BH+, *Pediatrics* 57, 529
(1968): Cochran M+, *Proc R Soc Med* 61, 656

(1967): Losada M+, *Rev Med Chil* (Spanish) 95, 380 (generalized)
(1965): Schütz E+, *Med Klin* (German) 60, 537
(1963): Jacobs JC, *Pediatrics* 32, 257
(1957): Lindquist T, *Acta Med Scand* 158, 131
(1957): Ruppli H+, *Schweiz Med Wochenschr* (German) 88, 1555
(1955): Capalbo EE+, *Rev Soc Argent Hemat* (Spanish) 5, 19
Pigmentation
(1964): Krebs A, *Schweiz Med Wochenschr* (German) 94, 748
(1964): Kuske H+, *Dermatologica* 129, 121
(1954): Dreyer R, *Dtsch Med Wochenschr* (German) 79, 1215
(Addison-like)
(1951): Hunter H+, *JAMA* 147, 744
Pruritus
(1954): Dreyer R, *Dtsch Med Wochenschr* (German) 79, 1215
Purpura
(1955): Capalbo EE+, *Rev Soc Argent Hemat* (Spanish) 5, 19
Scleroderma
(1990): May DG+, *Clin Pharmacol Ther* 28, 286
Side effects (sic)
(1951): Frankel AZ+, *Ohio State Med J* 47, 1013 (10%)
Stevens–Johnson syndrome
(1951): Frankel AZ+, *Ohio State Med J* 47, 1013
Toxic epidermal necrolysis
(1979): Pollack MA+, *Ann Neurol* 5, 262
(1976): Babala J+, *Acta Paediatr Acad Sci Hung* 17, 9
(1976): Nozickova M+, *Cesk Dermatol* (Czech) 51, 375
(1962): Walker J, *Med Proc* 8, 208
Urticaria
(1972): Levantine A+, *Br J Dermatol* 87, 646
(1951): Frankel AZ+, *Ohio State Med J* 47, 1013
(1951): Lindermayr W, *Hautarzt* (German) 2, 313

Hair

Hair – alopecia

Other

Gingival hyperplasia
Oral mucosal eruption
(1954): Dreyer R, *Dtsch Med Wochenschr* (German) 79, 1215
Polyarteritis nodosa
(1951): Frankel AZ+, *Ohio State Med J* 47, 1013
Stomatitis
(1996): Meloni G+, *Lancet* 347, 1691

MEPHOBARBITAL

Trade name: Mebaral (Sanofi-Synthelabo)
Other common trade name: *Prominal*
Indications: Epilepsy, anxiety
Category: Anticonvulsant; Barbiturate; Sedative
Half-life: 34 hours
**Clinically important, potentially hazardous interactions
with: alcohol**, anticoagulants, antihistamines, brompheniramine,
buclizine, chlorpheniramine, dicumarol, ethanolamine, imatinib,
warfarin

Reactions

Skin

Angioedema (<1%)
Exanthems
Exfoliative dermatitis (<1%)
Purpura
Rash (sic) (<1%)
Stevens–Johnson syndrome (<1%)
Urticaria

Other

Rhabdomyolysis
(1990): Larpin R+, *Presse Med* 19(30), 1403
Serum sickness
Thrombophlebitis (<1%)

MEPROBAMATE

Trade names: Equagesic (Women First); Miltown (Wallace)
Other common trade names: *Harmonin; Meditran; Meditrara;
Meprate; Meprospan; Miltaun; Neuramate; Praol; Probamyl; Urbilat;
Visanon*
Indications: Anxiety, insomnia
Category: Anxiolytic
Half-life: 10 hours

Reactions

Skin

Allergic reactions (sic)
(1955): Selling LS, *JAMA* 157, 1594 (1.1%)
Angioedema (<1%)
(1964): Welsh AL, *Med Clin North Am* 48, 459
(1958): Hollister LE, *Ann Intern Med* 49, 17
(1957): Bernstein C+, *JAMA* 163, 930
(1955): Selling LS, *JAMA* 157, 1594
Bullous eruption (<1%)
(1977): Varma AJ+, *Arch Intern Med* 137, 1208 (passim)
(1974): Tay C, *Asian J Med* 10, 223
Dermatitis (sic) (<1%)
Ecchymoses
Eczema (sic)
(1981): Edwards JG, *Drugs* 22, 495 (passim)
Erythema multiforme (<1%)
(1972): Kauppinen K, *Acta Derm Venereol* (Stockh) 52, 68
(1959): Wright W, *JAMA* 171, 1642
Erythema nodosum (<1%)
Exanthems
(1981): Edwards JG, *Drugs* 22, 495 (passim)
(1972): Kauppinen K, *Acta Derm Venereol* (Stockh) 52 (Suppl), 68
(1969): Savin JA, *Proc R Soc Med* 62, 349
(1967): Lockey SD, *Med Sci* 18, 43
(1966): Smith JW+, *Ann Intern Med* 65, 629 (2%)
(1965): Fellner MJ+, *Med Clin North Am* 49, 709
(1964): Welsh AL, *Med Clin North Am* 48, 459
(1959): Wright W, *JAMA* 171, 1642
(1958): Marcussen PV, *Acta Derm Venereol* (Stockh) 38, 398
(1957): Falk MS, *Arch Dermatol* 75, 437
(1956): Friedman HT+, *JAMA* 162, 628
Exfoliative dermatitis
Fixed eruption (<1%)
(1985): Kauppinen K+, *Br J Dermatol* 112, 575
(1984): Boyle J+, *BMJ* 289, 802
(1981): Edwards JG, *Drugs* 22, 495 (passim)
(1972): Kauppinen K, *Acta Derm Venereol* (Stockh) 52 (Suppl), 68
(1965): Gore HC+, *Arch Dermatol* 91, 627
Lupus erythematosus
(1957): Bernstein C+, *JAMA* 163, 930
Pemphigus
(1980): Godard W+, *Ann Dermatol Venereol* (French) 107, 1213
Pemphigus foliaceus
(1980): Godard W+, *Ann Dermatol Venereol* (French) 107, 1213
Peripheral edema (<1%)
Petechiae
(1956): Carmel WJ+, *N Engl J Med* 255, 770

Photosensitivity
 (1957): Bernstein C+, *JAMA* 163, 930
Pityriasis rosea
 (1959): Wright W, *JAMA* 171, 1642
Pruritus (<1%)
 (1970): Savin JA, *Br J Dermatol* 83, 546
 (1969): Savin JA, *Proc R Soc Med* 62, 349
 (1964): Welsh AL, *Med Clin North Am* 48, 459
 (1957): Falk MS, *Arch Dermatol* 75, 437
 (1956): Carmel WJ+, *N Engl J Med* 255, 770
 (1956): Friedman HT+, *JAMA* 162, 628
Purpura (<1%)
 (1993): Pang BK+, *Ann Acad Med Singapore* 22, 870
 (1985): Ambriz-Fernandez R+, *Rev Invest Clin* (Spanish) 37, 347
 (1981): Edwards JG, *Drugs* 22, 495 (passim)
 (1970): Savin JA, *Br J Dermatol* 83, 546
 (1969): Peterkin GAG+, *Practitioner* 202, 117
 (1969): Savin JA, *Proc R Soc Med* 62, 349
 (1967): Lockey SD, *Med Sci* 18, 43
 (1967): Peterson WC+, *Arch Dermatol* 95, 40
 (1957): Bernstein C+, *JAMA* 163, 930
 (1957): Falk MS, *Arch Dermatol* 75, 437
 (1957): Levan NE, *Arch Dermatol* 75, 437
 (1956): Carmel WJ Jr+, *N Engl J Med* 255, 770
 (1956): Friedman HT+, *JAMA* 162, 628
Rash (sic) (1–10%)
Side effects (sic)
 (1972): Kauppinen K, *Acta Derm Venereol* (Stockh) 52 (Suppl), 68 (2%)
 (1968): Montgomery DC+, *Can Med Assoc J* 99, 712 (2%)
Stevens–Johnson syndrome (<1%)
 (1972): Kauppinen K, *Acta Derm Venereol* (Stockh) 52 (Suppl), 68
 (1959): Wright W, *JAMA* 171, 1642
Toxic epidermal necrolysis (<1%)
 (1969): Sander-Jensen K, *Tidsskr Nor Laegeforen* (Norwegian) 89, 398
Toxic erythema
 (1974): Felix RH+, *Lancet* 1, 1017
Urticaria
 (1981): Edwards JG, *Drugs* 22, 495 (passim)
 (1972): Kauppinen K, *Acta Derm Venereol* (Stockh) 52 (Suppl), 68
 (1967): Lockey SD, *Med Sci* 18, 43
 (1966): Smith JW+, *Ann Intern Med* 65, 629 (2%)
 (1964): Welsh AL, *Med Clin North Am* 48, 459
 (1959): Wright W, *JAMA* 171, 1642
 (1958): Hollister LE, *Ann Intern Med* 49, 17
 (1957): Bernstein C+, *JAMA* 163, 930
 (1956): Friedman HT+, *JAMA* 162, 628
 (1955): Selling LS, *JAMA* 157, 1594
Vasculitis
 (1964): Welsh AL, *Med Clin North Am* 48, 459
 (1962): Schwank R, *Cesk Dermatol* 37, 6
 (1959): Wright W, *JAMA* 171, 1642
 (1958): von Marcussen P, *Acta Derm Venereol* (Stock) 38, 398
 (1957): Bernstein C+, *JAMA* 163, 930
 (1957): Falk MS, *Arch Dermatol* 75, 437
 (1957): Levan NE, *Arch Dermatol* 75, 437
 (1956): Carmel WJ+, *N Engl J Med* 255, 770

Other

Acute intermittent porphyria
 (1967): de Matteis F, *Pharmacol Rev* 19, 523
Anaphylactoid reactions
 (1974): Felix RH+, *Lancet* 1, 1017
Gynecomastia
Headache
Hypersensitivity
Oral mucosal eruption
 (1959): Wright W, *JAMA* 171, 1642

Oral ulceration
Paresthesias
Polyarteritis nodosa
 (1962): Schwank R, *Cesk Dermatol* 37, 6
Porphyria
 (1984): Magnus IA, *BMJ* 288, 1474
Rhabdomyolysis
 (1992): Bertran F+, *Therapie* 47(5), 444
Stomatitis (<1%)
 (1959): Brachfeld J+, *JAMA* 169, 1321
Xerostomia

MERCAPTOPURINE

Synonyms: 6-mercaptopurine; 6-MP
Trade name: Purinethol (GSK)
Other common trade names: *Classen; Ismipur; Leukerin; Puri-Nethol*
Indications: Leukemias
Category: Antimetabolite; Antineoplastic; Immunosuppressant
Half-life: triphasic: 45 minutes; 2.5 hours; 10 hours
Clinically important, potentially hazardous interactions with: aldesleukin, allopurinol, mycophenolate, olsalazine, vaccines

Reactions

Skin

Acral erythema
 (1991): Baack BR+, *J Am Acad Dermatol* 24, 457
Dermatitis (sic)
 (1968): Moore GE+, *Cancer Chemother Abstr* 52, 655 (2%)
Edema
Edema of foot
 (1987): Schmutz JL+, *Ann Dermatol Venereol* (French) 114, 569
 (1960): Ludwig GD+, *Clin Res* 8, 212
Exanthems
 (1989): Present DH+, *Ann Intern Med* 111, 641 (0.5%)
Herpes zoster
 (1999): Korelitz BI+, *Am J Gastroenterology* 94, 424
Lichenoid eruption
 (1973): Beylot C+, *Bull Soc Fr Dermatol Syphiligr* (French) 80, 190
Lupus erythematosus
 (1966): Lee SL+, *Arch Intern Med* 117, 620
Palmar–plantar erythema
 (1986): Cox GJ+, *Arch Dermatol* 122, 1413
Petechiae
Photosensitivity
 (1987): Schmutz JL+, *Ann Dermatol Venereol* (French) 114, 569
 (1960): Ludwig GD+, *Clin Res* 8, 212
Pigmentation (1–10%)
Pruritus
Purpura
Radiation recall
 (1975): Dreizen S+, *Postgrad Med* 58, 150
Rash (sic) (1–10%)
Toxic epidermal necrolysis
 (1969): Amerio PL+, *G Ital Dermatol Venereol* (Italian) 110, 514
Urticaria
 (1985): Sparling R+, *Clin Lab Haematol* 7, 184
Vasculitis
 (1997): Andersen JM+, *Pharmacotherapy* 17, 173

Hair

Hair – alopecia

Nails

Nails – loss (sic)

Other

Glossitis (<1%)
Lobular panniculitis
    (1997): Andersen JM+, *Pharmacotherapy* 17, 173
Mucositis (1–10%)
Oral mucosal lesions
    (1983): Bronner AK+, *J Am Acad Dermatol* 9, 645 (1–5%)
    (1968): Moore GE+, *Cancer Chemother Abstr* 52, 655 (2%)
Serum sickness
    (1997): Andersen JM+, *Pharmacotherapy* 17, 173
Stomatitis (1–10%)

MESALAMINE

Synonyms: 5-aminosalicylic acid; 5-ASA; fisalamine; mesalazine
Trade names: Asacol (Procter & Gamble); Canasa (Axcan
Scandipharm); Pentasa (Shire); Rowasa (Solvay)
Other common trade names: *Asacolitin; Claversal; Mesalazine;
Mesasal; Pentasa SR; Quintasa; Salofalk; Tidocol*
Indications: Ulcerative colitis
Category: anti-inflammatory; Bowel disease suppressant
Half-life: 0.5–1.5 hours

Reactions

Skin

Acne (1.2%)
Allergic reactions (sic) (<1%)
    (1990): Boulain T+, *Gastroenterol Clin Biol* (French) 14, 288
    (1989): Brogden RN+, *Drugs* 38, 500
Baboon syndrome
    (2002): Gallo R+, *Contact Dermatitis* 46(2), 110
Diaphoresis (3%)
Ecchymoses
Eczema (sic)
Edema (1.2%)
Erythema
    (1990): Boulain T+, *Gastroenterol Clin Biol* 14, 288 (rectal)
Erythema nodosum
Exanthems
    (1991): LeGros V+, *BMJ* 302, 970
    (1988): Fardy JM+, *J Clin Gastroenterol* 10, 635
    (1988): Gron I+, *Ugeskr Laeger* (Danish) 150, 32
Facial edema
    (1990): Boulain T+, *Gastroenterol Clin Biol* 14, 288 (rectal
        application)
Folliculitis
    (1996): Lizasoain J+, *Am J Gastroenterol* 91, 819
Lichen planus
    (1991): Alstead EM+, *J Clin Gastroenterol* 13, 335
Lupus erythematosus
    (1997): Timsit MA+, *Rev Rhum Engl Ed* 64, 586
    (1992): Pent MT+, *BMJ* 305, 159
Mucocutaneous lymph node syndrome (Kawasaki syndrome)
    (1991): Waanders H+, *Am J Gastroenterol* 86, 219
Peripheral edema (0.61%)
Photosensitivity
    (1999): Horiuchi Y+, *Am J Gastroenterol* 94, 3386
Pruritus (1.2%)

Psoriasis
Pustuloderma
    (2001): Gibbon KL+, *J Am Acad Dermatol* 45, S220–1
Pyoderma gangrenosum
Rash (sic) (3%)
    (1992): Giaffer MH+, *Aliment Pharmacol Ther* 6, 51
    (1992): Hautekeete ML+, *Gastroenterology* 103, 1925
    (1991): Lesur G+, *Gastroenterol Clin Biol* (French) 15, 457
Urticaria
Vasculitis
    (1994): Lim AG+, *BMJ* 308, 113
Xerosis

Hair

Hair – alopecia (0.86%)
    (1997): Timsit MA+, *Rev Rhum Engl Ed* 64, 586
    (1995): Netzer P, *Schweiz Med Wochenschr* (German) 125, 2438
    (1991): Hadjigogos K, *Ital J Gastroenterol* (Italian) 23, 257
    (1989): Brogden RN+, *Drugs* 38, 500
    (1982): Kutty PK+, *Ann Intern Med* 97, 785

Nails

Nails – changes (sic)

Other

Dysgeusia
Headache
Hypersensitivity (<1%)
    (2001): Safer L+, *Gastroenterol Clin Biol* 25(1), 104 (following
        severe allergic reaction to sulfasalazine)
    (2001): Sule A+, *J Assoc Physicians India* 49, 1120
    (1996): Aparicio J+, *Am J Gastroenterol* 91, 620
    (1992): Hautekeete ML+, *Gastroenterology* 103, 1925
Myalgia (3%)
Oral candidiasis
Oral lichenoid eruption
    (1991): Alstead EM+, *J Clin Gastroenterol* 13, 335
Oral ulceration
Paresthesias
Pseudotumor cerebri
    (2001): Rottembourg D+, *J Pediatr Gastroenterol Nutr* 33(3), 337
Tinnitus

MESNA

Trade name: Mesnex (Bristol-Myers Squibb)
Other common trade names: *Mexan; Uromitexan*
Indications: Hemorrhagic cystitis induced by ifosfamide
Category: Hemorrhagic cystitis prophylactic
Half-life: 24 minutes

Reactions

Skin

Allergic reactions (sic)
    (1991): D'Cruz D+, *Lancet* 338, 705
Angioedema
    (1998): Leal G, Fortaleza, Brazil (from Internet) (observation)
    (1992): Breathnach SM+, *Adverse Drug Reactions and the Skin*
        Blackwell, Oxford, 289
    (1992): Zonzits E+, *Arch Dermatol* 128, 80
Erythema
    (1992): Breathnach SM+, *Adverse Drug Reactions and the Skin*
        Blackwell, Oxford, 289
Exanthems
    (1998): Leal G, Fortaleza, Brazil (from Internet) (observation)

(1992): Breathnach SM+, *Adverse Drug Reactions and the Skin*
  Blackwell, Oxford, 289
(1992): Zonzits E+, *Arch Dermatol* 128, 80
Fixed eruption
  (1998): Leal G, Fortaleza, Brazil (from Internet) (observation) (2
    patients)
  (1992): Zonzits E+, *Arch Dermatol* 128, 80
Flushing
  (1992): Breathnach SM+, *Adverse Drug Reactions and the Skin*
    Blackwell, Oxford, 289
Pruritus (<1%)
Rash (sic) (<1%)
Urticaria
  (1998): Leal G, Fortaleza, Brazil (from Internet) (observation)
  (1992): Breathnach SM+, *Adverse Drug Reactions and the Skin*
    Blackwell, Oxford, 289
  (1992): Zonzits E+, *Arch Dermatol* 128, 80
  (1988): Pratt CB+, *Drug Intell Clin Pharm* 22, 913

Other
Dysgeusia (>17%)
Oral mucosal lesions
  (1988): Pralt CB+, *Drug Intell Clin Pharm* 22, 913
Oral mucosal ulceration
  (1992): Breathnach SM+, *Adverse Drug Reactions and the Skin*
    Blackwell, Oxford, 289

MESORIDAZINE

Trade name: Serentil (Boehringer Ingelheim)
Other common trade name: *Mesorin*
Indications: Schizophrenia
Category: Phenothiazine antipsychotic
Half-life: 24–48 hours
**Clinically important, potentially hazardous interactions
with:** antihistamines, arsenic, chlorpheniramine, dofetilide,
piperazine, quinolones, sparfloxacin

Reactions

Skin
Angioedema
Dermatitis
Eczema (sic)
Edema
Erythema
Exfoliative dermatitis
Flushing
Hypohidrosis (>10%)
Lupus erythematosus
Peripheral edema
Photosensitivity (1–10%)
Pigmentation (blue-gray) (<1%)
Pruritus
Rash (sic) (1–10%)
Seborrhea
Urticaria
Xerosis

Hair
Hair – alopecia

Other
Anaphylactoid reactions
Galactorrhea (<1%)

Gynecomastia
Hypertrophic papillae of tongue
Mastodynia (1–10%)
Paresthesias
Priapism (<1%)
Sialorrhea
Tremor
Xerostomia

METAXALONE

Trade name: Skelaxin (Elan)
Indications: Muscle spasm
Category: Skeletal muscle relaxant
Half-life: 2–3 hours

Reactions

Skin
Dermatitis (sic) (<1%)
Fixed eruption
  (2000): Mostow EN, Akron, OH (from Internet) (observation)
Pruritus
Rash (sic)
Urticaria

Other
Anaphylactoid reactions (<1%)
Headache

METFORMIN

Trade names: Avandamet; Glucophage (Bristol-Myers Squibb);
Glucovance (Bristol-Myers Squibb); Metaglip
Other common trade names: *Apo-Metformin; Diabex;
Diaformin; Diformin; Gen-Metformin; Glucomet; Metforal; Metomin;
Novo-Metformin*
Indications: Diabetes
Category: Antidiabetic
Half-life: 6.2 hours

Glucovance is metformin and glyburide

Reactions

Skin
Eczema (sic)
  (1970): Lawson AAH+, *Lancet* 2, 437
Erythema (transient)
  (1966): Berger W+, *Schweiz Med Wochenschr* (German)
    96, 1335
  (1966): Beurey J+, *Ann Dermatol Syphiligr* (French) 93, 13
    (French) 93,13
  (1964): Puchegger R+, *Wien Klin Wochenschr* (German) 76, 335
Exanthems
Grinspan's syndrome*
  (1990): Lamey PJ+, *Oral Surg Oral Med Oral Pathol* 70, 184
Lichenoid eruption
  (1970): Lawson AAH+, Lancet 2, 437
Photosensitivity (1–10%)
Pruritus
  (1964): Puchegger R+, *Wien Klin Wochenschr* (German) 76, 335
Purpura

(1966): Berger W+, *Schweiz Med Wochenschr* (German)
    96, 1335
Rash (sic) (1–10%)
Urticaria (1–10%)
    (1966): Berger W+, *Schweiz Med Wochenschr* (German)
        96, 1335
    (1966): Beurey J+, *Ann Dermatol Syphiligr* (French) 93, 13
    (1964): Puchegger R+, *Wien Klin Wochenschr* (German) 76, 335
Vasculitis
    (1986): Klapholz L+, *BMJ* 293, 483

Hair

Hair – alopecia
    (1999): Smith JG, Mobile, AL (from Internet) (2 observations)
    (1998): Klein AD, Statesboro, GA (from Internet) (observation)

Other

Death
    (2002): www.intellihealth.com (from Internet)
Dysgeusia (3%) (metallic taste)

*Note: Grinspan's syndrome: the triad of oral lichen planus, diabetes mellitus, and hypertension

METHADONE

Trade name: Dolophine (Roxane)
Other common trade names: *Eptadone; L-Polamidon; Mephenon; Metadon; Methadose; Physeptone*
Indications: Pain, narcotic addiction
Category: Antitussive; Narcotic analgesic; Suppressant (narcotic abstinence syndrome)
Half-life: 15–25 hours
Clinically important, potentially hazardous interactions with: diazepam, erythromycin, fluconazole

Reactions

Skin

Angioedema
Cellulitis
    (1988): Naschitz JE+, *Harefuah* (Hebrew) 115, 271
Diaphoresis
    (1973): Kreek MJ, *JAMA* 223, 665 (48%)
Edema (face)
Exanthems
Flushing
Pruritus (<1%)
Purpura
Rash (sic) (<1%)
Urticaria (<1%)

Other

Death
    (2002): Buster MC+, *Addiction* 97(8), 993 (overdose)
    (2001): Vormfelde SV+, *Pharmacopsychiatry* 34(6), 217
Headache
Injection-site burning
Injection-site induration
Injection-site pain (1–10%)
Rhabdomyolysis
    (1990): Larpin R+, *Presse Med* 19(30), 1403
Tremor
    (2001): Clark JD+, *Clin J Pain* 17(4), 375
Xerostomia (1–10%)

METHAMPHETAMINE

Trade name: Desoxyn (Abbott)
Indications: Attention deficit disorder, obesity
Category: Central nervous system stimulant; Recreational drug
Half-life: 4–5 hours
Clinically important, potentially hazardous interactions with: fluoxetine, fluvoxamine, MAO inhibitors, paroxetine, phenelzine, sertraline, tranylcypromine

Reactions

Skin

Acaraphobia
    (1971): Yaffee NS, *Arch Dermatol* 104, 687
Diaphoresis (1–10%)
Lichenoid eruption
    (1994): Deloach-Banta LJ, *Cutis* 53, 97
Pigmentation
    (1971): Yaffee NS, *Arch Dermatol* 104, 687
Rash (sic) (<1%)
Toxic epidermal necrolysis
    (2002): Yung A+, *Australas J Dermatol* 43(1), 35
Urticaria (<1%)

Other

Delusions of parasitosis
    (1999): Gregg LJ, Tulsa, OK, (from Internet) (4 observations)
Dysgeusia
Headache
Polyarteritis nodosa
    (1973): Koff RS+, *N Engl J Med* 288, 946
    (1970): Citron BP+, *N Engl J Med* 283, 1003
Rhabdomyolysis
    (1999): Richards JR+, *Am J Emerg Med* 17(7), 681 (43%)
    (1998): Kolecki P, *Pediatr Emerg Care* 14(6), 385
    (1998): Lan KC+, *J Formos Med Assoc* 97(8), 528
    (1994): Chan P+, *J Toxicol Clin Toxicol* 32(2), 147 (8 cases) (3 fatal)
    (1994): Sperling LS+, *Ann Intern Med* 121(12), 986
Tremor
Xerostomia (1–10%)

METHANTHELINE

Trade name: Banthine (Pharmacia)
Other common trade name: *Vagantin*
Indications: Duodenal ulcer
Category: Gastrointestinal anticholinergic
Half-life: N/A
Clinically important, potentially hazardous interactions with: anticholinergics, arbutamine

Reactions

Skin

Exanthems
Exfoliative dermatitis
Flushing
Hypohidrosis
Urticaria
Xerosis

Other
Ageusia
Anaphylactoid reactions
Dysgeusia
Sialopenia
Xerostomia

METHAZOLAMIDE

Trade name: Methazolamide
Indications: Glaucoma
Category: Carbonic anhydrase inhibitor; Sulfonamide diuretic
Half-life: ~14 hours

Reactions

Skin
Exanthems (<1%)
  (1998): Litt JZ, Beachwood, OH (personal case) (observation)
  (1993): Gandham SB+, Arch Ophthalmol 111, 370
Photosensitivity
Pruritus
Purpura
Rash (sic)
Stevens–Johnson syndrome
  (1998): Cotter JB, Arch Ophthalmol 116, 117
  (1997): Shirato S+, Arch Ophthalmol 115, 550
  (1995): Flach AJ+, Ophthalmology 102, 1677
Toxic epidermal necrolysis
Urticaria
  (1993): Gandham SB+, Arch Ophthalmol 111, 370
Vasculitis

Other
Anosmia (<1%)
Dysgeusia (>10%) (metallic taste)
Hypersensitivity (<1%)
Paresthesias (<1%)
Tinnitus
Trembling
Xerostomia (<1%)

METHENAMINE

Trade names: Hiprex (Aventis); Mandelamine (Warner Chilcott); Prosed (Star); Urised (PolyMedica); Uroqid
Other common trade names: Dehydral; Haiprex; Hip-Rex; Hipeksal; Hippramine; Reflux; Urasal; Urotractan
Indications: Urinary tract infections
Category: Urinary tract antibacterial
Half-life: 3–6 hours

Reactions

Skin
Edema
Erythema multiforme (<1%)
Exanthems
  (1976): Arndt KA+, JAMA 235, 918 (0.6%)
  (1968): Med Lett 10, 58
Fixed eruption (<1%)
  (1961): Welsh AL, Arch Dermatol 84, 1004

Photosensitivity
  (1994): Selvaag E+, Photodermatol Photoimmunol Photomed 10, 259
Pruritus (<1%)
Rash (sic) (3.5%)
Systemic eczematous contact dermatitis
Urticaria

Other
Headache
Stomatitis

METHICILLIN

Trade name: Staphcillin (Bristol-Myers Squibb)
Other common trade names: Estafcilina; Lucoperin; Mechicillin
Indications: Various infections caused by susceptible organisms
Category: Penicillinase-resistant penicillin
Half-life: 30 minutes
Clinically important, potentially hazardous interactions with: anticoagulants, cyclosporine, methotrexate, tetracycline

Reactions

Skin
Angioedema
Bullous eruption
  (1976): Schiffer CA+, Ann Intern Med 85, 338
Ecchymoses
Erythema multiforme
  (1969): Kaminska M+, Pediatr Pol (Polish) 44, 873
Erythema nodosum
Exanthems
  (1980): Fields DA, West J Med 133, 521
  (1978): Kancir LM+, Arch Intern Med 138, 909 (29%)
Exfoliative dermatitis
  (1966): Hadida E+, Bull Soc Fr Dermatol Syphiligr (French) 73, 497
Hematomas
Jarisch–Herxheimer reaction
Pruritus
Purpura
Pustular psoriasis
  (1966): Hadida E+, Bull Soc Fr Dermatol Syphiligr (French) 73, 497
Rash (sic) (1–10%)
Stevens–Johnson syndrome
Toxic epidermal necrolysis
Urticaria
Vasculitis

Other
Anaphylactoid reactions
Black tongue
Dysgeusia
Glossitis
Glossodynia
Hypersensitivity
Injection-site pain
Oral candidiasis
Phlebitis (<1%)
Serum sickness (<1%)
Stomatitis
Stomatodynia

Vaginitis
Xerostomia

METHIMAZOLE

Synonym: thiamazole
Trade name: Tapazole (Jones)
Other common trade names: *Strumazol; Thacapzol; Thiamazol; Thyrozol; Unimazole*
Indications: Hyperthyroidism
Category: Antithyroid
Half-life: 4–13 hours
Clinically important, potentially hazardous interactions with: anticoagulants, dicumarol, warfarin

Reactions

Skin
Edema (<1%)
Erythema nodosum
Exanthems
 (1986): Shiroozu A+, *J Clin Endocrinol Metab* 63, 125 (5–15%)
 (1972): Wiberg JJ+, *Ann Intern Med* 77, 414 (1–5%)
 (1970): Amrhein JA+, *J Pediatr* 76, 54
 (1951): Bartels EC+, *J Clin Endocrinol Metab* 11, 1057 (6%)
Exfoliative dermatitis
Fixed eruption
 (1984): Chan HL, *Int J Dermatol* 23, 607
Lupus erythematosus (1–10%)
 (1995): Kawachi Y+, *Clin Exp Dermatol* 20, 345
 (1994): Sato-Matsumura KC+, *J Dermatol* 21, 501
 (1987): Sakata S+, *Jpn J Med* 26, 373
 (1981): Searles RP+, *J Rheumatol* 8, 498
 (1981): Takuwa N+, *Endocrinol Jpn* 28, 663
 (1973): Hung W+, *J Pediatr* 82, 852
 (1970): Librik L+, *J Pediatr* 76, 64
Pigmentation
 (2000): Drayton G, Los Angeles, CA (from Internet)
   (observation)
Pruritus (3–5%)
 (1986): Shiroozu A+, *J Clin Endocrinol Metab* 63, 125 (2–3%)
 (1972): Wiberg JJ+, *Ann Intern Med* 77, 414 (1–5%)
Purpura
 (1972): Wiberg JJ+, *Ann Intern Med* 77, 414 (1%)
Rash (sic) (>10%)
Side effects (sic) (28% in high dosages)
 (1972): Wiberg JJ+, *Ann Intern Med* 77, 414 (1–5%)
Urticaria
 (1972): Wiberg JJ+, *Ann Intern Med* 77, 414 (>5%)
 (1970): Amrhein JA+, *J Pediatr* 76, 54
Vasculitis
 (1995): Kawachi Y+, *Clin Exp Dermatol* 20, 345

Hair
Hair – alopecia (<1%)

Other
Ageusia (1–10%)
Aplasia cutis congenita
 (1995): Vogt T+, *Br J Dermatol* 133, 994
 (1992): Martinez-Frias ML+, *Lancet* 339, 742
 (1985): Milham S, *Teratology* 32, 321
 (1984): Bachrach LK+, *Can Med Assoc J* 130, 1264
Dysgeusia
Headache
Myalgia

Oral ulceration
Paresthesias (<1%)
Polyarteritis nodosa
Scalp defects (sic)
 (1985): Milham S, *Teratology* 32, 321
Serum sickness
 (1983): Van Kuyk M+, *Acta Clin Belg* (French) 38, 68
Sialadenitis

METHOCARBAMOL

Trade name: Robaxin (Wyeth) (Elkins-Sinn)
Other common trade names: *Carbametin; Carxin; Delaxin; Lumirelax; Marbaxin; Miowas; Ortoton; Robinax; Robomol; Trolar*
Indications: Muscle spasm, tetanus
Category: Skeletal muscle relaxant
Half-life: 1–2 hours

Reactions

Skin
Allergic reactions (sic) (1–10%)
Exanthems
Flushing (1–10%)
Pruritus
Rash (sic)
Urticaria

Other
Anaphylactoid reactions
Dysgeusia
Headache
Injection-site pain (<1%)
Thrombophlebitis (<1%)

METHOHEXITAL

Trade name: Brevital (Jones)
Other common trade names: *Brevimytal; Brietal; Brietal Sodium*
Indications: General anesthesia
Category: Barbiturate; General anesthetic
Half-life: 4–8 minutes

Reactions

Skin
Angioedema
 (1972): Driggs RL+, *J Oral Surg* 30, 906
 (1972): Reichert EF+, *J Oral Surg* 30, 910
Erythema
Exanthems
 (1972): Driggs RL+, *J Oral Surg* 30, 906
Rash (sic)
Urticaria
 (1972): Driggs RL+, *J Oral Surg* 30, 906
 (1972): Reichert EF+, *J Oral Surg* 30, 910

Other
Anaphylactoid reactions
Injection-site edema
Injection-site pain (18%)
Injection-site phlebitis
 (1981): Clark RSJ, *Drugs* 27, 26

Rhabdomyolysis
  (1990): Larpin R+, *Presse Med* 19(30), 1403
Sialorrhea
Thrombophlebitis (<1%)
Tremor

METHOTREXATE

Synonyms: amethopterin; MTX
Trade name: Rheumatrex (Stada)
Other common trade names: *Farmitrexat; Lantarel;*
Ledertrexate; Maxtrex; Metex; Texate
Indications: Carcinomas, leukemias, lymphomas, psoriasis,
rheumatoid arthritis
Category: Antiarthritic; anti-inflammatory; Antineoplastic
Half-life: 3–10 hours
Clinically important, potentially hazardous interactions
with: acitretin, aldesleukin, aminoglycosides, amiodarone,
amoxicillin, ampicillin, aspirin, bacampicillin, bismuth, carbenicillin,
chloroquine, cisplatin, cloxacillin, co-trimoxazole, dapsone,
demeclocycline, diclofenac, dicloxacillin, etodolac, etretinate,
fenoprofen, flurbiprofen, folic acid antagonists, haloperidol,
ibuprofen, indomethacin, ketoprofen, ketorolac, lithium,
magnesium trisalicylate, meclofenamate, mefenamic acid,
methicillin, mezlocillin, minocycline, nabumetone, nafcillin,
naproxen, NSAIDs, omeprazole, oxaprozin, oxytetracycline,
paromomycin, penicillins, piperacillin, piroxicam, polypeptide
antibiotics, probenecid, procarbazine, rofecoxib, salicylates,
salsalate, sulfadiazine, sulfamethoxazole, sulfapyridine,
sulfasalazine, sulfisoxazole, sulindac, tetracycline, ticarcillin,
tolmetin, trimethoprim, **vaccines**

Reactions

Skin
Acne
Acral erythema
  (2003): Feizy V+, *Dermatol Online J* 9(1), 14 (bullous variety – on
    soles)
  (1996): Hellier I+, *Arch Dermatol* 132, 590 (bullous variety)
  (1989): Kampmann KK+, *Cancer* 63, 2482
  (1983): Doyle LA+, *Ann Intern Med* 98, 611
Allergic reactions (sic)
  (2000): Postovsky S+, *Med Pediatr Oncol* 35, 131
Bullous eruption
  (1987): Chang JC, *Arch Dermatol* 123, 990
  (1983): Reed KM+, *J Am Acad Dermatol* 8, 677
Burning (palms and soles)
  (1978): McDonald CJ+, *Cancer Treat Rep* 62, 1009
Candidiasis
  (1970): Baker H, *Br J Dermatol* 82, 65
Capillaritis
  (1978): McDonald CJ+, *Cancer Treat Rep* 62, 1009
  (1976): Jacobs SA+, *J Clin Invest* 57, 534
Carcinoma (sic)
  (1971): Craig LR+, *Arch Dermatol* 103, 505
Dermatitis (sic)
  (1996): Giordano N+, *Clin Exp Rheumatol* 14, 450
Ecchymoses
  (1998): Roenigk HH+, *J Am Acad Dermatol* 38, 478
Eccrine squamous syringometaplasia
  (1997): Valks R+, *Arch Dermatol* 133, 873
Erosion of psoriatic plaques (sic)
  (1996): Pearce HP+, *J Am Acad Dermatol* 35, 835

  (1988): Kaplan DL+, *Int J Dermatol* 27, 59
  (1988): Shupack JL+, *JAMA* 259, 3594
  (1987): Ng HW+, *BMJ* 295, 752
  (1984): Lawrence CM+, *J Am Acad Dermatol* 11, 1059
  (1983): Reed KM+, *J Am Acad Dermatol* 8, 677
  (1969): McDonald CJ+, *Arch Dermatol* 100, 655
Erosions
  (1996): Zackheim HS+, *J Am Acad Dermatol* 34, 626
Erythema (>10%)
Erythema multiforme
  (1989): Taylor SW+, *Gynecol Oncol* 33, 376
  (1978): Moe PJ+, *Acta Paediatr Scand* (French) 67, 265
Erythematous papules (sic)
  (1999): Goerttler E+, *J Am Acad Dermatol* 40, 702 (4 cases)
Erythroderma
  (2000): Alfaro J+, *Rev Med Chil* (Spanish) 128, 315
  (1996): Zackheim HS+, *J Am Acad Dermatol* 34, 626
Exanthems (15%)
  (2003): Feizy V+, *Dermatol Online J* 9(1), 14
  (1979): Stoller RG+, *Cancer Res* 39, 908
  (1971): Hansen HH+, *Br J Cancer* 25, 298
Folliculitis
  (1970): Baker H, *Br J Dermatol* 82, 65
Furunculosis
  (1996): Zackheim HS+, *J Am Acad Dermatol* 34, 626
Herpes simplex
  (1996): Vonderheid EC+, *J Am Acad Dermatol* 34, 470
Inflammation (sic) (reactivation)
  (1969): Möller H, *J Invest Dermatol* 52, 437
Melanoma
  (1984): Wemmer U, *Z Hautkr* (German) 59, 665
Necrolysis (sic)
  (1970): Baker H, *Br J Dermatol* 82, 65
Necrosis (sic)
  (1987): Harrison PV, *Br J Dermatol* 116, 867
  (1983): Reed KM+, *J Am Acad Dermatol* 8, 677
  (1982): Lawrence CM+, *Br J Dermatol* 107, 24
Nodules (sic)
  (2001): Ahmed SS+, *Medicine* (Baltimore) 80(4), 271
  (1998): Williams FM+, *J Am Acad Dermatol* 39, 359
  (1996): Muzaffer MA+, *J Pediatr* 128, 698
  (1996): Smith MD, *J Rheumatol* 23, 2004
  (1995): Berris B+, *J Rheumatol* 22, 2359
  (1995): Das SK+, *J Assoc Physicians India* 43, 651
  (1994): Abu-Shakra M+, *J Rheumatol* 21, 934
  (1994): Karam NE+, *J Rheumatol* 21, 1960
  (1994): Smith MD, *J Rheumatol* 22, 1439
  (1992): Kerstens PJSM+, *J Rheumatol* 19, 867
  (1988): Segal R+, *Arthritis Rheum* 31, 1182
Photo-recall phenomenon
  (2002): Thami GP+, *Postgrad Med J* 78(916), 116
Photosensitivity (5%)
  (2002): Thami GP+, *Postgrad Med J* 78(916), 116 (recall)
  (1996): Zackheim HS+, *J Am Acad Dermatol* 34, 626
  (1994): Oliver F, *The Schoch Letter* 44, 6 (observation)
  (1985): Neiman RA+, *J Rheumatol* 12, 354
  (1969): Möller H, *J Invest Dermatol* 52, 437
  (1969): Roenigk HH Jr+, *Arch Dermatol* 99, 86
  (1965): Vogler WR+, *Arch Intern Med* 115, 285
Pigmentation (1–10%)
Pruritus (1–5%)
  (1998): Roenigk HH+, *J Am Acad Dermatol* 38, 478
Purpura
Radiation recall
  (2001): Camidge DR, *Am J Clin Oncol* 24(2), 211
  (2000): Kharfan Dabaja MA+, *Am J Clin Oncol* 23(5), 531
  (1995): Guzzo C+, *Photodermatol Photoimmunol Photomed*
    11, 55 (sunburn)

Radiodermatitis (reactivation)
Rash (sic) (1–3%)
  (2000): Emery P+, *Rheumatology* (Oxford) 39(6), 655
  (1995): Copur S+, *Anticancer Drugs* 6, 154
Scabies (reactivation)
  (1975): Burrows D, *Br J Dermatol* 93, 219
Side effects (sic)
  (1997): Kasteler JS+, *J Am Acad Dermatol* 36, 67 (passim)
  (1996): Furuya T+, *Rymachi* (Japanese) 36, 746
Squamous cell carcinoma
  (1989): Jensen DB+, *Acta Derm Venereol* (Stockh) 69, 274
  (1971): Harris CC, *Arch Dermatol* 103, 501
Stevens–Johnson syndrome
  (2000): Hani N+, *Eur J Dermatol* 10(7), 548
  (1993): Cuthbert RJ+, *Ulster Med J* 62, 95
  (1978): Moe PJ+, *Acta Paediatr Scand* (French) 67, 265
Sunburn (reactivation)
  (2000): Khan AJ+, *Cutis* 66, 379
  (1998): Roenigk HH+, *J Am Acad Dermatol* 38, 478
  (1987): Westwick TJ+, *Cutis* 39, 49
  (1986): Mallory SB+, *Pediatrics* 78, 514
  (1981): Korossy KS+, *Arch Dermatol* 117, 310
Telangiectasia
Toxic epidermal necrolysis (<1%)
  (2000): Yang CH+, *Int J Dermatol* 39, 621 (with co-trimoxazole)
  (1997): Primka EJ+, *J Am Acad Dermatol* 36, 815 (fatal)
  (1970): Baker H, *Br J Dermatol* 82, 65
  (1967): Lyell A, *Br J Dermatol* 79, 367
Ulcerations
  (2001): Del Pozo J+, *Eur J Dermatol* 11(5), 450 (knuckles)
  (2000): Montero LC+, *J Rheumatol* 27(9), 2290
  (1998): Ben-Amitai D+, *Ann Pharmacother* 32, 651
  (1998): Roenigk HH+, *J Am Acad Dermatol* 38, 478 (of psoriatic lesions)
  (1970): Baker H, *Br J Dermatol* 82, 65
Urticaria
  (1998): Roenigk HH+, *J Am Acad Dermatol* 38, 478
  (1995): al-Lamki Z+, *Med Pediatr Oncol* 24, 137
  (1983): Bronner AK+, *J Am Acad Dermatol* 9, 645
Vasculitis (>10%)
  (2000): Borcea A+, *Br J Dermatol* 143, 203 (urticarial)
  (1998): Halevy S+, *J Eur Acad Dermatol Venereol* 10, 81
  (1997): Torner O+, *Clin Rheumatol* 16, 108
  (1995): Blanco R+, *Arthritis Rheum* 39, 1016
  (1989): Fondevila CG+, *Br J Haematol* 72, 591
  (1989): Jeurissen MEC+, *Clin Rheumatol* 8, 417
  (1986): Navarro M+, *Ann Intern Med* 105, 471
  (1984): Marks CR+, *Ann Intern Med* 100, 916

Hair

Hair – alopecia (1–3%)
  (2000): Emery P+, *Rheumatology* (Oxford) 39, 655
  (1998): Roenigk HH+, *J Am Acad Dermatol* 38, 478
  (1998): Zieglschmid ME+, *J Am Acad Dermatol* 38, 130
  (1997): Kasteler JS+, *J Am Acad Dermatol* 36, 67 (passim)
  (1996): Zackheim HS+, *J Am Acad Dermatol* 34, 626
  (1995): Zieglschmid-Adams ME+, *J Am Acad Dermatol* 32, 754
  (1989): Fehlauer CS+, *J Rheumatol* 16, 307
  (1988): Weinblatt ME+, *Arthritis Rheum* 31 (Suppl), s115
  (1982): Bachman DM, *Arthritis Rheum* 25, s65
  (1982): Bertino JR, *Med Pediatr Oncol* 10, 401
  (1971): Hansen HH+, *Br J Cancer* 25, 298
  (1969): Roenigk HH Jr+, *Arch Dermatol* 99, 86 (6%)
Hair – pigmented bands
  (1983): Wheeland RG+, *Cancer* 51, 1356

Nails

Nails – discoloration
Nails – onycholysis
  (1987): Chang JC, *Arch Dermatol* 123, 990

Nails – paronychia
  (1983): Wantzin GL+, *Arch Dermatol* 119, 623
Nails – pigmentation
  (1981): Nixon DW+, *Cutis* 27, 181

Other

Anaphylactoid reactions (1–10%)
  (1996): Alkins SA+, *Cancer* 77, 2123
  (1995): Lobelle C+, *Pediatr Hematol Oncol* 12, 213
  (1979): Gluck-Kuyt I+, *Cancer Treat Rep* 63, 797
  (1978): Goldberg NH+, *Cancer* 41, 52
Death
Dysgeusia
  (1988): Duhra P+, *Clin Exp Dermatol* 13, 126
Gingivitis (>10%)
Glossitis (>10%)
Gynecomastia
  (1995): Finger DR+, *J Rheumatol* 22, 796
  (1995): Thomas E+, *J Rheumatol* 22, 2189
  (1983): Del Paine DW+, *Arthritis Rheum* 26, 691
Headache
Hodgkin's disease (nodular sclerosing)
  (2000): Moseley AC+, *J Rheumatol* 27, 810
Malignant lymphoma
  (1997): Kamel OW, *Arch Dermatol* 133, 903
  (1996): Viraben R+, *Br J Dermatol* 135, 116
  (1994): Zimmer-Galler I+, *Mayo Clin Proc* 69, 258
  (1993): Kamel OW+, *N Engl J Med* 328, 1317
Mucositis
  (2000): Alfaro J+, *Rev Med Chil* (Spanish) 128, 315
Myalgia
Oral mucositis
  (1997): Plevova P+, *J Natl Cancer Inst* 89, 326
  (1996): Moe PJ, *Pediatr Hematol Oncol* 13, 313
  (1996): Rask C+, *Pediatr Hematol Oncol* 13, 359
  (1996): Zackheim HS+, *J Am Acad Dermatol* 34, 626
  (1979): Oliff A+, *Cancer Chemother Pharmacol* 2, 225
Oral ulceration
  (2001): Litt JZ, Beachwood, OH (personal case) (observation) (severe)
  (2001): Werth V, *Dermatology Times* 15
  (2000): Madinier I+, *Ann Med Interne* (Paris) (French) 151, 248
  (1986): Barrett AP, *J Periodontol* 57, 318
Peyronie's disease
  (1992): Phelan MJI, *Br J Rheumatol* 31, 425
Porphyria cutanea tarda
  (1983): Malina L+, *Z Hautkr* (German) 58, 241
Pseudolymphoma
  (1997): Flipo RM+, *J Rheumatol* 24, 809
  (1995): Delaporte E+, *Ann Dermatol Venereol* (French) 122, 521 (20 cases)
  (1994): Zimmer-Galler I+, *Mayo Clin Proc* 69, 258
  (1993): Kamel OW+, *N Engl J Med* 328, 1317
  (1993): Kerl H+, *Dermatology in General Medicine* McGraw-Hill, New York
  (1993): Shiroky JB+, *N Engl J Med* 329(22), 1657
  (1993): Taillan B+, *Rev Rhum Ed Fr* 60(3), 248
  (1992): Kingsmore SF+, *J Rheumatol* 19(9), 1462
  (1991): Ellman MH+, *J Rheumatol* 18(11), 1741
  (1991): Shiroky JB+, *J Rheumatol* 18(8), 1172
Stomatitis (3–10%)
  (1998): Roenigk HH+, *J Am Acad Dermatol* 38, 478 (ulcerative)
  (1998): Zieglschmid ME+, *J Am Acad Dermatol* 38, 130
  (1997): Kasteler JS+, *J Am Acad Dermatol* 36, 67 (passim)
  (1996): Vonderheid EC+, *J Am Acad Dermatol* 34, 470
  (1995): Zieglschmid-Adams ME+, *J Am Acad Dermatol* 32, 754
  (1994): Montecucco C+, *Arthritis Rheum* 37, 777
  (1978): Moe PJ+, *Acta Paediatr Scand* (French) 67, 265

Tendinitis
 (2001): Toverud EL+, *Med Pediatr Oncol* 37(2), 156 (Achilles; repeated)
Tinnitus

METHOXSALEN

Trade names: 8-MOP (ICN); Oxsoralen (ICN)
Other common trade names: *Geroxalen; Meladinine; Oxsoralon; Puvasoralen; Ultra-MOP*
Indications: Psoriasis, vitiligo
Category: Repigmenting agent
Half-life: 1.1 hours
Clinically important, potentially hazardous interactions with: caffeine, chloroquine, cyclosporine, fluoroquinolones, phenothiazines, sulfonamides

Reactions

Skin
Acne
 (1978): Nielsen EB+, *Acta Derm Venereol* (Stockh) 58, 374
Acute generalized exanthematous pustulosis (AGEP)
 (2002): Morant C+, *Ann Dermatol Venereol* 129(2), 234
Basal cell carcinoma
 (1996): Stern RS+, *J Pediatr* 129, 915
 (1995): Gritiyarangsan P+, *Photodermatol Photoimmunol Photomed* 11, 174
Bowen's disease
 (1979): Tam DW+, *Arch Dermatol* 115, 203
Bullous eruption (with UVA)
 (1982): Stüttgen G, *Int J Dermatol* 21, 198
 (1979): Abel EA+, *Arch Dermatol* 115, 988
 (1977): Melski JW+, *J Invest Dermatol* 68, 328
 (1976): Thomsen K+, *Br J Dermatol* 95, 568
Bullous pemphigoid
 (1996): Perl S+, *Dermatology* 193, 245
Burning
 (1996): Geary P, *Burns* 22, 636
 (1991): Boucaud C+, *Presse Med* (French) 20, 1945
 (1982): Stüttgen G, *Int J Dermatol* 21, 198 (passim) (1–10%)
Carcinoma (sic)
 (1995): Halder RM+, *Arch Dermatol* 131, 734
 (1984): Halprin KM+, *Natl Cancer Inst Monogr* 66, 185
 (1979): Morgan RW, *N Engl J Med* 301, 554
 (1979): Spellman CW, *N Engl J Med* 301, 554
 (1979): Stern RS+, *N Engl J Med* 301, 555
 (1976): Moller R+, *Arch Dermatol* 112, 1613 (multiple basal cell carcinomas)
Cheilitis (1–10%)
Dermatitis
 (1994): Korffmacher H+, *Contact Dermatitis* 30, 283
 (1991): Takashima A+, *Br J Dermatol* 124, 37
 (1980): Weissmann I+, *Br J Dermatol* 102, 113
 (1979): Saihan EM, *BMJ* 2, 20
Eczema (sic)
 (1979): Saihan EM, *BMJ* 2, 20
Edema (1–10%)
Erythema (1–10%)
Exanthems
 (2001): Ravenscroft J+, *J Am Acad Dermatol* 45, S2118–9
 (1986): Gisslen P+, *Photodermatol* 3, 308
Exfoliative dermatitis
Freckles (1–10%)

 (1995): Gritiyarangsan P+, *Photodermatol Photoimmunol Photomed* 11, 174
 (1995): Pierard GE+, *Dermatology* 190, 338
 (1984): Kietzmann E+, *Dermatologica* 168, 306
 (1983): Kanerva L+, *Dermatologica* 166, 281
 (1983): Kietzmann H+, *Ann Dermatol Venereol* (French) 110, 63
Granuloma annulare
 (1979): Dorval JC+, *Ann Dermatol Venereol* (French) 106, 79
Herpes simplex
 (1982): Stüttgen G, *Int J Dermatol* 21, 198
Herpes zoster
 (1982): Stüttgen G, *Int J Dermatol* 21, 198
 (1977): Roenigk HH+, *Arch Dermatol* 113, 1667
Hypopigmentation (1–10%)
Lupus erythematosus
 (1985): Bruze M+, *Acta Derm Venereol* (Stockh) 65, 31
 (1979): Eyanson S+, *Arch Dermatol* 115, 54
 (1978): Millns J+, *Arch Dermatol* 114, 1177
Miliaria
Pemphigus
 (1978): Robinson JK, *Br J Dermatol* 99, 709
Photodermatitis
 (1998): Clark SM+, *Contact Dermatitis* 38, 289
 (1991): Takashima A+, *Br J Dermatol* 124, 37
 (1990): Cox NH+, *Clin Exp Dermatol* 15, 75
Photosensitivity
 (2001): Tanew A+, *J Am Acad Dermatol* 44, 638
 (1992): Jeanmougin M+, *Ann Dermatol Venereol* (French) 119, 277
 (1991): Boucaud C+, *Presse Med* (French) 20, 1945
 (1989): Cox NH+, *Photodermatol* 6, 96
 (1978): Plewig G+, *Arch Derm Res* 261, 201
 (1968): Fulton JE+, *Arch Derm* 98, 445
Phototoxicity
 (1997): Morison WL+, *J Am Acad Dermatol* 36, 183
 (1993): Calzavara-Pinton PG+, *J Am Acad Dermatol* 28, 657
 (1989): Morison WL, *Arch Dermatol* 125, 433 (topical)
 (1985): Berakha GJ+, *Ann Plast Surg* 14, 458
 (1984): Meffert H+, *Photodermatol* 1, 191
 (1979): de Koning GA+, *Hautarzt* (German) 30, 27
 (1979): Swanbeck G+, *Clin Pharmacol Ther* 25, 478
Pigmentation
 (1989): Weiss E+, *Int J Dermatol* 28, 188
 (1987): Bruce DR+, *J Am Acad Dermatol* 16, 1087
 (1986): MacDonald KJS+, *Br J Dermatol* 114, 395
Porokeratosis (actinic)
 (1988): Beiteke U+, *Photodermatol* 5, 274
 (1985): Hazen PG+, *J Am Acad Dermatol* 12, 1077
 (1980): Reymond JL, *Acta Derm Venereol* (Stockh) 60, 539
Prurigo
 (1982): Stüttgen G, *Int J Dermatol* 21, 198 (passim)
Pruritus (>10%)
 (1982): Stüttgen G, *Int J Dermatol* 21, 198 (passim)
Purpura
 (1981): Barriere H+, *Nouv Presse Med* (French) 10, 337
Rash (sic) (1–10%)
Scleroderma
 (1976): Duperrat B+, *Bull Soc Franc Dermatol Syphiligr* (French) 83, 79
Seborrheic dermatitis
 (1983): Tegner E, *Acta Derm Venereol* (Stockh) Suppl 107, 5
Skin pain
 (1987): Norris PG+, *Clin Exp Dermatol* 12, 403
 (1983): Tegner E, *Acta Derm Venereol* (Stockh) Suppl 107, 5
Squamous cell carcinoma
 (1998): Stern RS+, *Arch Dermatol* 134, 1582 (with UVA)
 (1986): Kahn JR+, *Clin Exp Dermatol* 11, 398
 (1979): Tam DW+, *Arch Dermatol* 115, 203

(1979): Verdich J, *Arch Dermatol* 115, 1338
Urticaria
  (1994): Bech-Thomsen N+, *J Am Acad Dermatol* 31, 1063
Vasculitis
  (1981): Barriere H+, *Presse Med* (French) 10, 37
Vitiligo
  (1983): Tegner E, *Acta Derm Venereol* (Stockh) Suppl 107, 5
  (1976): Duperrat B+, *Bull Soc Franc Dermatol Syphiligr* (French) 83, 79
Warts
  (1982): Stüttgen G, *Int J Dermatol* 21, 198
Xerosis

Hair

Hair – hypertrichosis
  (1983): Rampen FHJ, *Br J Dermatol* 109, 657
  (1967): Singh G+, *Br J Dermatol* 79, 501
  (1959): Elliot JA, *J Invest Dermatol* 32, 311

Nails

Nails – photo-onycholysis
  (1990): Baran R+, *Ann Dermatol Venereol* (French) 117, 367
  (1984): Balato N+, *Photodermatol* 1, 202
  (1978): Rau RC+, *Arch Dermatol* 114, 448
  (1977): Vella-Briffa D+, *BMJ* 2, 1150
  (1977): Zala L+, *Dermatologica* 154, 203
Nails – pigmentation
  (1990): Trattner A+, *Int J Dermatol* 29, 310
  (1989): Weiss E+, *Int J Dermatol* 28, 188
  (1986): MacDonald KJS+, *Br J Dermatol* 114, 395
  (1982): Naik RPC+, *Int J Dermatol* 21, 275
  (1979): Naik RP+, *Br J Dermatol* 100, 229

Other

Anaphylactoid reactions
  (2001): Legat FJ+, *Br J Dermatol* 145(5), 821
Lymphoproliferative disease
  (1989): Aschinoff R+, *J Am Acad Dermatol* 21, 1134
Tumors (sic)
  (1988): Gupta AK+, *J Am Acad Dermatol* 19, 67
  (1987): Henseler T+, *J Am Acad Dermatol* 16, 108

METHOXYFLURANE

Trade name: Penthrane (Astral) (Ger)
Indications: Anesthesia
Category: Anesthesia adjunct
Half-life: N/A
Clinically important, potentially hazardous interactions with: cisatracurium, demeclocycline, doxacurium, doxycycline, gentamicin, kanamycin, minocycline, neomycin, oxytetracycline, pancuronium, rapacuronium, streptomycin, tetracycline

Reactions

Skin
None

Other
None

METHSUXIMIDE

Trade name: Celontin (Parke-Davis)
Other common trade name: *Petinutin*
Indications: Absence (petit-mal) seizures
Category: Succinimide anticonvulsant
Half-life: 2–4 hours

Reactions

Skin
Acanthosis nigricans
  (1972): Petko E+, *Arch Dermatol* 106, 918
Erythema multiforme
Exanthems
  (1972): Petko E+, *Arch Dermatol* 106, 918
Exfoliative dermatitis (<1%)
Lupus erythematosus (>10%)
Periorbital edema
Pruritus
Purpura
Rash (sic)
Stevens–Johnson syndrome (>10%)
Urticaria (<1%)

Hair
Hair – alopecia
Hair – hirsutism

Other
Gingival hyperplasia
Headache
Oral ulceration

METHYCLOTHIAZIDE

Trade names: Aquatensen (Wallace); Enduronyl (Abbott)
Other common trade names: *Enduron-M; Thiazidil; Urimor*
Indications: Hypertension
Category: Antihypertensive; Thiazide diuretic
Half-life: N/A
Clinically important, potentially hazardous interactions with: digoxin, lithium

Reactions

Skin
Erythema multiforme
Exanthems
Photosensitivity (<1%)
Purpura
Rash (sic) (<1%)
Stevens–Johnson syndrome
Urticaria

Other
Anaphylactoid reactions
Dysgeusia
Paresthesias (<1%)

*Note: Methyclothiazide is a sulfonamide and can be absorbed systemically. Sulfonamides can produce severe, possibly fatal, reactions such as toxic epidermal necrolysis and Stevens–Johnson syndrome

METHYLDOPA

Trade names: Aldoclor (Merck); Aldomet (Merck); Aldoril (Merck)
Other common trade names: *Amodopa; Densul; Dopamet; Equibar; Hydopa; Medimet; Nu-Medopa; Polinal; Presinol; Prodopa*
Indications: Hypertension
Category: Alpha-adrenoceptor blocker; Antihypertensive
Half-life: 1.7 hours
Clinically important, potentially hazardous interactions with: ephedrine

Aldoril is methyldopa and hydrochlorothiazide

Reactions

Skin

Ankle edema
  (1969): Varadi DP+, *Arch Intern Med* 124, 13
Cheilitis
  (1973): Almeyda J+, *Br J Dermatol* 88, 313
Eczema (sic)
  (1974): Church R, *Br J Dermatol* 91, 373
  (1969): Peterkin GAG, *Practitioner* 202, 117 (keratotic – palms and soles)
  (1965): Dollery CT, *Prog in Cardiovasc Dis* 8, 278
Edema
Erythema multiforme (<1%)
  (1985): Ting HC+, *Int J Dermatol* 24, 587
  (1975): Böttiger LE+, *Acta Med Scand* 198, 229
Erythema nodosum
  (1978): Furhoff AK, *Acta Med Scand* 203, 425
Exanthems
  (1986): Gidseg G, *South Med J* 79, 389
  (1978): Furhoff AK, *Acta Med Scand* 203, 425
  (1971): Perry HM+, *J Lab Clin Med* 78, 905 (3%)
Fixed eruption
  (1974): Burry JN+, *Br J Dermatol* 91, 475
Granulomas
  (1974): Wells JD+, *Ann Intern Med* 81, 701
Lichen planus
  (1994): Thompson DF+, *Pharmacotherapy* 14, 561
  (1979): Krebs A, *Hautarzt* (German) 30, 281
  (1974): Burry JN+, *Br J Dermatol* 91, 475
Lichenoid eruption
  (1986): Gonzalez JG+, *J Am Acad Dermatol* 15, 87
  (1982): Brooks SL, *J Oral Med* 37, 42
  (1982): Wiesenfeld D+, *Oral Surg Oral Med Oral Pathol* 54, 527
  (1980): *Med J Aust* 2, 130
  (1976): Burry JN, *Arch Dermatol* 112, 880 (ulcerative)
  (1974): Holt PJA+, *BMJ* 3, 234
  (1973): Almeyda J+, *Br J Dermatol* 88, 313
  (1971): Almeyda J+, *Br J Dermatol* 85, 604
  (1971): Stevenson CJ, *Br J Dermatol* 85, 600
Lupus erythematosus (<1%)
  (1995): Sakurai Y+, *Nippon Naika Gakkai Zasshi* (Japanese) 84, 2069
  (1994): Yung RL+, *Rheum Dis Clin North Am* 20, 61
  (1992): Skaer TL, *Clin Ther* 14, 496
  (1989): Nordstrom DM+, *Arthritis Rheum* 32, 205
  (1985): Cush JJ+, *Am J Med Sci* 290, 36
  (1985): Stratton MA, *Clin Pharm* 4, 657
  (1983): Homberg JC+, *J Pharmacol* (French) 14, 61
  (1982): Dupont A+, *BMJ* 2, 693
  (1981): Harrington TM+, *Chest* 79, 696
  (1977): Schubothe H+, *Immun Infekt* (German) 5, 142

  (1974): Gustavsen WR, *Tidsskr Nor Laegeforen* (Norwegian) 94, 22
  (1972): Dorfmann H+, *Nouv Presse Med* (French) 1, 2907
  (1967): Sherman JD+, *Arch Intern Med* 120, 321
Papulo-vesicular eruption
  (1977): Heid E+, *Ann Dermatol Venereol* (French) 104, 494
Peripheral edema (>10%)
Petechiae
  (1978): Furhoff AK, *Acta Med Scand* 203, 425
Photosensitivity
  (1988): Vaillant L+, *Arch Dermatol* 124, 326
  (1973): Almeyda J+, *Br J Dermatol* 88, 313
Pigmentation
  (1986): Brody HJ+, *Cutis* 38, 187
  (1973): Almeyda J+, *Br J Dermatol* 88, 313
  (1969): Varadi DP+, *Arch Intern Med* 124, 13
Pruritus
  (1973): Almeyda J+, *Br J Dermatol* 88, 313
Purpura
  (1971): Menohitharajah SM+, *BMJ* 1, 494
Rash (sic) (<1%)
Seborrheic dermatitis
  (1974): Burry JN+, *Br J Dermatol* 91, 475
  (1974): Church R, *Br J Dermatol* 91, 373
  (1973): Church R, *Br J Dermatol* 89, 10
Stevens–Johnson syndrome
  (1985): Ting HC+, *Int J Dermatol* 24, 587
Toxic epidermal necrolysis
Urticaria
  (1986): Gidseg G, *S Med J* 79, 389
  (1978): Furhoff AK, *Acta Med Scand* 203, 425
Vasculitis
  (1989): Matteson EL+, *Arthritis Rheum* 32, 356

Hair

Hair – alopecia

Other

Acute intermittent porphyria
Black tongue (<1%)
  (1986): Brody HJ+, *Cutis* 38, 137
Galactorrhea
  (1963): Pettinger WA+, *BMJ* 1, 1460
Glossodynia
Gynecomastia (<1%)
Headache
Hypersensitivity
  (1993): Wolf R+, *Ann Allergy* 71, 166
Myalgia
Oral lichenoid eruption
  (1988): Zain RB+, *Dent J Malays* 10, 15
  (1982): Brooks SL, *J Oral Med* 37, 42
Oral mucosal eruption
  (1973): Almeyda J+, *Br J Dermatol* 88, 313
Oral ulceration
  (1990): Espana A+, *Med Clin* (Barc) (Spanish) 94, 559 (lichenoid)
  (1980): McLellan GH+, *Clin Prevent Dent* 2, 18
  (1978): Hay KD+, *Br Dent J* 145, 195
  (1974): Burry JN+, *Br J Dermatol* 91, 475
  (1971): Stevenson CJ, *Br J Dermatol* 85, 600
  (1967): Mackie BS, *Br J Dermatol* 79, 106 (LIP)
Paresthesias (<1%)
Parkinsonism
Xerostomia (1–10%)
  (1969): Varadi DP+, *Arch Intern Med* 124, 13

METHYLPHENIDATE

Trade names: Concerta; Metadate CD (Celltech); Methylin (Mallinckrodt); Ritalin (Novartis)
Other common trade names: *Centedrin; Rilatine; Rubifen*
Indications: Attention deficit disorder, narcolepsy
Category: Central nervous system stimulant
Half-life: 2–4 hours
Clinically important, potentially hazardous interactions with: pimozide

Reactions

Skin
Angioedema
  (1977): Sverd J+, *Pediatrics* 59, 115
  (1972): Rothschild CJ+, *Can Med Assoc J* 106, 1064
Diaphoresis
Edema (eyelids)
  (1972): Rothschild CJ+, *Can Med Assoc J* 106, 1064
Eosinophilic syndrome
  (1978): Wolf J+, *Ann Intern Med* 89, 224
Erythema multiforme
Exanthems
  (1977): Sverd J+, *Pediatrics* 59, 115
Exfoliative dermatitis
  (1977): Sverd J+, *Pediatrics* 59, 115
  (1968): Weil AJ, *Ann Allergy* 26, 402
Fixed eruption
  (1992): Cohen HA+, *Ann Pharmacother* 26, 1378 (scrotum)
Photosensitivity
  (1977): Sverd J+, *Pediatrics* 59, 115
Pruritus
Purpura
  (1978): Wolf J+, *Ann Intern Med* 89, 224
Rash (sic) (<1%)
Urticaria
  (1977): Sverd J+, *Pediatrics* 59, 115
Vasculitis
  (1977): Sverd J+, *Pediatrics* 59, 115

Hair
Hair – alopecia

Other
Bruxism
  (2000): Gara L+, *J Child Adolesc Psychopharmacol* 10, 39 (with valproic acid)
Delusions of parasitosis
  (1999): Eisner J (from Internet) (observation)
Headache
Hypersensitivity (1–10%)
  (1990): Calis KA+, *Clin Pharm* 9, 632
Injection-site abscess
  (1976): Elenbaas RM+, *JACEP* 5, 977
Tourette's syndrome
Xerostomia
  (1993): Pataki CS+, *J Am Acad Child Adolesc Psychiatry* 32, 1065

METHYLTESTOSTERONE

Trade names: Android (ICN); Estratest (Solvay); Metandren; Oreton (ICN); Testred (ICN); Virilon (Star)
Other common trade names: *Androral; B; Enarmon; Teston; Testotonic 'B'; Testovis; Viromone*
Indications: Hypogonadism, impotence, metastatic breast cancer
Category: Androgen; Antineoplastic
Half-life: 2.5–3.5 hours
Clinically important, potentially hazardous interactions with: anticoagulants, cyclosporine, warfarin

Reactions

Skin
Acanthosis nigricans
  (1987): Shuttleworth D+, *Clin Exp Dermatol* 12, 288
Acne (>10%)
  (1992): Fryand O+, *Acta Derm Venereol* 72, 148
  (1990): Fuchs E+, *J Am Acad Dermatol* 23, 125
  (1989): Fryand O+, *Tidsskr Nor Laegeforen* (Norwegian) 109, 239
  (1989): Hartmann AA+, *Monatsschr Kinderheilkd* (German) 137, 466
  (1989): Heydenreich G, *Arch Dermatol* 125, 571 (fulminans)
  (1989): Scott MJ+, *Cutis* 44, 30
  (1989): von Muhlendahl KE+, *Dtsch Med Wochenschr* (German) 114, 712
  (1988): Traupe H+, *Arch Dermatol* 124, 414 (fulminans)
  (1987): Kiraly CL+, *Am J Dermatopathol* 9, 515
  (1984): Lamb DR, *Am J Sports Med* 12, 31
  (1965): Kennedy BJ, *J Am Geriatr Soc* 13, 230
  (1965): Rook A, *Br J Dermatol* 77, 115
Dermatitis
  (1989): Holdiness MR, *Contact Dermatitis* 20, 3 (from patch)
Edema (>10%)
Exanthems
Flushing (1–5%)
  (1965): Kennedy BJ, *J Am Geriatr Soc* 13, 230
Furunculosis
  (1989): Scott MJ+, *Cutis* 44, 30
Lichenoid eruption
  (1989): Aihara M+, *J Dermatol* (Tokio) 16, 330
Lupus erythematosus
  (1978): Robinson HM, *Z Haut* (German) 53, 349
Pruritus
Psoriasis
  (1990): O'Driscoll JB+, *Clin Exp Dermatol* 15, 68
Purpura
Seborrhea
Seborrheic dermatitis
  (1989): Scott MJ+, *Cutis* 44, 30
Striae
  (1989): Scott MJ+, *Cutis* 44, 30
Urticaria

Hair
Hair – alopecia
  (1989): Scott MJ+, *Cutis* 44, 30
  (1965): Kennedy BJ, *J Am Geriatr Soc* 13, 230
Hair – hirsutism (1–10%) (in females)
  (1994): Castillo-Ceballos A+, *Med Clin (Barc)* (Spanish) 102, 78
  (1991): Bates GW+, *Clin Obstet Gynecol* 34, 848
  (1991): No Author, *Obstet Gynecol* 78, 474
  (1991): Parker LU+, *Cleve Clin J Med* 58, 43
  (1991): Urman B+, *Obstet Gynecol* 77, 595

(1989): Scott MJ+, *Cutis* 44, 30
(1974): Baron J, *Zentralbl Gynakol* (German) 96, 129
(1971): Fusi S+, *Folia Endocrinol* (Italian) 24, 412
(1965): Kennedy BJ, *J Am Geriatr Soc* 13, 230

Other
Anaphylactoid reactions
Gynecomastia (<1%)
Headache
Hypersensitivity (<1%)
Injection-site pain
Mastodynia (>10%)
Paresthesias
Priapism (>10%)
Stomatitis

METHYSERGIDE

Trade name: Sansert (Novartis)
Other common trade names: *Deseril; Desernil; Deserril; Deseryl*
Indications: Vascular (migraine) headaches
Category: Ergot alkaloid; Vascular headache prophylactic
Half-life: 10 hours
Clinically important, potentially hazardous interactions with: almotriptan, amprenavir, clarithromycin, delavirdine, efavirenz, erythromycin, indinavir, naratriptan, nelfinavir, ritonavir, rizatriptan, saquinavir, sibutramine, sumatriptan, troleandomycin, zolmitriptan

Reactions

Skin
Adverse effects (sic)
  (1991): Mylecharane EJ, *J Neurol* 238, S45
Collagenosis (sic)
  (1973): Anker N, *Ugeskr Laeger* (Danish) 135, 2225
Exanthems
Flushing
  (1964): Graham JR, *N Engl J Med* 270, 67 (0.8%)
Hypermelanosis
  (1964): Graham JR, *N Engl J Med* 270, 67
Lupus erythematosus
  (1968): Racouchot J+, *Bull Soc Franc Dermatol Syphiligr* (French) 75, 513
  (1968): Racouchot J+, *Lyon Med* (French) 220, 1766
Orange-peel skin (sic)
  (1964): Graham JR, *N Engl J Med* 270, 67 (1%)
Peripheral edema (1–10%)
Pruritus
Rash (sic) (1–10%)
Raynaud's phenomenon
Scleroderma
  (1984): Garcia de Quesada FJ+, *Med Clin (Barc)* (Spanish) 82, 604
  (1980): Graham JR, *Trans Am Clin Climatol Assoc* 92, 122
  (1978): Goldberg NC+, *Arch Dermatol* 114, 550
Telangiectasia
Urticaria

Hair
Hair – alopecia
  (1991): Mylecharane EJ, *J Neurol* 238, S45
  (1974): Sadjadpour K, *JAMA* 229, 639
  (1964): Graham JR, *N Engl J Med* 270, 67 (1%)
  (1964): Leyton N, *Lancet* 1, 830 (0.4%)

Other
Headache
Hyperesthesia (<1%)
Myalgia
Paresthesias

METOCLOPRAMIDE

Trade name: Reglan (Elkins-Sinn) (Wyeth)
Other common trade names: *Apo-Metoclop; Duraclamid; Emex; Gastrocil; Gastronerton; Maxeran; Maxolon; Mygdalon; Primperan*
Indications: Gastroesophageal reflux
Category: Antiemetic; Dopaminergic blocking agent; Peristaltic stimulant
Half-life: 4–6 hours
Clinically important, potentially hazardous interactions with: sertraline, venlafaxine

Reactions

Skin
Allergic reactions (sic)
  (1986): Bigby M+, *JAMA* 256, 3358
Angioedema
  (1983): Pinder RM+, *Drugs* 25, 451
  (1976): Pinder RM+, *Drugs* 12, 81
Diaphoresis
  (2002): Fisher AA+, *Ann Pharmacother* 36(1), 67
Exanthems
  (1983): Pinder RM+, *Drugs* 25, 451
  (1976): Arndt KA+, *JAMA* 235, 918 (0.4%)
  (1976): Pinder RM+, *Drugs* 12, 81
Flushing
Rash (sic) (1–10%)
Urticaria
  (1983): Pinder RM+, *Drugs* 25, 451
  (1976): Pinder RM+, *Drugs* 12, 81

Other
Blue tongue
  (1989): Alroe C+, *Med J Aust* 150, 724
Galactorrhea
Gynecomastia
  (1997): Madani S+, *J Clin Gastroenterol* 24, 79
Mastodynia (1–10%)
Paresthesias
  (1997): du Bois A+, *Oncology* 54, 7
Parkinsonism
  (2002): Hoogendam A+, *Ned Tijdschr Geneeskd* 146(4), 175
Porphyria
  (1997): Gorchein A, *Lancet* 350, 1104
  (1981): Doss M+, *Lancet* 2, 91
Serotonin syndrome
  (2002): Fisher AA+, *Ann Pharmacother* 36(1), 67
  (2000): Vandermegel X+, *Rev Med Brux* 21(3), 161 (with sertaline)
Tardive dyskinesia
  (1990): Miller LG+, *South Med J* 83(5), 525 (8%)
Xerostomia (1–10%)

METOLAZONE*

Trade names: Mykrox (Celltech); Zaroxolyn (Celltech)
Other common trade names: *Barolyn; Diondel; Metenix 5; Normelan; Xuret*
Indications: Hypertension, edema
Category: Antihypertensive; Sulfonamide diuretic
Half-life: 6–20 hours
Clinically important, potentially hazardous interactions with: digoxin, lithium

Reactions

Skin
Chills (1–10%)
Edema (<2%)
Exanthems
Exfoliative dermatitis
Necrotizing angiitis
Photosensitivity (<2%)
Pruritus (<2%)
Purpura (<1%)
Rash (sic) (<2%)
Stevens–Johnson syndrome
Toxic epidermal necrolysis
  (1991): Lacy JA, *Nutr Clin Pract* 6, 18
Urticaria (<2%)
Vasculitis
  (1991): Cox NH+, *Postgrad Med J* 67, 860
  (1982): Weinrauch LA+, *Cutis* 30, 83
Xerosis (<2%)

Other
Anaphylactoid reactions (<2%)
Dysgeusia (<2%)
Headache
Paresthesias (<2%)
Tinnitus
Xanthopsia (<2%)
Xerostomia (<2%)

*Note: Metolazone is a sulfonamide and can be absorbed systemically. Sulfonamides can produce severe, possibly fatal, reactions such as toxic epidermal necrolysis and Stevens–Johnson syndrome

METOPROLOL

Trade names: Lopressor (Novartis); Toprol XL (AstraZeneca)
Other common trade names: *Beloc-Zoc; Betaloc; Betazok; Kenaprol; Mycol; Prolaken; Ritmolol; Seloken-Zok; Selozok*
Indications: Hypertension, angina pectoris
Category: Antihypertensive; Beta-adrenoceptor blocker
Half-life: 3–4 hours
Clinically important, potentially hazardous interactions with: clonidine, epinephrine, verapamil

Lopressor HCT is metoprolol and hydrochlorothiazide

Note: Cutaneous side effects of beta-receptor blockaders are clinically polymorphous. They apparently appear after several months of continuous therapy. Atypical psoriasiform, lichen planus-like, and eczematous chronic rashes are mainly observed. (1983): Hödl St, *Z Hautkr* (German) 58, 17

Reactions

Skin
Angioedema
  (1994): Krikorian RK+, *Chest* 106, 1922
Diaphoresis
Eczema (sic)
  (1981): Neumann HAM+, *Dermatologica* 162, 330
  (1979): Neumann HAM+, *Lancet* 2, 745
Edema
Erythema multiforme
Exanthems
  (1986): Benfield P+, *Drugs* 31, 376 (1.5%)
Exfoliative dermatitis
Hyperkeratosis (palms and soles)
Lichenoid eruption
  (1988): Kardaun SH+, *Br J Dermatol* 118, 545
  (1983): Hödl St, *Z Hautkr* (German) 58, 17
  (1978): Savage RL+, *BMJ* 1, 987
Lupus erythematosus
  (1981): Paladini G, *Int J Tissue React* 3, 95
Peripheral edema (1%)
Pigmentation
Pityriasis rubra pilaris
  (1978): Finlay AY+, *BMJ* 1, 987
Prurigo
  (1983): Hödl St, *Z Hautkr* (German) 58, 17
Pruritus (1–5%)
  (1994): Shelley WB+, *Cutis* 53, 39 (scalp) (observation)
  (1986): Benfield P+, *Drugs* 31, 376
Psoriasis (induction and aggravation of)
  (2002): Litt JZ, Beachwood, OH (personal case) (observation) (induction of)
  (1993): Litt JZ, Beachwood, OH (personal case) (observation)
  (1988): Heng MCY+, *Int J Dermatol* 27, 619 (pustular, generalized)
  (1987): Altomare GF+, *G Ital Dermatol Venereol* (Italian) 122, 531
  (1986): Abel EA+, *J Am Acad Dermatol* 15, 1007
  (1986): Czernielewski J+, *Lancet* 1, 808
  (1984): Arntzen N+, *Acta Derm Venereol* (Stockh) 64, 346
  (1981): Neumann HAM+, *Dermatologica* 162, 330
  (1979): Neumann HAM+, *Lancet* 2, 745
Purpura
Rash (sic) (<5%)
Raynaud's phenomenon (<1%)
  (1984): Eliasson K+, *Acta Med Scand* 215, 333
  (1976): Marshall AJ+, *BMJ* 1, 1498
Scleroderma

(1980): Graham JR, *Trans Am Clin Climatol Assoc* 92, 122
Toxic epidermal necrolysis
Urticaria
Xerosis

Hair

Hair – alopecia
  (1981): Graeber CW+, *Cutis* 28, 633

Nails

Nails – bluish
Nails – dystrophy
Nails – onycholysis
Nails – transverse depression (sic)
  (1981): Graeber CW+, *Cutis* 28, 633

Other

Dysgeusia
Gangrene (feet)
  (1979): Gokal R+, *BMJ* 19, 837
Headache
Oculo-mucocutaneous syndrome
  (1982): Cocco G+, *Curr Ther Res* 31, 362
Oral lichenoid eruption
Paresthesias
Peyronie's disease
  (1981): Jones HA+, *Med J Aust* 2, 514
  (1981): Neumann HAM+, *Dermatologica* 162, 330
  (1981): Paladini G, *Int J Tissue React* 3, 95
  (1979): Pryor JP+, *Lancet* 1, 331
  (1977): Yudkin JS, *Lancet* 2, 1355
Polymyalgia
  (1991): Snyder S, *Ann Intern Med* 114, 96
Scalp tingling
  (1979): Coulter DM, *N Z Med J* 90, 397
Tinnitus

METRONIDAZOLE

Trade names: Flagyl (Pharmacia); Helidac (Prometheus); Metrocream (Galderma); Metrogel (Galderma); Metrolotion (Galderma); Noritate (Dermik); Protostat; Satric
Other common trade names: *Arilin; Ariline; Asuzol; Clont; Fossyol; Milezzol; Nida Gel; Novo-Nidazol; Otrozol; Rozagel; Rozex; Trikacide; Zadstat*
Indications: Various infections caused by susceptible organisms, rosacea
Category: Antimicrobial; Antiprotozoal
Half-life: 6–12 hours
Clinically important, potentially hazardous interactions with: alcohol, anisindione, anticoagulants, dicumarol, disulfiram, fluorouracil, warfarin

Reactions

Skin

Acute generalized exanthematous pustulosis (AGEP)
  (1999): Watsky KL, *Arch Dermatol* 135, 93
  (1994): Manders SM+, *Cutis* 54, 194 (with cefazolin)
Angioedema
  (1978): Shevliakov LV, *Vestn Dermatol Venerol* (Russian) February, 49
Candidiasis (exacerbation)
  (1977): Maize JC+, *Arch Dermatol* 113, 1457 (passim)
Dermatitis
  (2002): Choudry K+, *Contact Dermatitis* 46(1), 60

  (1997): Vincenzi C+, *Contact Dermatitis* 36, 116
Erythema
Exanthems
  (1995): Litt JZ, Beachwood, OH (personal case) (observation)
  (1977): Swami B+, *Curr Med Res Opin* 5, 152 (1–5%)
  (1969): *Med Lett* 11, 27 (1–5%)
Fixed eruption
  (2002): Short KA+, *Clin Exp Dermatol* 27(6), 464
  (2002): Short KA, (London) (England) March AAD Poster (4 recurrences)
  (2002): Vila JB+, *Contact Dermatitis* 46(2), 122
  (2002): Walfish AE+, *Cutis* 69, 207 (doxycycline, in the same patient, also produced a fixed eruption)
  (2001): Gastaminza G+, *Contact Dermatitis* 44(1), 36
  (1998): Mahboob A+, *Int J Dermatol* 37, 833
  (1998): Thami GP+, *Dermatology* 196, 368
  (1990): Gaffoor PMA+, *Cutis* 45, 242
  (1990): Kanwar AJ+, *Dermatologica* 180, 277
  (1990): Mishra D+, *Int J Dermatol* 29, 740
  (1987): Shelley WB+, *Cutis* 39, 393
  (1977): Naik RPC+, *Dermatologica* 155, 59
Flushing
  (1992): Shelley WB+, *Advanced Dermatologic Diagnosis* WB Saunders, 582 (passim)
  (1977): Maize JC+, *Arch Dermatol* 113, 1457 (passim)
Linear IgA bullous dermatosis
Pityriasis rosea
  (1977): Maize JC+, *Arch Dermatol* 113, 1457
Pruritus (1–5%)
  (2001): Gastaminza G+, *Contact Dermatitis* 44(1), 36
  (1977): Maize JC+, *Arch Dermatol* 113, 1457 (passim)
  (1977): Swami B+, *Curr Med Res Opin* 5, 152 (10%)
  (1963): Foster SA+, *Am J Obstet Gynecol* 87, 1013
Rash (sic)
Toxic epidermal necrolysis
  (1999): Egan CA+, *J Am Acad Dermatol* 40, 458
  (1981): Titov RL, *Klin Med Mosk* (Russian) 59, 85
Urticaria
  (1997): Blumenthal HL, Beachwood, OH (personal case) (observation)
  (1977): Maize JC+, *Arch Dermatol* 113, 1457 (passim)
  (1963): Foster SA+, *Am J Obstet Gynecol* 87, 1013

Other

Acute intermittent porphyria
Disulfiram-like reaction
Dysgeusia (<1%) (metallic taste)
  (1997): Palop Larrea V+, *Aten Primaria* (Spanish) 20, 524
Glossitis
  (1987): Shelley WB+, *Cutis* 39, 393
Gynecomastia
  (1985): Fagan TC+, *JAMA* 254, 3217
Headache
Hypersensitivity (<1%)
Injection-site vasculitis
Oral mucosal eruption
  (1969): *Med Lett* 11, 27
Oral ulceration
Paresthesias
Serum sickness
  (1983): Weart CW+, *South Med J* 76, 410
Stomatitis
  (1987): Shelley WB+, *Cutis* 39, 393
Thrombophlebitis (<1%)
Tongue furry (<1%)
  (1987): Shelley WB+, *Cutis* 39, 393
  (1977): Maize JC+, *Arch Dermatol* 113, 1457 (passim)
Vaginal candidiasis (<1%)
Xerostomia (<1%)

MEXILETINE

Trade name: Mexitil (Boehringer Ingelheim)
Other common trade names: *Mexihexal; Mexilen; Mexitec*
Indications: Ventricular arrhythmias
Category: Antiarrhythmic class I B
Half-life: 10–12 hours
Clinically important, potentially hazardous interactions with: caffeine

Reactions

Skin
Acute generalized exanthematous pustulosis (AGEP)
  (2001): Sasaki K+, *Eur J Dermatol* 11, 469
Diaphoresis (<1%)
Edema (3.8%)
Exanthems
  (2001): Sasaki K+, *Eur J Dermatol* 11(5), 469
  (1997): Higa K+, *Pain* 73, 97
  (1996): Nagayama H+, *J Dermatol* 23, 899
  (1992): Habot B+, *Harefuah* (Hebrew) 123, 462
  (1991): Kikuchi K+, *Contact Dermatitis* 25, 70
  (1988): Kardaun SH+, *Br J Dermatol* 118, 545
  (1984): Ribera Pibernat M+, *Med Clin (Barc)* (Spanish) 83, 825
  (1979): Habeler G+, *Dtsch Med Wochenschr* (German) 104, 1244
Exfoliative dermatitis (<1%)
Facial edema
  (2001): Sasaki K+, *Eur J Dermatil* 11(5), 469
Hot flashes (<1%)
Lupus erythematosus (<1%)
Pruritus
  (1997): Higa K+, *Pain* 73, 97
Purpura
Rash (sic) (3.8%)
Stevens–Johnson syndrome (<1%)
Urticaria
  (1994): Yamazaki S+, *Br J Dermatol* 130, 538
  (1988): Kardaun SH+, *Br J Dermatol* 118, 545
Xerosis (<1%)

Hair
Hair – alopecia (<1%)

Other
Dysgeusia (<1%)
  (2000): Zervakis J+, *Physiol Behav* 68, 405
Headache
Paresthesias (3.8%)
Pseudolymphoma
  (1996): Magro CM+, *Hum Pathol* 27(2), 125
Salivary changes (sic) (<1%)
Tinnitus
Trembling (1–10%)
Tremor (12.6%)
Xerostomia (2.8%)

MEZLOCILLIN

Trade name: Mezlin (Bayer)
Other common trade name: *Baypen*
Indications: Various infections caused by susceptible organisms
Category: Beta-lactamase-sensitive penicillin
Half-life: 0.8–1.0 hours
Clinically important, potentially hazardous interactions with: anticoagulants, cyclosporine, demeclocycline, doxycycline, methotrexate, minocycline, oxytetracycline, tetracycline

Reactions

Skin
Allergic reactions (sic)
  (1994): Pleasants RA+, *Chest* 106, 1124 (in patients with cystic fibrosis)
Angioedema
Bullous eruption
Dermatitis
  (1992): Keller K+, *Contact Dermatitis* 27, 348
Ecchymoses
Erythema multiforme
Erythema nodosum
Exanthems
Exfoliative dermatitis (<1%)
Hematomas
Jarisch–Herxheimer reaction
Pruritus
Rash (sic) (<1%)
Stevens–Johnson syndrome
Toxic epidermal necrolysis
Urticaria
Vasculitis

Other
Anaphylactoid reactions
Black tongue
Dysgeusia
Glossitis
Glossodynia
Hypersensitivity
  (1992): Keller K+, *Contact Dermatitis* 27, 348
Injection-site pain
Oral candidiasis
Phlebitis
Serum sickness (<1%)
Stomatitis
Stomatodynia
Thrombophlebitis
Vaginitis
Xerostomia

MICONAZOLE

Trade names: Lotrimin (Schering); Monistat (Personal Products)
Other common trade names: *Aflorix; Aloid; Daktarin; Florid; Funcort; Fungoid Tincture; Micotef; Miracol; Monazole-7; Zole*
Indications: Fungal infections
Category: Imidazole antifungal
Half-life: initial: 40 minutes; terminal: 24 hours
Clinically important, potentially hazardous interactions with: anisindione, anticoagulants, dicumarol, vinblastine, vincristine, warfarin

Reactions

Skin
Angioedema
  (1983): Stevens DA, *Drugs* 26, 347 (2.4%)
Bullous eruption
  (1983): Stevens DA, *Drugs* 26, 347
Chills (>5%)
Dermatitis
  (1996): Fernandez L+, *Contact Dermatitis* 34, 217
  (1995): Goday JJ+, *Contact Dermatitis* 32, 370
  (1991): Baes H, *Contact Dermatitis* 24, 89
  (1988): Perret CM+, *Contact Dermatitis* 19, 75
  (1988): Raulin C+, *Contact Dermatitis* 18, 76
  (1984): Aldridge RD+, *Contact Dermatitis* 10, 58
  (1983): Frenzel UH+, *Contact Dermatitis* 9, 74
  (1982): Foged EK+, *Contact Dermatitis* 8, 284
  (1979): Wade TR+, *Contact Dermatitis* 5, 168
  (1977): Samsoen M+, *Contact Dermatitis* 3, 351
  (1975): Degreef H+, *Contact Dermatitis* 1, 269
Erythema
Exanthems
  (1987): Verhagen C+, *Eur J Haematol* 38, 225 (28%)
  (1983): Stevens DA, *Drugs* 26, 347 (2.4%)
  (1980): Heel RC+, *Drugs* 19, 7 (3–8%)
  (1977): Fischer TJ+, *J Pediatr* 91, 815 (10%)
  (1977): Sung JP+, *N Engl J Med* 297, 786 (87%)
Flushing (<1%)
  (1983): Stevens DA, *Drugs* 26, 347
  (1980): Heel RC+, *Drugs* 19, 7 (1–2%)
Pruritus (21%)
  (1983): Stevens DA, *Drugs* 26, 347 (36%)
  (1980): Heel RC+, *Drugs* 19, 7 (2–21%)
  (1977): Fischer TJ+, *J Pediatr* 91, 815 (21%)
Purpura
  (1980): Heel RC+, *Drugs* 19, 7 (3–8%)
Rash (sic) (9%)
Urticaria
  (1983): Stevens DA, *Drugs* 26, 347 (2.4%)
Xanthomas
  (1978): Barr RJ+, *Arch Dermatol* 114, 1544 (eruptive)

Other
Anaphylactoid reactions
Injection-site pain (>10%)
  (1980): Heel RC+, *Drugs* 19, 7 (0.5–2%)
Phlebitis (>5%)
  (1983): Stevens DA, *Drugs* 26, 347 (35%)
  (1980): Heel RC+, *Drugs* 19, 7 (6–28%)
  (1977): Fischer TJ+, *J Pediatr* 91, 815 (79%)

MIDAZOLAM

Trade name: Versed (Roche)
Other common trade name: *Dormicum*
Indications: Preoperative sedation
Category: Anesthetic; Benzodiazepine sedative-analgesic; Benzodiazepine sedative-hypnotic
Half-life: 1–4 hours
Clinically important, potentially hazardous interactions with: amprenavir, aprepitant, atazanavir, carbamazepine, chlorpheniramine, cimetidine, clarithromycin, clorazepate, CNS depressants, delavirdine, dexamethasone, efavirenz, erythromycin, esomeprazole, fluconazole, fluoxetine, griseofulvin, imatinib, indinavir, itraconazole, ivermectin, ketoconazole, nelfinavir, nevirapine, phenobarbital, phenytoin, primidone, rifabutin, rifampin, ritonavir, saquinavir, **St John's wort**

Reactions

Skin
Angioedema
  (1992): Yakel DL+, *Crit Care Med* 20, 307
Exanthems
Peripheral edema (<1%)
Pruritus (<1%)
  (1989): Yates A+, *Anaesthesia* 44, 449
Rash (sic) (<1%)
Urticaria (<1%)

Other
Anaphylactoid reactions (<1%)
Dysgeusia (<1%) (acid taste)
Headache
Injection-site pain (>10%)
  (1984): Dundee JW+, *Drugs* 28, 519 (26%)
Injection-site reactions (sic) (>10%)
Local reaction
  (1993): Kundrotas L+, *Gastrointest Endosc* 39, 109
Paresthesias
Sialorrhea (<1%)

MIDODRINE

Trade name: Proamatine (Shire)
Other common trade names: *Amatine; Gutron; Metligine; Midon*
Indications: Orthostatic hypotension, urinary incontinence
Category: Alpha agonist; Antihypotensive; Vasopressor
Half-life: ~3–4 hours

Reactions

Skin
Chills (5%)
Erythema multiforme
Flushing (1–10%)
Piloerection
  (1998): McClellan KJ+, *Drugs Aging* 12(1), 76
  (1989): McTavish D+, *Drugs* 38(5), 757
Pruritus (12.2%)
  (1998): McClellan KJ+, *Drugs Aging* 12(1), 76
  (1993): Jankovic J+, *Am J Med* 95(1), 38 (scalp) (13.5%)
Rash (sic) (2.4%)

Xerosis (2%)
Other
Aphthous stomatitis
Headache
Hyperesthesia
Pain (5%)
Paresthesias (18.3%)
  (1998): McClellan KJ+, *Drugs Aging* 12(1), 76
  (1997): Cruz DN+, *Am J Kidney Dis* 30(6), 772
  (1993): Jankovic J+, *Am J Med* 95(1), 38 (scalp) (13.5%)
Xerostomia (1–10%)

MIFEPRISTONE

Synonym: RU-486
Trade name: Mifeprex (Danco)
Indications: Medical termination of intrauterine pregnancy
Category: Abortifacient; Glucocorticoid antagonist
Half-life: ~20 hours

Reactions

Skin
Chills (3%)
Infections (sic)
  (2001): DeHart RM+, *Ann Pharmacother* 35(6), 707
Viral infections (4%)

Other
Headache
Vaginal bleeding (~100%)
Vaginitis (3%)

MIGLITOL

Trade name: Glyset (Pharmacia)
Indications: Non-insulin dependent diabetes type II
Category: Antidiabetic alpha-glucosidase inhibitor
Half-life: ~2 hours

Reactions

Skin
Rash (sic) (1–10%)

MILK THISTLE*

Scientific names: *Carduus marainum; Silibum marianum*
Family: Asteraceae; Compositae
Trade and other common names: Holy Thistle; Lady's Thistle; Marian Thistle; Mary Thistle; Silymarin
Category: anti-inflammatory; Hepatoprotective
Purported indications and other uses: Dyspepsia, liver protectant, hepatitis, loss of appetite, spleen diseases, supportive treatment for mushroom poisoning
Half-life: N/A

Reactions

Skin
Adverse effects (sic)
  (2000): *Evid Rep Technol* p(21), 1
  (1999): No Author, *Med J Aust* 170(5), 218
Allergic reactions (sic)
Diaphoresis
Rash (sic)
  (2001): Saller R+, *Drugs* 61(14), 2035
Urticaria
  (1990): Mironets VI+, *Vrach Delo* 7, 86

*Note: Seed as opposed to the 'aboveground parts'

MINOCYCLINE

Trade names: Arestin; Dynacin (Medicis); Minocin (Wyeth)
Other common trade names: *Alti-Minocycline; Apo-Minocycline; Mestacine; Minoclir 50; Minogalen; Minomycin; Mynocine; Syn-Minocycline*
Indications: Various infections caused by susceptible organisms
Category: Tetracycline antibiotic
Half-life: 11–23 hours
Clinically important, potentially hazardous interactions with: acitretin, aluminum salts, amoxicillin, ampicillin, antacids, bacampicillin, bismuth, calcium, carbenicillin, cloxacillin, digoxin, iron salts, isotretinoin, magnesium salts, methotrexate, methoxyflurane, mezlocillin, nafcillin, oxacillin, penicillins, piperacillin, ticarcillin, vitamin A, zinc salts

Reactions

Skin
Acute febrile neutrophilic dermatosis (Sweet's syndrome)
  (2002): Khan Durani+, *Br J Dermatol* 147(3), 558
  (1992): Thibault M-J+, *J Am Acad Dermatol* 27, 801
  (1991): Mensing H+, *Dermatologica* 182, 43
Acute generalized exanthematous pustulosis (AGEP)
  (1997): Yamamoto T+, *Acta Derm Venereol* (Stockh) 77, 168 (in a patient with pustular psoriasis)
Angioedema
  (1997): Shapiro LE+, *Arch Dermatol* 133, 1224
  (1994): Levy SB, Chapel Hill, NC (personal case) (reproducible) (observation)
  (1993): Litt JZ, Beachwood, OH (personal case) (observation)
Candidiasis
Cellulitis
  (1994): Kaufmann D+, *Arch Intern Med* 154, 1983
  (1989): Andreano JM+, *J Am Acad Dermatol* 20, 934
Elastolysis
  (2000): Ho NC+, *Am J Med* 109(4), 340

Eosinophilic pustular folliculitis (Ofuji's disease)
  (1989): Andreano JM+, J Am Acad Dermatol 20, 934
Erythema multiforme
  (1987): Shoji A+, Arch Dermatol 123, 18
Erythema nodosum
  (1990): Bridges AJ+, J Am Acad Dermatol 22, 959
Erythroderma
  (2002): Murray C+, World Congress Dermatol Poster, 0120
Exanthems
  (2002): Blumenthal HL, Beachwood, OH (personal case)
     (observation)
  (1996): Knowles SR+, Arch Dermatol 132, 934
  (1995): Karofsky PS+, Arch Pediatr Adolesc Med 149, 217
  (1995): Litt JZ, Beachwood, OH (2 personal cases) (mother and
     daughter) (observation)
  (1994): Kaufmann D+, Arch Intern Med 154, 1983
  (1975): Brogden RN+, Drugs 9, 251
  (1973): Shelley WB+, JAMA 224, 125
Exfoliative dermatitis (<1%)
  (1997): MacNeil M+, J Am Acad Dermatol 36, 347
  (1996): Knowles SR+, Arch Dermatol 132, 934
  (1989): Davies MG+, BMJ 298, 1523
Fixed eruption (<1%)
  (1999): Correia O+, Clin Exp Dermatol 24, 137 (genital) (with
     doxycycline)
  (1994): Chu P+, J Am Acad Dermatol 30, 802 (pigmentation)
  (1992): Ridgway HB+, Arch Dermatol 128, 565
  (1984): Bargman H, J Am Acad Dermatol 11, 900
  (1983): LePaw MI, J Am Acad Dermatol 8, 263
  (1978): Jolly HW+, Arch Dermatol 114, 1484
  (1977): Shimizu Y+, Jpn J Dermatol 4, 73
Folliculitis
  (1994): Kaufmann D+, Arch Intern Med 154, 1983 (pustular)
  (1989): Andreano JM+, J Am Acad Dermatol 20, 934
Lichenoid eruption
  (1993): Litt JZ, Beachwood, OH (personal case) (observation)
Livedo reticularis
  (2000): Schlienger RG+, Dermatology 200, 223
Lupus erythematosus
  (2002): Marai I+, Harefuah 141(2), 151
  (2001): Balestero S+, Int J Dermatol 40, 475
  (2001): Gordon MM+, J Rheumatol 28(5), 1004
  (2001): Graham LE+, Clin Rheumatol 20(1), 67
  (2001): Lawson TM+, Rheumatology (Oxford) 40(3), 329
  (2001): Marzo-Ortega H+, J Rheumatol 28(2), 377
  (2000): Choi HK+, Arthritis Rheum 43, 2488
  (2000): Colmegna I+, J Rheumatol 27, 1567
  (2000): Dunphy J+, Br J Dermatol 142, 461
  (2000): Schlienger RG+, Dermatology 200, 223 (57 cases)
  (1999): Angulo JM+, J Rheumatol 26, 1420
  (1999): Christodoulou CS+, Chest 115(5), 1471
  (1999): Dadamessi I+, Rev Med Interne (French) 20, 930
  (1999): Elkayam O+, Semin Arthritis Rheum 28, 392
  (1999): Katz R, Skin and Allergy News, May, 13
  (1999): Piette AM+, Rev Med Interne (French) 20, 869
  (1999): Sturkenboom MC+, Arch Intern Med 159, 493
  (1999): Thaler D, Monona, WI (from internet) (observation)
  (1999): Tournigand C+, Lupus 8, 773
  (1998): Akin E+, Pediatrics 101, 926
  (1998): Angulo JM+, Semin Arthritis Rheum 28, 187
  (1998): Blumenthal HL, Beachwood, OH (personal case)
     (observation)
  (1998): Knights SE+, Clin Exp Dermatol 16, 587
  (1997): Crosson J+, J Am Acad Dermatol 36, 867
  (1997): Emery P+, J Rheumatol 24, 1850
  (1997): Farver DK, Ann Pharmacother 31, 1160
  (1997): Golstein PE+, Am J Gastroenterol 92, 143
  (1997): Hoefnagel JJ+, Ned Tijdschr Geneeskd 141, 1424
  (1997): Pointud P, J Rheumatol 24, 1851

  (1997): Singer SJ+, JAMA 277, 295
  (1997): Wilde JL+, Arch Dermatol 133, 1344
  (1996): Gough A+, BMJ 312, 169 (18 cases)
  (1996): Hewack J, Gastroenterology 110, A1211
  (1996): Knowles SR+, Arch Dermatol 132, 934
  (1996): Masson C+, J Rheumatol 23, 2160
  (1995): Bulgen DY, Br J Rheumatol 34, 398
  (1995): Gendi NS+, Br J Rheumatol 34, 584
  (1995): Gordon P+, Br J Dermatol 132, 120
  (1994): Byrne PA+, Br J Rheumatol 33, 674
  (1994): Inoue CN+, Eur J Pediatr 153, 540
  (1994): Quilty B+, Br J Rheumatol 33, 1197
  (1992): Matsuura T+, Lancet 340, 1553
  (1984): Alston LL, The Schoch Letter 34, #8, Item 110
Lupus erythematosus
  (2003): Hill VA+, Br J Dermatol 148(5), 1056 (3 cases)
Nodules (sic) (facial, blue-gray)
  (1998): Dawe RS+, Arch Dermatol 134, 861
Petechiae
  (2000): Warshaw E, Minneapolis MN, The Schoch Letter 50,
     February #16
Photosensitivity (1–10%)
  (2002): Thaler D, Monona, WI (from Internet) (observation)
  (1996): Carrington PR, Little Rock, AR (from Internet)
     (observation) (from tanning bed)
  (1996): Goulden V+, Br J Dermatol 134, 693
  (1996): Uhlemann J, St. Charles, MO (from Internet)
     (observation)
  (1996): Wegman A, Sydney, Australia (from Internet)
     (observation)
  (1994): Litt JZ, Beachwood, OH (personal case) (observation)
  (1990): Black AK+, Br J Dermatol 123, 277
  (1985): Basler RSW, Arch Dermatol 121, 606
  (1972): Frost P+, Arch Dermatol 105, 681
Phototoxicity
  (2002): Sorkin M, Denver, CO (from Internet) (observation)
  (2002): Zabawski E, Longview, TX (from Internet) (observation)
Pigmentation
  (2003): Bock GN, Stockton, CA (from Internet) (observation)
  (2003): Condry PJ, Rochester, NY (from Internet) (observation)
  (2003): Crowe MA, Tacoma, WA (from Internet) (observation)
  (2003): Gregg LJ, Tulsa, OK (from Internet) (observation)
  (2003): Mitchell DF, Thomasville GA (from Internet)
     (observation) (nuchal area – blue)
  (2003): Nakamura S+, Br J Dermatol 148(5), 1073 (patient with
     atopic dermatitis)
  (2003): Sienkiewicz G, Johnson City, NY (from Internet) (2
     observations – slate-gray)
  (2003): Stafford S, Mt Pleasant SC (from Internet) (observation)
  (2003): Thaler D, Monona, WI (from Internet) (observation)
  (2002): Bloom E, Oakland, CA (from Internet) (observation)
     (shins)
  (2002): Jaffe P, Columbia, SC (from Internet) (observation) (gray-
     black on lower legs)
  (2002): Maffei KR, Athens, GA (from Internet) (observation)
  (2002): Spencer LV, Crawfordsville, IN (from Internet)
     (observation)
  (2002): Thaler D, Monona, WI (from Internet) (observation)
  (2001): Assad SA+, J Rheumatol 28(3), 679 (extensive)
  (2001): Bachelz H+, Arch Dermatol 137, 69 (grayish)
  (2001): Bressack M, Merrillville, IN (from Internet) (observation)
     (bluish)
  (2001): Ely H, Grass Valley, CA (from Internet) (observation)
  (2001): Mocci A, Panama (from Internet) ('deep blue spots on
     face') (observation)
  (2001): Werth V, Dermatology Times 18 (shins, ankles, arms)
  (2000): Chave TA+, Ann R Coll Surg Engl 82(5), 348
  (2000): Gregg LJ, Tulsa, OK (from Internet) (observation)
  (2000): Joseph WS+, J Am Podiatr Med Assoc 90, 268

(2000): Mouton RW, Poster Exhibit at University of Vienna clinical dermatology meeting (bluish)
(2000): Ozog DM+, *Arch Dermatol* 136, 1133 (7 cases; all with pemphigus or pemphigoid)
(1999): Aylesworth RJ, Rhinelander, WI (from Internet) (observation)
(1999): Drayton GE, Los Angeles, CA (from Internet) (observation)
(1999): Frederickson K, Novalo, CA (from Internet) (observation)
(1999): Gregg LJ, Tulsa, OK (from Internet) (observation)
(1999): Johnston AM+, *N Engl J Med* 340, 1597
(1999): Koester GA, Edmond, OK (from Internet) (observation)
(1999): Lycka BAS, Edmonton, Alberta (from Internet) (observation)
(1999): Messner E+, *J Clin Rheumatol* 5(5), 273
(1999): Pepper, M, *The Schoch Letter* 49, 25 Madison, WI (linear purple streaks of back)
(1998): Eisen D+, *Drug Saf* 18, 431
(1998): Greve B+, *Lasers Surg Med* 22, 223
(1998): Karrer S+, *Hautarzt* (German) 49, 219
(1998): Morrow GL+, *Am J Ophthalmol* 125, 396
(1998): Patel K+, *Br J Dermatol* 185, 560
(1998): Wasel NR+, *J Cutan Med Surg* 3, 105
(1998): Wood B+, *Br J Dermatol* 139, 562
(1997): Hoefnagel JJ+, *Ned Tijdschr Geneeskd* 141, 1424
(1997): Houck HE+, *Arch Dermatol* 133, 15
(1997): Rademaker M, New Zealand (eyelids) (from Internet) (observation)
(1997): Smith KC, Niagara Falls, Ontario (from Internet) (observation)
(1997): Wilde JL+, *Arch Dermatol* 133, 1344
(1996): Collins P+, *Br J Dermatol* 135, 317
(1996): Fleming CJ+, *Br J Dermatol* 134, 784
(1996): Goulden V+, *Br J Dermatol* 134, 693
(1996): Hardman CM+, *Clin Exp Dermatol* 21, 244
(1996): Knoell AG+, *Arch Dermatol* 132, 1251
(1996): Korbol M+, *J Am Podiatr Med Assoc* 76, 87
(1996): Tsao H+, *Arch Dermatol* 132, 1250
(1995): Hung PH+, *J Fam Pract* 41, 183
(1995): Meyer AJ+, *Arch Dermatol* 131, 1447
(1995): Poskitt L+, *Br J Dermatol* 132, 784
(1994): Miralles ES+, *J Dermatol* 21, 965
(1994): Siller GM+, *J Am Acad Dermatol* 30, 350
(1993): Dwyer CM+, *Br J Dermatol* 129, 158
(1993): Okada N+, *Br J Dermatol* 129, 403
(1993): Pepine M+, *J Am Acad Dermatol* 28, 295
(1993): Schofield JK+, *Br J Gen Pract* 43, 173
(1992): Altman DA+, *J Cutaneous Pathol* 19, 340 (in patients with bullous pemphigoid)
(1992): Fakhfakh AC+, *Ann Dermatol Venereol* (French) 119, 975
(1992): Ridgway HB+, *Arch Dermatol* 128, 565 ("pseudo-mongolian")
(1991): Eady DJ+, *Clin Exp Dermatol* 16, 55
(1991): Leffell DJ, *J Am Acad Dermatol* 24, 501
(1990): Bamberger N+, *Ann Dermatol Venereol* (French) 117, 299
(1990): Black AK+, *Br J Dermatol* 123, 277
(1990): Bridges AJ+, *J Am Acad Dermatol* 22, 959
(1989): Cataldo E+, *J Mass Dent Soc* 38, 5
(1989): Layton AM+, *J Dermatol Treatment* 1, 9
(1989): Okada N+, *Br J Dermatol* 121, 247
(1988): Serwatka LM, *J Assoc Military Derm* 14, 10
(1987): Angeloni VL+, *Cutis* 40, 229
(1987): Argenyi ZB+, *J Cutaneous Pathol* 14, 176
(1987): Zijdenbos AM+, *Ned Tijdschr Geneeskd* (Dutch) 131, 999
(1986): Prigent F+, *Ann Dermatol Venereol* (French) 113, 227
(1986): Shum DT+, *Arch Dermatol* 122, 18
(1985): Basler RSW, *Arch Dermatol* 121, 606
(1985): Basler RSW+, *J Am Acad Dermatol* 12, 577

(1985): Butler JM+, *Clin Exp Dermatol* 10, 432
(1985): Gordon G, *Arch Dermatol* 121, 618
(1985): Liu TTT+, *Cutis* 35, 254
(1984): Wolfe ID+, *Cutis* 33, 457
(1983): Verret JL+, *Ann Dermatol Venereol* (French) 110, 777
(1983): White SW+, *Arch Dermatol* 119, 1
(1982): Ridgway HA, *Br J Dermatol* 107, 95
(1981): Leroy JP+, *Ann Dermatol Venereol* (French) 108, 871
(1981): Sato S+, *J Invest Dermatol* 77, 264
(1980): Fenske NA+, *J Am Acad Dermatol* 3, 308
(1980): Fenske NA+, *JAMA* 244, 1103
(1980): McGrae JD+, *Arch Dermatol* 116, 1262
(1980): Simons JJ+, *J Am Acad Dermatol* 3, 244
(1979): Sauer GC+, *Schoch Letter* 29, 3
(1975): Brogden RN+, *Drugs* 9, 251
(1972): Velasco JE+, *JAMA* 220, 1323

Pruritus (<1%)
(2000): Bachelz H+, *Arch Dermatol* 137, 69
(1996): Goulden V+, *Br J Dermatol* 134, 693
(1996): Montemarano AD+, *J Am Acad Dermatol* 34, 253
(1973): Shelley WB+, *JAMA* 224, 125

Purpura
(2000): Warshaw E, Minneapolis MN, *The Schoch Letter* 50, February #16
(1995): Karofsky PS+, *Arch Pediatr Adolesc Med* 149, 217

Pustules (generalized)
(1999): Antunes A+, *Ann Dermatol Venereol* 126, 518

Rash (sic) (<1%)
(2000): Bachelz H+, *Arch Dermatol* 137, 69
(2000): Schlienger RG+, *Dermatology* 200, 223
(1997): Shapiro LE+, *Arch Dermatol* 133, 1224
(1995): Karofsky PS+, *Arch Pediatr Adolesc Med* 149, 217
(1994): Kaufmann D+, *Arch Intern Med* 154, 1983
(1994): Sitbon O+, *Arch Intern Med* 154, 1633

Raynaud's phenomenon
(2001): Gordon MM+, *J Rheumatol* 28(5), 1004
(1996): Hewack J, *Gastroenterology* 110, A1211

Stevens–Johnson syndrome
(1996): Knowles SR+, *Arch Dermatol* 132, 934
(1987): Shoji A+, *Arch Dermatol* 123, 18

Urticaria
(2003): Tuckman DJ, Sun City, AZ (from Internet) (observation)
(2001): Bark J, Lexington, KY (from Internet) (observation)
(1997): Shapiro LE+, *Arch Dermatol* 133, 1224
(1996): Goulden V+, *Br J Dermatol* 134, 693
(1996): Knowles SR+, *Arch Dermatol* 132, 934
(1996): Ottuso P, *The Schoch Letter* 46, 37 Vero Beach, FL (from generic)
(1995): Wallis M, *The Schoch Letter* 45, 38 (from generic)
(1994): Litt JZ, Beachwood, OH (personal case) (observation)
(1993): Litt JZ, Beachwood, OH (2 personal cases) (observation)
(1990): Puyana J+, *Allergy* 45, 313
(1975): Brogden RN+, *Drugs* 9, 251

Vasculitis
(2001): Schaffer JV+, *J Am Acad Dermatol* 44, 198 (necrotizing)
(2000): Choi HK+, *Arthritis Rheum* 43, 2488
(1999): Elkayam O+, *Semin Arthritis Rheum* 28, 392
(1999): Schrodt BJ, *Skin and Allergy News* April, 22 (2 cases)
(1999): Schrodt BJ+, *South Med J* 92, 502
(1998): Merkel PA, *Curr Opin Rheumatol* 10, 45

Hair
Hair – alopecia
(2000): Schlienger RG+, *Dermatology* 200, 223

Nails
Nails – onycholysis
Nails – photo-onycholysis
(1987): Baran R+, *J Am Acad Dermatol* 17, 1012 (passim)
(1981): Kestel JL, *Cutis* 28, 53

Nails – pigmentation (<1%)
  (2003): Mitchell DF, Thomasville, GA (from Internet)
    (observation)
  (2001): Gregg LJ, Tulsa, OK (from Internet) (observation)
  (2001): Werth V, *Dermatology Times* 18
  (1998): Morrow GL+, *Am J Ophthalmol* 125, 396
  (1995): Hung PH+, *J Fam Pract* 41, 183
  (1994): Mallon E+, *Br J Dermatol* 130, 794
  (1989): Berger RS+, *J Am Acad Dermatol* 21, 1300 (3–5%)
  (1988): Mooney E+, *J Dermatol Surg Oncol* 14, 1011
  (1987): Angeloni VL+, *Cutis* 40, 229
  (1985): Daniel CR III+, *Dermatol Clin* 3, 491 (longitudinal)
  (1985): Liu TTT+, *Cutis* 35, 254
  (1984): Wolfe ID+, *Cutis* 33, 457
  (1982): Litt JZ, *Diagnosis* 4, 23

Other

Anaphylactoid reactions (<1%)
  (1996): Okano M+, *Acta Derm Venereol* (Stockh) 76, 164
Arthralgia
  (2001): Emmet S, Solana Beach, CA (from Internet)
    (observation)
Black tongue
  (1995): Katz J+, *Arch Dermatol* 131, 620
  (1975): Brogden RN+, *Drugs* 9, 251
Conjuctival pigmentation
  (1981): Brothers DM+, *Opthalmology* 88, 1212
Galactorrhea (black)
  (1996): Hunt MJ+, *Br J Dermatol* 134, 943
  (1985): Basler RSW+, *Arch Dermatol* 121, 417
Gingival pigmentation
  (1989): Berger RS+, *J Am Acad Dermatol* 21, 1300 (8%)
Glossitis
Gynecomastia
  (1995): Davies JP+, *Br J Clin Pract* 49, 179
Headache
Hypersensitivity*
  (2002): Murray C+, *World Congress Dermatol* Poster, 0120
  (2001): Bachelz H+, *Arch Dermatol* 137, 69
  (2001): Colvin JH+, *Pediatr Dermatol* 18(4), 295
  (2000): Gil P, *Ann Dermatol Venereol* 127(10), 841
  (1999): Antunes A+, *Ann Dermatol Venereol* 126, 518
  (1999): Clayton BD+, *Arch Dermatol* 135, 139
  (1999): Lupton JR+, *Cutis* 64, 91 (infectious-mononucleosis-like)
  (1999): Piette AM+, *Rev Med Interne* (French) 20, 869
  (1998): Dutz J, Vancouver, Canada (from Internet) (observation)
  (1998): Schlienger RG+, *Epilepsia* 39, S3 (passim)
  (1997): Hoefnagel JJ+, *Ned Tijdschr Geneeskd* (Dutch) 141, 1424
  (1997): MacNeil M+, *J Am Acad Dermatol* 36, 347
  (1997): Shapiro LE+, *Arch Dermatol* 133, 1224
  (1995): Parneix-Spake A+, *Arch Dermatol* 131, 490
  (1994): Sitbon O+, *Arch Intern Med* 154, 1633
  (1973): Shelley WB+, *JAMA* 224, 125
Myalgia
  (2001): Gordon MM+, *J Rheumatol* 28(5), 1004
  (1998): Matteson EL+, *J Rheumatol* 25, 1653
Oral mucosal pigmentation
  (2002): Friedman IS+, *Dermatol Surg* 28(3), 205
  (2001): Werth V, *Dermatology Times* 18
Oral pigmentation
  (1998): Cockings JM+, *Aust Dent J* 43, 14
  (1998): Morrow GL+, *Am J Ophthalmol* 125, 396
  (1998): Patel K+, *Br J Dermatol* 185, 560
  (1997): Eisen D, *Lancet* 349, 379
  (1997): Smith KC, Niagara Falls, Ontario (from Internet)
    (observation) (blue on lips)
  (1995): Odell EW+, *Oral Surg Oral Med Oral Pathol Oral Radiol
    Endod* 79, 459
  (1994): Chu P+, *J Am Acad Dermatol* 30, 802

  (1994): Siller GM+, *J Am Acad Dermatol* 30, 350
  (1989): Berger RS+, *J Am Acad Dermatol* 21, 1300 (7%)
  (1989): Regezi JA+, *Oral Pathology* WB Saunders, 166
  (1986): Beehner ME+, *J Oral Maxillofac Surg* 44, 582
  (1985): Salman RA+, *J Oral Med* 40, 154
  (1984): Fendrich P+, *Oral Surg Oral Med Oral Pathol* 58 288
Oral ulceration
  (2000): Schlienger RG+, *Dermatology* 200, 223
Paresthesias (<1%)
  (1994): Blanchard L, *Schoch Letter* 44, #6 (observation)
Polyarteritis nodosa
  (2001): Schaffer JV+, *J Am Acad Dermatol* 44, 198
  (1999): Schrodt BJ+, *Pediatrics* 103, 503
Pseudo-mongolian spot (sic)
  (1992): Ridgway HB+, *Arch Dermatol* 128, 565
Pseudotumor cerebri
  (2002): Ang ERG+, *J Am Board Fam ract* 15, 229
  (2001): Oswald J+, *Schweiz Rundsch Med Prax* 90(39), 1691
  (2001): Weese-Mayer DE+, *Pediatrics* 108(2), 519
  (2000): Frederickson KS, Novato, CA (from Internet)
    (observation)
  (1998): Chiu AM+, *Am J Ophthalmol* 126, 116
  (1990): Delaney RA+, *Mil Med* 156, A5
  (1990): Shelley WB, *The Schoch Letter* 40, 27
  (1980): Beran RG, *Med J Aust* 1, 323
Rhabdomyolysis
  (2002): Rahman Z+, *Int J Dermatol* 41(8), 530
Scleral pigmentation
  (1998): Morrow GL+, *Am J Ophthalmol* 125, 396
  (1985): Liu TT+, *Cutis* 35, 254
Serum sickness
  (2001): *Arch Dermatol* 137, 100 (2 cases)
  (1999): Elkayam O+, *Semin Arthritis Rheum* 28, 392
  (1998): Martinez JA+, *Med Clin* (Barc) (Spanish) 111, 198
  (1997): Blumenthal HL, Beachwood, OH (personal case)
    (observation)
  (1997): Hoefnagel JJ+, *Ned Tijdschr Geneeskd* (Dutch) 141, 1424
  (1997): Shapiro LE+, *Arch Dermatol* 133, 1224
  (1997): Zabawski E, Dallas, TX (from Internet) (observation)
  (1996): Harel L+, *Ann Pharmacother* 30, 481
  (1996): Levenson T+, *Allergy Asthma Proc* 17, 79
  (1990): Puyana J+, *Allergy* 45, 313
Tongue discoloration
  (2000): Tanzi E+, *Arch Dermatol* 136, 427
  (1995): Katz J+, *Arch Dermatol* 131, 620
  (1995): Meyerson M+, *Oral Surg Oral Med Oral Pathol Oral Radiol
    Endod* 79, 180
Tongue pigmentation
  (2002): Friedman IS+, *Dermatol Surg* 28(3), 205
Tooth discoloration (>10%) (primarily in children)
  (2000): Bark JP, Lexington, KY (from Internet) (observation)
  (2000): McKenna BE+, *Dent Update* 26, 160 (in an adult)
  (2000): Thaler D, Monona, WI (from internet) (observation)
  (1999): Cheek CC+, *J Esthet Dent* 11, 43
  (1998): Dodd MA+, *Ann Pharmacother* 32, 887 (68–year-old
    woman)
  (1998): Morrow GL+, *Am J Ophthalmol* 125, 396
  (1998): Patel K+, *Br J Dermatol* 185, 560 (in an adult)
  (1997): Bowles WK+, *J Esthet Dent* 9, 30
  (1997): Smith KC, Niagara Falls, Ontario (from Internet)
    (observation)
  (1995): Hung PH+, *J Fam Pract* 41, 183
  (1994): Hofmann H, *Hautarzt* (German) 45, 803
  (1991): Allegue F+, *Actas Dermo-Sif* (Spanish) 82, 43
  (1989): Berger RS+, *J Am Acad Dermatol* 21, 1300 (3–5%)
  (1989): Regezi JA+, *Oral Pathology* WB Saunders, 166
  (1989): Rosen T+, *J Am Acad Dermatol* 21, 569
  (1988): Cale AE+, *J Periodontol* 59, 112
  (1985): Poliak SC+, *JAMA* 254, 2930

(1984): Wolfe ID+, *Cutis* 33, 457
(1980): Caro I, *J Am Acad Dermatol* 3, 317
(1979): Basler RSW, *Arch Dermatol* 115, 1391
Tooth pigmentation
(2001): Gregg LJ, Tulsa, OK (from Internet) (observation)

*Note: The antiepileptic drug hypersensitivity syndrome is a severe, occasionally fatal, disorder characterized by any or all of the following: pruritic exanthems, toxic epidermal necrolysis, Stevens–Johnson syndrome, exfoliative dermatitis, fever, hepatic abnormalities, eosinophilia, and renal failure

MINOXIDIL

Trade names: Loniten; Minoxidil (Par); Rogaine (topical) (Pharmacia)
Other common trade names: *Alopexy; Apo-Gain; Hairgaine; Lonolox; Lonoten; Minoximen; Regaine*
Indications: Hypertension, androgenetic alopecia
Category: Antihypertensive; Vasodilator
Half-life: 4.2 hours
Clinically important, potentially hazardous interactions with: alcohol, guanethidine

Note: For topical reaction patterns, I have added a bracket [T]

Reactions

Skin
Acne
(1985): Baral J, *J Am Acad Dermatol* 13, 1051 (scalp comedones)
Allergic reactions (sic) [T]
Ankle edema
Bullous eruption (<1%)
(1981): DiSantis DJ+, *Arch Intern Med* 141, 1515
(1978): Rosenthal T+, *Arch Intern Med* 138, 1856
Dermatitis (7.4%) [T]
(2002): Suzuki K+, *Am J Contact* 13(1), 45
(1998): Sanchez-Motilla J+, *Contact Dermatitis* 38, 283 (pustular)
(1995): Ebner H+, *Contact Dermatitis* 32, 316
(1992): Ruas E+, *Contact Dermatitis* 26, 57
(1992): Veraldi S+, *Contact Dermatitis* 26, 211
(1991): Wilson C+, *J Am Acad Dermatol* 24, 661
(1988): Alomar A+, *Contact Dermatitis* 18, 51
(1988): van Joost T, *Ned Tijdschr Geneeskd* (Dutch) 132, 1141
(1987): Valsecchi R+, *Contact Dermatitis* 17, 58
(1987): van der Willingen AH+, *Contact Dermatitis* 17, 44
(1985): Degreef H+, *Contact Dermatitis* 13, 194
(1985): Tosti A+, *Contact Dermatitis* 13, 275
Eczema (sic)
(1992): Ruas E+, *Contact Dermatitis* 26, 57
(1987): van der Willigen AH+, *Contact Dermatitis* 17, 44
Edema (>10%) [T]
(1977): Nawar T+, *Can Med Assoc J* 117, 1178
Erythema [T]
Erythema multiforme
(1981): DiSantis DJ+, *Arch Intern Med* 141, 1515
Erythroderma
(1988): Ackerman BH+, *Drug Intell Clin Pharm* 22, 703
Exanthems
(1988): Ackerman BH+, *Drug Intell Clin Pharm* 22, 703
(1981): Campese VM, *Drugs* 22, 257
(1981): DiSantis DJ+, *Arch Intern Med* 141, 1515
(1977): Nawar T+, *Can Med Assoc J* 117, 1178
Flushing [T]
Folliculitis [T]

(1996): Duvic M+, *J Am Acad Dermatol* 35, 74
Lupus erythematosus
(1987): Tunkel AR+, *Arch Intern Med* 147, 599
(1981): Mitas JA, *Arthritis Rheum* 24, 570
Peripheral edema (7%)
Pigmentation
Pruritus [T]
(1996): Duvic M+, *J Am Acad Dermatol* 35, 74
(1990): Colamarino R+, *Ann Intern Med* 113, 256
(1977): Nawar T+, *Can Med Assoc J* 117, 1178
Pyogenic granuloma
(1989): Baran R, *Dermatologica* 179(2), 76 (explosive, of the scalp)
Rash (sic) (<1%)
Seborrhea [T]
Stevens–Johnson syndrome (<1%)
(1981): DiSantis DJ+, *Arch Intern Med* 141, 1515
Sunburn (<1%)
Urticaria
Xerosis

Hair
Hair – alopecia [T]
(1987): Olsen EA, *J Am Acad Dermatol* 16, 145
(1983): Ingles RM+, *Int J Dermatol* 22, 120
Hair – hirsutism (in women)
(1981): Campese VM, *Drugs* 22, 257 (100%)
(1973): Pettinger WA+, *N Engl J Med* 289, 167
Hair – hypertrichosis (80%)
(2002): Litt JZ, Beachwood, OH (personal case) (observation)
(1997): Peluso AM+, *Br J Dermatol* 136, 118
(1995): Veyrac G+, *Therapie* (French) 50, 474 (in an infant)
(1994): Gonzalez M+, *Clin Exp Dermatol* 19, 157 [T]
(1990): Miwa LJ+, *Drug Intell Clin Pharm* 24, 365
(1989): Rousseau C+, *Dermatologica* 179, 221
(1988): Toriumi DN+, *Arch Otolaryngol Head Neck Surg* 114, 918
(1985): Bencini PL+, *G Ital Dermatol Venereol* (Italian) 120, 137
(1985): Lorette G+, *Ann Dermatol Venereol* (French) 112, 527
(1984): Henkes J+, *Med Clin* (Barc) (Spanish) 83, 89
(1983): Ingles RM+, *Int J Dermatol* 22, 120
(1983): Wilkin JK+, *Cutis* 31, 61
(1981): Campese VM, *Drugs* 22, 257 (100%)
(1981): Nielsen PG, *Lakartidningen* (Swedish) 78, 1891
(1980): Feldman HA+, *Curr Ther Res* 27, 205
(1980): Ryckmanns F, *Hautarzt* (German) 31, 205
(1979): Burton JL+, *Br J Dermatol* 101, 593
(1979): Pierard GE+, *Dermatologica* (French) 158, 17.5
(1977): Earhart RN+, *South Med J* 70, 442
(1977): Nawar T+, *Can Med Assoc J* 117, 1178
Hair – pigmentation
(1989): Rebora A+, *J Am Acad Dermatol* 21, 1314
(1983): Ingles RM+, *Int J Dermatol* 22, 120 (red)

Other
Anaphylactoid reactions
(2001): Blumenthal HL, Beachwood, OH (observation)
Anosmia
(1993): Litt JZ, Beachwood, OH (personal case) (observation)
Dysgeusia [T]
(1993): Litt JZ, Beachwood, OH (personal case) (observation)
Gynecomastia
Headache
Mastodynia (<1%)
Paresthesias
Polymyalgia
(1990): Colamarino R+, *Ann Intern Med* 113, 256
Tendinitis [T]

MIRTAZAPINE

Trade name: Remeron (Organon)
Indications: Depression
Category: Alpha-2-adrenoceptor blocker; Tetracyclic antidepressant
Half-life: 20–40 hours

Reactions

Skin

Acne
Cellulitis
Chills
Diaphoresis
  (1999): Leinonen E+, *Int Clin Psychopharmacol* 14, 329
Edema (1–10%)
Exfoliative dermatitis
Facial edema
Flu-like syndrome (sic) (1–10%)
  (2000): Benkert O+, *J Clin Psychiatry* 61, 656
Herpes simplex
Peripheral edema (1–10%)
  (2001): Kutscher EC+, *Ann Pharmacother* 35(11), 1494
Petechiae
Photosensitivity
Pruritus
Rash (sic) (1–10%)
Seborrhea
Ulcerations
Xerosis

Other

Ageusia
Aphthous stomatitis
Arthralgia
  (2001): Jolliet P+, *Eur Psychiatry* 16(8), 503
  (2000): Veyrac G+, *Therapie* 55(5), 652
Dysgeusia
Glossitis (1–10%)
Gynecomastia
Hyperesthesia
Mastodynia
Myalgia (1–10%)
  (2001): Jolliet P+, *Eur Psychiatry* 16(8), 503
Oral candidiasis
Paresthesias
  (2001): Ribeiro L+, *Braz J Med Biol Res* 34(10), 1303
Parosmia
Phlebitis
Restless legs syndrome
  (2002): Bahk WM+, *Psychiatry Clin Neurosci* 56(2), 209
Rhabdomyolysis
  (1998): Retz W+, *Int Clin Psychopharmacol* 13(6), 277
Serotonin syndrome
  (2002): Hernandez JL+, *Ann Pharmacother* 36(4), 641
  (2001): Demers JC+, *Ann Pharmacother* 35(10), 1217 (with
    fluvoxamine)
  (2001): Isbister GK+, *Ann Pharmacother* 35(12), 1674 (with
    fluvoxamine)
Sialorrhea
Stomatitis
Tendon rupture
Tongue discoloration
Tongue edema

Tremor (1–10%)
Vaginitis
Xerostomia (25%)
  (1995): Montgomery SA, *Int Clin Psychopharmacol* 10, 37

MISOPROSTOL

Trade names: Arthrotec (Pharmacia); Cytotec (Pharmacia)
Other common trade name: *Symbol*
Indications: Prevention of NSAID-induced ulcer
Category: Antiulcer; Synthetic prostaglandin E1 analog
Half-life: 20–40 minutes

Arthrotec is diclofenac and misoprostol

Reactions

Skin

Dermatitis (sic)
Diaphoresis
Exanthems
  (1987): Monk JP+, *Drugs* 33, 1
Rash (sic)
Shivering
  (2001): Elsheikh A+, *Arch Gynecol Obstet* 265(4), 204 (17.3%)
  (2001): Gulmezoglu AM+, *Lancet* 358, 689
  (2001): Li YT+, *Zhonghua Yi Xue Za Zhi* (Taipei) 64(12), 721
    (33%)
  (1999): Lumbiganon P+, *Br J Obstet Gynaecol* 106, 304

Hair

Hair – alopecia

Other

Anaphylactoid reactions
Gingivitis
Gynecomastia
  (1994): Garcia-Rodriguez LA+, *BMJ* 308, 503
Headache
Tinnitus

MISTLETOE

Scientific names: *Phoradendron flavescens; Phoradendron leucarpum; Phoradendron macrophyllum; Phoradendron rubrum; Phoradendron serotinum; Phoradendron tomentosum; Viscum album*
Family: Loranthacae; Viscaceae
Trade and other common names: ABNOBA viscum; All-heal; Devil's fuge; Eurixor; Folia Visci; Helixor; Herbe de la Croix; Iscador (Weleda); Isorel (Novipharm); Lektinol; Lignum Crucis; Stipites Visci; VaQuFrF (Labor Hiscia); Vysorel
Category: Adjuvant; Immune modulator
Purported indications and other uses: Injected: adjuvant tumor therapy. Oral: abortifacient, arteriosclerosis, arthritis, asthma, colds, depression, headache, HIV infection, hypertension, hypotension, hysteria, labor pain, lumbago, metrorrhagia, muscle spasms, otitis, whooping cough, hemorrhoids, internal bleeding, gout, sleep disorders, amenorrhea, liver and gallbladder conditions
Half-life: N/A
Clinically important, potentially hazardous interactions with: bepridil, corticosteroids, digoxin, diltiazem, immunosuppressants, MAO inhibitors, verapamil

Note: Purified extracts injected intramuscularly, subcutaneously or by intravenous infusion. Unless otherwise indicated, side effects listed are from injected preparations. The FDA considers *Viscum album* unsafe

Reactions

Skin
Adverse effects (sic)
  (1999): Stein GM+, *Eur J Med Res* 4(5), 169
  (1994): Stein G+, *Eur J Clin Phamacol* 47(1), 33
Allergic reactions (sic)
  (2000): Büssing A, *Mistletoe: The Genus Viscum* Harwood Academic Publishers
  (1994): Stein G+, *Eur J Clin Pharmacp;* 47(1), 33
  (1991): Pichler WJ+, *Dtsch Med Wochenschr* (German) 116(35), 1333
Chills
  (2000): Büssing A, *Mistletoe: The Genus Viscum* Harwood Academic Publishers
  (1995): Murray MT, *The Healing Power of Herbs* 253 Prima Publishing
Dermatitis (sic)
  (2000): Büssing A, *Mistletoe: The Genus Viscum* Harwood Academic Publishers
Edema of lip
  (1998): Hagenah W+, *Dtsch Med Wochenschr* (German) 123(34), 1001
Erythema
  (2001): Hutt N+, *Allergol Immunopathol* (Madr) 29(5), 201
  (1999): Stoss M+, *Arzneimittelforschung* 49(4), 366
  (1999): van Wely+, *Am J Ther* 6(1), 37
Flu-like syndrome
  (1999): Gorter RW+, *Altern Ther Health Med* 5(6), 37
  (1999): van Wely+, *Am J Ther* 6(1), 37
Nodules
  (1998): Hagenah W+, *Dtsch Med Wochenschr* (German) 123(34), 1001
Pruritus
  (1999): Stoss M+, *Arzneimittelforschung* 49(4), 366

Other
Anaphylactoid reactions
  (2001): Hutt N+, *Allergol Immunopathol* (Madr) 29(5), 201

  (1996): Friess H+, *Anticancer Res* 16(2), 915 (28%)
Death (low incidence – accidental ingestion)
  (1997): Krenzelok EP+, *Am J Emerg* 15(5), 516
  (1996): Spiller HA+, *J Toxicol Clin Toxicol* 34(4), 405
  (1995): Murray MT, *The Healing Power of Herbs* 253 Prima Publishing
  (1986): Hall AH+, *Annals Emergency Med* 15, 1320
Gingivitis
  (1999): Gorter RW+, *Altern Ther Health Med* 5(6), 37
  (1999): van Wely+, *Am J Ther* 6(1), 37
Injection-site edema
  (1999): Stoss M+, *Arzneimittelforschung* 49(4), 366
Injection-site inflammation
  (1999): Stein GM+, *Eur J Med Res* 4(5), 169
  (1999): Stoss M+, *Arzneimittelforschung* (German) 49(4), 366
  (1998): Gorter RW+, *Am J Ther* 5(3), 181
  (1998): Stoss M+, *Nat Immun* 16(5), 185
  (1995): Murray MT, *The Healing Power of Herbs* 253 Prima Publishing
  (1990): Kast A+, *Schweiz Rundsch Med Prax* (German) 79(10), 291

*Note: The well-known mistletoe is an evergreen parasitic plant, growing on the branches of some tree species

**Note: Shakespeare calls it 'the baleful mistletoe,' an illusion to the Scandinavian legend that Balder, the god of Peace, was slain with an arrow made of mistletoe

MITHRAMYCIN

(See PLICAMYCIN)

MITOMYCIN

Synonyms: mitomycin-C; MTC
Trade name: Mutamycin (Bristol-Myers Squibb)
Other common trade names: *Ametycine; Mitomycin; Mitomycin-C; Mitomycine*
Indications: Carcinomas
Category: Antineoplastic antibiotic
Half-life: 23–78 minutes
Clinically important, potentially hazardous interactions with: aldesleukin

Reactions

Skin
Angioedema
Bullous eruption
  (1984): Ritch PS+, *Cancer* 54, 32
Dermatitis (sic)
  (1997): Gomez Torrrijos E+, *Allergy* 52, 687
  (1993): Wahlberg JE+, *Lakartidningen* (Swedish) 90, 158
  (1992): Vidal C+, *Dermatology* 184, 208
  (1990): Colver GB+, *Br J Dermatol* 122, 217
  (1987): Sala F+, *G Ital Dermatol Venereol* (Italian) 122, 265
  (1984): Neild VJ+, *J R Soc Med* 77, 610
  (1981): Nissenkorn I+, *J Urol* 126, 596
  (1975): *Med Lett* 17, 62
Edema
Erythema
Erythema multiforme
  (1984): Spencer HJ, *J Surg Oncol* 26, 47
Exanthems
  (1995): Echechipia S+, *Contact Dermatitis* 33, 432

(1987): Sala F+, *G Ital Dermatol Venereol* (Italian) 122, 265
Exfoliative dermatitis
   (1987): Sala F+, *G Ital Dermatol Venereol* (Italian) 122, 265
   (1985): Bencini PL+, *Int J Dermatol* 24, 472
Necrosis
   (2000): Neulander EZ+, *J Urol* 164(4), 1306 (glans penis)
Palmar desquamation
   (1981): Nissenkorn I+, *J Urol* 126, 596
Photosensitivity
   (1981): Fuller B+, *Ann Intern Med* 94, 542
Pigmentation
   (1989): Kerker BJ+, *Semin Dermatol* 8, 173
Pityriasis rosea
   (1987): Sala F+, *G Ital Dermatol Venereol* (Italian) 122, 265
Pruritus (<1%)
Purpura
Rash (sic) (<1%)
   (1981): Nissenkorn I+, *J Urol* 126, 596 (generalized)
Thrombocytopenic purpura
   (2001): Medina PJ+, *Curr Opin Hematol* 8(5), 286
Ulcerations
   (1992): Ellsworth-Wolk J, *Oncol Nurs Forum* 19, 1554
Urticaria
   (1981): Weiss RB+, *Ann Intern Med* 94, 66

Hair

Hair – alopecia (1–10%)
   (1975): *Med Lett* 17, 62

Nails

Nails – pigmentation (purple) (1–10%)

Other

Injection-site cellulitis (>10%)
Injection-site extravasation
   (2000): Kassner E, *J Pediatr Oncon Nurs* 17, 135
Injection-site necrosis (>10%)
   (1987): Aizawa H+, *Acta Derm Venereol* (Stockh) 67, 364
   (1987): Dufresne RG, *Cutis* 39, 197
   (1987): Sala F+, *G Ital Dermatol Venereol* (Italian) 122, 265
Injection-site thrombophlebitis
Oral mucosal lesions
   (1987): Sala F+, *G Ital Dermatol Venereol* (Italian) 122, 265
   (1983): Bronner AK+, *J Am Acad Dermatol* 9, 645
   (1978): Levine N+, *Cancer Treat Rev* 5, 67 (2–8%)
   (1975): *Med Lett* 17, 62
Oral ulceration (1–10%)
   (1984): Spencer HJ, *J Surg Oncol* 26, 47
Paresthesias (1–10%)
Stomatitis (>10%)
Thrombophlebitis (<1%)

MITOTANE

Synonym: o,p'-DDD
Trade name: Lysodren (Bristol-Myers Squibb)
Other common trade name: *Opeprim*
Indications: Inoperable adrenocortical carcinoma
Category: Antiadrenal; Antineoplastic
Half-life: 18–159 days
Clinically important, potentially hazardous interactions with: aldesleukin, spironolactone

Reactions

Skin

Acral erythema
   (1991): Baack BR+, *J Am Acad Dermatol* 24, 457
   (1974): Zühlke RL, *Dermatologica* 148, 90
Angioedema (<1%)
Erythema multiforme
   (1978): Levine N+, *Cancer Treat Rev* 5, 67
   (1966): Hutter AM+, *Am J Med* 41, 581
Exanthems
   (1973): Lubitz JA+, *JAMA* 223, 1109 (9%)
   (1966): Hutter AM+, *Am J Med* 41, 581 (16%)
Flushing (1–10%)
Pigmentation
   (1973): Lubitz JA+, *JAMA* 223, 1109
   (1966): Hutter AM+, *Am J Med* 41, 581 (16%)
Pruritus
   (1974): Zühlke RL, *Dermatologica* 148, 90
Rash (sic) (15%)
Side effects (sic)
   (1973): Lubitz JA+, *JAMA* 223, 1109 (13%)
   (1966): Hutter AM+, *Am J Med* 41, 581 (17%)
Urticaria
   (1966): Hutter AM+, *Am J Med* 41, 581
Vasculitis (<1%)

Hair

Hair – alopecia
   (1973): Lubitz JA+, *JAMA* 223, 1109
   (1966): Hutter AM+, *Am J Med* 41, 581 (16%)

Other

Myalgia (1–10%)
Tremor (<1%)

MITOXANTRONE

Trade name: Novantrone (Immunex)
Indications: Acute myelogenous leukemia, multiple sclerosis, prostate cancer
Category: Synthetic antineoplastic antibiotic (parenteral)
Half-life: median terminal: 75 hours
Clinically important, potentially hazardous interactions with: aldesleukin

Reactions

Skin

Allergic reactions (sic) (<1%)
Chills (1–10%)
Diaphoresis (1–10%)
Ecchymoses (7%)

Edema (>10%)
Erythema
Fungal infections (>15%)
Infections (sic) (>66%)
Necrosis
Petechiae (>10%)
Pigmentation (bluish)
Purpura (>10%)
Rash (sic) (<1%)
Ulcerations
Urticaria
Vitiligo
  (2001): Schmid-Wendtner M-H+, *Lancet* 358, 1575

Hair
Hair – alopecia (20–60%)

MODAFINIL

Trade name: Provigil (Cephalon)
Other common trade name: *Alertec*
Indications: Narcolepsy
Category: Analeptic; Central nervous system stimulant
Half-life: ~15 hours

Reactions

Skin
Allergic reactions (sic) (>1%)
Chills (2%)
Diaphoresis (>1%)
Ecchymoses (>1%)
Edema (>1%)
Erythema
Herpes simplex (1%)
Hot flashes
Pruritus (>1%)
Psoriasis (>1%)
Rash (sic) (>1%)
Xerosis (1%)

Other
Dysgeusia (>1%)
Gingivitis (1%)
Headache
Myalgia (>1%)
Oral ulceration (1%)
Paresthesias (3%)
  (2002): Nieves AV+, *Clin Neuropharmacol* 25(2), 111
Sialorrhea
Tooth disorder (sic) (>1%)
Tremor (1%)
Xerostomia (5%)

MOEXIPRIL

Trade names: Uniretic (Schwartz); Univasc (Schwartz)
Indications: Hypertension
Category: Angiotensin-converting enzyme (ACE) inhibitor;
Antihypertensive
Half-life: 1 hour
**Clinically important, potentially hazardous interactions
with:** amiloride, spironolactone, triamterene

Uniretic is moexipril and hydrochlorothiazide

Reactions

Skin
Adverse effects (sic)
  (1994): White WB+, *J Human Hypertens* 8, 917
Angioedema (<1%)
  (2001): Cohen EG+, *Ann Otol Rhinol Laryngol* 110(8), 701 (64
  cases)
Diaphoresis (<1%)
Exanthems (1.6%)
Flushing (1.6%)
  (1995): Drayer JIM+, *Am J Ther* 2, 525
Pemphigus (<1%)
Pemphigus foliaceus
  (2000): Ong CS+, *Australas J Dermatol* 41(4), 242
Peripheral edema (1–10%)
  (1995): Drayer JIM+, *Am J Ther* 2, 525
Photosensitivity (<1%)
Pruritus (1–10%)
Rash (sic) (1.6%)
Urticaria (<1%)

Hair
Hair – alopecia (1–10%)

Other
Anaphylactoid reactions (<1%)
Cough
  (2001): Adigun AQ+, *West Afr J Med* 20(1), 46–7
  (2001): Lee SC+, *Hypertension* 38(2), 166
Dysgeusia (<1%)
Headache
Myalgia (1.3%)
Xerostomia (<1%)

MOLINDONE

Trade name: Moban (Endo)
Indications: Schizophrenia
Category: Antipsychotic
Half-life: 1.5 hours

Reactions

Skin
Allergic reactions (sic)
Edema
Hypohidrosis (<1%)
Peripheral edema
Photosensitivity (<1%)
Pigmentation (<1%)
Pruritus (<1%)
Rash (sic) (<1%)

Other
  Galactorrhea (<1%)
  Gynecomastia (1–10%)
  Sialorrhea
  Xerostomia (>10%)

MONTELUKAST

Trade name: Singulair (Merck)
Indications: Asthma
Category: Antiasthmatic
Half-life: 2.7–5.5 hours

Reactions

Skin
  Angioedema
    (1998): Condry P, Webster, NY (from Internet) (observation)
  Erythema nodosum
    (2000): Dellaripa PF+, *Mayo Clin Proc* 75(6), 643
  Flu-like syndrome (sic) (1–10%)
  Granulomatous dermatitis (Churg–Strauss syndrome)
    (2002): Alvarez-Fernandez JG+, *World Congress Dermatol*
      Poster, 0082
    (2002): Hammer HB+, *Tidsskr Nor Laegeforen* 122(5), 484
    (2002): Solans R+, *Thorax* 57(2), 183 (1 case)
    (2001): Donohue J, *Chest* 119(2), 668
    (2001): Hosker HS, *Thorax* 56(3), 244
    (2001): Kalyoncu A+, *Allergol Immunopathol* (Madr) 29(5), 185
    (2001): Lipworth BJ+, *Thorax* 56(3), 244
    (2001): Mukhopadhyay A+, *Postgrad Med J* 56(5), 417
    (2001): Sabio JM+, *Chest* 120(6), 2116
    (2001): Weschler M Thorax, *Thorax* 56(5), 417
    (2000): Price D, *Drugs* 59, 35 (passim)
    (2000): Trujillo-Santos AJ+, *Med Clin* (Barc) 115(15), 599
    (2000): Tuggey JM+, *Thorax* 55(9), 805
    (2000): Villena V+, *Eur Resp J* 15, 626
    (2000): Wechsler ME+, *Chest* 117. 708
  Pemphigus
    (2003): Cetkovska P+, *Clin Exp Dermatol* 28(3), 328
  Peripheral edema
    (2000): Geller M, *Ann Intern Med* 132, 924
  Rash (sic) (1.6%)
  Urticaria (1.6%)
    (1998): Jaffe P, Columbia, SC (from Internet) (observation)
    (1998): Knorr B+, *JAMA* 279, 1181

Other
  Cough
    (2001): Spector SL, *Ann Allergy Asthma Immunol* 86(6 Suppl 1), 18
  Headache
  Panniculitis
    (2000): Dellaripa PF+, *Mayo Clin Proc* 75(6), 643

MORICIZINE

Trade name: Ethmozine (Shire)
Indications: Ventricular arrhythmias
Category: Antiarrhythmic class I
Half-life: 3–4 hours

Reactions

Skin
  Diaphoresis (2–5%)
  Exanthems (<1%)
  Periorbital edema (1–10%)
  Pruritus (<2%)
  Rash (sic) (<1%)
  Urticaria (<2%)
  Xerosis (<2%)

Other
  Dysgeusia (<2%)
  Hyperesthesia (2–5%)
  Oral mucosal lesions
    (1990): Fitton A+, *Drugs* 40, 138
  Paresthesias (2–5%)
  Thrombophlebitis (<2%)
  Tinnitus
  Tongue edema (<2%)
  Xerostomia (2–5%)
    (1990): Carnes CA+, *Drug Intell Clin Pharm* 24, 745 (2–5%)
    (1990): Fitton A+, *Drugs* 40, 138 (2%)

MORPHINE

Trade names: Astramorph; Avinza (Ligand); Duramorph
(Baxter) (Elkins-Sinn); Infumorph (Elkins-Sinn); Kadian (Faulding);
MS Contin (Purdue Frederick); MS/S; MSIR Oral (Purdue
Frederick); OMS Oral; Oramorph SR; RMS; Roxanol (Elan)
Other common trade names: *Anamorph; Astramorph;
Contalgin; Epimorph; Morphine-HP; MOS; Moscontin; MS-IR; MST
Continus; Sevredol; Statex*
Indications: Severe pain, acute myocardial infarction
Category: Narcotic analgesic
Half-life: 2–4 hours
**Clinically important, potentially hazardous interactions
with:** buprenorphine, cimetidine, furazolidone, MAO inhibitors,
pentazocine

Reactions

Skin
  Diaphoresis
  Edema
  Exanthems
    (1977): Voorhorst R+, *Ned Tijdschr Geneeskd* (Dutch) 121, 737
  Flushing
  Pallor
  Peripheral edema
  Pruritus (<1%)
    (2002): Nakata K+, *J Clin Anesth* 14(2), 121
    (2001): Charuluxananan S+, *Anesth Analg* 93(1), 162
    (2001): Matsuda M+, *Masui* 50(10), 1096
    (2001): Mercadante S+, *Support Care Cancer* 9(6), 467
    (2001): Sakai T+, *Can J Anaesth* 48(8), 831

(2001): Subramaniam K+, *J Clin Anesth* 13(5), 339 (with ketamine)
(2000): Gunter JB+, *Paediatr Anaesth* 10, 167
(2000): Yeh HM+, *Anesth Analg* 91, 172
(1999): Joshi GP+, *Anesthesiology* 90(4), 1007
(1998): Thangaturai D+, *Anaesthesia* 43, 1055 (62%)
(1988): Gustafson LL+, *Drugs* 35, 597 (5–10%)
(1986): Attia J+, *Anesthesiology* 65, 590 (20%)
Pustular psoriasis
(1976): Lindgren S+, *Acta Derm Venereol* 56(2), 139
Rash (sic)

Other
Death
(2002): Byard RW, *J Forensic Sci* 47(1), 202
Gynecomastia
Hyperesthesia
Injection-site pain (>10%)
Rhabdomyolysis
(1985): Blain PG+, *Hum Toxicol* 4(1), 71
Trembling (1–10%)
Xerostomia (>10%)
(2002): Andersen G+, *Palliat Med* 16(2), 107
(1989): White JD+, *BMJ* 298, 1222 (75%)

MOXIFLOXACIN

Trade name: Avelox (Bayer)
Indications: Various infections caused by susceptible organisms
Category: Fluoroquinolone antibiotic
Half-life: 12 hours
Clinically important, potentially hazardous interactions with: amiodarone, arsenic, bepridil, bretylium, disopyramide, erythromycin, phenothiazines, procainamide, quinidine, sotalol, tricyclic antidepressants

Reactions

Skin
Allergic reactions (sic)
Burning
Candidiasis (<1%)
Chills (<1%)
Diaphoresis (<1%)
Edema
Exanthems
(2000): Litt JZ, Beachwood, OH (personal case; no pruritus)
Fixed eruption
(2001): Litt JZ, Beachwood, OH (personal case)
Peripheral edema (<1%)
Photosensitivity (<1%)
(2000): Balfour JA+, *Drugs* 59, 115
(2000): Stein GE+, *Inf Med* 17, 564
(2000): Traynor NJ+, *Toxicol Vitr* 14, 275
Pruritus (<1%)
Rash (sic) (<1%)
(2001): Culley CM+, *Am J Health-Syst Pharm* 58, 379
Urticaria (<1%)
Xerosis (<1%)

Other
Anaphylactoid reactions
(2001): Aleman A+, *J Allergy Clin Immunol* Feb, 107
Dysgeusia (>1%)
(2000): Stein GE+, *Inf Med* 17, 564

Glossitis (<1%)
Headache
Myalgia (<1%)
Paresthesias (<1%)
Stomatitis (<1%)
Tendinitis
Tendon rupture
Tremor (<1%)
Vaginitis (<1%)
(2000): Stein GE+, *Inf Med* 17, 564
Xerostomia (<1%)
(2001): Litt JZ, Beachwood, OH (personal case)

MUPIROCIN*

Trade name: Bactroban (GSK)
Other common trade names: *Bactoderm; Eismycin; Mupiderm*
Indications: Secondarily infected traumatic skin lesions due to susceptible strains of *Staphylococcus aureus* and *Streptococcus pyogenes*, Impetigo
Category: Anti-infective (topical or intranasal)
Half-life: N/A

*Note: Also known as *pseudomonic acid*, mupirocin is an antibacterial agent produced by fermentation using the organism *Pseudomonas fluorescens*

Reactions

Skin
Allergic reactions (sic)
(1999): Mylotte JM+, *Infect Control Hosp Epidemiol* 20(11), 741 (intranasal)
(1995): Eedy DJ, *Contact Dermatitis* 32(4), 240
Blepharitis (<1%) (intranasal)
Burning
(1997): Bertino JS, *Am J Health Sys Pharm* 54(19), 2185 (of nose) (intranasal)
Cellulitis (<1%)
Dermatitis (<1%)
(1997): Zappi EG+, *J Am Acad Dermatol* 36(2 Pt 1), 266
Edema
(1997): Bertino JS, *Am J Health Syst Pharm* 54(19), 2185 (of nose) (intranasal)
Erythema
(1997): Bertino JS, *Am J Health Syst Pharm* 54(19), 2185 (of nose) (intranasal)
Pruritus (1–2.4%)
(1997): Bertino JS, *Am J Health Syst Pharm* 54(19), 2185 (of nose) (intranasal)
Rash (sic) (1.1%)
Stinging
(1997): Bertino JS, *Am J Health Syst Pharm* 54(19), 2185 (of nose) (intranasal)
Xerosis
(1997): Bertino JS, *Am J Health Syst Pharm* 54(19), 2185 (of nose) (intranasal)

Other
Application-site burning (1–3.6%)
Cough (2%) (intranasal)
Dizziness (<1%)
Dysgeusia (3%) (intranasal)
Headache
Pharyngitis (intranasal (4%)

Stomatitis (<1%)
Xerostomia (<1%) (intranasal)

MYCOPHENOLATE

Synonym: mycophenolate mofetil
Trade name: CellCept (Roche)
Indications: Prophylaxis of organ rejection
Category: Immunosuppressant
Half-life: 18 hours
Clinically important, potentially hazardous interactions with: antacids, azathioprine, basiliximab, cholestyramine, corticosteroids, cyclophosphamide, cyclosporine, daclizumab, mercaptopurine, mofetil, mycophenolate, tacrolimus, **vaccines**

Reactions

Skin
Acne (>10%)
Bullous eruption
  (2000): Rault R, *Ann Intern Med* 133, 921 (hands)
Carcinoma (non-melanoma) (4%)
Dermatitis herpetiformis (aggravation)
  (2002): Gladstone GC, Worcester, MA (personal
    correspondence)
Diaphoresis
Edema (12.2%)
Herpes simplex
  (2000): Williams JV+, *Skin & Allergy News* September, 24
Infections (sic) (12–20%)

  (2002): Bernabeu-Wittel M+, *Eur J Clin Microbiol Infect Dis*
    21(3), 173
Peripheral edema (28.6%)
Pruritus
  (2002): Gladstone GC, Worcester, MA (personal
    correspondence)
Rash (sic) (7.7%)
Toxiderma (sic)
  (2002): Hafraoui S+, *Gastroenterol Clin Biol* 26(1), 17 (2 cases)

Hair
Hair – alopecia
  (2001): Zierhut M+, *Ophthalmologe* 98(7), 647

Nails
Nails – onycholysis
  (2000): Rault R, *Ann Intern Med* 133, 921

Other
Arthralgia
  (2002): Skelly MM+, *Inflamm Bowel Dis* 8(2), 93
Gingival hyperplasia
Gingivitis
Myalgia
  (2002): Greiner K+, *Ophthalmologe* 99(9), 691
Oral candidiasis (10.1%)
Oral ulceration
  (2001): Garrigue V+, *Transplantation* 72(5), 968
Paresthesias
Thrombophlebitis (1–10%)
Thrombosis (deep vein)
  (2001): Cherney DZI+, *Neph Dial Transp* 16, 1702
Tremor (11%)

NABUMETONE

Trade name: Relafen (GSK)
Other common trade names: *Arthaxan; Consolan; Nabuser; Prodac; Relif; Relifex; Unimetone*
Indications: Arthritis
Category: Nonsteroidal anti-inflammatory (NSAID)
Half-life: 22.5–30 hours
Clinically important, potentially hazardous interactions with: methotrexate

Reactions

Skin
Acne (<1%)
Adverse effects (sic)
  (1990): Fletcher AP, *Drugs* 40 (Suppl 5) 43
Angioedema (<1%)
  (1990): Jenner PN, *Drugs* 40 (Suppl 5), 80
Bullous eruption (<1%)
Diaphoresis (1–3%)
Edema (3–9%)
  (1990): Munzel P+, *Drugs* 40 (Suppl 5), 62
Erythema
  (1990): Alianti M+, *Clin Ter* (Italian) 133, 299
Erythema multiforme (<1%)
Exanthems (1.2%)
  (1999): Litt JZ, Beachwood, OH (personal case) (observation)
  (1988): Friedel HA+, *Drugs* 35, 504
Hot flashes (<1%)
Photosensitivity (<1%)
  (1998): Litt JZ, Beachwood, OH (personal case) (observation)
  (1994): Shelley WB+, *Cutis* 54, 70 (observation)
  (1993): Litt JZ, Beachwood, OH (personal case) (observation)
  (1989): Kaidbey KH+, *Arch Dermatol* 125, 783
  (1988): Friedel HA+, *Drugs* 35, 504
Phototoxicity
  (1989): Kaidbey KH+, *Arch Dermatol* 125, 783 and 824
Pruritus (3–9%)
  (1999): Litt JZ, Beachwood, OH (personal case) (observation)
  (1988): Friedel HA+, *Drugs* 35, 504
Rash (sic) (3–9%)
  (1988): Friedel HA+, *Drugs* 35, 504
  (1987): Jackson RE+, *Am J Med* 83, 115
  (1987): Jenner PN+, *Am J Med* 83, 110
  (1987): Mullen BJ, *Am J Med* 83, 70
Side effects (sic)
  (1991): Riccieri V+, *Clin Ter* (Italian) 137, 185
Stevens–Johnson syndrome (<1%)
  (1997): Sienkiewicz G, Johnson City, NY (from Internet) (observation)
Toxic epidermal necrolysis (<1%)
Urticaria (<1%)
Vasculitis (necrotizing)
  (1990): Willkins RF, *Drugs* 40 (Suppl 5), 34
Xerosis
  (1987): Mullen BJ, *Am J Med* 83, 70

Hair
Hair – alopecia (<1%)
  (1987): Mullen BJ, *Am J Med* 83, 70

Other
Anaphylactoid reactions (<1%)
Gingivitis (<1%)
Glossitis (<1%)

Headache
Myalgia
Oral ulceration
  (1989): Lussier A+, *J Clin Pharmacol* 29, 225
Paresthesias (<1%)
Parkinsonism
Porphyria cutanea tarda (<1%)
Pseudolymphoma
  (2001): Werth V, *Dermatology Times* 18
Pseudoporphyria
  (2000): Antony F+, *Br J Dermatol* 142, 1067
  (2000): Bergfeld W+, *Skin & Allergy News* December, 33
  (1999): Aylesworth R, Rhinelander, WI (from Internet) (observation)
  (1999): Krischer J+, *J Am Acad Dermatol* 40, 492
  (1999): Magro CM+, *J Cutan Pathol* 26, 42
  (1998): Varma S+, *Br J Dermatol* 138, 549
Sialorrhea
Stomatitis (1–3%)
Tinnitus
Xerostomia (1–3%)

NADOLOL

Trade names: Corigard; Corzide (Monarch)
Other common trade names: *Apo-Nadolol; Farmagard; Nadic; Solgol; Syn-Nadolol*
Indications: Hypertension, angina pectoris
Category: Antianginal; Antihypertensive; Beta-adrenoceptor blocker
Half-life: 10–24 hours
Clinically important, potentially hazardous interactions with: clonidine, epinephrine, verapamil

Corzide is nadolol and bendroflumethiazide*

Note: Cutaneous side effects of beta-receptor blockaders are clinically polymorphous. They apparently appear after several months of continuous therapy. Atypical psoriasiform, lichen planus-like, and eczematous chronic rashes are mainly observed. (1983): Hödl St, *Z Hautkr* (German) 58, 17

Reactions

Skin
Bullous pemphigoid
  (1984): Stage AH+, *Am J Obstet Gynecol* 150, 169
Diaphoresis (<1%)
  (1980): Heel RC+, *Drugs* 20, 1 (0.6%)
Eczema (sic)
Edema (1–5%)
Erythema multiforme
Exanthems
  (1980): Heel RC+, *Drugs* 20, 1 (0.4%)
Exfoliative dermatitis
Facial edema (<1%)
Hyperkeratosis (palms and soles)
Infiltrative dermatitis of the scalp (sic)
  (1985): Shelley ED+, *Cutis* 35, 148
Lichenoid eruption
  (1978): Savage RL+, *BMJ* 1, 987
Lupus erythematosus
Pityriasis rubra pilaris
  (1978): Finlay AY+, *BMJ* 1, 987
Pruritus (1–5%)

Psoriasis
  (1988): Gold MH+, *J Am Acad Dermatol* 19, 837 (aggravation of)
  (1988): Heng MCY+, *Int J Dermatol* 27, 619
  (1986): Czernielewski J+, *Lancet* 1, 808
  (1984): Arntzen N+, *Acta Derm Venereol* (Stockh) 64, 346
Pustules
  (1991): Bernard P+, *Dermatologica* 182, 115
Rash (sic) (1–5%)
Raynaud's phenomenon (2%)
  (1984): Eliasson K+, *Acta Med Scand* 215, 333
  (1976): Marshall AJ+, *BMJ* 1, 1498
Toxic epidermal necrolysis
Urticaria
Xerosis

Hair
Hair – alopecia
  (1985): Shelley ED+, *Cutis* 35, 148

Nails
Nails – bluish
Nails – dystrophy
Nails – onycholysis

Other
Dysgeusia
Headache
Numbness (fingers and toes) (>5%)
Oculo-mucocutaneous syndrome
  (1982): Cocco G+, *Curr Ther Res* 31, 362
Oral lichenoid eruption
Oral mucosal eruption
  (1980): Heel RC+, *Drugs* 20, 1 (0.6%)
Paresthesias (>5%)
Peyronie's disease
  (1979): Pryor JP+, *Lancet* 1, 331
Tinnitus
Xerostomia (<1%)
  (1980): Heel RC+, *Drugs* 20, 1

*Note: Bendroflumethiazide is a sulfonamide and can be absorbed systemically. Sulfonamides can produce severe, possibly fatal, reactions such as toxic epidermal necrolysis and Stevens–Johnson syndrome

NAFARELIN

Trade name: Synarel (Pharmacia)
Other common trade name: *Synarela*
Indications: Endometriosis
Category: Gonadotropin inhibitor; Posterior pituitary hormone
Half-life: ~3 hours

Reactions

Skin
Acne (>10%)
Chloasma (<1%)
Edema (1–10%)
Exanthems (<1%)
Flushing
  (1990): Chrisp P+, *Drugs* 39, 523 (90%)
  (1988): Henzl MR+, *N Engl J Med* 318, 485 (90%)
Hot flashes (>10%)
Pruritus (1–10%)
Rash (sic) (1–10%)

Seborrhea (1–10%)
Urticaria (1–10%)

Hair
Hair – hirsutism (1–10%)

Other
Gynecomastia (<1%)
Hypersensitivity (0.2%)
Mastodynia
Myalgia (>10%)
Paresthesias (<1%)
Vaginitis

NAFCILLIN

Trade name: Nafcil (Apothecon)
Other common trade name: *Vigopen*
Indications: Various infections caused by susceptible organisms
Category: Penicillinase-resistant penicillin
Half-life: 0.5–1.5 hours
Clinically important, potentially hazardous interactions with: anticoagulants, cyclosporine, demeclocycline, doxycycline, methotrexate, minocycline, oxytetracycline, tetracycline

Reactions

Skin
Allergic reactions (sic)
  (1994): Pleasants RA+, *Chest* 106, 1124 (in patients with cystic fibrosis)
Angioedema
Bullous eruption
Ecchymoses
Erythema multiforme
Exanthems
  (1978): Kancir LM+, *Arch Intern Med* 138, 909 (10%)
Exfoliative dermatitis
Hematomas
Jarisch–Herxheimer reaction
Pruritus
Rash (sic) (<1%)
  (2002): Maraqa NF+, *Clin Infect Dis* 34(1), 50 (32%)
Stevens–Johnson syndrome
Toxic epidermal necrolysis
Urticaria
Vasculitis

Other
Anaphylactoid reactions
Black tongue
Dysgeusia
Glossitis
Glossodynia
Hypersensitivity (<1%)
Injection-site necrosis
  (1987): Dufresne RG, *Cutis* 39, 197
  (1980): Tilden SJ+, *Am J Dis Child* 134, 1046
Injection-site pain
Oral candidiasis
Serum sickness
Stomatitis
Stomatodynia
Thrombophlebitis (<1%)
Vaginitis
Xerostomia

NALBUPHINE

Trade name: Nubain (Endo)
Other common trade names: *Bufigen; Nalcryn SP; Nubain SP*
Indications: Moderate to severe pain
Category: Narcotic agonist-antagonistic analgesic
Half-life: 5 hours
**Clinically important, potentially hazardous interactions
with:** CNS depressants, diazepam, pentobarbital, promethazine

Note: Nalbuphine contains sulfites

Reactions

Skin
Burning (<1%)
  (1995): Brenet O+, *Cah Anesthesiol* 43(3), 319
Clammy skin (9%)
Diaphoresis (9%)
Flushing (<1%)
Pruritus (<1%)
Urticaria (<1%)

Other
Blurred vision
Depression (<1%)
Dizziness (5%)
  (2001): Charuluxananan S+, *Anesth Analg* 93(1), 162
Dysgeusia (<1%)
Headache
Injection-site pain
  (2001): Charuluxananan S+, *Anesth Analg* 93(1), 162
  (1995): van den Berg+, *Eur J Anaesthesiol* 12(5), 513
Numbness
Paresthesias
Tingling
Xerostomia (4%)

NALIDIXIC ACID

Trade name: NegGram (Sanofi-Synthelabo)
Other common trade names: *Betaxina; Granexin; Mytacin;
Nalidixin; Negram; Nogram; Youdix*
Indications: Various urinary tract infections caused by
susceptible organisms
Category: Quinolone antibiotic; Urinary tract anti-infective
Half-life: 6–7 hours
**Clinically important, potentially hazardous interactions
with:** warfarin

Reactions

Skin
Angioedema (<1%)
Bullous eruption (<1%)
  (1981): Wolf A, *Z Hautkr* (German) 56, 109
  (1970): Brehm G+, *Med Welt* (German) 11, 423
  (1969): Birkett DA, *Br J Dermatol* 81, 342
  (1969): Puissant A+, *Bull Soc Fr Dermatol Syphiligr* (French)
    76, 84
  (1968): Baes H, *Dermatologica* 136, 61
  (1966): Burry JN+, *Med J Aust* 2, 243
Erythema multiforme (<1%)
  (1971): Alexander S+, *Br J Dermatol* 84, 429

Exanthems (>5%)
  (1971): Alexander S+, *Br J Dermatol* 84, 429
  (1969): Atlas E+, *Ann Intern Med* 70, 713 (7%)
  (1963): Barlow AM, *BMJ* 2, 1308 (3.5%)
  (1963): Lishman IV+, *Br J Urol* 35, 116
  (1962): Buchbinder M+, *Antimicrob Agents Chemother* 2, 308
Exfoliative dermatitis
  (1971): Alexander S+, *Br J Dermatol* 84, 429
Lupus erythematosus
  (1979): Rubinstein A, *N Engl J Med* 301, 1288
  (1971): Alexander S+, *Br J Dermatol* 84, 429
Photosensitivity (<1%)
  (1997): O'Reilly FM+, American Academy of Dermatology
    Meeting, Poster #14
  (1993): Wainwright NJ+, *Drug Saf* 9, 437
  (1990): Bilsland D+, *Br J Dermatol* 123, 548
  (1986): Ljunggren B+, *Photodermatol* 3, 26
  (1985): Epstein JH+, *Drugs* 30, 42
  (1982): Rosen K+, *Acta Derm Venereol* (Stockh) 62, 246
  (1981): Boisvert A+, *Drug Intell Clin Pharm* 15, 126
  (1981): Closas J+, *Rev Clin Esp* (Spanish) 162, 219
  (1980): Stern RS+, *Arch Dermatol* 116, 1269
  (1978): Fiocchi A+, *Minerva Pediatr* (Italian) 30, 585
  (1974): Ramsay CA+, *Br J Dermatol* 91, 523
  (1973): Ramsay CA, *Proc R Soc Med* 66, 747
  (1972): Jung EG, *Z Haut Geschlechtskr* (German) 47, 329
  (1971): Alexander S+, *Br J Dermatol* 84, 429
  (1970): Luscombe HA, *Arch Dermatol* 101, 122
  (1970): Neering KEHP, *Dermatologica* 141, 361
  (1970): No Author, *Tidsskr Nor Laegeforen* (Norwegian) 90, 2100
  (1970): Thivolet J+, *Bull Soc Fr Dermatol Syphiligr* (French)
    77, 286
  (1969): Garrett MH, *Med J Aust* 1, 83
  (1968): Baes H, *Dermatologica* 136, 61
  (1967): Haven E+, *Arch Belg Dermatol Syphiligr* (French) 23, 421
  (1966): Mathew FH, *Med J Aust* 53, 243
  (1965): Cahal DA, *BMJ* 1, 130
  (1965): Elmes PC, *Prescrib J* 5, 12
  (1965): Susskind W+, *BMJ* 1, 316
Phototoxic bullous eruption
  (1978): Brauer GJ, *Am J Med* 58, 576
  (1977): Hertzenberg S, *Tidsskr Nor Laegeforen* (Norwegian)
    97, 792
  (1976): Frodin T+, *Lakartidningen* (Swedish) 73, 3763
  (1976): Klaasen CH+, *Ned Tijdschr Geneeskd* (Dutch) 120, 247
  (1976): van Dijk E, *Ned Tijdschr Geneeskd* (Dutch) 120, 592
  (1975): Brauner GJ, *Am J Med* 58, 576
  (1974): Burry JN, *Arch Dermatol* 109, 263
  (1974): Ramsay CA+, *Br J Dermatol* 91, 523
  (1973): Louis P+, *Hautarzt* (German) 24, 445
  (1969): Birkett DA, *Br J Dermatol* 81, 342
  (1968): Baes H, *Dermatologica* 136, 61
  (1966): Burry JN+, *Med J Aust* 2, 243
  (1964): Zelickson AS, *JAMA* 190, 556
Pruritus (<1%)
  (1971): Alexander S+, *Br J Dermatol* 84, 429
  (1969): Atlas E+, *Ann Intern Med* 70, 713
Purpura
  (1971): Alexander S+, *Br J Dermatol* 84, 429
Rash (sic) (<1%)
Toxic epidermal necrolysis
  (1971): Alexander S+, *Br J Dermatol* 84, 429
Urticaria (<1%)
  (1985): Goolamali SK, *Postgrad Med J* 61, 925
  (1971): Alexander S+, *Br J Dermatol* 84, 429
  (1966): Beaty HN+, *Ann Intern Med* 65, 641

Hair
Hair – alopecia
  (1971): Alexander S+, *Br J Dermatol* 84, 429

Other

Acute intermittent porphyria
Anaphylactoid reactions
Arthralgia
  (1972): Bailey RR+, *Can Med Assoc* 107, 604 (passim)
Headache
Paresthesias
Porphyria cutanea tarda
  (1992): Shelley WB+, *Advanced Dermatologic Diagnosis* WB
    Saunders, 414 (passim)
  (1983): Goldsman CI+, *Cleve Clin Q* 50, 151
Pseudoporphyria
  (1990): Bilsland D+, *Br J Dermatol* 123, 547
  (1984): Harber LC+, *J Invest Dermatol* 82, 207
Pseudotumor cerebri
  (1998): Ryiaz A+, *J Indian Med Assoc* 96, 308

NALOXONE

Trade names: Narcan (Endo); Suboxone (Reckitt Benckiser);
Talwin-NX (Sanofi-Synthelabo)
Other common trade names: *Nalpin; Narcanti; Narcotan;*
Zynox
Indications: Narcotic overdose
Category: Opioid (narcotic) antagonist
Half-life: 1–1.5 hours

Reactions

Skin

Angioedema
  (1982): Smitz S+, *Ann Intern Med* 97, 788
Diaphoresis (1–10%)
Exanthems
Pruritus
  (1982): Smitz S+, *Ann Intern Med* 97, 788
Rash (sic) (1–10%)
Urticaria
  (1982): Smitz S+, *Ann Intern Med* 97, 788

Other

Headache

NALTREXONE

Trade names: Revex (Baker); ReVia (DuPont); Trexan
Other common trade names: *Antaxone; Celupan; Nalorex;*
Nemexin
Indications: Substance abuse, opioid dependence, alcohol
dependence
Category: Opioid antagonist
Half-life: 4 hours

Reactions

Skin

Acne (<1%)
Chills (<10%)
Diaphoresis
Edema (<1%)
Exanthems
  (1988): Ganzalez JP+, *Drugs* 35, 192
Eyelid edema (<1%)

Herpes simplex (<1%)
Herpes zoster (<1%)
Hot flashes
Pruritus (<1%)
  (1997): Sullivan JR+, *Australas J Dermatol* 38(4), 196
  (1990): Abboud TK+, *Anesthesiol* 72, 233
Purpura
Rash (sic) (<10%)
  (1988): Gonzalez JP+, *Drugs* 35, 192
Seborrhea (<1%)
Tinea pedis (<1%)

Hair

Hair – alopecia (<1%)

Other

Arthralgia (>10%)
  (1997): Ciraulo AM+, *Drugs & Ther Perspect* 10, 5
Death (in ultrarapid detoxification)
Depression (<1%)
  (1996): Berg BJ+, *Drug Saf* 15(4), 274
  (1988): Gonzalez JP+, *Drugs* 35, 192
Myalgia
Phlebitis (<1%)
Rhabdomyolysis
  (1999): Zaim S+, *Ann Pharmacother* 33(3), 312
Tinnitus
Tremor
Twitching
Xerostomia (<1%)

NAPROXEN

Trade names: Aleve; Naprosyn (Roche)
Other common trade names: *Aleve; Anaprox; Apranax;*
Dymenalgit; Flanax; Laraflex; Naprelan; Naprogesic; Napron X;
Naprosyne; Naxen; Novo-Naprox; Nu-Naprox; Supradol; Synflex;
Velsay
Indications: Pain, arthritis
Category: Nonsteroidal anti-inflammatory (NSAID)
Half-life: 13 hours
Clinically important, potentially hazardous interactions
with: methotrexate

Reactions

Skin

Angioedema (<1%)
  (2000): Ghislain PD+, *Ann Med Interne (Paris)* 151, 227 (nuchal
    scalp)
  (1984): Stern RS+, *JAMA* 252, 1433
Bullous eruption
  (1996): Gonzalo-Garijo MA+, *Allergol Immunopathol Madr*
    (Spanish) 24, 89
  (1990): Suarez SM+, *Arthritis Rheum* 33, 903
  (1989): Rivers JK+, *Med J Aust* 151, 167
  (1984): Stern RS+, *JAMA* 252, 1433
Diaphoresis (<3%)
  (1990): Todd PA+, *Drugs* 40, 91 (<3%)
  (1985): Bigby M+, *J Am Acad Dermatol* 12, 866
  (1982): Bailin PL+, *Clin Rheum Dis* 8, 493 (passim)
Ecchymoses (3–9%)
Edema (3–9%)
  (1978): Castles JJ+, *Arch Intern Med* 138, 362 (1–5%)
Edema of leg

(2002): Bandyopadhyay P+, *Int J Clin Pract* 56(2), 145
Erythema multiforme (<1%)
 (1985): Bigby M+, *J Am Acad Dermatol* 12, 866
 (1984): Stern RS+, *JAMA* 252, 1433
Erythema nodosum
 (1990): Todd PA+, *Drugs* 40, 91
Exanthems (>5%)
 (2002): Blumenthal HB, Beachwood, OH (personal case)
  (observation)
 (1994): Shelley WB+, *Cutis* 55, 21 (observation)
 (1990): Todd PA+, *Drugs* 40, 91
 (1985): Bigby M+, *J Am Acad Dermatol* 12, 866 (1–5%)
 (1984): Stern RS+, *JAMA* 252, 1433
 (1979): Brogden RN+, *Drugs* 18, 241
 (1978): Castles JJ+, *Arch Intern Med* 138, 362 (5.3%)
 (1976): Dyer HR, *Ann Intern Med* 84, 221
 (1975): Bowers DE+, *Ann Intern Med* 83, 470 (14%)
 (1975): Brigden RN+, *Drugs* 9, 326
Exfoliative dermatitis
Facial scarring
 (2001): Wallace CA+, *J Am Acad Dermatol* 45, 746 (in children)
Fixed eruption
 (2002): Li H+, *Int J Dermatol* 41(2), 96
 (2001): Gonzalo MA+, *Br J Dermatol* 144(6), 1291
 (2000): Ozkaya-Bayazit E+, *Eur J Dermatol* 10, 288
 (1998): Leal G, Fortaleza, Brazil (from internet) (observation)
 (1996): Enta T, *Can Fam Physician* 42, 1099
 (1996): Gonzalo-Garijo MA+, *Allergol Immunopathol Madr*
  (Spanish) 24, 89
 (1991): Shelley WB+, *Cutis* 48, 368 (observation)
 (1990): Black AK+, *Br J Dermatol* 123, 277 (observation)
 (1990): Todd PA+, *Drugs* 40, 91
 (1987): Habbema L+, *Dermatologica* 174, 184
 (1985): Bigby M+, *J Am Acad Dermatol* 12, 866
 (1984): Stern RS+, *JAMA* 252, 1433
Hot flashes (<1%)
Lichen planus
 (2002): Reed BR, Denver, CO (from Internet) (observation)
 (1999): *Acta Derm Venereol* (Stockh) 79, 329 (bullous)
 (1984): Heymann WR+, *J Am Acad Dermatol* 10, 299
Lichenoid eruption
 (1996): Shelley WB+, *Cutis* 60, 20
 (1990): Todd PA+, *Drugs* 40, 91
 (1985): Bigby M+, *J Am Acad Dermatol* 12, 866
Linear IgA bullous dermatosis
 (2000): Bouldin MB+, *Mayo Clin Proc* 75(9), 967
Lupus erythematosus
 (1992): Parodi A+, *JAMA* 268, 51
Peripheral edema
Photodermatitis (bullous)
 (1989): Rivers JK+, *Med J Aust* 151, 167
Photosensitivity (<1%)
 (1999): Litt JZ, Beachwood, OH (personal case) (observation)
 (1994): Berger TG+, *Arch Dermatol* 130, 609 (in HIV-infected)
 (1991): Allen R+, *J Rheumatol* 18, 893
 (1991): Lutzow-Holm C, *Tidsskr Nor Laegeforen* (Norwegian)
  111, 2739
 (1990): Suarez SM+, *Arthritis Rheum* 33, 903
 (1990): Todd PA+, *Drugs* 40, 91
 (1989): Kaidbey KH+, *Arch Dermatol* 125, 783
 (1987): Sterling JC+, *Br J Rheumatol* 26, 210
 (1986): Judd LE+, *Arch Dermatol* 122, 451
 (1986): Mayou S+, *Br J Dermatol* 114, 519
 (1986): Shelley WB+, *Cutis* 38, 169
 (1986): Szczeklik A, *Drugs* 32 (Suppl 4), 148
 (1985): Farr PM+, *Lancet* 1, 1166
 (1983): Diffey BL+, *Br J Rheumatol* 22, 239
Phototoxicity
 (1989): Kaidbey KH+, *Arch Dermatol* 125, 783

Pityriasis rosea
 (1993): Yosipovitch G+, *Harefuah* (Hebrew) 124, 198; 247
Pruritus (3–9%)
 (2002): Blumenthal HB, *Beachwood, OH* (personal case)
  (observation)
 (1990): Todd PA+, *Drugs* 40, 91 (1–5%)
 (1985): Bigby M+, *J Am Acad Dermatol* 12, 866 (14%)
 (1982): Bailin PL+, *Clin Rheum Dis* 8, 493 (passim)
 (1978): Castles JJ+, *Arch Intern Med* 138, 362
 (1975): Bowers DE+, *Ann Intern Med* 83, 470 (17%)
Pseudoreactions (sic)
 (1991): VanArsdel PP, *JAMA* 266, 3343
Purpura (<3%)
 (1985): Bigby M+, *J Am Acad Dermatol* 12, 866
 (1982): Bailin PL+, *Clin Rheum Dis* 8, 493 (passim)
 (1979): Brogden RN+, *Drugs* 18, 241
 (1975): Brogden RN+, *Drugs* 9, 326
Pustules
 (1989): Grattan CEH, *Dermatologica* 179, 57
 (1986): Page SR+, *BMJ* 293, 510
Pyogenic granuloma
 (1994): Shelley WB+, *Cutis* 53, 36 (observation)
Rash (sic) (3–9%)
 (2002): Bandyopadhyay P+, *Int J Clin Pract* 56(2), 145
 (1995): Knulst AC+, *Br J Dermatol* 133, 647
Side effects (sic)
 (1990): Todd PA+, *Drugs* 40, 91 (up to 9%)
 (1985): Bigby M+, *J Am Acad Dermatol* 12, 866 (up to 5%)
 (1974): Cuthbert MF, *Curr Med Res Opin* 2, 600 (5%)
Stevens–Johnson syndrome (<1%)
Toxic epidermal necrolysis (<1%)
 (1993): Correia O+, *Dermatology* 186, 32
Urticaria
 (2002): Litt JZ, Beachwood, OH (personal case) (observation)
 (1985): Bigby M+, *J Am Acad Dermatol* 12, 866 (1–5%)
 (1984): Stern RS+, *JAMA* 252, 1433
 (1979): Brogden RN+, *Drugs* 18, 241
 (1975): Brogden RN+, *Drugs* 9, 326
Vasculitis
 (1996): Lossos IS+, *Harefuah* (Hebrew) 130, 600
 (1992): Jahangiri M+, *Postgrad Med J* 68, 766
 (1992): Veraguth AJ+, *Schweiz Med Wochenschr* (German)
  122, 923
 (1990): Todd PA+, *Drugs* 40, 91 (1–5%) (necrotizing venulitis)
 (1989): Singhal PC+, *Ann Allergy* 63, 107
 (1985): Bigby M+, *J Am Acad Dermatol* 12, 866
 (1980): Mordes JP, *Arch Intern Med* 140, 985
 (1979): Brogden RN+, *Drugs* 18, 241
 (1979): Grennan DM+, *N Z Med J* 89, 48
Vesiculobullous eruption
 (1984): Stern RS+, *JAMA* 252, 1433

Hair
Hair – alopecia (<1%)
 (1990): Todd PA+, *Drugs* 40, 91 (<1%)
 (1989): Barter AC, *BMJ* 298, 325
 (1989): Barth JH, *BMJ* 298, 675

Other
Anaphylactoid reactions (<1%)
Aphthous stomatitis
 (2001): Vincent L+, *Ann Dermatol Venereol* (French) 128(1), 57
Headache
Hypersensitivity
 (2001): McMahon AD+, *J Clin Epidemiol* 54(12), 1271
Myalgia (<1%)
Oral ulceration
 (2000): Madinier I+, *Ann Med Interne (Paris)* (French) 151, 248
Porphyria cutanea tarda

(1992): Shelley WB+, *Advanced Dermatologic Diagnosis* WB
  Saunders, 414 (passim)
Pseudolymphoma
  (2001): Werth V, *Dermatology Times* 18
Pseudoporphyria
  (2002): Haber H, Cleveland, OH (Cleveland Dermatological
    Society)
  (2002): McNail S+, *Arch Dermatol* 138(12), 1607
  (2002): Schad SG+, *Hautarzt* 53(1), 51
  (2001): Maerker JM+, *Hautarzt* 52(11), 1026
  (2000): De Silva B+, *Pediatr Dermatol* 17, 480
  (1999): Al-Khenaizan S+, *J Cutan Med Surg* 3, 162
  (1995): Creemers MC+, *Scand J Rheumatol* 24, 185
  (1995): Girschick HJ+, *Scand J Rheumatol* 24, 108
  (1994): Lang BA+, *J Pediatr* 124, 639
  (1992): Cox NH+, *Br J Dermatol* 126, 86
  (1992): Petersen CS+, *Ugeskr Laeger* (Danish) 154, 1713
  (1991): Allen R+, *J Rheumatol* 18, 893
  (1990): Levy ML+, *J Pediatr* 117, 660
  (1990): Sternberg A, *Acta Derm Venereol* 70, 354
  (1990): Suarez SM+, *Arthritis Rheum* 33, 903
  (1990): Todd PA+, *Drugs* 40, 91
  (1989): Kaidbey KH+, *Arch Dermatol* 125, 783
  (1988): Diffey BL+, *Clin Exp Dermatol* 13, 207
  (1987): Burns DA, *Clin Exp Dermatol* 12, 296
  (1987): Nicholls D, *N Z Med J* 100, 427
  (1987): Shelley ED+, *Cutis* 40, 314
  (1987): Sterling JC+, *Br J Rheumatol* 26, 210
  (1987): Taylor BJ+, *N Z Med J* 100, 322
  (1986): Judd LE+, *Arch Dermatol* 122, 451
  (1986): Mayou S+, *Br J Dermatol* 114, 519
  (1985): Farr PM+, *Lancet* 1, 1166
  (1985): Howard AM+, *Lancet* 1, 819
Salivary gland enlargement
  (1995): Knulst AC+, *Br J Dermatol* 133, 647
Stomatitis (<3%)

Tinnitus
Xerostomia

NARATRIPTAN

Trade name: Amerge (GSK)
Indications: Acute migraine attacks
Category: Antimigraine; Serotonin agonist
Half-life: 6 hours
**Clinically important, potentially hazardous interactions
with:** dihydroergotamine, ergotamine, methysergide, rizatriptan,
sibutramine, **St John's wort**, sumatriptan, zolmitriptan

Reactions

Skin
Acne (<1%)
Allergic reactions (sic) (<1%)
Atypical sensations (sic) (<1)%
Dermatitis (sic) (<1%)
Diaphoresis (<1%)
Edema (<1%)
Erythema (<1%)
Exanthems (<1%)
Folliculitis (<1%)
Photosensitivity (<1%)
Purpura (<1%)
Rash (sic) (<1%)
Urticaria (<1%)
Xerosis (<1%)

Hair
Hair – alopecia (<1%)

Other
Dysgeusia (<1%)
Headache
Hyperesthesia (<1%)
Ocular pigmentation (<1%)
Paresthesias (2%)
Sialopenia (<1%)

NATEGLINIDE

Trade name: Starlix (Novartis)
Indications: Type 2 diabetes
Category: Short-acting insulin secretagogue antidiabetic
(phenylalanine derivative)
Half-life: 1.5 hours

Reactions

Skin
Exanthems
  (2002): Danby FW, Manchester, NH (from Internet)
    (observation)
Flu-like syndrome (4%)
Rash (sic)

NEBIVOLOL

Trade name: Nebilet (Menarini)
Indications: Hypertension
Category: Beta-adrenoceptor blocker
Half-life: 8 hours

Reactions

Skin
None

Other
Myalgia
Paresthesias
  (1999): McNeely W+, *Drugs* 57, 633

NEDOCROMIL

Trade names: Alocril (Allergan); Tilade (Monarch)
Other common trade names: *Mireze; Telavist; Tilade Mint*
Indications: Bronchial asthma, pruritus of allergic conjunctivitis
Category: Mast cell stabilizer
Half-life: 3.3 hours

Reactions

Skin
Rash (sic) (0.5%)
Upper respiratory infection (6.7%)

Other
Abdominal pain (1.9%)

Arthritis (<1%)
Cough (8.9%)
Dysgeusia (11.6%)
  (2002): Tauber J, *Adv Ther* 19(2), 73 (1.4%)
  (1995): Kjellman NI+, *Allergy* 50(21 Suppl), 14 (5%)
  (1993): Bailey CS+, *Eye* 7, 29
Fatigue (1%)
Headache
Ocular burning
  (2002): Tauber J, *Adv Ther* 19(2), 73 (2.7%)
  (1995): Kjellman NI+, *Allergy* 50(21 Suppl), 14
Ocular erythema
Ocular stinging
  (1995): Kjellman NI+, *Allergy* 50(21 Suppl), 14
  (1993): Bailey CS+, *Eye* 7, 29
Pharyngitis (7.6%)
Rhinitis (7.3%)
Tremor (<1%)
Xerostomia (1%)

NEFAZODONE

Trade name: Serzone (Bristol-Myers Squibb)
Indications: Depression
Category: Phenylpiperazine antidepressant
Half-life: 2–4 hours
Clinically important, potentially hazardous interactions
with: aprepitant, buspirone, isocarboxazid, MAO inhibitors,
phenelzine, pimozide, selegiline, sibutramine, sumatriptan,
tramadol, tranylcypromine, trazodone

Reactions

Skin
Acne (<1%)
Allergic reactions (sic) (<1%)
Burning (sic)
  (2000): Lerner V+, *J Clin Psychiatry* 61, 216
Cellulitis (<1%)
Ecchymoses (<1%)
Eczema (sic) (<1%)
Exanthems (<1%)
Facial edema (<1%)
Flu-like syndrome (sic) (1–10%)
Flushing (4%)
Infections (sic) (8%)
Peripheral edema (3%)
Photosensitivity (<1%)
Pruritus (2%)
Rash (sic) (2%)
Urticaria (<1%)
Vesiculobullous eruption (<1%)
Xerosis (<1%)

Hair
Hair – alopecia (<1%)
  (1998): Rademaker M, Hamilton, New Zealand (from Internet)
    (observation)
  (1997): Gupta S+, *J Fam Pract* 44, 20

Other
Ageusia (<1%)
Death
  (2003): Edwards IR, *Lancet* 361, 1240 (11 cases)
Dysgeusia (2%)

Foetor ex ore (halitosis) (<1%)
Gingivitis (<1%)
Glossitis (<1%)
Gynecomastia (<1%)
Headache
Hyperesthesia (<1%)
Mastodynia (1%)
Myalgia
Oral candidiasis (<1%)
Oral ulceration (<1%)
Paresthesias (4%)
  (1999): Litt JZ, Beachwood, OH (personal case) (observation)
Priapism (<1%)
  (1999): Brodie-Meijer CC+, *Int Clin Psychopharmacol* 14, 257
    (clitoral)
Rhabdomyolysis
  (2002): Thompson M+, *Am J Psychiatry* 159(9), 1607 (with
    simvastatin)
Sialorrhea (<1%)
Stomatitis (<1%)
Vaginitis (2%)
Xerostomia (25%)

NELFINAVIR

Trade name: Viracept (Pfizer)
Indications: HIV infection
Category: Antiretroviral; Protease inhibitor
Half-life: 3.5–5 hours
Clinically important, potentially hazardous interactions
with: benzodiazepines, chlordiazepoxide, clonazepam,
clorazepate, diazepam, dihydroergotamine, ergot alkaloids,
fentanyl, flurazepam, lorazepam, methysergide, midazolam, oral
contraceptives, oxazepam, phenytoin, pimozide, quazepam,
rifampin, sildenafil, **St John's wort**, temazepam

Reactions

Skin
Allergic reactions (sic) (<1%)
Dermatitis (sic) (<1%)
Diaphoresis (<1%)
Exanthems
  (1998): Bourezane Y+, *Clin Infect Dis* 27(5), 1321 (with
    indinavir)
Hyperhidrosis
  (2000): Bonfanti P+, *J Acquir Immune Defic Syndr* 23(3), 236
Lichenoid eruption
  (1998): Bourezane Y+, *Clin Infect Dis* 27(5), 1321
Palmar erythema
  (1998): Bourezane Y+, *Clin Infect Dis* 27(5), 1321 (with
    indinavir)
Pruritus (<1%)
Rash (sic) (1–10%)
  (2001): Abraham PE+, *Ann Pharmacother* 35(5), 553
  (2000): Fortuny C+, *AIDS* 14, 335
Urticaria (<1%)
  (1998): Demoly P+, *J Allergy Clin Immunol* 102(5), 875
Vasculitis
  (1998): Bourezane Y+, *Clin Infect Dis* 27(5), 1321

Other
DRESS syndrome
  (1998): Bourezane Y+, *Clin Infect Dis* 27, 1321

Gynecomastia
  (2001): Manfredi R+, *Ann Pharmacother* 35(4), 438
Headache
Hypersensitivity
  (1999): Demoly P+, *J Allergy Clin Immunol* 104 (2 Pt 1), 504
Myalgia (<1%)
Oral ulceration (<1%)
Paresthesias (<1%)
Perioral paresthesias
  (2001): McMahon D+, *Antivir Ther* 6(2), 105
Rhabdomyolysis
  (2002): Hare CB+, *Clin Infect Dis* 35(10), 111 (with simvastatin)

*Note: Protease inhibitors cause dyslipidemia which includes elevated triglycerides and cholesterol and redistribution of body fat centrally to produce the so-called "protease paunch," breast enlargement, facial atrophy, and "buffalo hump"

NEOMYCIN

Trade names: Cortosporin; Dexacine; Maxitrol (Monarch); Neosporin (Warner Lambert) (Monarch); Poly-Pred
Other common trade names: *Gemicina; Myciguent; Neomicina; Neomycine Diamant; Neosulf; Nivemycin*
Indications: Various infections caused by susceptible organisms
Category: Aminoglycoside antibiotic
Half-life: 3 hours
Clinically important, potentially hazardous interactions with: aldesleukin, aminoglycosides, atracurium, bumetanide, doxacurium, ethacrynic acid, furosemide, methoxyflurane, pancuronium, polypeptide antibiotics, rocuronium, succinylcholine, torsemide, vecuronium

Reactions

Skin

Allergic reactions (sic)
Angioedema
  (1959): Pirilä V+, *Acta Derm Venereol* (Stockh) 39, 1470
Bullous eruption
Dermatitis (sic) (1–10%)
  (2000): Hillen U+, *Hautarzt* 51, 239
  (1999): Giordano-Labadie F+, *Contact Dermatitis* 40, 192
    (2.6%) (in atopics)
  (1999): Lestringant GG+, *Int J Dermatol* 38, 181 (5.1%)
  (1998): Katsarou-Katsari A+, *J Eur Acad Dermatol Venereol* 11, 9
  (1998): Kimura M+, *Contact Dermatitis* 39, 148
  (1997): Dasaraju P+, *Clin Infect Dis* 25, 33
  (1996): Sheretz EF, *Arch Dermatol* 132, 461
  (1994): Fisher AA, *Cutis* 54, 300
  (1993): Lipozencic J+, *Arh Hig Rada Toksikol* (Serbo-Croatian-Roman) 44, 173
  (1991): Barros MA+, *Contact Dermatitis* 25, 156
  (1991): Mariani R+, *Contact Dermatitis* 24, 227
  (1990): Bouffioux B+, *Nouv Dermatol* (French) 9, 25
  (1990): Grandinetti PJ+, *J Am Acad Dermatol* 23, 646
  (1990): Smith IM+, *Clin Otolaryngol* 15, 155
  (1989): Guin JD+, *Cutis* 43, 564
  (1989): Massone L+, *Contact Dermatitis* 21, 344
  (1988): Shupp DL+, *Cutis* 42, 528
  (1987): Abdul-Gaffoor PM, *Indian J Dermatol* 32, 102
  (1986): Bajaj AK+, *Int J Dermatol* 25, 103
  (1986): Baldinger J+, *Ann Ophthalmol* 18, 95
  (1986): Rebandel P+, *Contact Dermatitis* 15, 92
  (1985): Fisher AA, *Cutis* 35, 315
  (1985): Fraki JE+, *Acta Otolaryngol Stockh* 100, 414
  (1985): Frenzel U+, *Phlebologie* (French) 38, 389
  (1985): Szarmach H+, *Przegl Dermatol* (Polish) 72, 521
    (disseminated)

(1984): Menne T+, *Hautarzt* (German) 35, 319
(1983): Macdonald RH+, *Clin Exp Dermatol* 8, 249
(1982): Fisher AA, *Ann Allergy* 49, 97
(1981): Fisher AA+, *Cutis* 28, 491
(1981): Gordon W, *S Afr Med J* 59, 212
(1981): LeRoy R+, *Derm Beruf Umwelt* (German) 29, 168
(1980): Epstein E, *Contact Dermatitis* 6, 219
(1979): Leyden JJ+, *JAMA* 242, 1276
(1979): Prystowsky SD+, *Arch Dermatol* 115, 713
(1979): Prystowsky SD+, *Arch Dermatol* 115, 959
(1978): Durocher LP, *Can Med Assoc J* (French) 118, 162
(1978): Forstrom L+, *Contact Dermatitis* 4, 312
(1977): Shouji A, *Nippon Rinsho* (Japanese) 35, 210
(1977): Sinka L+, *Bratisl Lek Listy* (Slovak) 67, 59
(1976): Carruthers JA+, *Contact Dermatitis* 2, 269
(1976): Fisher AA+, *Cutis* 18, 637
(1974): Bandmann HJ+, *Internist Berl* (German) 15, 47
(1974): Malten KE+, *Phlebologie* (French) 27, 417
(1974): Peterkin GA, *J Laryngol Otol* 88, 15
(1973): Ebner H, *Wien Klin Wochenschr* (German) 85, 203
(1973): *BMJ* 1, 250
(1973): Naess K, *Tidsskr Nor Laegeforen* (Norwegian) 93, 2498
(1972): Hadida ME+, *J Med Lyon* (French) 53, 1093
(1972): Hattori S, *Nippon Ika Daigaku Zasshi* (Japanese) 39, 23
(1971): Bielicky T+, *Z Haut Geschlechtskr* (German) 46, 771
(1971): EpsteinE, *Arch Dermatol* 103, 562
(1971): Foussereau J+, *Bull Soc Fr Dermatol Syphiligr* (French) 78, 457
(1970): Bandmann HJ, *Munch Med Wochenschr* (German) 112, 1125
(1970): Bowczyc J+, *Przegl Dermatol* (Polish) 57, 763
(1970): Chilvers AS+, *Lancet* 1, 402
(1969): Matner T, *Hautarzt* (German) 20, 446
(1969): Novak M+, *Cesk Dermatol* (Czech) 44, 177
(1968): Bartova J, *Cesk Dermatol* (Czech) 43, 271
(1968): Hiemisch I+, *Z Haut Geschlechtskr* (German) 43, 49
(1968): Hjorth N+, *Br J Dermatol* 80, 163
(1967): *Med Lett Drugs Ther* 9, 71
(1967): Pirila V+, *Acta Derm Venereol* (Stockh) 47, 419
(1967): Schwank R, *Cesk Dermatol* 42, 341
(1966): Jensen OC+, *JAMA* 195, 131
(1966): Pirila V+, *Acta Derm Venereol* (Stockh) 46, 489
(1965): Kirton V+, *Lancet* 1, 138
(1959): Pirilä V+, *Acta Derm Venereol* (Stockh) 39, 1470
Eczema (sic)
  (1969): Ekelund A+, *Acta Derm Venereol* (Stockh) 49, 422
Erythema multiforme
  (1986): Fisher AA, *Cutis* 37, 158
Exanthems
  (1990): Bouffioux B+, *Nouv Dermatol* (French) 9, 25
Fixed eruption
  (1985): Gomez B+, *Allergol Immunopathol Madr* (Spanish) 13, 87
Pruritus
Rash (sic) (1–10%)
Toxic epidermal necrolysis
  (1969): Muresan D+, *Viata Med* (Romanian) 16, 731
  (1959): Catto JVF, *BMJ* 2, 544
Ulcerations
Urticaria (1–10%)
  (1959): Pirilä V+, *Acta Derm Venereol* (Stockh) 39, 1470

Hair

Hair – alopecia

Other

Anaphylactoid reactions
  (1986): Goh CL, *Australian J Dermatol* 27, 125
Hypersensitivity
  (2001): Le Coz CJ, *Ann Dermatol Venereol* 128(12), 1359

NESIRITIDE

Trade name: Natrecor (Scios)
Indications: Acutely decompensated congestive heart failure
Category: Human B-type natriuretic peptide; Vasodilator
Half-life: 18 minutes

Reactions

Skin
Diaphoresis (>1%)
Pruritus (>1%)
Rash (sic) (>1%)

Other
Back pain
Cough (>1%)
Headache
Leg cramps (>1%)
Paresthesias (>1%)
Phlebitis
Tremor (>1%)

NEVIRAPINE

Trade name: Viramune (Boehringer Ingelheim)
Indications: HIV infections
Category: Antiretroviral non-nucleoside reverse transcriptase inhibitor (NNRTI)
Half-life: 45 hours
Clinically important, potentially hazardous interactions with: ketoconazole, midazolam, **St John's wort**

Reactions

Skin
Adverse effects (sic)
  (2001): *MMWR* 49, 1153
Exanthems
  (2000): Barreiro P+, *AIDS* 14(14), 2153
  (2000): Palacios Munoz R+, *Rev Clin Esp* (Spanish) 200(11), 635
Pruritus
Rash (sic) (<48%)
  (2001): Barreiro P+, *Lancet* 356(9239), 392
  (2001): Bersoff-Matcha SJ+, *Clin Infect Dis* 32(1), 124
  (2001): Colebundrs R+, *Lancet* 357, 392
  (2001): Wong KH+, *Clin Infect Dis* 33(12), 2096
  (2000): Bardsley-Elliot A+, *Paediatr Drugs* 2(5), 373
  (1999): Anton P+, *AIDS* 13, 524
  (1998): Barner A+, *Lancet* 351, 1133
  (1998): Bourezane Y+, *Clin Infect Dis* 27, 1321
  (1998): Ho TT+, *AIDS* 12, 2082
  (1996): Luzuriaga K+, *J Infect Dis* 174, 713
  (1995): Havlir D+, *J Infect Dis* 171, 537 (48%)
Stevens–Johnson syndrome (<1%)
  (2002): Dodi F+, *AIDS* 16(8), 1197 (2 cases)
  (2001): Fagot JP+, *AIDS* 15(14), 1843
  (2001): *MMWR* 49, 1153
  (2001): Metry DW+, *J Am Acad Dermatol* 44, 354
  (2001): Roujeau J-C+, *AIDS* 15, 1843
  (2000): Bardsley-Elliot A+, *Paediatr Drugs* 2(5), 373
  (2000): Garcia Fernandez D+, *Rev Clin Esp* (Spanish) 200, 179
  (1999): Wetterwald E+, *Br J Dermatol* 140, 980 (SJS/TEN overlap syndrome)

  (1998): McClain SA, SUNY Stony Brook, NY (from Internet) (observation)
  (1998): Warren KJ+, *Lancet* 351–567
Toxic epidermal necrolysis
  (2001): Fagot JP+, *AIDS* 15(14), 1843
  (2001): Roujeau J-C+, *AIDS* 15, 1843
  (1999): Descamps V+, *Lancet* 353, 1855
  (1999): Phan TG+, *Australas J Dermatol* 40, 153
  (1999): Wetterwald E+, *Br J Dermatol* 140, 980 (SJS/TEN overlap syndrome)

Other
DRESS syndrome*
  (2001): Claudio GA+, *Arch Intern Med* 161(20), 2501
  (2000): Sissoko D+, *Presse Med* (French) 29, 1041
  (1998): Bourezane Y+, *Clin Infect Dis* 27(5), 1321
Gingivitis (1–3%)
Headache
Hypersensitivity
  (2001): Wit FW+, *AIDS* 15(18), 2423
  (2000): Podzamczer D+, *AIDS* 14, 331
Lipodystrophy
  (2000): Lewis RH+, *J Acquir Immune Defic Syndrom* 23, 355
  (1999): Aldeen T+, *AIDS* 13, 865
Myalgia (1–10%)
Paresthesias (2%)
Ulcerative stomatitis (4%)

*****Note:** The DRESS syndrome consists of 'drug rash with eosinophilia and systemic symptoms'

NIACIN

Synonym: nicotinic acid
Trade names: Advicor (Kos); Niacor (Upsher-Smith); Niaspan (Kos); Nicobid; Nicolar (Aventis); Nicotinex; Slo-Niacin (Upsher-Smith)
Other common trade names: *Apo-Nicotinamide; I*; IV; Nia-Bid; Niac; Niacels; Nicobion; Nicotinex; Nicovital; Pepeom Amide; Vitamin B₃*
Indications: Hyperlipidemia
Category: Antihyperlipidemic
Half-life: 45 minutes
Clinically important, potentially hazardous interactions with: atorvastatin, selenium

Reactions

Skin
Acanthosis nigricans
  (2002): Burrall BA, Sacramento, CA (from Internet) (observation)
  (2002): Eisner J, Mt. Vernon, WA (from Internet) (observation)
  (2002): Liss WA, Pleasanton, CA (from Internet) (observation)
  (2002): Marmelzat, JA, Los Angeles, CA (from Internet) (observation)
  (1994): McKenney JM+, *JAMA* 271, 672
  (1994): Stals H+, *Dermatology* 189, 203
  (1993): Stone OJ, *Med Hypotheses* 40, 154
  (1992): Coates P+, *Br J Dermatol* 126, 412
  (1990): Audicana M+, *Contact Dermatitis* 22, 60
  (1990): Brown G+, *N Engl J Med* 323, 1289 (8.3%)
  (1989): Larmi E, *Int J Dermatol* 28, 609
  (1989): Ylipieti S+, *Contact Dermatitis* 21, 105
  (1981): Elgart ML, *J Am Acad Dermatol* 5, 709
  (1974): Pedro S, *N Engl J Med* 29, 422
  (1971): Curth HO, *Birth Defects* 7, 31

(1967): Branehog I+, *Lakartidningen* (Swedish) 64, 1449
(1964): Tromovitch TA+, *Arch Dermatol* 89, 222
Dermatitis
  (1995): Bilbao I+, *Contact Dermatitis* 33, 435
Erythema
  (1995): Fisher AA, *Cutis* 55, 132
Exanthems
  (1997): Blumenthal HL, Beachwood, OH (personal case)
    (observation)
  (1997): Litt JZ, Beachwood, OH (2 personal cases) (observation)
  (1990): Brown G+, *N Engl J Med* 323, 1289 (2.8%)
Fixed eruption (<1%)
  (1992): de la Hoz-Caballer B+, *Med Clin (Barc)* (Spanish) 98, 357
Flushing (1–10%)
  (2002): Kashyap ML+, *Am J Cardiol* 89(6), 672 (10%) (with
    lovastatin)
  (2002): Litt JZ, Beachwood, OH (personal case) (observation)
  (1998): Capuzzi DM+, *Am J Cardiol* 82, 74U
  (1998): Guyton JR+, *Am J Cardiol* 82, 737 (4.8%)
  (1998): Knopp RH, *Am J Cardiol* 82, 24U
  (1998): Morgan JM+, *Am J Cardiol* 82, 29U
  (1997): Jungnickel PW+, *J Gen Intern Med* 12, 591
  (1996): Crouse JR, *Coron Artery* 7, 321
  (1996): Glen AI+, *Prostaglandins Leukot Essent Fatty Acids* 55, 9
  (1994): Fivenson DP+, *Arch Dermatol* 130, 753
  (1994): McKenney JM+, *JAMA* 271, 672
  (1994): Sudan BJ, *Ann Pharmacother* 28, 1113
  (1993): Fisher AA, *Cutis* 51, 225
  (1992): Breathnach SM+, *Adverse Drug Reactions and the Skin*
    Blackwell, Oxford, 265 (passim)
  (1992): Whelan AM+, *J Fam Pract* 34, 165 (passim)
  (1989): Warady B+, *Perit Dial Int* 9, 81
  (1988): Figge HL+, *Pharmacotherapy* 8, 287
  (1985): Mooney E, *Int J Dermatol* 24, 549
  (1977): Estep DL+, *Clin Toxicol* 11, 325
  (1973): *Med Lett* 15, 102
  (1973): Levy RI+, *Drugs* 6, 12
Ichthyosis
  (1961): Berge KG+, *Am J Med* 31, 24
Keratoses, pigmented
  (1974): Wittenborn JR+, *Adv Biochem Psychopharmacol* 9, 295
Pigmentation
  (1992): Breathnach SM+, *Adverse Drug Reactions and the Skin*
    Blackwell, Oxford, 265 (passim)
Pruritus (1–5%)
  (2002): Kashyap ML+, *Am J Cardiol* 89(6), 672 (with lovastatin)
  (1997): Blumenthal HL, Beachwood, OH (personal case)
    (observation)
  (1997): Jungnickel PW+, *J Gen Intern Med* 12, 591
  (1994): Fivenson DP+, *Arch Dermatol* 130, 753
  (1994): McKenney JM+, *JAMA* 271, 672
  (1992): Breathnach SM+, *Adverse Drug Reactions and the Skin*
    (Oxford) 265 (passim)
  (1992): Whelan AM+, *J Fam Pract* 34, 165 (passim)
  (1977): Estep DL+, *Clin Toxicol* 11, 325
  (1973): *Med Lett* 15, 102
  (1973): Levy RI+, *Drugs* 6, 12
Rash (sic) (<1%)
  (2002): Kashyap ML+, *Am J Cardiol* 89(6), 672 (with lovastatin)
  (1994): McKenney JM+, *JAMA* 271, 672
  (1992): Breathnach SM+, *Adverse Drug Reactions and the Skin*
    Blackwell, Oxford, 265 (passim)
  (1988): Figge HL+, *Pharmacotherapy* 8, 287
Scaling (sic)
  (1992): Breathnach SM+, *Adverse Drug Reactions and the Skin*
    Blackwell, Oxford, 265 (passim)
Urticaria
  (1995): Fisher AA, *Cutis* 55, 132
Xerosis

Other
  Anaphylactoid reactions
  Burning mouth syndrome
    (1988): Haustein UF, *Contact Dermatitis* 19, 225
  Gingivitis
    (1998): Leighton RF+, *Chest* 114, 1472
  Headache
    (2002): Kashyap ML+, *Am J Cardiol* 89(6), 672 (with lovastatin)
  Myopathy
    (1994): Gharavi AG+, *Am J Cardiol* 74, 841
    (1989): Goldstein MR, *Am J Med* 87, 248
    (1989): Litin SC+, *Am J Med* 86, 481
  Paresthesias (1–10%)
    (1997): Jungnickel PW+, *J Gen Intern Med* 12, 591
    (1992): Whelan AM+, *J Fam Pract* 34, 165 (passim)
  Toothache (sic)
    (1998): Leighton RF+, *Chest* 114, 1472
  Xerostomia

NIACINAMIDE

Synonyms: nicotinamide; vitamin B$_3$
Trade name: Niacinamide
Indications: Prophylaxis and treatment of pellagra
Category: Water-soluble nutritional supplement
Half-life: 45 minutes
**Clinically important, potentially hazardous interactions
with:** primidone

Reactions

Skin
  Acanthosis nigricans
    (1984): Papa CM, *Arch Dermatol* 120, 281
  Pruritus (1–5%)
    (1981): Zackheim HS+, *J Am Acad Dermatol* 4, 736
    (1980): Bures FA, *J Am Acad Dermatol* 3, 530
  Rash (sic)

Other
  Paresthesias (1–10%)

NICARDIPINE

Trade name: Cardene (Roche)
Other common trade names: *Antagonil; Dagan; Loxen;
Nicardal; Nicodel; Ranvil; Ridene; Rydene*
Indications: Angina, hypertension
Category: Antianginal; Antimigraine; Calcium channel blocker
Half-life: 2–4 hours
**Clinically important, potentially hazardous interactions
with:** epirubicin, imatinib

Reactions

Skin
  Allergic reactions (sic)
  Edema (1%)
  Exanthems
  Flushing (5.6%)
    (1998): Knowles S+, *J Am Acad Dermatol* 38, 201 (passim)
    (1990): Webster J+, *Br J Clin Pharmacol* 29, 587P
  Peripheral edema (7.1%)

(1998): Knowles S+, *J Am Acad Dermatol* 38, 201 (passim)
(1990): Webster J+, *Br J Clin Pharmacol* 29, 587P (leg edema)
Rash (sic) (1.2%)
(1998): Knowles S+, *J Am Acad Dermatol* 38, 201 (passim)
(1985): Deedwania PC+, *Clin Pharmacol Ther* 37, 190
(1985): Gelman JS+, *Am J Cardiol* 56, 232
Side effects (sic)
(1993): Kitamura K+, *J Dermatol* 20, 279 (psoriasiform)
Urticaria
(1983): Brodmerkel GJ, *Ann Intern Med* 99, 415
(1983): Fisher JR+, *Ann Intern Med* 98, 671
(1982): Grunwald Z, *Drug Intell Clin Pharm* 16, 492

Other

Erythromelalgia
(1989): Drenth JH, *BMJ* 298, 1582
(1989): Levesque H+, *BMJ* 298, 1252
Gingival hyperplasia (<1%)
Headache
Myalgia (1%)
(1998): Knowles S+, *J Am Acad Dermatol* 38, 201 (passim)
Paresthesias (1%)
Parotitis
Tinnitus
Xerostomia (1.4%)

NICOTINE*

Trade names: Habitrol Patch (Novartis); Nicoderm (GSK); Nicorette (GSK); Nicotrol (Pharmacia)
Other common trade names: *Exodus; Nicabate; Nicolan; Nicorette Plus; Nicotinell-TTS; Nicotrans; Nikofrenon; Stubit*
Indications: Aid to smoking cessation
Category: Smoking deterrent
Half-life: varies with the delivery system*

Reactions

Skin

Dermatitis
(1993): Farm G, *Contact Dermatitis* 29, 214
Diaphoresis (1–3%)
Edema
Erythema (>10%)
Flushing
Pruritus (>10%)
Rash (sic)
Urticaria
Vasculitis
(1996): Van der Klauw MM+, *Br J Dermatol* 134, 361

Other

Application-site burning
Application-site erythema
Application-site pruritus
Dysgeusia
Headache
Hypersensitivity (<1%)
Myalgia (1–10%)
Paresthesias
Sialorrhea (>10%)
Stomatitis (>10%)
Tinnitus
Tremor

Xerostomia (1–3%)

*Note: Smoking cessation therapy has various delivery systems. These include: transdermal patches, chewing gum, nasal spray, inhaler, and oral forms

NIFEDIPINE

Trade names: Adalat (Bayer); Procardia (Pfizer)
Other common trade names: *Adalate; Apo-Nifed; Aprical; Calcilat; Coracten; Corogal; Corotrend; Nifecor; Nu-Nifed; Pidilat*
Indications: Angina, hypertension
Category: Antianginal; Antimigraine; Calcium channel blocker
Half-life: 2–5 hours
Clinically important, potentially hazardous interactions with: epirubicin, **grapefruit juice**, imatinib, rifampin, ritonavir

Reactions

Skin

Acute generalized exanthematous pustulosis (AGEP)
(1995): Moreau A+, *Int J Dermatol* 34, 263 (passim)
(1991): Roujeau J-C+, *Arch Dermatol* 127, 1333
Angioedema (<1%)
(1998): Knowles S+, *J Am Acad Dermatol* 38, 201 (passim)
(1989): Stern R+, *Arch Intern Med* 149, 829
Ankle edema
(1994): Mohammed KN, *Ann Pharmacother* 28, 967
(1991): Salmasi AM+, *Int J Cardiol* 30, 303
(1989): Williams SA+, *Eur J Clin Pharmacol* 37, 333
(1978): Bridgman JF, *BMJ* 276, 578
Bullous eruption
(1989): Stern R+, *Arch Intern Med* 149, 829
(1987): Alcalay J+, *Dermatologica* 175, 191
Chills (2%)
Dermatitis (sic) (<2%)
Diaphoresis (<2%)
(1989): Stern R+, *Arch Intern Med* 149, 829
(1983): Lewis JG, *Drugs* 25, 196
Edema
(1983): Lewis JG, *Drugs* 25, 196
(1978): Bridgman JF, *BMJ* 276, 578 (erythematous, of legs)
Erysipelas
(1988): Leibovici V+, *Cutis* 41, 367
(1983): Lewis JG, *Drugs* 25, 196
Erythema
(1998): Knowles S+, *J Am Acad Dermatol* 38, 201 (passim)
(1992): Gonzalez-Castro U+, *Med Clin (Barc)* (Spanish) 98, 759
Erythema multiforme
(1998): Knowles S+, *J Am Acad Dermatol* 38, 201 (passim)
(1997): Springuel P, *Can Med Assoc J* 156, 90
(1989): Stern R+, *Arch Intern Med* 149, 829
(1986): Myrhed M+, *Acta Pharmacol Toxicol* 58, 133
Erythema nodosum
(1998): Knowles S+, *J Am Acad Dermatol* 38, 201 (passim)
(1989): Stern R+, *Arch Intern Med* 149, 829
Exanthems
(1998): Knowles S+, *J Am Acad Dermatol* 38, 201 (passim)
(1995): Litt JZ, Beachwood, OH (personal case) (observation)
(1992): Parish LC+, *Cutis* 49, 113 (morbilliform)
(1989): Stern R+, *Arch Intern Med* 149, 829
(1987): Alcalay J+, *Dermatologica* 175, 191
(1985): Findlay GH, *S Afr Med J* 68, 176
(1983): Lewis JG, *Drugs* 25, 196 (1%)
(1982): Grunwald Z, *Drug Intell Clin Pharm* 16, 492
(1980): Antman E+, *N Engl J Med* 302, 1269 (1%)

Exfoliative dermatitis (<1%)
  (1994): Mohammed KN, *Ann Pharmacother* 28, 967
  (1993): Collins P, *Br J Dermatol* 129, 630 (passim)
  (1989): Reynolds HJ+, *Br J Dermatol* 121, 401
  (1989): Stern R+, *Arch Intern Med* 149, 829
  (1984): Scoble JE+, *Clin Nephrol* 21, 302
Facial edema (1%)
Fixed eruption
  (1993): Litt JZ, Beachwood, OH (personal case) (observation)
  (1987): Alcalay J+, *Dermatologica* 175, 191
  (1986): Alcalay J+, *BMJ* 292, 450
Flushing (3–25%)
  (2001): Rudolph RI, Wyomissing, PA (from Internet) (observation)
  (1992): Shelley WB+, *Advanced Dermatologic Diagnosis* WB
    Saunders, 582 (passim)
  (1985): Aberg H+, *Drugs* 29 (Suppl 2), 117 (22%)
  (1983): Lewis JG, *Drugs* 25, 196 (5–15%)
  (1980): Antman E+, *N Engl J Med* 302, 1269 (11%)
Lichenoid eruption
  (1989): Reynolds HJ+, *Br J Dermatol* 121, 401
  (1988): Leibovici V+, *Cutis* 41, 367
  (1984): Scoble JE+, *Clin Nephrol* 21, 302
Lupus erythematosus
  (2003): Gubinelli E+, *J Cutan Med Surg*
  (1998): Callen JP, Academy '98 Meeting
  (1997): Crowson AN+, *Hum Pathol* 28, 67
Painful edema of extremities
  (1985): Findlay GH, *S Afr Med J* 68, 176
  (1982): Grunwald Z, *Drug Intell Clin Pharm* 16, 492
Pemphigoid nodularis
  (2000): Ameen M+, *Br J Dermatol* 142, 575
Pemphigus foliaceus
  (1993): Kim S-C+, *Acta Derm Venereol* (Stockh) 73, 210
Periorbital edema (1%)
  (1985): Tordjman K+, *Am J Cardiol* 55, 1445
Peripheral edema (10–30%)
  (2002): No author, *Medscape Primary Care* 4
  (1996): Tailor SA+, *Arch Dermatol* 132, 350 (with itraconazole)
Photosensitivity
  (1996): Seggev JS+, *J Allergy Clin Immunol* 97, 852
  (1991): Zenarola P+, *Dermatologica* 182, 196
  (1990): Guarrera M+, *Photodermatology* 7, 25
  (1988): Zlotogorski A, *Dermatologica* 177, 249
  (1986): Thomas SE+, *BMJ* 292, 992
Prurigo nodularis
  (1992): Shelley WB+, *Cutis* 50, 179 (observation)
Pruritus (<2%)
  (1998): Knowles S+, *J Am Acad Dermatol* 38, 201 (passim)
  (1993): Collins P, *Br J Dermatol* 129, 630 (passim)
  (1989): Stern R+, *Arch Intern Med* 149, 829
Purpura (<2%)
  (1990): Regazzini R+, *Chron Derm* (Italian) 21, 225
  (1989): Oren R+, *Drug Intell Clin Pharm* 23, 88
  (1985): Findlay GH, *S Afr Med J* 68, 176
Rash (sic) (<3%)
  (1998): Knowles S+, *J Am Acad Dermatol* 38, 201 (passim)
  (1989): Stern R+, *Arch Intern Med* 149, 829
Shaking (sic) (2%)
Side effects (sic)
  (1993): Kitamura K+, *J Dermatol* 20, 279 (psoriasiform)
Stevens–Johnson syndrome
  (1998): Knowles S+, *J Am Acad Dermatol* 38, 201 (passim)
  (1993): Collins P, *Br J Dermatol* 129, 630 (passim)
  (1989): Stern R+, *Arch Intern Med* 149, 829
Telangiectasia
  (1994): Shelley WB+, *Cutis* 53, 40 (observation)
  (1993): Collins P, *Br J Dermatol* 129, 630 (photodistribution)
  (1992): Tsele E+, *Lancet* 339, 365

Toxic epidermal necrolysis
  (1998): Knowles S+, *J Am Acad Dermatol* 38, 201 (passim)
  (1993): Collins P, *Br J Dermatol* 129, 630 (passim)
Ulcerations
  (1999): Luca S+, *Minerva Cardioangiol* 47, 219
Urticaria (<1%)
  (1999): Luca S+, *Minerva Cardioangiol* 47, 219 (legs)
  (1998): Knowles S+, *J Am Acad Dermatol* 38, 201 (passim)
  (1991): Zenarola P+, *Dermatologica* 182, 196
  (1989): Stern R+, *Arch Intern Med* 149, 829
  (1988): Toner M+, *Chest* 93, 1320
  (1986): Myrhed M+, *Acta Pharmacol Toxicol* 58, 133
  (1978): Bridgman JF, *BMJ* 276, 578
Vasculitis
  (1989): Oren R+, *Drug Intell Clin Pharm* 23, 88
  (1987): Alcalay J+, *Dermatologica* 175, 191
  (1985): Brenner S+, *Harefuah* (Hebrew) 108, 139

Hair

Hair – alopecia (1%)
  (1998): Knowles S+, *J Am Acad Dermatol* 38, 201 (passim)
  (1993): Collins P, *Br J Dermatol* 129, 630 (passim)
  (1989): Reynolds HJ+, *Br J Dermatol* 121, 401
  (1989): Stern R+, *Arch Intern Med* 149, 829
Hair – pigmentation
  (1989): Stern R+, *Arch Intern Med* 149, 829

Nails

Nails – dystrophy
  (1989): Stern R+, *Arch Intern Med* 149, 829

Other

Dysgeusia (<1%)
Erythromelalgia (<0.5%)
  (1989): Stern R+, *Arch Intern Med* 149, 829
  (1987): Alcalay J+, *Dermatologica* 175, 191
  (1983): Brodmerkel GJ, *Ann Intern Med* 99, 415
  (1983): Fisher JR+, *Ann Intern Med* 98, 671
Gingival hyperplasia (>10%)
  (2001): Uzel MI+, *J Periodontol* 72(7), 921
  (2000): James JA+, *J Clin Periodontol* 27, 109 (with cyclosporine)
  (1999): Ellis JS+, *J Periodontol* 70, 63 (6.3%)
  (1998): Bokor-Bratic M+, *Med Pregl* (Serbo-Croatian [Roman])
    51, 445
  (1998): Desai P+, *J Can Dent Assoc* 64, 263
  (1998): Nakou M+, *J Periodontol* 69, 664
  (1998): Nohl F+, *Ther Umsch* (German) 55, 573
  (1997): Jackson C+, *N Y State Dent J* 63, 46
  (1997): Slezak R, *J West Soc Periodontal Periodontal Abstr* 45, 105
  (1997): Thomason JM+, *Clin Oral Investig* 1, 35
  (1997): Westbrook P+, *J Periodontol* 68, 645
  (1996): Abitbol TE+, *N Y State Dent J* 63, 34
  (1996): Ciantar M, *Dent Update* 23, 374
  (1996): Darbar UR+, *J Clin Periodontol* 23, 941
  (1996): Deen-Duggins L+, *Quintessence Int* 27, 163 (4 cases)
  (1996): Saito K+, *J Periodontol Res* 31, 545
  (1995): Harel-Raviv M+, *Oral Surg Oral Med Oral Pathol Oral
    Radiol Endoc* 79, 715
  (1995): Nery EB+, *J Periodontol* 66, 572
  (1995): Ramsdale DR+, *Br Heart J* 73, 115
  (1995): Silverstein LH+, *J Oral Implantol* 21, 116
  (1995): Wynn RL, *Gen Dent* 43, 218
  (1994): Henderson JS+, *Miss Dent Assoc J* 50, 12
  (1994): Shelley WB+, *Cutis* 53, 282 (passim)
  (1993): King GN+, *J Clin Periodontol* 20, 286
  (1993): Morisaki I+, *J Periodontal Res* 28, 396
  (1993): Steele RM+, *Arch Intern Med* 120, 663
  (1992): Hancock RH+, *J Clin Periodontol* 19, 12
  (1991): Nishikawa SJ+, *J Periodontol* 62, 30
  (1991): Wynn RL, *Gen Dent* 39, 240
  (1989): Veraldi S+, *Clin Exp Dermatol* 14, 93

(1988): Boisnic S+, *Ann Dermatol Venereol* (French) 115, 373
(1988): Zlotogorski A, *Dermatologica* 177, 249
(1986): Bencini PL+, *G Ital Dermatol Venereol* (Italian) 121, 29
(1986): Jones CM, *Br Dent J* 160, 416
(1985): Bencini PL+, *Acta Derm Venereol* (Stockh) 65, 362
(1985): Lucas RM+, *J Periodontol* 56, 211
(1984): Lederman D+, *Oral Surg Oral Med Oral Pathol* 57, 620
(1984): Ramon Y+, *Int J Cardiol* 5, 195
Gynecomastia (<1%)
  (1995): Marcos-Olea JL+, *Aten Primaria* (Spanish) 16, 115
  (1988): Zlotogorski A, *Dermatologica* 177, 249
  (1986): Clyne CAC, *BMJ* 292, 380
Headache
Myalgia (<1%)
Paresthesias (<3%)
  (1982): Macdonald JB, *BMJ* 285, 1744
Parosmia
Parotitis
Tinnitus
Tremor (2–8%)
Xerostomia (<3%)

NIMODIPINE

Trade name: Nimotop (Bayer)
Other common trade names: *Admon; Periplum; Vasotop*
Indications: Subarachnoid hemorrhage
Category: Calcium channel blocker
Half-life: 3 hours
Clinically important, potentially hazardous interactions with: epirubicin, imatinib

Reactions

Skin
Acne (<1%)
Acute generalized exanthematous pustulosis (AGEP)
  (1999): Zabawski E+, Dallas, TX (from Internet) (observation)
Diaphoresis (<1%)
Edema (2%)
Exanthems (2.4%)
  (1989): Langley MS+, *Drugs* 37, 669
Flushing (2.1%)
Peripheral edema
Pruritus (<1%)
Purpura
Rash (sic) (3%)

Hair
Hair – alopecia
  (1995): Daghfous R+, *Therapie* (French) 50, 590

Other
Headache

NISOLDIPINE

Trade name: Sular (First Horizon)
Other common trade names: *Baymycard; Syscor*
Indications: Hypertension
Category: Antihypertensive; Calcium channel blocker
Half-life: 7–12 hours
Clinically important, potentially hazardous interactions with: epirubicin, imatinib

Reactions

Skin
Acne (<1%)
Angioedema
Cellulitis (<1%)
Chills (<1%)
Diaphoresis (<1%)
Ecchymoses (<1%)
Exanthems (<1%)
  (1988): Friedel HA+, *Drugs* 36, 682 (0.7%)
Exfoliative dermatitis (<1%)
Facial edema (<1%)
Flu-like syndrome (sic) (<1%)
Flushing
  (1988): Friedel HA+, *Drugs* 36, 682 (13.21%)
Herpes simplex (<1%)
Herpes zoster (<1%)
Peripheral edema (22%)
  (2001): Lenz TL+, *Pharmacotherapy* 21(8), 898 (4 cases) (with amlodipine)
Petechiae (<1%)
Photosensitivity
Pigmentation (<1%)
Pruritus (<1%)
Pustules (<1%)
Rash (sic) (2%)
Side effects (sic)
  (1993): Kitamura K+, *J Dermatol* 20, 279
Ulcerations (<1%)
Urticaria (<1%)
Xerosis (<1%)

Hair
Hair – alopecia (<1%)

Other
Dysgeusia (<1%)
Gingival hyperplasia (<1%)
Glossitis (<1%)
Gynecomastia (<1%)
Headache
Hyperesthesia (<1%)
Hypersensitivity
Oral ulceration (<1%)
Paresthesias (<1%)
Tremor (<1%)
Vaginitis (<1%)
Xerostomia (<1%)

NITAZOXANIDE

Trade name: Alinia (Romark)
Other common trade name: *Cryptaz*
Indications: Diarrhea caused by *Cryptosporidium parvum* or *Giardia lamblia* (in children)
Category: Antiprotozoal

Reactions

Skin
Diaphoresis (<1%)
Infections (<1%)
Pruritus (<1%)

Other
Dizziness (<1%)
Rhinitis (<1%)
Salivary gland enlargement (<1%)
Scleral pigmentation (pale-yellow) (<1%)

NITISINONE

Trade name: Orfadin (Orphan Medical)
Indications: Hereditary tyrosinemia
Category: Metabolic enzyme; Tyrosine catabolism inhibitor
Half-life: 54 hours

Reactions

Skin
Blepharitis (1%)
Exanthems (1%)
Exfoliative dermatitis (1%)
Infections (<1%)
Pruritus (1%)
Rash (sic)
Xerosis (1%)

Hair
Hair – alopecia (1%)

Other
Brain tumor
Conjunctivitis (2%)
Death
Ocular irritation (1%)
Porphyria (1%)
Seizures (<1%)
Tooth discoloration (<1%)

NITROFURANTOIN

Trade names: Furadantin (First Horizon); Macrobid (Procter & Gamble); Macrodantin (Procter & Gamble)
Other common trade names: *Furadantina; Furadoine; Furalan; Furan; Furobactina; Infurin; Nephronex; Novo-Furan; Urofuran*
Indications: Various urinary tract infections caused by susceptible organisms
Category: Urinary tract antibiotic
Half-life: 20–60 minutes

Reactions

Skin
Acute febrile neutrophilic dermatosis (Sweet's syndrome)
  (1999): Retief CR+, *Cutis* 63, 177
Angioedema
  (1982): Penn RG+, *BMJ* 284, 1440
  (1981): Chisholm JC+, *J Nat Med Assoc* 73, 59 (passim)
  (1977): Delaney RA+, *Am J Pharm* 149, 26 (passim)
  (1971): Koch-Weser J+, *Ann Intern Med* 128, 399 (0.1%)
Bullous eruption
Chills
Dermatitis
  (1978): Novak M, *Cesk Dermatol* (Czech) 53, 128
  (1974): Bleumink E+, *Hautarzt* (German) 25, 403
  (1970): Laubstein H+, *Dermatol Monatsschr* (German) 156, 1
Eczema (sic)
  (1977): Delaney RA+, *Am J Pharm* 149, 26 (passim)
  (1976): Mitchell J+, *Modern Med* 44, 63
Erythema multiforme
  (1990): Chan HL+, *Arch Dermatol* 126, 43
  (1986): Chapman JA, *Ann Allergy* 56, 16
  (1971): Koch-Weser J+, *Ann Intern Med* 128, 399 (0.1%)
Erythema nodosum
  (1981): Chisholm JC+, *J Nat Med Assoc* 73, 59
Exanthems (1–5%)
  (2002): Blumenthal HL, Beachwood, OH (personal case)
    (observation)
  (1984): Paver R+, *Current Ther* 25, 55
  (1983): Swinyer LJ, *Dermatol Clin* 1, 417
  (1980): Calderwood SB+, *Surgical Clin N Amer* 60, 65
  (1980): Holmberg L+, *Am J Med* 69, 733 (28%)
  (1976): Stubb S, *Acta Derm Venereol* (Stockh) 56 (Suppl 76), 16
  (1974): Eggers B+, *Z Hautkr* (German) 49, 704
  (1972): Kauppinen K, *Acta Derm Venereol* (Stockh) 52 (Suppl), 68
  (1971): Bailey RR+, *Lancet* 2, 1112 (1%)
  (1971): Koch-Weser J+, *Ann Intern Med* 128, 399 (1%)
Exfoliative dermatitis
  (1984): Paver R+, *Current Ther* 25, 55
  (1983): Swinyer LJ, *Dermatol Clin* 1, 417
  (1972): Kauppinen K, *Acta Derm Venereol* (Stockh) 52 (Suppl), 68
Fixed eruption
  (1985): Kauppinen K+, *Br J Dermatol* 112, 575
Flushing
Lupus erythematosus
  (1986): Chapman JA, *Annals Allergy* 56, 16
  (1985): Stratton MA, *Clin Pharm* 4, 657
  (1981): Fleck RM, *Pennsylvania Med* 84, 36
  (1975): Selroos O+, *Acta Med Scand* 197, 125
  (1974): Back O+, *Lancet* 1, 930
Panniculitis, nodular nonsuppurative
  (1987): Sanford RG+, *Arthritis Rheum* 30, 1076
Photosensitivity
  (1987): Australian Drug Evaluation Committee, 61 (Oct 15)
Pruritus (<1%)
  (1987): Australian Drug Evaluation Committee, 61 (Oct 15)

(1981): Chisholm JC+, *J Nat Med Assoc* 73, 59 (passim)

Purpura
(1984): Paver R+, *Current Ther* 25, 55
(1983): Swinyer LJ, *Dermatol Clin* 1, 417

Rash (sic) (<1%)
(1982): Penn RG+, *BMJ* 284, 1440
(1977): Takala J+, *Acta Med Scand* 202, 75

Reticular hyperplasia
(1966): Korting GW+, *Dermatol Wochenschr* (German) 152, 257

Stevens–Johnson syndrome
(1971): Koch-Weser J+, *Ann Intern Med* 128, 399

Toxic epidermal necrolysis
(1993): Stables GI+, *Br J Dermatol* 128, 357
(1984): Kauppinen K+, *Acta Derm Venereol* (Stockh) 64, 320
(1983): Swinyer LJ, *Dermatol Clin* 1, 417
(1967): Duperrat B+, *Bull Soc Fr Dermatol Syphiligr* (French) 74, 423 (fatal)
(1963): Oswald FH, *Ned Tijdschr Geneesk* (Danish) 107, 999

Urticaria
(1999): Litt JZ, Beachwood, OH (personal case) (observation)
(1996): Blumenthal HL, Beachwood, OH (personal case) (observation)
(1983): Griffin JP, *Practitioner* 227, 1283
(1983): Swinyer LJ, *Dermatol Clin* 1, 417
(1982): Schneider RE, *Clin Ther* 4, 390
(1978): Watson B+, *Br J Dermatol* 99, 183
(1977): McLundie S, *Ann Allergy* 38, 71
(1972): Kauppinen K, *Acta Derm Venereol* (Stockh) 52 (Suppl), 68
(1971): Koch-Weser J+, *Ann Intern Med* 128, 399 (0.4%)
(1969): Aaronson CM, *JAMA* 210, 557

Hair

Hair – alopecia
(1983): No Author, *Lakartidningen* (Swedish) 80, 4040
(1983): Swinyer LJ, *Dermatol Clin* 1, 417
(1977): Delaney RA+, *Am J Pharm* 149, 26 (passim)
(1971): Coster C+, *Lakartidningen* (Swedish) 68, 3366
(1959): Johnson SH+, *J Urology* (Baltimore) 82, 162

Nails

Nails – onycholysis
(1982): Penn RG+, *BMJ* 284, 1440

Other

Anaphylactoid reactions
(1987): Australian Drug Evaluation Committee, 61 (Oct 15)
(1982): Penn RG+, *BMJ* 284, 1440
(1980): Calderwood SB+, *Surg Clin N Amer* 60, 65

Death

Galactorrhea
(1986): Auwaerter A+, *Krankenhausarzt* (German) 59, 766

Headache

Hypersensitivity
(1976): Fine SR, *Cutis* 17, 1171

Mastodynia
(1986): Auwaerter A+, *Krankenhausarzt* (German) 59, 766

Myalgia

Paresthesias (1–10%)

Pseudolymphoma
(1993): Kerl H+, *Dermatology in General Medicine* McGraw-Hill New York

Tooth discoloration

Xerostomia
(1977): Takala J+, *Acta Med Scand* 202, 75

NITROGLYCERIN

Synonyms: glyceryl trinitrate; nitroglycerol; NTG
Trade names:
  Buccal tablets: Nitrogard (Forest)
  Lingual aerosol: Nitrolingual (First Horizon)
  Oral capsules: Nitro-Bid (Fougera); Nitrocap; Nitrocine; Nitroglyn; Nitrospan
  Oral tablets: Klavikordal; Niong; Nitronet; Nitrong
  Parenteral: Nitro-Bid; Nitroject; Nitrol; Nitrostat; Tridil
  Sublingual tablets: Nitrostat (Parke-Davis)
  Topical ointment: Nitro-Bid (Fougera); Nitrol; Nitrong; Nitrostat
  Topical transdermal systems: Deponit; Minitran (3M); Nitrocine; Nitrodisc; Nitrodur (Schering); Transderm-Nitro. (Various pharmaceutical companies.)

Other common trade names: *Cardinit; Corditrine; Lenitral; Nitradisc; Nitroglin; Suscard; Sustac*
Indications: Acute angina
Category: Antianginal; Antihypertensive; Vasodilator
Half-life: 1–4 minutes
Clinically important, potentially hazardous interactions with: acetylcysteine, alteplase, sildenafil

Reactions

Skin

Allergic reactions (sic) (<1%)

Angioedema
(1998): Rademaker M+, *New Zealand Adverse Drug Reactions Committee*, April, 1998 (from Internet)

Cyanosis

Dermatitis (to topical systems) (<1%)
(2000): McKenna KE, *Contact Dermatitis* 42, 246
(1999): Machet L+, *Dermatology* 198, 106
(1994): de la Fuente-Prieto R+, *Ann Allergy* 72, 344
(1992): Torres V+, *Contact Dermatitis* 26, 53
(1991): Kanerva L+, *Contact Dermatitis* 24, 356
(1991): Laine R+, *Duodecim* (Finnish) 107, 41
(1990): Vaillant L+, *Contact Dermatitis* 23, 142
(1989): Carmichael AJ+, *Contact Dermatitis* 21, 113
(1989): Di Landro A+, *Contact Dermatitis* 21, 115
(1989): Holdiness MR, *Contact Dermatitis* 20, 3
(1988): Apted J, *Med J Aust* 148, 482
(1988): Niedner R, *Hautarzt* (German) 39, 761
(1987): Gupta AK+, *Arch Dermatol* 123, 295
(1987): Harari Z+, *Dermatologica* 174, 249
(1987): Topaz O+, *Ann Allergy* 59, 365
(1986): Schrader BJ+, *Pharmacotherapy* 6, 83
(1986): Weickel R+, *Hautarzt* (German) 37, 511
(1985): Fischer RG+, *South Med J* 78, 1523
(1984): Fisher AA, *Cutis* 34, 526
(1984): Letendre PW+, *Drug Intell Clin Pharm* 18, 69
(1984): Rosenfeld AS+, *Am Heart J* 108, 1061
(1983): Camarasa JG+, *Contact Dermatitis* 9, 320
(1979): Hendricks AA+, *Arch Dermatol* 115, 853

Diaphoresis (<1%)

Eczema (sic)
(1989): Carmichael AJ+, *Contact Dermatitis* 21, 113
(1987): Topaz O+, *Ann Allergy* 59, 365

Edema

Erythema (to transdermal delivery system)
(1990): Hogan JD+, *J Am Acad Dermatol* 22, 811

Erythema multiforme
(2001): Silvestre JF+, *Contact Dermatitis* 45(5), 299

Erythroderma
(1972): Ryan FP, *Br J Dermatol* 87, 498

Exanthems
Exfoliative dermatitis (1–10%)
  (1972): Ryan FP, *Br J Dermatol* 87, 498
Flushing (>10%)
  (1992): Shelley WB+, *Advanced Dermatologic Diagnosis* WB
    Saunders, 582 (passim)
Pallor
Peripheral edema (<1%)
Purpura
  (1989): Nishioka K+, *J Dermatol* 16, 220 (pigmented)
  (1955): Shmushkovich J+, *Br J Dermatol* 67, 299
Rash (sic) (1–10%)
Rosacea (exacerbation)
  (1980): Wilkin JK, *Arch Dermatol* 116, 598
Urticaria

Other

Anaphylactoid reactions (from perianal application)
  (1999): Pietroletti R+, *Am J Gastroenterol* 94, 292
Headache
Oral burn (from sublingual)
Xerostomia (<1%)

NIZATIDINE

Trade name: Axid (Reliant)
Other common trade names: *Apo-Nizatidine; Calmaxid;
Gastrax; Nizax; Nizaxid; Panaxid; Tazac; Zanizal*
Indications: Duodenal ulcer, gastroesophageal reflux disease
(GERD)
Category: Antihistamine H$_2$-blocker
Half-life: 1–2 hours

Reactions

Skin

Acne (<1%)
Allergic reactions (sic) (<1%)
Dermatitis
Diaphoresis (1%)
  (1988): Price AH+, *Drugs* 36, 521 (1%)
  (1987): Cloud ML, *Scand J Gastroenterol* 22, 39
Edema
Exanthems
Exfoliative dermatitis
Pruritus (1.7%)
  (1988): Price AH+, *Drugs* 36, 521
  (1987): Cloud ML, *Scand J Gastroenterol* 22, 39
Rash (sic) (1.9%)
  (1987): Cloud ML, *Scand J Gastroenterol* 22, 39
Urticaria (<1%)
  (1988): Price AH+, *Drugs* 36, 521 (0.5%)
Vasculitis
Xerosis (<1%)

Other

Gynecomastia
  (1987): Cloud ML, *Scand J Gastroenterol* 22, 39
Headache
Myalgia (1.7%)
Paresthesias (<1%)
Pseudolymphoma
  (1995): Magro CM+, *J Am Acad Dermatol* 32, 419
Serum sickness
Xerostomia (1.4%)

NORFLOXACIN

Trade names: Chibroxin (Merck); Noroxin (Merck) (Roberts)
Other common trade names: *Barazan; Chibroxine; Chibroxol;
Lexinor; Noroxine; Oranor; Utinor; Zoroxin*
Indications: Various urinary tract infections caused by
susceptible organisms, conjunctivitis
Category: Broad-spectrum quinolone antibiotic
Half-life: 2.3–4 hours
**Clinically important, potentially hazardous interactions
with:** amiodarone, arsenic, bepridil, bretylium, disopyramide,
erythromycin, phenothiazines, procainamide, quinidine, sotalol,
tricyclic antidepressants

Reactions

Skin

Angioedema
Bullous eruption
  (1993): Ramsey B+, *Br J Dermatol* 129, 500
Dermatitis
  (1998): Silvestre JF+, *Contact Dermatitis* 39, 83
Diaphoresis (<1%)
Edema
Erythema (sic) (<1%)
Erythema multiforme
Exanthems
  (1988): Wolfson JS+, *Ann Intern Med* 108, 238
  (1985): Holmes B+, *Drugs* 30, 482 (0.2%)
Exfoliative dermatitis
Fixed eruption
  (1997): Fenandez-Rivas M, *Allergy* 52, 477
Photosensitivity
  (1963): Oswald FH, *Ned Tijdschr Geneesk* (Dutch) 107, 999
Phototoxicity
  (2000): Traynor NJ+, *Toxicol Vitr* 14, 275
  (1998): Martinez LJ+, *Photochem Photobiol* 67, 399
  (1994): Fujita H+, *Photodermatol Photoimmunol Photomed*
    10, 202
  (1993): Ferguson J+, *Br J Dermatol* 128, 285
Pruritus (<1%)
  (1985): Holmes B+, *Drugs* 30, 482 (0.2%)
Pustules
  (1992): Allegue F+, *Med Clin (Barc)* (Spanish) 99, 274
Rash (sic) (<1%)
Stevens–Johnson syndrome
  (1992): Kubo-Shimasaki A+, *Rinsho Ketsueki* (Japanese) 33, 823
Stinging (from ophthalmic solution)
Subcorneal pustular dermatosis (Sneddon–Wilkinson)
  (1988): Shelley ED+, *Cutis* 42, 24
Toxic epidermal necrolysis
  (1993): Correia O+, *Dermatology* 186, 32
Toxic pustuloderma
  (1993): Tsuda S+, *Acta Derm Venereol* (Stockh) 73, 382 (passim)
Urticaria
Vasculitis

Nails

Nails – photo-onycholysis
  (1987): Baran R+, *J Am Acad Dermatol* 17, 1012
  (1986): Baran R+, *Dermatologica* 173, 185

Other

Anaphylactoid reactions
Dysgeusia (<1%) (bitter taste)
Headache

Myalgia
  (2001): Guis S+, *J Rheumatol* 28, 1405
Paresthesias
Rhabdomyolysis
  (2001): Guis S+, *J Rheumatol* 28, 1405
Stomatitis
Tendinitis
  (1983): Bailey RR+, *N Z Med J* 96, 590
Tendon rupture (<1%)
Tinnitus
Vaginal candidiasis
Xerostomia (<1%)

NORTRIPTYLINE

Trade names: Aventyl (Lilly); Pamelor (Mallinckrodt)
Other common trade names: *Allegron; Apo-Nortriptyline; Noritren; Norpress; Nortrilen; Paxtibi; Vividyl*
Indications: Depression
Category: Tricyclic antidepressant
Half-life: 28–31 hours
Clinically important, potentially hazardous interactions with: amprenavir, arbutamine, clonidine, epinephrine, fluoxetine, formoterol, guanethidine, isocarboxazid, linezolid, MAO inhibitors, phenelzine, quinolones, sparfloxacin, tranylcypromine

Reactions

Skin
Acne
Allergic reactions (sic) (<1%)
Diaphoresis (1–10%)
Edema
Erythema
Exanthems
Flushing
Petechiae
Photosensitivity (<1%)
  (1972): Macaione AS, *Bull Geisinger Med Cent* 24, 122
  (1972): Richards DL+, *Adverse Drug Reactions* Livingstone
Phototoxicity
Pruritus
Purpura
Rash (sic)
Urticaria
Vasculitis
Xerosis

Hair
Hair – alopecia (<1%)

Other
Acute intermittent porphyria
  (1986): Krummel SJ+, *Drug Intell Clin Pharm* 20, 487
Black tongue
  (1990): Vitiello B+, *Clin Pharm* 9, 421
Dysgeusia (>10%)
Galactorrhea (<1%)
Gynecomastia (<1%)
Paresthesias
Parkinsonism (1–10%)
Stomatitis
Tinnitus
Tongue edema
Tremor

Vaginitis
Xerostomia (>10%)
  (2001): Pomara N+, *Prog Neuropsychopharmacol Biol Psychiatry* 25(5), 1035

NYSTATIN

Trade names: Mycolog-11 (Apothecon); Mycostatin (Bristol-Myers Squibb)
Other common trade names: *Biofanal; Candio-Hermal; Mestatin; Moronal; Nistaquim; Nyaderm; Nystacid; Nystan; Nystex; Oranyst; Pedi-Dri*
Indications: Candidiasis
Category: Antifungal (anticandidal) antibiotic
Half-life: N/A

Reactions

Skin
Acrodermatitis perstans (exacerbation)
  (1971): Petrozzi JW+, *Arch Dermatol* 103, 442
Acute generalized exanthematous pustulosis (AGEP)
  (1999): Przybilla B+, *Hautarzt* (German) 50, 136
  (1998): Rosenberger A+, *Hautarzt* (German) 49, 492
  (1997): Kuchler A+, *Br J Dermatol* 137, 808 (3 cases)
Dermatitis (sic) (<1%)
  (1994): Fisher AA, *Cutis* 54, 300
  (1993): Hills RJ+, *Contact Dermatitis* 28, 48
  (1991): Quirce S+, *Contact Dermatitis* 25(3), 197 (generalized)
  (1990): de Groot AC+, *Dermatologic Clinics* 8, 153
  (1987): Lechner T+, *Mykosen* (German) 30, 143
  (1985): Lang E+, *Contact Dermatitis* 12, 182
  (1971): Chalmers D, *Arch Dermatol* 104, 437
  (1971): Coskey RJ, *Arch Dermatol* 103, 228
  (1971): Foussereau J+, *Bull Soc Fr Dermatol Syphiligr* (French) 78, 457
  (1971): Wasilewski C, *Arch Dermatol* 104, 437
  (1970): Wasilewski C, *Arch Dermatol* 102, 216
Eczema (sic)
  (1987): Lechner T+, *Mykosen* (German) 30, 143
  (1971): Coskey RJ, *Arch Dermatol* 103, 228
Erythema multiforme
  (1991): Garty BZ, *Arch Dermatol* 127, 741
Erythroderma
  (1980): Pareek SS, *Br J Dermatol* 103, 679
Exanthems
  (1991): Quirce S+, *Contact Dermatitis* 25, 197
Fixed eruption
  (1980): Pareek SS, *Br J Dermatol* 103, 679
  (1969): Kandil E, *Dermatologica* 139, 37
Pruritus
  (1987): Lechner T+, *Mykosen* (German) 30, 143
Rash (sic)
Stevens–Johnson syndrome (<1%)
  (1991): Garty BZ, *Arch Dermatol* 127, 741
Urticaria
Vulvovaginitis
  (2001): Dan M, *Am J Obstet Gynecol* 185(1), 254

Other
Hypersensitivity (<1%)
  (2001): Barranco R+, *Contact Dermatitis* 45(1), 60
Tongue edema
  (1991): Quirce S+, *Contact Dermatitis* 25, 197
Vaginitis
  (2001): Dan M, *Am J Obstet Gynecol* 185(1), 254

OCTREOTIDE

Trade name: Sandostatin (Novartis)
Other common trade names: *Sandostatina; Sandostatine*
Indications: Diarrhea
Category: Antihypoglycemic; Antihypotensive; Growth hormone suppressant; Somatostatin analog
Half-life: 1.5 hours

Reactions

Skin
Allergic reactions (sic)
Cellulitis (1–4%)
Diaphoresis
Edema (1–10%)
Exanthems
  (1990): Saltz L+, *Proc Am Soc Clin Oncol* 9, 97
Flushing (1–4%)
  (2000): Caplin ME+, *Nucl Med Commun* 21, 97
Granulomas
  (2001): Rideout DJ+, *Clin Nucl Med* 26, 650 (buttock)
Petechiae (1–4%)
Pruritus (1–4%)
Purpura (1–4%)
Rash (sic) (<1%)
Raynaud's phenomenon (1–4%)
Urticaria (1–4%)

Hair
Hair – alopecia (<1%)
  (1995): Nakauchi Y+, *Endocr J* 42, 385
  (1991): Jonsson A+, *Ann Intern Med* 115, 913

Other
Anaphylactoid reactions
Galactorrhea (1–4%)
Gynecomastia (1–4%)
Headache
Hyperesthesia (<1%)
Injection-site erythema (1%)
Injection-site granuloma
  (2001): Rideout DJ+, *Clin Nucl Med* 26(7), 650
Injection-site pain (7.5%)
Injection-site reaction (sic)
Thrombophlebitis (1–4%)
Vaginitis (1–4%)
Xerostomia

OFLOXACIN

Trade names: Floxin (Ortho-McNeil); Ocuflox (Allergan)
Other common trade names: *Bactocin; Exocine; Flobasin; Floxan; Floxil; Floxstat; Oflocet; Oflocin; Tabrin; Taravid*
Indications: Various infections caused by susceptible organisms
Category: Broad-spectrum fluoroquinolone antibiotic
Half-life: 4–8 hours
Clinically important, potentially hazardous interactions with: amiodarone, arsenic, bepridil, bretylium, disopyramide, erythromycin, phenothiazines, procainamide, quinidine, sotalol, tricyclic antidepressants

Reactions

Skin
Angioedema
  (1987): Jüngst G+, *Drugs* 34 (Suppl 1), 144
  (1987): Monk JP, *Drugs* 33, 346
Bullous eruption
Candidiasis (sic)
  (1987): Jüngst G+, *Drugs* 34 (Suppl 1), 144
Chills (<1%)
Dermatitis (sic)
  (2000): Litt JZ, Beachwood, OH (personal case) (observation)
  (1987): Monk JP, *Drugs* 33, 346
Diaphoresis
Ecchymoses
Edema (<1%)
Erythema multiforme
Erythema nodosum
Exanthems
  (1994): Shelley WB+, *Cutis* 54, 146 (observation)
  (1994): Shelley WB+, *Cutis* 55, 22 (observation)
  (1993): Litt JZ, Beachwood, OH (personal case) (observation)
  (1987): Jüngst G+, *Drugs* 34 (Suppl 1), 144
  (1987): Monk JP, *Drugs* 33, 346
  (1986): Baran R+, *Dermatologica* 173, 185
Exfoliative dermatitis
Fixed eruption
  (1996): Kawada A+, *Contact Dermatitis* 34, 427
  (1994): Kawada A+, *Contact Dermatitis* 31, 182
Petechiae
Photosensitivity (<1%)
  (2002): Trisciuoglio D+, *Toxicol In Vitro* 16(4), 449
  (1994): Fujita H+, *Photodermatol Photoimmunol Photomed* 10, 202
  (1993): Scheife RT+, *Int J Dermatol* 32, 413
  (1990): Przybilla G+, *Dermatologica* 181, 98
  (1988): Halkin H, *Rev Infect Dis* 10 (Suppl 1), 258
  (1987): Jensen T+, *J Antimicrob Chemother* 20, 585
  (1987): Jüngst G+, *Drugs* 34 (Suppl 1), 144
  (1986): Baran R+, *Dermatologica* 173, 185
Phototoxicity
  (2000): Traynor NJ+, *Toxicol Vitr* 14, 275
  (1998): Martinez LJ+, *Photochem Photobiol* 67, 399
Pigmentation
Pruritus (1–3%)
  (2000): Litt JZ, Beachwood, OH (personal case) (observation)
  (1987): Jüngst G+, *Drugs* 34 (Suppl 1), 144
  (1987): Monk JP, *Drugs* 33, 346
Pruritus vulvae (1–3%)
Purpura
Rash (sic) (1–10%)
  (1988): Kromann-Andersen B+, *J Antimicrob Chemother* 22 (Suppl C), 143

Side effects (sic) (0.4%)
(1988): Fostini R+, *Drug Exp Clin Res* 14, 393
(1987): Monk JP, *Drugs* 33, 346
Stevens–Johnson syndrome
Toxic epidermal necrolysis
(2001): Melde LM, *Ann Pharmacother* 35, 1388
Toxic pustuloderma
(1993): Tsuda S+, *Acta Derm Venereol* (Stockh) 73, 382
Urticaria (<1%)
(1987): Jüngst G+, *Drugs* 34 (Suppl 1), 144
(1987): Monk JP, *Drugs* 33, 346
Vasculitis (<1%)
(1996): Pipek R+, *Am J Med Sci* 311, 82
(1989): Huminer D+, *BMJ* 299, 303
(1989): Pace JL+, *BMJ* 299, 658
(1987): Jüngst G+, *Drugs* 34 (Suppl 1), 144

Nails

Nails – photo-onycholysis
(1987): Baran R+, *J Am Acad Dermatol* 17, 1012
(1986): Baran R+, *Dermatologica* 173, 185

Other

Anaphylactoid reactions
(1987): Jüngst G+, *Drugs* 34 (Suppl 1), 144
(1987): Monk JP, *Drugs* 33, 346
Death
(2001): Melde SL, *Ann Pharmacother* 35(11), 1388
Dysgeusia (1–3%)
(1995): Dark DS+, *Infections in Medicine* October, 551
Headache
Hypersensitivity
(1999): Desai C+, *J Assoc Physicians India* 47, 349
Injection-site pain (1–10%)
Myalgia (<1%)
Oral mucosal eruption
(1987): Jüngst G+, *Drugs* 34 (Suppl 1), 144
(1987): Monk JP, *Drugs* 33, 346
Paresthesias (<1%)
Parosmia
Serum sickness
Tendon rupture (<1%)
Tinnitus
Tourette's syndrome
Vaginitis (1–10%)
Xerostomia (1–3%)

OLANZAPINE

Synonym: LY170053
Trade name: Zyprexa (Lilly)
Indications: Psychotic disorders
Category: Benzodiazepine antipsychotic
Half-life: 21–54 hours

Reactions

Skin

Angioedema
(2001): Biswasl PN+, *J Psychopharmacol* 15(4), 265
Candidiasis (<1%)
Dermatitis (<1%)
Diaphoresis (>1%)
Ecchymoses (>1%)
Eczema (sic) (<1%)
Edema
Exanthems (<1%)
Facial edema (<1%)
Neuroleptic malignant syndrome
(2002): Aboraya A+, *W V Med* 98(2), 63 (with risperidone)
(2002): Malyuk R+, *Int J Geriatr Psychiatry* 17(4), 326
(2001): Biswasl PN+, *J Psychopharmacol* 15(4), 265
(2001): Philibert RA+, *Psychosomatics* 42(6), 528
Peripheral edema (2%)
(2000): Yovtcheva SP+, *Gen Hosp Psychiatry* 22, 290
Photosensitivity (<1%)
Pigmentation (<1%)
Pruritus (>1%)
Pustules
(1999): Adams BB+, *J Am Acad Dermatol* 41, 851
Rash (sic) (>1%)
(2001): Street JS+, *Int J Geriatr Psychiatry* 16(Suppl 1), S62
(1999): Green B, *Curr Med Res Opin* 15, 79 (2%)
Seborrhea (<1%)
Ulcerations (<1%)
Urticaria (<1%)
Vesiculobullous eruption (2%)
Xerosis (<1%)

Hair

Hair – alopecia (<1%)
(2000): Mercke Y+, *Ann Clin Psychiatry* 12, 35
Hair – hirsutism (<1%)

Other

Akathisia
(2001): Ishigooka J+, *Psychiatry Clin Neurosci* 55(4), 353
Aphthous stomatitis (<1%)
Dysgeusia (<1%)
Galactorrhea
(2002): Kingsbury SJ+, *Am J Psychiatry* 159(6), 1061
Gingivitis (<1%)
Glossitis (<1%)
Hyperesthesia (<1%)
Hypersensitivity
(2001): Raz A+, *Am J Med Sci* 321(2), 156
Myalgia (>1%)
(2001): Rosebraugh CJ+, *Ann Pharmacother* 35(9), 1020
Oral candidiasis (<1%)
Oral ulceration (<1%)
Parkinsonism (1–10%)
Priapism (<1%)
(2001): Compton MT+, *J Clin Psychiatry* 62(5), 363
(2001): Matthews SC+, *Psychosomatics* 42(3), 280
(2001): Songer DA+, *Am J Psychiatry* 158(12), 2087
(2000): Compton MT+, *Am J Psychiatry* 157, 659
(1999): Gordon M+, *J Clin Psychopharmacol* 19, 192
(1999): Green B, *Curr Med Res Opin* 15, 79 (0.1%)
(1998): Deirmenjian JM+, *J Clin Psychopharmacol* 18, 351
(1998): Heckers S+, *Psychosomatics* 39, 288
Rhabdomyolysis
(2001): Rosebraugh CJ+, *Ann Pharmacother* 35(9), 1020
(2000): Shuster J, *Nursing* 30(9), 87
(1999): Marcus EL+, *Ann Pharmacother* 33(6), 697
(1996): Meltzer HY+, *Neuropsychopharmacology* 15(4), 395
Sialorrhea (<1%)
(1998): Perkins DO+, *Am J Psychiatry* 155, 993
Stomatitis (<1%)
Tardive dyskinesia
(2003): Howard BG, Santa Maria, CA (from Internet)
(observation)
Tongue discoloration (<1%)

Tongue edema (<1%)
  (1997): Litt JZ, Beachwood, OH (personal case) (observation)
Tremor (1–10%)
  (2002): Tohen M+, *Arch Gen Psychiatry* 59(1), 62 (with lithium)
  (2001): Ishigooka J+, *Psychiatry Clin Neurosci* 55(4), 353
Twitching (2%)
Vaginitis (>1%)
Xerostomia (13%)
  (2002): Tohen M+, *Arch Gen Psychiatry* 59(1), 62 (with lithium)
  (1999): Green B, *Curr Med Res Opin* 15, 79 (7%)
  (1998): Bever KA+, *Am J Health Syst Pharm* 55, 1003

OLMESARTAN

Trade name: Benicar (Sankyo)
Indications: Hypertension
Category: Angiotensin II receptor antagonist
Half-life: ~13 hours
**Clinically important, potentially hazardous interactions
with:** ephedra, garlic, ginseng, lithium

Reactions

Skin
Angioedema
Facial edema
Flu-like syndrome (>1%)
Peripheral edema (>0.5)
Rash (sic) (0.5%)
Upper respiratory infection (>1%)

Other
Arthralgia (>0.5%)
Back pain (>1%)
Bone or joint pain (>0.5%)
Cough (0.7%)
Dizziness
  (2003): Gardner SF+, *Ann Pharmacother* 37(1), 99
Myalgia (>0.5%)
Pain (>0.5%)

OLOPATADINE

Trade name: Patanol (Alcon)
Indications: Pruritus due to allergic conjunctivitis
Category: Antihistamine H₁-blocker (ophthalmic)
Half-life: 3 hours

Reactions

Skin
Eyelid burning (<5%)
Eyelid edema (<5%)
Eyelid stinging (<5%)
Pruritus

Other
Dysgeusia
Headache

OLSALAZINE

Trade name: Dipentum (Celltech)
Indications: Ulcerative colitis
Category: Inflammatory bowel disease suppressant
Half-life: 0.9 hours
**Clinically important, potentially hazardous interactions
with:** azathioprine, mercaptopurine

Reactions

Skin
Acne
  (1990): Zinberg J+, *Am J Gastroenterol* 85, 562
Exanthems (0.4%)
  (1994): Shelley WB+, *Cutis* 53, 240 (observation)
  (1991): Wadworth AN+, *Drugs* 41, 647
Lupus erythematosus
  (1997): Gunnarsson I+, *Scand J Rheumatol* 26, 65
Pallor
Pruritus (1.1%)
Rash (sic) (2.3%)
  (1990): 28, 57
Urticaria (4.3%)
  (1987): Meyers S+, *Gastroenterology* 93, 1255

Other
Headache
Stomatitis (1%)
Tinnitus

OMEPRAZOLE

Trade name: Prilosec (AstraZeneca)
Other common trade names: *Antra; Audazol; Gastroloc;
Inhibitron; Logastric; Losec; Mopral; Omed; Ozoken; Parizac; Ulsen*
Indications: Duodenal ulcer, gastroesophageal reflux disease
(GERD)
Category: Antiulcer; Gastric acid secretion inhibitor; Proton
pump inhibitor
Half-life: 0.5–1 hour
**Clinically important, potentially hazardous interactions
with:** methotrexate

Reactions

Skin
Angioedema (<1%)
  (2002): Odeh M+, *Postgrad Med J* 78(916), 114 (passim)
  (1994): Bowlby HA+, *Pharmacotherapy* 14, 119
  (1992): Haeney MR, *BMJ* 305, 870
Bullous eruption
  (1995): Stenier C+, *Br J Dermatol* 133, 343
Bullous pemphigoid
  (1991): Chosidow O+, *Ann Dermatol Venereol* (French) 118, 45
  (1990): Joly P+, *Gastroenterol Clin Biol* (French) 14, 682
Burning (sic)
  (1984): Blanchi A+, *Gastroenterol Clin Biol* (French) 8, 943
Dermatitis
  (2002): Odeh M+, *Postgrad Med J* 78(916), 114 (passim)
Diaphoresis (<1%)
  (1989): Delchier JC+, *Gut* 30, 1173
Eczema (sic)

(1985): Classen M+, *Dtsch Med Wochenschr* (German) 110, 628 (scalp)

Edema (sic)
 (2000): Natsch S+, *Ann Pharmacother* MH(4), 474 (1–10%)
 (1989): Danish Omeprazole Study Group, *BMJ* 298, 645

Erythema (sic)
 (1984): Blanchi A+, *Gastroenterol Clin Biol* (French) 8, 943

Erythema multiforme (<1%)

Erythema nodosum
 (1996): Ricci RM+, *Cutis* 57, 434

Erythroderma
 (1999): Cockayne SE+, *Br J Dermatol* 141, 173

Exanthems
 (1991): Langman MSJ, *BMJ* 303, 481

Exfoliative dermatitis
 (1998): Rebuck JA+, *Pharmacotherapy* 18, 877
 (1995): Epelde-Gonzalo FD+, *Ann Pharmacother* 29, 82

Fixed eruption
 (1999): Kepekci Y+, *Int J Clin Pharmacol Ther* 37, 307 (hands)

Furunculosis
 (1998): West BC+, *Clin Infect Dis* 26, 1234

Lichen planus
 (1997): Litt JZ, Beachwood, OH (personal case) (observation)
 (1986): Pounder RE+, *Scand J Gastroenterol* 21, 108
 (1984): Sharma BK+, *Gut* 25, 957

Lichen spinulosus
 (2002): Odeh M+, *Postgrad Med J* 78(916), 114 (passim)
 (1989): Lee ML+, *Med J Aust* 150, 410

Lichenoid eruption
 (2000): Bong JL+, *BMJ* 320, 283

Lupus erythematosus
 (1994): Sivakumar K+, *Lancet* 344, 619

Pemphigus (exacerbation)
 (1992): Cox NH, *Lancet* 340, 857
 (1991): Chosidow D+, *Ann Dermatol Venereol* (French) 118, 45

Periorbital edema
 (2000): Natsch S+, *Ann Pharmacother* 34, 474

Peripheral edema (<1%)
 (2002): Chan FK+, *N Engl J Med* 347(26), 2104 (with diclofenac)
 (2001): Brunner G+, *Dig Dis Sci* 46(5), 993

Pityriasis rosea
 (1996): Buckley C, *Br J Dermatol* 135, 660

Pruritus (1–10%)
 (2000): Natsch S+, *Ann Pharmacother* 34, 474
 (1994): Bowlby HA+, *Pharmacotherapy* 14, 119
 (1989): Danish Omeprazole Study Group, *BMJ* 298, 645
 (1989): Lee ML+, *Med J Aust* 150, 410
 (1987): Bertaccini G+, *Clin Ter* (Italian) 121, 201
 (1987): Klinkenberg-Knol EC+, *Lancet* 1, 349
 (1986): Bardhan KD+, *J Clin Gastroenterol* 8, 408
 (1986): Rinetti M+, *Drugs Exp Clin Res* 12, 701

Psoriasis
 (1984): Blanchi A+, *Gastroenterol Clin Biol* (French) 8, 943

Purpura

Rash (sic) (1.5%)
 (2002): Odeh M+, *Postgrad Med J* 78(916), 114 (passim)
 (1989): Delchier JC+, *Gut* 30, 1173
 (1989): Lauritsen K+, *Aliment Pharmacol Ther* 3, 59
 (1988): Hirschowitz BI+, *Gastroenterol* 94, A188
 (1986): Bardhan KD+, *J Clin Gastroenterol* 8, 408

Stevens–Johnson syndrome (<1%)

Toxic epidermal necrolysis (<1%)
 (2002): Odeh M+, *Postgrad Med J* 78(916), 114 (passim)
 (1992): Cox NH, *Lancet* 340, 857

Urticaria (1–10%)
 (2002): Odeh M+, *Postgrad Med J* 78(916), 114 (passim)
 (1994): Bowlby HA+, *Pharmacotherapy* 14, 119
 (1994): Schneider S+, *Gastroenterol Clin Biol* (French) 18, 534

 (1993): Litt JZ, Beachwood, OH (personal case) (observation)
 (1992): Haeney MR, *BMJ* 305, 870

Vasculitis
 (2002): Odeh M+, *Postgrad Med J* 78(916), 114 (passim)

Xerosis (<1%)
 (1988): Marks IN+, *S Afr Med J* (Suppl), 54

Hair

Hair – alopecia (<1%)
 (2002): Litt JZ, Beachwood, OH (observation)
 (1999): Litt JZ, Beachwood, OH (2 personal cases) (observations)
 (1997): Borum ML+, *Am J Gastroenterol* 92, 1576
 (1994): Bowlby HA+, *Pharmacotherapy* 14, 119 (passim)

Hair – pigmentation

Other

Anaphylactoid reactions
 (2000): Natsch S+, *Ann Pharmacother* 34, 474
 (1999): Galindo PA+, *Ann Allergy Asthma Immunol* 82, 52

Dysesthesia (<1%)

Dysgeusia (1–10%)
 (1996): Markitziu A+, *Scand J Gastroenterol* 31, 624

Gynecomastia
 (2000): Hugues FC+, *Ann Med Interne (Paris)* (French) 151, 10 (passim)
 (1998): N Z Medicines Adverse Reactions Committee, (from Internet) (observation) (3 cases)
 (1995): Carvajal A+, *Am J Gastroenterol* 90, 1028
 (1995): Durand JM+, *Ann Med Interne (Paris)* (French) 146, 195
 (1994): Garcia-Rodriguez LA+, *BMJ* 308, 503
 (1994): Lindquist M+, *BMJ* 305, 451
 (1994): Pedrosa M+, *Med Clin (Barc)* (Spanish) 102, 435
 (1991): Convens C+, *Lancet* 338, 1153
 (1991): Santucci L+, *N Engl J Med* 324, 635

Headache

Myalgia (1–10%)

Oral candidiasis
 (1995): Anderson PC, *Arch Dermatol* 131, 966
 (1993): Mosimann F, *Transplantation* 56, 492
 (1992): Larner AJ+, *Gut* 33, 860

Paresthesias (<1%)
 (1986): Rinetti M+, *Drugs Exp Clin Res* 12, 701
 (1984): Blanchi A+, *Gastroenterol Clin Biol* (French) 8, 943

Tinnitus

Tremor (<1%)

Xerostomia (1–10%)
 (1985): Classen M+, *Dtsch Med Wochenschr* (German) 110, 628

ONDANSETRON

Trade name: Zofran (GSK)
Other common trade names: *Emeset; Oncoden; Zofron*
Indications: Nausea and vomiting
Category: Antiemetic; Serotonin antagonist
Half-life: 4 hours

Reactions

Skin

Angioedema
Chills (5–10%)
Exanthems
Fixed eruption
 (2000): Bernard S+, *Dermatology* 201, 184 (similar fixed eruption from acetaminophen)

(1995): Iglesias ME+, *Dermatology* 191, 270
Flushing
   (1994): Ahn MJ+, *Am J Clin Oncol* 17, 150
Pruritus (5%)
Rash (sic) (<1%)
Urticaria

Hair

Hair – alopecia

Other

Anaphylactoid reactions
   (2001): Weiss KS, *Arch Intern Med* 161(18), 2263
   (1998): Ross AK+, *Anesth Analg* 87, 779
   (1991): Milne RJ+, *Drugs* 41, 574
Dysgeusia
   (2000): Robbins L, *Headache* 11, 275
Headache
Hypersensitivity (<1%)
   (1996): Kataja V+, *Lancet* 347, 584
Injection-site burning
Injection-site erythema
Injection-site pain
Injection-site reactions (sic) (4%)
Paresthesias (2%)
Porphyria
   (1992): DeWet M+, *S Afr Med J* 82, 480
Sialopenia (1–5%)
Xerostomia (1–10%)
   (1994): Ahn MJ+, *Am J Clin Oncol* 17, 150
   (1991): Milne RJ+, *Drugs* 41, 574

ORAL CONTRACEPTIVES

Trade names: Alesse (Wyeth); Aviane (Barr); Brevicon (Watson); Demulen (Pharmacia); Desogen (Organon); Enovid (Ortho); Estrostep (Parke-Davis); Evra (Organon); Genora; Intercon; Jenest (Ortho); Levlen (Berlex); Levlite (Berlex); Levora (Watson); Lo/Ovral (Wyeth); Loestrin (Parke-Davis); Lunelle (Pharmacia); Mircette (Organon); Modicon (Ortho); Necon (Watson); NEE; Nelova; Nordette (Monarch); Norethin; Norinyl (Watson); Norlestrin (Parke-Davis); Ortho Tri-Cyclen (Ortho-McNeil); Ortho-Cept (Ortho-McNeil); Ortho-Cyclen (Ortho-McNeil); Ortho-Novum (Ortho-McNeil); Ovcon (Warner Chilcott); Ovral (Wyeth); Tri-Levlen (Berlex); Tri-Norinyl (Watson); Triphasil (Wyeth); Trivora (Watson); Yasmin (Berlex); Zovia (Watson)
Indications: Prevention of pregnancy
Clinically important, potentially hazardous interactions with: anticonvulsants, aprepitant, **cigarette smoking**, danazol, efavirenz, **licorice**, nelfinavir, rifabutin, rifampin, ritonavir, **saw palmetto**, selegiline, **St John's wort**, theophylline, troleandomycin, tuberculostatics

Reactions

Skin

Acanthosis nigricans
   (1975): Curth HO, *Arch Dermatol* 111, 1069
Acne
   (1987): Kovacs G+, *Australasian J Dermatol* 28, 86
   (1984): van der Meeren HL+, *Ned Tijdschr Geneeskd* (Dutch) 128, 1333
   (1981): Scholz C+, *Zentralbl Gynakol* (German) 103, 1158
   (1979): Harrison PV+, *BMJ* 2, 495

(1979): Marghescu S, *Ther Ggw* (German) 118, 2230
(1978): Amann W, *ZFA Stuttgart* (German) 54, 1809
(1974): Woodward RK, *Arch Dermatol* 110, 812
(1972): Gibbs WP, *Arch Dermatol* 109, 912
(1972): Kligman AM, *Arch Dermatol* 105, 298
(1972): Olson RL+, *Arch Dermatol* 105, 928
(1971): Dugois P+, *Ann Dermatol Syphiligr Paris* (French) 98, 479
(1971): Jelinek JE, *Am Fam Physician* 4, 68
(1971): Peterson WC, *Minn Med* 54, 836
(1971): Prenen M+, *Arch Belg Dermatol Syphiligr* (French) 27, 253
(1970): Jelinek JE, *Arch Dermatol* 101, 181
(1969): Chanial G+, *Bull Soc Fr Dermatol Syphiligr* (French) 76, 125
(1969): Racouchot J+, *Bull Soc Fr Dermatol Syphiligr* (French) 76, 132
Acute febrile neutrophilic dermatosis (Sweet's syndrome)
   (2002): Saez M+, *Dermatology* 204(1), 84
   (1991): Tefany FJ+, *Aust J Dermatol* 32, 55
Angioedema
   (2000): Bouillet L+, *Presse Med* (French) 29, 640
   (1990): Borradori L+, *Dermatologica* 181, 78
   (1967): Wolf RJ, *JAMA* 201, 982
Autoimmune dermatitis
   (1981): Stone J+, *Int J Dermatol* 20, 50
Bullous eruption
   (1981): Honeyman JF+, *Arch Dermatol* 117, 264
Candidiasis
   (1983): Lebherz TB+, *Clin Ther* 5, 409
   (1979): Marghescu S, *Ther Ggw* (German) 118, 1230
   (1976): Aron-Brunetiere R, *Contracept Fertil Sex* (Paris) (French) 4, 175
   (1971): Jelinek JE, *Am Fam Physician* 4, 68
   (1970): Jelinek JE, *Arch Dermatol* 101, 181
   (1969): Langer H, *Munch Med Wochenschr* (German) 111, 1748
   (1968): Walsh H+, *Amer J Obstet Gynec* 101, 991
   (1966): Catterall RD, *Lancet* 2, 830
   (1966): Porter PS+, *Arch Dermatol* 93, 402
Chloasma
   (1987): Kovacs G+, *Australasian J Dermatol* 28, 86
   (1977): Smith AG+, *J Invest Dermatol* 68, 169
   (1972): Ippen H, *Arch Dermatol Forsch* (German) 244, 500
   (1972): Ippen H+, *Hautarzt* (German) 23, 21
   (1972): Ippen H+, *Hautarzt* (German) 23, 235
   (1971): Amblard P+, *Bull Soc Fr Dermatol Syphiligr* (French) 78, 561
   (1969): Racouchot J+, *Bull Soc Fr Dermatol Syphiligr* (French) 76, 132
   (1968): Carruthers R, *Practitioner* 200, 564
   (1967): Basset H, *Bull Soc Fr Dermatol Syphiligr* (French) 74, 166
   (1967): Carruthers R, *BMJ* 3, 307
   (1967): Merklen FP+, *Bull Soc Fr Dermatol Syphiligr* (French) 74, 801
   (1967): Quamina DB, *BMJ* 2, 638
   (1966): Carruthers R, *Med J Aust* 2, 17
Cold urticaria
   (1983): Burns MR+, *Ann Intern Med* 98, 1025
Dermatitis herpetiformis
   (1972): Haim S+, *Dermatologica* 145, 199
Eczema (sic)
   (1988): Edman B, *Acta Derm Venereol* 68, 402 (palmar)
Edema
Erythema
   (1973): Delius L, *Dtsch Med Wochenschr* (German) 98, 1512 (flush-like)
Erythema multiforme
   (1973): Naess K, *Tidsskr Nor Laegeforen* (Norwegian) 93, 2498
   (1970): Savel H+, *Arch Dermatol* 101, 187
Erythema nodosum

(1981): Touboul JL+, *Nouv Presse Med* (French) 10, 712
(1980): Beaucaire G+, *Sem Hôp* (French) 56, 1426
(1980): Salvatore MA+, *Arch Dermatol* 116, 557
(1977): Bombardieri S+, *BMJ* 1, 1509
(1977): Taaffe A+, *BMJ* 2, 1353
(1976): Bernstein MZ+, *J Am Podiatry Assoc* 66, 417
(1976): Posternak F, *Rev Med Suisse Romande* (French) 96, 375
(1974): Berant N, *Harefuah* (Hebrew) 87, 19
(1974): Darlington LG, *Br J Dermatol* 90, 209
(1973): Elias PM, *Arch Dermatol* 108, 716
(1973): Kariher DH, *Obstet Gynecol* 42, 323
(1973): Stumbo WG, *J Ky Med Assoc* 71, 433
(1972): Kirby J+, *Obstet Gynecol* 40, 409
(1971): Jelinek JE, *Am Fam Physician* 4, 68
(1970): Jelinek JE, *Arch Dermatol* 101, 181
(1970): Savel H+, *Arch Dermatol* 101, 187
(1968): Baden HP+, *Arch Dermatol* 98, 634
(1967): Matz MH, *N Engl J Med* 276, 351

Exanthems
(1981): Scholz C+, *Zentralbl Gynakol* (German) 103, 1158
Fixed eruption
(1977): Coskey R, *Arch Dermatol* 113, 333
Fox-Fordyce disease
(1971): Jelinek JE, *Am Fam Physician* 4, 68
Herpes genitalis (sic)
(1981): Scholz C+, *Zentralbl Gynakol* (German) 103, 1158
Herpes gestationis
(1989): Kemper T+, *Akt Dermatol* (German) 15, 121
(1975): Kocsis M+, *Acta Derm Venereol* (Stockh) 55, 25
(1968): Morgan JK, *Br J Dermatol* 80, 456
Lichenoid eruption
(1977): Coskey R, *Arch Dermatol* 113, 333
Livedo racemosa (Sneddon's syndrome)
(1991): Berchtold B+, *Hautarzt* (German) 42, 328
Lupus erythematosus
(2001): Kakehasi AM+, *Arq Neuropsiquiatr* 59(3), 609
(1994): Hess EV+, *Curr Opin Rheumatology* 6, 474
(1994): Strom BL+, *Am J Epidemiol* 140, 632
(1994): Yung RL+, *Rheum Dis Clin North Am* 20, 61
(1993): Arden NK+, *Lupus* 2, 381
(1991): Furukawa F+, *J Dermatology* (Tokio) 18, 56
(1990): Franceschi S+, *Tumori* (Italian) 76, 439
(1990): Zanetti R+, *Int J Epidemiol* 19, 522
(1989): Beaumont V+, *Clin Physiol Biochem* 7, 263
(1989): Iskander MK+, *J Rheumatol* 16, 850
(1988): Mathur AK+, *J Rheumatology* 15, 1042
(1986): Asherson RA+, *Arthritis Rheum* 29, 1535
(1982): Jungers P+, *Arthritis Rheum* 25, 618
(1982): Jungers P+, *Nouv Presse Med* (French) 11, 3765
(1980): Condemi JJ, *Geriatrics* 35(3), 81
(1980): Garovich M+, *Arthritis Rheum* 23, 1396
(1975): Bielecka H, *Reumatologia* (Polish) 13, 223
(1974): Zurcher K+, *Dermatologica* 149, 321
(1973): Elias PM, *Arch Dermatol* 108, 716
(1972): Cordonnier V+, *J Sci Med Lille* (French) 90, 431
(1972): Dorfmann H+, *Nouv Presse Med* (French) 1, 2907
(1972): Tuffanelli DL, *Arch Dermatol* 106, 553
(1971): Chapel TA+, *Am J Obstet Gynecol* 110, 366
(1971): Cornet A+, *Ann Med Interne Paris* (French) 122, 1151
(1971): Laugier P+, *Bull Soc Fr Dermatol Syphiligr* (French) 78, 632
(1969): Rothfield NF, *Mayo Clin Proc* 44, 691
(1968): Dubois EL+, *Lancet* 2, 679
(1968): Pimstone BL, *Lancet* 1, 1153
(1968): Schleicher EM, *Lancet* 1, 821
Melanoma
(1992): Le MG+, *Cancer Causes Control* 3, 199
(1985): Bork K, *Hautarzt* (German) 36, 542
(1985): Gallagher RP+, *Br J Cancer* 52, 901
(1985): Green A+, *Med J Aust* 142, 446

(1985): Quencez E+, *Ann Dermatol Venereol* (French) 112, 341
Melasma
(1985): Lutfi RJ+, *J Clin Endocrinol Metab* 61, 28
(1981): Witkiewicz IM+, *Ned Tijdschr Geneeskd* (Dutch) 125, 609
(1970): Jelinek JE, *Arch Dermatol* 101, 181
(1968): *Northwest Med* 67, 251
(1967): Carruthers R, *BMJ* 3, 307
(1967): Resnick S, *JAMA* 199, 601
(1967): Resnick SS, *Trans N Engl Obstet Gynecol Soc* 21, 107
(1966): Resnick SS, *JAMA* 197, 25
Mucha–Habermann disease
(1973): Hollander A+, *Arch Dermatol* 107, 465
Perioral dermatitis
(1989): Ehlers G, *Hautarzt* (German) 20, 287
(1977): Kalkoff KW+, *Hautarzt* (German) 28, 74
(1975): Hornstein OP, *Internist Berl* (German) 16, 27
(1974): Buck A+, *Dtsch Med Wochenschr* (German) 99, 366
(1974): Reinken L+, *Int J Vitam Nutr Res* (German) 44, 75
(1972): Toyosi JO, *Hautarzt* (German) 23, 79
(1971): Kleine-Natrop HE, *Hautarzt* (German) 22, 508
(1969): Steigleder GK+, *Hautarzt* (German) 20, 288
Photosensitivity
(1994): Litt JZ, Beachwood, OH (personal case) (observation)
(1979): Marghescu S, *Ther Ggw* (German) 118, 1230
(1977): Roberts DT+, *Br J Dermatol* 96, 549
(1975): Horkay I+, *Arch Dermatol Res* 253, 53
(1973): Levantine A+, *Br J Dermatol* 89, 105
(1971): Elgart ML+, *Med Ann Dist Columbia* 40, 501
(1971): Jelinek JE, *Am Fam Physician* 4, 68
(1970): Jelinek JE, *Arch Dermatol* 101, 181
(1970): Mathison IW+, *Obstet Gynecol Surv* 25, 389
(1968): Erickson LR+, *JAMA* 203, 980
(1968): Oosterhuis WW, *Ned Tijdschr Geneeskd* (Dutch) 112, 2154
Pigmentation
(1981): Granstein RD+, *J Am Acad Dermatol* 5, 1
(1981): Scholz C+, *Zentralbl Gynakol* (German) 103, 1158
(1980): Hertz RS+, *J Am Dent Assoc* 100, 713
(1979): Marghescu S, *Ther Ggw* (German) 118, 1230
(1978): Harlap S, *Lancet* 2, 39
(1976): Aron-Brunetiere R, *Contracept Fertil Sex Paris* (French) 4, 175
(1972): Ippen H, *Arch Dermatol Forsch* (German) 244, 500
(1972): Leonhardi G, *Arch Dermatol Forsch* (German) 244, 495
(1971): Bazex A, *Rev Fr Gynecol Obset* (French) 66, 575
(1971): Dugois P+, *Ann Dermatol Syphiligr Paris* (French) 98, 479
(1971): Jelinek JE, *Am Fam Physician* 4, 68
(1971): Kleine-Natrop HE, *Dermatol Monatsschr* (German) 157, 549
(1970): Jelinek JE, *Arch Dermatol* 101, 181
(1969): Chanial G+, *Bull Soc Fr Dermatol Syphiligr* (French) 76, 125
(1968): Gotz H+, *Munch Med Wochenschr* (German) 110, 1913
(1968): Sotaniemi E+, *BMJ* 2, 120
(1967): No Author, *S Afr Med J* 41, 709
(1965): No Author, *BMJ* 5471, 1180
Polymorphous light eruption
(1989): Boonstra H+, *Photodermatol* 6, 55
(1988): Neumann R, *Photodermatol* 5, 40
Pruritus (<1%)
(1976): Medline A+, *Am J Gastroenterol* 65, 156
(1975): Gagnaire JC+, *Nouv Presse Med* (French) 4, 1105
(1971): Dugois P+, *Rev Fr Gynecol Obstet* (French) 66, 589
(1970): Dahl MG, *Trans St Johns Hosp Dermatol Soc* 56(1), 11
(1969): Baker H, *Br J Dermatol* 81, 946 (passim)
Psoriasis
(1981): Scholz C+, *Zentralbl Gynakol* (German) 103, 1158
Purpura
(1983): McShane PM+, *Am J Obstet Gynecol* 145, 762

(1971): Jelinek JE, *Am Fam Physician* 4, 68
(1970): Jelinek JE, *Arch Dermatol* 101, 181

Seborrhea
(1981): Scholz C+, *Zentralbl Gynakol* (German) 103, 1158 (seborrheic dermatitis)
(1979): Marghescu S, *Ther Ggw* (German) 118, 1230
(1969): Chanial G+, *Bull Soc Fr Dermatol Syphiligr* (French) 76, 125

Spider angiomas
(1970): Goldman L, *Lancet* 1, 108
(1970): Jelinek JE, *Arch Dermatol* 101, 181

Stevens–Johnson syndrome
(1972): O'Callaghan J+, *Med J Aust* 1, 695

Telangiectasia
(1983): Wilkin JK+, *J Am Acad Dermatol* 8, 468
(1971): Jelinek JE, *Am Fam Physician* 4, 68
(1970): Goldman L, *Lancet* 2, 108
(1970): Jelinek JE, *Arch Dermatol* 101, 181
(1968): Gotz H+, *Munch Med Wochenschr* (German) 110, 1913
(1964): Kopera H+, *Int J Fertil* 9, 69

Urticaria
(1981): Scholz C+, *Zentralbl Gynakol* (German) 103, 1158
(1970): Meyer-de-Schmid JJ+, *Bull Soc Fr Dermatol Syphiligr* (French) 77, 158

Varicosities

Hair

Hair – alopecia
(1989): Burke KE, *Postgrad Med* 85, 52
(1987): Kovacs G+, *Australasian J Dermatol* 28, 86
(1982): Hauser GA+, *Int J Tissue React* 4, 159
(1981): Scholz C+, *Zentralbl Gynakol* (German) 103, 1158
(1979): Marghescu S, *Ther Ggw* (German) 118, 1230
(1979): Price VH, *Int J Dermatol* 18, 95
(1978): Bergfeld W, *Cutis* 22, 190
(1978): Zaun H, *Dtsch Med Wochenschr* (German) 103, 240
(1974): Haim S, *Harefuah* (Hebrew) 86, 155
(1973): Griffiths WA, *Br J Dermatol* 88(1), 31
(1973): Levantine A+, *Br J Dermatol* 89, 549
(1973): No Author, *BMJ* 2, 499
(1973): Zaun H, *Z Geburtshilfe Perinatol* 177, 67
(1971): Dawber RP+, *BMJ* 4, 234
(1971): Prenen M+, *Arch Belg Dermatol Syphiligr* (French) 27, 253
(1970): Zaun H, *Dtsch Med Wochenschr* (German) 95, 1433
(1969): Chanial G+, *Bull Soc Fr Dermatol Syphiligr* (French) 76, 125
(1968): *BMJ* 1, 593
(1967): Cormia FE, *JAMA* 201, 635

Hair – alopecia areata
(1971): Jelinek JE, *Am Fam Physician* 4, 68
(1966): Orentreich N+, *BMJ* 5485, 483
(1965): *BMJ* 5470, 1124
(1965): Vallings R, *BMJ* 23, 1005

Hair – hirsutism
(1994): Burdova M+, *Ceska Gynekol* (Czech) 59, 62
(1987): Kovacs G+, *Australasian J Dermatol* 28, 86
(1981): Scholz C+, *Zentralbl Gynakol* (German) 103, 1158
(1979): Marghescu S, *Ther Ggw* (German) 118, 1230
(1973): Zaun H, *Hautarzt* (German) 24, 1
(1973): Zaun H, *Z Geburtshilfe Perinatol* (German) 177, 67
(1971): Dugois P+, *Ann Dermatol Syphiligr Paris* (French) 98, 479
(1971): Jelinek JE, *Am Fam Physician* 4, 68
(1971): Prenen M+, *Arch Belg Dermatol Syphiligr* (French) 27, 253
(1969): Chanial G+, *Bull Soc Fr Dermatol Syphiligr* (French) 76, 125
(1968): Gotz H+, *Munch Med Wochenschr* (German) 110, 1913
(1966): Carruthers R, *Med J Aust* 2, 17

Nails

Nails – onycholysis
(1976): Byrne JPH+, *Postgrad Med J* 52, 535

Other

Acute intermittent porphyria
(1979): Brinkmann OH+, *ZFA Stuttgart* (German) 55, 1227
(1978): Gerlis LS, *J Int Med Res* 6, 255
(1977): Tasic D+, *Med Pregl* (Serbo-Croatian) 30, 577
(1975): Schley G+, *Verh Dtsch Ges Inn Med* (German) 81, 1061
(1971): Contro L+, *Minerva Med* (Italian) 62, 2238

Application-site reactions
(2002): Sibai BM+, *Fertil Steril* 77(2 Suppl 2), S19 (patch) (92%)

Depression
(2001): Freeman MP, *JAMA* 286(6), 671

Galactorrhea
(1969): Friedman S+, *JAMA* 210, 1888

Gingival hyperplasia
(1967): Lindhe J+, *J Periodont Res* 2, 1
(1962): Sumner CF+, *J Periodont* 33, 344

Oral mucosal pigmentation
(1980): Hertz RS+, *J Am Dent Assoc* 100, 713 (gingival)

Porphyria cutanea prematura
(1977): Doss M, *Dtsch Med Wochenschr* (German) 102, 875
(1977): Leonhardi G+, *Dtsch Med Wochenschr* (German) 102, 160

Porphyria cutanea tarda
(2001): Emri G+, *Orv Hetil* 142(47), 2635
(1992): McKenna KE+, *Br J Dermatol* 127, 401
(1983): Doss M, *Dtsch Med Wochenschr* (German) 108, 1857
(1983): Zaumseil RP+, *Zentralbl Gynakol* (German) 105, 527
(1982): Zaumseil RP+, *Z Gesamte In Med* (German) 37, 703
(1981): Fiedler H+, *Dermatol Monatsschr* (German) 167, 481
(1979): Grossman ME+, *Am J Med* 67, 277
(1979): Willerson D+, *Ann Ophthalmol* 11, 409
(1977): Roberts DT+, *Br J Dermatol* 96, 549
(1976): Aron-Brunetiere R, *Contracept Fertil Sex Paris* (French) 4, 175
(1976): Byrne JPH+, *Postgrad Med J* 52, 536
(1976): Curtis P, *Br J Clin Pract* 30, 47
(1975): Austad WI+, *N Z Med J* 81, 8
(1974): Behm AR+, *Can Med Assoc J* 110, 1052
(1974): Le Reun M+, *Concours Med* (French) 96, 2697
(1974): Nuss A+, *Z Haut* (German) 49, 273
(1974): Vosmik F+, *Cesk Dermatol* (Czech) 49, 298
(1973): Constantinidis A+, *Minerva Ginecol* (Italian) 25, 192
(1973): Gajdos A+, *Nouv Presse Med* (French) 2, 1131
(1973): Gutzwiller P, *Dermatologia* (German) 146, 342
(1973): Palma-Carlos AG+, *Nouv Presse Med* (French) 1, 1996
(1973): Ruszczak Z+, *Wiad Lek* (Polish) 26, 2177
(1972): No Author, *BMJ* 3, 603
(1971): Goldswain PR+, *S Afr Med J* 25, 111
(1971): Jelinek JE, *Am Fam Physician* 4, 68
(1970): Roenigk HH+, *Arch Dermatol* 102, 260
(1969): Degos R+, *Ann Dermatol Syphiligr Paris* (French) 96, 5
(1967): Huber FB, *Schweiz Med Wochenschr* (German) 97, 1498

Porphyria variegata
(1975): Fowler CJ+, *BMJ* 1, 663
(1972): McKenzie AW+, *Br J Dermatol* 86, 453

Thrombophlebitis
(1967): Merklen FP+, *Bull Soc Fr Dermatol Syphiligr* (French) 74, 801

Tremor
(2001): Chetty M+, *Ther Drug Monit* 23(5), 556 (with chlorpromazine)

ORLISTAT

Trade name: Xenical (Roche)
Indications: Obesity, weight reduction
Category: Lipase inhibitor
Half-life: 1–2 hours
Clinically important, potentially hazardous interactions with: cyclosporine

Reactions

Skin
Dermatitis (sic)
Nodules
Rash (sic) (4.3%)
Xerosis

Other
Gingivitis (4.1%)
Headache
Myalgia (4.2%)
Tendinitis
Tooth disorder (sic) (4.3%)
Vaginitis (3.8%)

ORPHENADRINE

Trade names: Banflex (Forest); Norflex (3M)
Other common trade names: *Biorfen; Biorphen; Disipal; Distalene; Flexojet; Flexon; Myolin; Norgesic; Opheryl; Orfenace; Prolongatum*
Indications: Painful musculoskeletal conditions
Category: Skeletal muscle relaxant
Half-life: 14 hours

Reactions

Skin
Exanthems
Fixed eruption
  (1998): Mahboob A+, *Int J Dermatol* 37, 833
Flushing (1–10%)
Pigmentary changes (sic)
  (1978): Rebhun J, *Ann Allergy* 40, 44
Pruritus
Rash (sic) (1–10%)
Urticaria

Other
Anaphylactoid reactions
Embolia cutis medicamentosa (Nicolau syndrome)
  (1976): Brachtel R, *Med Klin* (German) 71, 504
Headache
Hypersensitivity
Paresthesias
Xerostomia

OSELTAMIVIR

Trade name: Tamiflu (Roche)
Indications: Influenza infection
Category: Antiviral (neuraminidase inhibitor)
Half-life: 6–10 hours

Reactions

Skin
Upper respiratory infection
  (2001): McNicholl IR+, *Ann Pharmacother* 35(1), 57

Other
Cough
  (2002): Bowles SK+, *J Am Geriatr Soc* 50(4), 608
Myalgia
  (2001): McNicholl IR+, *Ann Pharmacother* 35(1), 57

OXACILLIN

Trade name: Oxacillin
Other common trade names: *Bactocill; Bristopen; Prostaphlin; Stapenor*
Indications: Various infections caused by susceptible organisms
Category: Penicillinase-resistant penicillin
Half-life: 23–60 minutes
Clinically important, potentially hazardous interactions with: anticoagulants, cyclosporine, demeclocycline, doxycycline, methotrexate, minocycline, oxytetracycline, tetracycline

Reactions

Skin
Angioedema
Bullous eruption
  (1974): Hadida E+, *Bull Soc Fr Dermatol Syphiligr* (French) 81, 87
Ecchymoses
Erythema multiforme
Erythema nodosum
Exanthems
  (1978): Bruevich TS+, *Vestn Dermatol Venerol* (Russian) March, 74
  (1974): Spitzy KH, *Acta Med Austriaca* (German) 2, 46
Exfoliative dermatitis
Hematomas
Jarisch–Herxheimer reaction
Necrosis
  (1980): Tilden SJ+, *Am J Dis Child* 134, 1046
Pruritus
  (1998): Siegfried EC+, *J Am Acad Dermatol* 39, 797 (passim)
Rash (sic) (<1%)
  (2002): Maraqa NF+, *Clin Infect Dis* 34(1), 50 (22%)
Stevens–Johnson syndrome
  (1982): Sukovatykh TN+, *Pediatriia* (Russian) May, 76
Toxic epidermal necrolysis
Urticaria
  (1998): Siegfried EC+, *J Am Acad Dermatol* 39, 797 (passim)
Vasculitis
  (2001): Koutkia P+, *Diagn Microbiol Infect Dis* 46(5), 993

Other
Anaphylactoid reactions (0.04%)
  (1998): Siegfried EC+, *J Am Acad Dermatol* 39, 797 (passim)

Black tongue
Dysgeusia
Glossitis
Glossodynia
Hypersensitivity
Injection-site pain
Oral candidiasis
Phlebitis
Serum sickness (<1%)
Stomatitis
Stomatodynia
Thrombophlebitis
Tongue furry
Vaginitis
Xerostomia

OXALIPLATIN

Trade name: Eloxatin (Sanofi-Synthelabo)
Other common trade name: *Heloxatin*
Indications: Metastatic carcinoma of the colon or rectum (in combination with fluorouracil)
Category: Antineoplastic; Third-generation platinum agent
Half-life: 391 hours

Reactions

Skin

Allergic reactions (sic) (3%)
Angioedema
Diaphoresis (2–5%)
Edema (10%)
Erythema
  (2003): Thomas RR+, *Cancer* 97(9), 2301
Exanthems (2–5%)
Flushing (3%)
Hand-foot syndrome (1%)
Hot flashes (2–5%)
Peripheral edema (5%)
Pruritus (2–5%)
  (2003): Thomas RR+, *Cancer* 97(9), 2301
Purpura (2–5%)
Radiation recall
  (2001): Camidge R, *Clin Oncol* 13(3), 236
  (2001): Chan RT+, *Clin Oncol* 13(1), 55
Rash (sic) (5%)
Upper respiratory infection (7%)
Urticaria
  (2000): Petit-Laurent F+, *Gastroenterol Clin Biol* 24(8), 851
Xerosis (2–5%)

Hair

Hair – alopecia (3%)

Other

Anaphylactoid reactions
  (2001): Alliot C+, *Clin Oncol (R* 13(3), 236
  (2001): Arotcarena R+, *Gastroenterol Clin Biol* 25(2), 206
  (1999): Larzilliere I+, *Am J Gastroenterol* 94(11), 3387
  (1999): Medioni J+, *Ann Oncol* 10(5), 610
  (1998): Tournigand C+, *Eur J Cancer* 34(8), 1297
Angioedema
Anxiety (2–5%)
Arthralgia (7%)

Asthenia
  (2003): Mancuso A+, *Anticancer Res* 23(2C), 1917
Back pain (11%)
Conjunctivitis (2–5%)
Cough (11%)
Death
Depression (2–5%)
Dizziness (7%)
Dysesthesia (often cold-induced or cold-exacerbated)
  (2002): Gamelin E+, *Semin Oncol* 29(5 Suppl), 21
  (2002): Wilson RH+, *J Clin Oncol* 20(7), 1767
  (2001): Bugat R, *Bull Cancer* 88, S45
  (2001): Gent P+, *Int J Palliat Nurs* 7(7), 354
  (1998): Diaz-Rubio E+, *Ann Oncol* 9(1), 105
  (1998): Misset JL, *Br J Cancer* 77, 4 (distal & perioral)
Dysgeusia (5%)
Fatigue (61%)
  (1998): Gerard B+, *Anticancer Drugs* 9(4), 301 (also taking 5FU)
Fever (25%)
  (2003): Thomas RR+, *Cancer* 97(9), 2301
  (2000): Ulrich-Pur H+, *Oncology* 59(3), 187
Gingivitis (2–5%)
Hiccups (2%)
Hyperesthesia
Hypersensitivity
  (2003): Thomas RR+, *Cancer* 97(9), 2301
  (2002): Meyer L+, *J Clin Oncol* 20(4), 1146
  (2002): Wilson RH+, *J Clin Oncol* 20(7), 1767 (to cold)
Injection-site allergy (sic)
  (2003): Fracasso PM+, *Gynecol Oncol* 90(1), 177 (3 cases)
Injection-site edema
Injection-site erythema
Injection-site extravasation
Injection-site necrosis
Injection-site pain
  (2002): Wilson RH+, *J Clin Oncol* 20(7), 1767
Lacrimation
Mucositis (2%)
Myalgia (2–5%)
Neuropathy (48%)
Ocular irritation
  (2002): Wilson RH+, *J Clin Oncol* 20(7), 1767
Pain (14%)
  (2003): Mancuso A+, *Anticancer Res* 23(2C), 1917
Paresthesias
  (2002): Gamelin E+, *Semin Oncol* 29(5), 21
  (2002): Wilson RH+, *J Clin Oncol* 20(7), 1767
  (1998): Gerard B+, *Anticancer Drugs* 9(4), 301 (also taking 5FU)
  (1990): Extra JM+, *Cancer Chemother Pharmacol* 25(4), 299
Pharyngitis (2%)
Pneumonia (2–5%)
Rhinitis (6%)
Rigors (9%)
Stomatitis (14%)
  (2000): Haller DG, *Oncology* 14(12), 15
Xerostomia (2–5%)

OXAPROZIN

Trade name: Daypro (Pharmacia)
Other common trade names: *Deflam; Duraprox*
Indications: Arthritis
Category: Nonsteroidal anti-inflammatory (NSAID)
Half-life: 42–50 hours
Clinically important, potentially hazardous interactions with: methotrexate

Reactions

Skin
Angioedema (<1%)
Diaphoresis (<1%)
Ecchymoses (<1%)
Edema (<1%)
Erythema
Erythema multiforme (<1%)
 (1986): Todd PA+, *Drugs* 32, 291
Exanthems
 (1995): Litt JZ, Beachwood, OH (personal case) (observation)
 (1994): Litt JZ, Beachwood, OH (personal case) (observation)
 (1994): Shelley WB+, *Cutis* 54, 72 (eczematous eruption) (observation)
 (1983): Hubsher JA+, *Clin Pharmacol Ther* 33, 267
Exfoliative dermatitis (<1%)
Fixed eruption
 (1999): Blumenthal HL, Beachwood, OH (personal case) (observation)
Linear IgA dermatosis
 (1999): Abate KL+, *Arch Dermatol* 135, 81–86 (off-center fold)
Photosensitivity (<1%)
Phototoxicity
 (1995): Shelley WB+, *Cutis* 55, 143 (observation)
 (1986): Todd PA+, *Drugs* 32, 291
Pruritus (1–10%)
 (1994): Shelley WB+, *Cutis* 53, 284 (observation)
Purpura
Rash (sic) (>10%)
 (1983): Kahn SB+, *J Clin Pharmacol* 23, 139
 (1978): Jamar R+, *Curr Med Res Op* 5, 433
Stevens–Johnson syndrome (<1%)
 (1998): Bell MJ+, *J Rheumatol* 25, 2027
Toxic epidermal necrolysis
 (1999): Carucci JA+, *Int J Dermatol* 38, 233
 (1999): Egan CA+, *J Am Acad Dermatol* 40, 458
 (1998): Paul CD+, *J Burn Care Rehabil* 19, 321 (fatal)
Urticaria (<1%)
 (1997): Hicks A, Houston, TX (from Internet) (observation)
  (Note: Person is not a physician)
Vasculitis
 (1999): Reed BR, Denver, CO (from Internet) (observation)

Hair
Hair – alopecia

Other
Anaphylactoid reactions (<1%)
Death
Dysgeusia
Headache
Pseudolymphoma
 (2001): Werth V, *Dermatology Times* 18
Pseudoporphyria
 (1999): Al-Khenaizan S+, *J Cutan Med Surg* 3, 162

 (1996): Ingrish G+, *Arch Dermatol* 132, 1519
 (1996): Jaffe PG, Columbia, SC (from Internet) (observation)
Serum sickness (<1%)
Stomatitis (<1%)
Tinnitus

OXAZEPAM

Trade name: Serax (Faulding)
Other common trade names: *Adumbran; Apo-Oxazepam; Azutranquil; Durazepam; Murelax; Novoxapam; Oxpam; Praxiten; Serax; Serepax; Zapex*
Indications: Anxiety, depression
Category: Anticonvulsant; Benzodiazepine sedative-hypnotic
Half-life: 3–6 hours
Clinically important, potentially hazardous interactions with: amprenavir, chlorpheniramine, clarithromycin, efavirenz, esomeprazole, imatinib, nelfinavir

Reactions

Skin
Dermatitis (sic) (1–10%)
Diaphoresis (>10%)
Edema
Erythema multiforme
 (1986): McAlpine C, *BMJ* 293, 510
Exanthems
Fixed eruption
 (1996): Krischer J, *Arch Dermatol* 132, 718
Pruritus
Purpura
Rash (sic) (>10%)
Toxic epidermal necrolysis
 (2001): van der Meer JB+, *Clin Exp Dermatol* 26(8), 654
Urticaria

Other
Headache
Paresthesias
Sialopenia (>10%)
Sialorrhea (1–10%)
Tongue furry
Tremor
Xerostomia (>10%)

OXCARBAZEPINE

Synonym: GP 47680
Trade name: Trileptal (Novartis)
Indications: Partial epileptic seizures
Category: Anticonvulsant
Half-life: 1–2.5 hours

Reactions

Skin
Acne
Allergic reactions (sic) (2%)
 (1994): Dam M, *Epilepsia* 35, S23
 (1993): Beran RG, *Epilepsia* 34, 163
Angioedema

Dermatitis
Diaphoresis (3%)
Eczema
Edema (2%)
Erythema multiforme
Exanthems
  (1999): Ruble R+, *CNS Drugs* 12, 215
Facial rash (sic)
Folliculitis
Genital pruritus
Hot flashes (2%)
Infections (sic) (2%)
Lupus erythematosus
Photosensitivity
Purpura (2%)
Rash (sic) (4%)
  (1993): Friis ML+, *Acta Neurol Scand* 84, 224 (6%)
Sensitivity (sic)
  (1991): Watts D+, *Neurol Neurosurg Psychiatry* 54, 376
Stevens–Johnson syndrome
Toxic epidermal necrolysis
Vitiligo

Hair

Hair – alopecia

Other

Dysgeusia (5%)
Gingival hyperplasia
Headache
Hyperesthesia (3%)
Hypersensitivity
  (2001): No authors, *Prescrire Int* 10(56), 170
Priapism
Stomatitis
Toothache (2%)
Tremor (4–6%)
Ulcerative stomatitis
Vaginitis (2%)
Xerostomia (3%)

OXYBUTYNIN

Trade name: Ditropan (Ortho-McNeil)
Other common trade names: *Albert (Oxybutynin); Cystrin; Dridase; Novitropan; Oxyban; Tropax*
Indications: Neurogenic bladder, urinary incontinence
Category: Urinary antispasmodic
Half-life: 1–2.3 hours
Clinically important, potentially hazardous interactions with: anticholinergics, arbutamine

Reactions

Skin

Allergic reactions (sic) (<1%)
  (1993): Jonville AP+, *Arch Fr Pediatr* (French) 50, 27
  (1992): Jonville AP+, *Therapie* (French) 47, 389
Erythema multiforme
  (1992): Jonville AP+, *Therapie* (French) 47, 389
Flushing
Hot flashes (1–10%)
Hypohidrosis (>10%)
Pruritus

  (2001): Ho C, *Issues Emerg Health Technol* 24, 1 (18%)
Rash (sic) (1–10%)
Urticaria
Xerosis
  (1998): Arango Toro O+, *Actas Urol Esp* (Spanish) 22, 124 (6%)

Other

Anhidrosis
Headache
Sialopenia
  (1998): Arango Toro O+, *Actas Urol Esp* (Spanish) 22, 124 (42%)
  (1995): Loesche WJ+, *J Am Geriatr Soc* 43, 401
Xerostomia (>10%)
  (2002): Youdim K+, *Urology* 59(3), 428
  (2001): Crandall C, *J Womens Health Gend Based Med* 10(8), 735
  (2001): Davila GW+, *J Urol* 166(1), 140 (67–94%)
  (2001): Harvey MA+, *Am J Obstet Gynecol* 185, 56
  (2001): Ho C, *Issues Emerg Health Technol* 24, 1
  (2000): Versi E+, *Obstet Gynecol* 95, 718
  (1995): Loesche WJ+, *J Am Geriatr Soc* 43, 401

OXYCODONE

Trade names: Endocodone; OxyContin (Purdue); OxyIR (Purdue); Percodan (Endo); Percolone (Endo); Percoset (Endo); Roxicodone (Elan); Tylox (Ortho-McNeil)
Other common trade name: *Supeudol*
Indications: Pain
Category: Narcotic analgesic
Half-life: 4.6 hours
Clinically important, potentially hazardous interactions with: cimetidine

Oxycodone is often combined with acetaminophen (Percoset, Roxicet, Tylox) or aspirin (Percodan, Roxiprin)

Reactions

Skin

Diaphoresis
Pruritus
  (1999): Hale ME+, *Clin J Pain* 15, 179
  (1999): Salzman RT+, *J Pain Symptom Manage* 18, 271
Rash (sic) (<1%)
Urticaria (<1%)

Other

Headache
Injection-site pain (1–10%)
Xerostomia (1–10%)

OXYTETRACYCLINE

Trade name: Terramycin (Pfizer)
Other common trade names: *Aknin; Cotet; Macocyn; Oxacycle; Oxitraklin; Oxy; Rorap; Terramycine; Uri-Tet*
Indications: Various infections caused by susceptible organisms
Category: Antiprotozoal; Tetracycline antibiotic
Half-life: 6–10 hours
Clinically important, potentially hazardous interactions with: amoxicillin, ampicillin, antacids, bacampicillin, calcium, carbenicillin, cloxacillin, digoxin, methotrexate, methoxyflurane, mezlocillin, nafcillin, oxacillin, penicillins, piperacillin, ticarcillin

Reactions

Skin

Angioedema
Dermatitis
  (1976): Moller H, *Contact Dermatitis* 2, 289
  (1974): Bojs G+, *Berufsdermatosen* (German) 22, 202
  (1969): Walczynski Z+, *Wiad Lek* (Polish) 22, 929
Exanthems
Exfoliative dermatitis (<1%)
Fixed eruption
  (1985): Gomez B+, *Allergol Immunopathol Madr* (Spanish) 13, 87
  (1981): Shukla SR, *Dermatologica* 163, 160
  (1975): Giminez-Garcia RM+, *N Engl J Med* 292, 819
  (1970): Delaney TJ, *Br J Dermatol* 83, 357
  (1952): Dougherty JW, *Arch Dermatol* 65, 485
Lupus erythematosus

Photosensitivity (1–10%)
  (1987): Santucci B+, *G Ital Dermatol Venereol* (Italian) 122, IL-LII
  (1982): Hawk JL, *Clin Exp Dermatol* 7, 341
  (1977): Ramsay CA, *Clin Exp Dermatol* 2, 255
  (1963): Tromovitch TA+, *Ann Intern Med* 58, 529 (1–5%)
Pigmentation
Pruritus (<1%)
Purpura
  (1975): Kounis NG, *JAMA* 231, 734
Pustules
  (1971): Stevanovic DN, *Br J Dermatol* 85, 134
Sensitivity (sic)
  (1997): Rudzki E+, *Contact Dermatitis* 37, 136
Urticaria
Vasculitis

Nails

Nails – pigmentation (<1%)

Other

Anaphylactoid reactions (<1%)
Black tongue
  (1954): No Author, *Lancet* 2, 179
Hypersensitivity (<1%)
Oral mucosal lesions
  (1971): Merdi T+, *Czas Stomatol* (Polish) 24, 1309
Paresthesias (<1%)
Porphyria cutanea tarda
  (1982): Hawk JL, *Clin Exp Dermatol* 7, 341
Pseudotumor cerebri (<1%)
Thrombophlebitis (<1%)
Tooth discoloration (>10%) (in children)

PACLITAXEL

Trade name: Taxol (Bristol-Myers Squibb)
Other common trade name: *Paxene*
Indications: Metastatic carcinoma of the ovary
Category: Antineoplastic
Half-life: 5–17 hours

Reactions

Skin

Acral erythema
(1996): de Argila D+, *Dermatology* 192, 377
(1995): Zimmerman GC+, *Arch Dermatol* 131, 202
Allergic reactions (sic)
(2002): Cantu MG+, *J Clin Oncol* 20(5), 1232 (15%)
(2002): Feher O+, *Head Neck* 24(3), 228
(2001): Ansell SM+, *Cancer* 91(8), 1543
(2001): Hurwitz CA+, *J Pediatr Hematol Oncol* 23(5), 277
(2001): Sakai H+, *Cancer Chemother Pharmacol* 48(6), 499 (with cisplatin)
(1995): Link CJ+, *Invest New Drugs* 13, 261
Angioedema
(1990): Weiss RB+, *J Clin Oncol* 8, 1263
Edema (21%)
(2003): Kupfer I+, *J Am Acad Dermatol* 48(2), 279
Erythema
(2003): Kupfer I+, *J Am Acad Dermatol* 48(2), 279
(2001): Robinson JB+, *Gynecol Oncol* 82(3), 550
(1995): Berghmans T+, *Support Care Cancer* 3, 203
(1995): Zimmerman GC+, *Arch Dermatol* 131, 202
Erythrodysesthesia
(1994): Zimmerman GC+, *J Natl Cancer Inst* 86, 557
(1993): Vukelja SJ+, *J Natl Cancer Inst* 85, 1423
Exanthems (<1%)
(1990): Weiss RB+, *J Clin Oncol* 8, 1263
Fixed eruption
(2000): Baykal C+, *Eur J Gynaecol Oncol* 21, 190
(1996): Young PC+, *J Am Acad Dermatol* 34, 313 (bullous)
Flushing (28%)
(2001): Robinson JB+, *Gynecol Oncol* 82(3), 550
(1990): Weiss RB+, *J Clin Oncol* 8, 1263
Infections (sic) (>10%)
(2002): Souglakos J+, *Cancer* 95(6), 1326 (3%)
(2001): Fidias P+, *Clin Cancer Res* 7(12), 3942 (8.8%)
Photosensitivity
(2000): Mermershtain W+, *Ann Oncol* 11(suppl 4), 28 (with trastuzumab) (3 cases)
Pigmentation
(2003): Kupfer I+, *J Am Acad Dermatol* 48(2), 279
Pruritus (<1%)
(2001): Robinson JB+, *Gynecol Oncol* 82(3), 550
(1995): Freilich RJ+, *J Natl Cancer Inst* 87, 933
(1990): Weiss RB+, *J Clin Oncol* 8, 1263
Purpura
Pustules
(1997): Weinberg JM+, *Int J Dermatol* 36, 559
Radiation recall (<1%)
(1996): McCarty MJ+, *Med Pediatr Oncol* 27, 185
(1995): Phillips KA+, *J Clin Oncol* 13, 305
(1995): Schweitzer VG+, *Cancer* 76, 1069
(1994): Shenkier T+, *J Clin Oncol* 12, 439
(1993): Raghavan VT+, *Lancet* 341, 1354
Rash (sic) (12%)
Scleroderma
(2003): Kupfer I+, *J Am Acad Dermatol* 48(2), 279
(2002): Lauchli S+, *Br J Dermatol* 147(3), 619

Urticaria
(1990): Weiss RB+, *J Clin Oncol* 8, 1263

Hair

Hair – alopecia (87 – 100%)
(2002): *Lancet* 360(9332), 505 (with carboplatin)
(2002): Iwamoto S+, *Gan To Kagaku Ryoho* 29(6), 917
(2002): Sehouli J+, *Gynecol Oncol* 85(2), 321 (with carboplatin)
(2001): Rohl J+, *Gynecol Oncol* 81(2), 201
(2001): Sakai H+, *Cancer Chemother Pharmacol* 48(6), 499 (with cisplatin)
(2000): Oettle H+, *Anticancer Drugs* 11(8), 635
(1997): Jiang Z+, *Chung Hua Chung Liu Tsa Chih* (Chinese) 19, 445
(1995): Lemenager M+, *Lancet* 346, 371
(1990): McGuire WP+, *Ann Intern Med* 111, 273 (total) (100%) (between days 14 and 21; reversible)
Hair – alopecia areata
(2003): Motl SE+, *Pharmacotherapy* 23(1), 104 (recurrent) (with caboplatin)

Nails

Nails – changes (sic)
(1998): Luftner D+, *Ann Oncol* 9, 1139
Nails – onycholysis
(2003): Mackay-Wiggan J+, *Cutis* 71(3), 229
(2000): Almagro M+, *Eur J Dermatol* 10(2), 146 (2 cases)
(2000): Hussain S+, *Cancer* 88, 2367 (5 cases)
(1999): Flory SM+, *Ann Pharmacother* 33, 584
(1995): Link CJ+, *Invest New Drugs* 13, 261 (2 cases)
Nails – pigmentation (2%)
(1998): Auvinet M+, *Rev Med Interne* (French) 19, 353
Nails – thickening
(1995): Link CJ+, *Invest New Drugs* 13, 261 (2 cases)
Nails – transverse white bands
(1995): Link CJ+, *Invest New Drugs* 13, 261 (2 cases)

Other

Anaphylactoid reactions
(1999): Smith ME, *Oncol Nurs Forum* 26, 516
(1997): Ciesielski-Carlucci C+, *Am J Clin Oncol* 20(4), 373 (with cisplatin)
(1995): Rowinsky EK+, *N Engl J* 332(15), 1004
Arthralgia
(2003): Garrison JA+, *Oncology* (Huntingt) 17(2), 271
(2002): Hasegawa K+, *Gan To Kagaku Ryoho* 29(4), 569
(2001): Ansell SM+, *Cancer* 91(8), 1543
(2001): Ishikawa H+, *Int J Clin Oncol* 6(3), 128
Death
(2001): Fidias P+, *Clin Cancer Res* 7(12), 3942
(2001): Hurwitz CA+, *J Pediatr Hematol Oncol* 23(5), 277
Hypersensitivity (41%)
(2002): Denman JP+, *J Clin Oncol* 20(11), 2760
(2002): Kwon JS+, *Gynecol Oncol* 84(3), 420
(2002): Lehoczky O+, *Orv Hetil* 143(38), 2189
(2002): Myers JS, *Clin J Oncol Nurs* 6(3), 177
(2001): Kintzel PE, *Ann Pharmacother* 35(9), 1114
(2001): Koppler H+, *Onkologie* 24(3), 283
(2001): Robinson JB+, *Gynecol Oncol* 82(3), 550 (with carboplatin)
(2001): Szebeni J+, *Int Immunopharmacol* 1(4), 721
(2001): Yamada Y+, *Ann Oncol* 12(8), 1133 (15%)
(1998): Borovik R+, *Harefuah* (Hebrew) 134, 605
(1998): Lokich J+, *Ann Oncol* 9, 573
(1998): Tsavaris NB+, *Cancer Chemother Pharmacol* 42, 509
(1995): Del Priore G+, *Gynecol Oncol* 56, 316
(1994): Uziely B+, *Ann Oncol* 5, 474
(1993): Peereboom DM+, *J Clin Oncol* 11, 885
Injection-site cellulitis (>10%)
Injection-site extravasation (>10%)

(1997): Herrington JD+, *Pharmacotherapy* 17, 163
(1995): Berghmans T+, *Support Care Cancer* 3, 203
(1995): Raymond E+, *Rev Med Interne* (French) 16, 141
Injection-site pain (>10%)
Injection-site reactions (sic) (13%)
Mucocutaneous toxicity (sic)
  (1996): Payne JY+, *South Med J* 89, 542
Mucositis (>10%)
  (2002): Feher O+, *Head Neck* 24(3), 228
Myalgia (60%)
  (2003): Garrison JA+, *Oncology* (Huntingt) 17(2), 271
  (2002): Cantu MG+, *J Clin Oncol* 20(5), 1232 (19%)
  (2002): Hasegawa K+, *Gan To Kagaku Ryoho* 29(4), 569
  (2001): Ishikawa H+, *Int J Clin Oncol* 6(3), 128
  (1999): Markman M+, *Gynecol Oncol* 72, 100
  (1998): Savarese D+, *J Clin Oncol* 16, 3918
  (1997): Jiang Z+, *Chung Hua Chung Liu Tsa Chih* (Chinese)
    19, 445
Oral mucosal lesions
  (1990): McGuire WP+, *Ann Intern Med* 111, 273 (3–8%)
Paresthesias (>10%)
Phantom limb pain
  (2000): Khattab J+, *Mayo Clin Proc* 75, 740
Recall at site of prior extravasation
  (1996): du Bois A+, *Gynecol Oncol* 60, 94
  (1994): Meehan JL+, *J Natl Cancer Inst* 86, 1250
Stomatitis (39%)
  (2001): Miglietta L+, *Oncology* 60(2), 116

PALIVIZUMAB

Trade name: Synagis (MedImmune)
Indications: Prophylaxis of serious lower respiratory tract disease caused by RSV in pediatric patients
Category: Humanized monoclonal antibody
Half-life: 18 days

Reactions

Skin
Eczema (sic) (>1%)
Erythema
Flu-like syndrome (>1%)
Fungal dermatitis (sic) (>1%)
Infections (sic)
Rash (sic) (25.6%)
Seborrhea (>1%)

Other
Anaphylactoid reactions
  (2002): Medscape Medical News
Injection-site bruising
  (1999): Scott LJ+, *Drugs* 58, 305 (1–3%)
Injection-site edema
  (1999): Scott LJ+, *Drugs* 58, 305 (1–3%)
Injection-site erythema
  (1999): Scott LJ+, *Drugs* 58, 305 (1–3%)
  (1998): *Pediatrics* 102, 531
Injection-site induration
  (1999): Scott LJ+, *Drugs* 58, 305 (1–3%)
Injection-site pain (8.5%)
  (1999): Scott LJ+, *Drugs* 58, 305 (1–3%)
Injection-site reactions (sic)
  (1999): Sandritter T, *J Pediatr Health Care* 13, 191
Oral candidiasis (>1%)

PAMIDRONATE

Trade name: Aredia (Novartis)
Indications: Hypercalcemia, Paget's disease
Category: Antidote (hypercalcemia)
Half-life: 1.6 hours

Reactions

Skin
Angioedema (<1%)
Candidiasis
Edema (1%)
Exanthems
  (1984): Mantalen CA+, *BMJ* 288, 828 (1.2%)
Flu-like syndrome
  (2001): Body JJ, *Semin Oncol* 28(4 Suppl 11), 49
Rash (sic) (<1%)

Other
Conjunctivitis
  (2003): Frauenfelder FW+, *Am J Opthalmol* 135, 219
  (2003): Frauenfelder FW+, *N Engl J Med* 348, 1187
  (1994): Macarol V+, *Am J Ophthalmol* 118(2), 220
Dysgeusia (<1%)
Headache
Hypersensitivity (<1%)
Injection-site reactions (4%)
  (2001): Body JJ, *Semin Oncol* 28(4 Suppl 11), 49
Myalgia (1%)
Ocular irritation
  (2003): Frauenfelder FW+, *N Engl J Med* 348, 1187
Stomatitis (1%)

PANCURONIUM

Trade name: Pavulon (Organon)
Other common trade names: *Alpax; Bromurex; Curon-B; Panconium; Panslan*
Indications: Anesthesia adjunct, neuromuscular blockade, muscle relaxant
Category: Nondepolarizing neuromuscular blockade
Half-life: 89–161 minutes
Clinically important, potentially hazardous interactions with: aminoglycosides, cyclopropane, enflurane, gentamicin, halothane, isoflurane, kanamycin, methoxyflurane, neomycin, piperacillin, streptomycin, tobramycin

Reactions

Skin
Burning
Edema
Erythema
  (1989): Patriarca G+, *Br J Anaesth* 62(2), 210
Flushing
Pruritus
Rash (sic)

Other
Anaphylactoid reactions
  (1998): Sanchez-Guerrero IM+, *Eur J Anaesthesiol* 15(5), 613
  (1990): Moneret-Vautrin DA+, *Br J Anaesth* 64(6), 743
  (1989): Patriarca G+, *Br J Anaesth* 62(2), 210

(1986): Bonnet MC+, *Cah Anesthesiol* 34(3), 253
(1985): Conil C+, *Ann Fr Anesth Reanim* 4(2), 241
(1985): Galletly DC+, *Anaesthesia* 40(4), 329
(1985): Moneret-Vautrin DA+, *Anesth Analg* 64(9), 944
(1984): Mishima S+, *Anesth Analg* 63(9), 865
(1984): Pappagallo S+, *Minerva Anestesiol* 50(9), 481
Hypersensitivity
(1983): Nagao H+, *Br J Anaesth* 55(3), 253
Myalgia
Myopathy
(1994): Giostra E+, *Chest* 106(1), 210
(1993): De Smet, *Rev Neurol* 149(10), 573
(1993): Miyoshi T+, *Rinsho Shinkeigaku* 33(6), 620
Rhabdomyolysis
(1993): Clavelou P+, *Ann Fr Anesth Reanim* 12(3), 326
Sialorrhea

PANTOPRAZOLE

Trade name: Protonix (Wyeth)
Indications: Esophagitis associated with gastroesophageal reflux disease (GERD)
Category: Proton pump (gastric acid secretion) inhibitor
Half-life: 1 hour

Reactions

Skin
Abscess (<1%)
Acne (<1%)
Allergic reactions (sic) (<1%)
Angioedema (<1%)
Balanitis (<1%)
Dermatitis (<1%)
Diaphoresis (<1%)
(2000): Natsch S+, *Ann Pharmacother* 34, 474
Ecchymoses (<1%)
Eczema (<1%)
Edema (<1%)
Erythema multiforme (<1%)
Exanthems (<1%)
Facial edema (<1%)
Flu-like syndrome (sic) (1–10%)
Fungal infections (sic) (<1%)
Herpes simplex (<1%)
Herpes zoster (<1%)
Infections (sic) (1–10%)
Lichenoid eruption (<1%)
(2000): Bong JL+, *BMJ* 320, 283
Lupus erythematosus (discoid)
(2001): Correia O+, *Clin Exp Dermatol* 26(5), 455
Peripheral edema
(2001): Brunner G+, *Dig Dis Sci* 46(5), 993
(1994): Brunner G, *Aliment Pharmacol Ther* 8, 59
Photosensitivity
(2001): Correia O+, *Clin Exp Dermatol* 26(5), 455
Phototoxicity
(2001): Correia O+, *Clin Exp Dermatol* 26, 455
Pruritus (<1%)
(2000): Natsch S+, *Ann Pharmacother* 34, 474
Rash (sic) (<1%)
(2000): Avner DL, *Clin Ther* 22(10), 1169
(1992): Muller P+, *Z Gastroenterol* 30, 771
Stevens–Johnson syndrome (<1%)

Toxic epidermal necrolysis (<1%)
Ulcerations (<1%)
Urticaria (<1%)
(2000): Natsch S+, *Ann Pharmacother* 34, 474
Xerosis (<1%)
Hair
Hair – alopecia (<1%)
Other
Anaphylactoid reactions (<1%)
(2002): Fardet L+, *Am J Gastroenterol* 97(6), 1578
(2002): Kaatz M+, *Allergy* 57(2), 184
(2000): Natsch S+, *Ann Pharmacother* 3(4), 474
Aphthous stomatitis (<1%)
Dysgeusia (<1%)
Foetor ex ore (halitosis) (<1%)
Gingivitis (<1%)
Glossitis (<1%)
Headache
Hyperesthesia (<1%)
Mastodynia (<1%)
Myalgia (<1%)
Oral candidiasis (<1%)
Paresthesias (<1%)
Sialorrhea (<1%)
Stomatitis (<1%)
Thrombophlebitis (<1%)
Tongue edema
(2000): Natsch S+, *Ann Pharmacother* 34, 474
Tongue pigmentation (<1%)
Tremor (<1%)
Vaginitis (<1%)
Xerostomia (<1%)

PANTOTHENIC ACID

Trade name: Dexol
Indications: Vitamin B complex malabsorption
Category: Water-soluble vitamin
Half-life: N/A

Reactions

Skin
Exanthems
Pruritus
Urticaria

PAPAVERINE

Trade names: Genabid; Pavabid (Aventis); Pavatine
Other common trade names: *Angioverin; Optenyl; Pameion; Papaverine 60; Papaverini; Pavagen; Pavased*
Indications: Peripheral and cerebral ischemia
Category: Peripheral vasodilator
Half-life: 0.5–2 hours

Reactions

Skin
Diaphoresis (<1%)

Exanthems
Fixed eruption
  (1994): Kirby KA+, *Urology* 43, 886
Flushing (<1%)
Pruritus (<1%)
Pyogenic granuloma
  (1990): Summers JL, *J Urol* 143, 1227
Rash (sic)
Toxic epidermal necrolysis
  (1989): Simochkina ZA+, *Vrach Delo* (Russian) October, 91
Urticaria

Other
Headache
Injection-site thrombophlebitis (<1%)
Priapism
  (2001): Perimenis P+, *Urol Int* 66, 27 (5 cases)
  (2001): Secil M+, *J Urol* 165(2), 416 (11.1%)
  (1991): Schwarzer JU+, *J Urol* 146, 845
Xerostomia (<1%)

PARA-AMINOSALICYLIC ACID (PAS)

(See AMINOSALICYLATE SODIUM)

PARAMETHADIONE

Trade name: Paradione (Abbott)
Indications: Absence (petit-mal) seizures
Category: Anticonvulsant
Half-life: 12–24 hours

Reactions

Skin
Acne
Erythema multiforme
  (1972): Levantine A+, *Br J Dermatol* 87, 646
  (1961): Leblanc JL+, *Can Med Assoc J* 85, 200
Exanthems
Exfoliative dermatitis
  (1946): Lennox WG, *Am J Psychiatry* 103, 159
Lupus erythematosus
Pruritus

Hair
Hair – alopecia

Other
Gingivitis
Oral mucosal eruption
  (1946): Lennox WG, *Am J Psychiatry* 103, 159
Paresthesias

PARICALCITOL

Trade name: Zemplar (Abbott)
Indications: Secondary hyperparathyroidism associated with renal failure
Category: Vitamin D analog
Half-life: N/A
Clinically important, potentially hazardous interactions with: digitalis (with overdose of paricalcitol)

Reactions

Skin
Chills (5%)
Flu-like syndrome (5%)
Peripheral edema (7%)

Other
Xerostomia (3%)

PAROMOMYCIN

Trade name: Humatin (Monarch) (Aventis)
Other common trade names: *Gabbroral; Gabroral; Humagel; Sinosid*
Indications: Intestinal amebiasis
Category: Broad-spectrum antibacterial aminoglycoside amebicide
Half-life: N/A
Clinically important, potentially hazardous interactions with: methotrexate, succinylcholine

Reactions

Skin
Exanthems (<1%)
Pruritus (<1%)

PAROXETINE

Trade name: Paxil (GSK)
Other common trade name: *Aropax 20*
Indications: Depression
Category: Antidepressant; Selective serotonin reuptake inhibitor (SSRI)
Half-life: 21 hours
Clinically important, potentially hazardous interactions with: amphetamines, aprepitant, clarithromycin, dextroamphetamine, diethylpropion, erythromycin, isocarboxazid, linezolid, MAO inhibitors, mazindol, methamphetamine, phendimetrazine, phenelzine, phentermine, phenylpropanolamine, pseudoephedrine, selegiline, sibutramine, **St John's wort**, sumatriptan, sympathomimetics, tranylcypromine, trazodone, troleandomycin

Reactions

Skin
Acne (<1%)
Allergic reactions (sic) (<1%)
  (1998): Beauquier B+, *Encephale* (French) 24, 62

Angioedema (<1%)
  (1996): Mithani H+, J Clin Psychiatry 57, 486
Candidiasis
Dermatitis (<1%)
Diaphoresis (11.2%)
  (1998): Stein MB+, JAMA 280, 708
  (1997): Litt JZ, Beachwood, OH (personal case) (observation)
  (1992): Boyer WF+, J Clin Psychiatry 53, 61
  (1991): Dechant KL+, Drugs 41, 225
  (1990): Sindrup SH+, Pain 42, 135
  (1985): Laursen AL+, Acta Psychiatr Scand 71, 249
Ecchymoses (<1%)
  (1998): Cooper TA+, Am J Med 104, 197
Eczema (sic)
Edema (<1%)
Erythema multiforme
  (2000): Altman, EA, New York, NY (from Internet) (observation)
Erythema nodosum (<1%)
Exanthems (<1%)
Facial edema (<1%)
Flushing
  (2002): Salonia A+, J Urol 168(6), 2486 (with sildenafil)
Furunculosis (<1%)
Melanoma (<1%)
Peripheral edema (<1%)
Photosensitivity (<1%)
  (2001): Richard MA+, Ann Dermatol Venereol 128, 759
Pigmentation (<1%)
Pruritus (<1%)
  (1991): Dechant KL+, Drugs 41, 225
Purpura (<1%)
Rash (sic) (1.7%)
Toxic epidermal necrolysis
  (2000): Nelson RA+, Nashville, TN (Poster exhibit #16 from
    Academy 2000)
Urticaria (<1%)
Vasculitis
  (2001): Margolese HC+, Am J Psychiatry 158, 497
Xerosis (<1%)

Hair

Hair – alopecia (<1%)
  (2000): Umansky L+, Harefuah (Hebrew) 138, 547 ('massive')

Other

Ageusia (<1%)
  (1997): Litt JZ, Beachwood, OH (personal case) (observation)
Anosmia
  (1997): Litt JZ, Beachwood, OH (personal case) (observation)
Aphthous stomatitis (<1%)
Bruxism (<1%)
  (1996): Romanelli F+, Ann Pharmacother 30, 1246
Cough
  (2000): Hamel H+, Presse Med (French) 29, 1045
Dysgeusia (2.4%)
  (1998): Litt JZ, Beachwood, OH (personal case) (observation)
Galactorrhea
  (2001): Morrison J+, Can J Psychiatry 46, 88
Gingivitis (<1%)
Glossitis (<1%)
Headache
Lymphedema
Myalgia (1.7%)
Myopathy (1–10%)
Oral ulceration
Paresthesias (3.8%)
Priapism

(1996): Bertholon F+, Ann Med Psychol Paris (French) 154, 145
Serotonin syndrome
  (1999): Cavallazzi LO+, Arq Neuropsiq 57(3B), 886
Sialorrhea (<1%)
Stomatitis (<1%)
Tinnitus
Tongue edema (<1%)
  (1996): Mithani H+, J Clin Psychiatry 57, 486
Tremor (1–10%)
Vaginal candidiasis (<1%)
Vaginitis
Xerostomia (18.1%)
  (1998): Stein MB+, JAMA 280, 708
  (1992): Boyer WF+, J Clin Psychiatry 53, 61
  (1992): Claghorn JL, J Clin Psychiatry 53, 33
  (1992): Fabre LF, J Clin Psychiatry 53, 40
  (1992): Shrivastava RK+, J Clin Psychiatry 53, 48
  (1992): Smith WT+, J Clin Psychiatry 53, 36
  (1991): Dechant KL+, Drugs 1, 225
  (1991): Dunbar GC+, Br J Psychiatry 159, 394
  (1990): Cohn JB+, Psychopharmacol Bull 26, 185
  (1990): Sindrup SH+, Pain 42, 135

PEG-INTERFERON ALFA-2B

Trade name: PEG-Intron (Schering)
Indications: Chronic hepatitis C
Category: Interferon immunomodulator
Half-life: ~40 hours
**Clinically important, potentially hazardous interactions
with:** ACE inhibitors, melphalan, warfarin, zidovudine

Reactions

Skin

Abscess (~1%)
Angioedema (~1%)
Blistering
  (2003): Gallina K+, J Drugs Dermatol 2(1), 63
Dermatitis (sic) (7%)
Diaphoresis (6%)
Flu-like syndrome (46%)
  (2002): Gupta SK+, J Clin Pharmacol 42(10), 1109
Flushing (6%)
Pruritus (12%)
Psoriasis (~1%)
Purpura
Rash (sic) (6%)
Urticaria (~1%)
Viral infections (11%)
Xerosis (11%)

Hair

Hair – alopecia (22%)

Other

Anaphylactoid reactions (~1%)
Anxiety
  (2003): Alvarado Y+, Cancer Chemother Pharmacol 51(1), 81
Cough (6%)
Depression (16–29%)
  (2003): Alvarado Y+, Cancer Chemother Pharmacol 51(1), 81
Dysgeusia (1–10%)
Headache
  (2002): Gupta SK+, J Clin Pharmacol 42(10), 1109

Hypersensitivity (~1%)
Injection-site pain (2%)
Musculoskeletal pain (56%)
Myalgia (38–42%)
  (2001): Perry CM+, *Drugs* 61(15), 2263
Pain (12%)
Rigors (23–45%)

PEGFILGRASTIM

Synonym: G-CSF (PEG Conjugate)
Trade name: Neulasta (Amgen)
Indications: Myelosuppressive chemotherapy, decreases incidence of infection
Category: Colony stimulating factor; Hematopoietic
Half-life: 15–80 hours
Clinically important, potentially hazardous interactions with: lithium

Reactions

Skin
Allergic reactions (sic) (<1%)
Peripheral edema
Rash (sic) (<1%)
Urticaria (<1%)

Hair
Hair – alopecia

Other
Anaphylactoid reactions (<1%)
Arthralgia
Bone or joint pain (26%)
  (2002): Curran MP+, *Drugs* 62(8), 1207
Dysgeusia
Headache
Mucositis
Myalgia
Stomatitis

PEGVISOMANT

Synonyms: B2036-PEG; G120K-PEG; Trovert
Trade name: Somavert (Pharmacia)
Indications: Acromegaly
Category: An analog of human growth hormone (GH)
Clinically important, potentially hazardous interactions with: insulin, latex, opioids, oral hypoglycemics

Reactions

Skin
Edema
Flu-like syndrome (4%)
Infections (23%)
Peripheral edema (4–8%)
Pruritus

Other
Abdominal pain
Anaphylactoid reactions
Back pain (8%)

Chest pain (4%)
Dizziness (8%)
Hypersensitivity
Injection-site reactions (8–14%)
Pain (8%)
Paresthesias
Sinusitis (8%)

PEMIROLAST

Trade name: Alamast (Santen)
Other common trade name: *Alegysal*
Indications: Pruritus of allergic conjunctivitis
Category: Antiallergic ophthalmic; Mast cell stabilizer
Half-life: 4.5 hours

Reactions

Skin
Allergic reactions (sic)
Flu-like syndrome (10–25%)
Ocular burning
Ocular irritation (<5%)

Other
Back pain (<5%)
Dry eyes (sic)

PEMOLINE

Trade name: Cylert (Abbott)
Other common trade names: *Betanamin; Tradon*
Indications: Attention deficit disorder, narcolepsy
Category: Anorexiant; Central nervous system stimulant
Half-life: 9–14 hours
Clinically important, potentially hazardous interactions with: pimozide

Reactions

Skin
Exanthems (<1%)
  (1992): Zürcher K and Krebs A, *Cutaneous Drug Reactions* Karger, 280
Rash (sic) (>10%)

Other
Headache
Parkinsonism
Rhabdomyolysis
  (1988): Briscoe JG+, *Med Toxicol Adverse Drug Exp* 3(1), 72
Tourette's syndrome

PENBUTOLOL

Trade name: Levatol (Schwartz)
Other common trade names: *Betapresin; Betapressin*
Indications: Hypertension
Category: Antihypertensive; Beta-adrenoceptor blocker
Half-life: 5 hours
**Clinically important, potentially hazardous interactions
with:** clonidine, epinephrine, verapamil

Note: Cutaneous side effects of beta-receptor blockaders are
clinically polymorphous. They apparently appear after several months
of continuous therapy. Atypical psoriasiform, lichen planus-like, and
eczematous chronic rashes are mainly observed. (1983): Hödl St, *Z
Hautkr* (German) 1:58, 17

Reactions

Skin
Allergic reactions (sic)
  (1985): Marone C+, *Curr Med Res Opin* 9, 417 (1–5%)
Ankle edema
Diaphoresis (1.6%)
Exanthems
  (1985): Marone C+, *Curr Med Res Opin* 9, 417 (1–5%)
Flushing
  (1985): Marone C+, *Curr Med Res Opin* 9, 417 (1–5%)
Peripheral edema
Pruritus
Psoriasis
Purpura
Rash (sic)

Hair
Hair – alopecia

Nails
Nails – bluish

Other
Dysgeusia
Headache
Paresthesias
Peyronie's disease

PENICILLAMINE

Trade names: Cuprimine (Merck); Depen (Wallace)
Other common trade names: *Artamin; D-Penamine; Distamine;
Kelatin; Pendramine*
Indications: Wilson's disease, rheumatoid arthritis
Category: Antidote; Chelating agent
Half-life: 1.7–3.2 hours
**Clinically important, potentially hazardous interactions
with:** aluminum hydroxide, antacids, ascorbic acid, bone marrow
suppressants, chloroquine, cytotoxic agents, **food**, gold,
hydroxychloroquine, iron, magnesium, primaquine, probenecid

Note: For excellent reviews of many of the cutaneous manifestations
caused by penicillamine see (1983): Levy RS+, *J Am Acad Dermatol* 8,
548 and (1981): Sternlieb I+, *J Rheumatol* 8 (Suppl 7), 149

Reactions

Skin
Anetoderma
  (1977): Davis W, *Arch Dermatol* 113, 976
Atrophy
  (1982): Bailin PL+, *Clin Rheum Dis* 8, 493 (passim)
Bullous eruption
  (1996): Bialy-Golan A+, *J Am Acad Dermatol* 35, 732 (passim)
  (1982): Fulton RA+, *Br J Dermatol* 107 (Suppl 22), 95
  (1977): Stewart WM+, *Ann Dermatol Venereol* (French) 104, 542
Bullous pemphigoid
  (1998): Weller R+, *Ann Pharmacother* 32, 1368
  (1996): Weller R+, *Clin Exp Dermatol* 21, 121
  (1989): Rasmussen HB+, *J Cutan Pathol* 16, 154
  (1987): Brown MD+, *Arch Dermatol* 123, 1119
  (1986): Gall Y+, *Ann Dermatol Venereol* (French) 113, 55
Cutis laxa
  (2000): Werth V, *Dermatology Times* 18
  (1994): Amichai B+, *Isr J Med Sci* 30, 667
  (1983): Harpey JP+, *Lancet* 2, 858
  (1983): Levy RS+, *J Am Acad Dermatol* 8, 548
  (1982): Bailin PL+, *Clin Rheum Dis* 8, 493 (passim)
  (1979): Linares A+, *Lancet* 2, 43
  (1979): Walshe JM, *Lancet* 2, 144
  (1977): Solomon L+, *N Engl J Med* 296, 54
Cyst
  (1967): Katz R, *Arch Dermatol* 95, 196
Dermatitis
  (1993): De Moor A+, *Contact Dermatitis* 29, 155 (eyedrops)
  (1990): Coenraads PJ+, *Contact Dermatitis* 23, 371
Dermatomyositis
  (1992): Kolsi R+, *Rev Rhum Mal Osteoartic* (French) 59, 341
  (1991): Wilson CL+, *Int J Dermatol* 30, 148
  (1987): Carroll CG+, *J Rheumatol* 14, 995
  (1983): Doyle DR+, *Ann Intern Med* 98, 327
  (1983): Levy RS+, *J Am Acad Dermatol* 8, 548
  (1983): Lund HI+, *Scand J Rheumatol* 12, 350
  (1982): Bailin PL+, *Clin Rheum Dis* 8, 493 (passim)
  (1981): Major GA, *J R Soc Med* 74, 393
  (1980): Wojnarowska F, *J R Soc Med* 73, 884
  (1979): Simpson NB+, *Acta Derm Venereol* (Stockh) 59, 543
  (1978): Petersen J+, *Scand J Rheumatol* 7, 113
  (1977): Fernandes L+, *Ann Rheum Dis* 36, 94
Dermopathy
  (1987): Dootson G+, *Clin Exp Dermatol* 12, 66
Discoid lupus erythematosus
  (1978): Appelboom T+, *Scand J Rheumatol* 7, 64
Ecchymoses
Edema (1–10%)

(1986): Dijkstra JW, J Am Acad Dermatol 14, 687
(1986): Peyri J+, J Am Acad Dermatol 14, 681 (cicatricial)
(1986): Steen VD+, Ann Intern Med 104, 699
(1986): Tholen S, Z Hautkr (German) 61, 719
(1985): Ho VC+, J Rheumatol 12, 583
(1985): Lever LR+, Br J Dermatol 113, 88
(1985): Piette-Brion B+, Dermatologica (French) 170, 297
(1985): Shuttleworth D+, Br J Dermatol 113, 89
(1985): Shuttleworth D+, Clin Exp Dermatol 10, 392 (cicatricial)
(1985): Velthuis PJ+, Br J Dermatol 112, 615
(1984): Hashimoto K+, Arch Dermatol 120, 762
(1984): Venencie PY+, Ann Med Interne (Paris) (French) 135, 642
(1983): Doutre MS+, Rev Rhum Mal Osteoartic (French) 50, 167
(1983): Kaplan RP+, Clin Dermatol 1, 42
(1983): Levy RS+, J Am Acad Dermatol 8, 548
(1983): Tinozzi CC, G Ital Dermatol Venereol (Italian) 118, 45
(1982): Barety M+, Therapie (French) 37, 471
(1982): Benito-Urbino S+, Rev Clin Esp (Spanish) 166, 249
(1982): Fye KH+J, Rheumatol 9, 331
(1982): Ruocco V+, Arch Dermatol Res 274, 123
(1982): Ruocco V+, Dermatologica 164, 236
(1982): Yung CW+, J Am Acad Dermatol 6, 317 (pemphigus syndrome)
(1982): Zone J+, JAMA 247, 2705
(1981): Livden JK+, Scand J Rheumatol 10, 95
(1981): Santa-Cruz DJ+, Am J Dermatopathol 3, 85
(1981): Troy JL+, J Am Acad Dermatol 4, 547
(1981): Trunnell TN+, Cutis 27, 402 (pemphigus-like)
(1980): Chouyet B+, Dermatologica (French) 160, 297
(1980): Trau H+, Arch Dermatol 116, 721
(1979): Delcambre B+, Lille Med (French) 24, 283
(1979): Hill HF, Scand J Rheumatol Suppl 28, 94
(1978): Christoph R+, Med Welt (German) 29, 1761
(1977): Marsden RA+, Proc R Soc Med 70, 103
(1977): Stewart WM+, Ann Dermatol Venereol (French) 104, 542
(1976): Cairns RJ, Proc R Soc Med 69, 384
(1976): Colliard H+, Rev Stomatol Chir Maxillofac (French) 77, 741
(1976): Davies MG+, Arch Dermatol 112, 1308
(1976): From E+, Dermatologica 152, 358
(1976): Tan SG+, Br J Dermatol 95, 99 (pemphigus-like)
(1975): Asboe-Hansen G, Acta Derm Venereol 55, 461
(1975): Benveniste M+, Nouv Presse Med (French) 4, 3125
(1975): Hewitt J+, BMJ 3, 371
(1971): Hewitt J+, Ann Med Interne Paris (French) 122, 1003
(1969): Degos R+, Bull Soc Fr Dermatol Syphiligr (French) 76, 751

Pemphigus erythematosus (Senear–Usher)
(1990): Willemsen MJ+, Int J Dermatol 29, 193
(1985): Amerian ML+, Int J Dermatol 24, 16
(1985): Gibson LE+, J Am Acad Dermatol 12, 883
(1984): Amerian ML+, J Am Acad Dermatol 10, 215
(1982): Yung CW+, J Am Acad Dermatol 6, 317
(1980): Keilhauer A+, Z Hautkr (German) 55, 948
(1979): Thorvaldsen J, Dermatologica 159, 167
(1978): Fellner MJ+, Int J Dermatol 17, 308
(1977): Scherak O+, BMJ 1, 838

Pemphigus foliaceus
(2000): Elston DM+, Cutis 66, 375
(2000): Werth V, Dermatology Times 18
(1999): Toth GG+, Br J Dermatol 141, 583
(1998): Brenner S+, J Am Acad Dermatol 39, 137
(1997): McGovern TW+, Arch Dermatol 133, 499
(1997): Peñas PF+, J Am Acad Dermatol 37, 121
(1995): Brenner S+, American Academy of Dermatology Meeting, New Orleans (observation)
(1993): Zillikens D+, Hautarzt (German) 44, 167
(1986): Kohn SR, Arch Dermatol 122, 17 (fatal)
(1985): Bahmer FA+, Arch Dermatol 121, 665
(1984): Knezevic W+, Aust N Z J Med 14, 50
(1983): Brenner S+, Harefuah (Hebrew) 104, 94

(1982): Kohn SR, Dermatologic Capsule and Comment 4, 11
(1981): Matkaluk RM+, Arch Dermatol 117, 156
(1977): Kristensen JK+, Acta Derm Venereol (Stockh) 57, 69
(1976): Marsden RA+, BMJ 2, 1423

Pemphigus herpetiformis
(1988): Weltfriend S+, Hautarzt (German) 39, 587
(1980): Morioka S+, J Dermatol 7, 425
(1977): Marsden RA+, Br J Dermatol 97, 451

Pemphigus vulgaris
(2000): Werth V, Dermatology Times 18

Peripheral edema (1–10%)

Pruritus (44–50%)
(1982): Bailin PL+, Clin Rheum Dis 8, 493 (passim)
(1982): Yung CW+, J Am Acad Dermatol 6, 317 (passim)

Pseudoxanthoma elasticum
(2000): Werth V, Dermatology Times 18
(1998): Coatesworth AP+, J Clin Pathol 51, 169
(1992): Bolognia JL+, Dermatology (Basel) 184, 12
(1992): Narron GH+, Ann Plast Surg 29, 367
(1991): Buckley C+, Clin Exp Dermatol 16, 310
(1990): Dalziel KL+, Br J Dermatol 123, 305
(1988): Burge S+, Clin Exp Dermatol 13, 255
(1987): Dootson G+, Clin Exp Dermatol 12, 66
(1986): Light N+, Br J Dermatol 114, 381
(1985): Bentley-Phillips B, J R Soc Med 78, 787
(1985): Meyrick-Thomas RH+, Clin Exp Dermatol 10, 386

Psoriasis
(1987): Forgie JC+, BMJ 294, 1101
(1986): Daunt SON+, Br J Rheumatol 25, 74
(1983): Levy RS+, J Am Acad Dermatol 8, 548
(1981): Sternlieb I+, J Rheumatol 8, 149

Purpura
(1983): Trice JM+, Arch Intern Med 143, 1487
(1982): Bailin PL+, Clin Rheum Dis 8, 493 (passim)
(1982): Speth PA+, J Rheumatol 9, 812
(1964): Sternlieb I+, JAMA 189, 748

Rash (sic) (44–50%)
(2003): Corrigan JJ Jr+, Haemophilia 9(1), 64
(2000): Shannon MW+, Ann Pharmacother 34, 15
(1991): Barash J+, Clin Exp Rheumatol 9, 541
(1982): Kean WF+, J Am Geriatr Soc 30, 94
(1982): Smith PJ+, Br Med J (Clin Res Ed) 285, 595

Scleroderma
(1991): Bourgeois P+, Baillieres Clin Rheumatol 5, 13
(1987): Miyagawa S+, Br J Dermatol 116, 95
(1981): Bernstein RM+, Ann Rheum Dis 40, 42

Sjøgren's syndrome
(1996): Bialy-Golan A+, J Am Acad Dermatol 35, 732 (passim)

Stevens–Johnson syndrome
(1996): Kammler H-J, Jena, Germany (from Internet) (observation)

Toxic epidermal necrolysis (<1%)
(1984): Chan HL, J Am Acad Dermatol 10, 973
(1981): Ward K+, Ir J Med Sci 150, 252

Urticaria (44–50%)
(1983): Levy RS+, J Am Acad Dermatol 8, 548
(1979): Hill HFH, Scand J Rheumatol 28, 94

Vasculitis
(1998): Merkel PA, Curr Opin Rheumatol 10, 45
(1986): Gall Y+, Ann Dermatol Venereol (French) 113, 55
(1983): Banfi G+, Nephron 33, 56
(1983): Curran JJ+, J Rheumatol 10, 344
(1982): Bailin PL+, Clin Rheum Dis 8, 493 (passim)
(1974): Hill HFH, Curr Med Res Opin 2, 573

Vesicular eruptions
(1992): Godar JM+, Arch Dermatol 128, 977

Wrinkling (sic)
(1983): Levy RS+, J Am Acad Dermatol 8, 548

Xerosis
(1982): Yung CW+, J Am Acad Dermatol 6, 317 (passim)

Hair

Hair – alopecia
(1983): Levy RS+, *J Am Acad Dermatol* 8, 548
(1981): Sternlieb I+, *J Rheumatol* 8 (Suppl 7), 149
Hair – hirsutism
(1990): Rose BI+, *J Reprod Med* 35, 43
(1983): Levy RS+, *J Am Acad Dermatol* 8, 548

Nails

Nails – dystrophy
(1987): Brown MD+, *Arch Dermatol* 123, 1119 (passim)
Nails – elkonyxis (punched-out appearance of the nail at lunulae)
(1989): Bjellerup M, *Acta Derm Venereol (Stockh)* 69, 339
Nails – leukonychia
(1967): Thivolet J+, *Bull Soc Fr Dermatol* (French) 75, 61
Nails – longitudinal ridges
(1967): Thivolet J+, *Bull Soc Fr Dermatol* (French) 75, 61
Nails – onychoschizia
(1989): Bjellerup M, *Acta Derm Venereol (Stockh)* 69, 339
Nails – yellow
(1991): Ichikawa Y+, *Tokai J Exp Clin Med* 16, 203
(1989): Bjellerup M, *Acta Derm Venereol (Stockh)* 69, 339
(1983): Ilchyshyn A+, *Acta Derm Venereol (Stockh)* 63, 534
(1979): Lubach D+, *Hautarzt* (German) 30, 547

Other

Ageusia (12%)
(2002): ter Borg EJ+, *Neth J Med* 60(10), 402
(1982): Yung CW+, *J Am Acad Dermatol* 6, 317 (passim)
Aphthous stomatitis
(1983): Levy RS+, *J Am Acad Dermatol* 8, 548
Benign mucous membrane pemphigoid
(1985): Shuttleworth D+, *Clin Exp Dermatol* 10, 392
(1977): Pegum JS+, *BMJ* 1, 1473
Bromhidrosis
(1996): Bialy-Golan A+, *J Am Acad Dermatol* 35, 732 (passim)
Death
Dermatopathy with lymphangiectases
(1989): Goldstein JB+, *Arch Dermatol* 125, 92
Dysgeusia (metallic taste)
(1996): Bialy-Golan A+, *J Am Acad Dermatol* 35, 732 (passim)
(1983): Levy RS+, *J Am Acad Dermatol* 8, 548
(1982): Kean WF+, *J Am Geriatr Soc* 30, 94
(1980): Stein HB+, *Ann Intern Med* 92, 24
Gingivitis
Glossitis
(1967): Thivolet J+, *Bull Soc Fr Dermatol* (French) 75, 61
Guillain–Barré syndrome
(1984): Knezevic W+, *Aust N Z J Med* 14, 50
Gynecomastia
(1994): Desautels JE, *Can Assoc Radiol J* 45, 143 (gigantism)
(1985): Kahl LE+, *J Rheumatol* 12, 990
(1982): Reid DM+, *BMJ* 285, 1083
Hypersensitivity
(1999): Hsu HL+, *Taiwan Erh Ko I Hsueh Tsa Chih* 40, 448
(1994): Chan CY+, *Am J Gastroenterol* 89, 442
Hypogeusia (25–33%)
(1968): Keiser HR+, *JAMA* 203, 381
(1967): Henkin RI+, *Lancet* 2, 1268
Mucocutaneous reactions (sic)
(1982): Halla JT+, *Am J Med* 72, 423
Mucosal lesions (pemphigus-like)
(1981): Eisenberg E+, *Oral Surg Oral Med Oral Pathol* 51, 409
(1978): Hay KD+, *Oral Surg Oral Med Oral Pathol* 45, 385
Mucosal ulceration
(1981): Eisenberg E+, *Oral Surg* 51, 409
Oral lichenoid eruption
(1984): Blasberg B+, *J Rheumatol* 11, 348

Oral ulceration
(2000): Madinier I+, *Ann Med Interne (Paris)* (French) 151, 248
(1996): Bialy-Golan A+, *J Am Acad Dermatol* 35, 732 (passim)
(1982): Egeland T+, *J Oral Pathol* 11, 183
(1980): Stein HB+, *Ann Intern Med* 92, 24
(1964): Sternlieb I+, *JAMA* 189, 748
Polymyositis
(1996): Bialy-Golan A+, *J Am Acad Dermatol* 35, 732 (passim)
(1991): Santos JC+, *Clin Exp Dermatol* 16, 76
(1978): Petersen J+, *Scand J Rheumatol* 7, 113
Serum sickness
(1996): Bialy-Golan A+, *J Am Acad Dermatol* 35, 732 (passim)
Stomatitis
(1996): Bialy-Golan A+, *J Am Acad Dermatol* 35, 732 (passim)
(1982): Yung CW+, *J Am Acad Dermatol* 6, 317 (passim)
(1981): Sternlieb I+, *J Rheumatol* 8 (Suppl 7), 149 (passim)
(1980): Stein HB+, *Ann Intern Med* 92, 24
(1968): Thivolet J+, *Bull Soc Fr Dermatol Syphiligr* (French) 75, 61
Tinnitus

PENICILLINS

Generic names:
Amoxicillin
Trade names: Amoxil (GSK); Augmentin (GSK); Larotid; Polymox; Trimox (Geneva); Wymox
Ampicillin
Trade names: Omnipen (Wyeth); Olycillin; Principen (Geneva); Unasyn (Pfizer)
Azlocillin
Trade names: Azlin
Bacampicillin
Trade name: Spectrobid (Pfizer)
Carbenicillin
Trade name: Geopen
Cloxacillin
Trade names: Cloxapen (GSK); Tegopen (Bristol-Myers Squibb)
Cyclacillin
Trade name: none
Dicloxacillin
Trade names: Dycil; Dynapen (Bristol-Myers Squibb); Pathocil
Methicillin
Trade name: Staphcillin (Bristol-Myers Squibb)
Mexlocillin
Trade name: Mezlin (Bayer)
Nafcillin
Trade name: Unipen
Oxacillin
Trade names: Bactocill; Prostaphlin
Penicillin G
Trade names: Bicillin (Monarch); Crysticillin; Megacillin; Wycillin
Penicillin V
Trade names: Beepen; Betapen; Ledercillin; Pen Vee K; V-Cillin; etc.
Piperacillin
Trade name: Pipracil (Wyeth)
Ticarcillin
Trade name: Ticar (GSK)

Indications: Various infections caused by susceptible organisms
Category: Antibiotic
Half-life: varies
Clinically important, potentially hazardous interactions with: anisindione, anticoagulants, cyclosporine, demeclocycline, dicumarol, doxycycline, methotrexate, minocycline, oxytetracycline, tetracycline, warfarin

Note: 'Patients with a history of penicillin allergy are about ten times more likely than the general population to experience a potentially fatal reaction to subsequent therapy with most other haptenating drugs.' The degradation products of penicillin can bind with tissue or serum proteins to form an immunogenic complex that can elicit an immune response

Reactions

Skin
Acral numbness
  (1997): Takahashi H, *J Dermatol* 24, 50
Acute generalized exanthematous pustulosis (AGEP)
  (1995): Gebhardt M+, *Contact Dermatitis* 33, 204
  (1995): Moreau A+, *Int J Dermatol* 34, 263 (passim)
  (1994): Manders SM+, *Cutis* 54, 194
  (1991): Roujeau J-C+, *Arch Dermatol* 127, 1333
Allergic reactions (sic)
  (2003): Arroliga ME+, *Cleve Clin J Med* 70(4), 313
  (2003): Torres MJ+, *Clin Exp Allergy* 33(5), 714
  (2000): Lee CE+, *Arch Intern Med* 160, 2819
  (2000): Li JT+, *Mayo Clin Proc* 75, 902
  (1984): Cameron W+, *Ann Allergy* 53, 455
  (1984): Jolivet M+, *Union Med Can* (French) 113, 842
Angioedema
  (1988): Van Arsdel PP Jr, *JAMA* 260, 2572
  (1978): Girard JP, *Contact Dermatitis* 4, 309
  (1968): Rosenblum AH, *J Allergy* 42, 309
Baboon syndrome
  (1999): Panhans-Gross A+, *Contact Dermatitis* 41, 352
Bullous pemphigoid
  (1992): Shelley WB+, *Advanced Dermatologic Diagnosis* WB Saunders, 414 (passim)
  (1988): Alcalay J+, *J Am Acad Dermatol* 18, 345
Cutis laxa
  (1971): Reed WB+, *Arch Dermatol* 103, 661
Dermatitis (sic)
  (1991): Rudzki E+, *Contact Dermatitis* 25, 192
  (1990): Pecegueiro M, *Contact Dermatitis* 23, 190
  (1984): Beckerman A+, *Int J Dermatol* 23(2), 149
Diaphoresis
Eczema (sic)
Erythema annulare centrifugum
  (1978): Gupta HL+, *J Indian Med Assoc* 65, 307
  (1964): Shelley WB, *Arch Dermatol* 90, 54
Erythema multiforme
  (2000): Ibia EO+, *Arch Dermatol* 136, 849
  (1990): Garcia JJ+, *Clin Exp Allergy* 20 (Suppl 1), 121
  (1990): Staretz LR+, *JADA* 121, 436
  (1985): Huff JC, *Dermatologic Clinics* 3(1), 141
  (1983): Ansel J+, *Arch Dermatol* 119, 1006
Erythema nodosum
Exanthems
  (2002): Romano A+, *Int Arch Allergy Immunol* 129(2), 169
  (2000): Ibia EO+, *Arch Dermatol* 136, 849
  (2000): Schnyder B+, *Hautarzt* (German) 51, 46
  (1995): Romano A+, *Allergy* 50, 113
  (1986): de Haan P+, *Allergy* 41, 75
  (1976): Lackner F+, *Int J Clin Pharmacol Biopharm* (German) 13, 90
  (1976): Richter G, *Dermatol Monatsschr* (German) 162, 533
  (1974): Spitzy KH, *Acta Med Austriaca* (German) 2, 46
  (1970): Baer RL+, *Br J Dermatol* 83, 37
  (1970): Fellner MN+, *J Invest Dermatol* 55, 390
Exfoliative dermatitis
  (1986): Wengrower D+, *Respiration* 50, 301
Fixed eruption
  (1993): Inadomi T+, *Eur J Dermatol* 3, 674
  (1980): Haustein UF, *Dermatol Monatsschr* (German) 166, 680
  (1979): Pasricha JS, *Br J Dermatol* 100, 183

  (1975): Coskey RJ+, *Arch Dermatol* 111, 791
  (1970): Dennison WL+, *Arch Dermatol* 101, 594
  (1951): Canizares O, *Arch Dermatol* 63, 800
Jarisch–Herxheimer reaction (<1%)
  (2002): Silberstein P+, *J Clin Neurosci* 9(6), 689
  (2002): Whitley LS, Washington, DC (March AAD Poster)
  (1977): Pareek SS, *Br J Vener Dis* 53, 389
Linear IgA bullous dermatosis
  (1998): Wakelin SH+, *Br J Dermatol* 138, 310
  (1994): Kuechle MK+, *J Am Acad Dermatol* 30, 187
  (1993): Combemale P+, *Ann Dermatol Venereol* (French) 120, 847
Lupus erythematosus
  (1994): Yung RL+, *Rheum Dis Clin North Am* 20, 61
Pemphigus
  (1997): Brenner S+, *J Am Acad Dermatol* 36, 919
  (1991): Escallier F+, *Ann Dermatol Venereol* (French) 118, 381
  (1988): Alcalay J+, *J Am Acad Dermatol* 18, 345
  (1988): Duhra P+, *Br J Dermatol* 118, 307
  (1987): Brenner S+, *J Am Acad Dermatol* 17, 514
  (1987): Seidenbaum M+, *Drug Intell Clin Pharm* 21, 1012
  (1984): Ruocco V+, *Arch Dermatol Res* 274, 123
  (1980): Fellner MJ, *Int J Dermatol* 9, 392
  (1979): Ruocco V+, *Dermatologica* 159, 266
Pityriasis rosea
Pruritus
  (1995): Litt JZ, Beachwood, OH (personal case) (observation)
  (1970): Baer RL+, *Br J Dermatol* 83, 37
Purpura
Pustular psoriasis
  (1987): Katz M+, *J Am Acad Dermatol* 17, 918
  (1976): Lindgren S+, *Acta Derm Venereol* (Stockh) 56, 139
  (1971): Ryan TJ+, *Br J Dermatol* 85, 407
  (1969): Hadida E+, *Bull Soc Fr Dermatol Syphiligr* (French) 76, 1095
  (1969): Privat Y+, *Bull Soc Fr Dermatol Syphiligr* (French) 76, 505
Rash (sic) (<1%)
Stevens–Johnson syndrome
  (1997): Shoji T+, *J Am Acad Dermatol* 37, 337
  (1996): Kammler H-J, Jena, Germany (from Internet) (observation)
  (1993): Leenutaphong V+, *Int J Dermatol* 32, 428
  (1983): Herold M+, *Ethiop Med J* 21, 227
  (1983): Sullivan M, *Dent Health London* 22, 10
  (1971): Nava-Negrete A, *Alergia* (Spanish) 19, 29
Toxic epidermal necrolysis
  (1993): Leenutaphong V+, *Int J Dermatol* 32, 428
  (1983): Herold M+, *Ethiop Med J* 21, 227
  (1983): Tagami H+, *Arch Dermatol* 119, 910
  (1982): Herold M+, *Z Gesamte Inn Med* (German) 37, 706
  (1979): Frontera-Izquierdo P+, *An Esp Pediatr* 12, 703
  (1977): Ghosh JS, *Arch Dermatol* 113, 1162
  (1972): Carli-Basset C+, *Sem Hôp* (French) 48, 497
  (1969): Pustovaia AI+, *Vestn Dermatol Venerol* (Russian) 43, 73
  (1966): Ulcova I+, *Cesk Pediatr* (Czech) 21, 923
Toxic erythema
  (1995): Rademaker M, *N Z Med J* 108, 165 (with vancomycin)
Urticaria
  (2002): Romano A+, *Int Arch Allergy Immunol* 129(2), 169
  (2001): Torres MJ+, *Allergy* 56(9), 850
  (2000): Ibia EO+, *Arch Dermatol* 136, 849
  (1988): Sorensen HT+, *Ugeskr Laeger* (Danish) 150, 2913
  (1985): Rudzki E+, *Contact Dermatitis* 13, 192
  (1983): Fisher AA, *Cutis* 32, 314
  (1982): Boonk WJ+, *Br J Dermatol* 106, 183
  (1978): Girard JP, *Contact Dermatitis* 4, 309
  (1971): Van Hecke E, *Ann Dermatol Syphiligr* (Paris) (French) 98, 147
  (1970): Baer RL+, *Br J Dermatol* 83, 37

(1968): Rosenblum AH, *J Allergy* 42, 309
Vasculitis
Vesicular eruptions

Hair
Hair – alopecia
(1977): Pareek SS, *Br J Vener Dis* 53, 389

Other
Anaphylactoid reactions
(2001): Garvey LH+, *Acta Anaesthesiol Scand* 45(10), 1204
(2001): Kruszewski J+, *Wiad Lek* 54, 116 (recurrent)
(2001): Torres MJ+, *Allergy* 56(9), 850
(2000): Xi-Moy S+, *Anesthesiology* 93, 280
(1999): Dunn AB+, *J Reprod Med* 44, 381
(1993): van der Klauw MM+, *Br J Clin Pharmacol* 35, 400
(1977): Matveikov GP+, *Antibiotiki* (Russian) 22, 813
(1976): Kraus SJ+, *Cutis* 17, 765
(1972): Kelle L+, *Z Arztl Fortbild* (Jena) (German) 66, 538
(1969): Idsoe O+, *Schweiz Med Wochenschr* (German) 99, 1221
(151 deaths)
(1968): Bowszyc J, *Przegl Dermatol* (Polish) 55, 307
(1968): Rosenblum AH, *J Allergy* 42, 309
(1967): Fellner MJ+, *Arch Dermatol* 96, 687
(1953): Feinberg S+, *JAMA* 152, 114
Black tongue
Death
(2002): Gerber N+, *Otolaryngol Head Neck Surg* 126(3), 321
Dysgeusia
Embolia cutis medicamentosa (Nicolau syndrome)
(2003): Reding EL+, *J Am Acad Dermatol* 48(3), 472 (passim)
(2002): Poletti E+, *World Congress Dermatol* Poster, 0124
(1998): Saputo V+, *Pediatr Med Chir* (Italian) 20, 105
(1966): Deutsch J, *Dtsch Gesundheitw* (German) 21, 2433
Glossitis
Headache
Hypersensitivity (<1%)
(1998): Romano A, *Clin Exp Allergy* 28 (Suppl 4), 29
(1995): Bircher AJ, *Curr Probl Dermatol* 22, 31
(1988): Weiss ME+, *Clin Allergy* 18, 515
(1977): Reznikova ZT+, *Pediatriia* (Russian) April, 25
(1969): Leonhardi G+, *Hautarzt* (German) 20, 21
Injection-site aseptic necrosis
Injection-site reactions (sic) (1–10%)
(1990): Shen K, *Lancet* 336, 689
Injection-site urticaria
Lipoatrophy
(2000): Kuperman-Beade M+, *Pediatr Dermatol* 17, 302
Oral candidiasis (>10%)
Oral ulceration
(1990): Staretz LR+, *JADA* 121, 436
Pseudolymphoma
(1994): Rijlaarsdam JU+, *Semin Dermatol* 13(3), 187
(1993): Kerl H+, *Dermatology in General Medicine* McGraw-Hill
New York
(1990): Souteyrand P+, *Curr Probl Dermatol* 19, 176
Serum sickness
(2001): Tatum AJ+, *Ann Allergy Asthma Immunol* 86(3), 330 (3 cases)
(2000): Ibia EO+, *Arch Dermatol* 136, 849
(1990): Heckbert SR+, *Am J Epidemiol* 132, 336
(1980): Brandslund I+, *Haemostasis* 9, 193
(1967): Fellner MJ+, *Arch Dermatol* 96, 687
(1967): Fellner MJ+, *J Invest Dermatol* 48, 384
Stomatitis
Thrombophlebitis (<1%)
Tongue furry
Xerostomia

PENTAGASTRIN

Trade name: Peptavlon (Wyeth)
Other common trade name: *Gastrodiagnost*
Category: Diagnostic aid (gastric function)
Half-life: 10 minutes

Reactions

Skin
Angioedema
(1985): Arnved J+, *Lancet* 2, 1068
(1975): Wastell C+, *BMJ* 1, 334
Diaphoresis
Exanthems
(1975): Wastell C+, *BMJ* 1, 334
Flushing
(1975): Wastell C+, *BMJ* 1, 334
Pruritus
(1975): Wastell C+, *BMJ* 1, 334
Purpura
(1985): Arnved J+, *Lancet* 2, 1068
Rash (sic)
Urticaria

Other
Hypersensitivity
Injection-site pain
Paresthesias

PENTAMIDINE

Trade names: NebuPent (Fujisawa); Pentam-300 (Fujisawa)
Other common trade name: *Pentacarinat*
Indications: *Pneumocystis carinii* infection, trypanosomiasis
Category: Antiprotozoal antibiotic
Half-life: 9.1–13.2 hours (IM); 6.5 hours (IV)
**Clinically important, potentially hazardous interactions
with:** adefovir, sparfloxacin

Note: The rate of adverse side effects is increased in patients with
AIDS

Reactions

Skin
Bullous eruption
(1970): Wang JJ+, *J Pediatr* 77, 311
Edema
Erythema
Exanthems
(1992): Breathnach SM+, *Adverse Drug Reactions and the Skin*
Blackwell, Oxford, 179 (passim)
(1990): Leoung GS+, *N Engl J Med* 323, 769 (0.25%)
(1990): Monk JP+, *Drugs* 39, 741
(1990): Soo Hoo GW+, *Ann Intern Med* 113, 195 (1–5%)
(1989): Berger TG+, *Ann Intern Med* 110, 1035
(1988): Leen CLS+, *Lancet* 2, 1250
(1988): Sattler FR+, *Ann Intern Med* 109, 280 (15%)
(1987): Goa KL+, *Drugs* 33, 242 (1.5%)
(1984): Gordon FM+, *Ann Intern Med* 100, 495 (3%)
(1984): Kovacs JA+, *Ann Intern Med* 100, 663 (6%)
Jarisch–Herxheimer reaction (<1%)
(1987): Goa KL+, *Drugs* 33, 242
Pruritus

(1989): Berger TG+, *Ann Intern Med* 110, 1035
(1988): Leen CLS+, *Lancet* 2, 1250
Purpura
Rash (sic) (31–47%)
  (1993): Dohn M+, *Int Conf AIDS* 9, 372
  (1988): Leen CL+, *Lancet* 2, 1250
  (1984): Gordin FM+, *Ann Intern Med* 100, 495
  (1974): Walzer PD+, *Ann Intern Med* 80, 83 (1.5%)
Side effects (sic)
  (1989): Berger TG+, *Ann Intern Med* 110, 1035
Stevens–Johnson syndrome (0.2%)
Toxic epidermal necrolysis
  (1988): Leen CLS+, *Lancet* 2, 1250 (passim)
  (1987): Goa KL+, *Drugs* 33, 242
  (1985): Heng MCY, *Br J Dermatol* 113, 597
Ulcerations
  (1985): Gottlieb JR+, *Plast Reconstr Surg* 76, 630
Urticaria
  (1993): Belsito DV, *Contact Dermatitis* 29, 158 (contact)
  (1992): Breathnach SM+, *Adverse Drug Reactions and the Skin*
    Blackwell, Oxford, 179 (passim)
  (1988): Leen CLS+, *Lancet* 2, 1250
Vasculitis
Xerosis

Other
Ageusia
Anosmia
Dysgeusia (1.7%) (metallic taste)
  (2002): Lai A Fat E+, *Int J Dermatol* 41, 796
Gingivitis
Headache
Injection-site calcification
  (1987): Goa KL+, *Drugs* 33, 242
Injection-site irritation
  (1996): Andersen JM, *Am J Health Syst Pharm* 53, 185
  (1996): Herrero-Ambrosio A+, *Am J Health Syst Pharm* 53, 2881
Injection-site pain
  (2002): Lai A Fat E+, *Int J Dermatol* 41, 796
Injection-site reactions (sic) (>10%)
  (1992): Jones RS+, *Clin Infect Dis* 15, 561
Injection-site ulceration
  (1991): Bolognia JL, *Dermatologica* 183, 221
Myalgia (<5%)
Phlebitis
Rhabdomyolysis
  (1985): Sensakovic JW+, *Arch Intern Med* 145(12), 2247
Xerostomia

PENTAZOCINE

Trade name: Talwin (Sanofi-Synthelabo)
Other common trade names: *Fortral; Fortwin; Liticon;*
Ospronim; Pentafen; Sosegon; Susevin; Talacen
Indications: Pain
Category: Narcotic; Opioid analgesic; Sedative
Half-life: 2–3 hours
Clinically important, potentially hazardous interactions
with: cimetidine, morphine

Reactions

Skin
Cellulitis

(1992): Breathnach SM+, *Adverse Drug Reactions and the Skin*
    Blackwell, Oxford, 212 (passim)
Dermatitis (sic)
Diaphoresis
Exanthems
  (1987): Pedragosa R+, *Arch Dermatol* 123, 297
Facial edema
Flushing
  (1973): Brogden RN+, *Drugs* 5, 6
Generalized eruption (sic)
  (1992): Breathnach SM+, *Adverse Drug Reactions and the Skin*
    Blackwell, Oxford, 212 (passim)
Pigmentation (surrounding ulcers)
  (1990): Furner BB, *J Am Acad Dermatol* 694 (passim)
Pruritus (<1%)
Rash (sic) (1–10%)
Scleroderma
  (2000): D'Cruz D, *Toxicol Lett* 112 and 421
  (1991): Bourgeois P+, *Baillieres Clin Rheumatol* 5, 13
Sclerosis (sic)
  (1980): Palestine RF+, *J Am Acad Dermatol* 2, 47
  (1974): Beckner TF, *JAMA* 227, 1383
  (1973): Brogden RN+, *Drugs* 5, 6 (widespread)
Toxic epidermal necrolysis (<1%)
  (1987): Pedragosa R+, *Arch Dermatol* 123, 297 (passim)
  (1973): Hunter AAJ+, *Br J Dermatol* 88, 287
Tricotropism (sic)
  (1987): Pedragosa R+, *Arch Dermatol* 123, 297 (passim)
Ulcerations
  (1992): Breathnach SM+, *Adverse Drug Reactions and the Skin*
    Blackwell, Oxford, 212 (passim)
  (1990): Furner BB, *J Am Acad Dermatol* 694
  (1980): Palestine RF+, *J Am Acad Dermatol* 2, 47
  (1979): Padilla RS+, *Arch Dermatol* 115, 975 (punched-out
    ulcers)
  (1974): Winfield JB+, *South Med J* 67, 292
  (1973): Winfield JB+, *JAMA* 226, 189
Urticaria

Other
Dysgeusia
Embolia cutis medicamentosa (Nicolau syndrome)
  (1983): Bockers M+, *Med Welt* (German) 34, 1450
Fibrous myopathy
  (1976): Johnson KR+, *Arthritis Rheum* 19, 923
  (1975): Oh SJ+, *JAMA* 231, 271
Injection-site calcification
  (1991): Magee KL+, *Arch Dermatol* 127, 1591
  (1986): Hertzman A+, *J Rheumatol* 13, 210
Injection-site fibrosis
  (1979): Padilla RS+, *Arch Dermatol* 115, 975
Injection-site granuloma
  (1982): Menon PA, *J Assoc Military Dermatol* 2, 65
  (1972): Agache P+, *Bull Soc Fr Dermatol Syphiligr* (French) 79, 37
  (1971): Schlicher JE+, *Arch Dermatol* 104, 90
Injection-site induration and ulcers
  (1996): Bellman B+, *Arch Dermatol* 132, 1365
  (1996): Gillum P, Oklahoma City, OK (from Internet)
    (observation)
  (1984): Choucair AK+, *Neurology* 34, 524
  (1983): Adams EM+, *Arch Intern Med* 143, 2203
  (1977): Cosman A+, *Plast Reconstr Surg* 59, 255
  (1977): Schiff BL+, *JAMA* 238, 1542
  (1974): Seymour R+, *Am Surg* 40, 671
  (1973): Hönigsmann H+, *Hautarzt* (German) 24, 128
  (1971): Parks DL+, *Arch Dermatol* 104, 231
Injection-site pain
Injection-site pigmentation

(1980): Palestine RF+, *J Am Acad Dermatol* 2, 47
Lipogranulomas
  (1973): Hönigsmann H, *Dermatol Monatsschr* (German) 159, 146
Myofibrosis
  (1999): Jain A+, *J Dermatol* 26, 368
Panniculitis (chronic)
  (1992): Breathnach SM+, *Adverse Drug Reactions and the Skin*
    Blackwell, Oxford, 212 (passim)
Paresthesias
Phlebitis
  (1992): Breathnach SM+, *Adverse Drug Reactions and the Skin*
    Blackwell, Oxford, 212 (passim)
Soft tissue calcification
  (1990): Furner BB, *J Am Acad Dermatol* 694 (passim)
Tinnitus
Xerostomia (1–10%)

PENTOBARBITAL

Trade name: Nembutal (Abbott)
Other common trade names: *Medinox Mono; Mintal; Nova Rectal; Pentobarbitone; Prodromol; Sombutol*
Indications: Insomnia, sedation
Category: Anticonvulsant; Barbiturate sedative-hypnotic
Half-life: 15–50 hours
Clinically important, potentially hazardous interactions with: alcohol, anticoagulants, antihistamines, brompheniramine, buclizine, chlorpheniramine, dicumarol, ethanolamine, imatinib, nalbuphine, warfarin

Reactions

Skin
Acne
Angioedema (<1%)
Bullous eruption
  (1970): Groeschel D+, *N Engl J Med* 283, 409
Erythema multiforme
  (1975): Böttiger LE, *Acta Med Scand* 198, 229
Exanthems
  (1943): Davison TC, *Curr Res Anesth Analg* 22, 52
Exfoliative dermatitis (<1%)
  (1944): Potter JK+, *Ann Intern Med* 21, 1041
Fixed eruption
  (1970): Savin JA, *Br J Dermatol* 83, 546
Herpes simplex (activation)
Lupus erythematosus
  (1967): Williams DI, *Proc R Soc Med* 60, 299
  (1951): Grant Peterkin GA, *Edinb Med J* 58, 41
Necrosis
  (1972): Almeyda J+, *Br J Dermatol* 86, 313
Photosensitivity
  (1939): Stryker GV, *J Mo Med Assn* 36, 484
Pruritus
Purpura
  (1946): Grant Peterkin GA, *BMJ* 2, 52
Rash (sic) (<1%)
Stevens–Johnson syndrome (<1%)
Toxic epidermal necrolysis
  (1973): Stüttgen G, *Br J Dermatol* 88, 291
Urticaria
Vasculitis

Other
Headache

Hypersensitivity
Injection-site pain (1–10%)
Injection-site reactions (sic) (<1%)
Oral ulceration
Porphyria
  (1968): Lang PA+, *Tex Rep Biol Med* 26, 525
Porphyria variegata
Rhabdomyolysis
  (1990): Larpin R+, *Presse Med* 19(30), 1403
Thrombophlebitis (<1%)

PENTOSAN

Synonym: PPS
Trade name: Elmiron (Ortho-McNeil)
Indications: Bladder pain, interstitial cystitis
Category: Urinary analgesic
Half-life: 4.8 hours

Reactions

Skin
Allergic reactions (sic) (<1%)
Ecchymoses
Photosensitivity (<1%)
Pruritus (<1%)
Purpura (<1%)
Rash (sic) (1–10%)
Urticaria (<1%)

Hair
Hair – alopecia (1–10%)

Other
Gingivitis (<1%)
Headache
Oral ulceration (<1%)

PENTOSTATIN

Trade name: Nipent (SuperGen)
Indications: Hairy-cell leukemia
Category: Antimetabolite; Antineoplastic
Half-life: 5–15 hours
Clinically important, potentially hazardous interactions with: aldesleukin

Reactions

Skin
Acne (<3%)
Adverse effects (sic) (17%)
Allergic reactions (sic) (>10%)
Bullous eruption (3–10%)
Candidiasis (<3%)
Dermatitis (sic) (<1%)
Diaphoresis (3–10%)
Ecchymoses (3–10%)
Eczema (sic) (3–10%)
Erythema
Erythroderma
  (1999): Ghura HS+, *BMJ* 319, 549

Exanthems (3–10%)
  (1997): Greiner D+, J Am Acad Dermatol 36, 950
  (1989): O'Dwyer PJ+, Cancer Chemother Pharmacol 23, 173
Exfoliative dermatitis (<3%)
Facial edema (<3%)
Flushing (<3%)
Herpes simplex (3–10%)
Herpes zoster (3–10%)
Leukoplakia (<3%)
Peripheral edema (3–10%)
Petechiae (3–10%)
Photosensitivity (<3%)
Pigmentation (3–10%)
Pruritus (3–10%)
Psoriasis (<3%)
Purpura (<3%)
  (1999): Leach JW+, Am J Hematol 61, 268
Rash (sic) (26%)
Reactivation phenomenon (sic)
  (1989): Kerker BJ+, Semin Dermatol 8, 173
  (1985): Camisa C+, J Am Acad Dermatol 12, 1108
Seborrhea (3–10%)
Urticaria (<1%)
Xerosis (3–10%)

Hair
Hair – alopecia (<3%)

Other
Anaphylactoid reactions (<3%)
Dysgeusia (<3%)
Gingivitis (<3%)
Gynecomastia (<3%)
Headache
Injection-site hemorrhage (<3%)
Injection-site inflammation (<3%)
Myalgia (>10%)
Paresthesias (3–10%)
Stomatitis (1–10%)
Thrombophlebitis (3–10%)
Tinnitus
Vaginitis (<3%)

PENTOXIFYLLINE

Trade names: Pentoxil (Upsher-Smith); Trental (Aventis)
Other common trade names: Apo-Pentoxifylline; Artal; Azupentat; Elorgan; Hemovas; Pentoxi; Pexal; Torental
Indications: Peripheral vascular disease, intermittent claudication
Category: Blood viscosity reducing agent
Half-life: 0.4–0.8 hours

Reactions

Skin
Allergic reactions (sic)
  (1986): Bigby M+, JAMA 256, 3358
Angioedema (<1%)
  (1994): Samlaska CP+, J Am Acad Dermatol 30, 603 (passim)
Diaphoresis
Edema (<1%)
Exanthems
Flushing
  (1987): Ward A+, Drugs 34, 50 (2%)
  (1976): Drug Ther Bull 14, 59

Pruritus (<1%)
  (1994): Samlaska CP+, J Am Acad Dermatol 30, 603 (passim)
Purpura
Rash (sic) (<1%)
Urticaria

Nails
Nails – brittle (<1%)

Other
Dysgeusia (<1%)
Dysphagia
  (1997): Fetterman M, Miami, FL (from Internet) (observation)
  (1997): Puritz E, Smithtown, NY (from Internet) (observation)
Headache
Paresthesias
  (1994): Samlaska CP+, J Am Acad Dermatol 30, 603 (passim)
Serum sickness
  (1986): Panwalker AP+, Drug Intell Clin Pharm 20, 953
Sialorrhea (<1%)
Tremor
Xerostomia (<1%)
  (1994): Samlaska CP+, J Am Acad Dermatol 30, 603 (passim)

PEPPERMINT

Scientific name: Mentha piperita
Family: Labiatae
Trade and other common names: Aludrox; brandy mint; Colpermin; Enteroplant (peppermint and caraway oils); menthol; PCC
Category: Analgesic; Antemetic; Antiseptic; Carminative; Cholagogue; Choleretic; Diaphoretic; Disinfectant; Peripheral vasodilator; Spasmolytic
Purported indications and other uses: Dyspepsia, regress pancreatic, mammary, and liver tumors, irritable bowel syndrome, colonic spasm, colic, nausea, vomiting, biliary disorders, common cold, dysmenorrhoea, anxiolytic. Topical: pain, itching, inflammations, headaches, toothache, pruritus, urticaria, mosquito repellant. Vapor: bronchial catarrh, fever, influenza. Flavoring, cosmetics, toothpaste, mouthwash
Half-life: N/A
Clinically important, potentially hazardous interactions with: cisapride

Reactions

Skin
Adverse effects (sic)
  (1999): Madisch A+, Arzneimittelforschung 49(11), 925
  (1996): May B+, Arzneimittelforschung 46(12), 1149
Allergic reactions (sic)
  (1978): Andersen KE, Contact Dermatitis 4(4), 195
Burning (anal)
  (1987): Weston CF, Postgrad Med J 63(742), 717
Cheilitis
  (1995): Sainio EL+, Contact Dermatitis 33(2), 100
  (1984): Hausen BM, Dtsch Med Wochenschr 109(8), 300
Dermatitis
  (2002): Schempp CM+, Hautarzt 53(2), 93
  (1994): Wilkinson SM+, Contact Dermatitis 30(1), 42
  (1984): Mooller NE+, Acta Pharmacol Toxicol (Copenh) 55(2), 139 (occupational)
Lichenoid eruption
  (1995): Morton CA+, Contact Dermatitis 32(5), 281

Perioral dermatitis
   (1995): Sainio EL+, *Contact Dermatitis* 33(2), 100
Rash (sic)
   (1997): Liu JH+, *J Gastroenterol* 32(6), 765
Sensitivity
   (2001): Nair B, *Int J Toxicol* 20, 61
   (1995): Morton CA+, *Contact Dermatitis* 32(5), 281

Other

Burning mouth syndrome
   (1995): Morton CA+, *Contact Dermatitis* 32(5), 281
Gingivitis
   (1995): Sainio EL+, *Contact Dermatitis* 33(2), 100
Glossitis
   (1995): Sainio EL+, *Contact Dermatitis* 33(2), 100
Hypersensitivity
   (1995): Sainio EL+, *Contact Dermatitis* 33(2), 100
   (1977): Dooms-Goossens A+, *Contact Dermatitis* 3(6), 304
Oral mucosal ulceration
   (1999): Moghadam BK+, *Cutis* 64(2), 131 (mouthwash abuse)
   (1995): Morton CA+, *Contact Dermatitis* 32(5), 281
Side effects (sic)
   (1998): Belanger JT, *Altern Med Rev* 3(6), 448
   (1982): Jaffe G+, *J Int Med Res* 10(6), 437
Stomatitis
   (1995): Rogers SN+, *Dent Update* 22(1), 36
   (1995): Sainio EL+, *Contact Dermatitis* 33(2), 100
Toxicity
   (2001): Lazutka JR+, *Food Chem Toxicol* 39(5), 485

PERGOLIDE

Trade name: Permax (Amarin)
Other common trade names: *Celance; Parkotil; Pergolide*
Indications: Parkinsonism
Category: Antiparkinsonian; Dopamine receptor agonist; Ergot alkaloid
Half-life: 27 hours

Reactions

Skin

Acne
Chills (1–10%)
Diaphoresis (2.1%)
Discoloration (sic)
Edema (1.6%)
Exanthems
Facial edema (1.1%)
   (1993): Garcia-Escrig M+, *Medicina Clinica* (Spanish) 101, 275
Flu-like syndrome (sic) (1–10%)
Peripheral edema (1–10%)
Pruritus
Rash (sic) (3.2%)
Seborrhea
Ulcerations
Urticaria
Vasculitis
   (1989): Horn TD+, *Arch Dermatol* 125, 1512
Xerosis

Hair

Hair – alopecia
Hair – hirsutism

Other

Dysgeusia (1.6%)
Erythromelalgia
   (1989): Horn TD+, *Arch Dermatol* 125, 1512
   (1984): Monk BE+, *Br J Dermatol* 111, 97 (on shins)
Gingivitis (<1%)
Mastodynia
Myalgia (<1%)
Paresthesias (1.6%)
Priapism
Tinnitus
Tremor (1–10%)
Xerostomia (1–10%)

PERINDOPRIL

Trade name: Aceon (Solvay)
Other common trade names: *Acertil; Coversum; Coversyl; Prexum*
Indications: Hypertension
Category: Angiotensin-converting enzyme (ACE) inhibitor; Antihypertensive
Half-life: 1.5–3 hours

Reactions

Skin

Allergic reactions (sic) (1.3%)
   (1993): Desche P+, *Am J Cardiol* 71, 61E
Angioedema (<1%)
   (2001): Cohen EG+, *Ann Otol Rhinol Laryngol* 110(8), 701 (64 cases)
   (1998): Lapostolle F+, *Am J Cardiol* 81, 523 (lingual)
Chills (<1%)
Diaphoresis (0.3–1%)
Ecchymoses (0.3–1%)
Edema (3.9%)
Erythema (0.3–1%)
Exanthems
Facial edema (<1%)
Herpes simplex (0.3–1%)
Palmar–plantar pustulosis
   (1995): Eriksen JG+, *Ugeskr Laeger* (Danish) 157, 3335
Pemphigus foliaceus
   (2000): Ong CS+, *Australas J Dermatol* 41(4), 242
Pruritus (1–10%)
Psoriasis (<1%)
Purpura (<0.1%)
Rash (sic) (1–10%)
   (1991): Dratwa M+, *J Cardiovasc Pharmacol* 18, S40
Xerosis (0.3–1%)

Other

Anaphylactoid reactions (<1%)
   (1998): Speirs C+, *Br J Clin Pharmacol* 46, 63
Cough
   (2001): Adigun AQ+, *West Afr J Med* 20(1), 46–7
   (2001): Clark LT, *Am J Cardiol* 88(7), 36i
   (2001): Lee SC+, *Hypertension* 38(2), 166
Dysgeusia (<1%)
Headache
Myalgia (<1%)
Paresthesias (2.3%)
Vaginitis (0.3–1%)
Xerostomia (0.3–1%)

PERPHENAZINE

Trade names: Etrafon; Triavil (Lotus); Trilafon (Schering)
Other common trade names: *Apo-Perphenzine; Decentan; Fentazin; Leptopsique; Peratsin; Perphenan; Trilifan Retard; Triomin*
Indications: Psychotic disorders, nausea and vomiting
Category: Phenothiazine antipsychotic
Half-life: 9 hours
Clinically important, potentially hazardous interactions with: sparfloxacin

Etrafon and Triavil are combinations of perphenazine and amitriptyline

Reactions

Skin

Angioedema
Dermatitis
Diaphoresis
Eczema (sic)
Erythema
Exanthems
 (1976): Arndt KA+, *JAMA* 235, 918
 (1959): Wright W, *JAMA* 171, 1642
Exfoliative dermatitis
Lupus erythematosus
 (1988): Steen VD+, *Arthritis Rheum* 31, 923
 (1986): Gupta MA+, *J Am Acad Dermatol* 14, 638
 (1978): Gold MS+, *J Nerv Ment Dis* 166, 442
 (1971): Fabius AJM+, *Acta Rheum Scand* 17, 137
Peripheral edema
Photosensitivity
Pigmentation (blue-gray) (<1%)
Pruritus
Purpura
Rash (sic) (1–10%)
Seborrhea
Urticaria
 (1959): Wright W, *JAMA* 171, 1642
Xerosis

Other

Anaphylactoid reactions
Galactorrhea (black) (<1%)
 (1985): Basler RSW+, *Arch Dermatol* 121, 418
Gynecomastia
Headache
Mastodynia (1–10%)
Parkinsonism
Priapism (<1%)
Pseudolymphoma
 (1995): Magro CM+, *J Am Acad Dermatol* 32, 419
Rhabdomyolysis
 (1983): Caruana RJ+, *N C Med J* 44, 18 (with lorazepam and amitriptyline)
Sialorrhea
Tardive dyskinesia
 (1990): Miller LG+, *South Med J* 83(5), 525 (with amitriptyline) (30%)
Tinnitus
Xerostomia

PHELLODENDRON

Scientific names: *Phellodendron amurense; Phellodendron chinense; Phellodendron wilsonii*
Family: Rutaceae
Trade and other common names: Amur Cork-tree; Chuan huangbo; Cortex Phellodendri; Guan huangbo; Huang Bai; Nexrutine (Next Pharma); phellamurin. Ingredient in Oren-gedoku-to, zhi bai kuncao tang and Shangke Wangshui
Category: Antioxidant; Bactericide; COX-2 inhibitor; Immunosuppressant
Purported indications and other uses: anti-inflammatory, muscle and joint pain, gastroenteritis, abdominal pain, diarrhea, gastric ulcers, thrush, cholera, night sweats, fever, nocturnal emissions, dysentery, jaundice, leukorrhea, weakness and edema of legs, consumptive fever. Topical: sores, sores, skin infection with local redness and swelling, eczema with itching, periodontal disease (in dentifrice)
Half-life: N/A
Clinically important, potentially hazardous interactions with: aspirin, cyclosporine, NSAIDs

Reactions

Skin

Bleeding
Edema

Note: Should not be taken with impaired renal function, heart function, or hypertension

PHENAZOPYRIDINE

Trade names: Baridium; Geridium; Prodium; Pyridiate; Pyridium (Warner Chilcott)
Other common trade names: *Azodine; Eridium; Phenazo; Pyronium; Sedural; Urodine; Urogesic; Urohman; Uropyridin*
Indications: Urinary urgency, dysuria
Category: Urinary analgesic
Half-life: N/A

Reactions

Skin

Allergic reactions (sic)
 (1986): Bigby M+, *JAMA* 256, 3358 (0.88%)
Edema
Exanthems
 (1976): Arndt KA+, *JAMA* 235, 918 (0.6%)
Pigmentation (<1%)
 (1974): Eybel CE+, *JAMA* 228, 1027 (blue-gray; orange-yellow)
 (1970): Alano FA+, *Ann Intern Med* 72, 89
Pruritus
Rash (sic) (<1%)

Nails

Nails – yellow
 (1997): Amit G+, *Ann Intern Med* 127, 1137

Other

Anaphylactoid reactions
Headache

PHENDIMETRAZINE

Trade names: Bontril (Amarin); Prelu-2 (Roxane)
Other common trade name: *Obesan-X*
Indications: Obesity
Category: Appetite suppressant
Half-life: 5–12.5 hours
Clinically important, potentially hazardous interactions
with: fluoxetine, fluvoxamine, MAO inhibitors, paroxetine,
phenelzine, sertraline, tranylcypromine

Reactions

Skin
Diaphoresis
Flushing
Urticaria

Other
Dysgeusia
Headache
Xerostomia

PHENELZINE

Trade name: Nardil (Parke-Davis)
Other common trade name: *Nardelzine*
Indications: Depression
Category: Antidepressant; Monoamine oxidase (MAO) inhibitor
Half-life: N/A
Clinically important, potentially hazardous interactions
with: amitriptyline, amoxapine, amphetamines, bupropion,
citalopram, clomipramine, cyproheptadine, desipramine,
dextroamphetamine, dextromethorphan, diethylpropion,
dopamine, doxepin, entacapone, **ephedra**, ephedrine,
epinephrine, fluoxetine, fluvoxamine, **ginseng**, levodopa,
mazindol, meperidine, methamphetamine, nefazodone,
nortriptyline, paroxetine, phendimetrazine, phentermine,
phenylephrine, protriptyline, pseudoephedrine, rizatriptan,
sertraline, sibutramine, sumatriptan, sympathomimetics,
tramadol, tricyclic antidepressants, trimipramine, **tryptophan**,
venlafaxine, zolmitriptan

Reactions

Skin
Angioedema
  (1962): Busfield BL+, *J Nerv Ment Dis* 134, 339
Ankle edema
  (1977): Dunleavy DLF, *BMJ* 1, 1353
  (1970): Kelly D+, *Br J Psychiatry* 116, 387
Diaphoresis
  (1985): Levy AB+, *Can J Psychiatry* 30, 434
Edema
Exanthems
Lupus erythematosus
  (1978): Swartz C, *JAMA* 239, 2693
Peripheral edema (1–10%)
Photosensitivity
  (1988): Case JD+, *Photodermatology* 5, 101
  (1962): Busfield BL+, *J Nerv Ment Dis* 134, 339 (13%)
Pruritus (13%)
  (1962): Busfield BL+, *J Nerv Ment Dis* 134, 339

Rash (sic)
Telangiectasia
Urticaria

Other
Black tongue
Glossitis
  (1992): Zürcher K+, *Cutaneous Drug Reactions* Karger, Basel
    (passim)
Headache
Parkinsonism
Priapism
Rhabdomyolysis
  (1984): Linden CH+, *Ann Emerg Med* 13(12), 1137
Tremor
Twitching
Xerostomia (1–10%)
  (1962): Busfield BL+, *J Nerv Ment Dis* 134, 339 (20%)

PHENINDAMINE

Trade name: Nolahist (Carnrick)
Indications: Allergic rhinitis, urticaria, angioedema
Category: Antihistamine H_1-blocker
Half-life: N/A

Reactions

Skin
Angioedema
Dermatitis (sic)
Diaphoresis
Erythema
Flushing
Lupus erythematosus
Photosensitivity
Purpura
Rash (sic)
Urticaria

Other
Xerostomia

PHENOBARBITAL

Synonyms: phenobarbitone; phenylethylmalonylurea
Trade names: Barbita; Luminal (Sanofi-Synthelabo); Solfoton
(ECR)
Other common trade names: *Alepsal; Barbilixir; Barbital;*
Gardenal; Luminaletten; Phenaemal; Phenobarbitone
Indications: Insomnia, seizures
Category: Barbiturate sedative-hypnotic
Half-life: 2–6 days
Clinically important, potentially hazardous interactions
with: alcohol, anticoagulants, antihistamines, brompheniramine,
buclizine, chlorpheniramine, dicumarol, ethanolamine,
fluconazole, imatinib, meperidine, midazolam, warfarin

Reactions

Skin
Acne

(1992): Hesse S+, *Ann Dermatol Venereol* (French) 119, 655

Acute generalized exanthematous pustulosis (AGEP)
(1996): Wolkenstein P+, *Contact Dermatitis* 35, 234

Allergic reactions (sic)
(1987): Pigatto PD, *Contact Dermatitis* 16, 279
(1979): Montowska L+, *Pol Tyg Lek* (Polish) 34, 2029

Angioedema (<1%)

Bullous eruption
(1990): Dunn C+, *Cutis* 45, 43 (in coma)
(1970): Groeschel D+, *N Engl J Med* 283, 409
(1965): Beveridge GW+, *BMJ* 1, 835
(1940): Moss RE+, *Arch Dermatol* 46, 386
(1925): Birch CA, *Brit J Child Dis* 22, 280

Depigmentation
(1992): Mion N+, *Ann Dermatol Venereol* (French) 119, 927

Edema

Edema of foot
(1982): Stadler R+, *Hautarzt* (German) 33, 276

Erythema multiforme
(1994): Shelley WB+, *Cutis* 53, 162 (observation)
(1994): Stewart MG+, *Otolaryngol Head Neck Surg* 111, 236
(1990): Salomon D+, *Br J Dermatol* 123, 797
(1988): Shear NH+, *J Clin Invest* 82, 1826
(1986): Palomeque A+, *An Esp Pediatr* (Spanish) 34, 328
(1975): Böttiger LE, *Acta Med Scand* 198, 229
(1940): Moss RE+, *Arch Dermatol* 46, 386

Erythroderma
(1993): Sakai C+, *Intern Med* 32, 182

Exanthems
(2001): Hebert AA+, *J Clin Psychiatry* 62 (suppl 14), 22
(1997): Hyson C+, *Can J Neurol Sci* 24, 245
(1988): Shear NH+, *J Clin Invest* 82, 1826
(1986): Savich RD+, *Ill Med J* 169, 232
(1984): Fernandez de Corres L+, *Contact Dermatitis* 11, 319
(1979): Rudzki E, *Przegl Dermatol* (Polish) 66, 415
(1952): Sneddon IB+, *BMJ* 1, 1276
(1943): Davison TC, *Curr Res Anesth Analg* 22, 52
(1940): Moss RE+, *Arch Dermatol* 46, 386
(1925): Birch CA, *Brit J Child Dis* 22, 280

Exfoliative dermatitis (<1%)
(1993): Sakai C+, *Intern Med* 32, 182
(1986): Savich RD+, *Ill Med J* 169, 232
(1976): Weisburst M+, *South Med J* 69, 126
(1950): Welton DG, *JAMA* 143, 232
(1944): Potter JK+, *Ann Intern Med* 21, 1041
(1940): Moss RE+, *Arch Dermatol* 46, 386

Fixed eruption
(1998): Mahboob A+, *Int J Dermatol* 37, 833
(1989): Shiohara T+, *Arch Dermatol* 125, 1371
(1987): Savchak VI, *Vestn Dermatol Venerol* (Russian) 6, 62
(1979): Pasricha JS, *Br J Dermatol* 100, 183
(1974): Kuokkanen K, *Int J Dermatol* 13, 4 (genitalia and mucous membranes)
(1970): Savin JA, *Br J Dermatol* 83, 546
(1967): Schulz KH+, *Z Haut Geschlechtskr* (German) 42, 561

Graft-versus-host reaction
(1998): Jappe U+, *Hautarzt* (German) 49, 126 (passim)

Herpes simplex (activation)

Lupus erythematosus
(1967): Williams DI, *Proc R Soc Med* 60, 299
(1951): Grant Peterkin GA, *Edinb Med J* 58, 41

Necrosis
(1972): Almeyda J+, *Br J Dermatol* 86, 313

Pemphigus
(1986): Dourmishev AL+, *Dermatologica* 173, 256

Photosensitivity
(1939): Stryker GV, *J Mo Med Assn* 36, 484

Pruritus

(1994): Sigl B, *Hautarzt* (German) 45, 409

Purpura
(1952): Sneddon IB+, *BMJ* 1, 1276
(1946): Grant Peterkin GA, *BMJ* 2, 52

Pustules (generalized)
(1991): Kleier RS+, *Arch Dermatol* 127, 1361

Rash (sic) (<1%)

Stevens–Johnson syndrome (<1%)
(1999): Duncan KO, *J Am Acad Dermatol* 40, 493 (at sites of radiation therapy)
(1999): Rzany B+, *Lancet* 353, 2190
(1995): Labandiera-Garcia J, *An Med Interna* (Spanish) 12, 569
(1995): Wolkenstein P+, *Arch Dermatol* 131, 544
(1994): Koukoulis A+, *An Med Interna* (Spanish) 11, 311
(1993): Leenutaphong V+, *Int J Dermatol* 32, 428
(1992): Lleonart R+, *Med Clin (Barc)* (Spanish) 99, 474
(1985): Avery JK, *J Tenn Med Assoc* 78, 764
(1985): de Rego JA+, *Hillside J Clin Psychiatry* 7, 141
(1982): Brahams D, *Lancet* 2, 1474
(1982): Oles KS+, *Clin Pharm* 1, 565
(1971): Adeloye A+, *Ghana Med J* 10, 56

Toxic epidermal necrolysis
(2000): Devidal R+, *Therapie* 55, 225 (2 cases)
(1999): Rzany B+, *Lancet* 353, 2190
(1996): Blum L+, *J Am Acad Dermatol* 34, 1088
(1995): Wolkenstein P+, *Arch Dermatol* 131, 544
(1994): Errani A+, *Br J Dermatol* 131, 586
(1994): Shelley WB+, *Cutis* 53, 162 (observation)
(1993): Correia O+, *Dermatology* 186, 32
(1993): Leenutaphong V+, *Int J Dermatol* 32, 428
(1989): Dominguez-Perez F+, *Rev Esp Anestesiol Reanim* (Spanish) 36, 350
(1988): Shear NH+, *J Clin Invest* 82, 1826
(1987): Teillac D+, *Arch Fr Pediatr* (French) 44, 583
(1985): de Rego JA+, *Hillside J Clin Psychiatry* 7, 141
(1984): Chan HL, *J Am Acad Dermatol* 10, 973
(1975): Deviller G+, *Union Med Can* (French) 104, 399
(1975): Giallorenzi AF+, *Oral Surg Oral Med Oral Pathol* 40, 611
(1973): Stüttgen G, *Br J Dermatol* 88, 291
(1966): Campos EC de+, *An Bras Dermatol* (Portuguese) 41, 165
(1966): Haraszti A+, *Orv Hetil* (Hungarian) 107, 2133 (fatal)
(1966): Kaczorowska-Hanke H+, *Przegl Dermatol* (Polish) 53, 197

Toxicoderma (sic)
(1998): Arima M+, *Jpn Circ J* 62, 132

Urticaria
(1940): Moss RE+, *Arch Dermatol* 46, 386

Vasculitis

Hair

Hair – depigmentation
(1992): Mion N+, *Ann Dermatol Venereol* (French) 119, 927

Nails

Nails – hypoplasia
(1991): Thakker JC+, *Indian Pediatr* 28, 73
(1990): Holder M+, *Monatsschr Kinderheilkr* (German) 138, 34

Other

Acute intermittent porphyria
(2001): Sykes RM, *Seizure* 10(1), 64

Death

DRESS syndrome
(2001): Lachgar T+, *Allerg Immunol (Paris* (Paris) 33(4), 173
(1997): Descamps V+, *Br J Dermatol* 137, 605

Headache

Hypersensitivity (<1%)*
(2002): Metin A+, *World Congress Dermatol* Poster, 0116
(1999): Moss DM+, *J Emerg Med* 17, 503
(1998): Chapman MS+, *Br J Dermatol* 138, 710

(1998): Schlienger RG+, *Epilepsia* 39, S3 (passim)
(1997): Morkunas AR+, *Crit Care Clin* 13, 727
(1992): Nagata T+, *Jpn J Clin Oncol* 22, 421
(1984): Fonseca JC+, *Med Cutan Ibero Lat Am* (Spanish) 12, 187
Hypoplasia of phalanges
(1991): Thakker JC+, *Indian Pediatr* 28, 73
(1990): Holder M+, *Monatsschr Kinderheilkr* (German) 138, 34
Injection-site bullous eruption
(1987): Haroun M+, *Cutis* 39, 233
Injection-site pain (>10%)
Injection-site thrombophlebitis (>10%)
Oral ulceration
Porphyria cutanea tarda
(1966): Ziprkowski L+, *Isr J Med Sci* 2, 338
Porphyria variegata
Rhabdomyolysis
(1990): Larpin R+, *Presse Med* 19(30), 1403
Xerostomia
(1952): Sneddon IB+, *BMJ* 1, 1276

*Note: The antiepileptic drug hypersensitivity syndrome is a severe, occasionally fatal, disorder characterized by any or all of the following: pruritic exanthems, toxic epidermal necrolysis, Stevens–Johnson syndrome, exfoliative dermatitis, fever, hepatic abnormalities, eosinophilia, and renal failure

PHENOLPHTHALEIN

Trade names: Agoral; Alophen; Caroid; Correctol; Doxidan; Espotabs; Evac-U-Gen; Ex-Lax (Novartis); Feen-A-Mint; Medilax; Phenolax; Prulet; Trilax
Other common trade names: *Bom-Bon; Bonomint; Darmol; Easylax; Purganol; Ruguletts*
Indications: Constipation
Category: Laxative
Half-life: N/A

Reactions

Skin
Angioedema
(1972): Grillat JP+, *Rev Fr Allergie* (French) 12, 351
Bullous eruption
(1974): Magill M+, *Med J Aust* 1, 771
Diaphoresis
Erythema annulare (sic)
(1972): Grillat JP+, *Rev Fr Allergie* (French) 12, 351
Erythema multiforme
(1992): Breathnach SM+, *Adverse Drug Reactions and the Skin* Blackwell, Oxford, 344
(1972): Shelley WB+, *Br J Dermatol* 86, 118
Exanthems
(1972): Grilliat JP+, *Rev Fr Allergol* (French) 12, 351
(1969): Török H, *Dermatol Int* 8, 57
Exfoliative dermatitis
(1973): Nicolis GD+, *Arch Dermatol* 108, 788
Fixed eruption
(1997): Blumenthal HL, Beachwood, OH (personal case) (observation)
(1993): Zanolli MD+, *Pediatrics* 91, 1199
(1991): Smoller BR+, *J Cutan Pathol* 18, 13
(1990): Gaffoor PMA+, *Cutis* 45, 242
(1987): Stroud MB+, *Arch Dermatol* 123, 1227
(1986): Kanwar AJ+, *Dermatologica* 172, 315
(1985): Kauppinen K+, *Br J Dermatol* 112, 575

(1984): Chan HL, *Int J Dermatol* 23, 607
(1978): Sehgal VN+, *Int J Dermatol* 17, 78
(1972): Hunziker N, *Rev Med Suisse Romande* (French) 92, 237
(1972): Louis P, *Z Haut Geschlechtskr* (German) 47, 387
(1972): Shelley WB+, *Br J Dermatol* 86, 118 (bullous)
(1972): Wyatt E+, *Arch Dermatol* 106, 671
(1970): Savin JA, *Br J Dermatol* 83, 546
(1969): Török H, *Dermatol Int* 8, 57
(1967): Schulz KH+, *Z Haut Geschlechtskr* (German) 42, 561
(1964): Browne SG, *BMJ* 2, 1041
Lupus erythematosus
(1992): Breathnach SM+, *Adverse Drug Reactions and the Skin* Blackwell, Oxford, 344
Perianal irritation
Pigmentation
(1973): Levantine A+, *Br J Dermatol* 89, 105
Pruritus
(1972): Grillat JP+, *Rev Fr Allergie* (French) 12, 351
Stevens–Johnson syndrome
(1972): Monnat A, *Schweiz Med Wochenschr* (French) 102, 1876
Toxic epidermal necrolysis
(1997): Artymowicz RJ+, *Ann Pharmacother* 31, 1157
(1986): Kar PK+, *J Indian Med Assoc* 84, 189
(1973): Björnberg A, *Acta Dermatol Venereol* (Stockh) 53, 149
(1973): Khamadullin LG, *Vestn Dermatol Venerol* (Russian) 47, 67
(1972): Monnat A, *Schweiz Med Wochenschr* (French) 102, 1876
(1967): Lowney ED+, *Arch Dermatol* 95, 359
(1966): Témime P+, *Bull Soc Fr Dermatol Syphiligr* (French) 73, 305
(1961): Browne SG+, *BMJ* 1, 550
(1957): Lang R+, *S Afr Med J* 31, 713
Urticaria
(1972): Grillat JP+, *Rev Fr Allergie* (French) 12, 351

Nails
Nails – discoloration
(1984): Daniel CR+, *J Am Acad Dermatol* 10, 250

Other
Oral mucosal fixed eruption
Oral mucosal pigmentation
Oral mucosal ulceration

PHENOXYBENZAMINE

Trade name: Dibenzyline (Wellspring)
Other common trade names: *Dibenyline; Dibenzyran*
Indications: Pheochromocytoma
Category: Alpha-adrenoceptor blocker; Antihypertensive
Half-life: 24 hours
Clinically important, potentially hazardous interactions with: epinephrine

Reactions

Skin
Allergic reactions (sic)
(1973): Alexander SL+, *Lancet* 1, 317
Dermatitis
(1975): MitchellJC+, *Contact Dermatitis* 1, 363

Other
Priapism
(1974): Funderburk SJ+, *N Engl J Med* 290, 630
Xerostomia (1–10%)

PHENSUXIMIDE

Trade name: Milontin (Parke-Davis)
Indications: Petit mal seizures
Category: Anticonvulsant
Half-life: 5–12 hours

Reactions

Skin
Erythema multiforme (<1%)
Lupus erythematosus
Periorbital edema
Pruritus
Purpura
  (1980): Miescher PA+, *Clin Haematol* 9, 505
Rash (sic)
Stevens–Johnson syndrome

Hair
Hair – alopecia
Hair – hirsutism

Other
Acute intermittent porphyria
Gingival hyperplasia
Oral ulceration

PHENTERMINE

Trade names: Adipex-P (Gate); Fastin (GSK); Ionamin (Celltech)
Other common trade names: *Behapront; Diminex; Minobese-Forte; Panbesy; Panbesyl; Redusa; Umine; Zantryl*
Indications: Obesity
Category: Appetite suppressant (anorexiant)
Half-life: 19–24 hours
Clinically important, potentially hazardous interactions with: fluoxetine, fluvoxamine, MAO inhibitors, paroxetine, phenelzine, sertraline, tranylcypromine

Reactions

Skin
Diaphoresis (<1%)
Peripheral edema
Peripheral vasculopathy (sic)
  (1999): Jefferson HJ+, *Nephrol Dial Transplant* 14, 1761
Purpura
Rash (sic)
Raynaud's phenomenon
  (1990): Aeschlimann A+, *Scand J Rheumatol* 19, 87
Urticaria

Hair
Hair – alopecia (<1%)

Other
Dysgeusia
Headache
Myalgia (<1%)
Tremor
Xerostomia

PHENTOLAMINE

Trade name: Regitine (Novartis)
Other common trade names: *Regitin; Rogitene; Rogitine*
Indications: Hypertensive episodes in pheochromocytoma
Category: Alpha-adrenoceptor blocker; Antihypertensive; Diagnostic aid (pheochromocytoma)
Half-life: 19 minutes

Reactions

Skin
Flushing (1–10%)

Other
Priapism

PHENYLEPHRINE

Trade names: Dura-Vent (Biovail); IEntex (Elan); Neo-Synephrine (Sanofi-Synthelabo); Prolex-D (Blansett); Rynatan (Wallace); Tussi-12D (Wallace); Vasosulf (Novartis)
Other common trade names: *Dionephrine; Novahistine; Prefrin Liquifilm*
Indications: Nasal congestion, glaucoma, hypotension
Category: Alpha-adrenoceptor blocker; Mydriatic ophthalmic agent
Half-life: 2.5 hours
Clinically important, potentially hazardous interactions with: epinephrine, furazolidone, MAO inhibitors, phenelzine, tranylcypromine

Reactions

Skin
Dermatitis
  (2002): Erdmann SM+, *Am J Contact Dermat* 13(1), 37
  (1999): Resano A+, *J Invest Allergol Clin Immunol* 9, 55
    (blepharoconjunctivitis)
  (1998): Rafael M+, *Contact Dermatitis* 39, 143
    (blepharoconjunctivitis)
  (1998): Thomas P+, *Contact Dermatitis* 38, 41
    (blepharoconjunctivitis)
  (1998): Wigger-Alberti W+, *Allergy* 53, 217
    (blepharoconjunctivitis)
  (1997): Mancuso G+, *Contact Dermatitis* 36, 110
  (1997): Marcos ML+, *Contact Dermatitis* 37, 189
  (1997): Moreno-Ancillo M+, *Ann Allergy Asthma Immunol* 78, 569
    (periorbital)
  (1997): Ockenfels HM+, *Dermatology* 195, 119 (periorbital)
  (1995): Thomas P+, *Contact Dermatitis* 32, 249
  (1993): Wilkinson SM+, *Contact Dermatitis* 29, 100
  (1991): Anibarro B+, *Contact Dermatitis* 25, 323
    (blepharoconjunctivitis)
  (1991): Bardazzi F+, *Contact Dermatitis* 24, 56
  (1991): Okamoto H+, *Cutis* 47, 357
  (1990): Zucchi A+, *G Ital Dermatol Venereol* (Italian) 125, 155
  (1986): Ducombs G+, *Contact Dermatitis* 15, 107
  (1984): Camarasa JG, *Contact Dermatitis* 10, 182
  (1983): Hanna C+, *Am J Ophthalmol* 95, 703
  (1983): Rarber KA, *Contact Dermatitis* 9, 274 (periorbital)
  (1979): De Vita L+, *Minerva Pediatr* (Italian) 31, 535
  (1979): Mathias CG+, *Arch Ophthalmol* 97, 286
Pallor
Periorbital edema

(1998): Blum A+, *Hautarzt* (German) 49, 651
Stinging (from nasal or ophthalmic preparations) (1–10%)

Other
Headache
Hypersensitivity
(1991): Quirce Gancedo S+, *Med Clin (Barc)* (Spanish) 96, 317
Injection-site reactions
Paresthesias
Tremor

PHENYLPROPANOLAMINE

Synonym: PPA
Trade names: Acutrim; BC Cold Powder; Control; Dex-a-Diet; Dexatrim; Diet Gum; Genex; Maigret-50; Phenoxine; Phenyldrine; Prolamine; Propagest; Propandrine; Rhindecon; Spray-U-Thin; St. Joseph Aspirin-Free Cold Tablets (McNeil); Stay Trim; Unitrol; Westrim
Indications: Nasal decongestion, anorexiant
Category: Adrenergic agonist; Anorexiant; Nasal decongestant; Sympathomimetic
Half-life: 3–4 hours
Clinically important, potentially hazardous interactions with: caffeine, ephedra, ephedrine, fluoxetine, fluvoxamine, furazolidone, paroxetine, sertraline, tranylcypromine

Reactions

Skin
Fixed eruption
(2000): Heikkila H+, *Br J Dermatol* 142(4), 845
Pallor

Other
Death
(1984): Logie AW+, *Br Med J* 289(6445), 591
(1983): Mueller SM, *N Engl J* 308(11), 653
Depression
Rhabdomyolysis
(1983): Blewitt GA+, *JAMA* 249(22), 3017
(1983): Hampel G+, *Hum Toxicol* 2(2), 197
(1983): Rumpf KW+, *JAMA* 250(16), 2112
(1982): Swenson RD+, *JAMA* 248(10), 1216
Tremor
Xerostomia

PHENYTOIN

Synonyms: diphenylhydantoin; DPH; phenytoin sodium
Trade names: Dilantin (Parke-Davis); Phenytek (Bertek)
Other common trade names: *Di-Hydran; Diphenylan; Epanutin; Fenytoin; Phenhydan; Pyoredol; Zentropil*
Indications: Grand mal seizures
Category: Antiarrhythmic; Hydantoin anticonvulsant
Half-life: 7–42 hours (dose dependent)
Clinically important, potentially hazardous interactions with: amprenavir, aprepitant, calcium, chloramphenicol, cimetidine, clorazepate, cyclosporine, delavirdine, diazoxide, disulfiram, dopamine, fluconazole, fluoxetine, **ginkgo biloba**, imatinib, indinavir, isoniazid, itraconazole, meperidine, midazolam, nelfinavir, **primrose**, ritonavir, **sage**, saquinavir, **St John's wort**, sucralfate

An excellent overview of cutaneous reactions to phenytoin can be found in (1988): Silverman AK+, *J Am Acad Dermatol* 18, 721

Note: About 19% of patients receiving phenytoin develop skin reactions (1983): Rapp RP+, *Neurosurg* 13, 272. They typically develop 10 to 14 days following the start of treatment

Reactions

Skin
Acne
(1993): Shah M+, *Eur J Dermatol* 3, 576
(1990): Grunwald MH+, *Int J Dermatol* 29, 559
(1983): Greenwood R+, *Br Med J Clin Res Ed* 287, 1669
(1980): Stankler L+, *Br J Dermatol* 103, 453 (neonatal)
(1977): Frentz G, *Ugeskr Laeger* (Danish) 139, 338
(1972): Jenkins RB+, *N Engl J Med* 287, 148
(1964): Fegeler F, *Arch Klin Exp Derm* (German) 219, 335
Acute generalized exanthematous pustulosis (AGEP)
(2001): Burrow W, Jackson, MS (from Internet) (observation)
(1995): Moreau A+, *Int J Dermatol* 34, 263 (passim)
Angioedema
(1992): Schlaifer D+, *Eur J Hematol* 48, 274
(1967): Coleman WP, *Med Clin North Am* 51, 1073
Bullous eruption
(1988): Baird BJ+, *Int J Dermatol* 27, 170
Dermatomyositis
(1998): Dimachkie MM+, *J Child Neurol* 13, 577
Edema of feet
(2002): Kaur S+, *Pediatr Dermatol* 19(1), 93
Edema of foot
Eosinophilic fasciitis
(1980): Buchanan RR+, *J Rheumatol* 7, 733
Epidermolysis bullosa
(1982): Bergfeld WF+, *J Am Acad Dermatol* 7, 275
Erythema multiforme
(2001): Bravo F, Lima, Peru (from Internet) (observation)
(1999): Marinella MA, *Ann Pharmacother* 33, 748
(1999): Micali G+, *Pharmacotherapy* 19, 223 (with cranial irradiation)
(1995): Rodriguez-Castellanos M+, *Arch Dermatol* 131, 620
(1990): Giroud M+, *Therapie* (French) 45, 23
(1988): Delattre JY+, *Neurology* 38, 194
(1988): Shear NH+, *J Clin Invest* 82, 1826
(1986): Green ST, *Clin Neuropharmacol* 9, 561
(1985): Tucker MS+, *J Am Osteopath Assoc* 85, 511
(1972): Almeyda J+, *Br J Dermatol* 87, 646
(1967): Coleman WP, *Med Clin North Am* 51, 1073
Erythroderma
(1996): Chopra S+, *Br J Dermatol* 134, 1109

(1991): Yamashina T+, *Nippon Shokakibyo Gakkai Zasshi* (Japanese) 88, 1269
(1983): Lillie MA+, *Arch Dermatol* 119, 415
(1966): Fischbeck R+, *Dtsch Gesundheitsw* (German) 21, 1273

Exanthems
(2000): Cohen AD+, *Isr Med Assoc J* 1, 95
(1997): Hyson C+, *Can J Neurol Sci* 24, 245
(1996): Leong KP+, *Asian Pac J Allergy Immunol* 14, 65 (71.4%)
(1992): Tone T+, *J Dermatol* 19, 27
(1991): Pelekanos J+, *Epilepsia* 32, 554
(1988): Shear NH+, *J Clin Invest* 82, 1826
(1984): Chadwick D+, *J Neurol Neurosurg Psychiatry* 47, 642 (6%)
(1983): Rapp RP+, *Neurosurgery* 13, 272
(1978): Wilson JT+, *BMJ* 1, 1583
(1975): Weedon AP, *Aust NZ J Med* 5, 561
(1970): Robinson HM+, *Arch Dermatol* 101, 462
(1969): Levene G+, *Br J Dermatol* 81, 712
(1967): Coleman WP, *Med Clin North Am* 51, 1073

Exfoliative dermatitis
(1997): Westhoven GS+, *Arch Dermatol* 133, 494
(1996): Leong KP+, *Asian Pac J Allergy Immunol* 14, 65 (2.4%)
(1996): Sigurdsson V+, *J Am Acad Dermatol* 35, 53
(1989): Danno K+, *J Dermatol* (Tokio) 16, 392
(1985): Matson JR+, *Hum Pathol* 16, 94
(1983): Rapp RP+, *Neurosurgery* 13, 272
(1972): Almeyda J+, *Br J Dermatol* 87, 646
(1963): Beerman H+, *Arch Dermatol* 87, 783
(1958): Chaiken BH+, *N Engl J Med* 242, 897
(1956): Gropper AL, *N Engl J Med* 254, 522
(1948): Van Wyck JJ+, *Arch Intern Med* 81, 605
(1942): Ritchie EB+, *Arch Dermatol* 46, 856

Fixed eruption
(1997): Chan HL+, *J Am Acad Dermatol* 36, 259
(1988): Baird BJ+, *Int J Dermatol* 27, 170 (bullous)
(1963): Goldstein N+, *Arch Dermatol* 87, 612

Heel pad thickening
(1975): Kattan KR, *AJR* 124, 52

Lichen planus
(1991): MacLeod SP+, *Br Dent J* 171, 237

Lichenoid eruption
(1992): Tone T+, *J Dermatol* 19, 27

Linear IgA bullous dermatosis
(2002): Cohen LM+, *J Am Acad Dermatol* 46(2), S32 (passim)
(1998): Acostamadiedo JM+, *J Am Acad Dermatol* 38, 352
(1994): Kuechle MK+, *J Am Acad Dermatol* 30, 187

Lupus erythematosus
(2002): Ross S+, *Clin Exp Dermatol* 27(6), 474
(1993): Drory VE+, *Clin Neuropharmacol* 16, 19 (passim)
(1988): Jiang M, *Chung Kuo I Hsueh Ko Hsueh Yuan Hsueh Pao* (Chinese) 10, 379
(1985): Lovisetto P+, *Recenti Prog Med* (Italian) 76, 84
(1984): Wollina U, *Z Gesamte Int Med* (German) 39, 69
(1982): Gleichman H, *Arthritis Rheum* 25, 1387
(1981): Grossman J+, *Arthritis Rheum* 24, 927
(1977): Rybicka K+, *Pol Tyg Lek* (Polish) 32, 1269
(1976): Singsen BH+, *Pediatrics* 57, 529
(1974): Harpey JP, *Ann Allergy* 33, 256
(1970): Okuda M+, *Naika* (Japanese) 26, 989
(1967): Siegel M+, *Arthritis Rheum* 10, 407
(1966): Lee SL+, *Arch Intern Med* 117, 620
(1963): Goldstein N+, *Arch Dermatol* 87, 612
(1963): Jacobs JC, *Pediatrics* 32, 257
(1962): Benton JW+, *JAMA* 180, 115

Lymphoma (<1%)
(1985): Wolf R+, *Arch Dermatol* 121, 1181
(1978): Wilden JN+, *J Clin Pathol* 31, 761
(1975): Bichel J, *Acta Med Scand* 198, 327
(1975): Li FP+, *Cancer* 36, 1359
(1970): Anthony JJ, *Arch Neurol* 22, 450

Mucocutaneous lymph node syndrome
(1979): Anderson VM+, *Cutis* 23, 493

Mycosis fungoides
(1991): Rijlaarsdam U+, *J Am Acad Dermatol* 24(2 Pt 2), 216 (with carbamazepine)
(1990): Souteyrand P+, *Curr Probl Dermatol* 19, 176
(1985): Wolf R+, *Arch Dermatol* 121, 1181
(1982): Rosenthal CH+, *Cancer* 49, 2305

Necrosis
(2001): Bravo F, Lima, Peru (from Internet) (observation)

Pemphigus
(1988): Seghal VN+, *Int J Dermatol* 27, 258

Pigmentation
(1964): Kuske H+, *Dermatologica* 129, 121

Pruritus
(2002): Coplin WM+, *Neurol Res* 24(8), 842
(1997): Litt JZ, Beachwood, OH (personal case) (observation)
(1985): Rubinstein N+, *Int J Dermatol* 24, 54
(1967): Coleman WP, *Med Clin North Am* 51, 1073
(1963): Beerman H+, *Arch Dermatol* 87, 783

Pseudoacanthosis nigricans
(1972): Petko E+, *Arch Dermatol* 106, 918

Purple glove syndrome (sic)
(2001): Endoh T+, *No To Hattatsu* 33(5), 442
(2000): Schmutz J+, *Ann Dermatol Venereol* (French) 127, 548
(2000): Yoshikawa H+, *J Child Neurol* 15(11), 762
(1998): Cadenbach A+, *Dtsch Med Wochenschr* (German) 123, 318
(1994): Helfaer MA+, *J Neurosurg Anesthesiol* 6, 48

Purpura
(1975): Targan SR+, *Ann Intern Med* 83, 227 (fulminans)
(1967): Coleman WP, *Med Clin North Am* 51, 1073
(1963): Beerman H+, *Arch Dermatol* 87, 783
(1962): Weintraub RM+, *JAMA* 180, 528

Pustules
(1993): O'Brien TJ+, *Australas J Dermatol* 34, 128
(1991): Kleier RS, *Arch Dermatol* 127, 1361
(1978): Stanley J+, *Arch Dermatol* 114, 1350

Rash (sic) (1–10%)
(2001): Aihara M+, *Br J Dermatol* 144, 1231
(1999): Mamon HJ+, *Epilepsia* 40, 341 (with cranial radiation)
(1987): Maguire JH+, *Br J Clin Pharmacol* 24, 554

Reticular hyperplasia
(1975): Wasik F+, *Hautarzt* (German) 26, 273
(1966): Korting GW+, *Dermatol Wochenschr* (German) 152, 257

Rhinophyma
(2000): Jaramillo MJ+, *Br J Plast Surg* 53(6), 521

Scleroderma
(1974): Kashiwazaki S+, *Ryumachi* (Japanese) 14, 220

Sezary syndrome
(1994): Doyle MF+, *Acta Hematol* 92, 204

Sjøgren's syndrome
(1996): Chakravarty K+, *Br J Rheumatol* 35, 1033

Stevens–Johnson syndrome
(2001): Eralp Y+, *Am J Clin Oncol* 24(4), 347
(2000): Madnani NA, Mumbai, India (from Internet) (observation)
(1999): Khafaga YM+, *Acta Oncol* 38, 111 (with cranial irradiation)
(1999): Ruble R+, *CNS Drugs* 12, 215
(1999): Rzany B+, *Lancet* 353, 2190
(1996): Cockey G+, *Am J Clin Oncol* 19, 32 (with irradiation of brain)
(1996): Leong KP+, *Asian Pac J Allergy Immunol* 14, 65 (14.3%)
(1995): Borg M+, *Australas Radiol* 39, 42 (with irradiation of brain)
(1995): Cockey GH+, *Am J Clin Oncol* 19, 32
(1995): Wolkenstein P+, *Arch Dermatol* 131, 544
(1994): Marti J+, *An Med Interna* (Spanish) 11, 621

(1993): Janinis J+, *Eur J Cancer* 29A, 478 (with cranial irradiation)
(1993): Leenutaphong V+, *Int J Dermatol* 32, 428
(1993): Schlienger RG+, *Schweiz Rundsch Med Prax* (German) 82, 888
(1992): Tone T+, *J Dermatol* 19, 27
(1989): Kelly DF+, *Neurosurgery* 25, 976
(1988): Delattre JY+, *Neurology* 38, 194 (with cranial irradiation)
(1988): Shear NH+, *J Clin Invest* 82, 1826
(1985): Burge SM+, *J Am Acad Dermatol* 13, 665
(1985): de Rego JA+, *Hillside J Clin Psychiatry* 7, 141
(1985): Maiche A+, *Lancet* 2, 45 (with radiation therapy)
(1982): Oles KS+, *Clin Pharm* 1, 565
(1978): Assaad D+, *Can Med Assoc* 118, 154
(1976): Marg E, *Psychiatr Neurol Med Psychol Leipz* (German) 28, 436
(1971): Greenberg LM+, *Ann Ophthalmol* 3, 137
(1970): Rudner EJ, *Arch Dermatol* 102, 561

Toxic dermatitis (sic)
(1978): Huijgens PC+, *Acta Haematol* 59, 31

Toxic epidermal necrolysis
(2000): Cohen AD+, *Isr Med Assoc J* 1, 95 (2 patients)
(2000): Moussala M+, *J Fr Ophtalmol* (French) 23, 229
(1999): Cohen AD+, *Isr Med Assoc J* 1, 95 (2 cases)
(1999): Egan CA+, *J Am Acad Dermatol* 40, 458 (3 cases)
(1999): Ruble R+, *CNS Drugs* 12, 215
(1999): Rzany B+, *Lancet* 353, 2190
(1997): Jester BA+, American Academy of Dermatology Meeting (SF), Poster #163
(1997): Redondo Bellon P, *Rev Neurol* 25, S309
(1997): Sapadin A+, American Academy of Dermatology Meeting (SF), Poster #111 (with radiation)
(1996): Creamer JD+, *Clin Exp Dermatol* 21, 116
(1996): Frangogiannis NG+, *South Med J* 89, 1001
(1996): Leong KP+, *Asian Pac J Allergy Immunol* 14, 65 (2.4%)
(1995): Pion IA+, *N Engl J Med* 333, 1609
(1993): Janinis J+, *Eur J Cancer* 29A, 478
(1993): Leenutaphong V+, *Int J Dermatol* 32, 428
(1992): Tone T+, *J Dermatol* 19, 27
(1991): Rowe JE+, *Int J Dermatol* 30, 747
(1989): Kelly DF+, *Neurosurgery* 25, 976
(1989): Renfro L+, *Int J Dermatol* 28, 441
(1988): Dreyfuss DA+, *Ann Plast Surg* 20, 146
(1987): Birchall N+, *J Am Acad Dermatol* 16, 368
(1985): Burge SM+, *J Am Acad Dermatol* 13, 665
(1985): Muhar U, *Pediatr Dermatology* 3, 54
(1985): Sherertz EF+, *J Am Acad Dermatol* 12, 178
(1984): Chan HL, *J Am Acad Dermatol* 10, 973
(1984): Smith DA+, *J Am Acad Dermatol* 10, 106 (followed by universal depigmentation)
(1983): Schmidt D+, *Epilepsia* 24, 440 (fatal)
(1982): Peterson KA+, *Md State Med J* 31, 53
(1981): Spechler SJ+, *Ann Intern Med* 95, 455
(1979): Gately LE+, *Ann Intern Med* 91, 59
(1979): Lyell A, *Br J Dermatol* 100, 69
(1978): Assaad D+, *Can Med Assoc* 118, 154
(1975): Giallorenzi AF+, *Oral Surg Oral Med Oral Pathol* 40, 611
(1975): Schopf E+, *Z Hautkr* (German) 50, 865
(1968): Rodriguez-Adrados J+, *Rev Clin Esp* (Spanish) 110, 267
(1967): Coleman WP, *Med Clin North Am* 51, 1073
(1967): Vandvik IH, *Tidsskr Nor Laegeforen* (Norwegian) 87, 1068

Urticaria
(1995): Rodriguez-Castellanos M+, *Arch Dermatol* 131, 620
(1967): Coleman WP, *Med Clin North Am* 51, 1073
(1951): Jones DP, *BMJ* 1, 64

Vasculitis
(1999): Holt P, *N Z Med J* 112, 100
(1996): Leong KP+, *Asian Pac J Allergy Immunol* 14, 65 (2.4%)
(1996): Parry RG+, *Nephrol Dial Transplant* 11, 357
(1993): Drory VE+, *Clin Neuropharmacol* 16, 19 (passim)
(1983): Yermakov VM+, *Hum Pathol* 14, 182

(1967): Hass P, *Wiener Klin Wochenschr* (German) 75, 56

Warts
(1998): Kayal JD+, *Cutis* 61, 101

Hair

Hair – alopecia
(1984): Smith DA+, *J Am Acad Dermatol* 10, 106
(1973): Levantine A+, *Br J Dermatol* 89, 549

Hair – hirsutism
(1989): Backman K+, *Scand J Dent Res* 97, 222
(1989): Vivard P+, *Ann Dermatol Venereol* (French) 116, 562
(1972): Leng JJ+, *Pediatr Clin North Am* 19, 681
(1972): Levantine A+, *Br J Dermatol* 87, 646
(1970): Herberg KP, *South Med J* 70, 19

Hair – hypertrichosis
(2001): Oakley A, Hamilton, NZ (from Internet) (observation)
(1989): Rousseau C+, *Dermatologica* 179, 221

Nails

Nails – changes
(1981): Krebs A, *Schweiz Rundsch Med Prax* (German) 70, 1951
(1975): Hanson JW+, *J Pediatrics* 87, 285

Nails – hypoplasia
(1991): D'Souza SW+, *Arch Dis Child* 66, 320
(1981): Johnson RB+, *J Am Acad Dermatol* 5, 191
(1978): Prakash P+, *Indian Pediatr* 15, 866

Nails – onychopathy
(1988): Verdeguer JM+, *Pediatr Dermatol* 5, 56

Nails – pigmentation
(1981): Johnson RB+, *J Am Acad Dermatol* 5, 191

Other

Acromegaloid features
(1972): Lefebvre EB+, *N Engl J Med* 286, 1301

Acute intermittent porphyria
(1989): Herrick AL+, *Br J Clin Pharmacol* 27, 491

Ageusia
(1998): Henkin RI, *Lancet* 352, 68
(1998): Zeller JA+, *Lancet* 351, 1101

Coarse facies (sic)
(1973): Falconer MA+, *Lancet* 2, 1112
(1972): Lefebvre EB+, *Med Intell* 286, 1301

Death

Digital malformations
(1981): Johnson RB+, *J Am Acad Dermatol* 5, 191
(1978): Prakash P+, *Indian Pediatr* 15, 866
(1974): Barr M+, *J Pediatr* 84, 254 (hypoplasia)

Fetal hydantoin syndrome*
(1998): Ozkinay F+, *Turk J Pediatr* 40, 273 (2 siblings)
(1994): Buehler BA+, *Neurol Clin* 12, 741
(1989): Nanda A+, *Pediatr Dermatol* 6, 130
(1989): Nanda A+, *Pediatr Dermatol* 6, 66
(1988): Verdeguer JM+, *Pediatr Dermatol* 5, 56
(1983): Tomsick RS, *Cutis* 32, 535
(1981): Nagy R, *Arch Dermatol* 117, 593

Gingival hyperplasia (>10%)
(2001): Brunet L+, *Eur J Clin Invest* 31(9), 781
(2001): Uzel MI+, *J Periodontol* 72(7), 921
(1999): Kamali F+, *J Periodontal Res* 34, 145
(1999): Wood WH, San Jose, CA (from Internet) (observation)
(1998): Desai P+, *J Can Dent Assoc* 64, 263
(1998): Garzino-Demo P+, *Minerva Somatol* (Italian) 47, 387
(1998): Mattson JS+, *J Am Dent Assoc* 129, 78
(1998): Meraw SJ+, *Mayo Clin Proc* 73, 1196
(1997): Iacopino AM+, *J Periodontol* 68, 73
(1997): Mattioli A, *Minerva Stomatol* (Italian) 46, 525
(1997): Newland JR, *J Gt House Dent Soc* 69, 3
(1997): Silverstein LH+, *Gen Dent* 45, 371
(1996): Hayakawa I+, *Quintessence Int* 27, 235
(1996): Saito K+, *J Periodontol Res* 31, 545

(1995): Moghadam BKH+, *Cutis* 56, 46 (passim)
(1993): Lipton JM+, *J Indiana Dent Assoc* 72, 18
(1991): Hassell TM+, *Crit Rev Oral Biol Med* 2, 103
(1990): Hall WB, *Compendium* (Suppl) 14, 502
(1989): Backman K+, *Scand J Dent Res* 97, 222
(1989): Dooley G+, *J N Z Soc Periodontol* 68, 19
(1987): Norris JF+, *Int J Dermatol* 26, 602
(1987): Stinnett E+, *J Am Dent Assoc* 114, 814
(1976): Hassell TM+, *Proc Nat Acad Sci* 73, 2909
(1975): Angelopoulos AP, *J Can Dent Assoc* 2, 102

Gynecomastia
(1998): Ikeda A+, *J Neurol Neurosurg Psychiatry* 65, 803

Headache

Hypersensitivity syndrome**
(2002): Metin A+, *World Congress Dermatol* Poster, 0116
(2002): Nagai Y+, *J Dermatol* 29(10), 670
(2001): Aihara M+, *Br J Dermatol* 144, 1231
(2001): Bessmertny O+, *Ann Pharmacother* 35(5), 533
(2001): Gungor E+, *Neurol Sci* 22(3), 261
(2001): Klassen BD+, *Epilepsia* 42(3), 433
(2001): Nashed MH+, *Pharmacotherapy* 21(4), 502
(2000): Cohen AD+, *Isr Med Assoc J* 1, 95
(2000): Colombo-Arnet E, *Schweiz Rundsch Med Prax* (German) 89, 675
(2000): Lynfield Y, Brooklyn, NY (from Internet) (observation)
(2000): Moore SJ+, *J Med Genet* 37, 489
(2000): Troger U+, *Int J CLin Pharmacol Ther* 38(9), 452
(1999): Hamer HM+, *Seizure* 8, 190
(1999): Moss DM+, *J Emerg Med* 17, 503
(1999): Quinones MD+, *Allergy* 54, 83 (fatal)
(1998): Galindo Bonilla PA+, *J Investig Allergol Clin Immunol* 8, 186
(1997): Morkunas AR+, *Crit Care Clin* 13, 727
(1997): Redondo Bellon P, *Rev Neurol* 25, S309
(1997): Tennis P+, *Neurology* 49, 542
(1996): Chopra S+, *Br J Dermatol* 134, 1109
(1996): Conger LA+, *Cutis* 57, 223
(1994): Potter T+, *Arch Dermatol* 130, 856
(1993): Handfield-Jones SE+, *Br J Dermatol* 129, 175
(1984): Fonseca JC+, *Med Cutan Ibero Lat Am* (Portuguese) 12, 187
(1983): Rapp RP+, *Neurosurgery* 13, 272
(1978): Stanley J+, *Arch Dermatol* 114, 1350
(1975): Weedon AP, *Aust N Z J Med* 5, 561
(1973): Cohen BL+, *Clin Pediatr Phila* 12, 622
(1973): Sisca TS, *Am J Hosp Pharm* 30, 446

Injection-site extravasation
(2002): Edwards JJ+, *Anesth Analg* 94(3), 672

Injection-site necrosis
(1995): Hunt SJ, *Am J Dermatopathol* 17, 399
(1993): Hayes AG+, *J Am Acad Dermatol* 28, 360

Injection-site pain
(2002): Coplin WM+, *Neurol Res* 24(8), 842

Lymphadenopathy
(1971): Oates R+, *Med J Australia* 2/58, 371

Lymphoproliferative disease
(1992): Schlaifer D+, *Eur J Hematol* 48, 274

Mucocutaneous eruption
(1992): Tone T+, *J Dermatol* 19, 27
(1979): Pollack MA+, *Ann Neurol* 5, 262

Myopathy
(1986): Engel JN+, *Am J Med* 81, 928
(1983): Harney J+, *Neurology* 33, 790

Oral ulceration

Paresthesias (<1%)
(2002): Coplin WM+, *Neurol Res* 24(8), 842
(1995): Rodriguez-Castellanos M+, *Arch Dermatol* 131, 620

Periarteritis nodosa
(1967): Haas P, *Wiener Klin Wochenschr* (German) 75, 56

(1948): Van Wyk JJ+, *Arch Intern Med* 81, 605

Peyronie's disease

Polyfibromatosis
(1979): Pierard GE+, *Br J Dermatol* 100, 335

Polymyositis
(1983): Harney J+, *Neurology* 33, 790

Porphyria
(1980): Fuchs T+, *Int J Biochem* 12, 955

Porphyria cutanea tarda
(1996): Ruggian JC+, *J Am Soc Nephrol* 7, 397

Pseudolymphoma (<1%)
(2002): Lifshitz AY, Israel (from Internet) (observation) (solitary in infant)
(1998): Cooke LE+, *Clin Pharm* 7, 153
(1997): Gigli GL+, *Int J Neurosci* 87, 181
(1995): Wolkenstein P+, *Arch Dermatol* 131, 544
(1994): Rijlaarsdam JU+, *Semin Dermatol* 13(3), 187
(1993): Kerl H+, *Dermatology in General Medicine* McGraw-Hill New York
(1993): Sigal M+, *Ann Dermatol Venereol* (French) 120, 175
(1992): Braddock SW+, *J Am Acad Dermatol* 27, 337
(1992): D'Incan M+, *Arch Dermatol* 128, 1371
(1992): Harris DW+, *Br J Dermatol* 127, 403
(1991): Rijlaarsdam U+, *J Am Acad Dermatol* 24(2), 216
(1989): Torne R+, *Am J Dermatopathol* 11(6), 544
(1988): Cooke LE+, *Clin Pharm* 7, 153
(1988): Silverman AK+, *J Am Acad Dermatol* 18, 721
(1985): Brodell RT, *Dermatol Clin* 3, 719
(1985): Wolf R+, *Arch Dermatol* 121(9), 1181
(1983): Rapp RP+, *Neurosurgery* 13, 272
(1982): Rosenthal CJ+, *Cancer* 49, 2305
(1981): Adams JD, *Australas J Dermatol* 22, 28
(1980): Vellucci A+, *Clin Ter* (Italian) 94, 229
(1977): Charlesworth EN, *Arch Dermatol* 113, 477
(1977): Halevy S+, *Dermatologica* 155, 321
(1974): Dorfman RF+, *Hum Pathol* 5(5), 519
(1971): Oates RK+, *Med J Aust* 2, 371
(1968): Gams RA+, *Ann Intern Med* 69, 557
(1968): Schreiber MM+, *Arch Dermatol* 97, 297
(1963): Sparberg M, *Ann Intern Med* 59, 914
(1961): Rosenfeld S+, *JAMA* 176, 491
(1959): Salzstein SL+, *Cancer* 12, 164

Rhabdomyolysis
(1989): Korman LB+, *Clin Pharm* 8(7), 514
(1986): Engel JN+, *Am J Med* 81, 928

Serum sickness
(1981): Menitove JE+, *Am J Hematol* 10, 277
(1975): Zidar BL+, *Am J Med* 58, 704

Thrombophlebitis (<1%)

*Note: The fetal hydantoin syndrome (FHS) – children whose mothers receive phenytoin during pregnancy are born with FHS. The main features of this syndrome are mental and growth retardation, unusual facies, digital and nail hypoplasia, and coarse scalp hair. Occasionally neonatal acne will be present

**Note: The phenytoin hypersensitivity reaction (also known as the anticonvulsant hypersensitivity syndrome) is described in detail in (1978): Stanley J+, *Arch Dermatol* 114, 1350. The salient features of this reaction, which characteristically occur within the first 2 to 4 weeks of phenytoin therapy, are fever, generalized tender lymphadenopathy, hepatitis, leukocytosis, and a widespread, pruritic, irregular eruption consisting of ill-defined patches of macular erythema. Periorbital edema is common. The mucous membranes are frequently involved with erythema of the oral mucosa and pharynx. Papules, vesicles and pustules occasionally develop

PHYSOSTIGMINE

Synonyms: Eserine salicylates; Physostigmine salicylates; Physostigmine sulfate
Trade names: Antilirium (Forest); Isopto Eserine
Indications: Miotic in glaucoma treatment, reverses toxic CNS effects caused by anticholinergic drugs
Category: Anticholinesterase; Antidote; Antiglaucoma
Half-life: 15–40 minutes
Clinically important, potentially hazardous interactions with: bethanechol, corticosteroids, galantamine, methacholine, succinylcholine

Reactions

Skin
Burning (1–10%) (ophthalmic)
Diaphoresis (>10%)
Erythema (1–10%)
  (1995): Walter K+, *Br J Clin Pharmacol* 39(1), 59 (from transdermal patch)

Other
Death
Lacrimation (>10%) (ophthalmic)
Ocular irritation (>10%) (ophthalmic)
Seizures (1–10%)
  (1994): Amital D+, *Biol Psychiatry* 36(7), 498
  (1979): Stewart GO, *Anaesth Intensive Care* 7(3), 283
  (1976): Walker WE+, *JACEP* 5(6), 436
Sialorrhea (>10%)
Twitching (1–10%)

Note: Antilirium is a derivative of the Calabar bean, and its active moiety, physostigmine, is also known as eserine.

Note: Physostigmine is used to reverse the effect upon the nervous system caused by clinical or toxic dosages of drugs and herbs capable of producing the Anticholinergic syndrome.
Some of the drugs responsible are: amitriptyline, amoxapine, atropine, benztropine, biperiden, clidinium, cyclobenzaprine, desipramine, doxepin, hyoscyamine, imipramine, lorazepam, maprotiline, nortriptyline, protriptyline, propantheline, scopolamine, trimipramine. Some herbals that can elicit the anticholinergic syndrome are black henbane, deadly nightshade, Devil's apple, Jimson weed, Loco seeds or weeds, Matrimony vine, night blooming jessamine, stinkweed.

PHYTONADIONE

Synonyms: phylloquinone; phytomenadione; vitamin K₁
Trade names: AquaMEPHYTON (Merck); Konakion; Mephyton (Merck); Phytomenadione; Vitamin K (Abbott)
Other common trade names: *Kaywan; Vitak*
Indications: Coagulation disorders
Category: Fat-soluble nutritional supplement
Half-life: 2–4 hours
Clinically important, potentially hazardous interactions with: warfarin

Reactions

Skin
Allergic reactions (sic)
  (1999): Wong DA+, *Australas J Dermatol* 40, 147

  (1990): Pigatto PD+, *Contact Dermatitis* 22, 307
Dermatitis
  (1999): Drayton G, Los Angeles, CA (from Internet) (observation)
  (1995): Bruynzeel I+, *Contact Dermatitis* 32, 78
  (1995): Guy C+, *Therapie* (French) 50, 483
  (1988): Dinis A+, *Contact Dermatitis* 18, 170
  (1982): Camarasa JG+, *Contact Dermatitis* 8, 268
  (1980): Romaguera C+, *Contact Dermatitis* 6, 355
  (1979): Romaguera C+, *Actas Dermosifilogr* (Spanish) 70, 215
Diaphoresis (<1%)
Eczema
  (1992): Lee MM+, *Arch Dermatol* 128, 257
  (1988): Sanders MN+, *J Am Acad Dermatol* 19, 699
Erythema (annular)
  (1986): Kay MH+, *Cutis* 37, 445
Exanthems
  (1987): Finkelstein H+, *J Am Acad Dermatol* 16, 540
Flushing
Rash (sic)
Scleroderma
  (1995): Morell A+, *Int J Dermatol* 34, 201
  (1994): Guidetti MS+, *Contact Dermatitis* 31, 45
  (1992): Fitzpatrick JE, *Dermatol Clin* 10, 19
  (1989): Pujol RM+, *Cutis* 43, 365
  (1988): Brunskill NJ+, *Clin Exp Dermatol* 13, 276
  (1987): Finkelstein H+, *J Am Acad Dermatol* 16, 540
  (1985): Janin-Mercier A+, *Arch Dermatol* 121, 1421
  (1982): Rommel A+, *Ann Pediatr* (Paris) (French) 29, 64
  (1981): Jean-Pastor MJ+, *Therapie* (French) 36, 369
  (1975): Texier L+, *Bull Soc Fr Derm Syphiligr* (French) 82, 448
  (1972): Texier L+, *Ann Dermatol Syphiligr* (Paris) (French) 99, 363
  (1972): Texier L+, *Bord Med* (French) 5, 700
Urticaria
  (1993): Ford G, *J Paediatr Child Health* 29, 241
  (1988): Sanders MN+, *J Am Acad Dermatol* 19, 699
  (1987): Mosser C+, *Ann Dermatol Venereol* (French) 114, 243
  (1964): Piguet B+, *Bull Mem Soc Med Hop* (Paris) (French) 118, 1337
Vasculitis
  (1964): Piguet B+, *Bull Mem Soc Med Hop* (Paris) (French) 118, 1337

Other
Anaphylactoid reactions (<1%)
  (2001): Riegert-Johnson DL+, *Bone Marrow Transplant* 28(12), 1176
Dysgeusia (<1%)
Embolia cutis medicamentosa (Nicolau syndrome)
  (2003): Reding EL+, *J Am Acad Dermatol* 48(3), 472 (passim)
Headache
Hypersensitivity (<1%)
  (1998): Keogh GC+, *Cutis* 61, 81 (eczematous)
Injection-site eczematous eruption
  (1996): Moreau-Cabarrot A+, *Ann Dermatol Venereol* (French) 123, 177
  (1995): Keltz M+, American Academy of Dermatology Meeting, New Orleans (observation)
  (1994): Giudetti MS+, *Contact Dermatitis* 31, 45
  (1989): Allue-Bellosta L+, *Rev Clin Esp* (Spanish) 185, 217
  (1988): Joyce JP+, *Arch Dermatol* 124, 27
  (1988): Tsuboi R+, *J Am Acad Dermatol* 18, 386
  (1987): Finkelstein H+, *J Am Acad Dermatol* 16, 540
  (1978): Bullen AW+, *Br J Dermatol* 98, 561
  (1978): Robinson JW+, *Arch Dermatol* 114, 1790
  (1970): Anekoji K, *Chiryo* (Japanese) 52, 1577
  (1970): Honda M+, *Hifuka no Rinsho* (Japanese) 12, 295
Injection-site erythema

(1995): Keltz M+, American Academy of Dermatology Meeting, New Orleans (observation)
(1993): Lemlich G+, J Am Acad Dermatol 28, 345
(1992): Breathnach SM+, Adverse Drug Reactions and the Skin Blackwell, Oxford, 265 (passim)
Injection-site induration (Texier's syndrome) (<1%)
(2001): Jaffe PG, Columbia SC (from Internet) (observation)
(1999): Chung JY+, Cutis 63, 33 (2 cases)
(1996): Bourrat E+, Ann Dermatol Venereol (French) 123, 634 (6 cases)
(1996): Pang BK+, Australas J Dermatol 37, 44
(1995): Keltz M+, American Academy of Dermatology Meeting, New Orleans (observation)
(1994): Shelley WB+, Cutis 52, 203 (passim)
(1993): Lemlich G+, J Am Acad Dermatol 28, 345
(1993): Long CC+, BMJ 307, 336
(1992): Tuppal R+, J Am Acad Dermatol 27, 105
(1989): Pujol RM+, Cutis 43, 365
(1988): Brunskill NJ+, Clin Exp Dermatol 13, 276
(1988): Joyce JP+, Arch Dermatol 124, 27
(1988): Tsuboi R+, J Am Acad Dermatol 18, 386
(1977): Heydenreich G, Br J Dermatol 97, 697
(1976): Barnes HM+, Br J Dermatol 95, 653
(1972): Bazex A+, Bull Soc Fr Dermatol Syphiligr (French) 79, 578
(1972): Misson R+, Bull Soc Fr Dermatol Syphiligr (French) 79, 581

PILOCARPINE

Trade names: Adsorbocarbine; Akarpine; Isopto Carpine (Wyeth); Ocusert Pilo (Akorn); Pilocar (Novartis); Pilopin HS (Alcon); Pilopine (Alcon); Salagen (MGI); Storzine
Other common trade names: Diocarpine; Isopto Pilocarpine; Liocarpina; Miocarpine; Pilo Grin; Pilogel; Pilopt; Sno Pilo; Spersacarpine; Vistacarpin
Indications: Glaucoma, miosis induction, xerostomia
Category: Cholinergic parasympathomimetic
Half-life: N/A
Clinically important, potentially hazardous interactions with: galantamine

Reactions

Skin
Burning (1–10%)
(1996): Rattenbury JM+, Ann Clin Biochem 33, 456
Chills
Dermatitis
(2001): Holdiness MR, Am J Contact Dermat 12(4), 217
(1993): Cusano F+, Contact Dermatitis 29, 99
(1991): Helton J+, Contact Dermatitis 25, 133
(1991): Ortiz FJ+, Contact Dermatitis 25, 203
Diaphoresis (<1%)
Edema (4%)
Flushing
Photodermatitis
(1991): Helton J+, Contact Dermatitis 25, 133
Pruritus
Rash (sic)
Stinging (1–10%)
Urticaria
(1997): LeGrys VA+, Pediatr Pulmonol 24, 296

Other
Dysgeusia (2%)
Headache

Hypersensitivity (1–10%)
Myalgia (1%)
Ocular cicatricial pemphigoid
(2000): Plotkin A+, Arch Dermatol 136, 113
Sialorrhea (<1%)

PIMECROLIMUS

Synonym: ASM981
Trade name: Elidel (Novartis)
Indications: Atopic dermatitis
Category: Calcineurin inhibitor; Macrolactam ascomycin
Half-life: N/A

Reactions

Skin
Burning
(2002): Wahn U+, Pediatrics 110(1 Pt 1), e2 (10.5%)
Flu-like syndrome
Herpes simplex (1.2%)
Infections (sic) (5.4%)
(2002): Wahn U+, Pediatrics 110(1 Pt 1), e2 (12.4%)
Molluscum contagiosum (1.2%)
Upper respiratory infection (19.4%)

Other
Application-site burning (8–26%)
Application-site irritation (0.9%)
Application-site pruritus (0.6%)
Application-site reactions (sic) (2.1%)
Cough
(2002): Wahn U+, Pediatrics 110(1 Pt 1), e2
Headache

PIMOZIDE

Trade name: Orap (Gate)
Other common trade names: Frenal; Neurap; Pimodac
Indications: Tourette's syndrome, schizophrenia
Category: Antipsychotic-antidyskinetic (Tourette's syndrome); Neuroleptic agent
Half-life: 50 hours
Clinically important, potentially hazardous interactions with: amphetamines, aprepitant, atazanavir, azithromycin, azole antifungals, clarithromycin, dirithromycin, erythromycin, fluoxetine, **grapefruit juice**, imatinib, indinavir, itraconazole, ketoconazole, methylphenidate, nefazodone, nelfinavir, pemoline, phenothiazines, protease inhibitors, quinidine, ritonavir, saquinavir, sertraline, sparfloxacin, tricyclic antidepressants, troleandomycin, voriconazole, zileuton

Reactions

Skin
Diaphoresis
Exanthems
Facial edema (1–10%)
Periorbital edema
Photosensitivity
(1991): Opler LA+, J Clin Psychiatry 52, 221
Pigmentation

(1991): Opler LA+, *J Clin Psychiatry* 52, 221
Pruritus
Rash (sic) (8.3%)
Urticaria

Other
Death
  (2001): Glassman AH+, *Am J Psychiatry* 158(11), 1774
Dysgeusia
Galactorrhea
Gynecomastia (>10%)
Headache
Myalgia (2.7%)
Sialorrhea (13.8%)
  (1987): Shapiro AK+, *Pediatrics* 79, 1032
Tardive dyskinesia
  (2003): Howard BG, Santa Maria, CA (from Internet)
    (observation)
Tremor
Xerostomia (>10%)
  (1991): Opler LA+, *J Clin Psychiatry* 52, 221
  (1990): Sandor P+, *J Clin Psychopharmacol* 10, 197
  (1987): Shapiro AK+, *Pediatrics* 79, 1032

PINDOLOL

Trade name: Visken (Novartis)
Other common trade names: *Alti-Pindolol; Apo-Pindol; Barbloc; Durapindol; Gen-Pindolol; Nonspi; Pinbetol; Pinden; Syn-Pindol; Vypen*
Indications: Hypertension
Category: Antihypertensive; Beta-adrenoceptor blocker
Half-life: 3–4 hours
Clinically important, potentially hazardous interactions with: clonidine, epinephrine, verapamil

Note: Cutaneous side effects of beta-receptor blockaders are clinically polymorphous. They apparently appear after several months of continuous therapy. Atypical psoriasiform, lichen planus-like, and eczematous chronic rashes are mainly observed. (1983): Hödl St, *Z Hautkr* (German) 1:58, 17

Reactions

Skin
Diaphoresis (2%)
Eczema (sic)
Edema (6%)
Erythema multiforme
Exanthems
Exfoliative dermatitis
Hyperkeratosis (palms and soles)
Lichenoid eruption
  (1978): Savage RL+, *BMJ* 1, 987
  (1976): Palatsi R, *Ann Clin Res* 8, 239
Lupus erythematosus
  (1979): Bensaid J+, *BMJ* 1, 1603
Peripheral edema
Pityriasis rubra pilaris
  (1978): Finlay AY+, *BMJ* 1, 987
Pruritus (1–5%)
  (1976): Palatsi R, *Ann Clin Res* 8, 239
Psoriasis
  (1986): Abel EA+, *J Am Acad Dermatol* 15, 1007
  (1986): Czernielewski J+, *Lancet* 1, 808

  (1984): Arntzen N+, *Acta Derm Venereol* (Stockh) 64, 346
  (1976): Bonerandi JJ+, *Ann Dermatol Syphiligr* (Paris) (French) 103, 604
  (1976): Palatsi R, *Ann Clin Res* 8, 239
Purpura
Rash (sic) (1–10%)
Raynaud's phenomenon
  (1984): Eliasson K+, *Acta Med Scand* 215, 333
  (1976): Marshall AJ+, *BMJ* 1, 1498
Toxic epidermal necrolysis
Urticaria
Xerosis

Hair
Hair – alopecia

Nails
Nails – dystrophy
Nails – onycholysis

Other
Dysgeusia
Myalgia
Myopathy
  (1980): Uusitupa M+, *BMJ* 1, 183
Oculo-mucocutaneous syndrome
  (1982): Cocco G+, *Curr Ther Res* 31, 362
Oral lichenoid eruption
Paresthesias (3%)
Peyronie's disease
  (1979): Pryor JP+, *Lancet* 1, 331

PIOGLITAZONE

Trade name: Actos (Takeda)
Indications: Type 2 diabetes
Category: Thiazolidinedione antidiabetic
Half-life: 3–7 hours

Reactions

Skin
Angioedema
  (2002): Shadid S+, *Diabetes Care* 25(2), 405
Edema (4.8%)
  (2002): *Prescrire Int* 11(62), 170
  (2001): Chilcott J+, *Clin Ther* 23(11), 1792 (11.7%)
  (2001): Toyota T, *Nippon Rinsho* 59(11), 2211

Other
Headache
Myalgia (5.4%)
Tooth disorder (sic) (2.3%)

PIPECURONIUM

Trade name: Arduan (Organon)
Indications: Adjunct to general anesthesia
Category: Nondepolarizing neuromuscular blocking agent
Half-life: 2–3 hours
**Clinically important, potentially hazardous interactions
with:** anesthetics (inhalational), antibiotics, gentamicin,
magnesium salts, quinidine, succinylcholine

Reactions

Skin
Rash (sic) (<1%)
Urticaria (<1%)

Other
Hyperesthesia (<1%)
Muscle atrophy (<1%)

PIPERACILLIN

Trade names: Pipracil (Wyeth); Zosyn (Wyeth)
Other common trade names: *Avocin; Ivacin; Picillin; Pipcil;
Piperilline; Pipril; Piprilin; Pitamycin*
Indications: Various infections caused by susceptible organisms
Category: Beta-lactamase-sensitive penicillin
Half-life: 0.6–1.2 hours
**Clinically important, potentially hazardous interactions
with:** anisindione, anticoagulants, atracurium, cisatracurium,
demeclocycline, dicumarol, doxacurium, doxycycline,
methotrexate, minocycline, non-depolarizing muscle relaxants,
oxytetracycline, pancuronium, rapacuronium, reteplase,
tetracycline, warfarin

Zosyn is piperacillin and tazobactam

Reactions

Skin
Acute generalized exanthematous pustulosis (AGEP)
    (2003): Mysore V+, *J Dermatolog Treat* 14(1), 54
Allergic reactions (sic) (2–4%)
    (1994): Pleasants RA+, *Chest* 106, 1124 (in patients with cystic
        fibrosis)
    (1984): Holmes B+, *Drugs* 28, 375
Angioedema
Bullous eruption
Candidiasis
Ecchymoses
Edema
Erythema nodosum
Exanthems
    (2002): Romano A+, *Int Arch Allergy Immunol* 129(2), 169
    (1993): Warrington RJ+, *J Allergy Clin Immunol* 92, 626
    (1985): Mead GM+, *Lancet* 2, 499 (56%)
    (1985): No Author, *Lancet* 2, 723
    (1984): Holmes B+, *Drugs* 28, 375
Exfoliative dermatitis
Jarisch–Herxheimer reaction (<1%)
Pruritus
Purpura
    (2000): Yata Y+, *Ann Hematol* 79(10), 593
Radiation recall

(2001): Krishnan RS+, *J Am Acad Dermatol* 44, 1045 (with
    tobramycin & ciprofloxacin)
Rash (sic) (1%)
Stevens–Johnson syndrome
    (1995): Cheriyan S+, *Allergy Proc* 16, 85
Toxic epidermal necrolysis
Urticaria
    (2002): Romano A+, *Int Arch Allergy Immunol* 129(2), 169
    (1995): Moscato G+, *Eur Respir J* 8, 467
    (1984): Holmes B+, *Drugs* 28, 375
Vasculitis
Vesicular eruptions

Other
Anaphylactoid reactions (<1%)
Glossodynia
Headache
Hypersensitivity (<1%)
    (2002): Romano A+, *Allergy* 57(5), 459
    (1998): Cabanes R+, *Allergy* 53, 819
Injection-site pain (2%)
    (1984): Holmes B+, *Drugs* 28, 375
Injection-site phlebitis (2%)
    (1984): Holmes B+, *Drugs* 28, 375
Oral candidiasis
Serum sickness
Stomatodynia
Thrombophlebitis (<1%)
Tinnitus
Vaginitis

PIRBUTEROL

Trade name: Maxair (3M)
Other common trade names: *Exirel; Spirolair; Zeisin Autohaler*
Indications: Asthma, bronchospasm
Category: Beta-2-adrenoceptor blocker; Bronchodilator
Half-life: 2–3 hours

Reactions

Skin
Edema
Pruritus
Purpura (<1%)
Rash (sic)

Hair
Hair – alopecia

Other
Dysgeusia (1–10%)
Glossitis
Headache
Paresthesias (<1%)
Trembling (>10%)
Xerostomia

PIROXICAM

Trade name: Feldene (Pfizer)
Other common trade names: *Antiflog; Apo-Piroxicam; Baxo; Doblexan; Felden; Larapam; Nu-Pirox; Rogal; Sotilen; Zunden*
Indications: Arthritis
Category: Analgesic; Nonsteroidal anti-inflammatory (NSAID)
Half-life: 50 hours
Clinically important, potentially hazardous interactions with: methotrexate, ritonavir

Reactions

Skin

Allergic reactions (sic)
  (2001): Trujillo MJ+, *Allergol Immunopathol* (Madr) 29(4), 133 (with thimerosal)
Angioedema (<1%)
  (1987): Gerber D, *Drug Intell Clin Pharm* 21, 707 (passim)
Bullous dermatosis
  (1985): Guillaume JC+, *Ann Dermatol Venereol* (French) 112, 807
Dermatitis
  (1995): Valsecchi R+, *Contact Dermatitis* 32, 63
  (1993): Ophaswongse S+, *Contact Dermatitis* 29, 57
  (1993): Valsecchi R+, *Contact Dermatitis* 29, 167
  (1992): Green C+, *Contact Dermatitis* 27, 261 (to the gel)
  (1990): Serrano G+, *J Am Acad Dermatol* 23, 479
Diaphoresis (<1%)
  (1987): Gerber D, *Drug Intell Clin Pharm* 21, 707 (passim)
Dyshidrosis
  (1985): Braunstein BL, *Cutis* 35, 485
Ecchymoses (<1%)
Edema (>1%)
Erythema (<1%)
Erythema annulare centrifugum
  (1985): Hogan DJ+, *J Am Acad Dermatol* 13, 840
Erythema multiforme (<1%)
  (1987): Gerber D, *Drug Intell Clin Pharm* 21, 707 (passim)
  (1986): Penso D, *J Am Acad Dermatol* 14, 275
  (1986): Stern RS, *J Am Acad Dermatol* 14, 276
  (1985): Bigby M+, *J Am Acad Dermatol* 12, 866
  (1985): Guillaume JC+, *Ann Dermatol Venereol* (French) 112, 807
  (1985): O'Brien WM+, *J Rheumatol* 12, 13
  (1984): Brogden RN+, *Drugs* 28, 292
  (1984): Duro JC+, *J Rheumatol* 11, 554
  (1984): Stern RS+, *JAMA* 252, 1433
  (1982): Bertail MA, *Ann Dermatol Venereol* (French) 109, 261
  (1982): Faure M, *Ann Dermatol Venereol* (French) 109, 255
Erythroderma
  (1993): Sangla I+, *Rev Neurol* (Paris) (French) 149, 217
  (1985): Guillaume JC+, *Ann Dermatol Venereol* (French) 112, 807
Exanthems (>5%)
  (1994): Litt JZ, Beachwood, OH (personal case) (observation)
  (1987): Gerber D, *Drug Intell Clin Pharm* 21, 707 (passim)
  (1985): Bigby M+, *J Am Acad Dermatol* 12, 866 (2.4%)
  (1985): Guillaume JC+, *Ann Dermatol Venereol* (French) 112, 807
  (1984): Brogden RN+, *Drugs* 28, 292 (0.8%)
  (1984): Stern RS+, *JAMA* 252, 1433
  (1982): Faure M+, *Ann Dermatol Venereol* (French) 109, 255
  (1979): Dessain P+, *J Int Med Res* 7, 335
Exfoliative dermatitis (<1%)
  (1987): Gerber D, *Drug Intell Clin Pharm* 21, 707 (passim)
Fixed eruption
  (2003): Montoro J+, *Allergol Immunopathol* (Madr) 31(1), 53
  (1998): Leal G, Fortaleza, Brazil (from Internet) (observation) (2 cases)
  (1995): Ordoqui E+, *Allergy* 50, 741

(1994): Ordoqui E+, *J Allergy Clin Immunology* 93, 242
(1993): Gastaminza G+, *Contact Dermatitis* 28, 43
(1993): No Author, *Dermatology* 186, 164
(1990): de la Hoz B+, *Int J Dermatol* 29, 672
(1990): Stubb S+, *J Am Acad Dermatol* 22, 1111
(1989): Shiohara T+, *Arch Dermatol* 125, 1371
(1989): Valsecchi R+, *J Am Acad Dermatol* 21, 1300
Hot flashes (<1%)
Lichenoid eruption
  (1993): Veraldi S+, *Eur J Dermatol* 3, 156
  (1992): Vaillant L+, *Ann Dermatol Venereol* (French) 119, 936
  (1985): Guillaume JC+, *Ann Dermatol Venereol* (French) 112, 807
  (1984): Stern RS+, *JAMA* 252, 1433
Linear IgA bullous dermatosis
  (2001): Plunkett RW+, *J Am Acad Dermatol* 45(5), 691
  (1998): Camilleri M+, *J Eur Acad Dermatol Venereol* 10, 70
Lupus erythematosus
  (1991): Roura M+, *Dermatologica* 182, 56
Pemphigus
  (1985): Guillaume JC+, *Ann Dermatol Venereol* (French) 112, 807
  (1983): Martin RL, *N Engl J Med* 309, 795
Pemphigus foliaceus
  (1984): Brogden RN+, *Drugs* 28, 292
Peripheral edema
Petechiae (<1%)
Photodermatitis
  (2001): Trujillo MJ+, *Allergol Immunopathol* (Madr) 29(4), 133 (with thimerosal)
  (1992): Torinuki W, *Tohoku J Exp Med* 167, 267
Photosensitivity (<1%)
  (1998): Valentine M, Everett, WA (from Internet) (observation)
  (1998): Varela P+, *Acta Med Port* (Portuguese) 11, 997
  (1998): Varela P+, *Contact Dermatitis* 38, 229
  (1996): Stingeni L+, *Contact Dermatitis* 34, 60
  (1995): Gebhardt M+, *Z Rheumatol* (German) 54, 405
  (1995): Mammen L+, *Am Fam Physician* 52, 575
  (1994): Sassolas B+, *Clin Exp Dermatol* 19, 189
  (1993): Hariya T+, *J Dermatol Sci* 5, 165
  (1993): Youn JI+, *Clin Exp Dermatol* 18, 52
  (1992): Goncalo M+, *Contact Dermatitis* 27, 287
  (1992): Izekawa Z+, *J Invest Dermatol* 98, 918
  (1992): Serrano G+, *J Am Acad Dermatol* 26, 545
  (1991): de Castro JL+, *Contact Dermatitis* 24, 187
  (1991): Roura M+, *Dermatologica* 182, 56
  (1990): Black AK+, *Br J Dermatol* 123, 277
  (1990): Serrano G+, *J Am Acad Dermatol* 23, 479
  (1989): Cirne de Castro JL+, *J Am Acad Dermatol* 20, 706
  (1989): De la Cuadra J+, *Contact Dermatitis* 21, 349
  (1989): Kaidbey KH+, *Arch Dermatol* 125, 783
  (1989): Sunohara A, *Photodermatol* 6, 188
  (1987): Figueiredo A+, *Contact Dermatitis* 17, 73
  (1987): Gerber D, *Drug Intell Clin Pharm* 21, 707 (passim)
  (1987): Halasz CL, *Cutis* 39, 37
  (1987): Magana-Garcia M+, *Rev Invest Clin* (Spanish) 39, 177
  (1987): Morison WL+, *J Am Acad Dermatol* 17, 698
  (1986): Kochevar IE+, *Arch Dermatol* 122, 1283
  (1986): McKerrow KJ+, *J Am Acad Dermatol* 15, 1237
  (1985): Bigby M+, *J Am Acad Dermatol* 12, 866
  (1985): Braunstein BL, *Cutis* 35, 485
  (1985): Guillaume JC+, *Ann Dermatol Venereol* (French) 112, 807
  (1985): Serrano G+, *J Am Acad Dermatol* 11, 113
  (1985): Weigand DA, *J Am Acad Dermatol* 12, 373
  (1984): Brogden RN+, *Drugs* 28, 292
  (1984): Stern RS+, *JAMA* 252, 1433
  (1983): Diffey BL+, *Br J Rheumatol* 22, 239
  (1983): Fjellner B, *Acta Derm Venereol* (Stockh) 63, 557
  (1982): Faure M+, *Ann Dermatol Venereol* (French) 109, 255
Pruritus (1–10%)
  (1987): Gerber D, *Drug Intell Clin Pharm* 21, 707 (passim)

(1984): Brogden RN+, *Drugs* 28, 292
(1984): Stern RS+, *JAMA* 252, 1433
(1979): Dessain P+, *J Int Med Res* 7, 335
Purpura (<1%)
(1987): Gerber D, *Drug Intell Clin Pharm* 21, 707 (passim)
(1984): Brogden RN+, *Drugs* 28, 292
Rash (sic) (>10%)
Side effects (sic) (46.9%)
(1987): Gerber D, *Drug Intell Clin Pharm* 21, 707 (passim)
Stevens–Johnson syndrome (<1%)
(1995): Katoh N+, *J Dermatol* 22, 677
(1985): Guillaume JC+, *Ann Dermatol Venereol* (French) 112, 807
Toxic dermatitis (sic)
(1991): Chosidow O+, *Ann Dermatol Venereol* (French) 118, 903
Toxic epidermal necrolysis (<1%)
(2002): Correia O+, *Arch Dermatol* 138, 29 (two cases)
(1996): Blum L+, *J Am Acad Dermatol* 34, 1088
(1993): Correia O+, *Dermatology* 186, 32
(1990): Black AK+, *Br J Dermatol* 123, 277
(1987): Gerber D, *Drug Intell Clin Pharm* 21, 707 (passim)
(1987): Guillaume JC+, *Arch Dermatol* 123, 1166
(1986): Penso D+, *J Am Acad Dermatol* 14, 275 (letter)
(1986): Szczeklik A, *Drugs* 32 (Suppl 4), 148
(1985): Coscojuela C+, *Med Cutan Ibero Lat Am* (Spanish) 13, 291
(1985): Guillaume JC+, *Ann Dermatol Venereol* (French) 112, 807
(1982): Faure M+, *Ann Dermatol Venereol* (French) 109, 255
Urticaria (<1%)
(1987): Gerber D, *Drug Intell Clin Pharm* 21, 707 (passim)
(1985): Serrano G+, *J Am Acad Dermatol* 11, 113
(1984): Stern RS+, *JAMA* 252, 1433
(1982): Torras H+, *Med Cutan Ibero Lat Am* (Spanish) 10, 351
Vasculitis (<1%)
(1985): Bigby M+, *J Am Acad Dermatol* 12, 866
(1985): Guillaume JC+, *Ann Dermatol Venereol* (French) 112, 807
(1984): Stern RS+, *JAMA* 252, 1433
Vesicular eruptions (<1%)
(1986): Stern RS, *J Am Acad Dermatol* 14, 276 (letter)
(1984): Stern RS+, *JAMA* 252, 1433

Hair

Hair – alopecia
(1987): Gerber D, *Drug Intell Clin Pharm* 21, 707
(1985): Bigby M+, *J Am Acad Dermatol* 12, 866
(1984): Stern RS+, *JAMA* 252, 1433

Nails

Nails – onycholysis

Other

Anaphylactoid reactions (<1%)
Aphthous stomatitis
(2001): Vincent L+, *Ann Dermatol Venereol* 128(1), 57
(1991): Siegel MA+, *J Am Dent Assoc* 122, 75
Buccal ulceration
(1987): Gerber D, *Drug Intell Clin Pharm* 21, 707 (passim)
Death
(2002): Correia O+, *Arch Dermatol* 138, 29
Headache
Paresthesias
(1987): Gerber D, *Drug Intell Clin Pharm* 21, 707
Pseudoporphyria
(2000): De Silva B+, *Pediatr Dermatol* 17, 480
Serum sickness (<1%)
Stomatitis (>1%)
Tinnitus
Xerostomia (<1%)

PLICAMYCIN

Synonym: mithramycin
Trade name: Mithracin (Bayer)
Other common trade name: *Mithraline*
Indications: Paget's disease, malignant testicular tumors
Category: Antihypercalcemic; Antihypercalciuric; Antineoplastic; Bone resorption inhibitor
Half-life: 1 hour
Clinically important, potentially hazardous interactions with: aldesleukin

Reactions

Skin

Bleeding (5–12%)
Ecchymoses
(1970): Kennedy BJ, *Am J Med* 49, 494
Exanthems
Flushing (1–10%)
(1983): Bronner AK+, *J Am Acad Dermatol* 9, 645
(1982): Dunagin WG, *Semin Oncol* 9, 14
(1970): Kennedy BJ, *Am J Med* 49, 494 (35%)
Petechiae (1–10%)
Purpura
(1970): Kennedy BJ, *Am J Med* 49, 494 (10%)
Seborrheic keratoses (inflammation of)
(1987): Johnson TM+, *J Am Acad Dermatol* 17, 192
Toxic epidermal necrolysis
(1978): Purpora D+, *N Engl J Med* 299, 1412

Other

Dysgeusia (metallic taste)
Injection-site cellulitis (1–10%)
Injection-site erythema (1–10%)
Injection-site pain (1–10%)
Oral mucosal lesions
(1989): Kerker BJ+, *Semin Dermatol* 8, 173 (1–5%)
(1970): Kennedy BJ, *Am J Med* 49, 494 (15%)
Stomatitis (>10%)

POLYTHIAZIDE*

Trade names: Minizide (Pfizer); Renese (Pfizer)
Other common trade names: *Drenusil; Nephril*
Indications: Hypertension, edema
Category: Antihypertensive; Thiazide diuretic
Half-life: N/A
Clinically important, potentially hazardous interactions with: digoxin, lithium

Minizide is prazosin and polythiazide

Reactions

Skin

Exanthems
Photosensitivity (<1%)
Purpura
Rash (sic) (<1%)
Urticaria
Vasculitis

Other
Paresthesias

*Note: Polythiazide is a sulfonamide and can be absorbed systemically. Sulfonamides can produce severe, possibly fatal, reactions such as toxic epidermal necrolysis and Stevens–Johnson syndrome

POTASSIUM IODIDE

Synonyms: KI; Lugol's solution; strong iodine solution
Trade names: Kie (Laser); Pima (Fleming); SSKI (Upsher-Smith); Thyroid-Block
Other common trade names: *Jodatum; Jodid; Kalium*
Indications: Hyperthyroidism
Category: Antifungal; Antihyperthyroid; Expectorant
Half-life: N/A
Clinically important, potentially hazardous interactions with: ACE inhibitors, potassium-sparing diuretics, spironolactone, triamterene

Reactions

Skin
Acne (1–10%)
Angioedema (1–10%)
 (1979): Curd JG+, *Ann Intern Med* 91, 853
Bullous pemphigoid
 (1994): Piletta P+, *Br J Dermatol* 131, 145
Dermatitis herpetiformis
 (1989): Zone JJ+, *Immunol Ser* 46, 565
Diaphoresis
Exanthems
 (1981): Farkas J, *Dermatol Monatsschr* (German) 167, 579
Iododerma
 (1996): Alpay K+, *Pediatr Dermatol* 13, 51
 (1990): Soria C+, *J Am Acad Dermatol* 22, 418 (vegetating)
 (1989): Romanenko VN+, *Vestn Dermatol Venerol* (Russian) 12, 60
 (1987): O'Brien TJ, *Australas J Dermatol* 28, 119
 (1986): Raznatovskii IM+, *Vestn Dermatol Venerol* (Russian) 10, 71
 (1985): Stone OJ, *Int J Dermatol* 24, 565
 (1985): Wilkin JK+, *Cutis* 36, 335
 (1981): Huang TY+, *Ann Allergy* 46, 264
 (1978): Jezova J, *Cesk Dermatol* (Czech) 53, 240
 (1978): Labohm EB, *Ned Tijdschr Geneeskd* (Dutch) 122, 1291 (vegetating)
 (1974): Dienhart KJ, *N Engl J Med* 290, 521 (suppurative ulcerating)
 (1973): Khan F+, *N Engl J Med* 289, 1018 (suppurative ulcerating)
 (1971): Werbitt W, *J Am Osteopath Assoc* 70, 460
Lupus erythematosus
 (1979): Curd JG+, *Ann Intern Med* 91, 853
Purpura
Pustular psoriasis
 (1967): Shelley WB, *JAMA* 201, 1009
Rash (sic)
Systemic eczematous contact dermatitis
Urticaria (1–10%)
 (1979): Curd JG+, *Ann Intern Med* 91, 853
Vasculitis
 (1987): Eeckhout E+, *Acta Derm Venereol* (Stockh) 67, 362
 (1981): Zone JJ, *Arch Dermatol* 117, 758
 (1979): Curd JG+, *Ann Intern Med* 91, 853

Other
Dysgeusia (1–10%) (metallic taste)
Gingivitis
Paresthesias
Serum sickness
Sialorrhea
Stomatodynia

PRAMIPEXOLE

Trade name: Mirapex (Pharmacia)
Indications: Parkinsonism
Category: Antiparkinsonian
Half-life: ~8 hours

Reactions

Skin
Adverse effects (sic) (2%)
Allergic reactions (sic) (>1%)
Diaphoresis (>1%)
Edema (5%)
Peripheral edema (5%)
 (2000): Tan EK+, *Arch Neurol* 57, 729
Pruritus (>1%)
Rash (sic) (>1%)

Other
Dysgeusia (>1%)
Headache
Hyperesthesia (3%)
Myalgia (>1%)
Paresthesias (>1%)
Sialorrhea (>1%)
Tooth disorder (>1%)
Twitching (sic) (2%)
Xerostomia (7%)
 (1998): Dooley M+, *Drugs Aging* 12, 495

PRAVASTATIN

Trade name: Pravachol (Bristol-Myers Squibb)
Other common trade names: *Elisor; Lipostat; Pravasin; Pravasine; Selectin; Selektine; Selipran*
Indications: Hypercholesterolemia
Category: Antihyperlipidemic; HMG-CoA reductase inhibitor
Half-life: ~2–3 hours
Clinically important, potentially hazardous interactions with: azithromycin, clarithromycin, cyclosporine, erythromycin, gemfibrozil, imatinib

Reactions

Skin
Allergic reactions (sic)
 (1994): de Boer EM+, *Contact Dermatitis* 30, 238
Angioedema
Dermatomyositis
 (1992): Schalke BB+, *N Engl J Med* 327, 649
Eczema (generalized)
 (1993): Krasovec M+, *Dermatology* 186, 248
Erythema multiforme

Exanthems
Flu-like syndrome (sic)
Flushing
   (1990): Wiklund O+, *J Intern Med* 228, 241
Lichenoid eruption
   (1998): Keough GC+, *Cutis* 61, 98
   (1997): Anthony JL, Montgomery, AL (from Internet)
     (observation)
Lupus erythematosus
Neuroleptic malignant syndrome
   (2002): Tajima Y, *Rinsho Byori* 50(2), 133 (with loxapine)
Photosensitivity
Pruritus
   (1992): Yoshimura N+, *Transplantation* 53, 94
   (1991): Malini PL+, *Clin Ther* 13, 500
Purpura
Rash (sic) (1–10%)
   (1992): Betteridge DJ+, *BMJ* 304, 1335
   (1992): Jungnickel PW+, *Clin Pharm* 11, 677
   (1991): Crepaldi G+, *Arch Intern Med* 151, 146
   (1991): *Med Lett Drugs Ther* 33, 18
   (1991): McTavish D+, *Drugs* 42, 65
   (1991): Raasch RH, *Drug Intell Clin Pharm* 25, 388
   (1990): Hunninghake DB+, *Atherosclerosis* 85, 81 (3.4%)
Stevens–Johnson syndrome
Toxic epidermal necrolysis
Urticaria
Vasculitis

Hair

Hair – alopecia
   (1999): Oakley A, Hamilton, New Zealand (from Internet)
     (observation)
Hair – broken-off patches of scalp hair (sic) (greenish)
   (1998): Fixler R, Cincinnati, OH (personal communication)
     (observation)

Other

Anaphylactoid reactions
Dysgeusia (<1%)
Gynecomastia
   (1999): Aerts J+, *Presse Med* (French) 28, 787
Headache
Hypersensitivity
Myalgia (2.7%)
   (2003): Litt JZ, Beachwood, OH (personal case) (observation)
   (2002): Sinzinger H, *Wien Klin Wochenschr* 114(21), 943
   (2001): Rehbein H, Jacksonville, FL (from Internet) (observation)
Myopathy
   (1995): Garnett WR, *Am J Health Syst Pharm* 52(15), 1639
   (1992): Schalke BB+, *N Engl J Med* 327, 649
Paresthesias
Porphyria cutanea tarda
   (1994): Perrot JL+, *Ann Dermatol Venereol* (French) 121, 817
Rhabdomyolysis
   (2002): Cohen LH, *Ned Tijdschr Geneeskd* 146(9), 440
   (2002): Sica DA+, *Am J Geriatr Cardiol* 11(1), 48
   (2002): Sica DA+, *Curr Opin Nephrol Hypertens* 11(2), 123
   (2001): Borrego FJ+, *Nefrologia* 21(3), 309
   (1996): Ballantyne CM+, *Am J Cardiol* 78(5), 532
   (1995): Farmer JA+, *Baillieres Clin Endocrinol Metab* 9(4), 825
   (1995): Garnett WR, *Am J Health Syst Pharm* 52(15), 1639 (with
     either cyclosporine, erythromycin, gemfibrozil or niacin)
   (1992): Raimondeau J+, *Presse Med* 21(14), 663 (with
     fenofibrate)
Stomatitis

PRAZEPAM

Trade name: Centrax (Parke-Davis)
Other common trade names: *Centrac; Demetrin; Lysanxia; Prazene; Sedapran; Trepidan*
Indications: Anxiety, depression
Category: Antidepressant; Anxiolytic; Benzodiazepine sedative-hypnotic
Half-life: 30–100 hours

Reactions

Skin

Ankle edema
Dermatitis (sic) (1–10%)
Diaphoresis (>10%)
Exanthems
Facial edema
Pruritus
Purpura
Rash (sic) (>10%)
Urticaria

Hair

Hair – alopecia
Hair – hirsutism

Other

Gingivitis
Paresthesias
Sialopenia (>10%)
Sialorrhea (1–10%)
Xerostomia (>10%)

PRAZIQUANTEL

Trade name: Biltricide (Bayer)
Other common trade names: *Cisticid; Distocide; Flukacide; Kalcide; Prazite; Tecprazin; Teniken*
Indications: Helmintic infections
Category: Anthelmintic
Half-life: 0.8–1.5 hours

Reactions

Skin

Diaphoresis (1–10%)
Edema
   (1995): Stelma FF+, *Am J Trop Med Hyg* 53, 167
Pruritus (<1%)
Rash (sic) (<1%)
Urticaria (<1%)
   (1996): Jaoko WG+, *East Afr Med J* 73, 499
   (1995): Stelma FF+, *Am J Trop Med Hyg* 53, 167

Other

Headache

PRAZOSIN

Trade names: Minipress (Pfizer); Minizide (Pfizer)
Other common trade names: *Alti-Prazosin; Apo-Prazo; Duramipress; Eurex; Hypovase; Nu-Prazo; Peripress; Pratisol; Pressin*
Indications: Hypertension
Category: Alpha-adrenoceptor blocker; Antihypertensive
Half-life: 2–4 hours
Clinically important, potentially hazardous interactions with: epinephrine

Minizide is prazosin and polythiazide

Reactions

Skin
Angioedema
  (1983): Ruzicka T+, *Lancet* 1, 473
Diaphoresis (<1%)
  (1977): Lahon HFJ+, *Excerpta Med Int Congr* 431, 26
  (1975): Pitts NE, *Postgraduate Medicine, Prazosin Clinical Symposium Proceedings* 20
Edema (1–4%)
  (1975): Pitts NE, *Postgraduate Medicine, Prazosin Clinical Symposium Proceedings* 20
Exanthems (1–5%)
  (1977): Lahon HFJ+, *Excerpta Med Int Congr* 431, 26 (0.7%)
Lichen planus (<1%)
Lichenoid eruption
Lupus erythematosus
  (1979): Marshall AJ+, *BMJ* 1, 165
  (1979): Wilson JD+, *Clin Pharmacol Ther* 26, 209
Pruritus (<1%)
  (1975): Pitts NE, *Postgraduate Medicine, Prazosin Clinical Symposium Proceedings* 20
Rash (sic) (1–4%)
  (1983): Stanaszek WF+, *Drugs* 25, 339
  (1975): Pitts NE, *Postgraduate Medicine, Prazosin Clinical Symposium Proceedings* 20
Urticaria
  (1983): Ruzicka T+, *Lancet* 1, 473

Hair
Hair – alopecia (<1%)

Other
Anaphylactoid reactions
  (1983): Ruzicka T+, *Lancet* 1, 473
Headache
Myopathy
  (1977): Tomlinson IW+, *BMJ* 1, 1319
Paresthesias (<1%)
Priapism (<1%)
  (1980): Burke JR+, *Med J Aust* 1, 382
  (1975): Pitts NE, *Postgraduate Medicine, Prazosin Clinical Symposium Proceedings* 20
Tinnitus
Xerostomia (1–4%)
  (1983): Stanaszek WF+, *Drugs* 25, 339
  (1977): Lahon HFJ+, *Excerpta Med Int Congr* 431, 26 (5.6%)
  (1975): Pitts NE, *Postgraduate Medicine, Prazosin Clinical Symposium Proceedings* 20

PRIMAQUINE

Synonym: prymaccone
Trade name: Primaquine (Sanofi-Synthelabo)
Other common trade names: *Neo-Quipenyl; Palum*
Indications: Malaria
Category: Antimalarial; Antiprotozoal
Half-life: 4–10 hours
Clinically important, potentially hazardous interactions with: penicillamine

Reactions

Skin
Angioedema
  (1970): Stevenson DD+, *JAMA* 212, 624
Exanthems
  (1976): Arndt KA+, *JAMA* 235, 918 (5%)
Pallor
Pruritus (<1%)
Psoriasis
  (1963): Kirschenbaum MB, *JAMA* 185, 1044
Urticaria
  (1970): Stevenson DD+, *JAMA* 212, 624

PRIMIDONE

Trade name: Mysoline (Xcel)
Other common trade names: *Midone; Mylepsin; PMS Primidone; Prysoline; Sertan*
Indications: Seizures
Category: Anticonvulsant; Barbiturate
Half-life: 10–12 hours
Clinically important, potentially hazardous interactions with: alcohol, anticoagulants, antihistamines, brompheniramine, buclizine, chlorpheniramine, dicumarol, ethanolamine, imatinib, midazolam, niacinamide, warfarin

Reactions

Skin
Acne
Allergic reactions (sic)
  (1984): Steffan MA+, *Contact Dermatitis* 10, 184
Erythema multiforme (<1%)
  (2002): Krivo JM, Franklin Square, NY (from Internet) (observation)
  (1979): Pollack MA+, *Ann Neurol* 5, 262
  (1975): Böttiger LE+, *Acta Med Scand* 198, 229
Exanthems (1–5%)
  (1980): Marghescu S+, *Fortschr Med* (German) 98, 723
Exfoliative dermatitis
Lupus erythematosus (<1%)
  (1994): Yung RL+, *Rheum Dis Clin North Am* 20, 61
  (1993): Drory VE+, *Clin Neuropharmacol* 16, 19 (passim)
  (1980): Condemi JJ, *Geriatrics* 35(3), 81
  (1977): Schubothe H+, *Verh Dtsch Ges Inn Med* (German) 83, 727
  (1972): Levantine A+, *Br J Dermatol* 87, 646 (passim)
  (1966): Ahuja GK+, *JAMA* 198, 201
Rash (sic) (<1%)
Toxic epidermal necrolysis
  (1985): Muhar U+, *Pediatr Dermatol* 3, 54
  (1979): Pollack MA+, *Ann Neurol* 5, 262

(1973): Stüttgen G, *Br J Dermatol* 88, 291
(1970): Hermann WA, *Dermatologica* 141, 366
Urticaria
(1984): Steffan MA+, *Contact Dermatitis* 10, 184

Other

Acute intermittent porphyria
Gingival hyperplasia
Hypersensitivity*
(2002): Krivo JM, Franklin Square, NY (from Internet)
(observation)
(1998): Schlienger RG+, *Epilepsia* 39, S3 (passim)
Mucocutaneous syndrome
(1975): Böttiger LE+, *Acta Med Scand* 198, 229
Rhabdomyolysis
(1990): Larpin R+, *Presse Med* 19(30), 1403

*Note: The antiepileptic drug hypersensitivity syndrome is a severe, occasionally fatal, disorder characterized by any or all of the following: pruritic exanthems, toxic epidermal necrolysis, Stevens–Johnson syndrome, exfoliative dermatitis, fever, hepatic abnormalities, eosinophilia, and renal failure

PROBENECID

Trade names: Benemid (Merck); Col-Benemid (Merck); Probalan
Other common trade names: *Bencid; Benecid; Benuryl; Panuric; Procid; Solpurin; Urocid*
Indications: Gouty arthritis
Category: Uricosuric
Half-life: 6–12 hours (dose-dependent)
Clinically important, potentially hazardous interactions with: amphotericin B, benzodiazepines, ertapenem, ketoprofen, ketorolac, methotrexate, NSAIDs, penicillamine, salicylates, sulfonamides

Reactions

Skin

Allergic reactions (sic)
Dermatitis (sic)
Erythema multiforme
(1985): Ting HC+, *Int J Dermatol* 24, 587
Exanthems
Flushing (1–10%)
Pruritus (1–10%)
Rash (sic) (1–10%)
Urticaria (1–5%)

Hair

Hair – alopecia

Other

Anaphylactoid reactions (<1%)
Gingivitis (1–10%)
Hypersensitivity
(1998): Myers KW+, *Ann Allergy Asthma Immunol* 80, 416 (in AIDS)

PROCAINAMIDE

Trade names: Procan (Parke-Davis); Procanbid (Monarch); Pronestyl (Bristol-Myers Squibb); Rhythmin
Other common trade names: *Amisalen; Biocoryl; Procan SR; Promine; Ritmocamid*
Indications: Ventricular arrhythmias
Category: Antiarrhythmic class I A
Half-life: 2.5–4.5 hours
Clinically important, potentially hazardous interactions with: arsenic, ciprofloxacin, enoxacin, gatifloxacin, lomefloxacin, moxifloxacin, norfloxacin, ofloxacin, quinolones, sparfloxacin

Reactions

Skin

Angioedema (<1%)
(1985): Ponte CD+, *Drug Intell Clin Pharm* 19, 139
Chills (<1%)
Dermatitis (sic)
(1985): Gorsulowsky DC+, *J Am Acad Dermatol* 12, 245 (6%)
Eczema (sic)
Exanthems (1–5%)
(1999): Numata T+, *Sangyo Ika Daigaku Zasshi* (Japanese) 21, 235
(1985): Gorsulowsky DC+, *J Am Acad Dermatol* 12, 245 (8%)
(1984): Christensen DJ+, *Ann Intern Med* 100, 918
(1973): Kosowski BD+, *Circulation* 47, 1204 (5%)
(1972): Blomgren SE+, *Am J Med* 52, 338
Flushing (<1%)
Lichen planus
(1988): Sherertz EF, *Cutis* 42, 51
Lupus erythematosus (>10%)
(1998): Kameda H+, *Br J Rheumatol* 37, 1236
(1998): Ohtani Y+, *Nihon Kokyuki Gakkai Zasshi* (Japanese) 36, 535
(1997): Yung R+, *Arthritis Rheum* 40, 1436
(1996): Miyasaka N, *Intern Med* 35, 527
(1995): Finger DR+, *J Rheumatol* 22, 574
(1995): Muramatsu M+, *Nippon Naika Gakkai Zasshi* (Japanese) 84, 1736
(1995): Panine VV+, American Academy of Dermatology Meeting, New Orleans (observation)
(1995): Price EJ+, *Drug Saf* 12(4), 283
(1995): Rubin RL+, *J Immunol* 154, 2483
(1994): Cohen MG, *J Rheumatol* 21, 578
(1993): McDonald E+, *Hosp Pract Off ED* 28, 95
(1992): Klimas NG+, *Am J Med Sci* 303, 99
(1992): Rubin RL, *Clin Biochem* 25, 223
(1992): Rubin RL+, *J Clin Invest* 90, 165
(1992): Skaer TL, *Clin Ther* 14, 496
(1992): Stevens MB, *Hosp Pract Off Ed* 27, 27
(1990): Pauls JD+, *Mol Immunol* 27, 701
(1989): Adams LE+, *J Lab Clin Med* 113, 482
(1989): Asherson RA+, *Ann Rheum Dis* 48, 232
(1989): Mohindra SK+, *Crit Care Med* 17, 961
(1989): Nichols CJ+, *Ophthalmology* 96, 1535
(1989): Turgeon PW+, *Ophthalmology* 96, 68
(1989): Vivino FB+, *Arthritis Rheum* 32, 560
(1988): Agudelo CA+, *J Rheumatol* 15, 1431
(1988): Forrester J+, *J Rheumatol* 15, 1384
(1988): Hess E, *N Engl J Med* 318, 1460
(1988): No Author, *J Tenn Med Assoc* 81, 579
(1988): Sheretz EF, *Cutis* 42, 51
(1988): Totoritis MC+, *N Engl J Med* 318, 1431
(1988): Uetrecht JP, *Chem Res Toxicol* 1, 133
(1987): Craft JE+, *Arthritis Rheum* 30, 689

(1987): Shoenfeld Y+, *J Clin Immunol* 7, 410
(1986): Harle JR+, *Ann Med Interne Paris* (French) 137, 599
(1986): Jackson C+, *Clin Exp Rheumatol* 4, 290
(1986): Reidenberg MM+, *Angiology* 37, 968
(1986): Rubin RL+, *Am J Med* 80, 999
(1986): Vitas B+, *Lijec Vjesn* (Serbo-Croatian-Roman) 108, 137
(1986): Weisbart RH+, *Ann Intern Med* 104, 310
(1985): Amadio P+, *Ann Intern Med* 102, 419
(1985): Cush JJ+, *Am J Med Sci* 290, 36
(1985): Epstein A+, *Arthritis Rheum* 28, 158
(1985): Gorsulowsky DC+, *J Am Acad Dermatol* 12, 245 (>5%)
(1985): Kale SA, *Postgrad Med* 77, 231
(1985): Lovisetto P+, *Recenti Prog Med* (Italian) 76, 110
(1985): Rubin RL+, *Clin Immunol Immunopathol* 36, 49
(1985): Stratton MA, *Clin Pharm* 4, 657
(1985): Totoritis MC+, *Postgrad Med* 78, 149
(1984): Browning CA+, *Am J Cardiol* 53, 376
(1984): Goldberg SK+, *Am J Med* 76, 146
(1984): Tan EM+, *Allergy Clin Immunol* 74, 631
(1984): Wollina U, *Z Gesamte Inn Med* (German) 39, 69
(1982): Chokron R+, *Nouv Presse Med* (French) 11, 2568
(1982): Gupta AK+, *Indian J Dermatol* 27, 112
(1982): Harmon CE+, *Clin Rheum Dis* 8, 121
(1982): Hess EV, *Arthritis Rheum* 25, 857
(1982): Tannen RH+, *Immunol Commun* 11, 33
(1981): Edwards RL+, *Arch Intern Med* 141, 1688
(1981): Gonzalez ER, *JAMA* 246, 1634
(1981): Hess EV, *Arthritis Rheum* 24, vi
(1981): Reidenberg MM, *Arthritis Rheum* 24, 1004
(1981): Schoen RT+, *Am J Med* 71, 5
(1981): Sheikh TK+, *Am J Clin Pathol* 75, 755
(1981): Tan EM+, *Arthritis Rheum* 24, 1064
(1981): Uetrecht JP+, *Arthritis Rheum* 24, 994
(1980): Ahmad S, *Circulation* 61, 865
(1980): Chubick A, *Adv Intern Med* 26, 467
(1980): Condemi JJ, *Geriatrics* 35(3), 81
(1980): Dixon JA+, *J Rheumatol* 7, 544
(1980): Seligmann H+, *Harefuah* (Hebrew) 99, 166
(1980): Weinstein A, *Prog Clin Immunol* 4, 1
(1979): Bernstein RE, *Lancet* 2, 1076
(1979): Bluestein HG+, *Lancet* 2, 816
(1979): Foucar E+, *J Clin Lab Immunol* 2, 79
(1979): Hoff BH, *Chest* 75, 107
(1979): McLain DA+, *Arthritis Rheum* 22, 305
(1979): Sonnhag C+, *Acta Med Scand* 206, 245
(1979): Stec GP+, *Ann Intern Med* 90, 799
(1979): Stein HB+, *J Rheumatol* 6, 543
(1978): Jones WN+, *Ariz Med* 35, 16
(1978): Kaplan AI+, *Chest* 73, 875
(1978): Nick J+, *Ann Med Interne Paris* (French) 129, 259
(1978): Robinson HM, *Z Hautkr* (German) 53, 349
(1978): Wierzchowiecki M+, *Pol Arch Med Wewn* (Polish) 59, 197
(1978): Woosley RL+, *N Engl J Med* 298, 1157
(1978): Zeide MS+, *Clin Orthop* 134, 290
(1977): Bell WR+, *Arch Intern Med* 137, 1471
(1977): Carel RS+, *Chest* 72, 670
(1977): Healey LA, *Med Times* 105, 87
(1977): Homma M, *Nippon Rinsho* (Japanese) 35, 1330
(1977): Kahn MF+, *Sem Hôp* (French) 53, 2201
(1977): Sahenk Z+, *Ann Neurol* 1, 378
(1977): Schubothe H+, *Immun Infekt* 5, (German) 142
(1977): Schubothe H+, *Verh Dtsch Ges Inn Med* (German) 83, 727
(1977): Warner WA, *Ariz Med* 34, 172
(1977): Weiss RB, *W V Med J* 73, 101
(1976): Cohmen G, *Med Klin* (German) 71, 789
(1976): Demay-Wechsler P, *Rev Stomatol Chir Maxillofac* (French) 77, 727
(1976): Levo Y+, *Ann Rheum Dis* 35, 181

(1976): No Author, *Johns Hopkins Med J* 138, 289
(1976): Utsinger PD+, *Ann Intern Med* 84, 293
(1976): Whittle TS+, *Arch Pathol Lab Med* 100, 469
(1975): Dubois EL, *J Rheumatol* 2, 204
(1975): Falko JM+, *Ann Intern Med* 83, 832
(1975): Ghose MK, *Am J Med* 58, 581
(1975): Henningsen NC+, *Acta Med Scand* 198, 475 (>5%)
(1975): Lee SL+, *Semin Arthritis Rheum* 5, 83
(1975): Novack MA+, *JAMA* 232, 1269
(1975): Sunder SK+, *Am J Cardiol* 36, 960
(1974): Artinian B+, *Can Med Assoc J* 110, 314
(1974): Bareis RJ, *S D J Med* 27, 19
(1974): Frislid K+, *Tidsskr Nor Laegeforen* (Norwegian) 94, 1926
(1974): Harpey JP, *Ann Allergy* 33, 256
(1974): McEwen J, *Lancet* 2, 1570
(1974): No Author, *Med Lett Drugs Ther* 16, 34
(1974): No Author, *Va Med Mon* 101, 299
(1974): Winfield JB+, *Arthritis Rheum* 17, 325
(1974): Winfield JB+, *Arthritis Rheum* 17, 97
(1973): Auerbach RC+, *Radiology* 109, 287
(1973): Blomgren SE+, *Semin Hematol* 10, 345
(1973): Durand JP+, *Can Med* (French) 14, 9
(1973): Kosowski BD+, *Circulation* 47, 1204 (>5%)
(1973): Manigand G+, *Sem Hop* (French) 49, 3207
(1973): Rosenberg DS+, *South Med J* 66, 1294
(1973): Sokol SA, *J Maine Med Assoc* 64, 54
(1973): Swarbrick ET+, *Rheumatol Phys Med* 12, 94
(1972): Anastassiades TP+, *Can Med Assoc J* 107, 312
(1972): Blomgren SE+, *Am J Med* 52, 338
(1972): Donlan CJ+, *Chest* 61, 685
(1972): Dorfmann H+, *Nouv Presse Med* (French) 1, 2967
(1972): Hope RR+, *Med J Aust* 2, 298 (>5%)
(1972): Rasmussen K, *Tidsskr Nor Laegeforen* (Norwegian) 92, 709
(1972): Swarbrick ET+, *Br Heart J* 34, 284
(1971): Dabrowska B+, *Kardiol Pol* (Polish) 14, 316
(1971): Maxon HR+, *Mil Med* 136, 617
(1971): Sawaya J, *J Med Liban* (French) 24, 59
(1971): Wehr KL+, *N C Med J* 32, 56
(1970): Baker H+, *Br J Dermatol* 82, 320
(1970): Heymans G+, *Acta Cardiol* (French) 25, 404
(1970): Hopkins BE, *Med J Aust* 2, 734
(1970): Merwe JP van de, *Ned Tijdschr Geneeskd* (Dutch) 114, 105
(1970): Sheldon PJ+, *Ann Rheum Dis* 29, 236
(1970): Waagstein F, *Nord Med* (Swedish) 83, 468
(1970): Whittingham S+, *Australas Ann Med* 19, 358
(1969): Alarcon-Segovia D, *Mayo Clin Proc* 44, 664
(1969): Atkins CJ+, *Proc R Soc Med* 62, 197
(1969): Byrd RB+, *Dis Chest* 55, 170
(1969): Dubois EL, *Medicine* (Baltimore) 48, 217
(1969): Fellner MJ+, *Arch Belg Dermatol Syphiligr* (French) 25, 417
(1969): Gunther R+, *Dtsch Med Wochenschr* (German) 94, 2338
(1969): No Author, *JAMA* 208, 525
(1969): Russel AS+, *Ann Rheum Dis* 28, 328
(1968): Cohen AI+, *Ariz Med* 25, 565
(1968): Hunt WH, *Tex Med* 64, 54
(1968): Lappat EJ+, *Am J Med* 45, 846
(1968): Mehta BR, *Hawaii Med J* 28, 120
(1968): Petersen BN+, *Ugeskr Laeger* (Danish) 130, 2131
(1968): Puech P+, *Arch Mal Coeur Vaiss* (French) 61, 1550
(1968): Rutherford BD, *N Z Med J* 68, 235
(1967): Compton-Smith RN+, *Br J Clin Pract* 21, 248
(1967): Fakhro AM+, *Am J Cardiol* 20, 367 (>5%)
(1967): McDevitt DG+, *BMJ* 3, 780
(1967): Sanford HS+, *Dis Chest* 51, 172
(1966): Alarcon-Segovia D, *Rev Invest Clin* (Spanish) 18, 445
(1966): London BL+, *Am Heart J* 72, 806
(1966): Oster ZH, *Isr J Med Sci* 2, 354

(1966): Prockop LD, *Arch Neuron* 14, 326
(1965): Carabia AG+, *J Tenn Med Assoc* 58, 287
(1965): Paine R, *JAMA* 194, 23
(1962): Ladd AT, *N Engl J Med* 267, 1357
Pruritus (<1%)
Purpura
  (1984): Christensen DJ+, *Ann Intern Med* 100, 918
  (1976): Bluming AZ+, *JAMA* 236, 2521
  (1966): Stoffer RP, *J Kans Med Soc* 67, 20
Rash (sic) (<1%)
Sjøgren's syndrome
  (1968): Taylor JA, *Lancet* 1, 978
Urticaria (1–5%)
  (1988): Knox JP+, *Cutis* 42, 469
Vasculitis
  (1988): Knox JP+, *Cutis* 42, 469
  (1984): Ekenstam E+, *Arch Dermatol* 120, 484
  (1968): Dolan DL, *Mo Med* 65, 365
  (1967): Rosin JM, *Am J Med* 42, 625

Other
Dysgeusia (3–4%) (bitter taste)
  (2000): Zervakis J+, *Physiol Behav* 68, 405
Myalgia (<1%)
Myopathy (<1%)
  (1986): Lewis CA+, *BMJ* 292, 593
  (1968): Taylor JA, *Lancet* 1, 978
Oral mucosal eruption
  (1985): Gorsulowsky DC+, *J Am Acad Dermatol* 12, 245 (2%)
Pseudolymphoma
  (1996): Magro CM+, *Hum Pathol* 27(2), 125
Tremor (<1%)

PROCARBAZINE

Trade name: Matulane (Sigma-Tau)
Other common trade name: *Natulan*
Indications: Hodgkin's disease, lymphomas
Category: Antineoplastic
Half-life: 60 minutes
Clinically important, potentially hazardous interactions with: aldesleukin, methotrexate

Reactions

Skin
Allergic reactions (sic) (<1%)
Angioedema
  (1976): Glovsky MM+, *J Allergy Clin Immunol* 57, 134
Dermatitis (sic) (<1%)
Diaphoresis
Edema
Exanthems
  (1980): Andersen E+, *Scand J Haematol* 24, 149 (9%)
  (1972): Jones SE+, *Cancer* 29, 498
  (1966): Witte S+, *Schweiz Med Wochenschr* (German) 96, 93 (2%)
  (1965): Brunner KW+, *Ann Intern Med* 63, 69 (4%)
  (1965): Todd IDH, *BMJ* 1, 628
Exfoliative dermatitis
  (1976): Glovsky MM+, *J Allergy Clin Immunol* 57, 134
Fixed eruption
  (1988): Giguere JK+, *Med Pediatr Oncol* 16, 378
Flu-like syndrome (sic) (<1%)
Flushing
  (1966): Witte S+, *Schweiz Med Wochenschr* (German) 96, 93

(1965): Todd IDH, *BMJ* 1, 628
Herpes zoster
Petechiae
Photosensitivity
Pigmentation (1–10%)
Pruritus (<1%)
  (1965): Brunner KW+, *Ann Intern Med* 63, 69
Purpura
Rash (sic)
Toxic epidermal necrolysis
  (1980): Andersen E+, *Scand J Haematol* 24, 149
  (1969): Guerrin J+, *Rev Med Dijon* (French) 4, 523
Urticaria
  (1980): Andersen E+, *Scand J Haematol* 24, 149 (9%)
  (1976): Glovsky MM+, *J Allergy Clin Immunol* 57, 134
  (1972): Jones SE+, *Cancer* 29, 498

Hair
Hair – alopecia (1–10%)
  (1970): Stolinsky DC+, *Cancer* 26, 984
  (1965): Todd IDH, *BMJ* 1, 628

Other
Disulfiram-like reaction*
Gynecomastia
Headache
Hypersensitivity (2%)
  (1972): Jones SE+, *Cancer* 29, 498
Myalgia (<1%)
Oral mucosal lesions
  (1983): Bronner AK+, *J Am Acad Dermatol* 9, 645 (1–5%)
  (1970): Stolinsky DC+, *Cancer* 26, 984
Paresthesias (>10%)
Stomatitis (>10%)
Xerostomia

***Note:** Disulfiram-like reactions include headache, respiratory difficulties, nausea, vomiting, sweating, thirst, hypotension, and flushing

PROCHLORPERAZINE

Trade name: Compazine (GSK)
Other common trade names: *Edisylate; Novamin; Novomit; Pasotomin; Prorazin; Stella; Stemetil; Tementil; Vertigon*
Indications: Psychotic disorders
Category: Phenothiazine antipsychotic
Half-life: 23 hours
Clinically important, potentially hazardous interactions with: antihistamines, arsenic, chlorpheniramine, dofetilide, piperazine, quinolones, sparfloxacin

Reactions

Skin
Diaphoresis
Eczema (sic)
Erythema
Exanthems
  (1959): Wright W, *JAMA* 171, 1642
Exfoliative dermatitis
Fixed eruption (<1%)
  (1984): Reilly GD+, *Acta Derm Venereol* (Stockh) 64, 270
Hypohidrosis (>10%)
Lupus erythematosus
Peripheral edema

Photosensitivity (1–10%)
  (1997): O'Reilly FM+, American Academy of Dermatology
    Meeting, Poster #14
  (1988): Rasmussen HB+, *Ugeskr Laeger* (Danish) 150, 930
  (1964): Hartman DL+, *Skin* 3, 198
Phototoxicity
Pigmentation (<1%) (blue-gray)
Pruritus (1–10%)
Purpura
  (1965): Horowitz HI+, *Semin Hematol* 2, 287
Rash (sic) (1–10%)
Seborrhea
Toxic epidermal necrolysis
  (1986): Mérot Y+, *Arch Dermatol* 122, 455
  (1975): Benini G+, *Minerva Anestesiol* (Italian) 41, 314
Urticaria
Xerosis

Other
Anaphylactoid reactions (1–10%)
Blue tongue (sic)
  (1989): Alroe C+, *Med J Aust* 150, 724
Galactorrhea (<1%)
Gynecomastia (1–10%)
Headache
Lip ulceration
  (1984): Reilly GD+, *Acta Derm Venereol* (Stockh) 64, 270
Mastodynia
Parkinsonism
Priapism (<1%)
Sialorrhea
Tremor
Xerostomia (>10%)

PROCYCLIDINE

Trade name: Kemadrin (GSK)
Other common trade names: *Apricolin; Kemadren; Onservan; Procyclid*
Indications: Parkinsonism
Category: Anticholinergic; Antidyskinetic; Antiparkinsonian
Duration of action: 4 hours
Clinically important, potentially hazardous interactions with: anticholinergics, arbutamine

Reactions

Skin
Hypohidrosis (>10%)
Photosensitivity (1–10%)
Rash (sic) (<1%)
Urticaria
Xerosis (>10%)

Other
Xerostomia (>10%)

PROGESTINS

Generic names:
  Hydroxyprogesterone
    Trade names: Delta-Lutin; Duralutin; Hylutin; Pro-Depo;
      Prodrox
  Medroxyprogesterone
    Trade names: Amen (Carnick); Curretab; Cycrin (Wyeth);
      Provera (Pharmacia)
  Megestrol
    Trade name: Megace (Bristol-Myers Squibb)
  Norethindrone
    Trade names: Aygestin (Wyeth); Micronor (Ortho); Norlutin;
      Norlutate;
      Nor-QD
  Norgestrol
    Trade name: Ovrette (Wyeth)
  Progesterone
    Trade names: Gesterol 50; Progestaject (Various
      pharmaceutical companies.)
Category: Antineoplastic; Contraceptive (systemic); Progestin
Clinically important, potentially hazardous interactions with: acitretin, dofetilide

Reactions

Skin
Acne
  (1995): Freeman EW+, *JAMA* 274, 51
Acute generalized exanthematous pustulosis (AGEP)
  (1998): Kuno Y+, *Acta Derm Venereol* 78, 383
Angioedema
Ankle edema
Autoimmune dermatitis
  (2002): Oskay T+, *Eur J Dermatol* 12(6), 589
  (1997): Shahar E+, *Int J Dermatol* 36, 708
  (1991): Freychet F+, *Ann Dermatol Venereol* (French) 118, 551
  (1990): Teelucksingh S+, *J Intern Med* 227, 143
  (1985): Katayama I+, *Br J Dermatol* 112, 487
  (1984): Anderson RH, *Cutis* 33, 490
  (1978): Linse R+, *Dermatol Monatsschr* (German) 164, 656
  (1974): Hipkin LJ, *BMJ* 3, 575
  (1971): Farah FS+, *J Allergy Clin Immunol* 48, 257 (urticarial)
  (1967): Tromovitch TA+, *Calif Med* 106, 211 (urticarial)
Dermatitis (sic)
  (2001): Izu K+, *J UOEH* 23(4), 431
  (1974): Hipkin LJ, *BMJ* 3, 575
  (1964): Shelley WB+, *JAMA* 190, 35
Diaphoresis
  (1990): Willemse PHB+, *Eur J Cancer* 26, 337 (31%)
Edema
Erythema multiforme
  (1985): Wojnarowska F+, *J R Soc Med* 78, 407
Erythema nodosum
Exanthems
Flushing
  (1990): Willemse PHB+, *Eur J Cancer* 26, 337 (12%)
Hemorrhage (sic)
Melasma
Pruritus
Rash (sic)
Telangiectasia
  (1970): Aram H+, *Acta Derm Venereol* 50, 302
Urticaria
  (1995): Shelley WB+, *Cutis* 55, 282 (observation)
  (1994): Shelley WB+, *Cutis* 55, 21 (observation)
  (1994): Yee KC+, *Br J Dermatol* 130, 121

Hair
Hair – alopecia
Hair – hirsutism

Other
Anaphylactoid reactions
Galactorrhea
Gynecomastia (painful)

PROMAZINE

Trade name: Sparine (Wyeth)
Other common trade names: *Liranol; Prazine; Protactyl; Savamine; Talofen*
Indications: Psychotic disorders, schizophrenia
Category: Antiemetic; Phenothiazine antipsychotic
Half-life: 24 hours
Clinically important, potentially hazardous interactions with: sparfloxacin

Reactions

Skin
Dermatitis (sic)
Edema
Exanthems
   (1974): Rothstein E, *N Engl J Med* 290, 521
Hypohidrosis (>10%)
Photosensitivity (1–10%)
   (1964): Hartman DL+, *Skin* 3, 198
Phototoxicity
   (1985): Chignell CF+, *Environ Health Perspect* 64, 103
   (1985): Motten AG+, *Photochem Photobiol* 42, 9
Pigmentation (<1%) (slate-gray)
Purpura
Rash (sic) (1–10%)
Urticaria
Xerosis

Other
Galactorrhea (<1%)
Gynecomastia
Mastodynia (1–10%)
Parkinsonism
Priapism (<1%)
Xerostomia

PROMETHAZINE

Trade names: Anergan (Forest); Phenazine; Phenergan (Wyeth) (Elkins-Sinn)
Other common trade names: *Atosil; Bonnox; Closin; Goodnight; Histantil; Pentazine; Prometh-50; Prothiazine; Pyrethia*
Indications: Allergic rhinitis, urticaria
Category: Antivertigo; Phenothiazine
Half-life: 10–14 hours
Clinically important, potentially hazardous interactions with: antihistamines, arsenic, chlorpheniramine, dofetilide, nalbuphine, piperazine, quinolones, sparfloxacin

Reactions

Skin
Allergic reactions (sic) (<1%)
Angioedema (<1%)
Bullous eruption (<1%)
Chills
Dermatitis (sic)
   (1997): Varela P, Porto, Portugal (from Internet) (observation)
   (1970): Pirila V, *Allerg Asthma Leipz* (German) 16, 15 (endogenic)
   (1968): Periss Z, *Lijec Vjesn* (Serbo-Croat) 90, 15
   (1955): Sidi I+, *J Invest Dermatol* 24, 345
Diaphoresis
Eczema (sic)
   (1955): Sidi E+, *J Invest Dermatol* 24, 345
Erythema multiforme
   (1986): Dikland WJ+, *Pediatr Dermatol* 3, 135
   (1986): Fisher AA, *Cutis* 37, 158
Exanthems
   (1967): Lockey SD, *Med Sci* 18, 43
Fixed eruption
   (1984): Chan HL, *Int J Dermatol* 23, 607
Flushing
Jaundice
Lupus erythematosus
   (1971): Fabius AJM+, *Acta Rheumatol Scand* 17, 137
   (1965): Grupper C+, *Bull Soc Fr Dermatol Syphiligr* (French) 72, 714
Photosensitivity (<1%)
   (1997): Varela P, Porto, Portugal (from Internet) (observation)
   (1991): Bergner T+, *J Allergy Clin Immunol* 87, 278
   (1988): Menz J+, *J Am Acad Dermatol* 18, 1044
   (1982): Rosen K+, *Acta Derm Venereol* 62, 246
   (1982): Torinuki W+, *Tohoku J Exp Med* 138, 223
   (1974): Tay C, *Asian J Med* 10, 223
   (1970): Leong YO, *Acta Rheumatol Scand* 17, 137
   (1969): Kalivas J, *JAMA* 209, 1706
   (1967): Lockey SD, *Med Sci* 18, 43
   (1964): Hartman DL+, *Skin* 3, 198
   (1961): Stevanovic DV, *Br J Dermatol* 73, 233
   (1960): Newell RGD, *BMJ* 2, 359
   (1957): Epstein S+, *J Invest Dermatol* 29, 319
Pigmentation
Purpura
   (1967): Lockey SD, *Med Sci* 18, 43
   (1965): Horowitz HI+, *Semin Hematol* 2, 287
Rash (sic) (<1%)
   (1991): Blanc VF+, *Can J Anaesth* 38, 54
Stevens–Johnson syndrome
   (1972): Monnat A, *Schweiz Med Wochenschr* (German) 102, 1876
Systemic eczematous contact dermatitis
Toxic epidermal necrolysis (<1%)
   (1972): Monnat A, *Schweiz Med Wochenschr* (German) 102, 1876

(1959): Messaritakis J, *Ann Paediatr* (German) 207, 236
Urticaria
(1994): Myers P+, *Arch Ophthalmol* 112, 734
(1988): Mills PJ, *Anaesthesia* 43, 66 (with temazepam)
(1967): Lockey SD, *Med Sci* 18, 43

Other
Anaphylactoid reactions
(1988): Mills PJ, *Anaesthesia* 43, 66 (with temazepam)
Embolia cutis medicamentosa (Nicolau syndrome)
(1995): Faucher L+, *Pediatr Dermatol* 12, 187
Galactorrhea
Gynecomastia
Headache
Hypersensitivity
(1996): Palop V+, *Aten Primaria* (Spanish) 18, 47
Injection-site reactions
Mastodynia
Myalgia (<1%)
Oral ulceration
(1967): Mackie BS, *Br J Dermatol* 79, 106
Paresthesias (<1%)
Parkinsonism
Priapism
Tinnitus
Xerostomia (1–10%)
(1991): Blanc VF+, *Can J Anaesth* 38, 54

PROPAFENONE

Trade name: Rythmol (Abbott)
Other common trade names: *Arythmol; Norfenon; Normorytmin; Rythmex; Rytmonorm*
Indications: Ventricular arrhythmias
Category: Antiarrhythmic class I C
Half-life: 10–32 hours
Clinically important, potentially hazardous interactions with: digoxin, ritonavir

Reactions

Skin
Acne (1%)
Diaphoresis (1%)
Edema (<1%)
Exanthems
(1975): Harron DWG+, *Drugs* 34, 617
Flushing (<1%)
Lupus erythematosus (<1%)
(1986): Guindo J+, *Ann Intern Med* 104, 589
(1975): Harron DWG+, *Drugs* 34, 617
Pruritus (<1%)
Purpura (<1%)
Rash (sic) (1–3%)
Urticaria

Hair
Hair – alopecia (<1%)

Other
Dysgeusia (3–23%)
(2000): Zervakis J+, *Physiol Behav* 68, 405
Headache
Oral mucosal lesions
(1975): Harron DWG+, *Drugs* 34, 617 (>5%)

Paresthesias (<1%)
Parosmia (<1%)
Tinnitus
Tremor (<1%)
Xerostomia (2%)

PROPANTHELINE

Trade name: Propantheline
Other common trade names: *Bropantil; Corrigast; Ercoril; Ercotina; Norproban; Propantel*
Indications: Peptic ulcer
Category: Antispasmodic; Gastrointestinal anticholinergic
Half-life: 1.6 hours
Clinically important, potentially hazardous interactions with: anticholinergics, arbutamine, digoxin

Reactions

Skin
Allergic reactions (sic)
Dermatitis
(1996): Jansen T+, *Dtsch Med Wochenschr* (German) 121, 41
(1983): Przybilla B+, *Hautarzt* (German) 34, 459 (from antiperspirant)
(1982): Gall H+, *Derm Beruf Umwelt* (German) 30, 55 (from antiperspirant)
(1976): Agren-Jonsson S+, *Contact Dermatitis* 2, 79 (from antiperspirant)
(1975): Hannuksela M, *Contact Dermatitis* 1, 244
(1975): Osmundsen PE, *Contact Dermatitis* 1, 251
Diaphoresis (>10%)
Exanthems
Hypohidrosis
Rash (sic) (<1%)
Urticaria
Xerosis (>10%)

Other
Ageusia
Anaphylactoid reactions
Dysgeusia
Headache
Sialopenia
Xerostomia (>10%)

PROPOFOL

Trade name: Diprivan (AstraZeneca)
Indications: Induction and maintenance of anesthesia
Category: General anesthetic; Sedative
Half-life: initial: 40 minutes; terminal: 3 days

Reactions

Skin
Allergic reactions (sic)
(1988): Jamieson V+, *Anaesthesia* 43, 70
Edema (<1%)
Exanthems
(1987): Boittiaux P+, *Ann Fr Anesth Reanim* (French) 6, 324 (6.6%)

(1987): Coursange F+, *Ann Fr Anesth Reanim* (French) 6, 258
    (6.6%)
Fixed eruption (1%)
Flushing (>1%)
Pruritus (>1%)
    (1987): Coursange F+, *Ann Fr Anesth Reanim* (French) 6, 258
Rash (sic) (5%)
Raynaud's phenomenon
    (1999): Gilston A, *Anaesthesia* 54, 307
Urticaria
    (1988): Aitken HA, *Anaesthesia* 43, 170
    (1987): Coursange F+, *Ann Fr Anesth Reanim* (French) 6, 258

Hair

Hair – color change (sic)
    (1994): Motsch J+, *Eur J Anaesthesiol* 11, 499 (passim)
    (1992): Bublin JG+, *J Clin Pharm Ther* 17, 297

Other

Anaphylactoid reactions (1–10%)
    (2001): Girgis Y, *Anaesthesia* 56(10), 1016
    (2001): Knoarzewski W+, *Anaesthesia* 56(5), 497 (fatal) (with
        fentanyl)
    (2001): Lewis S+, *Anaesthesia* 56(11), 1128
    (2001): Tsai MH+, *J Formos Med Assoc* 100(6), 424
    (2000): Ducart AR+, *J Cardiothorac Vasc Anesth* 14(2), 200
Cough
    (2002): Maile CJ, *Anaesthesia* 57(2), 202
    (2001): Aly EE, *Anaesthesia* 56(10), 1016
Death
    (2002): Mertes PM+, *Anaesthesia* 57(8), 821 (with fentanyl)
    (2001): Cannon ML+, *J Neurosurg* 95(6), 1053
    (2001): Girgis Y, *Anaesthesia* 56(10), 1016
Dysgeusia (<1%)
Injection-site erythema (<1%)
Injection-site pain (>10%)
    (2002): Davies AF+, *Anaesthesia* 57(6), 557
    (2002): Grauers A+, *Acta Anaesthesiol Scand* 46(4), 361
    (2002): Lembert N+, *Ann Fr Anesth Reanim* 21(4), 263
    (2002): Suzuki S+, *Masui* 51(2), 140
    (2002): White PF, *Anesth Analg* 94(4), 1042
    (2001): Gupta S+, *Anaesthesia* 56(10), 1016
    (2001): Larsen B+, *Anaesthesist* 50(11), 842
    (2001): Larsen R+, *Anaesthesist* 50(9), 676
    (2001): Liljeroth E+, *Acta Anaesthesiol Scand* 45(7), 839
    (2001): Tsubokura H+, *Masui* 50(11), 1196
    (2000): Levecque JP+, *Can J Anaesth* (French) 47, 291
    (2000): Picard P+, *Anesth Analg* 90, 963
    (2000): Pickford A+, *Pediatr Anaesth* 10, 129
    (1998): Nathanson MH+, *Anaesthesia* 53, 608
    (1998): Ozturk E+, *Anesthesiology* 89, 1041
    (1998): Tan CH+, *Anaesthesia* 53, 468
    (1988): Langley MS+, *Drugs*
Injection-site pruritus (<1%)
Myalgia (>1%)
Phlebitis
Rhabdomyolysis
    (2001): Cannon ML+, *J Neurosurg* 95(6), 1053
Sialorrhea (>1%)
Tinnitus
Twitching (1–10%)
Xerostomia (<1%)

PROPOLIS

Scientific name: *Propolis*
Family: None
Trade and other common names: Bee Glue; Bee Propolis;
Hive Dross; Propolis Balsam; Propolis Resin; Propolis Wax;
Russian Penicillin
Category: antibacterial; Immune stimulant
Purported indications and other uses: Tuberculosis, bacterial,
fungal and protozoal infections, nasopharyngeal carcinoma,
duodenal ulcer, Helicobacter pylori infection, cold, wound
cleansing, mouth rinse, genital herpes. Ingredient in cosmetics
Half-life: N/A

Reactions

Skin

Allergic reactions (sic)
    (2002): Junghans V+, *Am J Contact Dermat* 13(2), 87
    (2001): Callejo A+, *Allergy* 56(6), 579
    (1996): Bellagrandi S+, *J Am Acad Dermatol* 35(4), 644 (in HIV-
        positive patient)
    (1988): Hausen BM+, *Contact Dermatitis* 19(4), 296
    (1988): Slezak R, *Prakt Zubn Lek* 36(7), 208
    (1987): Blanken R+, *Ned Tijdschr Geneeskd* 131(26), 1121
    (1987): Rudzki E+, *Przegl Dermatol* 19(4), 296
Cheilitis
    (1996): Bellegrandi S+, *J Am Acad Dermatol* 35, 644
Dermatitis (sic)
    (2003): Lombardi C+, *Allerg Immunol* (Paris) 35(2), 52
    (2002): Henschel R+, *Contact Dermatitis* 47(1), 52
    (2002): Lieberman HD+, *J Am Acad Dermatol* 46, S30
    (2001): Teraki Y+, *Br J Dermatol* 144(6), 1277 (granulomatous)
    (2000): Tumova L+, *Ceska Slov Farm* 49(6), 285
    (1998): Burdock GA, *Food Chem Toxicol* 36(4), 347
    (1998): Downs AM+, *Contact Dermatitis* 38(6), 359
        (occupational)
    (1998): Thomas P+, *Arch Dermatol* 134(4), 511
    (1997): Silvani S+, *Contact Dermatitis* 37(1), 48 (in patients with
        psoriasis)
    (1990): Hegyi E+, *Hautarzt* 41(12), 675 (0.64%)
    (1990): Raton JA+, *Contact Dermatitis* 22(3), 183
    (1988): Schuler TM+, *Hautarzt* 39(3), 139 (6 patients)
    (1987): Angelini G+, *Contact Dermatitis* 17(4), 251 (in psoriasis)
    (1987): Cirasino L+, *Contact Dermatitis* 16(2)
    (1987): Frosch PJ, *Z Haut* 62(23), 1631
    (1987): Hausen BM+, *Contact Dermatitis* 17(3), 163
    (1987): Kleinhaus D, *Contact Dermatitis* 17(3), 187 (airborne)
    (1987): Trevisan G+, *Contact Dermatitis* 16(1), 48
    (1985): Ayala F+, *Contact Dermatitis* 12(3), 181
    (1985): Machackova J, *Contact Dermatitis* 13(1), 43
    (1985): Rudzki E+, *Contact Dermatitis* 13(3), 198
    (1985): Tosti A+, *Contacr Dermatitis* 12(4), 227
    (1984): Bedello PG+, *G Ital Deramtol Venereol* 119(6), 431
    (1984): Pincelli C+, *Contact Dermatitis* 11(1), 49
    (1984): Valsecchi R+, *Contact Dermatitis* 11(5), 317
    (1983): Kokelj F+, *Contact Dermatitis* 9(6), 518
    (1983): Melli MC+, *Contact Dermatitis* 9(5), 427 (in a bee-
        keeper)
    (1983): Monti M+, *Contact Dermatitis* 9(2), 163 (occupational
        and cosmetic)
    (1983): Rudzki E+, *Contact Dermatitis* 9(1), 40
    (1983): Takahashi M+, *Contact Dermatitis* 9(6) (from honeybee
        royal jelly)
    (1982): Monti M+, *G Ital Dermatol Venereol* 117(2), 119
    (1982): Proserpio G, *G Ital Dermatol Venereol* 117(5), 316
    (1975): Camarasa G, *Contact Dermatitis* 1(2), 124 (from
        beeswax)

Erythroderma
  (2001): Horiuchi Y, *Br J Dermatol* 145, 691
Sensitivity (sic)
  (1988): Nakamura T, *Contact Dermatitis* 18(5), 313
  (1987): Young E, *Contact Dermatitis* 16(1), 49
  (1980): Bogdaszewska-Czabanowska J+, *Przegl Dermatol* 67(6), 747
  (1979): Grzywa Z+, *Przegl Dermatol* 66(6), 709

Other

Hypersensitivity (sic)
  (1987): Rudzki E+, *Pol Tyg Lek* (Polish) 42(2), 40
  (1984): Tosti A+, *G Ital Dermatol Venereol* 119(5)
  (1977): Peterson HO, *Contact Dermatitis* 3, 278
Lymphadenopathy
  (2001): Teraki Y+, *Br J Dermatol* 144(6), 1277
Mucositis
  (1990): Hay KD+, *Oral Surg Oral Med Oral Pathol* 70, 584
Oral ulceration
  (1990): Hay KD+, *Oral Surg Oral Med Oral Pathol* 70, 584
Stomatitis
  (1996): Bellegrandi S+, *J Am Acad Dermatol* 35, 644

PROPOXYPHENE

Trade names: Darvocet-N (Lilly); Darvon (Lilly); Darvon Compound (Lilly)
Other common trade names: *Algafan; Antalvic; Develin; Dolotard; Doloxene; Liberan; Parvon*
Indications: Pain
Category: Narcotic analgesic
Half-life: 8–24 hours
Clinically important, potentially hazardous interactions with: alcohol, alprazolam, ritonavir, warfarin

Darvocet is propoxyphene and acetaminophen; Darvon Compound is propoxyphene and aspirin

Reactions

Skin

Diaphoresis
Exanthems
  (1976): Arndt KA+, *JAMA* 235, 918
Facial edema
Flushing
Pruritus
Rash (sic) (<1%)
Urticaria (<1%)

Other

Ano-recto-vaginal ulcerations
  (1984): Laplanche G+, *Ann Dermatol Venereol* (French) 111, 347 (from suppositories)
Injection-site nodules (sic)
  (1987): Pedragosa R+, *Arch Dermatol* 123, 297
Injection-site pain (1–10%)
Trembling
Xerostomia (1–10%)

PROPRANOLOL

Trade names: Inderal (Wyeth) (Elkins-Sinn); Inderide (Wyeth)
Other common trade names: *Acifol; Apsolol; Betabloc; Cinlol; Detensol; Inderalici; Inderex; Novo-Pranol; Prosin; Sinal; Tesnol*
Indications: Hypertension, angina pectoris
Category: Antianginal; Antiarrhythmic class II; Antihypertensive; Beta-adrenoceptor blocker
Half-life: 2–6 hours
Clinically important, potentially hazardous interactions with: cimetidine, clonidine, epinephrine, haloperidol, insulin, insulin glargine, terbutaline, verapamil

Inderide is propranolol and hydrochlorothiazide

Note: Cutaneous side effects of beta-receptor blockaders are clinically polymorphous. They apparently appear after several months of continuous therapy. Atypical psoriasiform, lichen planus-like, and eczematous chronic rashes are mainly observed. (1983): Hödl St, *Z Hautkr* (German) 58, 17

Reactions

Skin

Acne
  (1973): Almeyda J+, *Br J Dermatol* 88, 313
Angioedema
  (1983): Hannaway PJ+, *N Engl J Med* 308, 1536
Bullous eruption
  (1979): Faure M+, *Ann Dermatol Venereol* (French) 106, 161
Dermatitis
  (1994): Valsecchi R+, *Contact Dermatitis* 30, 177 (occupational)
  (1990): Rebandel P+, *Contact Dermatitis* 23, 199
Diaphoresis
Eczema (sic)
  (1981): van Joost T+, *Arch Dermatol* 117, 600
  (1979): Faure M+, *Ann Dermatol Venereol* (French) 106, 161
Edema
Erythema multiforme
  (1969): Pimstone B+, *S Afr Med J* 43, 1203
Exanthems
  (1976): Jensen HA+, *Acta Med Scand* 199, 363
  (1974): Greenblatt DJ+, *Drugs* 7, 118. (0.8%)
  (1973): Almeyda J+, *Br J Dermatol* 88, 313
  (1966): Stephen SA+, *Am J Cardiol* 18, 463 (0.4%)
Exfoliative dermatitis
  (1976): Jensen HA+, *Acta Med Scand* 199, 363
Flushing
  (1973): Almeyda J+, *Br J Dermatol* 88, 313
  (1966): Stephen SA+, *Am J Cardiol* 18, 463
Hyperkeratosis (palms and soles)
Lichenoid eruption
  (1991): Massa MC+, *Cutis* 48, 41
  (1980): Hawk JLM, *Clin Exp Dermatol* 5, 93
  (1976): Cochran REI+, *Arch Dermatol* 112, 1173
Lupus erythematosus
  (1982): Hughes GRV, *BJM* 284, 1358
  (1976): Harrison T+, *Postgrad Med* 59, 241
Necrosis
Pemphigus
  (1982): Ruocco V+, *Arch Dermatol Res* 274, 123
  (1980): Godard W+, *Ann Dermatol Venereol* (French) 107, 1213
Peripheral edema
Peripheral skin necrosis (sic)
  (1979): Gokal R+, *BMJ* 1, 721
  (1979): Hoffbrand BI, *BMJ* 1, 1082
Photosensitivity

(1979): Faure M+, *Ann Dermatol Venereol* (French) 106, 161
Phototoxicity
　(1992): Shelley WB+, *Cutis* 50, 182 (observation)
Pruritus
　(1973): Almeyda J+, *Br J Dermatol* 88, 313
Psoriasis
　(1993): Halevy S+, *J Am Acad Dermatol* 29, 504
　(1992): Raychaudhuri SP+, *J Am Acad Dermatol* 27, 787
　(1990): Halevy S+, *Arch Dermatol Res* 283, 472
　(1988): Heng MCY+, *Int J Dermatol* 27, 619
　(1987): Altomare GF+, *G Ital Dermatol Venereol* (Italian) 122, 531
　(1987): Savola J+, *BMJ* 295, 637
　(1986): Abel EA+, *J Am Acad Dermatol* 15, 1007
　(1986): Czernielewski J, *Lancet* 1, 808 (exacerbation)
　(1984): Arntzen K+, *Acta Derm Venereol* (Stockh) 64, 346
　(1983): Kaur S+, *Indian Heart J* 35, 181
　(1979): Faure M+, *Ann Dermatol Venereol* (French) 106, 161
　(1979): Halevy S+, *Cutis* 24, 95
　(1976): Enger E, *Tidsskr Nor Laegeforen* (Norwegian) 96, 1103
　(1976): Jensen HA+, *Acta Med Scand* 199, 363
　(1976): Wadskov S+, *Ugeskr Laeger* (Danish) 138, 784
　(1975): Padfield PL+, *BMJ* 1, 626
Purpura
　(1966): Harris A, *Am J Cardiol* 18, 431
Pustular psoriasis
　(1988): Heng MCY+, *Int J Dermatol* 27, 619
　(1985): Hu C-H+, *Arch Dermatol* 121, 1326
Rash (sic) (1–10%)
Raynaud's phenomenon
　(1976): Marshall AJ+, *BMJ* 1, 1498 (59%)
Sclerosis
　(1980): Graham JR, *Trans Am Clin Climatol Assoc* 92, 122
Stevens–Johnson syndrome
　(1990): Zukervar P+, *J Toxicol Clin Exp* (French) 10, 169
　(1989): Mukul+, *J Assoc Physicians India* 37, 797
Systemic erythematous eruption (sic)
　(1975): Felix RH+, *BMJ* 1, 626
Toxic epidermal necrolysis
　(1977): van Ketel WG+, *Ned Tijdschr Geneeskd* (Dutch) 121, 1475
Toxicoderma
　(1981): Danilov LN, *Vestn Dermatol Venerol* (Russian) January 42
Urticaria
　(1983): Hannaway PJ+, *N Engl J Med* 308, 1536
　(1983): Oliver R, *Cent Afr J Med* 29, 91
　(1975): Seides SF+, *Chest* 67, 496
Xerosis

Hair

Hair – alopecia
　(1994): Friedman M, *J Fam Pract* 39, 114
　(1983): Hödl ST, *Z Hautkr* (German) 58, 17.
　(1982): England JRF+, *Aust Fam Physician* 11, 225
　(1979): Hilder RJ, *Cutis* 24, 63
　(1977): Scribner MD, *Arch Dermatol* 113, 1303
　(1973): Martin CM+, *Am Heart J* 86, 236
Hair – alopecia areata
　(2001): Vinson RP, El Paso, TX (from Internet) (observation) (from a single dose)

Nails

Nails – discoloration
　(1976): Jensen HA+, *Acta Med Scand* 199, 363
Nails – onycholysis
　(1983): Hödl ST, *Z Hautkr* (German) 58, 17.
Nails – pitting (psoriasiform)
　(1976): Jensen HA+, *Acta Med Scand* 199, 363
Nails – thickening

(1983): Hödl ST, *Z Hautkr* (German) 58, 17.
(1979): Faure M+, *Ann Dermatol Venereol* (French) 106, 161

Other

Anaphylactoid reactions
　(1983): Hannaway PJ+, *N Engl J Med* 308, 1536
Cheilostomatitis (sic)
　(1977): Tangsrud SE+, *BMJ* 2, 1385
Dupuytren's contracture
　(1966): Coupland WW, *Med J Aust* 2, 137
Dysgeusia
　(2000): Zervakis J+, *Physiol Behav* 68, 405
Headache
Myalgia
Myopathy
　(1980): Uusitupa M+, *BMJ* 1, 183
Oral ulceration
　(1980): Hawk JLM, *Clin Exp Dermatol* 5, 93
Paresthesias
Peyronie's disease
　(1981): Neumann HAM+, *Dermatologica* 162, 330
　(1979): Pryor JP+, *Lancet* 1, 824
　(1977): Osborne DR, *Lancet* 1, 1111
　(1977): Wallis AA+, *Lancet* 2, 980
　(1977): Yudkin JS, *Lancet* 2, 1355 (passim)
　(1966): Coupland WW, *Med J Aust* 2, 137
Serum sickness
　(1983): Yen MC+, *Postgrad Med* 74, 291
Tongue pigmentation
　(1975): Raleigh F, *Drug Intell Clin Pharm* 9, 455
Xerostomia

PROPYLTHIOURACIL

Trade name: Propylthiouracil (Wyeth)
Other common trade names: *Propacil; Propycil; Propyl-Thyracil; Tiotil*
Indications: Hyperthyroidism
Category: Antithyroid
Half-life: 1–5 hours
Clinically important, potentially hazardous interactions with: anticoagulants, dicumarol, warfarin

Reactions

Skin

Acne
　(1980): Vasily DB+, *JAMA* 243, 458
Adverse effects (sic)
　(1982): Pacini F+, *J Endocrinol Invest* 5, 403
Angioedema
　(1980): Vasily DB+, *JAMA* 243, 458
　(1970): Amrhein JA+, *J Pediatr* 76, 54 (1%)
　(1965): Shelley WB, *Arch Dermatol* 91, 165
Dermatitis (sic)
　(1993): Elias AN+, *J Am Acad Dermatol* 29, 78
Edema (<1%)
Erythema nodosum
　(1985): Keren G+, *Isr J Med Sci* 21, 62
Exanthems
　(1987): Wing SS+, *Can Med Assoc J* 136, 121
　(1982): Gammeltoft M+, *Acta Dermatol Venereol* (Stockh) 62, 171 (3–5%)
　(1980): Vasily DB+, *JAMA* 243, 458
　(1972): Wiberg JJ+, *Ann Intern Med* 77, 414
　(1970): Amrhein JA+, *J Pediatr* 76, 54

Exfoliative dermatitis (<1%)
Lichenoid eruption
  (1967): Coleman WP, *Med Clin North Am* 51, 1073
Lupus erythematosus (1–10%)
  (1994): Sato-Matsumura KC+, *J Dermatol* 21, 501
  (1992): Skaer TL, *Clin Ther* 14, 496
  (1991): Alarcon-Segovia D+, *Baillieres Clin Rheumatol* 5, 1
  (1989): Horton RC+, *Lancet* 2, 568
  (1987): Wing SS+, *Can Med Assoc J* 136, 121 (20% ANA)
  (1985): Bulvik S+, *Harefuah* (Hebrew) 109, 13
  (1983): Berkman EM+, *Transfusion* 23, 135
  (1981): Searles RP+, *J Rheumatol* 8, 498
  (1981): Takuwa N+, *Endocrinol* (Jpn) 28, 663
  (1980): Condemi JJ, *Geriatrics* 35(3), 81
  (1973): Hung W+, *J Pediatr* 82, 852
  (1970): Amrhein JA+, *J Pediatr* 76, 54
  (1966): Faber V+, *Acta Med Scand* 179, 257
  (1964): Best MM+, *J Ky Med Assoc* 62, 47
Photosensitivity
  (1997): Ohtsuka M+, *Eur Resp J* 10, 1405
Pigmentation
Pruritus (<1%)
  (1980): Vasily DB+, *JAMA* 243, 458
Purpura
  (1987): Wing SS+, *Can Med Assoc J* 136, 121
  (1962): Walzer RA, *Arch Dermatol* 86, 826
Pyoderma gangrenosum
  (1999): Darben T+, *Australas J Dermatol* 40, 144
Rash (sic) (>10%)
Rosacea
  (1980): Vasily DB+, *JAMA* 243, 458
Ulcerations
  (2002): Helfgott SM+, *N Engl J Med* 347(2), 122
  (1987): Wing SS+, *Can Med Assoc J* 136, 121
Urticaria (<1%)
  (1980): Vasily DB+, *JAMA* 243, 458
  (1970): Amrhein JA+, *J Pediatr* 76, 54
Vasculitis (<1%)
  (2002): Helfgott SM+, *N Engl J Med* 347(2), 122
  (2000): Lopez-Marina V+, *Med Clin (Barc)* (Spanish) 114, 398
  (2000): Otsuka S+, *Br J Dermatol* 142(4), 828
  (1999): Gunton JE+, *J Clin Endocrinol Metab* 84(1), 13
  (1998): Harper L+, *Nephrol Dial Transplant* 13, 455
  (1998): Merkel PA, *Curr Opin Rheumatol* 10, 45
  (1998): Miller RM+, *Australas J Dermatol* 39, 96
  (1997): Kitahara T+, *Clin Nephrol* 47, 336
  (1997): Yarman S+, *Int J Clin Pharm Ther* 35, 282
  (1993): Dolman KM+, *Lancet* 342, 651
  (1992): Stankus SJ+, *Chest* 102, 1595
  (1992): Wolf D+, *Cutis* 49, 253
  (1987): Carrasco MD+, *Arch Intern Med* 147, 1677
  (1987): Wing SS+, *Can Med Assoc J* 136, 121
  (1986): Gleisner A+, *Rev Child Pediatr* (Spanish) 57, 64
  (1985): Cox NH+, *Clin Exp Dermatol* 10, 292
  (1982): Gammeltoft M+, *Acta Dermatol Venereol* (Stockh) 62, 171
  (1982): Reidy TJ+, *South Med J* 75, 1297
  (1980): Vasily DB+, *JAMA* 243, 458
  (1979): Houston BD+, *Arthritis Rheum* 22, 925
  (1978): Griswold WR+, *West J Med* 128, 543
  (1973): Hung W+, *J Pediatr* 82, 852
  (1965): McCombs RP, *JAMA* 194, 1059
  (1965): Shelley WB, *Arch Dermatol* 91, 165
  (1962): Walzer RA, *Arch Dermatol* 86, 826
Vesicular eruptions (in newborn)
  (1980): Vasily DB+, *JAMA* 243, 458
  (1977): Caplan RH+, *Wis Med J* 76, S88

Hair
Hair – alopecia (<1%)
  (1997): Ohtsuka M+, *Eur Resp J* 10, 1405
  (1980): Vasily DB+, *JAMA* 243, 458
  (1951): Clarke MLB, *JAMA* 147, 1711
Hair – depigmentation
  (1980): Vasily DB+, *JAMA* 243, 458

Other
Ageusia (1–10%)
Dysgeusia (1–10%) (metallic taste)
  (1993): Elias AN+, *J Am Acad Dermatol* 29, 78
Headache
Hypersensitivity
  (1999): Chastain MA+, *J Am Acad Dermatol* 41, 757
  (1991): Fong PC+, *Horm Res* 35, 132
  (1963): Walzer RA+, *JAMA* 184, 743
Myalgia
Oral mucosal lesions
  (1970): Amrhein JA+, *J Pediatr* 76, 54
Oral ulceration
  (1979): Houston BD+, *Arthritis Rheum* 22, 925
  (1970): Amrhein JA+, *J Pediatr* 76, 54
Paresthesias (<1%)
Polyarthritis
  (2002): Helfgott SM+, *N Engl J Med* 347(2), 122

PROTAMINE

Indications: Heparin overdose
Category: Heparin antagonist
Duration of action: 2 hours

Reactions

Skin
Angioedema
  (1991): Roelofse JA+, *Anesth Prog* 38, 99
Exanthems
  (1989): Weiss ME+, *N Engl J Med* 320, 886
Flushing (<1%)
Urticaria
  (1989): Weiss ME+, *N Engl J Med* 320, 886

Other
Anaphylactoid reactions
  (1991): Roelofse JA+, *Anesth Prog* 38, 99
  (1988): Oswald-Mammosser M+, *Rev Fr Allergol* (French) 28, 173
Death
  (2002): Kimmel SE+, *Anesth Analg* 94(6), 1402
Hypersensitivity (<1%)

PROTAMINE SULFATE

Indications: Heparin overdosage
Category: Anticoagulant; Coagulant
Half-life: N/A

Reactions

Skin
Adverse effects (sic)
  (1993): Cormack JG+, *Coron Artery Dis* 4(5), 420

Allergic reactions (sic)
(2002): Lee AY+, *Acta Derm Venereol* 82(2), 114
(2000): Ralley FE+, *J Cardiothorac Vasc Anesth* 14(6), 710
(1999): Bollinger ME+, *J Allergy Clin Immunol* 104(2), 462
(1999): Petays T+, *Duodecim* 115(5), 517 (immediate)
(1999): Porsche R+, *Heart Lung* 28(6), 418
(1995): Hughes C+, *CRNA* 6, 172
(1995): Hynynen M+, *Duodecim* 111(20), 1969
(1994): Pharo GH+, *Anesth Analg* 78(1), 181
(1993): Sticco SL, *CRNA* 4(3), 144
(1986): Bruni S+, *Diabetes Care* 9(5), 552
(1983): Watson RA+, *Urology* 22(5), 493
(1982): Sanchez MB+, *Lancet* 1(8283), 1243

Angioedema
(1999): Bollinger ME+, *J Allergy Clin Immunol* 104(2), 462
(1993): Kim R, *Del Med J* 65(1), 17
(1991): Roelofse JA+, *Anesth Prog* 38, 99

Erythema
(1992): Neidhart PP+, *Eur Heart J* 13(6), 856

Flushing

Rash (sic)
(1991): Weiss ME+, *Clin Rev Allergy* 9(3), 339
(1990): Weiss ME+, *Clin Exp Allergy* 20(6), 713

Urticaria
(1993): Kim R, *Del Med J* 65(1), 17
(1991): Weiss ME+, *Clin Rev Allergy* 9(3), 339
(1990): Weiss ME+, *Clin Exp Allergy* 20(6), 713
(1988): Gottschlich GM+, *Ann Allergy* 61(4), 277 (passim)

Other

Anaphylactoid reactions (sic)
(2002): Lee AY+, *Acta Derm Venereol* 82(2), 114
(2000): Peng CH+, *Acta Anaesthesiol Sin* 38(2), 97
(1999): Ravi R+, *Heart Dis* 1(5), 289
(1997): Abe K+, *Can J Anaesth* 44(6), 662 (2 cases)
(1996): Takenoshita M+, *Anesthesiology* 84(1), 233
(1995): Hruby M+, *Rozhl Chir* 74(6), 282
(1994): Dykewicz MS+, *J Allergy Clin Immunol* 93(1), 117 (2 cases)
(1993): Kim R, *Del Med J* 65(1), 17
(1993): Mezt S, *Anesthesiology* 79(3), 617
(1992): Neidhart PP+, *Eur Heart J* 13(6), 856
(1991): Hobbhahn J+, *Anaesthesist* 40(7), 365
(1991): Hobbhahn J+, *Anaesthesist* 40(8), 421
(1991): Roelofse JA+, *Anesth Prog* 38, 99
(1991): Vincent GM+, *Cathet Cardiovasc Diagn* 23(3), 164
(1989): Gupta SK+, *J Vasc Surg* 9(2), 342 (11 cases)
(1989): Kambam JR+, *Can J Anaesth* 36(4), 463 (2 cases)
(1989): Zhang ZY+, *Proc Chin Med Sci Peking Union Med Coll* 4(2), 117
(1988): Gottschlich GM+, *Ann Allergy* 61(4), 277 (passim)
(1988): Shikuma LR+, *Drug Intell Clin Pharm* 22(3), 211
(1985): Horrow JC, *Int Anesthesiol Clin* 23(3), 133
(1985): Mingi CL+, *Ma Zui Xue Za Zhi* 23(4), 220
(1985): Sharath MD+, *J Thorac Cardiovasc Surg* 90(1), 86
(1985): Weiler JM+, *J Allergy Clin Immunol* 75(2), 297
(1985): Westaby S+, *Br Heart J* 53(5), 574
(1984): Holland CL+, *Clin Cardiol* 7(3), 157 (4 cases)
(1984): Stewart WJ+, *Circulation* 70(5), 788 (patient allergic to fish)
(1984): Walker WS+, *Br Heart J* 52(1), 112 (2 patients)
(1983): Best N+, *Br J Anaesth* 55(11), 1149
(1983): Vierthaler LD+, *J Kans Med Soc* 84(9), 454
(1982): Vontz FK+, *Am Surg* 48(10), 549
(1981): Doolan L+, *Anaesth Intensive Care* 9(2), 147 (3 cases)
(1981): Knape JT+, *Anesthesiology* 55(3), 324 (patient allergic to fish)
(1980): Moorthy SS+, *Anesth Analg* 59(1), 77
(1978): Lakin JD+, *J Allergy Clin Immunol* 61(2), 102
(1978): Nordstrom L+, *Acta Anaesthesiol Scand* 22(3), 195

Back pain

Death
(2002): Kimmel SE+, *Anesth Analg* 94(6), 1402
(2000): Hakala T+, *Ann Chir Gynaecol* 89(2), 150
(2000): Peng CH+, *Acta Anaesthesiol Sin* 38(2), 97
(1991): Hobbhahn J+, *Anaesthesist - 0370525* 40(7), 365
(1991): Weiss ME+, *Clin Rev Allergy* 9(3), 339
(1989): Gupta SK+, *J Vasc Surg* 9(2), 342 (11 cases)
(1988): Gottschlich GM+, *Ann Allergy* 61(4), 277 (passim)
(1984): Holland CL+, *Clin Cardiol* 7(3), 157 (4 cases)
(1984): Just-Viera JO+, *Am Surg* 50(1), 52
(1984): Stewart WJ+, *Circulation* 70(5), 788 (patient allergic to fish)

Headache

Hypersensitivity
(1993): Kim R, *Del Med J* 65(1), 17
(1992): Hulshof MM+, *Br J Dermatol* 127(3), 286 (granulomatous)
(1991): Kollner A+, *Dtsch Med Wochenschr* 116(33), 1234
(1989): Lindblad B, *Eur J Vasc Surg* 3, 195
(1986): Tsuji Y+, *Kyobu Geka* 39(12), 973
(1984): Campbell FW+, *Anesthesiology* 61(6), 761

Malignant hyperthermia
(1997): Abe K+, *Can J Anaesth* 44(6), 662 (2 cases)

Rhabdomyolysis
(1999): Lobato EB+, *Anesthesiology* 91(1), 303

PROTEASE INHIBITORS*

Generic names:
Amprenavir
Trade name: Agenerase (GSK)
Indinavir
Trade name: Crixivan (Merck)
Nelfinavir
Trade name: Viracept (Agouron)
Ritonavir
Trade name: Norvir (Abbott)
Saquinavir
Trade names: Invirase (Roche); Fortovase (Roche)

Indications: HIV infection
Half-life: varies
Clinically important, potentially hazardous interactions with: pimozide, rifampin

Reactions

Skin

Acanthosis nigricans
(2002): Mellor-Pita S+, *Clin Infect Dis* 34(5), 716
Acute generalized exanthematous pustulosis (AGEP)
(1998): Aquilina C+, *Arch Intern Med* 158, 2160
Angiolipomas
(2002): Dauden E+, *AIDS* 16(5), 805
Angiolipomatosis
(2000): Dank JP+, *J Am Acad Dermatol* 42(1), 129
Striae
(1999): Darvay A+, *J Am Acad Dermatol* 41, 467

Nails

Nails – ingrown
(2000): Miot HA, Sao Paulo, Brazil (from Internet) (observation)
Nails – paronychia
(2000): Panse I+, *Br J Dermatol* 142, 496

Other

Buffalo hump

(2000): Carr A+, *AIDS* 14, F25
(1998): De Luca A+, *Lancet* 352, 320
(1998): Dieleman JP+, *Ned Tijdschr Geneeskd* (Dutch) 142, 2856
(3 patients)
(1998): Lo JC+, *Lancet* 351, 867 (8 patients)
(1998): Saint-Marc T+, *Lancet* 352, 319
(1998): Schindler JT+, *Ann Intern Med* 129, 164

Buffalo neck
(1999): Milpied-Homsi B+, *Ann Dermatol Venereol* (French)
126, 254

Bull neck (sic)
(1998): Meinrenken S, *Dtsch Med Wochenschr* (German) 123, A9

Fat distribution abnormality
(1999): Mann M+, *Aids Patient Care* 13, 287
(1998): Ho TT+, *Lancet* 351, 1736
(1998): Mishriki YY, *Postgrad Med* 104, 45 ('bulging belly')
(1998): Wurtz R, *Lancet* 351, 1735

Galactorrhea
(2000): Hutchinson J+, *Lancet* 356(9234), 1003

Hypersensitivity
(1997): Bonfanti P+, *AIDS* 11, 1301

Lipoatrophy
(2000): Carr A+, *AIDS* 14, F25
(2000): Panse I+, *Br J Dermatol* 142, 496

Lipodystrophy
(2002): James J+, *Dermatol Surg* 28(11), 979
(2001): Allan DA+, *Int J STD AIDS* 12(8), 532
(2001): Djokic M+, *Vojnosanit Pregl* 58(4), 433
(2000): Behrens GM+, *MMM Fortschr Med* (German) 142, 68
(2000): Graham NM, *J Acquir Immune Defic Syndr* 25(Suppl 1), S4
(2000): Hartmann M+, *Hautarzt* 51, 159
(2000): Lyon DE+, *J Assoc Nurses AIDS Care* 11, 36
(2000): Panse I+, *Br J Dermatol* 142, 496
(2000): Paparizos VA+, *AIDS* 14, 903
(2000): Reus S+, *An Med Interna* (Spanish) 17, 123
(1999): Madge S+, *AIDS* 13(6), 735
(1999): Mercie P+, *Lancet* 354(9181), 867
(1999): Ponce-de-Leon S+, *Lancet* 353, 1244
(1999): Williamson K+, *J Am Acad Dermatol* 40(4), 635
(1999): Yanovski JA+, *J Clin Endocrinol Metab* 84, 1925
(1998): Carr A+, *AIDS* 12, F51
(1998): Carr A+, *Lancet* 351(9119), 1881
(1998): Carr A+, *N Engl J Med* 339, 1296
(1998): Dieleman JP+, *Ned Tijdschr Geneeskd* (Dutch) 142, 2856
(3 patients)
(1998): Fischer T+, *Dtsch Med Wochenschr* (German) 123, 1512
(1998): Hengel RL+, *Conference on Retroviruses and Opportunistic
Infections* 156 (Abstract 407)
(1998): *Drugs and Ther Perspect* 12, 11
(1998): Lipsky J, *Lancet* 351, 847
(1998): Mann M+, *Conference on Retroviruses and Opportunistic
Infections* (Abstract 412)
(1998): Miller KD+, *Lancet* 351, 871 (indinavir)
(1998): Rosenberg HE+, *Conference on Retroviruses and
Opportunistic Infections* (Abstract 408)
(1998): Striker R+, *Clin Infect Dis* 27(1), 218
(1998): Wurtz R, *Lancet* 351, 1735

Note: Protease inhibitors cause dyslipidemia which includes elevated
triglycerides and cholesterol and redistribution of body fat centrally
to produce the so-called 'protease paunch,' breast enlargement, facial
atrophy, and 'buffalo hump'

*Note: Please see individual generic drugs for more references

PROTRIPTYLINE

Trade name: Vivactil (Merck) (Odessey)
Other common trade names: *Concordin; Triptil*
Indications: Depression
Category: Tricyclic antidepressant
Half-life: 54–92 hours
**Clinically important, potentially hazardous interactions
with:** amprenavir, arbutamine, clonidine, epinephrine,
formoterol, guanethidine, isocarboxazid, linezolid, MAO
inhibitors, phenelzine, quinolones, sparfloxacin, tranylcypromine

Reactions

Skin
Acne
Allergic reactions (sic) (<1%)
Angioedema
Dermatitis (sic) (3%)
(1967): Gilbert MM, *Int J Neuropsychiatry* 3, 36
Diaphoresis (1–10%)
Edema
Erythema
Exanthems
Flushing
Petechiae
Photosensitivity (<1%)
(1972): Bruinsma W, *Dermatologica* 145, 377
Phototoxicity
(1980): Kochevar IE, *Toxicol App Pharmacol* 54, 258
Pruritus (1–5%)
(1967): Gilbert MM, *Int J Neuropsychiatry* 3, 36
Purpura
Rash (sic)
Urticaria
Vasculitis
Xerosis

Hair
Hair – alopecia (<1%)

Other
Black tongue
Death
Dysgeusia (>10%)
Galactorrhea (<1%)
Glossitis
Gynecomastia (<1%)
Headache
Oral mucosal eruption
Paresthesias
Parkinsonism (1–10%)
Rhabdomyolysis
(1974): Greenblatt DJ+, *JAMA* 229(5), 556 (overdose) (fatal)
Stomatitis
Tinnitus
Tremor
Xerostomia (>10%)

PSEUDOEPHEDRINE

Trade names: Allegra-D (Aventis); Aquatab DM (Adams); Benadryl (Warner Lambert); Bromfed (Muro); Clatitin-D (Schering); Deconsal (Celltech); Entex (Elan); Robitussin-CF (Wyeth); Sudafed (Warner Lambert); Trinalin (Schering)
Other common trade names: *Balminil; Eltor 120; Maxiphed; Robidrine*
Indications: Nasal congestion
Category: Adrenergic agonist; Nasal decongestant; Sympathomimetic
Half-life: 9–16 hours
Clinically important, potentially hazardous interactions with: bromocriptine, fluoxetine, fluvoxamine, furazolidone, MAO inhibitors, paroxetine, phenelzine, sertraline, tranylcypromine

Reactions

Skin
Angioedema
 (1997): Rademaker M, Hamilton, New Zealand (3 personal cases) (observation)
 (1993): Cavanah DK+, *Ann Intern Med* 119, 302
Baboon syndrome
 (2000): Sanchez TS+, *Contact Dermatitis* 42, 312
Dermatitis (sic)
 (1998): Downs AM+, *Contact Dermatitis* 39, 33
 (1998): Vega F+, *Allergy* 53, 218
Diaphoresis (1–10%)
Eczema (sic)
 (1991): Tomb RR+, *Contact Dermatitis* 24, 86
Eruptions
 (1994): Shelley WB+, *Cutis* 52, 203 (observation)
 (1993): Cavanah DK+, *Ann Intern Med* 119, 302
Erythema multiforme
 (2002): Fontaine JF+, *Allerg Immunol (Paris* 34(7), 230
Exanthems
 (1995): Rochina A+, *J Invest Allergol Clin Immunol* 5, 235
 (1994): Shelley WB+, *Cutis* 52, 203 (observation)
 (1993): Cavanah DK+, *Ann Intern Med* 119, 302 (generalized)
 (1978): Frankland AW, *Practitioner* 211, 828
Exfoliative dermatitis
 (1993): Cavanah DK+, *Ann Intern Med* 119, 302
Fixed eruption
 (2001): Cowen E, *Dermatology Online Journal* 7, 23C
 (2001): Cowen E, *Dermatology Online Journal* 7, 24C (disseminated bullous)
 (1998): Anibarro B+, *Allergy* 53, 902
 (1998): Hindioglu U+, *J Am Acad Dermatol* 38, 499 (non-pigmenting solitary)
 (1998): Litt JZ, Beachwood, OH (personal case) (observation)
 (1998): Vidal C+, *Ann Allergy Asthma Immunol* 80, 309 (non-pigmenting)
 (1997): Garcia Ortiz JC+, *Allergy* 52, 229 (non-pigmenting)
 (1996): Alanko K+, *J Am Acad Dermatol* 35, 647
 (1996): Quan MB+, *Int J Dermatol* 35, 367 (non-pigmenting)
 (1994): Hauken M, *Ann Intern Med* 120, 442
 (1994): Krivda SJ+, *J Am Acad Dermatol* 31, 291 (non-pigmenting)
 (1994): Shelley WB+, *Cutis* 53, 116 (observation)
 (1994): Shelley WB+, *Cutis* 54, 240 (observation)
 (1988): Camisa C, *Cutis* 41, 339
 (1987): Shelley WB+, *J Am Acad Dermatol* 17, 403 (non-pigmenting)
 (1968): Brownstein MH, *Arch Dermatol* 97, 115
Pallor
Pseudo-scarlatina (sic)

 (1988): Taylor BJ+, *Br J Dermatol* 118, 827
Systemic contact dermatitis
 (1991): Tomb RR+, *Contact Dermatitis* 24, 86
Toxic erythema
 (1999): Oakley A, (from Internet) (2 observations)
Urticaria
 (1997): Rademaker M, Hamilton, New Zealand (3 personal cases) (observation)
 (1994): Shelley WB+, *Cutis* 54, 375 (observation)

Other
Headache
Tinnitus
Trembling
Tremor
Xerostomia

PSORALENS

Trade names: 8-MOP (ICN); Oxsoralen (ICN); Trisoralen (ICN)
Indications: Vitiligo
Category: Repigmenting agent
Half-life: 2 hours

Reactions

Skin
Acne
 (1978): Nielsen EB+, *Acta Derm Venereol (Stockh)* 58, 374
Basal cell carcinoma
 (2002): Katz KA+, *J Invest Dermatol* 118(6), 1038
 (1999): Hannuksela-Svahn A+, *J Am Acad Dermatol* 40, 694
Blistering (sic)
 (1993): Sheehan MP+, *Br J Dermatol* 129, 431 (PUVA)
 (1991): No Author, *Ned Tijdschr Geneeskd* (Dutch) 135, 1764
Bowen's disease
 (1979): Hofmann C+, *Br J Dermatol* 101, 685
Bullous pemphigoid (with UVA)
 (1996): George PM, *Photodermatol Photoimmunol Photomed* 11, 185
 (1996): Perl S+, *Dermatology* 193, 245
 (1994): Fryer EJ+, *J Am Acad Dermatol* 30, 651 (passim)
 (1989): Weber PJ+, *Arch Dermatol* 125, 690
 (1985): Grunwald MH+, *J Am Acad Dermatol* 13, 224
 (1982): Stüttgen G, *Int J Dermatol* 21, 198
 (1979): Abel EA+, *Arch Dermatol* 115, 988
 (1978): Robinson JK, *Br J Dermatol* 99, 709
 (1977): Melski JW+, *J Invest Dermatol* 68, 328
 (1976): Thomsen K+, *Br J Dermatol* 95, 568
Burning (1–10%)
 (2000): Al-Qattan MM, *Burns* 26(7), 653 (children)
 (1996): Nettelblad H+, *Burns* 22, 633
 (1982): Stüttgen G, *Int J Dermatol* 21, 198 (passim)
Cheilitis (1–10%)
Dermatitis
 (1994): Korffmacher H+, *Contact Dermatitis* 30, 283
 (1991): Takashima A+, *Br J Dermatol* 124, 37
 (1990): Fleming D+, *Allergy Proc* 11, 125
 (1990): Moller H, *Photodermatol Photoimmunol Photomed* 7, 43
 (1979): Saihan EM, *BMJ* 2, 20
Eczema (sic)
 (1994): Korffmacher H+, *Contact Dermatitis* 30, 283
 (1979): Saihan EM, *BMJ* 2, 20
Edema (1–10%)
Erythema
 (2000): Yeo UC+, *Br J Dermatol* 142, 733

Other

Anaphylactoid reactions
(2001): Legat FJ+, *Br J Dermatol* 145(5), 821
Lymphoproliferative disease
(1989): Aschinoff R+, *J Am Acad Dermatol* 21, 1134
Tumors (for the most part malignant)
(1995): Weinstock MA+, *Arch Dermatol* 131, 701
(1994): Altman JS+, *J Am Acad Dermatol* 31, 505
(1994): Lever LR+, *Clin Exp Dermatol* 19, 443 (malignant)
(1994): Lewis FM+, *Lancet* 344, 1157
(1993): Lindelof B+, *Br J Dermatol* 129, 39
(1990): Young AR, *J Photochem Photobiol B* 6, 237
(1989): Hannuksela M+, *J Am Acad Dermatol* 21, 813
(1989): Stern RS+, *Carcinog Compr Surv* 11, 85
(1988): Gupta AK+, *J Am Acad Dermatol* 19, 67
(1987): Henseler T+, *J Am Acad Dermatol* 16, 108
(1983): Farber EM+, *Arch Dermatol* 119, 426
(1983): Shafrir A, *Harefuah* (Hebrew) 104, 364
(1981): No Author, *Br Med J Clin Red Ed* 283, 335
(1980): Brown FS+, *J Am Acad Dermatol* 2, 393
(1980): Halprin KM+, *J Am Acad Dermatol* 2, 334
(1980): Halprin KM+, *J Am Acad Dermatol* 2, 432
(1978): Bridges BA, *Clin Exp Dermatol* 3, 349

PYRAZINAMIDE

Trade names: Pyrazinamide (Wyeth); Rifater (Aventis)
Other common trade names: *Braccopril; Dipimide; Isopas; Lynamide; Pirilene; Pyrazide; Rozide; Tebrazid; Zinastat*
Indications: Tuberculosis
Category: Antibacterial; Antitubercular
Half-life: 9–10 hours
Clinically important, potentially hazardous interactions with: rifampin

Reactions

Skin

Acne (<1%)
Edema of foot
(1983): Jorgensen J, *Int J Dermatol* 22, 44
Erythema multiforme
(1996): Perdu D+, *Allergy* 51, 340
Exanthems
(1990): Goday J+, *Contact Dermatitis* 22, 181
Fixed eruption
(1990): Goday J+, *Contact Dermatitis* 22, 181
Flushing
Photoallergic reaction
(2001): Maurya V+, *Int J Tuberc Lung Dis* 5(11), 1075
Photodermatitis (<1%)
(1999): Choonhakarn C+, *J Am Acad Dermatol* 40, 645 (lichenoid)
Pruritus (<1%)
Purpura
Rash (sic) (<1%)
(2000): Gordin F+, *JAMA* 283, 1445
(1998): Olivier C+, *Arch Pediatr* (French) 5, 289
(1998): Radal M+, *Rev Mal Respir* (French) 15, 305 (3 cases)
Side effects
(2002): Papastavros T+, *CMAJ* 167(2), 131 (with levofloxacin) (14 cases)
Urticaria

Other

Acute intermittent porphyria

(1976): Treece GL+, *Am Rev Respir Dis* 113, 233
Death
(2002): Medinger A, *Chest* 121(5), 1710 (with rifampin)
(2001): No authors, *Can Commun Dis Rep* 27(13), 114 (with rifampin)
(2001): No authors, *JAMA* 286(12), 1445 (with rifampin)
(2001): No authors, *MMWR Morb Mortal Wkly Rep* 50(34), 733 (with rifampin)
Hypersensitivity
Myalgia (1–10%)
(2002): Papastavros T+, *CMAJ* 167(2), 131 (with levofloxacin) (14 cases)
Oral mucosal lesions
Porphyria cutanea tarda (<1%)
Tinnitus

PYRIDOXINE

Synonym: vitamin B$_6$
Trade names: Hexabetalin (Lilly); Nestrex
Other common trade names: *B(6)-Vicotrat; Beesix; Benadon; Godabion B6; Hexa-Betalin*
Indications: Pyridoxine deficiency
Category: Water-soluble nutritional supplement
Half-life: 15–20 days
Clinically important, potentially hazardous interactions with: levodopa

Reactions

Skin

Acne
(1991): Sherertz EF, *Cutis* 48, 119
(1976): Braun-Falco O+, *MMW Münch Med Wochenschr* (German) 118, 155
(1964): Fegeler F, *Arch Klin Exp Dermatol* (German) 219, 335
Allergic reactions (sic) (<1%)
Bullous eruption
(1984): Ruzicka T+, *Hautarzt* (German) 35, 197
Dermatitis
(2001): Bajaj AK+, *Contact Dermatitis* 44(3), 184 (occupational)
(1990): Camarasa JG+, *Contact Dermatitis* 23, 115
(1985): Yoshikawa K+, *Contact Dermatitis* 12, 55
(1983): Fujita M+, *Contact Dermatitis* 9, 61
Fixed eruption
(1972): Kuokkanen K, *Acta Allergol* 27, 407
Photosensitivity
(2001): Bajaj AK+, *Contact Dermatitis* 44(3), 184 (occupational)
(1998): Murata Y+, *J Am Acad Dermatol* 39, 314 (2 cases)
(1996): Tanaka M+, *J Dermatol* 23, 708
Purpura
Rosacea fulminans
(2001): Jansen T+, *J Eur Acad Dermatol Venereol* 15(5), 484
Toxic epidermal necrolysis
(1980): Andriushchenko OM+, *Klin Med Mosk* (Russian) 58, 101
Vasculitis
(1984): Ruzicka T+, *Hautarzt* (German) 35, 197
Vesicular eruptions
(1986): Friedman MA+, *J Am Acad Dermatol* 14, 915

Hair

Hair – pigmentation
(1972): Shelley WB+, *Arch Dermatol* 106, 228

Other

Hypersensitivity

(1969): Zheltakov MM+, *Vestn Dermatol Venerol* (Russian) 43, 62
Injection-site burning
Injection-site pain
Paresthesias (<1%)
Porphyria cutanea tarda
  (1992): Shelley WB+, *Advanced Dermatologic Diagnosis* WB
    Saunders, 414 (passim)
Pseudoporphyria
  (1984): Baer RL+, *J Am Acad Dermatol* 10, 527

PYRILAMINE

Indications: Allergic rhinitis
Category: Antihistamine H$_1$-blocker
Half-life: N/A

Reactions

Skin
Angioedema
Dermatitis (sic)
Diaphoresis
Flushing
Lupus erythematosus
Photosensitivity
Purpura
Rash (sic)
Urticaria

Other
Anaphylactoid reactions
Gynecomastia
Paresthesias
Stomatitis
Tinnitus
Xerostomia

PYRIMETHAMINE

Trade names: Daraprim (GSK); Fansidar (Roche)
Other common trade names: *Erbaprelina; Malocide;*
Pirimecidan
Indications: Malaria
Category: Antimalarial
Half-life: 80–95 hours
**Clinically important, potentially hazardous interactions
with:** dapsone

Fansidar is pyrimethamine and sulfadoxine

Reactions

Skin
Acute generalized exanthematous pustulosis (AGEP)
  (1995): Moreau A+, *Int J Dermatol* 34, 263 (passim)
Angioedema
  (1992): Breathnach SM+, *Adverse Drug Reactions and the Skin*
    Blackwell, Oxford, 176 (passim)
Bullous eruption
  (1992): Breathnach SM+, *Adverse Drug Reactions and the Skin*
    Blackwell, Oxford, 176 (passim)
  (1989): Caumes E+, *Presse Med* (French) 18, 1708
Dermatitis (sic) (<1%)

Erythema multiforme (<1%)
  (1993): Sturchler D+, *Drug Saf* 8, 160
  (1991): Porteous DM+, *Arch Dermatol* 127, 740 (in HIV+
    patients)
  (1987): Hellgren U+, *Br Med J Clin Res Ed* 295, 365
  (1986): Miller KD+, *Am J Trop Med Hyg* 35, 451
Exanthems
  (2002): Thong BY+, *Ann Allergy Asthma Immunol* 88(5), 527
    (with dapsone)
  (1989): Ortel B+, *Dermatologica* 178, 39 (papular)
  (1987): Groth H+, *Schweiz Rundsch Med Prax* (German) 76, 570
Exfoliative dermatitis
  (1987): Elsas T+, *Tidsskr Nor Laegeforen* (Norwegian) 107, 1231
  (1986): Langtry JA+, *Br Med J Clin Res Ed* 292, 1107
Fixed eruption
  (1988): Tham SN+, *Singapore Med J* 29, 300
Lichenoid eruption
  (1989): Zain RB, *Southeast Asian J Trop Med Public Health* 20, 253
    (oral)
  (1980): Cutler TP, *Clin Exp Dermatol* 5, 253
Lymphoma
  (1997): Costello JM+, *N Z Med J* 86, 430
Photosensitivity (>10%)
  (1992): Breathnach SM+, *Adverse Drug Reactions and the Skin*
    Blackwell, Oxford, 176 (passim)
  (1989): Ortel B+, *Dermatologica* 178, 39
  (1974): Craven SA, *BMJ* 2, 556
Pigmentation (<1%)
  (1991): Poizot-Martin I+, *Presse Med* (French) 20, 632
  (1990): Poizot-Martin I+, *Int Conf AIDS* 6, 357
  (1977): Costello JM+, *N Z Med J* 86, 430
  (1965): TenPas A+, *Am J Med Sciences* 249, 448
Pruritus
  (1987): Groth H+, *Schweiz Rundsch Med Prax* (German) 76, 570
Purpura
  (1965): TenPas A+, *Am J Med Sciences* 249, 448
Pustules
  (1973): Macmillan AL, *Dermatologica* 146, 285 (generalized)
Rash (sic) (<1%)
Stevens–Johnson syndrome (1–10%)
  (1995): Caumes E+, *Clin Infect Dis* 21, 656
  (1993): Schlienger RG+, *Schweiz Rundsch Med Prax* (German)
    82, 888
  (1993): Sturchler D+, *Drug Saf* 8, 160
  (1992): Breathnach SM+, *Adverse Drug Reactions and the Skin*
    Blackwell, Oxford, 176 (passim)
  (1991): Porteous DM+, *Arch Dermatol* 127, 740 (in HIV+
    patients)
  (1990): Thiel HJ+, *Klin Monatsbl Augenheilkd* (German) 197, 142
  (1989): Ortel B+, *Dermatologica* 178, 39
  (1989): Phillips-Howard PA+, *Lancet* 2, 803
  (1988): Mimoun G+, *Bull Soc Ophtalmol Fr* (French) 88, 961
  (1987): Hellgren U+, *Br Med J Clin Res Ed* 295, 365
  (1987): Lenox-Smith I, *J Infect* 14, 90 (fatal)
  (1987): Lyn PC+, *Med J Aust* 146, 335
  (1986): Bamber MG+, *J Infect* 13, 31 (fatal)
  (1986): Gascon-Brustenga J+, *Med Clin (Barc)* (Spanish) 87, 821
  (1986): Miller KD+, *Am J Trop Med Hyg* 35, 451
  (1985): Adams SJ+, *Postgrad Med J* 61, 263
  (1985): Clareus BW+, *Lakartidningen* (Swedish) 82, 4211
  (1983): Ligthelm RJ+, *Ned Tijdschr Geneeskd* (Dutch) 127, 1735
  (1982): Hornstein OP+, *N Engl J Med* 307, 1529
Toxic dermatitis (sic)
  (1995): Piketty C+, *Presse Med* (French) 24, 1710
Toxic epidermal necrolysis (<1%)
  (1998): Moussala M+, *J Fr Ophtalmol* (French) 21, 72
  (1998): Schmidt-Westhausen A+, *Oral Dis* 4, 90
  (1995): Caumes E+, *Clin Infect Dis* 21, 656
  (1993): Sturchler D+, *Drug Saf* 8, 160

(1992): Breathnach SM+, *Adverse Drug Reactions and the Skin*
    Blackwell, Oxford, 176 (passim)
(1991): Kimura S+, *Jpn J Med* 30, 553
(1990): Ward DJ+, *Burns* 16, 97
(1988): *Morb Mortal Wkly Rep* 37, 571
(1988): Phillips-Howard PA+, *Br Med J Clin Res Ed* 296, 1605
(1988): Raviglione MC+, *Arch Intern Med* 148, 2683 (fatal)
(1987): Hellgren U+, *Br Med J Clin Res Ed* 295, 365
(1986): Miller KD+, *Am J Trop Med Hyg* 35, 451
Urticaria
Vasculitis

Hair
Hair – alopecia

Other
Anaphylactoid reactions (<1%)
Death
Dysgeusia
Glossitis (<1%) (atrophic)
Hypersensitivity (>10%)
  (2002): Thong BY+, *Ann Allergy Asthma Immunol* 88(5), 527
    (with dapsone)
Lymphoproliferative disease
  (1977): Costello JM+, *N Z Med J* 86, 430
Tinnitus
Xerostomia (<1%)

QUAZEPAM

Trade name: Doral (Wallace)
Other common trade names: *Oniria; Pamerex; Quazium; Quiedorm; Selepam; Temodal*
Indications: Insomnia
Category: Antidepressant; Benzodiazepine sedative-hypnotic
Half-life: 25–41 hours
Clinically important, potentially hazardous interactions with: amprenavir, chlorpheniramine, clarithromycin, efavirenz, esomeprazole, imatinib, indinavir, nelfinavir, ritonavir

Reactions

Skin
Dermatitis (sic) (1–10%)
Diaphoresis (>10%)
Pruritus
  (1991): Roth T+, *J Clin Psychiatry* 52 Suppl 38–41
Purpura
Rash (sic) (>10%)
  (1991): Roth T+, *J Clin Psychiatry* 52 Suppl 38–41
Urticaria

Hair
Hair – alopecia
Hair – hirsutism

Other
Dysgeusia
Headache
Oral ulceration
Paresthesias
Sialopenia (>10%)
Sialorrhea (1–10%)
Xerostomia (1–5%)
  (1991): Roth T+, *J Clin Psychiatry* 52 Suppl 38–41

QUETIAPINE

Trade name: Seroquel (AstraZeneca)
Indications: Psychotic disorders, schizophrenia
Category: Antipsychotic
Half-life: ~6 hours

Reactions

Skin
Angioedema
  (1999): Drayton G, Los Angeles, CA (from Internet) (observation) (patient is also allergic to sulfa)
Candidiasis (<1%)
Diaphoresis (1–10%)
Edema
Facial edema (<1%)
Neuroleptic malignant syndrome
  (2002): Bourgeois JA+, *J Neuropsychiatry Clin neurosci* 14(1), 87
  (2002): Sing KJ+, *Am J Psychiatry* 159(1), 149
Photosensitivity (<1%)
Rash (sic) (4%)
Xerosis (<1%)

Other
Bruxism (<1%)

Gingivitis (<1%)
Glossitis (<1%)
Headache
Myalgia (<1%)
Oral ulceration (<1%)
Paresthesias (1%)
Priapism
  (2001): Pais VM+, *Urology* 58(3), 462
Sialorrhea (<1%)
Stomatitis (<1%)
Thrombophlebitis (<1%)
Tongue edema (<1%)
Xerostomia (7%)
  (2001): Mullen J+, *Clin Ther* 23(11), 1839 (14.5%)
  (2000): Matheson AJ+, *CNS Drugs* 14(2), 157

QUINACRINE

Trade name: Atabrine (Sanofi-Synthelabo)
Other common trade name: *Atabil*
Indications: Various infections caused by susceptible helminths
Category: Anthelmintic; Antimalarial
Half-life: 4–10 hours

Reactions

Skin
Dermatitis
Erythema dyschromicum perstans
  (1970): Tolman MM, *Arch Dermatol* 102, 113
Erythematous plaques
  (1981): Bauer F, *J Am Acad Dermatol* 4, 239
Exanthems
  (1981): Bauer F, *J Am Acad Dermatol* 4, 239 (eczematous) (80%)
  (1963): Nagy E+, *Dermatologica* (German) 126, 13 (1.4%)
  (1955): Alexander HL, *Reactions with Drug Therapy* Philadelphia, WB Saunders
  (1953): Zeller F, *Hautarzt* (German) 4, 384
Exfoliative dermatitis
  (1981): Bauer F, *J Am Acad Dermatol* 4, 239 (8%)
  (1967): Lockey SD, *Med Sci* 18, 43
  (1955): Alexander HL, *Reactions with Drug Therapy* Philadelphia, WB Saunders
Fixed eruption
  (1967): Lockey SD, *Med Sci* 18, 43
  (1964): Browne SG, *BMJ* 2, 1041
  (1961): Welch AL+, *Arch Dermatol* 84, 1004
  (1955): Alexander HL, *Reactions with Drug Therapy* Philadelphia, WB Saunders
Hypomelanosis
  (1967): Lockey SD, *Med Sci* 18, 43
Keratoderma
  (1978): Bauer F, *Aust J Dermatol* 19, 9
Lichenoid eruption
  (1981): Bauer F, *J Am Acad Dermatol* 4, 239 (12%)
  (1979): Callaway JL, *J Am Acad Dermatol* 1, 456
  (1978): Bauer F, *Aust J Dermatol* 19, 9
  (1971): Almeyda J+, *Br J Dermatol* 85, 604
  (1964): Baker H, *Br J Dermatol* 76, 186
  (1963): Nagy E+, *Dermatologica* (German) 126, 13 (1.4%)
  (1955): Alexander HL, *Reactions with Drug Therapy* Philadelphia, WB Saunders
Ochronosis
  (1976): Egorin MJ+, *JAMA* 236, 385
  (1976): Tuffanelli DL, *JAMA* 236, 2491

Photosensitivity
(1997): Hindson C, *The Schoch Letter* 47, 53
Pigmentation
(1982): Sokol RJ+, *Pediatrics* 69, 232 (yellow)
(1981): Koranda FC, *J Am Acad Dermatol* 4, 650
(1981): Zuehlke RL+, *Int J Dermatol* 20, 57
(1979): Leigh IM+, *Br J Dermatol* 101, 147
(1978): Bauer F, *Aust J Dermatol* 19, 9
(1969): *Med Lett* 11, 27 (yellowish)
Pruritus (<1%)
Squamous cell carcinoma
(1979): Callaway JL, *J Am Acad Dermatol* 1, 456
(1978): Bauer F, *Aust J Dermatol* 19, 9
Urticaria
(1969): *Med Lett* 11, 27 (1–5%)
(1955): Alexander HL, *Reactions with Drug Therapy* Philadelphia,
WB Saunders

Hair

Hair – alopecia
(1981): Bauer F, *J Am Acad Dermatol* 4, 239 (eczematous) (80%)
(1978): Bauer F, *Aust J Dermatol* 19, 9

Nails

Nails – changes (sic)
(1978): Bauer F, *Aust J Dermatol* 19, 9
Nails – pigmentation
(1969): *Med Lett* 11, 27
Nails – pigmentation (ala nasi) (blue-gray)
(2000): Kleinegger CL+, *Oral Surg Oral Med Oral Pathol Oral
Radiol Endod* 90, 189

Other

Oral mucosal pigmentation
(2000): Kleinegger CL+, *Oral Surg Oral Med Oral Pathol Oral
Radiol Endod* 90, 189
Oral pigmentation
(1970): Brynolf I, *Sven Tandlak Tidskr* (Swedish) 63, 585

QUINAPRIL

Trade name: Accupril (Parke-Davis)
Other common trade names: *Accuprin; Accupro; Acuitel;
Acupril; Asig; Korec; Quinazil*
Indications: Hypertension
Category: Angiotensin-converting enzyme (ACE) inhibitor;
Antihypertensive
Half-life: 1–2 hours
**Clinically important, potentially hazardous interactions
with:** amiloride, spironolactone, triamterene

Reactions

Skin

Angioedema (<1%)
(2001): Cohen EG+, *Ann Otol Rhinol Laryngol* 110(8), 701 (64
cases)
(1997): Sigler C+, *Arch Dermatol* 113, 972
(1996): Boxer M, *J Allergy Clin Immunol* 98, 471
(1995): Maier C, *Anaesthesist* (German) 44, 875
(1994): Cosano L+, *Med Clin* (Barc) (Spanish) 102, 275
(1993): Mendez-Mora JL+, *Med Clin* (Barc) (Spanish) 101, 76
(1992): Materson BJ, *Am J Cardiol* 69, 46C
(1989): Sedman AJ+, *Angiology* 40 (4 Pt 2), 360
Ankle edema
(1992): Bahena JH+, *Clin Ther* 14, 527
Bullous eruption

(1998): Sienkiewicz G, Johnson City, NY (from Internet)
(observation)
Diaphoresis (<1%)
(1991): Morant J+, *Arzneimittel-Kompendium der Schweiz*
(German) Basel, Documed, 1990
(1989): Frank GJ+, *Angiology* 40 (4 Pt 2), 405
(1989): Maclean D, *Angiology* 40 (4 Pt 2), 370
Edema
(1989): Frank GJ+, *Angiology* 40 (4 Pt 2), 405
(1989): Frank GJ, *Cardiology* 76 (Suppl 2), 56
Exanthems
(1991): Morant J+, *Arzneimittel-Kompendium der Schweiz*
(German) Basel, Documed, 1990
Exfoliative dermatitis (<1%)
Facial edema (sic)
(1989): Sedman AJ+, *Angiology* 40 (4 Pt 2), 360
Flushing (<1%)
Pemphigus (<1%)
Pemphigus foliaceus
(2000): Ong CS+, *Australas J Dermatol* 41(4), 242
Pemphigus vulgaris
(2000): Ong CS+, *Australas J Dermatol* 41(4), 242
Peripheral edema (<1%)
(1991): Wadworth AN+, *Drugs* 41, 378
Photosensitivity (<1%)
(1989): Maclean D, *Angiology* 40 (4 Pt 2), 370
Pruritus (<1%)
(1991): Cetnarowski-Cropp AB, *Drug Intell Clin Pharm* 25, 499
(1991): Morant J+, *Arzneimittel-Kompendium der Schweiz*
(German) Basel, Documed, 1990
(1990): Frishman WH, *Clin Cardiol* 13 (Suppl 7), VII19
(1990): Swartz RD+, *J Clin Pharmacol* 30, 1136
(1989): Frank GJ+, *Angiology* 40 (4 Pt 2), 405
(1989): Frank GJ, *Cardiology* 76 (Suppl 2), 56
(1989): Maclean D, *Angiology* 40 (4 Pt 2), 370
Rash (sic) (1.2%)
(1992): Materson BJ, *Am J Cardiol* 69, 46C
(1989): Frank GJ+, *Angiology* 40 (4 Pt 2), 405
(1989): Frank GJ, *Cardiology* 76 (Suppl 2), 56
(1989): Maclean D, *Angiology* 40 (4 Pt 2), 370
(1989): Taylor SH, *Angiology* 40 (4 Pt 2), 382
Urticaria (<1%)
Vasculitis (<1%)

Hair

Hair – alopecia (<1%)

Other

Cough
(2002): Culy CR+, *Drugs* 62(2), 339 (2–4%)
(2001): Adigun AQ+, *West Afr J Med* 20(1), 46–7
(2001): Lee SC+, *Hypertension* 38(2), 166
Dysgeusia
(1991): Cetnarowski-Cropp AB, *Drug Intell Clin Pharm* 25, 499
(1989): Taylor SH, *Angiology* 40 (4 Pt 2), 382
Headache
Hypersensitivity
Myalgia (1.5%)
Paresthesias (<1%)
Xerostomia (<1%)

QUINESTROL

Trade name: Estrovis
Indications: Atrophic vaginitis, menopausal symptoms
Category: Estrogen
Half-life: 120 hours

Reactions

Skin
Angioedema
  (1970): Aitken DA+, *BMJ* 2, 177
Chloasma (<1%)
Edema (<1%)
Erythema
Melasma (<1%)
Peripheral edema (>10%)
Photosensitivity
Rash (sic) (<1%)
Urticaria
  (1970): Aitken DA+, *BMJ* 2, 177

Other
Acute intermittent porphyria
Gynecomastia (>10%)
Mastodynia (>10%)
Thrombophlebitis

QUINETHAZONE

Trade name: Hydromox (Wyeth)
Other common trade name: *Aquamox*
Indications: Hypertension, edema
Category: Sulfonamide diuretic
Half-life: N/A
**Clinically important, potentially hazardous interactions
with:** digoxin, lithium

Reactions

Skin
Bullous eruption (<1%)
  (1966): Miller RC+, *Arch Dermatol* 93, 346
Exanthems
  (1966): Miller RC+, *Arch Dermatol* 93, 346
Photosensitivity (<1%)
  (1969): Kalivas J, *JAMA* 209, 1706
  (1966): Miller RC+, *Arch Dermatol* 93, 346
Pruritus
  (1969): Kalivas J, *JAMA* 209, 1706
Purpura
Rash (sic) (<1%)
Urticaria
Vasculitis

Other
Hypersensitivity
Paresthesias
Xanthopsia
Xerostomia

*Note: Quinethazone is a sulfonamide and can be absorbed
systemically. Sulfonamides can produce severe, possibly fatal,
reactions such as toxic epidermal necrolysis and Stevens–Johnson
syndrome

QUINIDINE

Trade names: Cardioquin (Purdue Frederick); Cin-Quin;
Quinaglute (Berlex); Quinalan; Quinidex (Wyeth); Quinora
Other common trade names: *Cardine; Gluquine; Kinidin;
Quinate; Quini Durules*
Indications: Tachycardia, atrial fibrillation
Category: Antiarrhythmic class I A
Half-life: 6–8 hours
**Clinically important, potentially hazardous interactions
with:** amiloride, amiodarone, amprenavir, anisindione,
anticoagulants, aripiprazole, arsenic, ciprofloxacin, delavirdine,
dicumarol, digoxin, enoxacin, gatifloxacin, itraconazole,
lomefloxacin, moxifloxacin, norfloxacin, ofloxacin, pimozide,
pipecuronium, quinolones, ritonavir, **senna**, sparfloxacin,
verapamil, voriconazole, warfarin

Reactions

Skin
Acne
  (1981): Burkhart CG, *Arch Dermatol* 117, 603
Acute generalized exanthematous pustulosis (AGEP)
  (1995): Moreau A+, *Int J Dermatol* 34, 263 (passim)
  (1991): Roujeau J-C+, *Arch Dermatol* 127, 1333
Allergic reactions (sic)
  (1986): Bigby M+, *JAMA* 256, 3358 (1.34%)
Angioedema (<1%)
Bullous eruption
Dermatitis
  (1985): Fowler JF, *Contact Dermatitis* 13, 280
  (1981): Wahlberg JE+, *Contact Dermatitis* 7, 27 (occupational)
  (1965): Fernstrom AI, *Acta Derm Venereol* 45, 129
Eczema (sic)
Erythema multiforme
  (1989): Alanko K, *Acta Derm Venereol* (Stockh) 69, 223
Exanthems
  (1990): Lou CP+, *Postgrad Med J* 66, 406
  (1985): Bruce S+, *J Am Acad Dermatol* 12, 332
  (1982): Holt RJ, *Drug Intell Clin Pharm* 16, 615
  (1980): Harrison DC+, *Am Heart J* 100, 1046 (16.6%)
  (1976): Arndt KA+, *JAMA* 235, 918 (generalized) (1.2%)
  (1976): Geltner D+, *Gastroenterology* 70, 650 (0.8%)
Exfoliative dermatitis (<1%)
  (1996): Sigurdsson V+, *J Am Acad Dermatol* 35, 53
  (1987): Bellogini GC+, *Minerva Cardioangiol* (Italian) 35, 457
  (1985): Bruce S+, *J Am Acad Dermatol* 12, 332
  (1965): Gouffault J+, *Sem Hôp* (French) 41, 1350
  (1951): Taylor DR+, *JAMA* 145, 641
Exudative dermatitis (sic)
  (1942): Goldschlag F, *Med J Australia* 2, 501
Fixed eruption
  (1960): Engelhardt AW, *Hautarzt* (German) 11, 49
Flushing (<1%)
  (1991): Ross EV+, *J Assoc Military Dermatol* XVII (1), 16
  (1985): Bruce S+, *J Am Acad Dermatol* 12, 332
Granuloma annulare
  (1991): Ross EV+, *J Assoc Military Dermatol* XVII (1), 16
Lichen planus
  (1994): Thompson DF+, *Pharmacotherapy* 14, 561
  (1985): Bruce S+, *J Am Acad Dermatol* 12, 332 (passim)
  (1985): Rebondy JP+, *Ann Dermatol Venereol* (French) 112, 989
  (1980): Maltz BL+, *Int J Dermatol* 19, 96
  (1967): Anderson TE, *Br J Dermatol* 79, 500
  (1967): Sarkany I, *Br J Dermatol* 79, 123
  (1954): Wechsler HL, *Arch Dermatol* 69, 741

Lichenoid eruption
  (1988): de Larrard G+, *Ann Dermatol Venereol* (French)
    115, 1172
  (1987): Jeanmougin M+, *Ann Dermatol Venereol* (French)
    114, 1397 (photosensitive)
  (1982): Berger TC+, *Cutis* 29, 595
  (1981): Haim S+, *Harefuah* (Hebrew) 101, 310
  (1976): Gammer S+, *Cutis* 17, 72
  (1968): Pegum JS, *Br J Dermatol* 80, 343
Livedo reticularis (<1%)
  (1989): Manzi S+, *Arch Dermatol* 125, 417 (photosensitive)
  (1985): Bruce S+, *J Am Acad Dermatol* 12, 332 (photosensitive)
  (1977): Cohen IS+, *Prog Cardiovasc Dis* 20, 151
  (1974): de Groot WP+, *Dermatologica* 148, 371 (photosensitive)
  (1973): Marion DF+, *Arch Dermatol* 108, 100 (photosensitive)
Lupus erythematosus (<1%)
  (1996): Rich MW, *Postgrad Med* 100, 299
  (1995): Alloway JA+, *Semin Arthritis Rheum* 24, 315
  (1994): Yung RL+, *Rheum Dis Clin North Am* 20, 61
  (1992): Rubin RL, *Clin Biochem* 25, 223
  (1992): Rubin RL+, *J Clin Invest* 90, 165
  (1992): Skaer TL, *Clin Ther* 14, 496
  (1991): Alarcon-Segovia D+, *Baillieres Clin Rheumatol* 5, 1
  (1991): Tebas P+, *Rev Clin Esp* (Spanish) 189, 123
  (1989): Cohen MG, *Geriatric Med Today* 8, 95
  (1988): Cohen MG+, *Ann Intern Med* 108, 369
  (1988): Schmid FR, *Ann Intern Med* 109, 247
  (1988): Webb J+, *Med J Aust* 149, 53
  (1987): Sukenik S+, *Isr J Med Sci* 23, 1232
  (1986): Bar-El Y+, *Am Heart J* 111, 1209
  (1985): Amadio P+, *Ann Intern Med* 102, 419
  (1985): Gastineau DA+, *Arch Intern Med* 145, 1926
  (1985): Krainin MJ+, *Arch Intern Med* 145, 1740
  (1985): Lavie CJ+, *Arch Intern Med* 145, 446
  (1985): McCormack GD+, *Semin Arthritis Rheum* 15, 73
  (1985): Rebondy JP+, *Ann Dermatol Venereol* (French) 112, 989
  (1985): Stratton MA, *Clin Pharm* 4, 657
  (1984): West SG+, *Ann Intern Med* 100, 840
  (1982): Chagnon A+, *Nouv Presse Med* (French) 11, 2020
  (1981): Barrier J+, *Nouv Presse Med* (French) 10, 2991
  (1980): Condemi JJ, *Geriatrics* 35(3), 81
  (1978): Robinson HM, *Z Hautkr* (German) 53, 349
  (1977): Cohen IS+, *Prog Cardiovasc Dis* 20, 151
  (1977): Tweed JM, *N Z Med J* 86, 40
  (1976): Yudis M+, *JAMA* 235, 2000
  (1974): Donoho CR+, *Arthritis Rheum* 17, 322
  (1973): Hanauer LB, *Ann Intern Med* 78, 308
  (1973): Marion DF+, *Arch Dermatol* 108, 100
  (1972): Anderson FP+, *Conn Med* 36, 84
  (1970): Kendall MJ+, *Postgrad Med J* 46, 729
Palmar–plantar keratoderma
  (1988): De Larrard G+, *Ann Dermatol Venereol* (French)
    115, 1172
Photosensitivity (<1%)
  (1992): Schürer NY+, *Photodermatol Photoimmunol Photomed*
    9, 78
  (1991): Schürer NY+, *Hautarzt* (German) 42, 158
  (1990): Fertin C+, *Nouv Dermatol* (French) 9, 446
  (1989): Rosen C, *Semin Dermatol* 8, 149
  (1988): De Larrard G+, *Ann Dermatol Venereol* (French)
    115, 1172
  (1987): Bonnetblanc JM+, *Ann Dermatol Venereol* (French)
    114, 957 (lichenoid)
  (1987): Ferguson J+, *Br J Dermatol* 117, 631
  (1987): Wolf R+, *Dermatologica* 174, 285 (lichenoid and
    eczematous)
  (1986): Jeanmougin M+, *Ann Dermatol Venereol* (French)
    113, 985
  (1986): Ljunggren B+, *Photodermatol* 3, 26
  (1985): Armstrong RB+, *Arch Dermatol* 121, 525

  (1985): Bonnetblanc JM+, *Ann Dermatol Venereol* (French)
    112, 671
  (1985): Rebondy JP+, *Ann Dermatol Venereol* (French) 112, 989
  (1984): Fisher DA, *Arch Dermatol* 120, 298
  (1983): Lang PS, *J Am Acad Dermatol* 9, 124
  (1983): Marx JL+, *Arch Dermatol* 119, 39
  (1982): Berger TC+, *Cutis* 29, 595 (lichenoid)
  (1976): Bogoch ER+, *Arch Dermatol* 112, 559
  (1976): Gammer S+, *Cutis* 17, 72
  (1976): Pariser RJ+, *Arch Dermatol* 112, 1610
  (1975): Pariser DM+, *Arch Dermatol* 111, 1440
Pigmentation (<1%)
  (1996): Conroy EA+, *Cutis* 57, 425
  (1996): Messina JL+, *J Geriatr Dermatol* 4, 198
  (1995): Rippis G+, American Academy of Dermatology Meeting,
    New Orleans (observation)
  (1986): Mahler R+, *Arch Dermatol* 122, 1062
Pruritus (<1%)
  (1985): Bruce S+, *J Am Acad Dermatol* 12, 332 (passim)
  (1982): Holt RJ, *Drug Intell Clin Pharm* 16, 615
  (1976): Geltner D+, *Gastroenterology* 70, 650 (0.8%)
Psoriasis (<1%)
  (1998): Smith KC, Niagara Falls, Canada (from Internet)
    (observation)
  (1993): Brenner S+, *Arch Dermatol* 129, 1331
  (1986): Abel EA+, *J Am Acad Dermatol* 15, 1007
  (1983): Harwell WB, *J Am Acad Dermatol* 9, 278
  (1977): Cohen IS+, *Prog Cardiovasc Dis* 20, 151 (with
    erythroderma)
  (1973): Almeyda J+, *Br J Dermatol* 88, 313 (with erythroderma)
Purpura
  (1993): Kaufman DW+, *Blood* 82, 2714
  (1991): Salom IL, *JAMA* 266, 1220 (letter)
  (1988): Reid DM+, *Ann Intern Med* 108, 206
  (1981): Barrier J+, *Nouv Presse Med* (French) 10, 2991
  (1981): Conri C+, *Nouv Presse Med* (French) 7, 3361
  (1980): Miescher PA+, *Clin Haematol* 9, 505
  (1976): Geltner D+, *Gastroenterology* 70, 650 (1.4%)
  (1976): Khaleeli AA, *BMJ* 2, 562
  (1962): Weintraub RM+, *JAMA* 180, 528
  (1959): Bishop RC+, *Ann Intern Med* 50, 1227
  (1958): Shaftel N+, *Angiology* 9, 34
  (1956): Bolton FG, *Blood* 11, 547
  (1956): Freedman AL+, *J Lab Clin Med* 48, 205
Pustules
  (1951): Taylor DR+, *JAMA* 145, 641
Rash (sic) (1–10%)
Side effects (sic)
  (1977): Cohen IS+, *Prog Cardiovasc Dis* 20, 151 (1%)
Subcorneal pustular dermatosis (Sneddon–Wilkinson)
  (1983): Halevy S+, *Acta Derm Venereol* (Stockh) 63, 441
Toxic epidermal necrolysis
  (2000): Adornato MC, *N Y State Dent J* 66, 38
  (1974): Callaway JL+, *Arch Dermatol* 109, 909
Urticaria (<1%)
  (1985): Bruce S+, *J Am Acad Dermatol* 12, 332
Vasculitis (<1%)
  (1990): Zax RH+, *Arch Dermatol* 126, 69
  (1989): Cohen MG, *Geriatric Med Today* 8, 99
  (1988): Quin J+, *Med J Aust* 148, 145 (allergic granulomatous)
  (1985): Shalit M+, *Arch Intern Med* 145, 2051

Hair
Hair – alopecia
  (1988): de Larrard G+, *Ann Dermatol Venereol* (French)
    115, 1172

Other
Dysgeusia (>10%) (bitter taste)
Headache

Hypersensitivity
  (1966): Martt JM+, *Mo Med* 63, 908
Lymphoproliferative disease
  (1987): Gay RG+, *Am J Med* 82, 143
Myalgia (<1%)
Oral mucosal eruption
  (1988): De Larrard G+, *Ann Dermatol Venereol* (French) 115, 1172
  (1958): Shaftel N+, *Angiology* 9, 34
Oral mucosal pigmentation
  (1988): Birek C+, *Oral Surg Oral Med Oral Pathol* 66, 59
Oral ulceration
Polymyalgia
  (1995): Alloway JA+, *Semin Arthritis Rheum* 24, 315
Porphyria
  (1971): Sayag J+, *Bull Soc Franc Dermatol Syphiligr* (French) 78, 664
Pseudoporphyria
  (1992): Petersen CS+, *Ugeskr Laeger* (Danish) 154, 1713
Sicca syndrome (<1%)
  (1983): Naschitz JE+, *J Toxicol Clin Toxicol* 20, 367
Tinnitus
Tremor (2%)

QUININE

Trade names: Formula-Q; Legatrin (Columbia); M-KYA; Q-Vel; Quiphile (Geneva)
Other common trade names: *Adaquin; Chinine; Genin; Quinoctal; Quinsan; Quinsul*
Indications: Malaria, nocturnal leg cramps
Category: Antiprotozoal
Half-life: 8–14 hours
Clinically important, potentially hazardous interactions with: anisindione, anticoagulants, dicumarol, warfarin

Reactions

Skin
Acne
  (1981): Burkhart CC, *Arch Dermatol* 117, 603
  (1967): Hitch JM, *JAMA* 200, 879
Acral erythema
  (2000): Abreu-Gerke L+, *Hautarzt* 51(5), 332
Acral necrosis
  (2000): Abreu-Gerke L+, *Hautarzt* 51(5), 332
Angioedema (<1%)
Bullous eruption
Dermatitis
  (1994): Dias M+, *Contact Dermatitis* 30, 121
  (1994): Isaksson M+, *Acta Derm Venereol* 74, 286
  (1994): Tapadinhas C+, *Contact Dermatitis* 31, 127 (from hair lotion)
  (1978): Calnan CD+, *Contact Dermatitis* 4, 58
  (1978): Hardie RA+, *Contact Dermatitis* 4, 121 (occupational)
  (1961): Calnan CD+, *BMJ* 2, 1750
Diaphoresis
Eczema (sic)
Erythema
Erythema multiforme (<1%)
  (2000): Abreu-Gerke L+, *Hautarzt* 51(5), 332 (passim)
  (1967): Coleman WP, *Med Clin North Am* 51, 1073
Exanthems (1–5%)
  (2000): Abreu-Gerke L+, *Hautarzt* 51(5), 332 (passim)
  (1969): Török H, *Dermatol Int* 8, 57

Exfoliative dermatitis
  (1975): Jarratt M+, *Arch Dermatol* 111, 132
  (1974): Callaway JL+, *Arch Dermatol* 109, 909
Facial edema
Fixed eruption
  (2000): Litt JZ, Beachwood, OH (personal case) (observation)
  (1993): Litt JZ, Beachwood, OH (from quinine water) (personal case) (observation)
  (1990): Gaffoor PMA+, *Cutis* 45, 242 (passim)
  (1974): Kuokkanen K, *Int J Dermatol* 13, 4
  (1970): Savin JA, *Br J Dermatol* 83, 546
  (1967): Kogoj F, *Med Glas* (Serbo-Croatian-Roman) 21, 351
  (1961): Welsh AL+, *Arch Dermatol* 84, 1004
  (1960): Engelhardt AW, *Hautarzt* (German) 11, 49
Flushing (<1%)
Lichen planus
  (1994): Litt JZ, Beachwood, OH (personal case) (observation)
  (1986): Dawson TAJ, *Clin Exp Dermatol* 11, 670
  (1986): Meyrick-Thomas RH+, *Clin Exp Dermatol* 11, 97 (photosensitive distribution)
  (1979): Krebs A, *Hautarzt* (German) 30, 281
Lichenoid eruption
  (1995): Dawson TA, *BMJ* 310, 738
  (1989): Tan SV+, *Clin Exp Dermatol* 14, 335
  (1987): Ferguson J+, *Br J Dermatol* 117, 631
Livedo racemosa (photosensitive)
  (1988): Diffey BL+, *Br J Dermatol* 118, 679
  (1974): de Groot WP+, *Dermatologica* 148, 371
  (1973): Marion DF, *Arch Dermatol* 108, 100
Lupus erythematosus
  (1996): Rosa-Re D+, *Ann Rheum Dis* 55, 559
Ochronosis
  (1986): Bruce S+, *J Am Acad Dermatol* 15, 357
Photosensitivity
  (2000): Abreu-Gerke L+, *Hautarzt* 51(5), 332 (passim)
  (1998): Rademaker M, Hamilton, New Zealand (from Internet) (observation)
  (1995): Dawson TA, *BMJ* 310, 738
  (1995): Delmas A+, *Presse Med* (French) 24, 1707
  (1994): Isaksson M+, *Acta Derm Venereol* 74, 286
  (1994): Litt JZ, Beachwood, OH (personal case) (observation)
  (1994): Okun MM+, *Clin Exp Dermatol* 19, 246 (mycosisfungoides-like)
  (1994): Wagner GH+, *Br J Dermatol* 131, 734 (from tonic water)
  (1992): Fitzpatrick JE, *Dermatol Clin* 10, 19
  (1992): Ljunggren B+, *Contact Dermatitis* 26, 1
  (1990): Guzzo C+, *Photodermatol Photoimmunol Photomed* 7, 166
  (1988): Diffey BL+, *Br J Dermatol* 118, 679
  (1987): Ferguson J+, *Br J Dermatol* 117, 631
  (1986): Dawson TAJ, *Clin Exp Dermatol* 11, 670 (lichenoid)
  (1986): Ljunggren B+, *Arch Dermatol* 122, 909
  (1986): Ljunggren B+, *Photodermatol* 3, 26
  (1984): Jeanmougin M+, *Ann Dermatol Venereol* (French) 11, 565
  (1978): Calnan CD+, *Contact Dermatitis* 4, 58
  (1975): Johnson BE+, *Br J Dermatol* 93 (Suppl 11), 21
  (1969): Kalivas J, *JAMA* 209, 1706
Pigmentation
  (1999): Rosen T+, Houston, TX (personal case) (observation)
  (1994): Litt JZ, Beachwood, OH (personal case) (observation)
  (1986): Bruce S+, *J Am Acad Dermatol* 15, 357 (from injections)
  (1986): Mahler R+, *Arch Dermatol* 122, 1062
  (1964): Dummett CO, *J Oral Ther Pharmacol* 1, 106
  (1963): Tuffanelli D+, *Arch Dermatol* 88, 419
Pruritus (<1%)
  (2000): Abreu-Gerke L+, *Hautarzt* 51(5), 332 (passim)
Psoriasis
  (1998): Smith KC, Niagara Falls, Canada (from Internet) (observation)

Purpura
 (2000): Abreu-Gerke L+, *Hautarzt* 51(5), 332 (passim)
 (1993): Kaufman DW+, *Blood* 82, 2714
 (1985): Ambriz-Fernandez R+, *Rev Invest Clin* (Spanish) 37, 347
 (1980): Miescher PA+, *Clin Haematol* 9, 505
 (1969): Török H, *Dermatol Int* 8, 57
 (1967): Belkin CA, *Ann Intern Med* 66, 583
 (1967): Helmly RB+, *Arch Intern Med* 120, 59
 (1965): Horowitz HI+, *Semin Hematol* 2, 287
 (1962): Weintraub RM+, *JAMA* 180, 528
 (1952): Lincoln RB+, *Am Pract* 3, 42
 (1946): Schrager J+, *Am J Med Sci* 212, 54
Rash (sic) (<1%)
 (1993): Siderov J, *J Am Geriatr Soc* 41, 498
Stevens–Johnson syndrome
 (1986): Gascon-Brustenga J+, *Med Clin (Barc)* (Spanish) 87, 821
 (1967): Coleman WP, *Med Clin North Am* 51, 1073
Thrombocytopenic purpura
 (2001): *Ann Intern Med* 135(12), S
 (2001): Medina PJ+, *Curr Opin Hematol* 8(5), 286
Toxic epidermal necrolysis (<1%)
 (1975): Jarratt M+, *Arch Dermatol* 111, 132
 (1974): Callaway JL+, *Arch Dermatol* 109, 909 (tonic water)
Urticaria
 (2000): Abreu-Gerke L+, *Hautarzt* 51(5), 332 (passim)
 (1969): Török H, *Dermatol Int* 8, 57
Vasculitis
 (1992): Price EJ+, *Br J Clin Pract* 46, 138
 (1991): Harland CC+, *BMJ* 302, 295
 (1990): Mathur S+, *BMJ* 300, 613
 (1968): Rockl H+, *Munch Med Wochenschr* (German) 110, 2549
 (1952): Lincoln RB+, *Am Pract* 3, 42
Vitiligo
 (1998): Rademaker M, Hamilton, New Zealand (from Internet)
   (observation) (following photosensitivity)

Nails
Nails – photo-onycholysis
 (1989): Tan SV+, *Clin Exp Dermatol* 14, 335

Other
Headache
Hypersensitivity (<1%)
 (1998): Schattner A, *Am J Med* 104–488
Oral mucosal eruption
 (1964): Dummett CO, *J Oral Ther Pharmacol* 1, 106
Oral ulceration
Porphyria
 (1971): Sayag J+, *Bull Soc Franc Dermatol Syphiligr* (French)
   78, 664
Tinnitus

QUINUPRISTIN/DALFOPRISTIN

Synonyms: pristinamycin; RP59500
Trade name: Synercid (Monarch)
Indications: Serious life-threatening bacterial infections
Category: Streptogramin antibiotic
Half-life: 1.3–1.5 hours

Reactions

Skin
Allergic reactions (sic) (<1%)
Candidiasis (<1%)
Diaphoresis (<1%)
Exanthems (<1%)
Peripheral edema (<1%)
Pruritus (1.5%)
Rash (sic) (2.5%)
 (2001): Allington DR+, *Clin Ther* 23(1), 24 (2.5–4.6%)
Ulcerations (<1%)
Urticaria (<1%)

Other
Anaphylactoid reactions (<1%)
Arthralgia
 (2001): Allington DR+, *Clin Ther* 23(1), 24
 (2001): Manzella JP, *Am Fam Physician* 64(11), 1863
 (2001): Olsen KM+, *Clin Infect Dis* 32(4), 83
 (2000): Delgado G+, *Pharacotherapy* 20(12), 1469
Injection-site edema (17.3%)
 (2001): Allington DR+, *Clin Ther* 23(1), 24
Injection-site extravasation (42%)
 (2001): Allington DR+, *Clin Ther* 23(1), 24
Injection-site pain (40%)
 (2001): Allington DR+, *Clin Ther* 23(1), 24
 (2000): Delgado G+, *Pharmacotherapy* 20(12), 1469
Injection-site reactions (sic) (13.4%)
Myalgia (<1–5%)
 (2001): Allington DR+, *Clin Ther* 23(1), 24
 (2001): Manzella JP, *Am Fam Physician* 64(11), 1863
 (2001): Olsen KM+, *Clin Infect Dis* 32(4), 83
 (2000): Delgado G+, *Pharmacotherapy* 20(12), 1469
Oral candidiasis (<1%)
Paresthesias (<1%)
Phlebitis (<1%)
Stomatitis (<1%)
Thrombophlebitis (2.4%)
 (2001): Allington DR+, *Clin Ther* 23(1), 24
Tremor (<1%)
Vaginitis (<1%)

RABEPRAZOLE

Synonym: pariprazole
Trade name: Aciphex (Eisai) (Janssen)
Indications: Gastroesophageal reflux disease (GERD)
Category: Proton pump (gastric acid secretion) inhibitor
Half-life: 1–2 hours

Reactions

Skin
Allergic reactions (sic) (<1%)
Chills (<1%)
Diaphoresis (<1%)
Ecchymoses (<1%)
Edema
Eruptions (sic) (<1%)
Facial edema (<1%)
Herpes zoster (<1%)
Peripheral edema (<1%)
Photosensitivity (<1%)
Pigmentation (<1%)
Pruritus (<1%)
Psoriasis (<1%)
Purpura
Rash (sic) (<1%)
Urticaria (<1%)
Xerosis (<1%)

Hair
Hair – alopecia (<1%)

Other
Gingivitis (<1%)
Glossitis (<1%)
Gynecomastia (<1%)
Headache
Myalgia (<1%)
Oral ulceration
Paresthesias (<1%)
Rhabdomyolysis
  (2002): Bourlon S+, *Therapie* 57(6), 597
Stomatitis (<1%)
  (2003): Stoecker WV, MO (from Internet) (observation)
Thrombophlebitis (<1%)
Tongue edema
  (2003): Stoecker WV, MO (from Internet) (observation)
Tremor (<1%)
Twitching (<1%)
Xerostomia (<1%)

RALOXIFENE

Synonym: Keoxifene
Trade name: Evista (Lilly)
Indications: Osteoporosis
Category: Selective estrogen receptor modulator
Half-life: 27.7 hours
Clinically important, potentially hazardous interactions with: cholestyramine

Reactions

Skin
Diaphoresis (3.1%)
Edema
Flu-like syndrome (sic) (~2%)
Hot flashes (24.6%)
  (2002): Kinsinger LS+, *Ann Intern Med* 137(1), 59
  (2001): Seeman E, *J Bone Miner Metab* 19, 65 (406%)
  (2000): Eriksen EF, *Ugeskr Laeger* (Danish) 162, 4182
  (2000): Snyder KR+, *Am J Health Syst Pharm* 57, 1669
  (1999): Ettinger B+, *JAMA* 282, 637 (10%)
  (1999): Scott JA+, *Am Fam Physician* 60, 1131
  (1998): Walsh BW+, *JAMA* 279, 1445 (22%)
Infections (sic) (~2%)
Peripheral edema (3.3%)
  (2000): Eriksen EF, *Ugeskr Laeger* (Danish) 162, 4182
  (1999): Cummings SR+, *JAMA* 281, 2189
  (1999): Ettinger B+, *JAMA* 282, 637 (5%)
Rash (sic) (5.5%)
Vitiligo
  (2002): Litt JZ, Beachwood, OH (personal case) (observation)
    (after 3 weeks of raloxifene, patient developed leukoderma
    over exposed areas of chest and forearms after sun
    exposure)

Other
Leg cramps
  (2001): Seeman E, *J Bone Miner Metab* 19, 65 (2–4%)
Mastodynia (4.4%)
  (1999): Cummings SR+, *JAMA* 281, 2189
  (1998): Walsh BW+, *JAMA* 279, 1445 (4%)
Myalgia (7.7%)
Vaginitis (4.3%)

RAMIPRIL

Trade name: Altace (Monarch)
Other common trade names: *Delix; Hytren; Pramace; Quark; Ramace; Triatec; Tritace; Unipril*
Indications: Hypertension
Category: Angiotensin-converting enzyme (ACE) inhibitor; Antihypertensive
Half-life: 3–17 hours
Clinically important, potentially hazardous interactions with: amiloride, spironolactone, triamterene

Reactions

Skin
Acne
  (1987): Predel HG+, *Am J Cardiol* 59, 143D
Angioedema (0.3%)
  (2002): Kaur S+, *J Dermatol* 29(6), 336

(2001): Cohen EG+, *Ann Otol Rhinol Laryngol* 110(8), 701 (64 cases)
(1995): Epeldo-Gonzalo F+, *Ann Pharmacother* 29, 431
(1990): Todd PA+, *Drugs* 39, 110
Dermatitis (sic) (<1%)
Diaphoresis (<1%)
(1988): Zabludowski J+, *Curr Med Res Opin* 11, 93
(1987): Walter U+, *Am J Cardiol* 59, 125D
Dry feeling on face (sic)
(1987): Fukiyama K+, *Am J Cardiol* 59, 121D
Edema (<1%)
(1990): Todd PA+, *Drugs* 39, 110
Erythema (sic) (circumscribed)
(1987): Predel HG+, *Am J Cardiol* 59, 143D
Erythema multiforme (<1%)
Exanthems
(1990): Todd PA+, *Drugs* 39, 110
Flushing
(1988): Zabludowski J+, *Curr Med Res Opin* 11, 93
(1987): Kaneko Y+, *Am J Cardiol* 59, 86D
Lichen planus pemphigoides
(1997): Ogg GS+, *Br J Dermatol* 136, 412
Pemphigus (<1%)
(1996): Vignes S+, *Br J Dermatol* 135, 657
Pemphigus foliaceus
(2000): Ong CS+, *Australas J Dermatol* 41(4), 242
Photosensitivity (<1%)
(2000): Wagner SN+, *Contact Dermatitis* 43(4), 245 (with hydrochlorothiazide)
(1994): Shelley WB+, *Cutis* 53, 39 (observation)
(1993): Shelley WB+, *Cutis* 52, 81 (observation)
Pruritus (<1%)
(1990): Todd PA+, *Drugs* 39, 110
(1987): Predel HG+, *Am J Cardiol* 59, 143D
(1987): Walter U+, *Am J Cardiol* 59, 125D
Purpura (<1%)
Rash (sic) (<1%)
(1990): Janka HU+, *Arzneimittelforschung* (German) 40, 432
(1990): Todd PA+, *Drugs* 39, 110
(1987): Ball SG+, *Am J Cardiol* 59, 23D
(1987): Walter U+, *Am J Cardiol* 59, 125D
Urticaria (<1%)
Vasculitis (<1%)

Hair

Hair – alopecia (1–10%)

Other

Ageusia (<1%)
Anaphylactoid reactions (<1%)
Cough
(2001): Adigun AQ+, *West Afr J Med* 20(1), 46–7
(2001): Lee SC+, *Hypertension* 38(2), 166
Dysgeusia (<1%)
(1990): Todd PA+, *Drugs* 39, 110
Headache
Hypersensitivity (<1%)
Paresthesias (<1%)
(1987): Walter U+, *Am J Cardiol* 59, 125D
Sialorrhea (<1%)
Tinnitus
Tremor (<1%)
Xerostomia (<1%)

RANITIDINE

Trade name: Zantac (GSK)
Other common trade names: *Apo-Ranitidine; Axoban; Azantac; Nu-Ranit; Raniben; Raniplex; Ranisen; Sostril; Zantab; Zantac-C; Zantic*
Indications: Duodenal ulcer
Category: Antihistamine H_2-blocker; Antiulcer
Half-life: 2.5 hours
Clinically important, potentially hazardous interactions with: alfentanil, **devil's claw**, fentanyl

Note: Ranitidine is present in mother's milk in relatively large amounts. It is thought that gynecomastia develops as a result of ranitidine blocking the androgen receptors at the end organs

Reactions

Skin

Acute generalized exanthematous pustulosis (AGEP)
(1996): Sawhney RA+, *Int J Dermatol* 35, 826
Angioedema (<1%)
Dermatitis
(2003): Ryan PJ+, *Contact Dermatitis* 48(2), 67
(1988): Romaguera C+, *Contact Dermatitis* 18, 177
(1987): Alomar A+, *Contact Dermatitis* 17, 54
(1984): Goh CL+, *Contact Dermatitis* 4, 252
(1983): Rycroft RJ, *Contact Dermatitis* 9, 456 (occupational)
Eczema (sic)
(1992): Juste S+, *Contact Dermatitis* 27, 339
(1988): Romaguera C+, *Contact Dermatitis* 18, 177
Erythema multiforme
Exanthems
(1993): Devuyst O+, *Acta Clin Belg* 48, 109
(1989): Grant SM+, *Drugs* 37, 801
(1988): Haboubi N+, *Br Med J Clin Res Ed* 296, 897
(1984): Khandheria BK, *JAMA* 253, 3252
Fixed eruption
(1990): Black AK+, *Br J Dermatol* 123, 277
Lichenoid eruption
(1996): Horiuchi Y+, *J Dermatol* 23, 510
Lupus erythematosus
(1999): Crowson AN+, *J Cutan Pathol* 26, 95 (subacute cutaneous)
Photosensitivity
(2000): Kondo S+, *Dermatology* 201, 71
(1995): Todd P+, *Clin Exp Dermatol* 20, 146
Pruritus (<1%)
(1985): Classen M+, *Dtsch Med Wochenschr* (German) 110, 628
Psoriasis
(1991): Andersen M, *Ugeskr Laeger* (Danish) 153, 132
Purpura
(1989): Gafter U+, *Gastroenterol* 84, 560
(1987): Gafter U+, *Ann Intern Med* 106, 477
Pustules
Rash (sic) (1–10%)
(1988): Haboubi N+, *Br Med J Clin Res Ed* 296, 897
Stevens–Johnson syndrome
(2001): Lin C-C+, *Gastroenterol Hepatol* 16, 481
Toxic epidermal necrolysis
(2000): Velez A+, *J Am Acad Dermatol* 42, 305
(1995): Miralles ES+, *J Am Acad Dermatol* 32, 133
Urticaria
(1997): Sancho Calabuig A+, *Aten Primaria* 20, 396
(1989): Grant SM+, *Drugs* 37, 801
(1984): Khandheria BK, *JAMA* 253, 3252
(1983): Picardo M+, *Contact Dermatitis* 4, 327

Vasculitis
    (1988): Haboubi N+, *BMJ* 296, 897
Xerosis

Hair

Hair – alopecia
    (1995): Shelley WB+, *Cutis* 55, 148 (observation)

Other

Anaphylactoid reactions
    (1993): Lazaro M+, *Allergy* 48, 385
    (1993): Powell JA+, *Anaesth Intensive Care* 21, 702
Dysgeusia
    (1985): Classen M+, *Dtsch Med Wochenschr* (German) 110, 628
Gynecomastia (>1%)
    (1994): Garcia-Rodriguez LA+, *BMJ* 308, 503
    (1984): Bianchi Porro G+, *It J Gastroenterol* (Italian) 16, 56
    (1982): Tosi S+, *Lancet* 2, 160
Headache
Hypersensitivity
    (1996): Gonzalo-Garijo MA+, *Allergy* 51, 659
Injection-site burning
Injection-site pain
Myalgia
Porphyria
    (1988): Bhadoria DP+, *J Assoc Physicians India* 36, 295
    (1988): Pratap D+, *J Assoc Physicians India* 36, 237
    (1988): Tripathi SK, *J Assoc Physicians India* 36, 680
Pseudolymphoma
    (1995): Magro CM+, *J Am Acad Dermatol* 32, 419
    (1988): Kardaun SH+, *Br J Dermatol* 118(4), 545

RAPACURONIUM

Trade name: Raplon (Organon)
Indications: To facilitate tracheal intubation
Category: Anesthesia adjunct; Nondepolarizing neuromuscular blockade
Half-life: ~22 days
Clinically important, potentially hazardous interactions with: aminoglycosides, cyclopropane, enflurane, halothane, isoflurane, methoxyflurane, piperacillin

Reactions

Skin

Diaphoresis (~1%)
Edema (~1%)
Erythema
    (1999): Abouleish EI+, *Br J Anaesth* 83, 862
Exanthems (>1%)
Flushing
Non-inflammatory swelling (sic)
Peripheral edema (~1%)
Pruritus
Purpura (~1%)
Rash (sic) (~1%)
Urticaria (~1%)

Other

Hyperesthesia (~1%)
Injection-site pain (~1%)
Injection-site reactions (sic) (~1%)
    (1999): Onrust SV+, *Drugs* 58, 887
Myalgia (~1%)

Sialorrhea (~1%)
    (2000): Meakin GH+, *Anesthesiology* 92, 1002
Thrombophlebitis (~1%)
Tooth disorder (sic) (~1%)

RASBURICASE

Trade name: Elitek (Sanofi-Synthelabo)
Indications: Hyperuricemia (secondary to cancer chemotherapy), tumor lysis syndrome
Category: Enzyme (metabolic); Uricolytic
Half-life: 16–21 hours (pediatric patients)

Reactions

Skin

Cellulitis (<1%)
Edema
    (2001): Pui CH+, *Leukemia* 15(10), 1505 (%)
Hot flashes (<1%)
Infections (<1%)
Rash (sic) (13%)
    (2002): Brant JM, *Clin J Oncol Nurs* 6(1), 12
    (2002): Goldman S+, *38th Annual Meeting of the Proceedings of the ASCO* 21, 399a
    (2001): Easton J+, *Paediatr Drugs* 3(6), 433
    (1998): Lascombes F+, *Blood* 92(10 Suppl 1), 237B
    (1997): Landman-Parker J+, *Med Pediatr Oncol* 29(5), 339
    (1997): Schaison G+, *Proceedings Am Assoc Cancer Res* 38, 223

Other

Anaphylactoid reactions (<1%)
Headache
Hypersensitivity
    (2002): Goldman S+, *38th Annual Meeting of the Proceedings of the ASCO* 21, 399a
    (2001): Pui C-H+, *J Clin Oncol* 19, 697
    (2001): Pui C-H, *Leukemia* 15, 1505 (%)
    (1998): Lascombes F+, *Blood* 92(10 Suppl 1), 237B
Mucositis (2–15%)
    (2002): Brant JM, *Clin J Oncol Nurs* 6(1), 12
    (2002): Pui C-H+, *38th Annual Meeting of the Proceedings of the ASCO* 21, 370a
Myalgia
    (2001): Pui CH+, *Leukemia* 15(10), 1505 (%)
Pain
    (2002): Pui C-H+, *38th Annual Meeting of the Proceedings of the ASCO* 21, 370a
Paresthesias (<1%)
Rigors
Thrombophlebitis (<1%)

RASPBERRY LEAF

Scientific name: *Rubus idaeus*
Family: Rosaceae
Trade and other common names: Braamboss; Bramble of Mount Ida; Hindberry; Hindebar; Raspis
Category: Dietary supplement
Purported indications and other uses: Astringent, stimulant, gargle for sore throat, mouth ulcers, bleeding gums, diarrhea, morning sickness, to shorten labor, menstrual complaints, respiratory tract infections, fever, dysmenorrhea, menorrhagia, rash
Half-life: N/A
Clinically important, potentially hazardous interactions with: atropine, codeine, theophylline

Reactions

Skin
Allergic reactions (sic)

RED CLOVER

Scientific name: *Trifolium pratense*
Family: Leguminosae
Trade and other common names: Coumestrol; Cow Clover; Cowgrass; Meadow Clover; Menoflavon (Pascoe); Pavine Clover; Promensil (Novogen); Purple Clover; Three-Leaved Grass
Category: Phytoestrogen
Purported indications and other uses: Menopausal symptoms, hot flashes, muscle spasms, hypercholesterolemia, breast pain, osteoporosis, diuretic, expectorant, mild antispasmodic, sedative, blood purifier, bladder infections, liver disorders. Ointment for acne, eczema, psoriasis and other rashes
Half-life: N/A
Clinically important, potentially hazardous interactions with: conjugated estrogens, heparin, ticlopidine, warfarin

Reactions

Skin
Mutagen
 (2001): Domon OE+, *Mutat Res* 474(1), 129

Note: Red clover contains phytoestrogens that bind to estrogen and progesterone receptors, potentially adversely affecting breast tissue

REPAGLINIDE

Trade name: Prandin (Novo Nordisk)
Indications: Non-insulin dependent diabetes type II
Category: Antidiabetic
Half-life: 1 hour

Reactions

Skin
Allergic reactions (sic) (2%)

Other
Anaphylactoid reactions (<1%)
Headache
Paresthesias (3%)
Tooth disorder (sic)

RESERPINE

Trade names: Resa; Ser-Ap-Es (Novartis); Serpalan; Serpasil (Novartis); Serpatabs
Other common trade names: *Anserpin; Inerpin; Novo-Reserpine; Reserfia; Sedaraupin; Serpasol; Tionsera*
Indications: Hypertension
Category: Nondiuretic antihypertensive; Rauwolfia alkaloid
Half-life: 50–100 hours

Ser-Ap-Es is reserpine, hydralazine and hydrochlorothiazide

Reactions

Skin
Ankle edema
Bullous eruption
 (1994): Watanabe S+, *Reg Anesth* 19, 59 (following intravenous block)
Edema
Exanthems
Flushing
Lupus erythematosus (exacerbation)
 (1963): Rivero I+, *Arthritis Rheum* 6, 293
Peripheral edema (1–10%)
Pruritus
Purpura
Rash (sic) (<1%)
Toxic epidermal necrolysis
 (1979): Kats GL+, *Vrach Delo* (Russian) November, 97
Urticaria

Other
Gynecomastia
Headache
Parkinsonism
Sialorrhea
Xerostomia (>10%)

RETEPLASE

Synonyms: recombinant plasminogen activator; r-PA
Trade name: Retavase (Centocor)
Indications: Acute myocardial infarction
Category: Thrombolytic; Tissue plasminogen activator
Half-life: 13–16 minutes
Clinically important, potentially hazardous interactions with: abciximab, aspirin, bivalirudin, dipyridamole, piperacillin, salicylates

Reactions

Skin
Allergic reactions (sic) (<1%)
Bleeding
Ecchymoses
Purpura

Other
Anaphylactoid reactions (<1%)
Headache
Injection-site bleeding (1–10%)

RIBAVIRIN

Synonyms: RTCA; tribavirin
Trade names: Copegus; Rebetol (Schering); Rebetron (Schering); Virazole (ICN)
Other common trade names: *Viramid; Virazid*
Indications: Respiratory syncytial viral infections
Category: Antiviral (against respiratory syncytial virus [RSV])
Half-life: 24 hours
Clinically important, potentially hazardous interactions with: zidovudine

Rebetron is interferon and ribavirin

Reactions

Skin
Eczema
  (2002): Dereure O+, *Br J Dermatol* 147(6), 1142 (with
    interferons alfa-2)
Erythema multiforme
  (1960): Heijer A+, *Acta Derm Venereol* (Stockh) 40, 35
Exanthems
  (2002): Farady KK, Austin, TX* (from Internet) (observation)
  (1990): Janai HK+, *Pediatr Infect Dis J* 9, 209 (0.5%)
Flu-like syndrome (sic) (10%)*
Grover's disease
  (2000): Antunes I+, *Br J Dermatol* 142, 1257
Herpes simplex (activation)
Photosensitivity
  (2002): Castillo R+, *World Congress Dermatol* Poster, 0091
  (2002): Dereure O+, *Br J Dermatol* 147(6), 1142 (with
    interferons alfa-2)
  (1999): Stryjek-Kaminska D+, *Am J Gastroenterol* 94, 1686
Pruritus (>10%)*
  (1999): Stryjek-Kaminska D+, *Am J Gastroenterol* 94, 1686
Rash (sic) (<10%)*
  (2001): Karim A+, *Am J Med Sci* 322(4), 233
Sarcoidosis
  (2002): Cogrel O+, *Br J Dermatol* 146(2), 320 *
  (2002): Wendling J+, *Arch Dermatol* 138, 546 * (2 cases)
Urticaria
  (1999): Stryjek-Kaminska D+, *Am J Gastroenterol* 94, 1686

Hair
Hair – alopecia (>10%)*
  (2001): Zucker DM+, *Gastroenterol Nurs* 24(4), 192 (with
    interferon alpha)

Other
Arthralgia
  (2001): Zucker DM+, *Gastroenterol Nurs* 24(4), 192 *
Cough
  (2001): Karim A+, *Am J Med Sci* 322(4), 233
Depression
  (2001): Karim A+, *Am J Med Sci* 322(4), 233
Dysgeusia (1–10%)*
Headache
Myalgia (>10%)*

*****Note:** The reaction patterns with an asterisk occurred while
receiving combination therapy with interferon alpha 2-B

RIBOFLAVIN

Synonyms: Lactoflavin; Vitamin B$_2$; Vitamin G
Trade name: Riobin
Indications: Riboflavin deficiency
Category: Water-soluble nutritional supplement
Half-life: 66–84 minutes

Reactions

Skin
Acne
  (1964): Fegeler F, *Arch Klin Exp Dermatol* (German) 219, 335
Allergic reactions (sic)
  (1975): Soloshenko EN+, *Sov Med* (Russian) October, 141
Angioedema
  (1972): Kuokkanen K, *Acta Allergol* 27, 407
Ichthyosis
  (1985): Spirov G+, *Dermatol Venereol* (Sofia) 24, 50
Urticaria
  (1972): Kuokkanen K, *Acta Allergol* 27, 407

Other
Anaphylactoid reactions
  (2001): Ou LS+, *Ann Allergy Asthma Immunol* 87(5), 430

RIFABUTIN

Trade name: Mycobutin (Pharmacia)
Indications: Prevention of disseminated *Mycobacterium avium*
infection
Category: Antitubercular antibiotic
Half-life: 45 hours
**Clinically important, potentially hazardous interactions
with:** amiodarone, anisindione, anticoagulants, corticosteroids,
cyclosporine, dapsone, dicumarol, midazolam, oral
contraceptives, ritonavir, tacrolimus, voriconazole

Reactions

Skin
Lupus erythematosus
  (1997): Berning SE+, *Lancet* 349, 1521
Pigmentation
  (1995): Smith JF+, *Clin Infect Dis* 21, 1515
Rash (sic) (11%)
Urticaria

Other
Ageusia
  (1993): Morris JT+, *Ann Intern Med* 119, 171
Discolored sputum (sic)
Dysgeusia (3%)
Headache
Myalgia (2%)
Paresthesias (<1%)
Polyarthalgia-arthritis syndrome
  (2000): Curino C+, *Presse Med* 29(28), 1563

RIFAMPIN

Synonym: rifampicin
Trade names: Rifadin (Aventis); Rimactane (Geneva) (Novartis)
Other common trade names: *Abrifam; Corifam; Ramicin; Rifaldin; Rifamed; Rimpin; Rimycin; Rofact*
Indications: Tuberculosis
Category: Tuberculostatic
Half-life: 3–5 hours
Clinically important, potentially hazardous interactions with: amiodarone, amprenavir, anisindione, antacids, anticoagulants, aprepitant, atazanavir, atovaquone, corticosteroids, cyclosporine, dapsone, delavirdine, dicumarol, digoxin, halothane, imatinib, isoniazid, itraconazole, ketoconazole, midazolam, nelfinavir, nifedipine, oral contraceptives, protease inhibitors, pyrazinamide, ritonavir, saquinavir, tacrolimus, triazolam, voriconazole, warfarin

Reactions

Skin

Acne
  (1990): Mimouni A+, *Drug Intell Clin Pharm* 24, 947
  (1985): Holdiness MR, *Int J Dermatol* 24, 280
  (1974): Nwokolo U, *BMJ* 3, 473 (1–5%) (only men)
Allergic reactions (sic)
  (1973): Nessi R+, *Scand J Respir Dis* 84, 15
Angioedema
  (1989): Holdiness MR, *Med Toxicol Adv Drug Exp* 4, 444 (72%)
Bullous eruption (<1%)
Dermatitis
  (1991): Guerra L+, *Contact Dermatitis* 25, 328
  (1986): Holdiness MR, *Contact Dermatitis* 15, 282
  (1986): Milpied B+, *Contact Dermatitis* 14, 252
Diaphoresis (1–10%)
Erythema multiforme (<1%)
  (1990): Mimouni A+, *Drug Intell Clin Pharm* 24, 947
  (1988): Hira SK+, *J Am Acad Dermatol* 19, 451 (in AIDS patients)
  (1979): Nigam P+, *Lepr India* 51, 249
  (1977): Nyirenda R+, *BMJ* 2, 1189
Exanthems (1–5%)
  (1998): Zimmerli W+, *JAMA* 279, 1537
  (1989): Wurtz RM+, *Lancet* 1, 955 (in AIDS patients)
  (1985): Holdiness MR, *Int J Dermatol* 24, 280
  (1976): Mangi RJ, *N Engl J Med* 294, 113 (3%)
  (1971): Esposito R+, *Lancet* 2, 491 (1–5%)
  (1971): Poole G+, *BMJ* 3, 343 (1–5%)
Exfoliative dermatitis
  (1987): Goldin HM+, *Ann Intern Med* 107, 789
Facial edema
Fixed eruption
  (2001): Goel A+, *Indian J Lepr* 73(2), 159 (bullous, necrotizing)
  (2000): Jaiswal AK+, *Lepr Rev* 71, 217
  (1998): John SS, *Lepr Rev* 69, 397
  (1993): Pavithran K, *Indian J Lepr* 65, 339
  (1990): Mimouni A+, *Drug Intell Clin Pharm* 24, 947
  (1985): Naik RPC+, *Indian J Lepr* 57, 648
Flushing
  (1995): Hoss DM+, *Arch Dermatol* 131, 647
  (1993): Tsankov NK+, *Int J Dermatol* 32, 401 (passim)
  (1990): Mimouni A+, *Drug Intell Clin Pharm* 24, 947
  (1985): Holdiness MR, *Int J Dermatol* 24, 280
  (1982): Girling DJ, *Drugs* 23, 56 (5%)
  (1976): Mangi RJ, *N Engl J Med* 294, 113 (7%)
  (1972): Girling HM+, *BMJ* 1, 765
  (1971): Girling DJ+, *BMJ* 4, 231

Linear IgA bullous dermatosis
  (2002): Cohen LM+, *J Am Acad Dermatol* 46, S32 (passim)
  (1994): Kuechle MK+, *J Am Acad Dermatol* 30, 187
Lupus erythematosus
  (2001): Patel GK+, *Clin Exp Dermatol* 26(3), 260
Pemphigus
  (1995): Hoss DM+, *Arch Dermatol* 131, 647
  (1993): Tsankov NK+, *Int J Dermatol* 32, 401 (passim)
  (1987): Honeybourne D+, *Br J Clin Pract* 41, 937
  (1986): Miyagawa S+, *Br J Dermatol* 114, 729 (exacerbation)
  (1984): Lee CW+, *Br J Dermatol* 111, 619 (foliaceus)
  (1982): Ruocco V+, *Arch Dermatol Res* 274, 123
  (1976): Gange RW+, *Br J Dermatol* 95, 445
Pruritus (<1%)
  (1995): Hoss DM+, *Arch Dermatol* 131, 647
  (1995): Walker-Renard P, *Ann Pharmacother* 29, 267
  (1993): Tsankov NK+, *Int J Dermatol* 32, 401 (passim)
  (1989): Holdiness MR, *Med Toxicol Adv Drug Exp* 4, 444 (62%)
  (1987): Goldin HM+, *Ann Intern Med* 107, 789
  (1972): Girling HM+, *BMJ* 1, 765
  (1971): Girling DJ+, *BMJ* 4, 231
Purpura
  (1980): Miescher PA+, *Clin Haematol* 9, 505
  (1972): Girling HM+, *BMJ* 1, 765 (0.5–1%)
  (1971): Esposito R+, *Lancet* 2, 491
  (1971): Girling DJ+, *BMJ* 4, 231 (0.5–1%)
  (1971): Poole G+, *BMJ* 3, 343
  (1970): Blajckman MA+, *BMJ* 3, 24
Rash (sic) (1–5%)
  (2000): Gordin F+, *JAMA* 283, 1445
  (1995): Chaisson RE, *Infections in Medicine* 12, 48
Red man syndrome
  (1995): Dayavathi+, *J Assoc Physicians India* 43, 724
  (1992): Gupta M+, *Indian Pediatr* 29, 1315
  (1989): Holdiness MR, *Med Toxicol Adv Drug Exp* 4, 444
  (1988): Gross DJ+, *Cutis* 42, 175 (red/orange person syndrome)
  (1986): Bolan G+, *Pediatrics* 77, 633
  (1980): Meisel S+, *Ann Intern Med* 92, 262
  (1975): Newton RW+, *Scott Med J* 20, 55
Side effects (sic)
  (1985): Holdiness MR, *Int J Dermatol* 24, 280 (5%)
Stevens–Johnson syndrome
  (1994): Marfatia YS, *Arch Dermatol* 130, 1074 (passim)
  (1993): Tsankov NK+, *Int J Dermatol* 32, 401 (passim)
  (1988): Hira SK+, *J Am Acad Dermatol* 19, 451 (in AIDS patients)
  (1977): Nyirenda R+, *BMJ* 2, 1189
Toxic epidermal necrolysis
  (1996): Blum L+, *J Am Acad Dermatol* 34, 1088
  (1994): Marfatia YS, *Arch Dermatol* 130, 1074 (passim)
  (1990): Prazuck T+, *Scand J Infect Dis* 22, 629
  (1987): Guillaume JC+, *Arch Dermatol* 123, 1166
  (1987): Okano M+, *J Am Acad Dermatol* 17, 303
Urticaria
  (1997): Sharma VK+, *Lepr Rev* 68, 331
  (1987): Grob JJ+, *Contact Dermatitis* 16(5), 284
  (1987): Gupta CM+, *Lepr Rev* 58, 308
  (1985): Holdiness MR, *Int J Dermatol* 24, 280
  (1972): Girling HM+, *BMJ* 1, 765
  (1971): Girling DJ+, *BMJ* 4, 231
Vasculitis
  (1995): Hoss DM+, *Arch Dermatol* 131, 647
  (1990): Chan CH+, *Tubercle* 71, 297
  (1989): Iredale JP+, *Chest* 96, 215

Hair

Hair – alopecia areata
  (2001): McMillen R+, *J Am Acad Dermatol* 44(1), 142 (in 2 sisters)

Other
Anaphylactoid reactions
(1999): Garcia F+, *Allergy* 54, 527 (to topical)
(1999): Magnan A+, *J Allergy Clin Immunol* 103, 954
(1998): Erel F+, *Ann Allergy Asthma Immunol* 81, 257
(1995): Cardot E+, *J Allergy Clin Immunol* 95, 1
(1989): Piazza I, *Allergologia* 12, 96 (suppl)
(1989): Wurtz RM+, *Lancet* 1, 955 (in AIDS patients)
Death
(2002): Medinger A, *Chest* 121(5), 1710 (with pyrazinamide)
(2001): No authors, *Can Commun Dis Rep* 27(13), 114 (with pyrazinamide)
(2001): No authors, *JAMA* 286(12), 1445 (with pyrazinamide)
(2001): No authors, *MMWR Morb Mortal Wkly Rep* 50(34), 733 (with pyrazinamide)
Glossodynia
Headache
Injection-site erythema
(1988): Fan-Havard P+, *Clin Pharm* 7, 616
Mucosal bleeding (sic)
(1971): Poole G+, *BMJ* 3, 343
Myalgia
Myopathy
Oral mucosal eruption
(1971): Poole G+, *BMJ* 3, 343
Porphyria
(1985): Holdiness MR, *Int J Dermatol* 24, 280
(1982): Igual JP+, *Presse Med* (French) 11, 2846
Porphyria cutanea tarda
(1980): Millar JW, *Br J Dis Chest* 74, 405
Serum sickness
(1994): Parra FM+, *Ann Allergy* 73, 123
Stomatitis (<1%)

RIFAPENTINE

Trade name: Priftin (Aventis)
Indications: Tuberculosis
Category: Antitubercular antibiotic
Half-life: 14–17 hours
Clinically important, potentially hazardous interactions with: amiodarone, anisindione, anticoagulants, corticosteroids, cyclosporine, dicumarol, ritonavir, tacrolimus, warfarin

Reactions

Skin
Acne (1–10%)
Peripheral edema (<1%)
Pigmentation (<1%)
Pruritus (1–10%)
Purpura (<1%)
Rash (sic) (1–10%)
Urticaria (<1%)

Other
Headache

RILUZOLE

Synonym: Rilutek (Aventis)
Indications: Amyotrophic lateral sclerosis (ALS)
Category: Amyotrophic lateral sclerosis (ALS) agent
Half-life: N/A

Reactions

Skin
Candidiasis
Cellulitis
Chills
Eczema (sic) (1.6%)
Edema
Exfoliative dermatitis
Facial edema
Granulomas (sic)
Peripheral edema (3%)
Petechiae
Photosensitivity
Pruritus
Purpura

Hair
Hair – alopecia (1%)

Other
Dysgeusia
Gingival hemorrhage
Glossitis
Headache
Hyperesthesia
Injection-site reactions (sic)
Mastodynia
Oral candidiasis (0.6%)
Paresthesias
Phlebitis (1%)
Stomatitis (1%)
Tongue discoloration
Tooth disorder (sic) (1%)
Vaginal candidiasis
Xerostomia (3.5%)

RIMANTADINE

Trade name: Flumadine (Forest)
Other common trade name: *Ruflual*
Indications: Various infections caused by influenza virus
Category: Antiviral
Half-life: 25–30 hours

Reactions

Skin
Edema (pedal) (1–10%)
Rash (sic) (<1%)
(1989): Hayden FG+, *N Engl J Med* 321, 1696 (1%)

Other
Ageusia (<0.3%)
Dysgeusia
Headache

Hyperesthesia
Parosmia (<0.3%)
Stomatitis
Xerostomia (1.6%)

RISEDRONATE

Trade name: Actonel (Procter & Gamble)
Indications: Paget's disease of bone, postmenopausal osteoporosis
Category: Biphosphonate
Half-life: terminal: 220 hours

Reactions

Skin
Ecchymoses (4.3%)
Edema
Flu-like syndrome (sic) (9.8%)
Peripheral edema (8.2%)
Pruritus (3.0%)
Rash (sic) (11.5%)

Other
Conjunctivitis
   (2003): Frauenfelder FW+, *N Engl J Med* 348, 1187
Glossitis (<1%)
Headache
Myalgia (6.6%)
Paresthesias (2.1%)
Tendon disorder (sic) (3.0%)
Tooth disorder (sic) (2.1%)

RISPERIDONE

Trade name: Risperdal (Janssen)
Indications: Psychotic disorders
Category: Antipsychotic
Half-life: 3–30 hours
Clinically important, potentially hazardous interactions with: clozapine

Reactions

Skin
Acne (<1%)
Allergic reactions (sic) (<1%)
   (1998): Terao T+, *J Clin Psychiatry* 59, 82
Angioedema
   (2001): Kores Plesnicar B+, *Eur Psychiatry* 16(8), 506
   (1995): Cooney C+, *BMJ* 311, 1204
Bullous eruption (<1%)
Bullous pemphigoid
   (1996): Wijeratne C+, *Am J Psychiatry* 153, 735
Dermatitis (sic)
Diaphoresis (<1%)
Edema
   (2001): Ravasia S, *Can J Psychiatry* 46(5), 453
   (1996): Baldassano CF+, *J Clin Psychiatry* 57, 422 (generalized)
Exfoliative dermatitis (0.1–1%)
Flushing (<1%)
   (2001): Masi G+, *J Child Neurol* 16(6), 395

Furunculosis (<1%)
Hyperkeratosis (sic) (<1%)
Hypohidrosis (<1%)
Irritation (sic)
   (2002): McCracken JT+, *N Engl J Med* 347(5), 314 (22%)
Lichenoid eruption (<1%)
Neuroleptic malignant syndrome
   (2002): Aboraya A+, *W V Med J* 98(2), 63 (with olanzapine)
   (2002): Beauchemin MA+, *Can J Psychiatry* 47(9), 886
   (2002): Bottlender R+, *Pharmacopsychiatry* 35(3), 119
Peripheral edema
   (2001): Hwang JP+, *J Clin Psychopharmacol* 21(6), 583 (16.4%)
Photosensitivity (1–10%)
   (1998): Almond DS+, *Postgrad Med J* 74, 252
Pigmentation (1%)
Pruritus (<1%)
Psoriasis (<1%)
Purpura (<1%)
Rash (sic) (5%)
Seborrhea
Ulcerations (<1%)
Urticaria (<0.1%)
Warts (<1%)
Xerosis (2%)

Hair
Hair – alopecia (<1%)
   (2000): Mercke Y+, *Ann Clin Psychiatry* 12, 35
Hair – hypertrichosis (<1%)

Other
Akathisia
   (2002): Wetter TC+, *Pharmacopsychiatry* 35(3), 109
Anaphylactoid reactions
Death
Dysgeusia (<1%)
Dysphagia
   (2001): Nair S+, *Gen Hosp Psychiatry* 23(4), 231
Galactorrhea (1–10%)
   (2001): Gupta S+, *J Am Acad Dermatol* 40(5), 504
   (1998): Popli A+, *Ann Clin Psychiatry* 10, 31
Gingivitis (<1%)
Gynecomastia (1–10%)
   (1999): Benazzi F, *Pharmacopsychiatry* 32, 41
Headache
Hyperesthesia (<1%)
Mastodynia (<1%)
Muscle rigidity
   (2002): McCracken JT+, *N Engl J Med* 347(5), 314 (10%)
Myalgia (<1%)
Paresthesias (<1%)
Parkinsonism
   (2001): Takahashi H+, *Clin Neuropharmacol* 24(6), 358
Priapism (1–10%)
   (2003): Bourgeois JA+, *J Clin Psychiatry* 64(2), 218
   (2003): Relan P+, *J Clin Psychiatry* 64(4), 482
   (2002): Freudenreich O, *J Clin Psychiatry* 63(3), 249 (with citalopram)
   (2002): Reeves RR+, *Pharmacotherapy* 22(8), 1070
   (2001): Compton MT+, *J Clin Psychiatry* 62(5), 363 (passim)
Restless legs syndrome
   (2002): Wetter TC+, *Pharmacopsychiatry* 35(3), 109
Rhabdomyolysis
   (2002): Giner V+, *J Intern Med* 251(2), 177 (with cerivastatin)
   (1996): Meltzer HY+, *Neuropsychopharmacology* 15(4), 395
Sialopenia (5%)
Sialorrhea (2%)

(2001): Gajwani P+, *Psychosomatics* 42(3), 276
Stomatitis (<1%)
Stutter
  (2001): Lee HJ+, *J Clin Psychopharmacol* 21(1), 115
Thrombophlebitis (<1%)
Tinnitus
Tongue edema (<1%)
Tongue pigmentation (<1%)
Tremor
  (2002): McCracken JT+, *N Engl J Med* 347(5), 314 (14%)
Xerostomia (1–10%)
  (2002): McCracken JT+, *N Engl J Med* 347(5), 314 (18%)
  (2001): Hodge CH+, *Vet Hum Toxicol* 43(6), 339 (2 cases)
  (2001): Mullen J+, *Clin Ther* 23(11), 1839 (6.9%)

RITODRINE

Trade names: Pre-Par; Yutopar (AstraZeneca)
Indications: Preterm labor
Category: Adrenergic agonist; Tocolytic (uterine relaxant)
Half-life: 1.3–12 hours

Reactions

Skin
Chills (3–10%)
Diaphoresis (1–3%)
  (1978): Hauser GA, *Ther Umsch* (German) 35, 422 (3–14%)
Erythema (10–15%)
Erythema multiforme
  (1988): Beitner O+, *Drug Intell Clin Pharm* 22, 724
Exanthems
Pustules (in a pregnant woman with psoriasis)
  (1998): D'Incan M+, *J Eur Acad Dermatol Venereol* 11, 91
Rash (sic) (1–3%)
  (2001): Yamada T+, *Arch Gynecol Obstet* 264(4), 218
Urticaria
Vasculitis
  (1991): Bosnyak S+, *Am J Obstet Gyn* 165, 427

Other
Anaphylactoid reactions (1–3%)
Headache
Tremor (>10%)

RITONAVIR

Trade name: Norvir (Abbott)
Indications: HIV infection
Category: Antiretroviral; Protease inhibitor
Half-life: 3–5 hours
**Clinically important, potentially hazardous interactions
with:** alfentanil, alprazolam, amiodarone, aprepitant, bepridil,
bupropion, buspirone, chlordiazepoxide, clozapine, cyclosporine,
diazepam, dihydroergotamine, ergot alkaloids, estazolam,
fentanyl, flecainide, flurazepam, halazepam, ketoconazole,
meperidine, methysergide, midazolam, nifedipine, oral
contraceptives, phenytoin, pimozide, piroxicam, propafenone,
propoxyphene, quazepam, quinidine, rifabutin, rifampin,
rifapentine, saquinavir, sildenafil, simvastatin, **St John's wort**,
triazolam, zolpidem

Reactions

Skin
Acne (<2%)
Allergic reactions (sic) (<2%)
Angioedema
Bullous eruption (<2%)
Cheilitis (<2%)
  (2000): Bonfanti P+, *J Acquir Immune Defic Syndr* 23(3), 236
Dermatitis (<2%)
Diaphoresis (1–10%)
Ecchymoses (<2%)
Eczema (sic) (<2%)
Edema
Exanthems (<2%)
  (1997): Bachmeyer C+, *Dermatology* 195, 301 (2 HIV patients)
Facial edema (<2%)
Folliculitis (<2%)
Granulomas
  (2002): Kawsar M+, *Int J STD AIDS* 13(4), 273
Peripheral edema (<2%)
Photosensitivity (<2%)
Pruritus (<2%)
Psoriasis (<2%)
Rash (sic) (1–10%)
Seborrhea (<2%)
Stevens–Johnson syndrome
Urticaria (<2%)
Xerosis (<2%)

Hair
Hair – alopecia
  (2002): Ginarte M+, *AIDS* 16(12), 1695 (with indinavir)

Nails
Nails – ingrown
  (2001): James CW+, *Ann Pharmacother* 35(7), 881 (with
    indinavir)

Other
Ageusia (<2%)
Anaphylactoid reactions
Dysgeusia (10.3%)
Gingivitis (<2%)
Gynecomastia
  (2001): Manfredi R+, *Ann Pharmacother* 35(4), 438
  (2000): Bonfanti P+, *J Acquir Immune Defic Syndr* 23(3), 236
Headache

Hyperesthesia (<2%)
Lipodystrophy
  (2002): Reid S, *Can Adv Drug Reaction Newsletter* 12, 5
  (2001): van der Valk M+, *AIDS* 15(7), 847
Myalgia (1–10%)
Oral candidiasis (<2%)
Oral ulceration (<2%)
Paresthesias (2.6%)
  (2001): Scully C+, *Oral Dis* 7(4), 205 (circumoral) (passim)
Parkinsonism
  (2003): Clay PG+, *Ann Pharmacother* 37(2), 202 (with
    busipirone)
Parosmia (<2%)
Perioral paresthesias
  (2001): McMahon D+, *Antivir Ther* 6(2), 105
Rhabdomyolysis
  (2003): Mah Ming+, *AIDS Patient Care STDS* 17(5), 207 (with
    atorvastatin, and clarithromycin)
Thrombophlebitis
  (2000): Bonfanti P+, *J Acquir Immune Defic Syndr* 23(3), 236
Xerostomia (<2%)

*Note: Protease inhibitors cause dyslipidemia which includes
elevated triglycerides and cholesterol and redistribution of body fat
centrally to produce the so-called 'protease paunch,' breast
enlargement, facial atrophy, and 'buffalo hump'

RITUXIMAB

Trade name: Rituxan (Genentech)
Indications: Non-Hodgkin's lymphoma
Category: Antineoplastic; Monoclonal antibody
Half-life: 60 hours (after first infusion)

Reactions

Skin
Angioedema (>10%)
Chills (10%)
  (2003): Boye J+, *Ann Oncol* 14(4), 520
  (2003): *Prescrire Int* 12(66), 125
  (2003): Rehwald U+, *Blood* 101(2), 420
  (2002): Salopek TG+, *J Am Acad Dermatol* 47(5), 785
Diaphoresis
Exanthems (10%)
Flushing (<5%)
Maculopapular rash
  (2002): Lowndes S+, *Ann Oncol* 13(12), 1948
Peripheral edema
Pruritus (10%)
  (2002): Salopek TG+, *J Am Acad Dermatol* 47(5), 785
Rash (sic) (10%)
Stevens–Johnson syndrome
  (2002): Lowndes S+, *Ann Oncol* 13(12), 1948
Urticaria (10%)

Other
Cytomegalovirus infection (reactivation)
  (2001): Suzan F+, *N Engl J Med* 345, 1000
Death
  (2003): Sirvent-Von Bueltzingsloewen A+, *Med Pediatr Oncol*
    40(6), 408
  (2001): Huhn D+, *Blood* 98(5), 1326
  (2001): Suzan F+, *N Engl J Med* 345(13), 1000
Fever
  (2003): Boye J+, *Ann Oncol* 14(4), 520

  (2003): *Prescrire Int* 12(66), 125
  (2003): Rehwald U+, *Blood* 101(2), 420
Headache
Injection-site reactions (sic)
  (2002): Meo P+, *Recenti Prog Med* 93(7), 421
  (2002): Motto DG+, *Isr Med Assoc J* 4(11), 1006
  (2001): Stasi R+, *Blood* 98(4), 952
  (2001): Wood AM, *Am J Health Syst Pharm* 58(3), 215
Myalgia (7%)
Orogenital ulceration
  (2002): Lowndes S+, *Ann Oncol* 13(12), 1948
Rhinitis
  (2003): Rehwald U+, *Blood* 101(2), 420
Rigors
  (2003): Boye J+, *Ann Oncol* 14(4), 520
Serum sickness
  (2002): Herishanu Y, *Am J Hematol* 70(4), 329
  (2001): D'Arcy CA+, *Arthritis Rheum* 44, 1717

RIVASTIGMINE

Trade name: Exelon (Novartis)
Indications: Alzheimer's disease and dementia
Category: Acetylcholinesterase inhibitor; Cholinergic
Half-life: 1–2 hours
**Clinically important, potentially hazardous interactions
with:** galantamine

Reactions

Skin
Allergic reactions (sic) (~1%)
Bullous eruption (~1%)
Cellulitis (~1%)
Clammy skin (~1%)
Dermatitis (~1%)
Diaphoresis (10%)
Edema (~1%)
Exanthems (~1%)
  (2001): Monastero R+, *Am J Med* 111(7), 583
Exfoliative dermatitis (~1%)
Facial edema (~1%)
Flushing (~1%)
Herpes simplex (~1%)
Hot flashes (~1%)
Infections (sic) (~2%)
Periorbital edema (~1%)
Peripheral edema (~2%)
Psoriasis (~1%)
Purpura (~1%)
Rash (sic) (~2%)
Ulcerations (~1%)
Urticaria (~1%)

Hair
Hair – alopecia (~1%)

Other
Ageusia (~1%)
Dysgeusia (~1%)
Foetor ex ore (halitosis) (~1%)
Gingivitis (~1%)
Glossitis (~1%)
Headache
Hyperesthesia (~1%)

Mastodynia (~1%)
Myalgia (20%)
Paresthesias (~1%)
Sialorrhea (~1%)
Thrombophlebitis (<2%)
Tremor (4%)
Ulcerative stomatitis (~1%)
Vaginitis (~1%)
Xerostomia (~1%)

RIZATRIPTAN

Synonym: MK462
Trade name: Maxalt (Merck)
Indications: Migraine
Category: Antimigraine; Serotonin agonist
Half-life: 2–3 hours
Clinically important, potentially hazardous interactions
with: dihydroergotamine, ergot-containing drugs, isocarboxazid,
MAO inhibitors, methysergide, naratriptan, phenelzine,
sibutramine, **St John's wort**, sumatriptan, tranylcypromine,
zolmitriptan

Reactions

Skin
Chills (<1%)
Diaphoresis (<1%)
Facial edema (<1%)
Flushing (1–10%)
Hot flashes (1–10%)
Pruritus (<1%)

Other
Dizziness
  (2003): Christie S+, *Eur Neurol* 49(1), 20 (6.7%)
Headache
Hyperesthesia
Myalgia (<1%)
Paresthesias
Tongue edema
Xerostomia (<5%)

ROFECOXIB

Trade name: Vioxx (Merck)
Indications: Osteoarthritis, acute pain
Category: Nonsteroidal anti-inflammatory (Cox-2 inhibitor)
analgesic
Half-life: 17 hours
Clinically important, potentially hazardous interactions
with: anisindione, anticoagulants, dicumarol, lithium,
methotrexate, warfarin

Reactions

Skin
Abrasion (<2%)
Allergic reactions (sic) (<2%)
Angioedema
  (2002): Kumar NP+, *Postgrad Med J* 78(921), 439
  (2001): Kelkar PS+, *J Rheumatol* 28(11), 2553

(2000): Medicines Control Agency and Committee on Safety of
    Medicines Reports (5 cases)
Atopic dermatitis (<2%)
Basal cell carcinoma (<2%)
Bullous eruption (<2%)
Cellulitis (<2%)
Dermatitis (<2%)
Diaphoresis (<2%)
Edema (3.7%)
  (2002): Carder KR+, *Pediatr Dermatol* 19(4), 353 (palms & soles)
  (2000): Medicines Control Agency and Committee on Safety of
    Medicines Reports (101 cases)
Erythema (<2%)
  (2000): Wright WL, Castro Valley, CA (from Internet)
    (observation) (after the second day)
Exanthems
  (2000): Blumenthal HL, Beachwood, OH (personal case)
    (observation)
Fixed eruption
  (2002): Nederost ST+, *Cutis* 70, 125
  (2001): Kaur C+, *Dermatology* 203(4), 351 (with sulfonamides)
  (2000): Conners RC, Greenwich, CT (personal communication)
Flu-like syndrome (sic) (2.9%)
Flushing (<2%)
Fungal infections (<2%)
Granuloma annulare
  (2000): Rotman H, Houston, TX (personal communication)
    (observation)
Herpes simplex (<2%)
Herpes zoster (<2%)
Peripheral edema (6%)
  (2001): Litt JZ, Beachwood, OH (2 personal cases)
  (2000): Litt JZ, Beachwood, OH (personal case)
Photosensitivity
  (2001): Klein AD, Statesboro, GA (from Internet) (observation)
  (2000): Valentine M, Everett, WA (from Internet) (observation)
  (1999): Gregg LJ, Tulsa, OK (from Internet) (observation)
Phototoxicity
  (2001): Klein AD, Statesboro, GA (from Internet) (observation)
Pruritus (<2%)
Psoriasis
  (2003): Clark DW+, *Arch Dermatol* 139(9), 1223
Purpura
  (2001): Litt JZ, Beachwood, OH (personal case)
  (2000): Litt JZ, Beachwood, OH (personal case)
Rash (sic) (<2%)
Urticaria (<2%)
  (2002): Nettis E+, *Ann Allergy Asthma* 88(3), 331
  (2001): Kelkar PS+, *J Rheumatol* 28(11), 2553
  (2000): Wright WL, Castro Valley, CA (from Internet) (2
    observations) (after the second day)
Vasculitis
  (2002): Reed BR, Denver, CO (from Internet) (observation)
Wrinkling
  (2002): Carder KR+, *Pediatr Dermatol* 19(4), 353 (aquagqnic –
    palms & soles)
Xerosis (<2%)

Hair
Hair – alopecia (<2%)

Nails
Nails – changes (sic) (<2%)

Other
Aphthous stomatitis (<2%)
Death
  (2002): Kumar NP+, *Postgrad Med J* 78(921), 439

(2001): Weaver J+, *Am J Gastroenterol* 96(12), 3449
Dizziness
    (2003): Bannwarth B+, *Drug Saf* 26(1), 49 (2.1%)
Headache
Hyperesthesia (<2%)
Myalgia (<2%)
Oral ulceration (<2%)
Paresthesias (<2%)
Tendinitis (<2%)
Tinnitus
    (2001): Litt JZ, Beachwood, OH (personal case)
Xerostomia (<2%)

ROPINIROLE

Trade name: Requip (GSK)
Indications: Parkinsonism
Category: Antiparkinsonian; Dopamine agonist
Half-life: ~6 hours

Reactions

Skin
Balanoposthitis (<1%)
Basal cell carcinoma (>1%)
Cellulitis (<1%)
Dermatitis (sic) (<1%)
Diaphoresis (6%)
Eczema (sic) (<1%)
Edema (<1%)
Exanthems (<1%)
Flushing (3%)
Fungal dermatitis (sic) (<1%)
Furunculosis (<1%)
Herpes simplex (<1%)
Herpes zoster (<1%)
Hyperkeratosis (<1%)
Hypertrophy (sic) (<1%)
Peripheral edema (<1%)
Photosensitivity (<1%)
Pigmentation (<1%)
Pruritus (<1%)
Psoriasis (<1%)
Purpura (<1%)
Rash (sic) (>1%)
Ulcerations (<1%)
Urticaria (<1%)
Viral infections

Hair
Hair – alopecia (<1%)

Other
Dizziness
    (2003): Im JH+, *J Neurol* 250(1), 90
Dyskinesia
    (2003): Im JH+, *J Neurol* 250(1), 90
Gingivitis (>1%)
Glossitis (<1%)
Gynecomastia (<1%)
Headache
Hyperesthesia (4%)

Mastitis (<1%)
Paresthesias (5%)
Peyronie's disease (<1%)
Sialorrhea (>1%)
Stomatitis (<1%)
Thrombophlebitis (<1%)
Tongue edema (<1%)
Tremor (6%)
Ulcerative stomatitis (<1%)
Vaginal candidiasis (<1%)
Xerostomia (5%)

ROSIGLITAZONE

Trade names: Avandamet (GSK); Avandia (GSK)
Indications: Type 2 diabetes
Category: Thiazolidinedione antidiabetic
Half-life: 3.5 hours

Reactions

Skin
Ankle edema
    (2002): Niemeyer NV+, *Pharmacotherapy* 22(7), 924
Edema (4.8%)
    (2002): *Prescrire Int* 11(62), 170
    (2002): Kuschel U+, *Med Klin* 97(9), 553
    (2001): Werner AL+, *Pharmacotherapy* 21(9), 1082
Edema of hand
    (2002): Niemeyer NV+, *Pharmacotherapy* 22(7), 924
Exanthems
    (1999): Rehbein HM, Jacksonville, FL (from Internet)
        (observation)
Exfoliative dermatitis
    (2000): Vinson RP, El Paso, TX (from Internet) (observation)
Facial edema
    (2002): Niemeyer NV+, *Pharmacotherapy* 22(7), 924

Other
Headache

RUE

Scientific names: *Ruta chalepensis; Ruta corsica; Ruta graveolens; Ruta montana*
Family: Rutaceae
Trade and other common names: Country man's treacle; Herb of grace; Herbygrass; ruda
Category: Antispasmodic; Emmenagogue
Purported indications and other uses: Hysteria, coughs, croup, colic, flatulence, mild stomachic, insomnia, abdominal cramps, nervous headache, giddiness, hysteria, palpitation, abortifacient, cysticide, vermifuge, insecticide. Topical: irritant, rubefacient for eczemas, psoriasis and rheumatic pain, sciatica, headache, chronic bronchitis. Flavoring in alcoholic beverages, salads, meats and cheeses
Half-life: N/A

Reactions

Skin
Blistering
(1985): Brener S+, *Contact Dermatitis* 12(4), 230
(1983): Heskel NS+, *Contact Dermatitis* 9(4), 278

Bullous dermatitis
(1999): Schempp CM+, *Hautarzt* 50(6), 432
(1968): Hanslian L+, *Cesk Farm* 17(6), 293
Clammy skin
Dermatitis
Edema
Erythema
(1985): Brener S+, *Contact Dermatitis* 12(4), 230
(1983): Heskel NS+, *Contact Dermatitis* 9(4), 278
Mutagen
(1987): Paulini H+, *Mutagenesis* 2(4), 271
Photodermatitis
(1999): Schempp CM+, *Hautarzt* 50(6), 432
(1999): Wessner D+, *Contact Dermatitis* 41(4), 232
(1995): Ortiz-Frutos FJ+, *Contact Dermatitis* 33(4), 284
(1990): Ena P+, *Contact Dermatitis* 22(1), 63
(1989): Goncalo S+, *Contact Dermatitis* 21(3), 200
(1985): Brener S+, *Contact Dermatitis* 12(4), 230
(1983): Gawkrodger DJ+, *Contact Dermatitis* 9(3), 224
(1983): Heskel NS+, *Contact Dermatitis* 9(4), 278

Other
Death
Seizures

SACCHARIN

Trade names: Saccharin; Sweet 'n Low
Indications: Sugar substitute
Category: Sulfonamide sweetener
Half-life: N/A

Reactions

Skin
Dermatitis (sic)
  (1989): Birbeck J, *N Z Med J* 102, 24
  (1972): Gordon H, *Am J Obstet Gynecol* 15, 1145
  (1972): Gordon H, *Cutis* 10, 77
Exanthems
  (1965): Boros E, *JAMA* 194, 571
  (1965): Fujita H+, *Acta Derm* 60, 303
Fixed eruption
  (1956): Stritzler C+, *Arch Dermatol* 74, 433
Notalgia paresthetica
  (1986): Fishman HC, *J Am Acad Dermatol* 15, 1304
Photosensitivity
  (1972): Gordon H, *Cutis* 10, 77
  (1972): Taub SJ, *Eye Ear Nose Throat Mon* 51, 405
  (1961): Kennedy B+, *J Louisiana Med Soc* 113, 365
Pruritus
  (1989): Birbeck J, *N Z Med J* 102, 24
  (1972): Gordon H, *Cutis* 10, 77
  (1965): Boros E, *JAMA* 194, 571
Sensitivity (sic)
  (1966): Kingsley HJ, *Cent Afr J Med* 12, 243
Urticaria
  (1989): Birbeck J, *N Z Med J* 102, 24
  (1974): Miller R+, *J Allergy Clin Immunol* 53, 240
  (1972): Gordon H, *Cutis* 10, 77
  (1956): Stritzler C+, *Arch Dermatol* 74, 433
  (1955): Stritzler C+, *New York J Med* 55, 3479

Other
Dysgeusia
  (1965): Boros E, *JAMA* 194, 571

*****Note:** Saccharin is a sulfonamide and can be absorbed systemically. Sulfonamides can produce severe, possibly fatal, reactions such as toxic epidermal necrolysis and Stevens–Johnson syndrome

SALMETEROL

Trade names: Advair (GSK); Serevent (GSK)
Other common trade names: *Salmeter; Serobid; Zantirel*
Indications: Asthma
Category: Adrenergic agonist; Sympathomimetic bronchodilator
Half-life: 3–4 hours

Reactions

Skin
Angioedema
Eczema (sic)
  (1997): Leal GB, Fortaleza, Brazil (from Internet) (observation)
Exanthems
Infections (sic) (12%)
  (2000): Beeh KM+, *Pneumologie* (German) 54, 225 (2.7%)
Pruritus
Rash (sic) (1–3%)

(1994): D'Alonzo GE+, *JAMA* 271, 1412
(1991): Hatton MQ+, *Lancet* 337, 1169
Urticaria (1–3%)
  (1991): Hatton MQF+, *Lancet* 337, 1169

Other
Death
  (2003): *Prescrire Int* 12(66), 142
Headache
Hypersensitivity (<1%)
Myalgia (1–3%)
Oral candidiasis
  (2002): Beeh KM+, *Pneumologie* 56(2), 91
Paresthesias
Trembling
Tremor (1–10)
  (2001): Shrewsbury S+, *Ann Allergy Asthma Immunol* 87(6), 465 (5.7%)
  (2000): Beeh KM+, *Pneumologie* (German) 54, 225

SALSALATE

Synonyms: disalicylic acid; salicylic acid
Trade names: Disalcid (3M); Mono-Gesic (Schwartz); Salflex (Carnrick); Salsitab (Upsher-Smith)
Other common trade names: *Argesic-SA; Artha-G; Atisuril; Disalgesic; Marthritic; Nobegyl; Salgesic; Salina; Umbradol*
Indications: Arthritis
Category: Nonsteroidal anti-inflammatory (NSAID) analgesic; Salicylate
Half-life: 7–8 hours
Clinically important, potentially hazardous interactions with: methotrexate

Reactions

Skin
Angioedema
Dermatitis (sic)
Exanthems
Lichenoid eruption
  (2001): Powell MI+, *J Am Acad Dermatol* 45, 616
Pruritus
Purpura
Rash (sic) (1–10%)
Urticaria
  (1986): Chudwin DS+, *Ann Allergy* 57, 133

Nails
Nails – onychoschizia
  (2001): Powell MI+, *J Am Acad Dermatol* 45, 616

Other
Anaphylactoid reactions (1–10%)
Tinnitus

SAQUINAVIR

Trade names: Fortovase (Roche); Invirase (Roche)
Indications: Advanced HIV infection
Category: Antiretroviral; Protease inhibitor
Half-life: 12 hours
Clinically important, potentially hazardous interactions with: alprazolam, clindamycin, dihydroergotamine, eplerenone, ergot derivatives, fentanyl, **garlic**, ketoconazole, methysergide, midazolam, phenytoin, pimozide, rifampin, ritonavir, sildenafil, **St John's wort**

Reactions

Skin
Acne (<2%)
Bullous eruption
Candidiasis (<2%)
Cheilitis (<2%)
Dermatitis (sic) (<2%)
Diaphoresis (<2%)
Eczema (sic) (<2%)
Erythema (<2%)
Erythema multiforme
  (1998): Garat H+, *Ann Dermatol Venereol* (French) 125, 42
Exanthems (<2%)
Fixed eruption
  (2000): Smith KJ+, *Cutis* 66, 29 (2 cases)
Folliculitis (<2%)
Furunculosis
Herpes simplex (<2%)
Herpes zoster (<2%)
Papulo-vesicular eruptions
  (2000): Smith KJ+, *Cutis* 66, 29 (2 cases)
Photosensitivity (<2%)
  (1997): Winter AJ+, *Genitourin Med* 73, 323
Pigmentary changes (<2%)
  (2000): Smith KJ+, *Cutis* 66, 29 (2 cases)
Pruritus
  (2000): Smith KJ+, *Cutis* 66, 29 (2 cases)
Psoriasis
  (2000): Bonfanti P+, *J Acquir Immune Defic Syndr* 23(3), 236
Rash (sic) (1.3%)
Seborrheic dermatitis (<2%)
Stevens–Johnson syndrome
Ulcerations (<2%)
Urticaria (<2%)
Warts (<2%)
Xerosis (<2%)
  (2000): Bonfanti P+, *J Acquir Immune Defic Syndr* 23(3), 236

Hair
Hair – alopecia
Hair – changes (sic) (<2%)

Other
Dysesthesia (<2%)
Dysgeusia (<2%)
Gingivitis (<2%)
Glossitis (<2%)
Guillain–Barré syndrome
Gynecomastia
  (2000): Bonfanti P+, *J Acquir Immune Defic Syndr* 23(3), 236
  (1999): Donovan B+, *Int J STD AIDS* 10, 49
Headache

Hyperesthesia (<2%)
Lingual lesions (sic)
  (1998): Ruscin JM+, *Ann Pharmacother* 32, 1248
Lipodystrophy
  (2002): Reid S, *Can Adv Drug Reaction Newsletter* 12, 5
Oral ulceration (2.5%)
Paresthesias (2.6%)
Perioral paresthesias
  (2001): McMahon D+, *Antivir Ther* 6(2), 105
Stomatitis (<2%)
Tendon xanthomata
  (2001): Leung N+, *Diabetes* 50(Suppl.2), 452
Xerostomia (<2%)

*Note: Protease inhibitors cause dyslipidemia which includes elevated triglycerides and cholesterol and redistribution of body fat centrally to produce the so-called 'protease paunch,' breast enlargement, facial atrophy, and 'buffalo hump'

SARGRAMOSTIN

(See GRANULOCYTE COLONY-STIMULATING FACTOR [GCSF])

SARSAPARILLA

Scientific names: *Smilax aristolochiaefolia; Smilax febrifuga; Smilax glabra; Smilax japicanga; Smilax officinalis; Smilax ornata; Smilax regelii; Smilax rotundifolia*
Family: Smilacaceae
Trade and other common names: Greenbriar; Horsebrier; jupicanga; khao yen; Round-leaf; Salsaparrilha; saparna; smilace; smilax; zarzaparilla
Category: Anti-inflammatory; Antioxidant; Immunomodulator
Purported indications and other uses: blood purifier, general tonic, gout, syphilis, gonorrhea, rheumatism, wounds, arthritis, fever, cough, scrofula, hypertension, digestive disorders, psoriasis, skin diseases, cancer
Half-life: N/A
Clinically important, potentially hazardous interactions with: digoxin

Reactions

Skin
None

Note: Sarsaparilla vine should not be confused with sasparilla and sassafras (the root and bark of which were once used to flavor root beer). Sarsaparilla is only used in root beer and other beverages for its foaming properties

SAW PALMETTO

Scientific names: *Sabal serrulata; Serenoa repens; Serenoa serrulata*
Family: Arecaceae; Palmae
Trade and other common names: American Dwarf Palm Tree; Cabbage Palm; Ju-Zhong; Palmier Nain; Sabal Fructus
Category: Anti-inflammatory; Antiseptic
Purported indications and other uses: Benign prostatic hyperplasia, diuretic, sedative, prostate cancer (with other herbs), aphrodisiac, hair growth, colds, coughs, sore throat, asthma, chronic bronchitis, migraine
Half-life: N/A
Clinically important, potentially hazardous interactions with: oral contraceptives, warfarin

Reactions

Skin

Adverse effects (sic)
(2002): Ernst E, *Ann Intern Med* 136(1), 42
(2002): Mattsson K+, *Lakartidningen* 99(50), 5095
(2002): Wilt T+, *Cochrane Database Syst Rev* imed(3), CD00
Hemorrhage
(2001): Cheema P+, *J Intern Med* 250(2), 167
Sensitization
(2002): Sinclair RD+, *Australas J Dermatol* 43(4), 311

SCOPOLAMINE

Trade names: Isopto Hyoscine Ophthalmic*; Scopase; Transderm-Scop Patch (Novartis)
Other common trade names: *Scopace; Scopoderm-TTS; Transdermal-V*
Indications: Nausea and vomiting, excess salivation
Category: Anticholinergic; Antispasmodic
Half-life: 8 hours
Clinically important, potentially hazardous interactions with: anticholinergics, arbutamine

Reactions

Skin

Allergic reactions (sic)
(2001): Decraene T+, *Contact Dermatitis* 45(5), 309
Dermatitis (sic) (transdermal patch and ophthalmic)
(1990): Hogan DJ+, *J Am Acad Dermatol* 22, 811
(1989): Gordon CR+, *BMJ* 298(6682), 1220
(1989): Holdiness MR, *Contact Dermatitis* 20, 3
(1988): van der Willigen AH+, *J Am Acad Dermatol* 18, 146
(1985): Clissold SP+, *Drugs* 29, 189
(1985): Trozak DJ, *J Am Acad Dermatol* 13, 247
(1984): Fisher AA, *Cutis* 34, 526
Edema (<1%) (ophthalmic)
Erythema
Erythema multiforme
(1986): Fisher AA, *Cutis* 37, 158; 262
(1979): Guill MA+, *Arch Dermatol* 115, 742
Exanthems
(1985): Clissold SP+, *Drugs* 29, 189 (transdermal patch)
Fixed eruption
(1981): Kanwar AJ+, *Dermatologica* 162, 378
Flushing

Hypohidrosis (>10%)
Photosensitivity (1–10%)
Rash (sic) (<1%)
Urticaria
Xerosis (>10%)

Other

Anaphylactoid reactions
(1995): Manhart AR+, *J Toxicol Clin Toxicol* 33, 189 (fatal)
(1994): Watanabe F+, *J Toxicol Clin Toxicol* 32, 593 (fatal)
Death
Dizziness
(2002): Kranke P+, *Anesth Analg* 95(1), 133
Headache
Injection-site irritation (>10%)
Oral mucosal lesions
(1985): Clissold SP+, *Drugs* 29, 189 (transdermal patch) (>5%)
Xerostomia (>60%)
(2002): Kranke P+, *Anesth Analg* 95(1), 133
(1985): Clissold SP+, *Drugs* 29, 189 (transdermal patch) (66%)
(1981): Price NM+, *Clin Pharmacol Ther* 29, 414

*****Note:** Systemic adverse effects have been reported following ophthalmic administration

SECOBARBITAL

Synonym: quinalbarbitone
Trade name: Seconal (Lilly)
Other common trade names: *Immenoctal; Novo-Secobarb; Secanal*
Indications: Insomnia
Category: Short-acting barbiturate sedative-hypnotic
Half-life: 15–40 hours
Clinically important, potentially hazardous interactions with: alcohol, anticoagulants, antihistamines, brompheniramine, buclizine, chlorpheniramine, dicumarol, ethanolamine, imatinib, warfarin

Reactions

Skin

Angioedema (<1%)
Exanthems
Exfoliative dermatitis (<1%)
Purpura
Rash (sic) (<1%)
Stevens–Johnson syndrome (<1%)
Urticaria

Other

Headache
Hypersensitivity
Injection-site pain (>10%)
Rhabdomyolysis
(1990): Larpin R+, *Presse Med* 19(30), 1403
Serum sickness
Thrombophlebitis (<1%)

SECRETIN

Trade name: Secretin-Ferring (Ferring)
Indications: Diagnosis of gastrinoma (Zollinger–Ellison syndrome)
Category: Gastrointestinal peptide hormone
Half-life: N/A

Reactions

Skin

Allergic reactions (sic)
Urticaria
  (1975): Baenkler HW+, *BMJ* 2, 747

Other

Injection-site reactions (sic)
  (1975): Baenkler HW+, *BMJ* 2, 747

SELEGILINE

Synonyms: deprenyl; L-deprenyl
Trade name: Eldepryl (Somerset)
Other common trade names: *Apo-Selegiline; Carbex; Eldeprine; Jumex; Movergan; Novo-Selegiline; Plurimen*
Indications: Parkinsonism
Category: Antiparkinsonian; Monoamine oxidase (MAO) inhibitor
Half-life: 9 minutes
Clinically important, potentially hazardous interactions with: carbidopa, citalopram, doxepin, **ephedra**, ephedrine, escitalopram, fluoxetine, fluvoxamine, levodopa, meperidine, nefazodone, oral contraceptives, paroxetine, sertraline, venlafaxine

Reactions

Skin

Diaphoresis
Peripheral edema
Photosensitivity
Rash (sic)

Hair

Hair – alopecia
Hair – hypertrichosis (facial)

Other

Application-site reactions
  (2002): Bodkin JA+, *Am J Psychiatry* 159(11), 1869
Bruxism (1–10%)
Death
  (2002): *Prescrire Int* 11(60), 108
Dysgeusia
Headache
Paresthesias
Serotonin syndrome
  (2002): *Prescrire Int* 11(60), 108
Tinnitus
Tremor
Xerostomia (>10%)
  (1988): Golbe LI+, *Clin Neuropharmacol* 11, 45

SELENIUM

Trade names: Bio-Active Selenium (Solaray); Exsel Shampoo; Head & Shoulders Intensive Treatment Dandruff Shampoo (Procter & Gamble); SelenoMax (Source Naturals); Selsun Blue (Abbott); Selsun Shampoo (Abbott); Vpak51
Other common trade names: *Selenate; Selenite; selenium dioxide; selenium sulfide; selenocysteine; selenomethionine*
Indications: Anticancer (stomach, colorectal, lung, prostate), arthritis, asthma, heart disease, HIV inhibitor. Treatment of dandruff, fungal infections (tinea versicolor), and seborrhea
Category: Essential micronutrient
Half-life: 12–41 hours; Selenomethionine: 252 days, Selinite: 102 days
Clinically important, potentially hazardous interactions with: cholesterol-lowering drugs, cisplatin, clozapine, niacin, oral corticosteroids, simvastatin

Reactions

Skin

Adverse effects (sic)
  (1994): Yang G+, *J Trace Elem Electrolytes Health Dis* 8(3–4), 159 (chronic exposure)
  (1989): Stacchini A+, *J Trace Elem Electrolytes Health Dis* 3(4), 193
Allergic reactions (sic)
Carcinoma
  (2001): Vinceti M+, *Rev Environ Health* 16(4), 233 (chronic exposure)
  (2000): Vinceti M+, *J Clin Epidemiol* 53(10), 1062 (chronic exposure)
  (2000): Vinceti M+, *Sci Total Environ* 250(1–3), 1 (chronic exposure)
  (1999): Barceloux DG, *J Toxicol Clin Toxicol* 37(2), 145 (deficiency)
  (1997): Foster LH+, *Crit Rev Food Sci Nutr* 37(3), 211 (deficiency)
Dermatitis
  (2001): Vinceti M+, *Rev Environ Health* 16(4), 233 (chronic exposure)
Diaphoresis
Erythema chronicum persistans
  (2003): Smith S, Louisville, KY (from Internet) (observation)
Flushing
Infections
Lupus erythematosus (deficiency)
Melanoma
  (1998): Vinceti M+, *Cancer Epidemiol Biomarkers Prev* 7(10), 853 (chronic exposure)
Photodermatitis
Pruritus
Rash (sic)
Scleroderma (deficiency)

Hair

Hair – alopecia
  (2001): Vinceti M+, *Rev Environ Health* 16(4), 233 (chronic exposure)
  (1996): Whanger P+, *Ann Clin Lab Sci* 26(2), 99 (chronic exposure)
Hair – brittle
  (1994): Yang G+, *J Trace Elem Electrolytes Health Dis* 8(3–4), 159 (chronic exposure)
Hair – changes (sic)

(1999): Barceloux DG, *J Toxicol Clin Toxicol* 37(2), 145 (chronic exposure)

(1997): Hathcock JN, *Am J Clinical Nutrition* 66, 427

Hair – color change

Nails

Nails – brittle

(1997): Hathcock JN, *Am J Clinical Nutrition* 66, 427

(1996): Whanger P+, *Ann Clin Lab Sci* 26(2), 99 (chronic exposure)

(1995): Yang GQ+, *Biomed Environ Sci* 8(3), 187 (deficiency)

(1994): Yang G+, *J Trace Elem Electrolytes Health Dis* 8(3–4), 159 (chronic exposure)

Nails – loss

(2001): Vinceti M+, *Rev Environ Health* 16(4), 233 (chronic exposure)

Nails – paronychia

Nails – white streaking

Other

Amyotrophic lateral sclerosis

(2001): Vinceti M+, *Rev Environ Health* 16(4), 233 (chronic exposure)

(1996): Vinceti M+, *Epidemiology* 7(5), 529 (chronic exposure)

(1993): Moriwaka F+, *J Neurol Sci* 118(1), 38 (chronic exposure)

(1977): Kilness AW+, *JAMA* 237(26), 2843 (chronic exposure)

Arthritis (deficiency)

Death (overdose)

Dysgeusia (metallic taste)

Myalgia

Paresthesias

Sialorrhea

Tooth disorder (sic)

Tremor

Note: Selenium is an essential component of glutathione peroxidase. Inadequate concentrations of dietry selenium account, in part, for Keshan disease (a fatal cardiomyopathy)

SENNA

Scientific names: *Cassia acutifolia; Cassia angustifolia; Cassia obtusifloia; Cassia senna; Cassia tora; Senna alexandrina; Senna obtusifolia; Senna tora*

Family: Caesalpiniaceae; Fabaceae

Trade and other common names: Agiolax; Agoral (Numark); Alesandrian; Black-Draught (Monticello); Cassia leaf; Ex-Lax (Novartis); Fletcher's Castoria (Mentholatum); Gentlax ; Glysennid; Goldline Senna; Herbal Trim Tea; Khartoum senna; Laci Le Beau Corp; Manevac; Perdiem (Novartis); PMS-Sennosides; Prodiem Plus (Novartis); Riva-Senna; Senexon; Senna alenxandrina; Senna Lax; Senna-Gen; Sennatab; Senokot; Senolax; Super Dieter's Tea; X-Prep

Category: Anthraquinone stimulant laxative

Purported indications and other uses: Laxative, cathartic, cholagogue, purgative

Half-life: N/A

Clinically important, potentially hazardous interactions with: digoxin, quinidine

Part used: Leaves and/or seed pods

Reactions

Skin

Adverse effects (sic)

(1996): Sykes NP, *J Pain Symptom Manage* 11(6), 363

(1993): Passmore AP+, *Pharmacology* 47, 249

(1988): Jagjivan B+, *Br J Radiol* 61(729), 853

Allergic reactions (sic)

(1991): Marks GB+, *Am Rev Respir Dis* 144(5), 1065

Bullous eruption

(2003): Spiller HA+, *Ann Pharmacother* 37(5), 636

Dermatitis

(2001): Leventhal JM+, *Pediatrics* 107(1), 178

Edema

Pruritus

Rash (sic)

Rhinoconjunctivitis (occupational exposure)

Side effects (sic)

(1977): Perkin JM, *Curr Med Res* 4(8), 540

Other

Arthopathy (from abuse)

(1988): Fichter M+, *Nervenarzt* (German) 59(4), 244

(1981): Armstrong RD+, *Br Med J* (Clin Res Ed) 282(6279), 1836

Death (from abuse)

Finger clubbing (from abuse) (reversible)

(1980): Malmquist J+, *Postgrad Med J* 56(662), 862

(1978): Prior J+, *Lancet* 2(8096), 947

(1975): Silk DB+, *Gastroenterology* 68, 790

Note: Prolonged or excessive laxative use can lead to electrolyte and fluid disturbances, development of carthartic colon, and possible increased risk of colorectal cancer. Treatment should be limited to 8 to 10 days

SERMORELIN

Trade name: Geref (Serono)

Other common trade name: *Gerel*

Category: Human growth hormone-releasing factor

Half-life: ~12 minutes

Clinically important, potentially hazardous interactions with: aspirin, drugs affecting pituitary secretion of somatotropin, glucocorticoids, indomethacin, insulin

Reactions

Skin

Flushing

Pallor

Pruritus

Urticaria

Other

Dizziness

Dysgeusia

Dysphagia

Injection-site edema

Injection-site erythema

Injection-site pain

SERTRALINE

Trade name: Zoloft (Roerig)
Other common trade name: *Atruline*
Indications: Depression, panic disorders, obsessive compulsive disorders
Category: Antidepressant; Selective serotonin reuptake inhibitor (SSRI)
Half-life: 24–26 hours
Clinically important, potentially hazardous interactions with: amphetamines, clarithromycin, dextroamphetamine, diethylpropion, erythromycin, isocarboxazid, linezolid, MAO inhibitors, mazindol, methamphetamine, metoclopramide, phendimetrazine, phenelzine, phentermine, phenylpropanolamine, pimozide, pseudoephedrine, selegiline, sibutramine, **St John's wort**, sumatriptan, sympathomimetics, tranylcypromine, trazodone, troleandomycin

Reactions

Skin
Acne (<1%)
Allergic reactions (sic)
  (1998): Beauquier B+, *Encephale* (French) 24, 62
  (1991): Guthrie SK, *Drug Intell Clin Pharm* 25, 952
Angioedema
  (2001): Adson DE+, *Ann Pharmacother* 35(11), 1375
  (1994): Gales BJ+, *Am J Hosp Pharm* 51, 118
Balanoposthitis (<1%)
Bullous eruption (<1%)
Dermatitis (sic) (<1%)
Diaphoresis (8.4%)
  (2002): Ahmed A, *Am J Geriatr Psychiatry* 10(4), 484
  (2002): Fisher AA+, *Ann Pharmacother* 36(1), 67
  (2000): Henney JE, *JAMA* 283, 596
  (1991): Guthrie SK, *Drug Intell Clin Pharm* 25, 952
  (1990): Reimherr FW+, *J Clin Psychiatry* 51, 18
  (1988): Doogan DP+, *J Clin Psychiatry* 49, 46
Discoloration (sic) (<1%)
Edema (<1%)
Erythema
Erythema multiforme (<1%)
  (1994): Gales BJ+, *Am J Hosp Pharm* 51, 118
Exanthems (<1%)
  (2000): Fernandes B+, *Contact Dermatitis* 42, 287
  (2000): Kittay SA, (from Internet) (observation)
  (1999): Blumenthal HL, Beachwood, OH (personal case) (observation)
  (1998): Litt JZ, Beachwood, OH (personal case) (observation)
Fixed eruption
  (1997): Sawada KY, Wheat Ridge, CO (from Internet) (observation)
Flushing (2.2%)
Lupus erythematosus
  (1998): Hill VA+, *J R Army Med Corps* 144, 109
Night sweats
  (2002): Ahmed A, *Am J Geriatr Psychiatry* 10(4), 484
Periorbital edema (<1%)
Photosensitivity (<1%)
Pruritus (<1%)
  (1999): Blumenthal HL, Beachwood, OH (personal case) (observation)
Purpura (<1%)
Rash (sic) (2.1%)

Stevens–Johnson syndrome
  (1999): Jan V+, *Acta Derm Venereol* 79, 401
Urticaria (<1%)
Xerosis (<1%)

Hair
Hair – abnormal texture (sic) (<1%)
Hair – alopecia (<1%)
  (1996): Bourgeois JA, *J Clin Psychopharmacol* 16, 91
Hair – hirsutism (<1%)

Other
Akathisia
  (2002): Walker L, *Psychiatr Serv* 53(11), 1477
Aphthous stomatitis (<1%)
Bromhidrosis (<1%)
Bruxism (<1%)
Death
  (2002): Musshoff F+, *Arch Kriminol* 210(1), 51
  (2001): Fartoux-Heymann L+, *J Hepatol* 35(5), 683
  (2001): Gillespie JA, *Ann Pharmacother* 35(12), 1671
  (2001): Hoehns JD+, *Ann Pharmacother* 35(7), 862 (with clozapine)
Dysgeusia
Dystonia
  (2002): Walker L, *Psychiatr Serv* 53(11), 1477
Foetor ex ore (halitosis) (<1%)
Galactorrhea
  (1993): Bronzo MR+, *Am J Psychiatry* 150, 1269
Gingival hyperplasia (<1%)
Glossitis (<1%)
Gynecomastia (<1%)
Headache
Hyperesthesia (<1%)
Paresthesias (2%)
Priapism
  (1998): Rand EH, *J Clin Psychiatry* 59, 538
Serotonin syndrome
  (2002): Fisher AA+, *Ann Pharmacother* 36(1), 67
  (2001): Adson DE+, *Ann Pharmacother* 35(11), 1375
  (2000): Vandermegel X+, *Rev Med Brux* (French) 21(3), 161 (with metoclopramide)
  (2000): Voirol P+, *J Clin Psychopharmacol* 20(6), 713
Sialorrhea (<1%)
Stomatitis (<1%)
Tinnitus
Tongue edema (<1%)
Tongue ulceration (<1%)
Tremor (1–10%)
  (2002): No Author, *Prescrire Int* 11(59), 69
Vaginitis (atrophic)
Xerostomia (16.3%)
  (2000): Brady K+, *JAMA* 283, 1837
  (1992): Berman H+, *Hosp Community Psychiatry* 43, 671
  (1991): Guthrie SK, *Drug Intell Clin Pharm* 25, 952
  (1990): Reimherr FW+, *J Clin Psychiatry* 51, 18
  (1988): Doogan DP+, *J Clin Psychiatry* 49, 46

SIBERIAN GINSENG

Scientific names: *Acanthopanax senticosus; Eleutherococcus senticosus*
Family: Araliaceae
Trade and other common names: Ciwuija; Devil's root; Eleuthero; Ezoukogi; Medexport; Shigoka; Taiga Wurzel; Touch-me-not
Category: Adaptogen; Antidementia; Emmenagogue; Immunoregulator
Purported indications and other uses: Alzheimer's disease, anaphylaxis, arthritis, colds, depression, fatigue, flu, impotence, infertility, menopause, multiple sclerosis, osteoporosis, perimenopause, PMS, stress
Half-life: N/A
Clinically important, potentially hazardous interactions with: antihypertensives, digoxin

Reactions

Skin
None

Other
Headache
Mastalgia

Note: Eleutherococcus may prevent biotransformation of some drugs to less toxic compounds

SIBUTRAMINE

Trade name: Meridia (Abbott)
Indications: Obesity
Category: Anorexiant; Obesity management
Half-life: 1.1 hours
Clinically important, potentially hazardous interactions with: dextromethorphan, dihydroergotamine, **ephedra**, ergot, fluoxetine, fluvoxamine, isocarboxazid, linezolid, lithium, MAO inhibitors, meperidine, methysergide, naratriptan, nefazodone, paroxetine, phenelzine, rizatriptan, sertraline, sumatriptan, tranylcypromine, **tryptophan**, venlafaxine, verapamil, zolmitriptan

Reactions

Skin
Acne (1.0%)
Allergic reactions (sic) (1.5%)
Diaphoresis (2.5%)
Ecchymoses (0.7%)
Edema (2%)
Flu-like syndrome (sic) (1–10%)
Herpes simplex (1.3%)
Peripheral edema (>1%)
Pruritus (>1%)
Rash (sic) (3.8%)

Other
Death
   (2002): London, *Reuters Health Information* 3-26-02 (2 cases)
Dysgeusia (2.2%)
Headache
Myalgia (1.9%)

Paresthesias (2.0%)
Tooth disorder (sic)
Vaginal candidiasis (1.2%)
Xerostomia (17.2%)
   (2001): Scheen AJ, *Rev Med Liege* 56(9), 656

SILDENAFIL

Trade name: Viagra (Pfizer)
Indications: Erectile dysfunction
Category: Phosphodiesterase (type 5) enzyme inhibitor
Half-life: 4 hours
Clinically important, potentially hazardous interactions with: amprenavir, amyl nitrite, atazanavir, erythromycin, indinavir, isosorbide dinitrate, isosorbide mononitrate, itraconazole, ketoconazole, nelfinavir, nitrates, nitroglycerin, ritonavir, saquinavir

Reactions

Skin
Allergic reactions (sic) (<2%)
Dermatitis (<2%)
Diaphoresis (<2%)
Edema (<2%)
Exfoliative dermatitis (<2%)
   (2002): Smith JG, Mobile, AL (from Internet) (observation)
Facial edema (<2%)
Fixed eruption (urticarial)
   (1998): Reed BR, Denver, CO (from Internet) (observation)
Fixed eruption (glans penis)
   (2002): Panagotacos P, San Francisco, CA (from Internet) (observation)
Flushing (10%)
   (2002): Becher E+, *Int J Impot Res* 14, S33
   (2002): Coelho OR, *Int J Impot Res* 14, S54
   (2002): Fink HA+, *Arch Intern Med* 162(12), 1349 (12%)
   (2002): Glina S+, *Int J Impot Res* 14, S27
   (2002): Lim PH+, *Ann N Y Acad Sci* 962, 378
   (2002): Salonia A+, *J Urol* 168(6), 2486 (with paroxetine)
   (2001): Chen KK+, *Int J Impot Res* 13(4), 221 (25%)
   (2001): Rosenkranz S+, *Dtsch Med Wochenschr* 126(41), 1144
   (2001): Steers W+, *Int J Impot Res* 13(5), 261
Genital edema (<2%)
Herpes simplex (<2%)
Lichenoid eruption
   (2000): Goldman BD, *Cutis* 66, 282
Peripheral edema (<2%)
Photosensitivity (<2%)
Pruritus (<2%)
Rash (sic) (2%)
Ulcerations (<2%)
Urticaria (<2%)

Other
Death
   (2002): Dumestre-Toulet V+, *Forensic Sci Int* 126(1), 71
Dyschromatopsia (3%) (blue-green vision)
   (2002): Coelho OR, *Int J Impot Res* 14, S54
   (2002): Laties A+, *Prog Retin Eye Res* 21(5), 485
   (1998): Craig D+, *Cleveland Clinic Foundation* 52, 963 (11%)
Gingivitis (<2%)
Glossitis (<2%)
Gynecomastia (<2%)
Headache

Hyperesthesia (<2%)
Myalgia (<2%)
Ocular pigmentation (<2%)
Paresthesias (<2%)
Priapism
    (2002): Goldmeier D+, *BMJ* 324(7353), 1555
    (2000): Sur RL+, *Urology* 55, 950
Seizures
    (2002): Gilad R+, *BMJ* 325(7369), 869
Stomatitis (<2%)
Visual halos
    (2002): Potter MJ+, *Ophthalmology* 109(5), 823
Xerostomia (<2%)

SIMVASTATIN

Trade name: Zocor (Merck)
Other common trade names: *Denan; Lipex; Liponorm; Lodales; Simovil; Sivastin; Zocord*
Indications: Hypercholesterolemia
Category: Antihyperlipidemic (cholesterol-lowering); HMG-CoA reductase inhibitor
Half-life: 1.9 hours
Clinically important, potentially hazardous interactions with: atazanavir, azithromycin, bosentan, clarithromycin, cyclosporine, diltiazem, erythromycin, gemfibrozil, imatinib, itraconazole, ritonavir, selenium, tacrolimus, verapamil

Reactions

Skin
Actinic dermatitis (sic)
    (1998): Granados MT+, *Contact Dermatitis* 38, 294
Angioedema
Ankle edema
    (1991): Borland Y+, *Nephron* 57, 365
Cheilitis
    (1998): Mehregan DR+, *Cutis* 62, 197
Dermatomyositis
    (1994): Khattak FH+, *Br J Rheumatol* 32(2), 199
Diaphoresis
    (1991): Scott RS+, *N Z Med J* 104, 493
Eczema (sic)
    (1995): Proksch E, *Hautarzt* (German) 46, 76
    (1991): Steyn K+, *S Afr Med J* 79, 639
Eczema (generalized)
    (1993): Feldmann R+, *Dermatology* 186, 272
    (1993): Krasovec M+, *Dermatology* 186, 248
Eosinophilic fasciitis
    (2001): Choquet-Kastylevsky G+, *Arch Intern Med* 161(11), 1456
Erythema multiforme
Erythematous plaques
    (1993): Feldmann R+, *Dermatology* 186, 272
Exanthems
    (1991): McDowell IF+, *Br J Clin Pharmacol* 31, 340
Flushing
Lichen planus
    (1991): Steyn K+, *S Afr Med J* 79, 639
Lichenoid eruption
    (1994): Roger D+, *Clin Exp Dermatol* 19, 88
Lupus erythematosus
    (2000): Ahmad A+, *Tenn Med* 93(1), 21
    (1998): Hanson J+, *Lancet* 352, 1070
    (1998): Khosia R+, *South Med J* 91, 873

(1992): Bannwarth B+, *Arch Intern Med* 152, 1093
Petechiae
    (1997): Horiuchi Y+, *J Dermatol* 24, 549
Photosensitivity
    (1995): Morimoto K+, *Contact Dermatitis* 33, 274
    (1991): Brocard JJ+, *Schweiz Med Wochenschr* (German) 121, 977
Pruritus
    (1993): Feldmann R+, *Dermatology* 186, 272
    (1991): Steyn K+, *S Afr Med J* 79, 639
Purpura
    (1998): Koduri PR, *Lancet* 352, 2020
    (1991): Steyn K+, *S Afr Med J* 79, 639
Pustules
Radiation recall
    (1995): Abadir R+, *Clin Oncol R Coll Radiol* 7, 325
Rash (sic) (1–10%)
    (2001): Coverman M, *The Schoch Letter* 51, 23 (with atorvastatin)
    (1993): Feldmann R+, *Dermatology* 186, 272
    (1990): Ziegler O+, *Cardiology* 77 (Suppl 4), 50
Rosacea
    (1991): Brocard JJ+, *Schweiz Med Wochenschr* (German) 121, 977
Stevens–Johnson syndrome
Thrombocytopenic purpura
    (1998): McCarthy LJ+, *Lancet* 352, 1284
Toxic epidermal necrolysis
Urticaria
Vasculitis

Hair
Hair – alopecia
    (1999): Litt JZ, Beachwood, OH (personal case) (observation)
    (1998): Robb-Nicholson C, *Harv Womens Health Watch* 5, 8 (anecdote)
    (1997): Shelley WB+, *Cutis* 60, 20 (observation)
    (1995): Litt JZ, Beachwood, OH (personal case) (observation)
    (1994): Litt JZ, Beachwood, OH (personal case) (observation)

Other
Anaphylactoid reactions
Death
    (2001): Federman DG+, *South Med J* 94(10), 1023
Dysgeusia (<1%)
    (1991): Saito Y+, *Arterioscler Thromb* 11, 816
Gynecomastia
Headache
Hypersensitivity
Myalgia (1.6%)
    (2003): Litt JZ, Beachwood, OH (personal case) (observation)
    (2003): Olsson AG+, *Clin Ther* 25(1), 119 (2.4%)
    (2002): Litt JZ, Beachwood, OH (personal observation)
    (2002): Sinzinger H, *Wien Klin Wochenschr* 114(21), 943
    (2001): Litt JZ, Beachwood, OH (personal case)
    (2001): Rehbein H, Jacksonville, FL (from Internet) (observation)
    (1998): Galper JB, *Am J Cardiol* 81(2), 259
Myopathy (1–10%)
    (2002): Hsu WC+, *Clin Neuropharmacol* 25(5), 266 (with colchicine)
    (2002): Udawat H+, *J Assoc Physicians India* 50, 439
    (1995): Garnett WR, *Am J Health Syst Pharm* 52(15), 1639
    (1994): al-Jubouri MA+, *BMJ* 308, 588
    (1991): Deslypere JP+, *Ann Intern Med* 114, 342
    (1990): Bilheimer DW, *Cardiology* 77 (Suppl 4), 58
Paresthesias
Porphyria cutanea tarda
    (1994): Perrot JL+, *Ann Dermatol Venereol* (French) 121, 817
Rhabdomyolysis

(2002): Hare CB+, *Clin Infect Dis* 35(10), 111 (with nelfinavir)
(2002): Rhodes CA+, *Clin Nucl Med* 27(11), 793
(2002): Thompson M+, *Am J Psychiatry* 159(9), 1607 (with nefazodone)
(2001): Borrego FJ+, *Nefrologia* 21(3), 309
(2001): Federman DG+, *South Med J* 94(10), 1023 (with gemfibrozil)
(2001): Kanathur N+, *Tenn Med* 94(9), 339 (with diltiazem)
(2001): Lee AJ, *Ann Pharmacother* 35(1), 26 (with clarithromycin)
(2001): Peces R+, *Nephron* 89(1), 117 (with diltiazem)
(2001): Reed BR, Denver, CO (from internet) (observation)
(2001): Stirling CM+, *Nephrol Dial Transplant* 16(4), 873
(2000): Al Shohaib, *Am J Nephrol* 20(3), 212
(2000): Davidson MH, *Curr Atheroscler Rep* 2(1), 14
(2000): Kusus M+, *Am J Med Sci* 320(6), 394 (with cyclosporine, digoxin and verapamil)
(2000): Oldemeyer JB+, *Cardiology* 94(2), 127 (with gemfibrozil)
(1999): Bottorff M, *Atherosclerosis* 147(Suppl 1), S23
(1999): Corsini A+, *Pharmacol Ther* 84, 413 (with either cyclosporine, mibefradil or nefazodone)
(1996): Ballantyne CM+, *Am J Cardiol* 78(5), 532
(1995): Farmer JA+, *Baillieres Clin Endocrinol Metab* 9(4), 825
(1995): Garnett WR, *Am J Health Syst Pharm* 52(15), 1639 (with either cyclosporine, erythromycin, gemfibrozil or niacin)
(1995): Meier C+, *Schweiz Med Wochenschr* 125(27), 1342 (with cyclosporine)
(1992): Blaison G+, *Rev Med Interne* 13(1), 61 (with cyclosporine)
Tendinopathy
(2001): Chazerain P+, *Joint Bone Spine* 68(5), 430

SIROLIMUS

Synonym: Rapamycin
Trade name: Rapamune (Wyeth)
Indications: Prophylaxis of organ rejection in renal transplants
Category: Immunosuppressant
Half-life: 62 hours
Clinically important, potentially hazardous interactions with: St John's wort, voriconazole

Reactions

Skin
Abscess (3–20%)
Acne (20–31%)
(2001): Reitamo S+, *Br J Dermatol* 145(3), 438 (13%) (with cyclosporine)
(2000): Vasquez EM, *Am J Health Syst Pharm* 57, 437
Cellulitis (3–20%)
Chills (3–20%)
Dermatitis (sic)
Dermatitis herpetiformis (aggravation)
(2002): Gladstone GC, Worcester, MA (personal correspondence)
Diaphoresis (3–20%)
Ecchymoses (3–20%)
Edema (16–24%)
Eyelid edema
(2001): Mohaupt MG+, *Transplantation* 72(1), 162 (40%)
Facial edema (3–20%)
Flu-like syndrome (sic) (3–20%)
Fungal dermatitis (3–20%)
Hot flashes
(2001): Reitamo S+, *Br J Dermatol* 145(3), 438 (12%) (with cyclosporine)

Hypertrophy (3–20%)
Infections (sic)
(2002): *Prescrire Int* 11(62), 165
Peripheral edema (54–64%)
Pruritus (3–20%)
(2002): Gladstone GC, Worcester, MA (personal correspondence)
Purpura (3–20%)
Rash (sic) (10–20%)
(2000): Vasquez EM, *Am J Health Syst Pharm* 57, 437
Scrotal edema
Ulcerations (3–20%)
Upper respiratory infection (20–26%)

Hair
Hair – hirsutism (3–20%)

Other
Aphthous stomatitis
(2001): Reitamo S+, *Br J Dermatol* 145(3), 438 (9%) (with cyclosporine)
Arthralgia (25–31%)
(2000): Vasquez EM, *Am J Health Syst Pharm* 57, 437
Depression (3–20%)
Dysgeusia
(1999): Watson CJ+, *Transplantation* 67, 505
Gingival hyperplasia (3–20%)
Gingivitis (3–20%)
Headache
Hyperesthesia (3–20%)
Myalgia (3–20%)
Oral candidiasis (3–20%)
Oral ulceration (3–20%)
Paresthesias (3–20%)
Stomatitis (3–20%)
Thrombophlebitis (3–20%)
Tinnitus (3–20%)
Tremor (21–31%)
(1999): Groth CG+, *Transplantation* 67, 1036

SMALLPOX VACCINE

Trade name: Dryvax (Wyeth)
Indications: Prevention of smallpox (variola)
Category: Vaccine
Half-life: ~5 years
Clinically important, potentially hazardous interactions with: corticosteroids

Reactions

Skin
Acne vaccinatum
(1971): Schmitt BS+, *Pediatrics* 48(5), 815
Allergic reactions (sic)
(1967): De Carlo M+, *Arch Ital Sci Med Trop Parassitol* 48(1), 51
(1965): Keller W, *Monatsschr Kinderheilkd* 113(6), 394
Basal cell carcinoma
(1988): Ribeiro R+, *Med Cutan Ibero Lat Am* 16(2), 137
(1970): Riley KA, *Arch Dermatiol* 101, 416
(1968): Marmelzat W, *Arch Dermatol* 97, 400 (at vaccination scar) (5 cases)
(1968): Zelickson AS, *Arch Dermatol* 98(1), 35 (at vaccination site)
Bullous eruption

(1971): Martin J+, *Schweiz Med Wochensch* 101, 1446
(1963): Weber G+, *Dtsch Med Wochenschr* 88, 1878

Carcinoma
(1980): Gecht ML, *JAMA* 244(15), 1675
(1968): Bazex A+, *Bull Soc Fr Dermatol Syphiligr* 75(6), 743 (in scar)

Chills
(2002): Frey SE+, *N Engl J Med* 346, 1265

Dermatofibrosarcoma protuberans
(2003): Green JJ+, *J Am Acad Dermatol* 48, S54 (in scar)

Eczema vaccinatum
(1974): Kage K+, *Rinsho Byori* 22 (10 Suppl), 353
(1972): Heitmann HJ, *Fortschr Med* 90(14), 530
(1971): Cherniaeva TV, *Vopr Okhr Materin Det* 16(8), 82
(1970): Gol'dshtein LM+, *Pediatriia* 49(11), 77
(1970): Grosfeld JC+, *Dermatologica* 141(1), 1
(1970): Hicks R+, *Ann Allergy* 28(10), 491
(1969): Castrow FF+, *Tex Med* 65(2), 48
(1969): Fierens F, *Arch Belg Dermatol Syphiligr* 25(3), 367
(1968): Hoede N+, *Med Welt* 4, 268
(1968): Piriatinskaia RG, *Vestn Dermatol Venerol* 42(8), 73
(1967): Gomez-Orozco L+, *Alergia* 14(4), 123
(1967): Kubiska E+, *Med Welt* 40, 2336
(1966): Tidstrom B, *Ugeskr Laeger* 128(1), 18

Erythema multiforme
(1975): Goldstein JA+, *Pediatrics* 55(3), 342
(1973): Patrone P+, *Archo Ital Dermatol Venereol* 38, 34
(1971): Martin J+, *Schweiz Med Wochenschr* 101, 1446
(1970): Coskey RJ+, *Cutis* 6, 761
(1969): Loeffler A+, *Dermatologica* 138 (Suppl), 1
(1969): Scott EG+, *J Miss State Med Assoc* 10(2), 41
(1963): Weber G+, *Dtsch Med Wochenschr* 88, 1878

Erythema nodosum
(1971): Mattheis H, *Dermatologica* 142, 340

Exanthems
(1975): Goldstein JA+, *Pediatrics* 55(3), 342
(1973): Patrone P+, *Archo Ital Dermatol Venereol* 38, 34
(1971): Martin J+, *Schweiz Med Wochenschr* 101, 1446
(1971): Mattheis H, *Dermatologica* 142, 340
(1965): Cherry JD+, *J Pediatr* 67(4), 679
(1963): Weber G+, *Dtsch Med Wochenschr* 88, 1878

Exfoliative dermatitis
(1963): Weber G+, *Dtsch Med Wochenschr* 88, 1878

Herpes simplex
(1982): Mintz L, *JAMA* 247(19), 2704 (recurrent) (at site)
(1973): Patrone P+, *Archo Ital Dermatol Venereol* 38, 34

Herpes zoster
(1974): Verbov J, *Br J Dermatol* 90(1), 110
(1973): Patrone P+, *Archo Ital Dermatol Venerol* 38, 34

Histiocytoma, malignant fibrous
(1981): Slater DN+, *Br J Dermatol* 105(2), 215

Jadassohn-Borst epithelioma
(1972): Porter E+, *Br J Dermatol* 86, 177

Kaposi's varicelliform eruption
(1970): Proenca N+, *An Bras Dermatol* 45(4), 353

Keratoacanthoma
(1974): Haider S, *Br J Dermatol* 90(6), 689 (in vaccination site)

Lichen vaccinatus
(1963): Weber G+, *Dtsch Med Wochenschr* 88, 1878

Lupus erythematosus (discoid)
(1987): Lupton GP, *J Am Acad Dermatol* 17, 688 (in vaccination scar)

Melanoma
(1973): de Oreo G, *Int J Dermatol* 12, 217 (15 cases)
(1968): Marmelzat W, *Arch Dermatol* 97, 400 (in vaccination scar) (6 cases)

Photosensitivity
(1970): Coskey RJ+, *Cutis* 6, 761
(1969): Pace BF+, *Cutis* 5, 850

Pigmentation
(1978): Helman J, *S Afr Med J* 53(12), 430 (in scars)

Purpura
(1981): Burke PJ+, *Pa Med* 84(9), 49
(1971): Monuiko O+, *Pediatr Pol* 45, 919
(1971): Wong KY, *Hawaii Med J* 30(5), 388 (anaphylactoid)
(1970): Coskey RJ+, *Cutis* 6, 761
(1969): Casteles-Van Daele M, *N Engl J Med* 280(14), 781
(1969): Feyling T+, *Tidsskr Nor Laegeforen* 89(10), 725
(1969): Lane JM, *N Engl J Med* 280(14), 781
(1969): Wasser S+, *Kinderarztl Prax* 37(7), 299
(1968): Jiminez EL+, *N Engl J Med* 279(21), 1171
(1965): Hofele U, *Arch Kinderheilkd* 173(2), 175
(1963): Weber G+, *Dtsch Med Wochenschr* 88, 1878

Pustular vaccina
(1967): Epshtein AB+, *Gig Tr Prof Zabol* 11(4), 53 (occupational)

Pyogenic granuloma
(1974): Zayid I+, *Br J Dermatol* 90(3), 293

Rash (sic)
(2002): Frey SE+, *N Engl J Med* 346, 1265 (site other than vaccination site)
(1978): Lakotkina EA+, *Pediatriia* 12, 49

Scar
(1968): Kumar LR+, *Indian J Pediatr* 35(245), 283 (pigmented & hairy)

Side effects (sic) (0.01%)
(1973): Patrone P+, *Archo Ital Dermatol Venereol* 38, 34

Stevens–Johnson syndrome
(1975): Goldstein JA+, *Pediatrics* 55(3), 342

Toxic epidermal necrolysis
(1978): Kacprzyk-Bergman I+, *Pediatr Pol* 63, 393 (patient had a rubeola infection)
(1971): Martin J+, *Schweiz Med Wochenschr* 101(40), 1446
(1970): Czarnecki L+, *Pol Tyg Lek* 25(26), 982
(1969): Debenedetti L, *Minerva Pediatr* 21(45), 2136
(1968): Kushner PG+, *J Am Osteopath Assoc* 67(10), 1134

Urticaria
(1975): Goldstein JA+, *Pediatrics* 55(3), 342
(1973): Patrone P+, *Archo Ital Dermatol* 38, 34
(1970): Coskey RJ+, *Cutis* 6, 761
(1963): Weber G+, *Dtsch Med Wochenschr* 88, 1878
(1955): Alexander HL, *Reactions with Drug Therapy* Philadelphia, Saunders

Vaccinia
(1979): Datta KK+, *Indian J Public Health* 23(2), 106 (generalized)
(1978): Pasternak J+, *Rev Inst Med Trop Sao Paulo* 20(6), 359 (progressive & fatal)
(1977): Robinson MJ+, *Aust Paediatr* 13(2), 125
(1977): Verret JL+, *Ann Dermatol Venereol* 104(3), 251
(1976): Beliaev NV, *Vestn Dermatol Venerol* 2, 63 (ulcerative)
(1975): Goldstein JA+, *Pediatrics* 55(3), 342 (generalizes)
(1974): Kulesza MO, *J Obstet Gynaecol Br Commonw* 81(3), 251
(1974): Russell G, *Tandlaegebladet* 78(2), 59 (oral)
(1972): Meyer A, *Dtsch Med Wochenschr* 97(28), 1073
(1968): Aitkens GH+, *Med J Aust* 2(4), 173 (fetal)
(1967): Abrassart C+, *Rev Med Liege* 22(1), 6
(1966): Green DM+, *Lancet* 1(7450), 1296 (generalized)
(1965): Chatterjee SN+, *Bull Calcutta Sch Trop Med* 13(4), 136 (generalized)

Vaccinia (face, eyelids, nose, mouth, genitalia & rectum)
(1980): Kanra G+, *Cutis* 26, 267 (vulva from 7–month-old daughter's vaccination)
(1976): Haim S, *Cutis* 17(2), 308 (vulva from heteroinoculation)
(1971): Polk LD, *Clin Pediatr* 10, 486
(1969): Andreev VC+, *Dermatol Int* 8(1), 5
(1969): Jelinek JE, *Arch Dermatol* 99(4), 504 (eye)
(1953): Berkowitz J, *Am J Surg* 86, 549

Vaccinia (generalized)

Vaccinia gangrenosum
  (1973): Raff MJ, *J Ky Med Assoc* 71(2), 92
  (1967): Van Rooyen CE+, *Can Med Assoc J* 97(4), 160
  (1966): Hansson O+, *Acta Pediatr Scand* 55(3), 264
Vaccinia maculata
  (1988): Landthaler M+, *Hautarzt* 39, 322
Vaccinia necrosum
  (1982): *MMWR Morb Mortality Wkly Rep* 31(36), 501
  (1981): Funk EA+, *South Med J* 74(3), 383
  (1977): Turkel SB+, *Cancer* 40(1), 226
  (1972): Freed ER+, *Am J Med* 52(3), 411
  (1970): Neff JM+, *JAMA* 213(1), 123
  (1968): Colon VF+, *Geriatrics* 23(12), 81

Other
Death
  (1979): Du Mont GC+, *BMJ* 1(6175), 1398 (3 cases)
  (1979): Frongillo RF, *Ann Sclavo* 21(6), 856
  (1977): Feery BJ, *Med J Aust* 2(6), 180
  (1970): Lane JM+, *JAMA* 212(3), 441
  (1966): Ehrengut W+, *Dtsch Med Wochenschr* 91(52), 2339
Fever
Headache
Injection-site pain
  (2002): Frey SE+, *N Engl J Med* 346, 1265
Kerato-uveitis
  (1994): Lee SF+, *Am J Opthalmol* 117(4), 480 (autoinoculation)
Lymphadenitis
  (1972): Charlebois G+, *Union Med Can* 101(8), 1587
  (1968): Hartsock RJ, *Cancer* 21(4), 632
Myalgia
  (2002): Frey SE+, *N Engl J Med* 346, 1265
Tumors
  (1971): Mattheis H, *Dermatologica* 142, 340
  (1968): Marmelzat W, *Arch Dermatol* 97, 400 (in vaccination scar) (24 cases) (malignant)
  (1968): Reed WB+, *Arch Dermatol* 98, 132 (malignant)

SODIUM CROMOGLYCATE

(See CROMOLYN)

SODIUM OXYBATE

Synonyms: Gamma Hydroxybutyrate; GHB
Trade name: Xyrem (Orphan Medical)
Indications: Cataplexy (in patients with narcolepsy)
Category: Anesthetic; Anticataplectic; CNS depressant; Dietary supplement
Half-life: 0.3–1 hour
Clinically important, potentially hazardous interactions with: alcohol, hypnotics, sedatives

Reactions

Skin
Diaphoresis
  (2001): Bowles TM+, *Pharmacotherapy* 21(2), 254 (following withdrawal)
  (2001): Dyer JE+, *Ann Emerg Med* 37(2), 147 (following withdrawal)
  (2000): Craig K+, *J Emerg Med* 18(1), 65 (following withdrawal)
Flu-like syndrome
Infections
Upper respiratory infection

Other
Back pain
Death
  (2002): Smith KM+, *Am J Health Syst Pharm* 59(11), 1067
  (2001): Dyer JE+, *Ann Emerg Med* 37(2), 147 (following withdrawal)
  (2001): Kalasinsky KS+, *J Forensic Sci* 46(3), 728
  (2001): Nini A+, *Harefuah* 140(12), 1148
  (2001): Okun MS+, *J Pharm Pharm Sci* 4(2), 167
  (2001): Persson SA+, *Lakartidningen* 98(38), 4026
  (2000): Timby N+, *Am J Med* 108(6), 518
  (1998): Li J+, *Ann Emerg Med* 31(6), 729
  (1995): Ferrara SD+, *J Forensic Sci* 40(3), 501 (also taking IV heroin)
Depression
Pain
Porphyria
Rhabdomyolysis
Seizures
  (2002): Smith KM+, *Am J Health Syst Pharm* 59(11), 1067
  (1998): Hovda KE+, *Tidsskr Nor Laegeforen* 118(28), 4390
  (1998): Kam PC+, *Anaesthesia* 53(12), 1195
  (1997): Galloway GP+, *Addiction* 92(1), 89
  (1995): Steele MT+, *Mo Med* 92(7), 354
  (1992): Adornato BT+, *West J Med* 157(4), 471
  (1991): Dyer JE, *Am J Emerg Med* 9(4), 321
Sialorrhea
Sinusitis
Tremor
  (2001): Dyer JE+, *Ann Emerg Med* 37(2), 147 (following withdrawal)
  (2000): Craig K+, *J Emerg Med* 18(1), 65 (following withdrawal)
  (1998): Hovda KE+, *Tidsskr Nor Laegeforen* 118(28), 4390 (following withdrawal)
  (1997): Galloway GP+, *Addiction* 92(1), 89 (following withdrawal)

Note: Sodium Oxybate is a class of drugs that are also known as: 'Designer drugs'; Party drugs; Club drugs; Recreational drugs; 'Rave' drugs; Fantasy drugs; Date rape drugs; abuse drugs

SOTALOL

Trade name: Betapace (Berlex)
Other common trade names: *Beta-Cardone; Betades; Cardol; Sotacor; Sotacor; Sotahexal; Sotalex*
Indications: Ventricular arrhythmias
Category: antiarrhythmic class III; Beta-adrenoceptor blocker
Half-life: 7–18 hours
Clinically important, potentially hazardous interactions with: arsenic, ciprofloxacin, enoxacin, gatifloxacin, lomefloxacin, moxifloxacin, norfloxacin, ofloxacin, quinolones, sparfloxacin

Reactions

Skin
Cold extremities (sic)
Cutaneous thickening (sic)
Diaphoresis (<1%)
  (1995): Schmutz JL+, *Dermatology* 190, 86
Edema (5%)
Exanthems
Irritation (sic)
Lichenoid eruption
  (1994): O'Brien TJ+, *Australas J Dermatol* 35, 93
Peripheral edema

Photosensitivity (<1%)
Pruritus (1–10%)
Psoriasis
  (1988): Heng MCY+, *Int J Dermatol* 27, 619
  (1986): Czernielewski J+, *Lancet* 1, 808
  (1984): Arntzen N+, *Acta Derm Venereol* (Stockh) 64, 346
Rash (sic) (3%)
Raynaud's phenomenon (<1%)
Scleroderma
  (1988): Ahmad N+, *Scott Med J* 33, 210
  (1979): Bonnetblanc JM+, *Ann Dermatol Venereol* (French)
    106, 927
  (1979): Michel JP+, *Lancet* 1, 54
Urticaria
Vasculitis
  (1998): Rustmann WC+, *J Am Acad Dermatol* 38, 111

Hair
Hair – alopecia (<1%)

Other
Dysgeusia
Headache
Injection-site extravasation (<1%)
Myalgia (<1%)
Myopathy
  (1979): Forfar JC+, *BMJ* 2, 1331
Paresthesias (3%)
Phlebitis (<1%)
Xerostomia (<1%)

SPARFLOXACIN

Trade name: Zagam (Bertek)
Other common trade names: *Spara; Sparlox; Torospar*
Indications: Community-acquired pneumonia
Category: Quinolone antibiotic
Half-life: 16–30 hours
**Clinically important, potentially hazardous interactions
with:** amiodarone, amitriptyline, amoxapine, arsenic, bepridil,
bretylium, calcium, chlorpromazine, clomipramine, desipramine,
disopyramide, doxepin, erythromycin, fluphenazine, imipramine,
iron salts, magnesium, mesoridazine, nortriptyline, pentamidine,
perphenazine, phenothiazines, pimozide, procainamide,
prochlorperazine, promazine, promethazine, protriptyline,
quinidine, sotalol, sucralfate, thioridazine, tricyclic
antidepressants, trifluoperazine, trimipramine, zinc salts

Reactions

Skin
Acne (<1%)
Allergic reactions (sic) (<1%)
Angioedema (<1%)
Bullous eruption (<1%)
Cellulitis (<1%)
Dermatitis (<1%)
Diaphoresis (<1%)
Ecchymoses (<1%)
Edema (<1%)
Erythema nodosum
Exanthems (<1%)
Exfoliative dermatitis (<1%)
Facial edema (<1%)

Fixed eruption
  (2001): Sharma R, Aligarh, India (from Internet) (observation)
    (recurrence with ciprofloxacin)
Furunculosis (<1%)
Herpes simplex (<1%)
Lichenoid eruption
  (1998): Hamanaka H+, *J Am Acad Dermatol* 38, 945
Peripheral edema (<1%)
Petechiae (<1%)
Photosensitivity (3.6%)
  (2000): Schentag JJ, *Clin Ther* 22, 372
  (1999): Hamanaka H, *J Dermatol Sci* 21, 27
  (1999): Lipsky BA+, *Clin Ther* 21, 148
  (1998): Hamanaka H+, *J Am Acad Dermatol* 38, 945
  (1997): Burrow WH, Jackson, MS (from Internet) (observation)
  (1996): Tokura Y+, *Arch Dermatol Res* 288, 45
  (1995): Hamanaka H+, *Jpn J Dermatol* 105, 601
  (1995): Hiramoto T+, *Rinsho Dermatol* (Japanese) 37, 1681
Phototoxicity (7.9%)
  (2000): Pierfitte C+, *Br J Clin Pharmacol* 49, 609
  (1999): Blondeau JM, *Clin Ther* 21, 6
  (1996): Tokura Y+, *Arch Dermatol Res* 288, 45
Pigmentation (<1%)
Pruritus (3.3%)
Purpura
Pustules (<1%)
Rash (sic) (1.1%)
Stevens–Johnson syndrome
Toxic epidermal necrolysis
Urticaria (<1%)
Vasculitis
Xerosis (<1%)

Hair
Hair – alopecia (<1%)

Other
Anaphylactoid reactions (<1%)
Anosmia
Dysgeusia (1.4%)
  (1999): Lipsky BA+, *Clin Ther* 21, 148
Gingivitis (<1%)
Headache
Hyperesthesia (<1%)
Hypersensitivity
Mastodynia (<1%)
Myalgia (<1%)
Oral candidiasis (<1%)
Oral ulceration (<1%)
Paresthesias (<1%)
Serum sickness
Stomatitis (<1%)
Tendon rupture
Tongue disorder (<1%)
Torsades de pointes
  (2002): Kakar A+, *J Assoc Physicians India* 50, 1077
Vaginal candidiasis (2.8%)
Vaginitis (<1%)
Xerostomia (1.4%)

SPECTINOMYCIN

Trade name: Trobicin (Pharmacia)
Other common trade name: *Spectam*
Indications: Gonorrhea
Category: Antibiotic
Half-life: 1–3 hours

Reactions

Skin

Chills
Dermatitis
  (1994): Dal-Monte A+, *Contact Dermatitis* 31, 204
     (occupational)
  (1991): Vilaplana J+, *Contact Dermatitis* 24, 225
Exanthems
Pruritus (<1%)
  (1974): Bogden C+, *Schweiz Med Wochenschr* (German) 104, 46
Rash (sic) (<1%)
Urticaria (<1%)
  (1971): *Med Lett* 13, 105

Other

Anaphylactoid reactions
  (1977): Raab W, *Z Hautkr* (German) 9, 14
Hypersensitivity
  (1977): Raab W, *Z Hautkr* (German) 9, 14
Injection-site induration
Injection-site pain (<1%)
Oral mucosal lesions

SPIRONOLACTONE

Trade names: Aldactazide (Pharmacia); Aldactone (Pharmacia)
Other common trade names: *Aldopur; Almatol; Diram; Merabis; Novo-Spiroton; Osiren; Spiroctan; Tensin*
Indications: Hyperaldosteronism, hirsutism, hypertension
Category: Diuretic; Potassium-sparing antihypertensive diuretic
Half-life: 78–84 minutes
Clinically important, potentially hazardous interactions with: ACE inhibitors, **alcohol**, amiloride, barbiturates, benazepril, captopril, cyclosporine, enalapril, fosinopril, **juniper**, lisinopril, mitotane, moexipril, narcotics, NSAIDs, potassium chloride, potassium iodide, quinapril, ramipril, trandolapril, triamterene

Aldactazide is spironolactone and hydrochlorothiazide

Reactions

Skin

Bullous pemphigoid
  (2002): Modeste AB+, *Ann Dermatol Venereol* 129(1), 56
Chills
Chloasma
  (1988): Hughes BR+, *Br J Dermatol* 118, 687
Dermatitis
  (1996): Corazza M+, *Contact Dermatitis* 35, 365
  (1994): Aguirre A+, *Contact Dermatitis* 30, 312
  (1994): Balato N+, *Contact Dermatitis* 31, 203
  (1994): Fernandez-Vozmediano JM+, *Contact Dermatitis* 30, 118
  (1993): Vincenzi C+, *Contact Dermatitis* 29, 277 (from anti-acne cream)

  (1984): Klijn J, *Contact Dermatitis* 10, 105
Diaphoresis
Eczema (sic)
  (1994): Balato N+, *Contact Dermatitis* 31, 203
  (1994): Fernandez-Vozmediano JM+, *Contact Dermatitis* 30, 118
Erythema
Erythema annulare centrifugum
  (1987): Carsuzaa F+, *Ann Dermatol Venereol* (French) 114, 375
Erythema multiforme
  (1986): Greenberger PA+, *N Engl Reg Allergy Proc* 7, 343
Exanthems
  (1994): Gupta AK+, *Dermatol* 189, 402
  (1988): Hughes BR+, *Br J Dermatol* 118, 687 (9.3%)
  (1986): Wathen CG+, *Lancet* 1, 919
  (1979): Uddin MS+, *Cutis* 24, 198 (passim)
  (1977): Ferguson RK+, *Clin Pharmacol Ther* 21, 62 (1–5%)
  (1973): Greenblatt DJ+, *JAMA* 225, 40 (0.5%)
Facial edema
  (1998): Lubbos HG+, *Arch Dermatol* 134, 1163
Flushing (<1%)
Graft-versus-host reaction
  (1998): Jappe U+, *Hautarzt* (German) 49, 126 (passim)
Lichen planus
  (1978): Downham TF, *JAMA* 240, 1138
Lichenoid eruption
  (1998): Clark C+, *Clin Exp Dermatol* 23, 43
  (1994): Schon MP+, *Acta Derm Venereol* 74, 476
Lupus erythematosus
  (2002): Boye T+, *World Congress Dermatol* Poster, 0088
  (1987): Leroy D+, *Ann Dermatol Venereol* (French) 114, 1237
Melasma
  (2000): Shaw JC, *J Am Acad Dermatol* 43, 498
  (1979): Uddin MS+, *Cutis* 24, 198
Necrotizing angiitis
Pemphigus
  (2002): Karam A+, *World Congress Dermatol* Poster, 0328
  (1997): Grange F+, *Ann Dermatol* (French) 124, 700
Photosensitivity
Pigmentation
  (1988): Hughes BR+, *Br J Dermatol* 118, 687 (chloasma-like)
  (1988): Hughes BR, *Dermatology Times* June, 10 (chloasma-like)
  (1983): Luderschmidt C, *Dtsch Med Wochenschr* (German) 108, 1922
  (1975): Davies DL+, *Drugs* 9, 214
Pruritus
  (1988): Hughes BR, *Dermatology Times* June, 10
  (1986): Wathen CG+, *Lancet* 1, 919
Purpura
Rash (sic) (1–10%)
  (1988): Hughes BR, *Dermatology Times* June, 10
  (1973): Greenblatt DJ+, *JAMA* 225, 40
Raynaud's phenomenon
  (1975): Davies DL+, *Drugs* 9, 214
Side effects (sic)
  (1973): Almeyda J+, *Br J Dermatol* 88, 313
Urticaria
  (1988): Helfer EL+, *J Clin Endocrinol Metab* 66, 208
  (1979): Uddin MS+, *Cutis* 24, 198 (passim)
Vasculitis
  (1984): Phillips GWL+, *BMJ* 288, 368
Xerosis
  (2000): Shaw JC, *J Am Acad Dermatol* 43, 498
  (1988): Hughes BR+, *Br J Dermatol* 118, 687 (40%)
  (1988): Hughes BR, *Dermatology Times* June, 10

Hair

Hair – alopecia
  (1988): Helfer EL+, *J Clin Endocrinol Metab* 66, 208

(1975): Davies DL+, *Drugs* 9, 214
Hair – hirsutism

Other

Acute intermittent porphyria
Ageusia
Anaphylactoid reactions
Gynecomastia (<1%)
  (2001): Yamamoto S, *Intern Med* 40(6), 550
  (2000): Hugues FC+, *Ann Med Interne (Paris)* (French) 151, 10
    (passim)
  (1994): Dove F, *Hosp Pract Off Ed* 29, 27
  (1994): *BMJ* 308, 503
  (1993): Thompson DF+, *Pharmacotherapy* 13, 37
  (1988): Hughes BR+, *Br J Dermatol* 118, 687
  (1977): Rose LI+, *Ann Intern Med* 87, 398
  (1976): Loriaux DL, *Ann Intern Med* 85, 630
  (1973): Greenblatt DJ+, *JAMA* 225, 40 (passim)
  (1965): Clark E, *JAMA* 193, 163
  (1963): Mann NM, *JAMA* 190, 160
Headache
Mastodynia
  (2000): Shaw JC, *J Am Acad Dermatol* 43, 498
Oral lichen planus
  (1990): Lamey PJ+, *Oral Surg Oral Med Oral Pathol* 70, 184
Paresthesias
Xerostomia

ST JOHN'S WORT

Scientific name: *Hypericum perforatum*
Family: Hypericaceae
Trade and other common names: Amber; Demon Chaser;
Fuga Daemonum; Goatweed; Hardhay; Hypereikon; Hypericum;
Johns Wort; Klamath Weed; Rosin Rose; Tipton Weed
Category: Anti-anxiety
Purported indications and other uses: Depression, dysthymic
disorder, fatigue, insomnia, loss of appetite, anxiety, obsessive-
compulsive disorders, mood disturbances, migraine headaches,
neuralgia, fibrositis, sciatica, palpitations, exhaustion, headache,
muscle pain, vitiligo, diuretic, bruises, abrasions, first degree
burns, hemorrhoids
Half-life: N/A
**Clinically important, potentially hazardous interactions
with:** amitriptyline, amprenavir, atazanavir, bosentan,
carbamazepine, citalopram, cyclosporine, digoxin, eplerenone,
eplerenone, escitalopram, escitalopram, etoposide, fluoxetine,
fluvoxamine, imatinib, indinavir, irinotecan, loperamide,
midazolam, naratriptan, nelfinavir, nevirapine, oral contraceptives,
paroxetine, phenobarbitone, phenytoin, quinolones ritonavir,
rizatriptan, saquinavir, sertraline, sirolimus, SSRIs, sumatriptan,
tetracyclines, theophylline, tricyclic antidepressants, warfarin,
zolmitriptan

Reactions

Skin

Adverse effects (sic)
  (2002): Ernst E, *Ann Intern Med* 136(1), 42
  (2002): Haller CA+, *Adverse Drug React Toxicol Rev* 21(3), 143
Allergic reactions (sic)
  (1994): Woelk H+, *J Geriatr Psychiatry Neurol* 7 (Suppl 1), S34
Irritation (sic)
Photosensitivity
  (2000): Lane-Brown MM, *Med J Aust* 172(6), 302

(2000): Schulz V, *Schweiz Rundsch Med Prax* 89(50), 2131
(1999): Gulick RM+, *Ann Intern Med* 130, 510
(1997): Brockmoller J+, *Pharmacopsychiatry* 30, 94
(1997): Golsch S+, *Hautarzt* (German) 48, 249
Pruritus
  (1997): Golsch S+, *Hautarzt* 48, 249

Hair

Hair – alopecia
  (2001): Parker V+, *Can J Psychiatry* 46(1), 77

Other

Bleeding
  (2001): Izzo AA+, *Drugs* 61(15), 2163 (intermenstrual)
Delirium
  (2001): Izzo AA+, *Drugs* 61(15), 2163
Erythroderma
  (2000): Holme SA+, *Br J Dermatol* 143(5), 1127
Hypersensitivity
Mania
  (2001): Boniel T+, *Harefuah* 140(8), 780
Paresthesias
  (1998): Ernst E+, *Eur J Clin Pharmacol* 54, 589
Serotonin syndrome
  (2001): Izzo AA+, *Drugs* 61(15), 2163
  (2001): Parker V+, *Can J Psychiatry* 46(1), 77
  (2000): Brown TM, *Am J Emerg Med* 18, 231
Side effects
  (1999): Tinsley JA, *Minn Med* 82(5), 29
Xerostomia
  (1997): *Med Lett Drugs Ther* 39, 107

Note: St. John's wort is a natural source of flavoring in Europe.
Although not indigenous to Australia, and long considered a weed, St.
John's wort is now grown there as a cash crop and produces 20% of
the world's supply

STANOZOLOL

Trade name: Winstrol (Sanofi-Synthelabo)
Other common trade names: *Menabol; Stromba*
Indications: Hereditary angioedema
Category: Anabolic steroid; Androgen
Half-life: N/A
**Clinically important, potentially hazardous interactions
with:** anticoagulants, warfarin

Reactions

Skin

Acne (>10%)
  (1995): Helfman T+, *J Am Acad Dermatol* 32, 254
Chills (1–10%)
Edema
Exanthems
Folliculitis
  (1995): Helfman T+, *J Am Acad Dermatol* 32, 254
Pigmentation (1–10%)
Rosacea
  (1995): Helfman T+, *J Am Acad Dermatol* 32, 254
Seborrheic dermatitis
  (1995): Helfman T+, *J Am Acad Dermatol* 32, 254
Urticaria

Hair

Hair – alopecia (in women)
Hair – hirsutism (in women)

(1995): Helfman T+, *J Am Acad Dermatol* 32, 254
(1987): Sheffer AL+, *J Allergy Clin Immunol* 80, 855

Other
Gynecomastia (>10%)
  (1995): Helfman T+, *J Am Acad Dermatol* 32, 254
Priapism (>10%)

STAVUDINE

Synonym: d4T
Trade name: Zerit (Bristol-Myers Squibb)
Indications: Human immunodeficiency virus (HIV)
Category: Antiretroviral; Nucleoside reverse transcriptase inhibitor (NRTI)
Half-life: 1.44 hours

Reactions

Skin
Allergic reactions (sic) (9%)
Chills (50%)
Diaphoresis (19%)
Neutrophilic eccrine hidradenitis
  (1998): Krischer J+, *J Dermatol* 25, 199
Rash (sic) (~40%)

Other
Buffalo hump
Death
  (2001): Hwang SW+, *Singapore Med J* 42(6), 247 (2 cases) (with didanosine)
Gynecomastia
  (2001): Aquilina C+, *Int J STD AIDS* 12(7), 481 (with didanosine)
  (2001): Manfredi R+, *Ann Pharmacother* 35(4), 438 (with didanosine)
  (2001): Manfredi R+, *Ann Pharmacother* 35(4), 438 (with lamivudine) (3 cases)
  (1998): Melbourne KM+, *Ann Pharmacother* 32, 1108
Headache
Lipoatrophy
  (2001): Lichtenstein KA+, *AIDS* 15(11), 1389
Lipodystrophy
  (2002): Bernasconi E+, *J Acquir Immune Defic Syndr* 31(1), 50
  (2002): Reid S, *Can Adv Drug Reaction Newsletter* 12, 5
  (2001): Aquilina C+, *Int J STD AIDS* 12(7), 481 (with didanosine)
  (2001): Arpadi SM+, *J Acquir Immune Defic Syndr* 27(1), 30
  (2001): Bogner JR+, *J Acquir Immune Defic Syndr* 27(3), 237
  (2001): van der Valk M+, *AIDS* 15(7), 847
  (1999): Ruel M+, *Ann Med Interne (Paris)* (French) 150, 269
Myalgia (32%)
  (2000): Miller KD+, *Ann Intern Med* 133, 192
Paresthesias
Tendon xanthomata
  (2001): Leung N+, *Diabetes* 50(Suppl.2), 452

STREPTOKINASE

Trade names: Kabikinase (Pharmacia); Streptase (AstraZeneca)
Indications: Pulmonary embolism, acute myocardial infarction
Category: Thrombolytic
Half-life: 83 minutes
Clinically important, potentially hazardous interactions with: bivalirudin

Reactions

Skin
Allergic reactions (sic) (4.4%)
  (2001): Toquero J+, *Rev Esp Cardiol* 54(10), 1225
  (1998): Stephens MB+, *Postgrad Med* 103, 89
  (1997): Cannas S+, *G Ital Cardiol* (Italian) 27, 278
Angiitis
  (1988): Sorber WA+, *Cutis* 42, 57
Angioedema (>10%)
  (1994): Cooper JP+, *Postgrad Med J* 70, 592
Bleeding
  (1990): Goa KL+, *Drugs* 39, 693 (3.6%)
Diaphoresis (1–10%)
Ecchymoses
Exanthems (1–5%)
  (1990): Goa KL+, *Drugs* 39, 693
  (1976): Kohner GM+, *BMJ* 1, 550
Flushing (<1%)
Periorbital edema (>10%)
Pruritus (1–10%)
Purpura
Rash (sic) (1–10%)
Urticaria (1–5%)
  (1990): Goa KL+, *Drugs* 39, 693
Vasculitis
  (1994): Penswick J+, *BMJ* 309, 378
  (1991): Patel A+, *J Am Acad Dermatol* 24, 652
  (1988): Davidson JR+, *Clin Exp Rheumatol* 6, 381
  (1988): Ong AC+, *Int J Cardiology* 21, 71
  (1986): Manoharan A+, *Aust N Z J Med* 16, 815
  (1985): Thompson RF+, *Clin Pharm* 4, 383

Other
Anaphylactoid reactions (<1%)
  (1993): Hohage H+, *Wien Klin Wochenschr* (German) 105, 176
Back pain
  (2002): Pinheiro RF+, *Arq Bras Cardiol* 78(2), 230 (infusion)
Headache
Injection-site bleeding
  (1990): Goa KL+, *Drugs* 39, 693 (3%)
Injection-site phlebitis
Serum sickness
  (1995): Creamer JD+, *Clin Exp Dermatol* 20, 468
  (1994): Proctor BD+, *N Engl J Med* 330, 576
  (1991): Patel A+, *J Am Acad Dermatol* 24, 652
  (1984): Alexopoulos D+, *Eur Heart J* 5, 1010
  (1982): Totty WG+, *Am J Roentgenol* 138, 143
Stomatitis (following local application)
Tongue edema (with hemorrhagic swelling)

STREPTOMYCIN

Trade name: Streptomycin (Pfizer)
Indications: Tuberculosis
Category: Aminoglycoside antibiotic; Tuberculostatic
Half-life: 2–5 hours
**Clinically important, potentially hazardous interactions
with:** aldesleukin, aminoglycosides, atracurium, bumetanide, doxacurium, ethacrynic acid, furosemide, methoxyflurane, non-depolarizing muscle relaxants, pancuronium, polypeptide antibiotics, rocuronium, succinylcholine, torsemide, vecuronium

Reactions

Skin

Acute generalized exanthematous pustulosis (AGEP)
  (1995): Moreau A+, *Int J Dermatol* 34, 263 (passim)
Allergic reactions (sic)
  (1961): Chakravarty S+, *Acta Tuberc Pneumol Scand* 41, 144
    (11%)
  (1947): Steiner K+, *Arch Dermatol* 56, 511 (18%)
Angioedema (<1%)
  (1959): Bereston ES, *J Invest Dermatol* 33, 427
Bullous eruption (<1%)
Cheilitis (2%)
  (1949): Cohen AC+, *Arch Dermatol* 60, 373
Dermatitis
  (1988): Holdiness MR, *Contact Dermatitis* 15, 282
  (1983): Fisher AA, *Cutis* 32, 314
Eczema (sic)
  (1958): Wilson HT, *BMJ* 1, 1378
Edema
Erythema multiforme (<1%)
  (1988): Hira SK+, *J Am Acad Dermatol* 19, 451 (in AIDS patient)
  (1985): Holdiness MR, *Int J Dermatol* 24, 280 (1–5%)
  (1985): Ting HC+, *Int J Dermatol* 24, 587
  (1947): Steiner K+, *Arch Dermatol* 56, 511
Erythema nodosum (<1%)
Exanthems (>5%)
  (1968): Sarkany I, *Proc R Soc Med* 61, 891
  (1966): Smith JW+, *Ann Intern Med* 65, 629
  (1961): Gupta SK, *Indian J Dermatol* 6, 115
  (1960): Heijer A+, *Acta Derm Venereol* (Stockh) 40, 35
  (1955): Yow EM, *Ann Intern Med* 43, 323 (10%)
  (1949): Bunn PA+, *Streptomycin* Williams and Wilkins, Baltimore,
    524
  (1949): Cohen AC+, *Arch Dermatol* 60, 373 (11%)
  (1948): Keefer CS+, *The Therapeutic Value of Streptomycin*
    Edwards, Ann Arbor
  (1947): Steiner K+, *Arch Dermatol* 56, 511
Exfoliative dermatitis
  (1992): Matsuzawa Y+, *Kekkaku* (Japanese) 67, 413
  (1986): Sehgal VN+, *Dermatologica* 173, 278
  (1985): Holdiness MR, *Int J Dermatol* 24, 280
  (1973): Nicolis GD+, *Arch Dermatol* 108, 788
  (1972): Kauppinen K, *Acta Derm Venereol* (Stockh) 52, 68
  (1969): Agrawal R, *BMJ* 4, 540
  (1965): McQueen A, *N Z Med J* 64, 663
  (1961): Gupta SK, *Indian J Dermatol* 6, 115
  (1959): Bereston ES, *J Invest Dermatol* 33, 427
  (1949): Bunn PA+, *Streptomycin* Williams and Wilkins, Baltimore,
    524
  (1949): Cohen AC+, *Arch Dermatol* 60, 373
  (1948): Coombs FC+, *N Y State J Med* 48, 2024
Fixed eruption (<1%)
Follicular pustular eruption (sic)
  (1981): Kushimoto H+, *Arch Dermatol* 117, 444

Lichenoid eruption
  (1958): Renkin A, *Arch Belg Dermatol Syph* (French) 14, 185
Lupus erythematosus
  (1993): Toyoshima M+, *Kekkaku* (Japanese) 68, 319
  (1986): Layer P+, *Dtsch Med Wochenschr* (German) 111, 1603
  (1980): Agarwal MB+, *J Postgrad Med* 26, 263
  (1980): Condemi JJ, *Geriatrics* 35(3), 81
  (1959): Popkhristov P+, *Surv Med* (Sofia) 10, 81
Photosensitivity
  (1971): Girard JP, *Helv Med Acta* 36, 3
Pruritus (<1%)
  (1972): Levantine A+, *Br J Dermatol* 86, 651
Purpura
  (1969): Peterkin GAG+, *Practitioner* 202, 117
  (1965): Horowitz HI+, *Semin Hematol* 2, 287
  (1955): Yow EM, *Ann Intern Med* 43, 323 (10%)
  (1949): Bunn PA+, *Streptomycin* Williams and Wilkins, Baltimore,
    524
Pustules
  (1981): Kushimoto H+, *Arch Dermatol* 117, 444
Rash (sic) (<1%)
Stevens–Johnson syndrome
  (1988): Hira SK+, *J Am Acad Dermatol* 19, 451 (in AIDS patient)
  (1985): Holdiness MR, *Int J Dermatol* 24, 280
  (1982): Sarkar SK+, *Tubercle* 63, 137
Systemic eczematous contact dermatitis
Toxic epidermal necrolysis
  (1994): *Drug Facts and Comparisons* 1926
  (1988): Fesenko IP+, *Vrach Delo* (Russian) April, 93
  (1980): Jain VK+, *Indian J Chest Dis Allied Sci* 22, 73
  (1979): Frontera-Izquierdo P+, *An Esp Pediatr* (Spanish) 12, 703
  (1979): Odinokova VA+, *Arkh Patol* (Russian) 41, 37
  (1974): Ruiz-Maldonado R+, *Bol Med Hosp Infant Mex* (Spanish)
    31, 1201
  (1973): Sehgal VN+, *Indian J Chest Dis* 15, 57
  (1967): Lowney ED+, *Arch Dermatol* 95, 359
Toxic erythema (sic)
  (1981): Kushimoto H+, *Arch Dermatol* 117, 444
Urticaria
  (1961): Gupta SK, *Indian J Dermatol* 6, 115
  (1960): Heijer A+, *Acta Derm Venereol* (Stockh) 40, 35
  (1949): Bunn PA+, *Streptomycin* Williams and Wilkins, Baltimore,
    524
  (1949): Cohen AC+, *Arch Dermatol* 60, 373 (11%)
Vasculitis
  (1971): Girard JP, *Helv Med Acta* 36, 3
  (1949): Bunn PA+, *Streptomycin* Williams and Wilkins, Baltimore,
    524

Hair

Hair – hypertrichosis
  (1992): Shelley WB+, *Advanced Dermatologic Diagnosis* WB
    Saunders, 725 (passim)

Other

Anaphylactoid reactions
  (1969): Levene GM+, *Trans St Johns Hosp Dermatol Soc* 55, 184
Black tongue
  (1954): No Author, *Lancet* 2, 179
Embolia cutis medicamentosa (Nicolau syndrome)
  (2003): Reding EL+, *J Am Acad Dermatol* 48(3), 472
  (1972): Labouche F+, *Bull Soc Fr Dermatol Syphiligr* (French)
    79, 559
Glossitis (2%)
  (1949): Cohen AC+, *Arch Dermatol* 60, 373
Headache
Injection-site granuloma
Injection-site reactions (sic)
Oral mucosal eruption

(1972): Levantine A+, *Br J Dermatol* 86, 651
(1964): Dummett CO, *J Oral Ther Pharmacol* 1, 106
Oral ulceration
Paresthesias (<1%)
Stomatitis
(1964): Dummett CO, *J Oral Ther Pharmacol* 1, 106
(1948): Beham H+, *JAMA* 138, 495
Tinnitus
Tremor (<1%)

STREPTOZOCIN

Trade name: Zanosar (Pharmacia)
Indications: Carcinoma of the pancreas, carcinoid tumor,
Hodgkin's disease
Category: Antineoplastic
Half-life: 35 minutes
**Clinically important, potentially hazardous interactions
with:** aldesleukin

Reactions

Skin
Edema
Exanthems
(1978): Levine N+, *Cancer Treat Rev* 5, 67
Pruritus
(1978): Levine N+, *Cancer Treat Rev* 5, 67
Purpura
Toxic epidermal necrolysis
(1975): Hadida E+, *Bull Soc Fr Dermatol Syphiligr* (French) 81, 76

Other
Injection-site erythema
Injection-site necrosis
(1987): Dufresne RG, *Cutis* 39, 197
Injection-site pain (1–10%)

SUCCINYLCHOLINE

Synonym: suxamethonium
Trade name: Anectine (GSK)
Indications: Skeletal muscle relaxation during general anesthesia
Category: Cholinergic; Skeletal muscle relaxant
Half-life: N/A
**Clinically important, potentially hazardous interactions
with:** amikacin, aminoglycosides, galantamine, gentamicin,
kanamycin, neomycin, paromomycin, physostigmine,
pipecuronium, streptomycin, tobramycin, vancomycin

Reactions

Skin
Dermatitis
(1996): Delgado J+, *Contact Dermatitis* 35, 120
Erythema (<1%)
(1975): Fisher MMcD, *Anaesth Intensive Care* 3, 180
Exanthems
Flushing
Pruritus (<1%)
Rash (sic) (<1%)
Urticaria

Other
Anaphylactoid reactions
(1999): Porter JM+, *Ir J Med Sci* 168, 99
(1999): Villas Martinez F+, *J Investig Allergol Clin Immunol* 9, 126
(1998): Tresch K+, *Ann Fr Anesth Reanim* (French) 17, 1181
(1990): Moneret-Vautrin DA+, *Br J Anaesth* 64(6), 743
(1981): Moneret-Vautrin DA+, *Clin Allergy* 11, 175 (13 cases)
(1975): Mandappa JM+, *Br J Anaesth* 47, 523 (2 cases)
Hypersensitivity
(1983): Yamaya R+, *Masui* (Japanese) 32, 1464
Myalgia (<1%)
(2002): Amornyotin S+, *J Med Assoc Thai* 85, S969
(1996): van den Berg AA+, *Anaesth Intensive Care* 24, 116
Myopathy
(1990): Shoji S, *Nippon Rinsho* (Japanese) 48, 1517
Rhabdomyolysis
(2001): Gronert GA, *Anesthesiology* 94(3), 523
(2000): Le Puura+, *Acta Anaesthesiol Belg* 51(1), 51
(2000): Matthews JM, *Anesth Analg* 91(6), 1552
(2000): Shaaban MJ+, *Middle East J Anesthesiology* 15(6), 681
(1996): Fiacchino F, *Anesthesiology* 84(2), 480
(1996): Pedrozzi NE+, *Pediatr Neurol* 15(3), 254 (2 cases)
(1996): Perret D+, *Ann Fr Anesth Reanim* 15(8), 1193
(1996): Takamatsu F+, *Masui* 45(11), 1406
(1995): Friedman S+, *Anesth Analg* 81(2), 422
(1994): Sullivan M+, *Can J Anaesth* 41(6), 497
(1993): Bhave CG+, *J Postgrad Med* 39(3), 157
(1992): Bakshi KK, *J Assoc Physicians India* 40(8), 549
(1991): Gokhale YA+, *J Assoc Physicians India* 39(12), 968
(1987): Lee SC+, *J Oral Maxillofac Surg* 45(9), 789 (with
    enflurane)
(1987): Lee SC+, *Ma Zui Xue Za Zhi* 25(2), 97
(1985): Hawker F+, *Anaesth Intensive Care* 13(2), 208
(1985): Sodano R+, *Minerva Anestesiol* 51(3), 109
(1984): Blumberg A+, *Schweiz Med Wochenschr* 114(30), 1068 (2
    cases)
(1984): Hool GJ+, *Anaesth Intensive Care* 12(4), 360
(1981): Lewandowski KB, *Br J Anaesth* 53(9), 981
(1979): Bomholt A, *Ugeskr Laeger* 141(14), 925
(1978): Gibbs JM, *Anaesth Intensive Care* 6(2), 141
(1976): Moore WE+, *Anesth Analg* 55(5), 680 (with halothane)
Sialorrhea (1–10%)

SUCRALFATE

Trade name: Carafate (Aventis)
Other common trade names: *Antepsin; Sucrabest; Sulcrate;
Ulcar; Ulcogant; Ulcyte; Urbal*
Indications: Duodenal ulcer
Category: Antiulcer; Gastric mucosa protectant
Half-life: N/A
**Clinically important, potentially hazardous interactions
with:** ciprofloxacin, clorazepate, ketoconazole, lansoprazole,
lomefloxacin, phenytoin, sparfloxacin, tetracycline

Reactions

Skin
Angioedema
Exanthems
(1984): Brogden RN+, *Drugs* 17, 233
Facial edema
Pruritus (<0.5%)
Rash (sic) (<0.5%)
Urticaria

Other

Headache
Xerostomia (<1%)

SUFENTANIL

Trade name: Sufenta (Taylor)
Indications: Epidural and general anesthesia
Category: Narcotic analgesic
Half-life: 152 minutes
Clinically important, potentially hazardous interactions with: cimetidine

Reactions

Skin

Chills
Cold, clammy skin (<1%)
Erythema
Pruritus (25%)
Rash (sic) (<1%)
Urticaria (<1%)

Other

Dysesthesia (<1%)

SULFACETAMIDE

Trade names: Ak-Sulf (Akorn); Albucid; Antebor; Bleph-10 (Allergan); Blephamide (Allergan); Blephamide (Allergan); Cetasil; Colirio Sulfacetamido Kriya; Covosulf; Dansemid; Dayto-Sulf; Diosulf; FML-S (Allergan); I-Sulfacet; Isopto Cetapred (Alcon); Klaron (Dermik); Lersa; Novacet; Ocu-Sulf; Ophthacet; Optamide; Optin; Optisol; Ovace (Healthpoint); Plexion (Medicis); Prontamid; Rosula (Doak); Sodium Sulamyd (Schering); Sodium Sulfacetamide; Spectro-Sulf; Spersacet; Storz-Sulf; Sulf-10; Sulfac; Sulfacel-15; Sulfacet Sodium (Dermik); Sulfacet-R (Dermik); Sulfair; Sulfamide; Sulfex; Sulphacalre; Vasocidin (Novartis); Vasosulf (Novartis)
Indications: Infectious conjunctivitis, acne vulgaris, seborrheic dermatitis
Category: Anti-acne; Sulfonamide antibiotic (ophthalmic)
Half-life: 7–13 hours
Clinically important, potentially hazardous interactions with: anticoagulants, cyclosporine, silver salts

Reactions

Skin

Allergic reactions (sic)
  (2002): Smith JG, Mobile, AL (from Internet) (observations 2 cases) (Klaron & Sulfacet-R)
  (2000): Blumenthal HL, Beachwood, OH (personal case) (observation) (Novacet Lotion)
Edema
Erythema
Erythema multiforme
  (1985): Genvert GI+, *Am J Ophthalmol* 99(4), 465 (topical)
Exfoliative dermatitis (1–10%)
Infections (sic)
Lupus erythematosus – dermatomyositis (sic)
  (1979): Mackie BS+, *Australas J Dermatol* 20(1), 49 (eye-drops)

Ocular burning
Photosensitivity
Pruritus
Stevens–Johnson syndrome (1–10%)
  (1977): Rubin Z, *Arch Dermatol* 113(2), 235 (ophthalmic)
  (1976): Gottschalk HR+, *Arch Dermatol* 112(4), 513 (ophthalmic) (previous bullous eruption to a sulfonamide)
Toxic epidermal necrolysis (1–10%)
  (2003): Spencer L, Crawfordsville, IN (from Internet) (observation) (from topical Silvadene)

Other

Death
Hypersensitivity
Ocular irritation
Ocular stinging

SULFADIAZINE

Trade name: Microsulfon
Other common trade name: *Coptin*
Indications: Various infections caused by susceptible organisms
Category: Sulfonamide antibiotic
Half-life: 17 hours
Clinically important, potentially hazardous interactions with: anticoagulants, cyclosporine, methotrexate

Reactions

Skin

Allergic reactions (sic)
  (1991): de la Hoz Caballer B+, *J Allergy Clin Immunol* 88, 137
Argyria
  (2002): Maitre S+, *Ann Dermatol Venereol* 129(2), 217 (topical silver sulfadiazine)
  (2001): Thomas K+, *BJOG* 108(8), 890
  (1992): Fraser-Moodie A, *Burns* 18, 74 (from silver sulfadiazine)
  (1992): Payne CM+, *Lancet* 340, 126 (from silver sulfadiazine)
Chills
Erythema multiforme
  (1983): Lockhart SP+, *Burns Incl Therm Inj* 10, 9
Exanthems
  (1984): Finland M+, *JAMA* 251, 1467
Exfoliative dermatitis
Fixed eruption
  (1991): Thankappen TP+, *Int J Dermatol* 30, 867 (12.4%)
Lupus erythematosus
Periorbital edema
Photosensitivity (>10%)
Pigmentation
  (1985): Dupuis LL+, *J Am Acad Dermatol* 12, 1112
Pruritus (>10%)
Purpura
Rash (sic) (>10%)
Stevens–Johnson syndrome (1–10%)
  (1999): Carrion-Carrion C+, *Ann Pharmacother* 33, 379 (fatal) (in AIDS patient)
  (1965): Sharma R+, *J Assoc Physicians India* 13, 727
Toxic epidermal necrolysis (1–10%)
  (1993): Correia O+, *Dermatology* 186, 32
Urticaria

Other

Anaphylactoid reactions
  (2001): Stephens R+, *Br J Anaesth* 87(2), 306 (with chlorhexidine)

Death
Hypersensitivity
  (2001): Morand JJ+, *Ann Dermatol Venereol* 128(12), 1351
  (1987): Volckaert A+, *Acta Clin Belg* 42, 381
  (1985): Jia XM, *Chung Hua Cheng Hsing Shao Shang Wai Ko Tsa Chih* (Chinese) 1, 232
Serum sickness (<1%)
Stomatitis
Tinnitus

*Note: Sulfadiazine is a sulfonamide and can be absorbed systemically. Sulfonamides can produce severe, possibly fatal, reactions such as toxic epidermal necrolysis and Stevens–Johnson syndrome

SULFADOXINE

Trade name: Fansidar (Roche)
Other common trade names: *Cryodoxin; Malocide; Methipox*
Indications: Malaria
Category: Folate antagonist; Sulfonamide antimalarial
Half-life: 5–8 days

Fansidar is sulfadoxine and pyrimethamine (this combination is almost always prescribed)

Reactions

Skin

Bullous eruption
  (1985): Hernborg A, *Lancet* 1, 1072
Erythema multiforme (<1%)
  (1993): Sturchler D+, *Drug Saf* 8, 160
  (1989): Ortel B+, *Dermatologica* 178, 39
  (1986): Miller KD+, *Am J Trop Med Hyg* 35, 451
Exanthems
  (1987): Groth H+, *Schweiz Rundsch Med Prax* (German) 76, 570
Exfoliative dermatitis
  (1987): Elsas T+, *Tidsskr Nor Laegeforen* (Norwegian) 107, 1231
  (1987): Zitelli BJ+, *Ann Intern Med* 106, 393
  (1986): Langtry JA+, *Br Med J Clin Res Ed* 292, 1107
Lupus erythematosus
Necrosis (<1%)
Periorbital edema
Photosensitivity (>10%)
  (1989): Ortel B+, *Dermatologica* 178, 39
  (1985): Hernborg A, *Lancet* 1, 1072 (passim)
Pruritus
  (1987): Groth H+, *Schweiz Rundsch Med Prax* (German) 76, 570
Purpura
  (1985): Hernborg A, *Lancet* 1, 1072 (passim)
Pustules
Rash (sic) (<1%)
Stevens–Johnson syndrome (1–10%)
  (1993): Sturchler D+, *Drug Saf* 8, 160
  (1990): Thiel HJ+, *Klin Monatsbl Augenheilkd* (German) 197, 142
  (1989): Ortel B+, *Dermatologica* 178, 39
  (1989): Phillips-Howard PA+, *Lancet* 2, 803
  (1987): Hellgren U+, *Br Med J Clin Res Ed* 295, 365
  (1987): Lenox-Smith I, *J Infect* 14, 90 (fatal)
  (1986): Bamber MG+, *J Infect* 13, 31 (fatal)
  (1986): Gascon-Brustenga J+, *Med Clin* (Barc) (Spanish) 87, 821
  (1986): Jeffrey RF, *Postgrad Med J* 62, 893
  (1986): Miller KD+, *Am J Trop Med Hyg* 35, 451
  (1986): Steffen R+, *Lancet* 1, 610
  (1985): Adams SJ+, *Postgrad Med J* 61, 263
  (1985): Clareus BW+, *Lakartidningen* (Swedish) 82, 4211
  (1985): Hernborg A, *Lancet* 2, 1072
  (1985): Navin TR+, *Lancet* 1, 1332
  (1983): Ligthelm RJ+, *Ned Tijdschr Geneeskd* (Dutch) 127, 1735
  (1982): Aberer W+, *Hautarzt* (German) 33, 484
  (1982): Hornstein OP+, *N Engl J Med* 307, 1529
  (1982): Olsen VV+, *Lancet* 2, 994
Toxic epidermal necrolysis
  (2000): Moussala M+, *J Fr Ophtalmol* (French) 23, 229
  (1998): Moussala M+, *J Fr Ophtalmol* (French) 21, 72
  (1998): Schmidt-Westhausen A+, *Oral Dis* 4, 90
  (1993): Correia O+, *Dermatology* 186, 32
  (1993): Sturchler D+, *Drug Saf* 8, 160
  (1991): Kimura S+, *Jpn J Med* 30, 553
  (1990): Ward DJ+, *Burns* 16, 97
  (1989): Caumes E+, *Presse Med* (French) 18, 1708 (fatal)
  (1988): No Author, *JAMA* 260, 2193 (fatal)
  (1988): No Author, *Morb Mortal Wkly Rep* 37, 571 (fatal)
  (1988): Raviglione MC+, *Arch Intern Med* 148, 2863 (fatal)
  (1986): Miller KD+, *Am J Trop Med Hyg* 35, 451
  (1984): Chan HL, *J Am Acad Dermatol* 10, 973
  (1983): Ghinelli F+, *Acta Biomed Ateneo Parmense* (Italian) 54, 363
Urticaria

Other

Ageusia
Anaphylactoid reactions
Death
Glossitis (>10%)
Hypersensitivity (>10%)
Oral lichenoid eruption
  (1989): Zain RB, *Southeast Asian J Trop Med Public Health* 20, 253
Oral ulceration
  (1985): Hernborg A, *Lancet* 1, 1072
Stomatitis
  (1985): Hernborg A, *Lancet* 1, 1072 (passim)
Tinnitus
Tremor (>10%)
Urogenital ulceration
  (1985): Hernborg A, *Lancet* 1, 1072

*Note: Sulfadoxine is a sulfonamide and can be absorbed systemically. Sulfonamides can produce severe, possibly fatal, reactions such as toxic epidermal necrolysis and Stevens–Johnson syndrome

SULFAMETHOXAZOLE

Trade names: Bactrim (Women First); Septra (Monarch)
Other common trade names: *Sinomin; Urobak*
Indications: Various infections caused by susceptible organisms
Category: Antibacterial
Half-life: 7–12 hours
Clinically important, potentially hazardous interactions with: anticoagulants, cyclosporine, methotrexate, warfarin

Note: Sulfamethoxazole is commonly used in conjunction with trimethoprim (see co-trimoxazole)

Reactions

Skin

Acute febrile neutrophilic dermatosis (Sweet's syndrome)
  (1996): Walker DC+, *J Am Acad Dermatol* 34, 918
  (1989): Cobb MW, *J Am Acad Dermatol* 21, 339 (passim)
  (1986): Su WPD+, *Cutis* 37, 167
Acute generalized exanthematous pustulosis (AGEP)

(2003): Anliker MD+, *J Investig Allergol Clin Immunol* 13(1), 66
(1995): Moreau A+, *Int J Dermatol* 34, 263 (passim)

Angioedema
(1988): Fihn SD+, *Ann Intern Med* 108, 350 (1–5%)

Bullous eruption
(1989): Caumes E+, *Presse Med* (French) 18, 1708

Dermatitis (sic)
(1989): Atahan IL+, *Br J Radiol* 62, 1107 (at previously irradiated area)
(1987): Vukelja SJ+, *Cancer Treat Rep* 71, 668 (at previously irradiated area)
(1984): Shelley WB+, *J Am Acad Dermatol* 11, 53 (at site of previous sunburn)
(1971): Cotterill JA+, *Br J Dermatol* 84, 366

Erythema multiforme
(1997): Rieder MJ+, *Pediatr Infect Dis J* 16, 1028 (70% in children with HIV)
(1991): Tilden ME+, *Arch Ophthalmol* 109, 67
(1990): Chan HL+, *Arch Dermatol* 126, 43
(1989): Alanko K+, *Acta Derm Venereol* (Stockh) 69, 223
(1988): Hira SK+, *J Am Acad Dermatol* 19, 451
(1988): Platt R+, *J Infect Dis* 158, 474
(1987): Penmetcha M, *BMJ* 295, 556
(1987): Schöpf E, *Infection* 15 (Suppl 5P), S254
(1985): Heer M+, *Gastroenterology* 88, 1954
(1982): Brettle RP+, *J Infect* 4, 149
(1979): Beck MH+, *Clin Exp Dermatol* 4, 201
(1978): Assaad D+, *Can Med Assoc J* 118, 154
(1978): Azinge NO+, *J Allergy Clin Immunol* 62, 125
(1975): Bernstein LS, *Can Med Assoc J* 112 (Suppl), 96
(1971): Koch-Weser J+, *Arch Intern Med* 128, 399 (0.15%)

Erythema nodosum
(1974): Delaney TJ+, *Br J Dermatol* 90, 205
(1971): Koch-Weser J+, *Arch Intern Med* 128, 399

Erythroderma
(1979): Kennedy C+, *BMJ* 1, 1356

Exanthems
(1998): Hattori N+, *J Dermatol* 25, 269
(1997): Caumes E+, *Arch Dermatol* 133, 465
(1995): Hertl M+, *Br J Dermatol* 132, 215
(1995): Wolkenstein P+, *Arch Dermatol* 131, 544
(1994): Litt JZ, Beachwood, OH (personal case) (observation)
(1993): Agarwal BR+, *Indian Pediatr* 30, 1026
(1993): Litt JZ, Beachwood, OH (personal case) (observation)
(1993): Malnick SDH+, *Ann Pharmacotherapy* 27, 1139
(1990): Medina I+, *N Engl J Med* 323, 776 (47% in AIDS patients)
(1988): DeRaeve L+, *Br J Dermatol* 119, 521 (in AIDS patient)
(1988): Fihn SD+, *Ann Intern Med* 108, 350 (1–5%)
(1988): Sattler FR+, *Ann Intern Med* 109, 280 (44% in AIDS patients)
(1988): Weinke T+, *Dtsch Med Wochenschr* (German) 113, 1129 (25% in AIDS patients)
(1987): Goa KL+, *Drugs* 33, 242 (65% in AIDS patients)
(1987): Schöpf E, *Infection* 15 (Suppl 5P), S254
(1986): Sonntag MR+, *Schweiz Med Wochenschr* (German) 116, 142
(1985): DeHovitz JA+, *Ann Intern Med* 103, 479
(1985): Maayan S+, *Arch Intern Med* 145, 1607
(1984): Gordon FM+, *Ann Intern Med* 100, 495 (51% in AIDS patients)
(1984): Kovacs JA+, *Ann Intern Med* 100, 663 (29% in AIDS patients)
(1983): Mitsuyasu R+, *N Engl J Med* 308, 1535 (69% in AIDS patients.)
(1982): Goetz MB+, *JAMA* 247, 3118
(1980): Fennell RS+, *Clin Pediatr* 19, 124
(1979): Abengowe CU, *Curr Med Res Opin* 5, 749 (3.2%)
(1977): Taylor B+, *BMJ* 2, 552 (12%)
(1976): Arndt KA+, *JAMA* 235, 918 (5.9%)

(1976): Gower PE+, *BMJ* 1, 684 (>5%)
(1975): Bernstein LS, *Can Med Assoc J* 112 (Suppl), 96 (1.9%)
(1975): Gleckman RA, *JAMA* 233, 427 (0.84%)
(1975): Sallam MA+, *Curr Med Res Opin* 3, 229 (3.4%)
(1972): Halpern GM, *BMJ* 1, 691
(1971): Koch-Weser J+, *Arch Intern Med* 128, 399 (1%)

Exfoliative dermatitis
(1990): Ponte CD+, *Drug Intell Clin Pharm* 24, 140 (feet)
(1975): Bernstein LS, *Can Med Assoc J* 112 (Suppl), 96
(1971): Koch-Weser J+, *Arch Intern Med* 128, 399

Fixed eruption
(1997): Gruber F+, *Clin Exp Dermatol* 22, 144
(1996): Sharma VK+, *J Dermatol* 23, 530
(1995): Wolkenstein P+, *Arch Dermatol* 131, 544
(1993): Oleaga JM+, *Contact Dermatitis* 29, 155
(1993): Ramam M+, *Indian Pediatr* 30, 110 (in an infant)
(1992): Lim JT+, *Ann Acad Med Singapore* 21, 408
(1991): Jain VK+, *Ann Dent* 50, 9 (oral mucous membrane)
(1991): Smoller BR+, *J Cutan Pathol* 18, 13
(1990): Gaffoor PMA+, *Cutis* 45, 242 (genitalia)
(1989): Basomba A+, *J Allergy Clin Immunol* 84, 409
(1989): Bharija SC+, *Australas J Dermatol* 30, 43
(1989): Gupta R, *Indian J Dermatol* 55, 181 (in an infant)
(1989): Varsano I+, *Dermatologica* 178, 232
(1988): Baird BJ+, *Int J Dermatol* 27, 170 (bullous and generalized)
(1988): Bharija SC+, *Dermatologica* 176, 108 (in an infant)
(1987): Amir J+, *Drug Intell Clin Pharm* 21, 41
(1987): Hughes BR+, *Br J Dermatol* 116, 241
(1987): Van Voorhees A+, *Am J Dermatopathol* 9, 528
(1986): Kanwar AJ+, *Dermatologica* 172, 230
(1985): Gomez B+, *Allergol Immunopathol Madr* (Spanish) 13, 87
(1984): Pandhi RK+, *Sex Transm Dis* 11, 164
(1982): Gibson JR, *BMJ* 284, 1529
(1980): Talbot MD, *Practitioner* 224, 823
(1978): Verbov J, *Arch Dermatol* 114, 963
(1972): Aoyama H+, *Jpn J Dermatol* 82, 16

Flushing
(1984): Jick SS+, *Lancet* 2, 631

Lichenoid eruption
(1994): Berger TG+, *Arch Dermatol* 130, 609

Linear IgA bullous dermatosis
(1994): Kuechle MK+, *J Am Acad Dermatol* 30, 187

Lupus erythematosus
(1985): Stratton MA, *Clin Pharm* 4, 657
(1975): Grennan DM+, *BMJ* 4, 385

Photosensitivity (>10%)
(1994): Berger TG+, *Arch Dermatol* 130, 609 (in HIV-infected) (4 cases)
(1994): Shelley WB+, *Cutis* 53, 162 (observation)
(1987): Schöpf E, *Infection* 15 (Suppl 5P), S254
(1986): Chandler MJ, *J Infect Dis* 153, 1001

Pruritus (>10%)
(1997): Caumes E+, *Arch Dermatol* 133, 465
(1997): Thaler D, Monona, WI (from internet) (observation)
(1996): Litt JZ, Beachwood, OH (personal case) (observation)
(1990): Medina I+, *N Engl J Med* 323, 776 (1–5%)
(1987): Colebunders R+, *Ann Intern Med* 107, 599 (4% in AIDS patients)
(1986): Sher MR, *J Allergy Clin Immunol* 77, 133
(1984): Kramer BS+, *Cancer* 53, 329
(1975): Gleckman RA, *JAMA* 233, 427 (0.84%)
(1971): Koch-Weser J+, *Arch Intern Med* 128, 399 (0.15%)

Pruritus vulvae
(1981): *Modern Medicine* 49, 111

Psoriasis
(1979): Kennedy C+, *BMJ* 1, 1356

Purpura
(1993): Kaufman DW+, *Blood* 82, 2714

(1989): Saxena SK, *J Assoc Physicians India* 37, 479
(1971): Koch-Weser J+, *Arch Intern Med* 128, 399
Pustules
    (1994): Spencer JM+, *Br J Dermatol* 130, 514
    (1990): Guy C+, *Nouv Dermatol* (French) 9, 540
    (1989): Grattan CEH, *Dermatologica* 179, 57 (passim)
    (1986): Macdonald KJS+, *BMJ* 293, 1279
    (1978): Braun-Falco O+, *Hautarzt* (German) 29, 371
    (1977): Knudsen L+, *Ugeskr Laeger* (Danish) 139, 1007
Radiation recall
    (1990): Leslie MD+, *Br J Radiol* 63, 661
    (1987): Vukelja SJ+, *Cancer Treat Rep* 71, 668 (at previously
        irradiated area)
    (1984): Shelley WB+, *J Am Acad Dermatol* 11, 53 (at site of
        previous sunburn)
Rash (sic) (>10%)
    (1995): Williams JW+, *JAMA* 273, 1015
    (1993): Malnick SD+, *Ann Pharmacother* 27, 1139
Side effects (sic)
    (1994): Roudier C+, *Arch Dermatol* 130, 1383 (48% in AIDS
        patients)
    (1971): Koch-Weser J+, *Arch Intern Med* 128, 399 (2.1%)
Stevens–Johnson syndrome (1–10%)
    (1997): Douglas R+, *Clin Infect Dis* 25, 1480
    (1997): Rieder MJ+, *Pediatr Infect Dis J* 16, 1028 (10% in
        children with HIV)
    (1996): Caumes E, *Rev Mal Respir* (French) 13, 101
    (1996): McCarty J, Fort Worth, TX (from Internet) (observation)
    (1995): Kuper K+, *Ophthalmologe* (German) 92, 823
    (1995): Sharma VK+, *Pediatr Dermatol* 12, 178
    (1995): Wolkenstein P+, *Arch Dermatol* 131, 544
    (1994): Shelley WB+, *Cutis* 53, 159 (observation)
    (1993): Litt JZ, Beachwood, OH (personal case) (observation)
    (1990): Chan HL+, *Arch Dermatol* 126, 43
    (1988): Platt R+, *J Infect Dis* 158, 474
    (1985): Heer M+, *Gastroenterology* 88, 1954
    (1982): Brettle RP+, *J Infect* 4, 149
    (1979): Beck MH+, *Clin Exp Dermatol* 4, 201
    (1978): Azinge NO+, *J Allergy Clin Immunol* 62, 125
    (1978): Kikuchi S+, *Lancet* 2, 580
    (1978): Thorpe JA+, *Lancet* 1, 276 (fatal)
    (1975): Bernstein LS, *Can Med Assoc J* 112 (Suppl), 96
    (1970): Shaw DJ+, *Johns Hopkins Med J* 126, 130
Toxic epidermal necrolysis (1–10%)
    (2002): Nassif A+, *J Invest Dermatol* 118(4), 728
    (2001): See S+, *Ann Pharmacother* 35(6), 694
    (2000): Moussala M+, *J Fr Ophtalmol* (French) 23, 229
    (1996): Caumes E, *Rev Mal Respir* 13, 101
    (1996): Rehbein H, Jacksonville, FL (from Internet) (observation)
    (1995): Sharma VK+, *Pediatr Dermatol* 12, 178
    (1995): Wolkenstein P+, *Arch Dermatol* 131, 544 (7 cases)
    (1993): Correia O+, *Dermatology* 186, 32
    (1990): Chan HL+, *Arch Dermatol* 126, 43
    (1990): Kobza Black A+, *Br J Dermatol* 123, 277
    (1990): Roujeau JC+, *Arch Dermatol* 126, 37
    (1990): Ward DJ+, *Burns* 16, 97
    (1989): Carmichael AJ+, *Lancet* 2, 808
    (1989): Whittington RM, *Lancet* 2, 574
    (1988): De Raeve L+, *Br J Dermatol* 119, 521 (passim)
    (1987): Guillaume JC+, *Arch Dermatol* 123, 1166
    (1987): Schöpf E, *Infection* 15 (Suppl 5P), S254
    (1986): Miller KD+, *Am J Trop Med Hyg* 33, 451
    (1986): Revuz J, *J Dermatol Paris* 153
    (1986): Roman O+, *Rev Pediatr Obstet Ginecol Pediatr*
        (Romanian) 35, 261
    (1984): Fong PH+, *Singapore Med J* 25, 184
    (1984): Westly ED+, *Arch Dermatol* 120, 721
    (1983): Petersen P+, *Ugeskr Laeger* (Danish) 145, 3345
    (1982): Ortiz JE+, *Ann Plast Surg* 9, 249

(1978): Assaad D+, *Can Med Assoc J* 118, 154
(1978): Petricevic I+, *Lijec Vjesn* (Serbo-Croatian-Roman)
    100, 596
(1975): Bernstein LS, *Can Med Assoc J* 112 (Suppl), 96
(1973): Beyvin AJ+, *Anesth Analg Paris* (French) 30, 767
(1972): Chanial G+, *J Med Lyon* (French) 53, 859
(1971): Chanial G+, *Bull Soc Fr Dermatol Syphiligr* (French)
    78, 565
Urticaria
    (1994): Blumenthal HL, Beachwood, OH (personal case)
        (observation)
    (1993): Litt JZ, Beachwood, OH (personal case) (observation)
    (1991): Greenberger PA, *JAMA* 265, 458
    (1987): Schöpf E, *Infection* 15 (Suppl 5P), S254
    (1985): Goolamali SK, *Postgrad Med J* 61, 925
    (1985): Maayan S+, *Arch Intern Med* 145, 1607
    (1984): Kramer BS+, *Cancer* 53, 329
    (1981): Abi-Mansur P+, *Am J Gastroenterol* 76, 356
    (1971): Koch-Weser J+, *Arch Intern Med* 128, 399
Vasculitis (<1%)
    (1989): Verne-Pignatelli J+, *Postgrad Med J* 65, 51
    (1987): Schöpf E, *Infection* 15 (Suppl 5P), S254
    (1978): Braun-Falco O+, *Hautarzt* (German) 29, 371
    (1978): Coquin Y+, *Nouv Presse Med* (French) 7, 3145
    (1976): Wåhlin A+, *Lancet* 2, 1415
    (1971): Koch-Weser J+, *Arch Intern Med* 128, 399
Vulvovaginitis
    (1985): Wong ES+, *Ann Intern Med* 102, 302

Other

Anaphylactoid reactions
    (1988): Arnold PA+, *Drug Intell Clin Pharm* 22, 43
    (1985): Gossius G+, *Scand J Infect Dis* 16, 373
Aphthous stomatitis
    (1981): *J Antimicrob Chemother* 7, 179
Black tongue
    (1993): Blumenthal HL, Beachwood, OH (personal case)
        (observation)
Death
Dysgeusia
    (1988): Fischl MA+, *JAMA* 259, 1185
Glossitis
Hypersensitivity
    (1998): Chen D, Chicagi, IL (from Internet) (observation)
    (1997): Hicks ME+, *Ann Pharmacother* 31, 1259
    (1993): Marinac JS+, *Clin Infect Dis* 16, 178
    (1993): Martin GJ+, *Clin Infect Dis* 16, 175
    (1993): Mathelier-Fusade P+, *Presse Med* (French) 22, 1363
    (1993): Mehta J+, *J Assoc Physicians India* 41, 235
Mucocutaneous syndrome
    (1982): Brettle RP+, *J Infect* 4, 149
Oral mucosal eruption
    (1991): Tilden ME+, *Arch Ophthalmol* 109, 67
    (1988): Fihn SD+, *Ann Intern Med* 108, 350 (1–5%)
Oral ulceration
    (1987): Hughes WT+, *N Engl J Med* 316, 1627
    (1981): Orenstein WA+, *Am J Med Sci* 282, 27
Pseudolymphoma
    (1978): Laugier P+, *Z Hautkr* (German) 53, 353
Serum sickness (<1%)
    (1988): Platt R+, *J Infect Dis* 158, 474
Stomatitis
Tongue ulceration
    (1981): *J Antimicrob Chemother* 7, 179

*Note: Sulfamethoxazole is a sulfonamide and can be absorbed systemically. Sulfonamides can produce severe, possibly fatal, reactions such as toxic epidermal necrolysis and Stevens–Johnson syndrome

SULFASALAZINE

Synonym: salicylazosulfapyridine
Trade name: Azulfidine (Pharmacia)
Other common trade names: Colo-Pleon; Salazopyrin; Salisulf; Saridine; SAS-500; Sulfazine; Ulcol
Indications: Inflammatory bowel disease, ulcerative colitis, rheumatoid arthritis
Category: Sulfonamide
Half-life: 5–10 hours
Clinically important, potentially hazardous interactions with: cholestyramine, methotrexate

Reactions

Skin

Acute generalized exanthematous pustulosis (AGEP)
  (1999): Kawaguchi M+, J Dermatol 26, 359
  (1998): Mitchell D, Thomasville, GA (from Internet)
    (observation)
  (1993): Marce S+, Presse Med (French) 22, 271
  (1993): Wainwright NJ+, Drug Saf 9, 437
Adverse effects (sic)
  (1993): Gran JT+, Scand J Rheumatol 22, 229
Angioedema
  (1990): Donovan S+, Br J Rheumatol 29, 201
  (1990): Petterson T+, Br J Rheumatol 29, 239
Bullous eruption
Bullous pemphigoid
  (1970): Bean SF+, Arch Dermatol 102, 205
Cheilitis
  (1986): Farr M+, Drugs 32 (Suppl 1), 49
Dermatitis (sic)
  (2001): Lau G+, Forensic Sci Int 122(2), 79
  (1989): Challier P+, Presse Med (French) 18, 778
Diaphoresis
  (1986): Farr M+, Drugs 32 (Suppl 1), 49
Eczema (sic)
  (1947): Sulzberger MB+, J Allergy 18, 92
Erythema multiforme
  (1987): Penmetcha M, BMJ 295, 556
  (1986): Garcia e Silva L, Acta Med Port (Portuguese) 7, 71
  (1985): Heer M+, Gastroenterology 88, 1954
  (1985): Hernborg A, Lancet 2, 1072
  (1985): Huff JC, Dermatol Clin 3, 141
  (1982): Hornstein OP+, N Engl J Med 307, 1529
  (1979): Beck MH+, Clin Exp Dermatol 4, 201
  (1966): Cameron HA+, BMJ 2, 1174
Erythema nodosum
  (1986): Areias E+, Ann Dermatol Venereol (French) 113, 197
  (1971): Koch-Weser J+, Arch Intern Med 128, 399
Erythroderma
  (1984): Sala F+, Cronica Dermatol (Italian) 15, 209
Exanthems
  (1995): Wolkenstein P+, Arch Dermatol 131, 544
  (1994): Akahoshi K+, J Gastroenterol 29, 772
  (1992): Bodokh I+, Presse Med (French) 21, 630
  (1991): Hertzberger-ten-Cate R+, Clin Exp Rheumatol 9, 85
  (1990): Donovan S+, Br J Rheumatol 29, 201 (4.1%)
  (1990): Gupta AK+, Arch Dermatol 126, 487 (23%)
  (1990): Petterson T+, Br J Rheumatol 29, 239
  (1989): Alanko K+, Acta Derm Venereol (Stockh) 69, 223
  (1989): Gremse DA+, J Pediatr Gastroenterol Nutr 9, 261
  (1988): Williams HJ+, Arthritis Rheum 31, 702 (7%)
  (1986): Farr M+, Drugs 32 (Suppl 1), 49
  (1986): Poland GA+, Am J Med 81, 707
  (1985): Maayan S+, Arch Intern Med 145, 1607

(1984): Iwatsuki K+, Arch Dermatol 120, 964
(1984): Peppercorn MA, Ann Intern Med 101, 377
(1984): Purdy BH+, Ann Intern Med 100, 512
(1982): Goetz MB+, JAMA 247, 3118
(1980): Fennell RS+, Clin Pediatr 19, 124
(1976): Arndt KA+, JAMA 235, 918 (2%)
(1973): Das KM+, N Engl J Med 289, 491 (2%)
(1972): Halpern GM, BMJ 1, 691
(1968): Baron JH+, Lancet 1, 1094
(1962): Truelove SC+, BMJ 2, 1708 (3%)
Exfoliative dermatitis
  (1990): Donovan S+, Br J Rheumatol 29, 201
  (1984): Sala F+, Cronica Dermatol (Italian) 15, 209
  (1978): Mihas AA+, JAMA 239, 2590
  (1975): Bernstein LS, Can Med Assoc J 112, 96S
  (1971): Koch-Weser J+, Arch Intern Med 128, 399
Fixed eruption
  (1996): Kawada A+, Contact Dermatitis 34, 155
  (1988): Bharija SC+, Dermatologica 176, 108
  (1987): Hughes BR+, Br J Dermatol 116, 241
  (1987): Kanwar AJ+, Dermatologica 174, 104
  (1986): Kanwar AJ+, Dermatologica 172, 230
  (1982): Gibson JR, BMJ 284, 1529
  (1980): Talbot MD, Practitioner 224, 823
Flushing
  (2000): Jung JH+, Clin Exp Rheumatol 18, 245
  (1984): Jick SS+, Lancet 2, 631
Lichen planus
  (1995): Kaplan S+, J Rheumatol 22, 191
  (1991): Alstead EM+, J Clin Gastroenterol 13, 335
Lupus erythematosus
  (2002): Angelova I+, World Congress Dermatol Poster, 0083
    (patient has psoriasis)
  (2002): Tsai WC+, Clin Rheumatol 21(4), 339
  (2000): Gunnarsson I+, Rheumatology (Oxford) 39(8), 886
  (1997): Gunnarsson I+, Br J Rheumatol 36, 1089
  (1996): Khattak FH+, Br J Rheumatol 35, 104
  (1995): Veale DJ+, Br J Rheumatol 34, 383
  (1994): Borg AA+, Clin Rheumatol 13, 522
  (1994): Bray VJ+, J Rheumatol 21, 2157
  (1994): Caulier M+, J Rheumatol 21, 750
  (1994): Fritzler MJ, Lupus 3, 455
  (1994): Mongey AB+, Br J Rheumatol 33, 789
  (1994): Walker EM+, Br J Rheumatol 33, 175
  (1993): Siam AR+, J Rheumatol 20, 207
  (1993): Wildhagen K+, Clin Rheumatol 12, 265
  (1992): Skaer TL, Clin Ther 14, 496
  (1991): Alarcon-Segovia D+, Baillieres Clin Rheumatol 5, 1
  (1989): Deboever G+, Am J Gastroenterol 84, 85
  (1989): Sugimoto M+, Nippon Naika Gakkai Zasshi (Japanese)
    78, 583
  (1988): Clementz GL+, Am J Med 84, 535
  (1987): Hobbs RN+, Ann Rheum Dis 46, 408
  (1985): Lovisetto P+, Recenti Prog Med (Italian) 76, 110
  (1985): Stratton MA, Clin Pharm 4, 657
  (1983): Vanheule BA+, Eur J Pediatr 140, 66
  (1982): Carr-Locke DL, Am J Gastroenterol 77, 614
  (1980): Crisp AJ+, J R Soc Med 73, 60
  (1980): Rouleau L+, Union Med Can (French) 109, 1326
  (1979): Weiller PJ+, Ann Med Interne Paris (French) 130, 665
  (1978): Jaup BH, Dtsch Med Wochenschr (German) 103, 1211
  (1977): Griffiths ID+, BMJ 2, 1188
  (1969): Alarcon-Segovia D, Mayo Clin Proc 44, 664
  (1966): Cohen P+, JAMA 197, 817
Necrosis
  (1988): Krakamp B+, Med Klin (German) 83, 611
Periorbital edema
Photosensitivity (>10%)
  (1999): Bouyssou-Gauthier ML, Dermatology 198, 388
  (1994): Shelley WB+, Cutis 53, 240 (observation)

(1990): Petterson T+, *Br J Rheumatol* 29, 239
(1975): Delage C+, *Union Med Can* (French) 104, 579
Stomatitis
(1993): Gran JT+, *Scand J Rheumatol* 22, 229
Tongue ulceration
(1981): *J Antimicrob Chemother* 7, 179
Xerostomia
(1990): Donovan S+, *Br J Rheumatol* 29, 201

*Note: Sulfasalazine is a sulfonamide and can be absorbed systemically. Sulfonamides can produce severe, possibly fatal, reactions such as toxic epidermal necrolysis and Stevens–Johnson syndrome

SULFINPYRAZONE

Trade name: Anturane (Novartis)
Other common trade names: *Antazone; Antiran; Anturan; Anturano; Enturen; Falizal; Novopyrazone*
Indications: Gouty arthritis
Category: Antigout; Antihyperuricemic sulfonamide
Half-life: 2–7 hours
Clinically important, potentially hazardous interactions with: anisindione, anticoagulants, dicumarol, warfarin

Reactions

Skin

Dermatitis (sic) (1–10%)
Edema
Exanthems (<3%)
Flushing (<1%)
Purpura
Rash (sic) (1–10%)

*Note: Sulfinpyrazone is a sulfonamide and can be absorbed systemically. Sulfonamides can produce severe, possibly fatal, reactions such as toxic epidermal necrolysis and Stevens–Johnson syndrome

SULFISOXAZOLE

Trade name: Pediazole (Ross)
Other common trade names: *Isoxazine; Novo-Soxazole; Oxazole; Sulfazin; Sulfazole; Sulizole; Thiazin; Urazole*
Indications: Various infections caused by susceptible organisms
Category: Urinary tract antibacterial-antiprotozoal sulfonamide
Half-life: 3–7 hours
Clinically important, potentially hazardous interactions with: anticoagulants, cyclosporine, methotrexate, warfarin

Reactions

Skin

Allergic reactions (sic)
(1971): Koch-Weser J+, *Arch Intern Med* 128, 399 (2.8%)
Angioedema (<1%)
(1971): Koch-Weser J+, *Arch Intern Med* 128, 399 (0.15%)
Bullous eruption (<1%)
(1966): Falk AB+, *Arch Dermatol* 94, 249
Eczema (sic)
(1947): Sulzberger MB+, *J Allergy* 18, 92
Erythema multiforme (<1%)
(1987): Penmetcha M, *BMJ* 295, 556

(1985): Heer M+, *Gastroenterology* 88, 1954
(1985): Hernborg A, *Lancet* 2, 1072
(1979): Beck MH+, *Clin Exp Dermatol* 4, 201
(1975): Bernstein LS, *Can Med Assoc J* 112, 96S
(1971): Koch-Weser J+, *Arch Intern Med* 128, 399 (0.15%)
(1970): Shaw DJ+, *Johns Hopkins Med J* 126, 130
Erythema nodosum
(1971): Koch-Weser J+, *Arch Intern Med* 128, 399
Exanthems (1–5%)
(1985): Maayan S+, *Arch Intern Med* 145, 1607
(1982): Goetz MB+, *JAMA* 247, 3118
(1980): Fennell RS+, *Clin Pediatr* 19, 124
(1976): Arndt KA+, *JAMA* 235, 918 (1.7%)
(1972): Halpern GM, *BMJ* 1, 691
(1972): Kauppinen K, *Acta Derm Venereol* (Stockh) 52 (Suppl), 68
(1971): Koch-Weser J+, *Arch Intern Med* 128, 399 (1%)
(1967): Lehr D, *Ann N Y Acad Sci* 69, 417 (2%)
(1956): Davis JB, *JAMA* 161, 228
Exfoliative dermatitis
(1975): Bernstein LS, *Can Med Assoc J* 112, 96S
(1971): Koch-Weser J+, *Arch Intern Med* 128, 399
Fixed eruption (<1%)
(1988): Bharija SC+, *Dermatologica* 176, 108
(1987): Hughes BR+, *Br J Dermatol* 116, 241
(1986): Kanwar AJ+, *Dermatologica* 172, 230
(1982): Gibson JR, *BMJ* 284, 1529
(1980): Talbot MD, *Practitioner* 224, 823
(1968): Sarkany I, *Proc R Soc Med* 61, 891
Flushing
(1984): Jick SS+, *Lancet* 2, 631
Linear IgA bullous dermatosis
(1981): Safai B+, *J Am Acad Dermatol* 4, 435
Lupus erythematosus
(1975): Grossman J+, *Am J Dis Child* 129, 123
(1966): Cohen P+, *JAMA* 197, 817
Periorbital edema
Photosensitivity (>10%)
(1986): Chandler MJ, *J Infect Dis* 153, 1001
(1981): Flach AJ+, *Arch Ophthalmol* 100, 1206 (from topical application)
(1981): Flach AJ+, *Arch Ophthalmol* 99, 609 (from topical application)
(1972): Kauppinen K, *Acta Derm Venereol* (Stockh) 52 (Suppl), 68
Phototoxicity
(1982): Flach AJ+, *Arch Ophthalmol* 100, 1286 (from topical application)
Pruritus (>10%)
(1987): Colebunders R+, *Ann Intern Med* 107, 599
(1986): Sher MR, *J Allergy Clin Immunol* 77, 133
(1984): Kramer BS+, *Cancer* 53, 329
(1971): Koch-Weser J+, *Arch Intern Med* 128, 399 (0.15%)
Pruritus vulvae
(1981): *Modern Medicine* 49, 111
Purpura
(1980): Miescher PA+, *Clin Haematol* 9, 505
(1977): Cimo PL+, *Am J Hematol* 2, 65
(1956): Green TW+, *JAMA* 161, 1563
(1951): Gale GL, *Can Med Assoc J* 64, 252
Pustules
Rash (sic) (>10%)
Side effects (sic)
(1971): Koch-Weser J+, *Arch Intern Med* 128, 399 (2.1%)
Stevens–Johnson syndrome (1–10%)
(1983): Fischer PR+, *Am J Dis Child* 137, 914
(1970): Shaw DJ+, *Johns Hopkins Med J* 126, 130
(1956): Davis JB, *JAMA* 161, 228
Toxic epidermal necrolysis (1–10%)
(1995): Raymond F+, *Arch Pediatr* (French) 2, 494
(1990): Jacqz-Aigrain E+, *Lancet* 336, 1010

(1989): Alanko K+, *Acta Derm Venereol* (Stockh) 69, 223
(1975): Bernstein LS, *Can Med Assoc J* 112, 96S
(1972): Kauppinen K, *Acta Derm Venereol* (Stockh) 52 (Suppl), 68
Urticaria
(1985): Maayan S+, *Arch Intern Med* 145, 1607
(1984): Kramer BS+, *Cancer* 53, 329
(1981): Abi-Mansur P+, *Am J Gastroenterol* 76, 356
(1971): Koch-Weser J+, *Arch Intern Med* 128, 399 (0.04%)
Vasculitis (<1%)
(1971): Koch-Weser J+, *Arch Intern Med* 128, 399
(1967): Lee DK+, *JAMA* 200, 720
(1965): McCombs RP, *JAMA* 194, 1059
Vulvovaginitis
(1985): Wong ES+, *Ann Intern Med* 102, 302

Hair

Hair – alopecia
(1975): Grossman J+, *Am J Dis Child* 129, 123

Other

Anaphylactoid reactions
(1988): Arnold PA+, *Drug Intell Clin Pharm* 22, 43
(1985): Gossius G+, *Scand J Infect Dis* 16, 373
Aphthous stomatitis
(1981): *J Antimicrob Chemother* 7, 179
Dysgeusia
(1988): Fischl MA+, *JAMA* 259, 1185
Glossitis
Headache
Hypersensitivity
Myalgia
Oral psoriasis (sic)
(1974): Yaffee HS, *Int J Dermatol* 13, 185
Oral ulceration
(1987): Hughes WT+, *N Engl J Med* 316, 1627
(1981): Orenstein WA+, *Am J Med Sci* 282, 27
Serum sickness (<1%)
(1969): Mukherjee DN, *J Indian Med Assoc* 52, 225
Stomatitis
Temporal arteritis
(1967): Lee DK+, *JAMA* 200, 720
Tinnitus
Tongue ulceration
(1981): *J Antimicrob Chemother* 7, 179

*Note: Sulfisoxazole is a sulfonamide and can be absorbed systemically. Sulfonamides can produce severe, possibly fatal, reactions such as toxic epidermal necrolysis and Stevens–Johnson syndrome

SULINDAC

Trade name: Clinoril (Merck)
Other common trade names: *Aflodac; Algocetil; APO-Sulin; Arthrocine; Mobilin; Novo-Sundac; Sulene; Sulic; Suloril*
Indications: Arthritis
Category: Nonsteroidal anti-inflammatory (NSAID) analgesic
Half-life: 7.8–16.4 hours
Clinically important, potentially hazardous interactions with: methotrexate, warfarin

Reactions

Skin

Angioedema (<1%)
Dermatitis (sic)

(1991): Renaut JJ, *Allerg Immunol Paris* (French) 23, 365
Diaphoresis
Ecchymoses (<1%)
Edema
Erythema
(1991): Renaut JJ, *Allerg Immunol Paris* (French) 23, 365
Erythema multiforme (<1%)
(1987): Jeanmougin M+, *Ann Dermatol Venereol* (French) 114, 1400
(1985): Bigby M+, *J Am Acad Dermatol* 12, 866
(1985): O'Brien WM+, *J Rheumatol* 12, 13
(1984): Stern RS+, *JAMA* 252, 1433
(1982): Park GD+, *Arch Intern Med* 142, 1292
(1981): Husain Z+, *J Rheumatol* 8, 176
(1981): Maguire FW, *Del Med J* 53, 193
(1980): Russell IJ, *Ann Intern Med* 92, 716
Exanthems (1–5%)
(1993): Litt JZ, Beachwood, OH (personal case) (observation)
(1991): Hyson CP+, *Arch Intern Med* 151, 387
(1987): Jeanmougin M+, *Ann Dermatol Venereol* (French) 114, 1400
(1985): Bigby M+, *J Am Acad Dermatol* 12, 866
(1984): Stern RS+, *JAMA* 252, 1433
(1982): Park GD+, *Arch Intern Med* 142, 1292
(1981): Dhand A+, *Gastroenterology* 80, 585
(1980): Russell IJ, *Ann Intern Med* 92, 716
(1979): Anderson R, *N Engl J Med* 300, 735
(1977): Calabro JJ+, *Clin Pharmacol Ther* 22, 358 (3%)
Exfoliative dermatitis (<1%)
Exfoliative erythroderma
(1984): Stern RS+, *JAMA* 252, 1433
Facial erythema
(1979): Anderson R, *N Engl J Med* 300, 735
Fixed eruption (<1%)
(1987): Jeanmougin M+, *Ann Dermatol Venereol* (French) 114, 1400
(1986): Bruce DR+, *Cutis* 38, 323
(1985): Bigby M+, *J Am Acad Dermatol* 12, 866
(1984): Aram H, *Int J Dermatol* 23, 421
(1984): Stern RS+, *JAMA* 252, 1433
Hot flashes (<1%)
Jaundice
(1979): Wolfe PB, *Ann Intern Med* 91, 656
Lichen planus
(1983): Hamburger J+, *BMJ* 287, 1258
Pernio
(1981): Reinertsen JL, *Arthritis Rheum* 24, 1215
Photosensitivity (<1%)
(1987): Jeanmougin M+, *Ann Dermatol Venereol* (French) 114, 1400
(1984): Stern RS+, *JAMA* 252, 1433
Phototoxicity
Pruritus (1–10%)
(1987): Jeanmougin M+, *Ann Dermatol Venereol* (French) 114, 1400
(1985): Bigby M+, *J Am Acad Dermatol* 12, 866
(1984): Stern RS+, *JAMA* 252, 1433
(1982): Park GD+, *Arch Intern Med* 142, 1292
(1980): Russell IJ, *Ann Intern Med* 92, 716
Purpura (<1%)
(1987): Jeanmougin M+, *Ann Dermatol Venereol* (French) 114, 1400
(1984): Stern RS+, *JAMA* 252, 1433
Rash (sic) (>10%)
Raynaud's phenomenon
(1981): Reinertsen JL, *Arthritis Rheum* 24, 1215 (passim)
Skin pain (sic)
(1984): Stern RS+, *JAMA* 252, 1433

Stevens–Johnson syndrome (<1%)
  (1993): Awaya N+, *Ryumachi* (Japanese) 33, 432
  (1983): Klein SM+, *J Rheumatol* 10, 512
  (1981): Husain Z+, *J Rheumatol* 8, 176
  (1981): Maguire FW, *Del Med J* 53, 193
  (1980): Levitt L+, *JAMA* 243, 1262
Toxic epidermal necrolysis (<1%)
  (1990): Hovde O, *Tidsskr Nor Laegeforen* (Norwegian) 110, 2537
  (1988): Small RE+, *Clin Pharm* 7, 766
  (1987): Ikeda N+, *Z Rechtsmed* (German) 98, 141
  (1987): Jeanmougin M+, *Ann Dermatol Venereol* (French) 114, 1400
  (1986): Rodt SA+, *Tidsskr Nor Laegeforen* (Norwegian) 106, 2982
  (1985): Bigby M+, *J Am Acad Dermatol* 12, 866
  (1985): Chevrant-Breton JC, *Therapie* (French) 40, 67
  (1985): Heng MCY, *Br J Dermatol* 113, 597
  (1984): Stern RS+, *JAMA* 252, 1433
  (1983): Klein SM+, *J Rheumatol* 10, 512
  (1982): Park GD+, *Arch Intern Med* 142, 1292
  (1980): Levitt L+, *JAMA* 243, 1262
  (1980): Russell IJ, *Ann Intern Med* 92, 716
Urticaria (<1%)
  (1987): Jeanmougin M+, *Ann Dermatol Venereol* (French) 114, 1400
  (1985): Bigby M+, *J Am Acad Dermatol* 12, 866
  (1984): Stern RS+, *JAMA* 252, 1433
  (1981): Burrish G+, *Ann Emerg Med* 10, 154
Vasculitis (<1%)

Hair

Hair – alopecia (<1%)

Other

Ageusia (<1%)
Anaphylactoid reactions (<1%)
  (1991): Hyson CP+, *Arch Intern Med* 151, 387
  (1985): O'Brien WM+, *J Rheumatol* 12, 13
  (1981): Burrish G+, *Ann Emerg Med* 10, 154
  (1980): Smith F+, *JAMA* 244, 269
Aphthous stomatitis
Death
Dysesthesia
  (1980): Russell IJ, *Ann Intern Med* 92, 716
Dysgeusia (<1%)
Glossitis (<1%)
Gynecomastia
  (1983): Kapoor A, *JAMA* 250, 2284
Headache
Hypersensitivity (<1%) (potentially fatal)
Oral lichenoid eruption
  (1983): Hamburger J+, *BMJ* 287, 1258
Oral mucosal eruption
  (1985): Bigby M+, *J Am Acad Dermatol* 12, 866
  (1977): Calabro JJ+, *Clin Pharmacol Ther* 22, 358 (3%)
Oral mucosal erythema
  (1979): Anderson RJ, *N Engl J Med* 300, 735
Oral ulceration
Paresthesias (<1%)
Pseudolymphoma
  (2000): Werth V, *Dermatology Times* 18
Rectal mucosal ulceration
  (2002): Cruz-Correa M+, *Gastroenterology* 122(3), 641
Serum sickness
  (1984): Stern RS+, *JAMA* 252, 1433

Stomatitis (<1%)
  (1991): Renaut JJ, *Allerg Immunol Paris* (French) 23, 365
  (1978): Brogden R+, *Drugs* 16, 97
Tinnitus
Xerostomia
  (1980): Smith F+, *JAMA* 244, 269
  (1978): Huskinson L+, *Ann Rheum Dis* 37, 89

SUMATRIPTAN

Trade name: Imitrex (GSK)
Other common trade name: *Imigrane*
Indications: Migraine attacks
Category: Antimigraine; Serotonin agonist
Half-life: 2.5 hours
Clinically important, potentially hazardous interactions with: citalopram, dihydroergotamine, ergot-containing drugs, escitalopram, fluoxetine, fluvoxamine, isocarboxazid, MAO inhibitors, methysergide, naratriptan, nefazodone, paroxetine, phenelzine, rizatriptan, sertraline, sibutramine, **St John's wort**, tranylcypromine, venlafaxine, zolmitriptan

Reactions

Skin

Angioedema
  (1995): Dachs R+, *Am J Med* 99, 684
Burning (sic) (1–10%)
Diaphoresis (1.6%)
Erythema (<1%)
Exanthems
Flushing (6.6%)
Hot flashes (>10%)
Hot sensations
  (1991): Multiple authors, *N Engl J Med* 325, 316
Photosensitivity (<1%)
Pruritus (<1%)
Rash (sic) (<1%)
Raynaud's phenomenon (<1%)
Sensitivity (sic)
  (1994): Black P+, *N Z Med J* 107, 20
Urticaria
  (1996): Pradalier A+, *Cephalalgia* 16, 280

Other

Anaphylactoid reactions
Dysesthesia (<1%)
Dysgeusia (<1%)
  (2001): Hershey AD+, *Headache* 41, 693
Glossodynia
Headache
Hyperesthesia (<1%)
Injection-site reactions (sic) (58%)
  (1991): Multiple authors, *N Engl J Med* 325, 316 (10–20%)
Myalgia (1.8%)
Parageusia (<1%)
Paresthesias (13.5%)
Parosmia (<1%)
Xerostomia

TACRINE

Synonym: THA
Trade name: Cognex (First Horizon)
Indications: Dementia of Alzheimer's disease
Category: Anticholinesterase; Cholinergic
Half-life: 1.5–4 hours
Clinically important, potentially hazardous interactions with: fluvoxamine, galantamine

Reactions

Skin
Acne (<1%)
Basal cell carcinoma
Bullous eruption
Cellulitis
Cyst (sic)
Dermatitis (sic) (<1%)
Desquamation (sic)
Diaphoresis
Eczema (sic)
Edema (<1%)
Exanthems (7%)
Facial edema (<1%)
Flushing (3%)
Furunculosis (<1%)
Herpes simplex (<1%)
Herpes zoster (<1%)
Melanoma (<1%)
Necrosis (<1%)
Peripheral edema (<1%)
Petechiae
Pruritus (7%)
Psoriasis (<1%)
Purpura (2%)
Rash (sic) (7%)
Seborrhea
Squamous cell carcinoma
Ulcerations (<1%)
Urticaria (7%)
Xerosis (<1%)

Hair
Hair – alopecia (<1%)

Other
Dysgeusia (<1%)
Gingivitis (<1%)
Glossitis (<1%)
Headache
Myalgia (9%)
Paresthesias (<1%)
Parkinsonism
  (1999): Cabeza-Alvarez CI+, *Neurologia* (Spanish) 14, 96
Sialorrhea (<1%)
Stomatitis (<1%)
Tremor (1–10%)
Xerostomia (<1%)

TACROLIMUS

Synonym: FK506
Trade names: Prograf (Fujisawa); Protopic (Fujisawa)
Indications: Prophylaxis of organ rejection, atopic dermatitis (topical)
Category: Immunosuppressant; Topical for atopic dermatitis
Half-life: ~8.7 hours
Clinically important, potentially hazardous interactions with: beta-blockers, cyclosporine, danazol, erythromycin, **grapefruit juice**, HMG-CoA reductase inhibitors, ibuprofen, immunosuppressants, ketoconazole, lovastatin, mycophenolate, potassium, potassium-sparing diuretics, rifabutin, rifampin, rifapentine, simvastatin, **vaccines**

Reactions

Skin
Burning
  (2002): Rozycki TW+, *J Am Acad Dermatol* 46, 27
  (2002): Russell JJ, *Am Fam Physician* 66(10), 1899
  (2001): Goldman D, *J Am Acad Dermatol* 44, 995 (transient, localized)
  (2000): Reitamo S+, *Arch Dermatol* 136, 999 (46.8%)
  (1999): Ruzicka R+, *Arch Dermatol* 135, 574
  (1998): Alaiti S+, *J Am Acad Dermatol* 38, 69
Connective tissue nevi (sic)
  (1999): Reed BR, Denver, CO (from Internet) (observation) (confirmed by biopsies)
Diaphoresis (>3%)
Ecchymoses (>3%)
Edema (>10%)
Erythema
  (2000): Reitamo S+, *Arch Dermatol* 136, 999 (12.3%)
Erythema (facial)
  (2001): Bohannon JS, Midlothian, VA (from Internet) (observation) (from topical) (following wine)
Exanthems
  (2001): Takamatsu Y+, *Bone Marrow Transplant* 28(4), 421 (with cyclosporine)
  (2000): Reitamo S+, *Arch Dermatol* 136, 999 (4.1%)
Flushing
  (2000): Reitamo S+, *Arch Dermatol* 136, 999
  (1997): Sandborn WJ, *Am J Gastroenterol* 92, 876
Folliculitis
  (2000): Reitamo S+, *Arch Dermatol* 136, 999 (10.8%)
Herpes simplex
  (2000): Reitamo S+, *Arch Dermatol* 136, 999 (13%)
Infections (sic) (>10%)
Irritation
  (2002): Rozycki TW+, *J Am Acad Dermatol* 46(1), 27
Peripheral edema (26%)
Photosensitivity (>3%)
Pigmentation
  (2002): Phillips R, Melbourne, AU (from Internet) (observation)
Pruritus (36%)
  (2002): Russell JJ, *Am Fam Physician* 66(10), 1899
  (2000): Emre S+, *Transpl Int* 13, 73
  (2000): Reitamo S+, *Arch Dermatol* 136, 999 (25.3%)
Purpura
  (1996): Nash RA+, *Blood* 88, 3634
Pustules
  (2000): Reitamo S+, *Arch Dermatol* 136, 999 (6.3%)
Rash (sic) (24%)
Squamous cell carcinoma
  (2001): Otley CC+, *Arch Dermatol* 137, 459

Urticaria
  (2001): Takamatsu Y+, *Bone Marrow Transplant* 28(4), 421 (with cyclosporine)

Hair

Hair – alopecia (>3%)
  (1999): Ushigome H+, *Transplant Proc* 31, 2885 (2 cases)
  (1998): Shapiro R+, *Transplantation* 65, 1284
  (1997): Talbot D+, *Transplantation* 64, 1631
Hair – growth (sic)
  (1994): Yamamoto S+, *J Dermatol Sci* 7, S47
Hair – hirsutism

Other

Anaphylactoid reactions (<1%)
  (2001): Takamatsu Y+, *Bone Marrow Transplant* 28(4), 421 (with cyclosporine)
Application-site burning
  (1997): Ruzicka T+, *N Engl J Med* 337, 816
Dysphagia (>3%)
  (2001): Hernandez G+, *Oral Surg Oral Med Oral Pathol Oral Radiol Endod* 92(5), 526
Gingival hyperplasia
  (2000): Schmutz J+, *Ann Dermatol Venereol* (French) 127, 646
  (1998): Basile C+, *Nephrol Dial Transplant* 13, 2980
Headache
Hyperesthesia
Myalgia (>3%)
Oral candidiasis (>3%)
Oral ulceration
  (2001): Hernandez G+, *Oral Surg Oral Med Oral Pathol Oral Radiol Endod* 92(5), 526
  (2001): Macario-Barrel A+, *Ann Dermatol Venereol* 128(12), 1327
Paresthesias (40%)
  (1997): Sandborn WJ, *Am J Gastroenterol* 92, 876
  (1996): *Arch Dermatol* 132, 419
Tremor (>10%)

TAMOXIFEN

Trade name: Nolvadex (AstraZeneca)
Other common trade names: *Apo-Tamox; Bilim; Istubol; Kessar; Mamofen; Novofen; Tamaxin; Tamofen; Tamoxan; Taxus; Valodex*
Indications: Advanced breast cancer
Category: Antiestrogen; Antineoplastic estrogen receptor
Half-life: 7 days
Clinically important, potentially hazardous interactions with: black cohosh, dong quai, ginseng

Reactions

Skin

Dermatomyositis
  (1982): Harris AL+, *BMJ* 284, 1674
Diaphoresis
  (1986): Buchanan RB+, *J Clin Oncology* 4, 1326
  (1980): Pritchard KI+, *Cancer Treat Rep* 64, 787
Edema (3.8%)
  (1986): Buchanan RB+, *J Clin Oncology* 4, 1326
  (1978): Heel RC+, *Drugs* 16, 1 (2–6%)
Exanthems
  (1999): Descamps V+, *Ann Dermatol Venereol* (French) 126, 716
  (1980): Pritchard KI+, *Cancer Treat Rep* 64, 787
  (1978): Heel RC+, *Drugs* 16, 1 (3.6%)
Flushing (>10%)
  (1999): Drayton G, Los Angeles, CA (from Internet) (observation)
  (1992): Shelley WB+, *Advanced Dermatologic Diagnosis* WB Saunders, 583 (passim)
  (1989): Buckley MMT+, *Drugs* 37, 451 (10–20%)
  (1986): Buchanan RB+, *J Clin Oncology* 4, 1326
  (1981): Ingle JN+, *N Engl J Med* 304, 16 (29%)
  (1980): Pritchard KI+, *Cancer Treat Rep* 64, 787
  (1978): Heel RC+, *Drugs* 16, 1 (14%)
  (1977): Kiang DT+, *Ann Intern Med* 87, 687 (21%)
  (1973): Ward HWC, *BMJ* 1, 13 (12%)
Hot flashes
  (2002): Kinsinger LS+, *Ann Intern Med* 137(1), 59
  (2001): Vogel NE+, *Ned Tijdschr Geneeskd* 145(22), 1041
Peripheral edema
Pruritus
  (1980): Pritchard KI+, *Cancer Treat Rep* 64, 787
Pruritus vulvae
  (1980): Pritchard KI+, *Cancer Treat Rep* 64, 787
  (1978): Heel RC+, *Drugs* 16, 1 (2–3%)
Purpura
  (1978): Heel RC+, *Drugs* 16, 1
Radiation recall
  (1999): Bostrom A+, *Acta Oncol* 38, 955
  (1992): Parry BR, *Lancet* 340, 49
Rash (sic) (1–10%)
Urticaria
Vaginal pruritus
Vasculitis
  (1994): Rzany B+, *J Am Acad Dermatol* 30, 509
  (1990): Drago F+, *Ann Intern Med* 112, 965
Xerosis
  (1978): Heel RC+, *Drugs* 16, 1 (7%)

Hair

Hair – alopecia
  (2001): Puglisi F+, *Ann Intern Med* 134(12), 1154 (total)
  (1993): Litt JZ, Beachwood, OH (personal case) (observation)
  (1980): Pritchard KI+, *Cancer Treat Rep* 64, 787
  (1978): Heel RC+, *Drugs* 16, 1 (2%)
Hair – color change (sic)
  (1995): Hampson JP+, *Br J Dermatol* 132, 483
Hair – hirsutism
  (1980): Pritchard KI+, *Cancer Treat Rep* 64, 787
Hair – hypertrichosis

Other

Depression
  (2001): Day R+, *J Natl Cancer Inst* 93(21), 1615
Dysgeusia
Galactorrhea (1–10%)
Headache
Myopathy
  (1982): Harris AL+, *BMJ* 284, 1674
Thrombophlebitis
  (1996): Zimmet S, *The Schoch Letter* 46, 22 (#86) (observation)
Xerostomia
  (1978): Heel RC+, *Drugs* 16, 1 (7%)

TAMSULOSIN

Trade name: Flomax (Boehringer Ingelheim)
Indications: Benign prostatic hypertrophy
Category: Selective alpha-blocker
Half-life: 9–13 hours

Reactions

Skin
Angioedema
Eczema (sic)
  (2000): Frederickson KS, Novalo, CA (from Internet)
    (observation)
Erythema multiforme
  (1999): Reed BR, Denver, CO (from Internet) (observation)
Pruritus
Rash (sic)

Other
Headache
Tooth disorder (sic)

TARTRAZINE

Synonyms: Acid Yellow T; Acilan Yellow GG; Cake Yellow;
Tartar Yellow S; Wool Yellow
Trade names: E102; FD&C yellow No.5
Category: Food colorant
Half-life: N/A

Reactions

Skin
Adverse effects (sic)
  (1986): Stevenson DD+, *J Allergy Clin Immunol* 78(1 Pt 2), 182
  (1982): Rosenhall L, *Eur J Respir Dis* 63(5), 410
  (1981): Neumann CJ+, *Am J Hosp Pharm* 38(6), 790, 792
Allergic reactions (sic)
  (2000): Bhatia MS, *J Clin Psychiatry* 61(7), 473
  (1989): Pollock I+, *BMJ* 299(6700), 649
  (1988): McLean JD, *Can J Psychiatry* 33(4), 331
  (1987): Pohl R+, *Am J Psychiatry* 144(2), 237 (in antidepressents)
  (1982): MacCara ME, *Can Med Assoc J* 126(8), 910
  (1979): Pellegrin A, *Ann Med Interne* (Paris) (French) 130(4), 211
  (1977): Zlotlow MJ+, *Am J Clin Nutr* 30(7), 1023 (aspirin
    intolerance)
Angioedema
  (1996): Jimenez-Aranda GS+, *Rev Alerg Mex* (Spanish) 43(6), 152
  (1992): Novembre E+, *Pediatr Med Chir* (Italian) 14(1), 39
    (passim)
  (1989): Hong SP+, *Yonsei Med J* 30(4), 339
  (1989): Montano Garcia ML+, *Rev Alerg Mex* (Spanish) 36(1), 15
  (1989): Montano Garcia ML, *Rev Alerg Mex* (Spanish) 36(3), 107
  (1985): Collins-Williams C, *J Asthma* 22(3), 139 (aspirin
    intolerance)
  (1984): Diez Gomez ML+, *Allergol Immunopathol* (Madr)
    (Spanish) 12(3), 179
  (1981): Alvarez Cuesta E+, *Allergol Immunopathol* (Madr)
    (Spanish) 9(1), 45
  (1980): Makol GM+, *Ariz Med* 37(2), 79
  (1978): Mikkelsen H+, *Arch Toxicol Suppl* Suppl 1, 141
Atopic dermatitis
  (2001): Worm M+, *Clin Exp Allergy* 31(2), 265
  (1992): Devlin J+, *Arch Dis Child* 67(6), 709

Dermatitis
  (1990): Dipalma JR, *Am Fam Physician* 42(5), 1347
Edema
  (1989): Pachor ML+, *Oral Surg Oral Med Oral Pathol* 67(4), 393
Fixed eruption
  (1997): Orchard DC+, *Australas J Dermatol* 38(4), 212
Photosensitivity
  (1978): Meneghini CL+, *Z Hautkr* (German) 53(10), 329
Pruritus
  (1981): Alvarez Cuesta E+, *Allergol Immunopathol* (Madr)
    (Spanish) 9(1), 45
  (1978): Neuman I+, *Clin Allergy* 8(1), 65
Purpura
  (1999): Kalinke DU+, *Hautarzt* (German) 50(1), 47
  (1993): Wuthrich B, *Ann Allergy* 71(4), 379
  (1990): Dipalma JR, *Am Fam Physician* 42(5), 1347
  (1985): Parodi G+, *Dermatologica* 171(1), 62
  (1981): Alvarez Cuesta E+, *Allergol Immunopathol* (Madr)
    (Spanish) 9(1), 45
Rash (sic)
  (1995): Thuvander A, *Lakartidningen* (Swedish) 92(4), 296
Urticaria (often related to aspirin intolerance)
  (1996): Jimenez-Aranda GS+, *Rev Alerg Mex* (Spanish) 43(6), 152
  (1993): Wuthrich B, *Ann Allergy* 71(4), 379
  (1992): Novembre E+, *Pediatr Med Chir* (Italian) 14(1), 39
  (1990): Dipalma JR, *Am Fam Physician* 42(5), 1347
  (1989): Baumgardner DJ, *Postgrad Med* 85(6), 265
  (1989): Hong SP+, *Yonsei Med J* 30(4), 339
  (1989): Montano Garcia ML+, *Rev Alerg Mex* (Spanish) 36(1), 15
  (1989): Montano Garcia ML, *Rev Alerg Mex* (Spanish) 36(3), 107
  (1989): Wilson N+, *Clin Exp Allergy* 19(3), 267
  (1987): Settipane GA, *N Engl Reg Allergy Proc* 8(1), 39 (aspirin
    intolerance)
  (1986): Chudwin DS+, *Ann Allergy* 57(2), 133 (aspirin
    intolerance)
  (1986): Simon RA, *N Engl Reg Allergy Proc* 7(6), 533
  (1986): Warrington RJ+, *Clin Allergy* 16(6), 527
  (1985): Collins-Williams C, *J Asthma* 22(3), 139 (aspirin
    intolerance)
  (1985): Podell RN, *Postgrad Med* 78(8), 83, 87, 92
  (1984): Diez Gomez ML+, *Allergol Immunopathol* (Madr)
    (Spanish) 12(3), 179
  (1984): Royal College of Physicians and the British Nutrition
    Foundation, *J Royal College of Physicians of London* 18(2)
  (1982): Ortolani C+, *Ann Allergy* 48(1), 50
  (1982): Warin RP+, *Br Med J* (Clin Res Ed) 284(6327), 1443
  (1981): Alvarez Cuesta E+, *Allergol Immunopathol* (Madr)
    (Spanish) 9(1), 45
  (1981): Juhlin L, *Br J Dermatology* 104, 369
  (1981): Wuthrich B+, *Schweiz Med Wochenschr* 111(39), 1445
    (6.1%)
  (1980): Makol GM+, *Ariz Med* 37(2), 79
  (1980): Valverde E+, *Clin Allergy* 10(6), 691
  (1979): Lindemayr H+, *Wien Klin Wochenschr* (German)
    91(24), 817
  (1978): Mikkelsen H+, *Arch Toxicol Suppl* 1, 141
  (1978): Neuman I+, *Clin Allergy* 8(1), 65
  (1977): Lockey SD Sr, *Ann Allergy* 38(3), 206 (aspirin intolerance)
  (1977): Warin RP, *Hautarzt* (German) 28(10), 511
  (1976): Settipane GA+, *J Allergy Clin Immunol* 57(6), 541 (aspirin
    intolerance)
  (1975): Doeglas HM, *Br J Dermatol* 93(2), 135 (aspirin
    intolerance)
  (1974): Noid HE+, *Arch Dermatology* 109, 866
  (1972): Juhlin L+, *Allergy and Clin Immunol* 50, 92
Vasculitis
  (1999): Kalinke DU+, *Hautarzt* (German) 50(1), 47
  (1993): Wuthrich B, *Ann Allergy* 71(4), 379
  (1990): Dipalma JR, *Am Fam Physician* 42(5), 1347

Other

Anaphylactoid reactions
(1993): Wuthrich B, *Ann Allergy* 71(4), 379
(1989): Montano Garcia ML, *Rev Alerg Mex* (Spanish) 36(3), 107
(1981): Desmond RE+, *Ann Allergy* 46(2), 81
(1981): Schneiweiss F, *Ann Allergy* 46(5), 294
(1980): Kallos P+, *Med Hypotheses* 6(5), 487
(1978): Trautlein JJ+, *Ann Allergy* 41(1), 28
(1977): Morris SJ+, *Arch Intern Med* 137(9), 1222

Arthralgia
(1992): Novembre E+, *Pediatr Med Chir* (Italian) 14(1), 39

Asthenia
(1978): Neuman I+, *Clin Allergy* 8(1), 65

Depression
(1992): Novembre E+, *Pediatr Med Chir* (Italian) 14(1), 39

Gingival hypertrophy
(1989): Pachor ML+, *Oral Surg Oral Med Oral Pathol* 67(4), 393

Hypersensitivity
(1995): Sakakibara H+, *Nihon Kyobu Shikkan Gakkai Zasshi* (Japanese) 33, 106
(1995): Thuvander A, *Lakartidningen* (Swedish) 92(4), 296
(1980): Weliky N+, *Clin Allergy* 10(4), 375
(1979): Weliky N+, *Immunol Commun* 8(1), 65
(1978): Berglund F, *Arch Toxicol Suppl* 1, 33
(1978): Mikkelsen H+, *Arch Toxicol Suppl* 1, 141
(1976): Rosenhall L+, *Bull Int Union Tuberc* 51(1), 515 (aspirin intolerance)
(1976): Stenius BS+, *Clin Allergy* 6(2), 119 (aspirin intolerance)
(1975): Rosenhall L+, *Tubercle* 56(2), 168 (aspirin intolerance)

Paresthesias
(1981): Alvarez Cuesta E+, *Allergol Immunopathol* (Madr) (Spanish) 9(1), 45

Serum sickness
(1978): Wolfe MS+, *Am J Trop Med Hyg* 27(4), 762

Note: Tartrazine intolerance has been estimated to affect between 0.01% and 0.1% of the population. Adverse reactions are most common in people who are sensitive to aspirin. Banned in Norway and Austria

TEA TREE

Scientific names: *Cordyline australis; Leptospermum scoparium; Melaleuca alternifolia; Melaleuca cajeputi; Melaleuca dissitifolia; Melaleuca linafolia*

Family: Myrtaceae

Trade and other common names: Amber Gold; Australian Tea Tree; Burnaid; Cajuput; Dessert Essence; Melasol; New Zealand Manuka,; New Zealand Ti-Tree; Teatree oil

Category: Acaricide; Antifungal; Antimicrobial; Antiviral; Topical antiseptic

Purported indications and other uses: Gram-negative and Gram-positive bacteria, acne, vaginal infection, burns, onychomycosis, tinea pedis, bruises, insect bites, skin infections, mouthwash, genital herpes, antiperspirant, gingivitis, disinfectant, scabies

Half-life: N/A

Clinically important, potentially hazardous interactions with: colophony, turpentine

Reactions

Skin

Adverse effects
(2002): Haller CA+, *Adverse Drug React Toxicol Rev* 21(3), 143

Allergic reactions (sic)
(2002): Haller CA+, *Adverse Drug React Toxicol Rev* 21(3), 143
(2000): Ernst E+, *Forsch Komplementarmed Klass Naturheilkd* 7(1), 17
(2000): Thomson KF+, *Br J Dermatol* 142, 84
(2000): Varma S+, *Contact Dermatitis* 42(5), 309
(1997): Hackzell-Bradley M+, *Lakartidningen* 94(47), 4359
(1994): Selvaag E+, *Contact Dermatitis* 31(2), 124
(1993): de Groot AC+, *Contact Dermatitis* 28(5), 309

Burning
(2002): Groppo FC+, *Int Dent J* 52(6), 433

Dermatitis
(2003): Perrett CM+, *Clin Exp Dermatol* 28(2), 167
(2002): Schempp CM+, *Hautarzt* 53(2), 93
(2001): Fritz TM+, *Ann Dermatol Venereol* 128(2), 123 (7 cases)
(2000): Khanna M+, *Am J Contact Dermat* 11(4), 238
(1999): Bruynzeel DP, *Trop Med Int Health* 4(9), 630
(1999): Greig JE+, *Contact Dermatitis* 41(6), 354
(1999): Hausen BM+, *Am J Contact Dermat* 10(2), 68
(1998): Rubel DM+, *Australas J Dermatol* 39(4), 244
(1998): Wolner-Hanssen P+, *Lakartidningen* 95(30), 3309
(1997): Bhushan M+, *Contact Dermatitis* 36(2), 117
(1997): Kranke B, *Hautarzt* 48(3), 203
(1996): De Groot AC, *Contact Dermatitis* 35(5), 304
(1994): Knight TE+, *J Am Acad Dermatol* 30(3), 423
(1994): van der Valk PG+, *Ned Tijdschr Geneeskd* 138(16), 823 (4 cases)
(1992): de Groot AC+, *Contact Dermatitis* 27(4), 279
(1991): Apted JH, *Australas J Dermatol* 32(3), 177

Eczema
(2002): Dharmagunawardena B+, *Contact Dermatitis* 47(5), 288

Erythema multiforme
(2000): Khanna M+, *Am J Contact Dermat* 11(4), 238

Inflammation
(1999): Syed TA+, *Trop Med Int Health* 4(4), 284 (4 cases) (with butenafine)

Linear IgA dermatosis
(2003): Perrett CM+, *Clin Exp Dermatol* 28(2), 167

Pruritus
(1998): Wolner-Hanssen P+, *Lakartidningen* 95(30), 3309

Rash (sic)

Sensitization
(1999): Hausen BM+, *Am J Contact Dermat* 10(2), 68

Toxicity (sic)
(1995): Carson CF+, *J Toxicol Clin Toxicol* 33(2), 193

Other

Ataxia
(1995): Del Beccaro, *Vet Hum Toxicol* 37(6), 557 (ingested)

Confusion
(1994): Jacobs MR+, *J Toxicol Clin Toxicol* 32(4), 461 (ingested)

Depression
(1994): Villar D+, *Vet Hum Toxicol* 36(2), 139 (ingested)

Hypersensitivity
(2003): Mozelsio NB+, *Allergy Asthma Proc* 24(1), 73
(2001): Fritz TM+, *Ann Dermatol Venereol* 128(2), 123 (7 cases)

Side effects
(2000): Ernst E, *Br J Dermatol* 143(5), 923

Tremor
(1994): Villar D+, *Vet Hum Toxicol* 36(2), 139

Note: Tea tree oil in bottles may undergo photooxidation, and degradation products are moderate to strong sensitizers.

The plant was discovered and named by Captain James Cook of the Royal Navy in 1770, who found groves of trees with sticky, aromatic leaves that, when boiled, made a spicy tea

TEGASEROD

Trade name: Zelnorm (Novartis)
Indications: Irritable bowel syndrome
Category: Serotonin 5-HT4 receptor agonist
Half-life: 11±5 hours

Reactions

Skin
Diaphoresis
Facial edema
Flushing
Pruritus

Other
Back pain (5%)
Breast carcinoma
Depression
Dizziness (4%)
Headache
   (2003): Kellow J+, *Gut* 52(5), 671 (12%)
Limb pain (1%)
Mouth vesiculation
Pain

TELMISARTAN

Trade name: Micardis (Boehringer Ingelheim)
Indications: Hypertension
Category: Angiotensin II receptor antagonist; Antihypertensive
Half-life: 24 hours

Reactions

Skin
Allergic reactions (sic) (<1%)
Angioedema (>0.3%)
Dermatitis (sic) (>0.3%)
Diaphoresis (>0.3%)
Eczema (sic) (>0.3%)
Edema
   (2001): Lacourciere Y+, *J Hum Hypertens* 15(11), 763
Edema of leg (>0.3%)
Flu-like syndrome (sic) (1%)
Flushing (>0.3%)
Fungal infections (sic) (>0.3%)
Peripheral edema (1%)
Pruritus (>0.3%)
Rash (sic) (>0.3%)

Other
Hyperesthesia (>0.3%)
Myalgia (1%)
Paresthesias (>0.3%)
Xerostomia (>0.3%)

TEMAZEPAM

Trade names: Restoril (Mallinckrodt); Temazepam
Other common trade names: *Apo-Temazepam; Cerepax; Euhypnos; Lenal; Levanxene; Normison; Nu-Temazepam; Planum*
Indications: Insomnia, anxiety
Category: Benzodiazepine sedative-hypnotic
Half-life: 8–15 hours
Clinically important, potentially hazardous interactions with: amprenavir, chlorpheniramine, clarithromycin, efavirenz, esomeprazole, imatinib, nelfinavir

Reactions

Skin
Adverse effects (sic)
   (1984): Stricker BH, *Ned Tijdschr Geneeskd* (Dutch) 128, 870
Bullous eruption
   (1999): Verghese J+, *Acad Emerg Med* 6, 1071
Dermatitis (sic) (1–10%)
Diaphoresis (>10%)
Exanthems
Fixed eruption
   (1988): Archer CB+, *Clin Exp Dermatol* 13, 336
Lichenoid eruption
   (1986): Norris P+, *BMJ* 293, 510
Pruritus
Purpura
Rash (sic) (>10%)
Urticaria

Other
Anaphylactoid reactions
   (1988): Mills PJ, *Anaesthesia* 43, 66
Dysgeusia
Headache
Paresthesias
Sialopenia (>10%)
Sialorrhea (1–10%)
Tremor (<1%)
Xerostomia (1.7%)

TEMOZOLOMIDE

Trade name: Temodar (Schering)
Indications: Anaplastic astrocytoma
Category: Antineoplastic
Half-life: 1.8 hours

Reactions

Skin
Edema
   (2003): Hwu W-J, *J Drugs Dermatol* 2, 53 (with thalidomide)
Infections (sic)
   (2003): Hwu W-J, *J Drugs Dermatol* 2, 53 (with thalidomide)
Peripheral edema (11%)
Pruritus (8%)
Rash (sic) (8%)
   (2003): Hwu W-J, *J Drugs Dermatol* 2, 53 (with thalidomide)
Viral infections (sic) (11%)

Other
Headache

Mastodynia (6%)
Myalgia (5%)
Paresthesias (9%)
Tremor
  (2003): Hwu W-J, *J Drugs Dermatol* 2, 53 (with thalidomide)

TENECTEPLASE

Trade name: TNKase (Genentech)
Indications: Acute myocardial infarction
Category: Recombinant tissue plasminogen activator;
Thrombolytic
Half-life: 90–130 minutes
**Clinically important, potentially hazardous interactions
with:** bivalirudin

Reactions

Skin
Angioedema (<1%)
Ecchymoses
Hematomas (local) (12%)
Livedo reticularis (<1%)
Purple glove syndrome (<1%)
Purpura
Rash (sic) (<1%)
Urticaria (<1%)

Other
Anaphylactoid reactions (<1%)
Gangrene (<1%)
Rhabdomyolysis (<1%)

TENOFOVIR

Synonyms: PMPA; TDF
Trade name: Viread (Gilead)
Indications: Management of HIV Infections in combination with
at least two other antiretroviral agents
Category: Antiretroviral; Nucleotide reverse transcriptase
inhibitor (NRTI)
Half-life: 12.0–14.4 hours
**Clinically important, potentially hazardous interactions
with:** acyclovir, cidofovir, didanosine, valganciclovir

Reactions

Skin
Chills
Flu-like syndrome
Purpura
Rash (sic)

Other
Headache
Pain (fingers or toes)
Paresthesias
Tremor

TERAZOSIN

Trade name: Hytrin (Abbott)
Other common trade names: *Heitrin; Hitrin; Hytrine; Hytrinex;
Itrin; Vicard*
Indications: Hypertension, benign prostatic hypertrophy
Category: Alpha-adrenoceptor blocker; Antihypertensive
Half-life: 12 hours

Reactions

Skin
Diaphoresis (>1%)
Edema (1–10%)
Exanthems
  (1998): Hernandez-Cano N+, *Lancet* 352, 202 (generalized)
  (1998): Rosen R, (from Internet) (observation) (following PUVA)
Facial edema (>1%)
Flu-like syndrome (sic) (<1%)
Lichenoid eruption
  (1993): Shelley WB+, *Cutis* 52, 88 (observation)
Peripheral edema (5.5%)
Phototoxicity
  (1993): Shelley WB+, *Cutis* 52, 259 (observation)
Pruritus (>1%)
  (1998): Hernandez-Cano N+, *Lancet* 352, 202
Rash (sic) (>1%)

Other
Anaphylactoid reactions
Headache
Myalgia (>1%)
Paresthesias (2.9%)
Priapism (<1%)
  (1998): Vaidyanathan S+, *Spinal Cord* 36, 805
Tinnitus
Xerostomia (1–10%)

TERBINAFINE

Trade name: Lamisil (Novartis)
Indications: Fungal infections of the skin and nails
Category: Antifungal
Half-life: 22–26 hours

Reactions

Skin
Acute generalized exanthematous pustulosis (AGEP)
  (2001): Rogalski C+, *Hautarzt* 52(5), 444
  (2000): Hall AP+, *Australas J Dermatol* 41, 42
  (1998): Condon CA+, *Br J Dermatol* 138, 709
  (1997): Kempinaire A+, *J Am Acad Dermatol* 37, 653
  (1996): Dupin N+, *Arch Dermatol* 132, 1253 (2 cases)
Allergic reactions (sic) (1–10%)
  (1989): Savin R, *Clin Exp Dermatol* 14, 116
Angioedema
  (1997): Hall M+, *Arch Dermatol* 133, 1213
Baboon syndrome
  (2001): Weiss JM+, *Hautarzt* 52(12), 1104
Dermatitis (1–10%)
Desquamation (sic)
  (1995): Wachs F+, *Arch Dermatol* 131, 960 (passim)
Eczema (sic)

(1997): Hall M+, *Arch Dermatol* 133, 1213 (0.2%)
(1990): Villars V+, *J Dermatol Treat* 1, 33

Erythema multiforme
(1998): Gupta AK+, *Br J Dermatol* 138, 529 (5 patients)
(1997): Hall M+, *Arch Dermatol* 133, 1213
(1995): Todd P+, *Clin Exp Dermatol* 20, 247
(1995): Tramaloni S+, *Therapie* (French) 50, 594
(1994): Carstens J+, *Acta Derm Venereol* (Stockh) 74, 391
(1994): McGregor JM+, *Br J Dermatol* 131, 587
(1994): Rzany B+, *J Am Acad Dermatol* 30, 509

Erythroderma
(1998): Gupta AK+, *Br J Dermatol* 138, 529
(1996): Mitchell D, Charleston, SC (from Internet) (observation)
(1990): Villars V+, *J Dermatol Treat* 1, 33

Exanthems
(2001): Weiss JM+, *Hautarzt* 52(12), 1104
(1999): Valentine MC, Everett, WA (from Internet) (observation)
(1997): Sidhu JS, Malaysia (from Internet) (observation)
(1995): Hofmann H+, *Arch Dermatol* 131, 919
(1995): Wachs F+, *Arch Dermatol* 131, 960 (passim)
(1990): Villars V+, *J Dermatol Treat* 1, 33

Fixed eruption
(1995): Munn SE+, *Br J Dermatol* 133, 815

Lichenoid eruption
(2002): McCarty JR, Fort Worth, TX (from Internet) (observaion) (3 cases)

Lupus erythematosus
(2001): Bonsmann G+, *J Am Acad Dermatol* 44, 925 (subacute cutaneous) (4 cases)
(2001): Callen JP, *Arch Dermatol* 137, 1196
(2000): Callen JP, *Skin & Allergy News* March, 23 (subacute)
(2000): Gruchalla RS, *Lancet* 356, 1505
(2000): Reed BR, Denver, CO (personal communication) (from a meeting presented by Callen JP, Louisville, KY) (4 cases)
(1999): *Ann Dermatol Venereol* (French) 126, 463
(1999): Poster Exhibit #239, AAD Meeting, March 1999 (reported by ED and WB Shelley) (3 patients)
(1998): Brooke R+, *Br J Dermatol* 139, 1132
(1998): Holmes S+, *Br J Dermatol* 139, 1133
(1998): Murphy M+, *Br J Dermatol* 138, 708
(1997): Crowson AN+, *Hum Pathol* 28, 67 (subacute cutaneous)

Peripheral edema
(1997): Hall M+, *Arch Dermatol* 133, 1213

Photosensitivity
(1998): Litt JZ, Beachwood, OH (personal case) (observation)
(1997): Sidhu JS, Malaysia (from Internet) (observation)

Pityriasis rosea
(1998): Gupta AK+, *Br J Dermatol* 138, 529

Pruritus (2.8%)
(2001): Chambers WM+, *Eur J Gastroenterol Hepatol* 13, 1115
(1998): Litt JZ, Beachwood, OH (personal case) (observation)
(1997): Hall M+, *Arch Dermatol* 133, 1213 (0.3%)
(1995): Wachs F+, *Arch Dermatol* 131, 960 (passim)
(1990): Villars V+, *J Dermatol Treat* 1, 33

Psoriasis
(1998): Gupta AK+, *Br J Dermatol* 138, 529 (2 patients)
(1997): Gupta AK+, *J Am Acad Dermatol* 36, 858
(1995): Wachs F+, *Arch Dermatol* 131, 960 (erythema annulare centrifugum-like [sic])

Pustular psoriasis
(2000): Le Guyadec T+, *Ann Dermatol Venereol* (French) 127, 279
(1998): Papa CA+, *J Am Acad Dermatol* 39, 115
(1998): Wilson NJ+, *Br J Dermatol* 139, 168
(1997): Gupta AK+, *J Am Acad Dermatol* 36, 858
(1995): Gupta AK+, unpublished findings

Pustules
(1999): Bennett ML+, *Int J Dermatol* 38, 596

Rash (sic) (5.6%)

(1995): Haroon TS+, *Br J Dermatol* 135, 86

Side effects (sic) (2.7%)
(1990): Villars V+, *J Dermatol Treat* 1, 33

Stevens–Johnson syndrome
(1999): Rosen R, (from Internet) (observation)
(1994): Rzany B+, *J Am Acad Dermatol* 30, 509

Toxic epidermal necrolysis
(1996): White SI+, *Br J Dermatol* 134, 188
(1994): Carstens J+, *Acta Derm Venereol* (Stockh) 74, 391
(1993): Beutler M+, *BMJ* 307, 26

Toxicoderma
(1997): Hall M+, *Arch Dermatol* 133, 1213

Urticaria (1.1%)
(1998): Gupta AK+, *Br J Dermatol* 138, 529
(1998): Rademaker M+, *New Zealand Adverse Drug Reactions Committee*, April, 1998 (from Internet)
(1997): Billon S, *The Schoch Letter* 47, 32 (observation)
(1997): Hall M+, *Arch Dermatol* 133, 1213 (0.3%)
(1995): Wachs F+, *Arch Dermatol* 131, 960 (passim)
(1990): Savin RC, *J Am Acad Dermatol* 23, 807
(1990): Villars V+, *J Dermatol Treat* 1, 33

Hair
Hair – alopecia (1–10%)
(2001): Richert B+, *Br J Dermatol* 145(5), 842
Hair – alopecia areata
(1990): Del Palacio Hernanz A+, *Clin Exp Dermatol* 15, 210

Nails
Nails – onychocryptosis
(2000): Weaver TD+, *Cutis* 66, 211
(1995): Arenas R+, *Int J Dermatol* 34, 138

Other
Ageusia
(2000): Schmutz JL+, *Ann Dermatol Venereol* (French) 127, 341 (persistent)
(1999): Private Patient Query (from Internet)
(1999): Villota Hoyos R+, *Aten Primaria* (Spanish) 23, 102
(1998): Bong JL+, *Br J Dermatol* 139, 747
(1997): Hall M+, *Arch Dermatol* 133, 1213 (0.3%)
(1995): Haroon TS+, *Br J Dermatol* 135, 86
(1995): Martinez-Yelamos S+, *Med Clin* (Barc) (Spanish) 105, 276
(1994): Cribier B+, *Ann Dermatol Venereol* (French) 121, 15
(1993): Stricker BHC, *Ned Tijdschr Geneeskd* 137, 617
(1992): Back D, *Lancet* 340, 252
(1992): Juhlin L, *Lancet* 339, 1483
(1992): Ottervanger JP+, *Lancet* 340, 728
(1992): Stricker BHC, *Ned Tijdschr Geneeskd* 136, 2438

Anaphylactoid reactions

Anosmia
(1993): Beutler M+, *BMJ* 307, 26

Aphthous stomatitis
(1998): Litt JZ, Beachwood, OH (personal case) (observation)

Depression
(2001): Richert B+, *Br J Dermatol* 145(5), 842

Dyschromatopsia (green vision)
(1996): Gupta AK+, *Arch Dermatol* 132, 845

Dysgeusia (2.8%) (metallic taste)
(2001): Lemont H+, *J Am Podiatr Med Assoc* 91(10), 540
(2000): Duxbury AJ+, *Br Dent J* 188, 295 ('persistent')
(2000): Marmelzat J, Los Angeles, CA (from Internet) (observation)
(1999): Marmelzat J, Los Angeles, CA (from Internet) (observation) (lasted for 6 months)
(1997): Danby FW, Kingston, Ontario (from Internet) (observation)
(1997): Hall M+, *Arch Dermatol* 133, 1213 (0.4%)
(1997): Marmelzat J, Los Angeles, CA (from Internet) (observation)

(1997): Sidhu JS, Malaysia (from Internet) (observation)
(1993): Beutler M+, *BMJ* 307, 26
(1992): Ottervanger JP+, *Lancet* 340, 728
Gingivitis
(1998): Gupta AK+, *J Am Acad Dermatol* 38, 765
Headache
Hypersensitivity*
(1998): Gupta AK+, *Australas J Dermatol* 39, 171
(1998): Schlienger RG+, *Epilepsia* 39, S3 (passim)
(1997): Gupta AK+, *J Am Acad Dermatol* 36, 1018
(1996): Gupta AK+, London, Ontario (observation)
(1996): Marmelzat J, Los Angeles, CA (from Internet)
(observation)
(1996): Uhleman J, St. Charles, MO (from Internet)
(observation)
Hypogeusia
(1992): Ottervanger JP+, *Lancet* 340, 728
Hyposmia
(1999): Villota Hoyos R+, *Aten Primaria* (Spanish) 23, 102
Parosmia
(1997): Hall M+, *Arch Dermatol* 133, 1213 (0.02%)
Parotid gland swelling
(1998): Torrens JK+, *BMJ* 316, 440
Serum sickness
(1995): Kruczynski K+, *Can J Clin Pharmacol* 2, 1
Stomatitis
(1998): Gupta AK+, *J Am Acad Dermatol* 38, 765
Tongue pigmentation
(1992): Ottervanger JP+, *Lancet* 340, 728

***Note:** The antiepileptic drug hypersensitivity syndrome is a severe, occasionally fatal, disorder characterized by any or all of the following: pruritic exanthems, toxic epidermal necrolysis, Stevens–Johnson syndrome, exfoliative dermatitis, fever, hepatic abnormalities, eosinophilia, and renal failure

TERBUTALINE

Trade names: Brethaire (Novartis); Brethine (Neosan); Bricanyl (Aventis)
Other common trade names: *Ataline; Brothine; Bucaril; Butaline; Convon; Respirol; Vacanyl*
Indications: Bronchospasm
Category: Beta-2-adrenergic bronchodilator; Sympathomimetic; Tocolytic
Half-life: 11–16 hours
Clinically important, potentially hazardous interactions with: beta-blockers, epinephrine, propranolol, sympathomimetics

Reactions

Skin
Dermatitis (irritant)
(1988): Eedy DJ+, *Postgrad Med J* 64, 306
Diaphoresis (1–10%)
Exanthems
(1996): Drugge R, Stamford, CT (from Internet) (observation)
Flushing
Pruritus
(1996): Drugge R, Stamford, CT (from Internet) (observation)
Urticaria
Vasculitis
(1988): Enat R+, *Ann Allergy* 61, 275

Other
Dysgeusia (1–10%)
Headache
Oral ulceration
(1987): High S, *BMJ* 294, 375
Rhabdomyolysis
(1989): Blake PG+, *Nephron* 53(1), 76
Xerostomia (1–10%)

TERCONAZOLE

Synonym: triaconazole
Trade name: Terazol (Ortho-McNeil)
Other common trade names: *Fungistat; Gyno-Terazol; Tercospor*
Indications: Vulvovaginal candidiasis
Category: Antifungal
Half-life: N/A

Reactions

Skin
Chills
Pruritus (2.3%)
Toxic epidermal necrolysis
(1998): Searles GE+, *J Cutan Med Surg* 3, 85 (from vaginal suppository)

Other
Headache
Vulvovaginal burning (1–10%)

TERFENADINE*

Other common trade names: *Alergist; Allerplus; Cyater; Ferdin; Teldane; Teldanex; Triludan*
Category: Antihistamine H$_1$-blocker
Half-life: 16–22 hours
Clinically important, potentially hazardous interactions with: aprepitant, **devil's claw**, erythromycin

Reactions

Skin
Angioedema (<1%)
(1986): Stricker BHC+, *BMJ* 293, 536
Atopic dermatitis (exacerbation)
(1986): Goodfield MJD+, *BMJ* 293, 1103
Diaphoresis
Exanthems
(1986): Stricker BHC+, *BMJ* 293, 536
Exfoliation (sic)
(1986): Stricker BHC+, *BMJ* 293, 536
Fixed eruption
(1994): Gani F+, *Ann Allergy* 72, 76
Flushing
Lupus erythematosus
Photosensitivity (<1%)
(1994): Berger TG+, *Arch Dermatol* 130, 609 (in HIV-infected) (2 cases)
(1994): Shelley WB+, *Cutis* 53, 121 (observation)
(1986): Fenton D+, *BMJ* 293, 823
(1986): Stricker BHC+, *BMJ* 293, 536

Pruritus
Psoriasis (exacerbation)
 (1990): Navaratnam AE+, *Clin Exp Dermatol* 15, 78
 (1988): Harrison PV+, *Clin Exp Dermatol* 13, 275
Purpura
Rash (sic) (<1%)
Side effects (sic)
 (1995): McClintock AD+, *N Z Med J* 108, 208
Urticaria
 (1986): Stricker BHC+, *BMJ* 293, 536

Hair
Hair – alopecia
 (1993): Shelley WB+, *Cutis* 52, 81 (observation)
 (1992): Frazier CA, *N C Med J* 53, 390
 (1985): Jones SK+, *BMJ* 291, 940

Other
Anaphylactoid reactions
Galactorrhea
Gynecomastia
Myalgia (<1%)
Oral mucosal eruption
 (1990): McTavish D+, *Drugs* 39, 552
Paresthesias (<1%)
Pseudolymphoma
 (1995): Magro CM+, *J Am Acad Dermatol* 32, 419
Stomatitis
Xerostomia (1–10%)
 (1990): McTavish D+, *Drugs* 39, 552

*Note: Terfenadine has been withdrawn in the USA

TERIPARATIDE

Trade name: Forteo (Lilly)
Indications: Postmenopausal osteoporosis
Category: Recombinant segment of human parathyroid hormone
Half-life: 1 hour
Clinically important, potentially hazardous interactions with: digoxin

Reactions

Skin
Allergic reactions (sic)
Diaphoresis
Rash (sic)

Other
Arthralgia
Asthenia
Cough
Depression
Dizziness
Dysgeusia (<2%)
Headache
Injection-site edema
Injection-site erythema
Injection-site pain (<2%)
Leg cramps
Pain
Paresthesias (<2%)
Pharyngitis
Rhinitis
Tooth disorder (sic)

TESTOSTERONE

Trade names: Andro-L.A; Androderm (Watson); AndroGel (Unimed); Andronaq; Delatest; Delatestryl (BTG); depAndro; Duratest; Testim (Auxilium); Testoderm (Ortho-McNeil)
Other common trade names: *Malogen; Testandro; Testex; Testopel*
Indications: Androgen replacement, hypogonadism, postpartum breast pain
Category: Androgen
Half-life: 10–100 minutes
Clinically important, potentially hazardous interactions with: anisindione, anticoagulants, cyclosporine, dicumarol, warfarin

Reactions

Skin
Acne (>10%)
 (1998): Kwon PS+, *Arch Dermatol* 134, 376
 (1995): Tabata N+, *J Am Acad Dermatol* 33, 676 (infantile)
 (1992): Fyrand O+, *Acta Derm Venereol* 72, 148
 (1990): Fuchs E+, *J Am Acad Dermatol* 23, 125
 (1989): Fyrand O+, *Tidsskr Nor Laegeforen* (Norwegian) 109, 239
 (1989): Hartmann AA+, *Monatsschr Kinderheilkd* (German) 137, 466
 (1989): Heydenreich G, *Arch Dermatol* 125, 571 (fulminans)
 (1989): Scott MJ+, *Cutis* 44, 30
 (1989): von Muhlendahl KE+, *Dtsch Med Wochenschr* (German) 114, 712
 (1988): Traupe H+, *Arch Dermatol* 124, 414 (fulminans)
 (1987): Kiraly CL+, *Am J Dermatopathol* 9, 515
 (1984): Lamb DR, *Am J Sports Med* 12, 31
 (1965): Kennedy BJ, *J Am Geriatr Soc* 13, 230
 (1965): Rook A, *Br J Dermatol* 77, 115
Dermatitis (4%)
 (1998): Buckley DA+, *Contact Dermatitis* 39, 91 (from patch)
 (1989): Holdiness MR, *Contact Dermatitis* 20, 3 (from patch)
Edema (1–10%)
Exanthems
 (2001): McGriff NJ+, *Pharmacotherapy* 21(11), 1425
Flushing (1–10%)
 (1965): Kennedy BJ, *J Am Geriatr Soc* 13, 230
Folliculitis
 (1998): Kwon PS+, *Arch Dermatol* 134, 376
Furunculosis
 (1989): Scott MJ+, *Cutis* 44, 30
Lichenoid eruption
 (1989): Aihara M+, *J Dermatol* (Tokio) 16, 330
Lupus erythematosus
 (1978): Robinson HM, *Z Haut* (German) 53, 349
Peripheral edema
Pruritus
 (2001): McGriff NJ+, *Pharmacotherapy* 21(11), 1425
Psoriasis
 (1990): O'Driscoll JB+, *Clin Exp Dermatol* 15, 68
Rash (sic) (2%)
Seborrhea (sic) (<1%)
Seborrheic dermatitis
 (1989): Scott MJ+, *Cutis* 44, 30
Striae
 (1989): Scott MJ+, *Cutis* 44, 30
Urticaria

Hair

Hair – alopecia (<1%)
  (1989): Scott MJ+, *Cutis* 44, 30
  (1965): Kennedy BJ, *J Am Geriatr Soc* 13, 230
Hair – hirsutism (1–10%)
  (1994): Castillo-Ceballos A+, *Med Clin (Barc)* (Spanish) 102, 78
  (1991): Bates GW+, *Clin Obstet Gynecol* 34, 848
  (1991): No Author, *Obstet Gynecol* 78, 474
  (1991): Parker LU+, *Cleve Clin J Med* 58, 43
  (1991): Urman B+, *Obstet Gynecol* 77, 595
  (1989): Scott MJ+, *Cutis* 44, 30
  (1974): Baron J, *Zentralbl Gynakol* (German) 96, 129
  (1971): Fusi S+, *Folia Endocrinol* (Italian) 24, 412
  (1965): Kennedy BJ, *J Am Geriatr Soc* 13, 230

Other

Anaphylactoid reactions (<1%)
Application-site bullae (12%)
Application-site burning (3%)
Application-site erythema (7%)
Application-site induration (3%)
Application-site pruritus (37%)
Application-site vesicles (6%)
Gynecomastia (<1%)
Headache
Hypersensitivity (<1%)
Injection-site pain
  (2002): Amory JK+, *J Androl* 23(1), 84
Mastodynia (>10%)
Paresthesias (<1%)
Priapism (>10%)
  (2001): Madrid Garcia+, *Arch Esp Urol* 54(7), 703
Stomatitis

TETRACYCLINE

Trade names: Achromycin V (Wyeth); Ala-Tet (Del-Ray); Helidac (Prometheus); Panmycin (Pharmacia); Robitet (Wyeth); Sumycin (Par)
Other common trade names: *Apo-Tetra; Economycin; Florocycline; Steclin; Teflin; Teline; Tetramig; Topicycline (Topical); Zorbenal-G*
Indications: Various infections caused by susceptible organisms
Category: Antibiotic
Half-life: 6–11 hours
Clinically important, potentially hazardous interactions with: acitretin, aluminum hydroxide, amoxicillin, ampicillin, antacids, bacampicillin, bismuth, calcium, carbenicillin, cholestyramine, cloxacillin, corticosteroids, **dairy products**, dicloxacillin, didanosine, digoxin, **food**, iron, isotretinoin, methicillin, methotrexate, methoxyflurane, mezlocillin, nafcillin, oxacillin, penicillins, piperacillin, retinoids, sucralfate, ticarcillin, vitamin A, zinc

Reactions

Skin

Acne
  (1971): Bean SF, *Br J Dermatol* 85, 585
  (1969): Weary PE+, *Arch Dermatol* 100, 179
Angioedema
  (1997): Shapiro LE+, *Arch Dermatol* 133, 1224
  (1978): Jolly HW+, *Arch Dermatol* 114, 1485
Bullous eruption
  (1971): Benazeraf C+, *Bull Soc Fr Dermatol Syphiligr* (French) 78, 19

Candidiasis
  (1970): Lehner T+, *Br J Dermatol* 83, 161 (oral)
  (1965): Clendenning WE, *Arch Dermatol* 91, 628
Cheilitis
  (1978): Jolly HW+, *Arch Dermatol* 114, 1485
Dermatitis (sic)
  (1970): Chilvers AS+, *Lancet* 1, 402 (leg)
Diaphoresis
Eczema (sic)
Erythema multiforme
  (1988): Lewis-Jones MS+, *Clin Exp Dermatol* 13, 245
  (1987): Curley RK+, *Clin Exp Dermatol* 12, 124
  (1987): Leroy D+, *Photodermatol* 4, 52 (photodistributed)
  (1987): Shoji A+, *Arch Dermatol* 123, 18
  (1983): Albengres E+, *Therapie* (French) 38, 577
  (1968): Bianchine JR+, *Am Med J* 44, 390
  (1965): Clendenning WE, *Arch Dermatol* 91, 628
Exanthems
  (1993): Chaffins ML+, *J Am Acad Dermatol* 28, 988
  (1979): Patriarca G+, *Boll Ist Sieroter Milan* (Italian) 57, 805 (fixed)
  (1978): Jolly HW+, *Arch Dermatol* 114, 1485
Exfoliative dermatitis (<1%)
  (1978): Jolly HW+, *Arch Dermatol* 114, 1485
  (1972): Kauppinen K, *Acta Derm Venereol* (Stock) 52, 68
Fixed eruption
  (2003): Marmelzat J, los Angeles, CA (from Internet) (observation)
  (1998): Leal G, Fortaleza, Brazil (from Internet) (observation) (pulsating)
  (1998): Mahboob A+, *Int J Dermatol* 37, 833
  (1994): Bielan B, *Dermatol Nurs* 6, 198
  (1991): Thankappen TP+, *Int J Dermatol* 30, 867 (15.9%)
  (1990): Gaffoor PMA+, *Cutis* 45, 242
  (1988): Chan HL+, *Ann Acad Med Singapore* 17, 514
  (1986): Sehgal VH+, *Genitourin Med* 62, 56 (genital)
  (1985): Chan HL+, *J Am Acad Dermatol* 13, 302
  (1985): Dodds PR+, *J Urol* 133, 1044 (balanitis)
  (1985): Kauppinen K+, *Br J Dermatol* 112, 575
  (1985): Pandhi RK+, *Australas J Dermatol* 26, 88
  (1984): Chan HL, *Int J Dermatol* 23, 607
  (1984): Kanwar AJ+, *J Dermatol* 11, 383
  (1984): Pandhi RK+, *Sex Transm Dis* 11, 164 (male genitalia)
  (1982): Kanwar AJ+, *Dermatologica* 164, 115
  (1981): Bhargava NC+, *Int J Dermatol* 20, 435
  (1981): Fiumara NJ+, *Sex Transm Dis* 8, 258
  (1981): Fiumara NJ+, *Sex Transm Dis* 8, 23 (penile)
  (1979): Pasricha JS, *Br J Dermatol* 100, 183
  (1979): Pasricha JS, *Br J Dermatol* 101, 361
  (1979): Patriarca G+, *Boll Ist Sieroter Milan* (Italian) 57, 805
  (1978): Jolly HW+, *Arch Dermatol* 114, 1485
  (1978): Parish LC+, *Acta Derm Venereol* (Stockh) 58, 545 (pulsating)
  (1976): Epstein JH+, *Arch Dermatol* 112, 661 (porphyria-like)
  (1976): Farkas J, *Dermatol Monatsschr* (German) 162, 250
  (1974): Brown ST, *JAMA* 227, 801 (balanitis)
  (1974): Sehgal VN, *Dermatologica* 148, 120
  (1973): Armati RP, *Australas J Dermatol* 14, 75
  (1971): Csonka GW+, *Br J Ven Dis* 47, 42 (balanitis)
  (1970): Brodin MB, *Arch Dermatol* 101, 621
  (1970): Delaney TJ, *Br J Dermatol* 83, 357
  (1970): Duricic S, *Med Arh* (Serbo-Croatian-Roman) 24, 143
  (1970): Savin JA, *Br J Dermatol* 83, 546
  (1970): Tarnowski WM, *Acta Derm Venereol* (Stockh) 50, 117
  (1970): Tarnowski WM, *Arch Dermatol* 102, 234
  (1969): Kandil E, *Dermatologica* 139, 37
  (1969): Minkin W+, *Arch Dermatol* 100, 749
  (1963): Reiner E+, *Arch Dermatol* 88, 465
  (1962): Post CF+, *Arch Dermatol* 86, 678
  (1961): Welsh AL+, *Arch Dermatol* 84, 1004

(1952): Dougherty JW, *Arch Dermatol* 65, 485
(1950): Peck SM+, *JAMA* 142, 1137
Granulomas
(1979): Hagedorn M+, *Dermatologica* 158, 93 (multiple and pyogenic)
Lichenoid eruption
(1974): Maibach HI+, *Arch Dermatol* 109, 97
(1974): Tay C, *Asian J Med* 10, 223
(1971): Almeyda J+, *Br J Dermatol* 85, 604
Lupus erythematosus
(1999): Sturkenboom MCJM+, *Arch Int Med* 159, 493
(1985): Stratton MA, *Clin Pharm* 4, 657
(1980): Condemi JJ, *Geriatrics* 35(3), 81
(1964): Sulkowski SR+, *JAMA* 189, 152
(1959): Domz CA+, *Ann Intern Med* 50, 1217
Lymphoepithelioma
(1973): Sadoff L+, *Lancet* 1, 675
Photosensitivity (1–10%)
(1997): Shapiro LE+, *Arch Dermatol* 133, 1224
(1993): Wainwright NJ+, *Drug Saf* 9, 437
(1989): Rosen C, *Semin Dermatol* 8, 149
(1977): Epstein E, *Arch Dermatol* 113, 236
(1975): Breit R, *Munch Med Wochenschr* (German) 117, 23
(1969): Levene G+, *Br J Dermatol* 81, 712
(1969): Moller H, *Lakartidningen* (Swedish) 66, 1446
(1967): Ippen H, *Z Haut Geschlechtskr* (German) 42, 47
(1967): Tarsitani F+, *Policlinico Prat* (Italian) 74, 329
(1966): Cullen SI+, *Arch Dermatol* 93, 77
(1965): Clendenning WE, *Arch Dermatol* 91, 628
Phototoxicity
(2002): Sorkin M, Denver, CO (from Internet) (observation)
(1980): Stern RS+, *Arch Dermatol* 116, 1269
(1975): Breit R, *Munch Med Wochenschr* (German) 117, 23
Pigmentation
(2001): Dereure O, *Am J Clin Dermatol* 2(4), 253
(1983): White SW+, *Arch Dermatol* 119, 1
(1981): Brothers DM+, *Ophthalmology* 88, 1212 (conjunctival)
(1981): Granstein RD+, *J Am Acad Dermatol* 5, 1 (blue-black)
Pruritus (<1%)
(1995): Nowakowski J+, *J Am Acad Dermatol* 32, 223
Pruritus ani
Psoriasis (exacerbation)
(1990): Bergner T+, *J Am Acad Dermatol* 23, 770
(1988): Tsankov N+, *J Am Acad Dermatol* 19, 629
Purpura
(1965): Horowitz HI+, *Semin Hematol* 2, 287
Pustules
(1973): Thomsen K+, *Br J Dermatol* 89, 293 (palms and soles)
Rash (sic)
(1997): Shapiro LE+, *Arch Dermatol* 133, 1224
Stevens–Johnson syndrome
(1997): Shoji T+, *J Am Acad Dermatol* 37, 337
(1993): Leenutaphong V+, *Int J Dermatol* 32, 428
(1985): Burge SM+, *J Am Acad Dermatol* 13, 665
(1968): Bianchine JR+, *Am Med J* 44, 390
Sunburn (exaggerated)
(1965): Clendenning WE, *Arch Dermatol* 91, 628
Toxic epidermal necrolysis
(1993): Leenutaphong V+, *Int J Dermatol* 32, 428
(1989): Davies MG+, *BMJ* 298, 1523
(1988): Gimova EK+, *Sov Med* (Russian) 6, 119
(1987): Curley RK+, *Clin Exp Dermatol* 12, 124
(1985): Burge SM+, *J Am Acad Dermatol* 13, 665
(1985): Tatnall FM+, *Br J Dermatol* 113, 629
(1984): Chan HL, *J Am Acad Dermatol* 10, 973
(1979): Izmailov GA+, *Khirurgiia Mosk* (Russian) September 102
(1974): Maibach HI+, *Arch Dermatol* 109, 97
(1970): Ocheret'ko MP, *Pediatriia* (Russian) 49, 86
(1967): Lowney ED+, *Arch Dermatol* 95, 359

(1966): Messaritakis J, *Ann Paediatr* 207, 236
(1959): Evans C, *BMJ* 2, 827
Urticaria
(1997): Shapiro LE+, *Arch Dermatol* 133, 1224
(1978): Jolly HW+, *Arch Dermatol* 114, 1485
(1977): McLundie S, *Ann Allergy* 38, 71
Vasculitis
(1960): Calnan CD+, *Trans A Rep St John's Hosp Derm Soc* (London) 44, 69
Warts (flat)
(1975): Gould WM, *Arch Dermatol* 111, 930

Nails

Nails – discoloration (<1%)
(1980): Hendricks AA, *Arch Dermatol* 116, 438 (yellow lunulae)
Nails – onycholysis
(1979): Kanwar AJ+, *Cutis* 23, 657
(1976): Sanders CV+, *South Med J* 69, 1090
(1974): Merrill RH, *South Med J* 67, 677
(1972): Kestel JL, *Arch Dermatol* 106, 766
(1965): Clendenning WE, *Arch Dermatol* 91, 628
Nails – photo-onycholysis
(2002): Rudolph RI, Wyomissing, PA (from Internet) (observation)
(1987): Baran R+, *J Am Acad Dermatol* 17, 1012
(1983): Ibsen HH+, *Acta Derm Venereol* 63, 555
(1978): Hatch DJ+, *J Am Podiatry Assoc* 68, 172
(1978): Lasser AE+, *Pediatrics* 61, 98
(1977): Rothstein MS, *Arch Dermatol* 113, 520
(1973): Verma KC+, *Indian J Dermatol* 18, 23
(1971): Frank SB+, *Arch Dermatol* 103, 520

Other

Anaphylactoid reactions (<1%)
(1965): Clendenning WE, *Arch Dermatol* 91, 628
Black tongue
(1954): Annotations, *Lancet* 2, 179
Fixed intraoral eruption
(1982): Murray VK+, *J Periodontology* 53, 267
Gingivitis
Glossitis
(1978): Jolly HW+, *Arch Dermatol* 114, 1485
Headache
Hypersensitivity (<1%)
(1997): Shapiro LE+, *Arch Dermatol* 133, 1224
(1972): No Author, *Tidsskr Nor Laegeforen* (Norwegian) 92, 1478
Mucocutaneous febrile syndrome
(1972): *Tidsskr Nor Laegeforen* (Norwegian) 92, 175
Mucous membrane pigmentation
Oral ulceration
Paresthesias (<1%)
(1996): Sorkin M, *The Schoch Letter* 45 (5), 18 (observation)
(1994): Blanchard L,, *The Schoch Letter* 44, 6 (observation)
Porphyria cutanea tarda
(1992): Shelley WB+, *Advanced Dermatologic Diagnosis* WB Saunders, 414 (passim)
Pseudoporphyria
(1976): Epstein JH+, *Arch Dermatol* 112, 661
Pseudotumor cerebri
(1999): Quinn AG+, *J Aapos* 3, 53
(1998): Noll K, La Crosse, WI (from Internet) (observation)
(1995): Lee AG, *Cutis* 55, 165
(1986): Pierog SH+, *J Adolesc Health Care* 7, 139
(1981): Steigleder GK, *Z Haut* 56, 839
(1978): Stuart BH+, *J Pediatr* 92, 679
Serum sickness
(1997): Shapiro LE+, *Arch Dermatol* 133, 1224
Thrombophlebitis (<1%)
Tinnitus

Tongue pigmentation
Tooth discoloration (commonly in under 8–year-olds)
(>10%)
  (2002): Kugel G+, *Compend Contin Educ Dent* 23(1A), 29
  (2001): Fukuta Y+, *J Oral Sci* 43(3), 213
  (1998): Livingston HM+, *Ann Pharmacother* 32, 607
  (1994): Hofmann H, *Hautarzt* (German) 45, 803
  (1979): Jackson R, *Cutis* 23, 613
  (1974): Moffitt JM+, *J Am Dent Ass* 88, 547
  (1971): Grossman ER+, *Pediatrics* 47, 567
  (1970): Conchie JM+, *Can Med Ass J* 103, 351
  (1968): *Med Lett<D 10, 76*
  (1964): Stewart DJ, *Br J Dermatol* 76, 374
  (1962): Wallman IS+, *Lancet* 1, 827 (>5%)
Vaginitis
  (1977): Hall JH+, *Cutis* 20, 97
  (1972): Gilgor RS, *N C Med J* 33, 331
  (1972): Litt IF, *Pediatrics* 49, 637

THALIDOMIDE

Trade names: Contergan; Distaval; Kevadon; Thalidomid
(Celgene)
Indications: Graft-versus-host reactions, recalcitrant aphthous
stomatitis
Category: Graft-versus-host disease; Immunosuppressant
Half-life: 8.7 hours

Reactions

Skin
Bullous eruption
  (1975): Sheskin J, *Hautarzt* (German) 26, 1 (5%)
Burning
  (1989): Gutierrez-Rodriguez O+, *J Rheumatol* 16, 158
Dermatitis (sic)
  (1971): Waters MFR, *Lepr Rev* 42, 26
Diaphoresis
  (1978): Smithells RW, *Lancet* 1, 1042
Edema
  (2003): Hwu W-J, *J Drugs Dermatol* 2, 53 (with temozolomide)
  (2000): Oliver SJ+, *Clin Immunol* 97(2), 109
  (1997): Duran McKinster C, *Skin and Allergy News* August, 37
  (1996): Tseng S+, *J Am Acad Dermatol* 35, 969 (passim)
  (1989): Grinspan D+, *J Am Acad Dermatol* 20, 1060
  (1984): Gutierrez-Rodriguez O, *Arthritis Rheum* 27, 1118
Erythema
  (1989): Gutierrez-Rodriguez O+, *J Rheumatol* 16, 158
Erythema nodosum
  (2000): Gardener-Merwin JM+, *Ann Rheum Dis* 53, 828
  (1988): Viraben R+, *Dermatologica* 176, 107
Erythroderma
  (1996): Tseng S+, *J Am Acad Dermatol* 35, 969 (passim)
  (1994): Bielsa I+, *Dermatology* (Basel) 189, 178
Exanthems
  (2000): Camisa C+, *Arch Dermatol* 136, 1442
  (1999): Burrow WH, Jackson, MS (from Internet) (observation)
  (1991): Williams I+, *Lancet* 337, 436 (37% in AIDS patients)
Exfoliative dermatitis
  (1996): Tseng S+, *J Am Acad Dermatol* 35, 969 (passim)
  (1988): Salafia A+, *Int J Lepr Other Mycobact Dis* 56, 625
Facial erythema
  (1989): Gutierrez-Rodriguez O+, *J Rheumatol* 16, 158
  (1975): Sheskin J, *Hautarzt* (German) 26, 1 (1–5%)
Infections
  (2003): Hwu W-J, *J Drugs Dermatol* 2, 53 (with temozolomide)

Nodules
  (2000): Bahl S+, *Skin and Aging,* May, 41
Peripheral edema
  (2000): Camisa C+, *Arch Dermatol* 136, 1442
  (2000): Gardener-Merwin JM+, *Ann Rheum Dis* 53, 828
Pruritus
  (1996): Tseng S+, *J Am Acad Dermatol* 35, 969 (passim)
  (1989): Gutierrez-Rodriguez O+, *J Rheumatol* 16, 158
Psoriasis
  (2003): Dobson CM+, *Br J Dermatol* 149(2), 432
Purpura
  (1996): Tseng S+, *J Am Acad Dermatol* 35, 969 (passim)
Pustuloderma
  (1999): Rua-Figuero I+, *Lupus* 8, 248
Rash (sic)
  (2003): Hwu W-J, *J Drugs Dermatol* 2, 53 (with temozolomide)
  (2002): Baughman RP+, *Chest* 122(1), 227
  (2002): Steins MB+, *Blood* 99(3), 834
  (2002): Tosi P+, *Haematologica* 87(4), 408 (11%)
  (2001): Rajkumar SV, *Oncology* (Huntingt) 15(7), 867
  (2001): Singhal S+, *BioDrugs* 15(3), 163 (30%)
  (2000): Gardener-Merwin JM+, *Ann Rheum Dis* 53, 828
  (2000): Oliver SJ+, *Clin Immunol* 97(2), 109
  (2000): Rajkumar SV, *Oncology* (Huntingt) 14(12), 11
  (1997): Haslett P+, *Infect Med* 14, 393
  (1997): Jacobson JM+, *New Engl J Med* 336, 1487 (>50%)
  (1993): Holm AL+, *Arch Dermatol* 129, 1548 (passim)
  (1986): Hamza MH, *Clin Rheumatol* 5, 365
Red palms
  (1996): Tseng S+, *J Am Acad Dermatol* 35, 969 (passim)
Shaking (sic)
  (1999): Duong DJ, *Arch Dermatol* 135, 1079
Stevens–Johnson syndrome
  (2001): Clark TE+, *Drug Saf* 24(2), 87
Toxic epidermal necrolysis
  (2001): Diggle GE, *Int J Clin Pract* 55(9), 627
  (2000): Rajkumar SV+, *N Engl J Med* 343(13), 972
  (1999): Horowitz SB+, *Pharmacotherapy* 19, 1177
Toxic pustuloderma
  (1997): Darvay A+, *Clin Exp Dermatol* 22, 297
Ulcerations
  (2001): Schlossberg H+, *Bone Marrow Transplant* 27, 229
    (serious)
Urticaria
  (1975): Sheskin J, *Hautarzt* (German) 26, 1 (3%)
Vasculitis
  (1996): Tseng S+, *J Am Acad Dermatol* 35, 969 (passim)
Xerosis
  (2002): Bariol C+, *J Gastroenterol Hepatol* 17(2), 135
  (2000): Bahl S+, *Skin and Aging* May, 41
  (2000): Oliver SJ+, *Clin Immunol* 97(2), 109
  (1989): Gutierrez-Rodriguez O+, *J Rheumatol* 16, 158

Hair
Hair – alopecia
  (1989): Gutierrez-Rodriguez O+, *J Rheumatol* 16, 158

Nails
Nails – brittle
  (1996): Tseng S+, *J Am Acad Dermatol* 35, 969 (passim)

Other
Death
  (2001): Diggle GE, *Int J Clin* 55(9), 627
Dysesthesia
  (1989): Grinspan D+, *J Am Acad Dermatol* 20, 1060
Galactorrhea
  (1996): Tseng S+, *J Am Acad Dermatol* 35, 969 (passim)
Gynecomastia

(2002): Pulik M+, *Am J Hematol* 70(3), 265
Headache
Hyperesthesia
  (2000): Bahl S+, *Skin and Aging,* May, 41
Hypersensitivity
  (2002): Kane S+, *J Clin Gastroenterol* 35(2), 149
Paresthesias
  (2002): Baughman RP+, *Chest* 122(1), 227
  (2000): Bahl S+, *Skin and Aging,* May, 41
  (2000): Ordi-Ros J+, *J Rheumatol* 27, 1429
  (1999): Duong DJ, *Arch Dermatol* 135, 1079
  (1998): Lee JB+, *J Am Acad Dermatol* 39, 835
Tremor
  (2003): Hwu W-J, *J Drugs Dermatol* 2, 53 (with temozolomide)
Xerostomia
  (2002): Bariol C+, *J Gastroenterol Hepatol* 17(2), 135
  (2000): Bahl S+, *Skin and Aging* May, 41
  (1999): Monastirli A+, *Skin Pharmacol Appl Skin Physiol* 12(6), 305
  (1996): Tseng S+, *J Am Acad Dermatol* 35, 969 (passim)
  (1994): Gardener-Merwin JM+, *Ann Rheum Dis* 53, 828
  (1989): Grinspan D+, *J Am Acad Dermatol* 20, 1060
  (1989): Gutierrez-Rodriguez O+, *J Rheumatol* 16, 158

THEOPHYLLINE

(See AMINOPHYLLINE)

THIABENDAZOLE

Synonym: tiabendazole
Trade name: Mintezol (Merck)
Other common trade name: *Triasox*
Indications: Various infections caused by susceptible helminths
Category: Anthelmintic
Half-life: 1.2 hours

Reactions

Skin

Angioedema
Dermatitis
  (1994): Mancuso G, *Contact Dermatitis* 31, 207
  (1993): Izu R+, *Contact Dermatitis* 28, 243 (photoaggravated)
  (1968): De Irureta-Goyena A, *Arch Dermatol* 97, 348
Erythema multiforme (<1%)
  (2003): Johnson-Reagan L+, *Allergy* 58(5), 445 (similar eruptions in 2 siblings)
  (1988): Humphreys F+, *Br J Dermatol* 118, 855
  (1988): Kardaun SH+, *Br J Dermatol* 118, 545
Exanthems (>5%)
  (1982): Sanchez del Rio J+, *Actas Dermosifiliogr* (Spanish) 73, 125
  (1977): Casado-Jiminez M+, *Actas Dermosifiliogr* (Spanish) 68, 675
  (1976): Marron-Gasca J+, *Actas Dermosifiliogr* (Spanish) 67, 701
  (1965): Bowen J+, *Arch Dermatol* 91, 425
Fixed eruption (<1%)
  (1976): Marron-Gasca J+, *Actas Dermosifiliogr* (Spanish) 67, 701
Flushing
Jarisch–Herxheimer reaction
Perianal rash
Pruritus (<1%)
  (1965): Bowen J+, *Arch Dermatol* 91, 425
Psoriasis (exacerbation)
Rash (sic) (1–10%)

Sjøgren's syndrome
  (1995): Bion E+, *J Hepatol* 23, 672
  (1979): Fink AI+, *Ophthalmology* 86, 1892
Stevens–Johnson syndrome (1–10%)
  (2003): Johnson-Reagan L+, *Allergy* 58(5), 445 (similar eruptions in 2 siblings)
Toxic epidermal necrolysis (<1%)
  (1993): Correia O+, *Dermatology* 186, 32
  (1976): Robinson HM+, *Arch Dermatol* 112, 1757
Urticaria (1–5%)
  (1970): Tanowitz HB+, *J Trop Med Hyg* 73, 141

Other

Anaphylactoid reactions
Dry mucous membranes (sic)
Headache
Hypersensitivity (<1%)
Paresthesias
Tinnitus
Xanthopsia (<1%)
Xerostomia
  (1979): Fink AI+, *Ophthalmology* 86, 1892

THIAMINE

Synonym: vitamin B$_1$
Trade names: Betalin; Thiamilate
Other common trade names: *Actamin; Beneuril; Betabion; Betamin; Betaxin; Bewon; Biamine; Thiamilate; Tiamina; Vitantial*
Indications: Thiamine deficiency
Category: Nutritional supplement; Water-soluble vitamin
Half-life: N/A

Reactions

Skin

Allergic reactions (sic)
  (1969): Zheltakov MM+, *Vestn Dermatol Venerol* (Russian) 43, 62
Angioedema (<1%)
Dermatitis
  (1989): Ingemann-Larsen A+, *Contact Dermatitis* 20, 387
  (1958): Hjorth N, *J Invest Dermatol* 30, 261
Diaphoresis
Eczema (sic)
  (1958): Hjorth N, *J Invest Dermatol* 30, 261
Exanthems
  (1980): Kolz R+, *Hautarzt* (German) 31, 657
Pruritus (<1%)
Purpura
  (1989): Nishioka K+, *J Dermatol* 16, 220
  (1980): Nishioka K+, *Clin Exp Dermatol* 5, 213
Rash (sic) (<1%)
Systemic eczematous contact dermatitis
Urticaria
Vasculitis
  (1989): Nishioka K+, *J Dermatol* 16, 220

Other

Anaphylactoid reactions
  (2000): Johri S+, *Am J Emerg Med* 18(5), 642
  (1998): Morinville V+, *Schweiz Med Wochenschr* 128, 1743
  (1997): Fernandez M+, *Allergy* 52, 958
Foetor ex ore (halitosis)
Injection-site reactions (sic)
Paresthesias (<1%)

THIMEROSAL

Trade names: Aeroaid; Mersol; Merthiolate
Other common trade names: *Curativ; Merseptyl; Topicaldermo; Vitaseptol*
Indications: Antiseptic, bacteriostatic, fungistatic
Category: Organomercurial antiseptic
Half-life: N/A

Reactions

Skin

Allergic reactions (sic)
  (2001): Suneja T+, *J Am Acad Dermatol* 45(1), 23
  (2001): Trujillo MJ+, *Allergol Immunopathol* (Madr) 29(4), 133 (with piroxicam)
  (2000): Kiec-Swierczynska M+, *Int J Occup Med Environ Health* 13(3), 179
  (1997): Rees S+, *Br Dent J* 183, 395 (in health care workersr)
  (1997): Wray D, *Br Dent J* 183, 316 (in health care workers)
  (1995): Barbaud A+, *Ann Dermatol Venereol* 122(3), 129
  (1993): Pirker C+, *Contact Dermatitis* 29(3), 152
  (1992): Wonk WK+, *Contact Dermatitis* 26(3), 195
Atopic dermatitis
  (1999): Patrizi A+, *Contact Dermatitis* 40(2), 94
  (1998): Romaguera C+, *Contact Dermatitis* 39(6), 277
Cheilitis
  (1999): Kanthraj GR+, *Contact Dermatitis* 40(5), 285
Dermatitis (sic)
  (2001): Suneja T+, *J Am Acad Dermatol* 45(1), 23
  (2000): Kiec-Swierczynska M+, *Int J Occup Med Environ Health* 13(3), 179
  (2000): Schafer MP+, *Contact Dermatitis* 43(3), 150
  (2000): Westphal GA+, *Int Arch Occup Environ Health* 73(6), 384
  (1999): Lebrec H+, *Cell Biol Toxicol* 15(1), 57
  (1999): McKenna KE, *Contact Dermatitis* 40(3), 158
  (1999): Sertoli A+, *Am J Contact Dermat* 10(1), 18
  (1999): Wolfe, S, Statesville, NC (from Internet) (observation) (eyelids)
  (1998): Ramsay HM+, *Contact Dermatitis* 39(4), 205
  (1998): Romaguera C+, *Contact Dermatitis* 39(6), 277
  (1998): Santucci B+, *Contact Dermatitis* 38(6), 325
  (1997): Luka RE+, *J Allergy Clin Immunol* 100(1), 138
  (1995): Aberer W+, *Contact Dermatitis* 32(6), 367
  (1995): Schafer T+, *Contact Dermatitis* 32(2), 114
  (1995): Zenarola P+, *Contact Dermatitis* 32(2), 107 (systemic)
  (1994): Meding B+, *Contact Dermatitis* 30(3), 129
  (1994): Wantke F+, *Contact Dermatitis* 30(2), 115
  (1994): Zemstov A+, *Contact Dermatitis* 30(1), 57 (bullous)
  (1991): Oritz FJ+, *Contact Dermatitis* 25(3), 203
  (1990): de Groot AC+, *Contact Dermatitis* 23(3), 168 (eyelids, from contact lens fluid)
  (1990): Landa A+, *Contact Dermatitis* 22(5), 290
  (1990): Wekkeli M+, *Contact Dermatitis* 22(5), 295
  (1989): Seidenari S+, *G Ital Dermatol Venereol* 124(7–8), 335
  (1987): Bardazzi F+, *Contact Dermatitis* 16(5), 298
  (1987): Smith JM+, *Practitioner* 231, 579
  (1987): Tosti A+, *Contact Dermatitis* 15, 187
  (1987): Tosti A+, *G Ital Dermatol Venereol* 122(10), 543
  (1986): Melino M+, *Contact Dermatitis* 14(2), 125
  (1986): Moeller H, *Acta Derm Venereol* (Stockh) 57(6), 509 (3.7%)
  (1986): Novak M+, *Contact Dermatitis* 15(5), 309 (in infants)
  (1985): Fisher AA, *Cutis* 36(3), 209
  (1985): Whittington CV, *Contact Dermatitis* 13(3), 186 (eye cream)
  (1984): Miller JR, *West J Med* 140(5), 791 (contact lens solution)
  (1984): Stolman LP+, *N Engl J Med* 311(23), 1521 (contact lens)

  (1982): Rietschel RL+, *Arch Dermatol* 118(3), 147 (contact lens)
  (1981): Fisher AA, *Cutis* 27(6), 580 (merthiolate)
  (1980): Miranda A+, *Actas Dermatosifiliogr* 71(7–8), 301
  (1980): Moller H, *Int J Dermatol* 19(1), 29
  (1980): Sertoli A+, *Contact Dermatitis* 6(4), 292 (soft contact lens)
  (1979): Wllkinson DS, *Contact Dermatitis* 5(1), 58
  (1978): Moriearty PL+, *Contact Dermatitis* 4(4), 185
  (1978): Novak M+, *Cesk Dermatol* (Czech) 53(5), 313
  (1976): Hannuksela M+, *Contact Dermatitis* 2(2), 105
  (1975): *Contact Dermatitis* 1(5), 277
Eczema
  (1999): Patrizi A+, *Contact Dermatitis* 40(2), 94
  (1998): Romaguera C+, *Contact Dermatitis* 39(6), 277
Lichen planus
  (2001): Scalf LA+, *Am J Contact Dermat* 12(3), 146
Lichenoid eruption
  (1984): Lindemayr H+, *Hautarzt* 35, 192
Photoallergic reaction
  (1993): de la Cuadra J, *Ann Dermatol Venereol* 120(1), 37 (with piroxicam)
  (1991): de Castro JL+, *Contact Dermatitis* 24(3), 187 (with piroxicam)
  (1989): de la Cuadra J+, *Contact Dermatitis* 21(5), 349 (with piroxicam)
Photodermatitis
  (2001): Trujillo MJ+, *Allergol Immunopathol* (Madr) 29(4), 133 (with piroxicam)
Urticaria
  (1987): Lohiya G+, *West J Med* 147(3), 341
  (1984): Lindemayr H+, *Hautarzt* 35, 192

Other

Conjunctivitis (allergic contact)
  (1998): *Allergy* 53(3):333
  (1988): Tosti A+, *Contact Dermatitis* 18(5), 268 (eye drops)
  (1980): van Ketel WG+, *Contact Dermatitis* 6(5), 321 (soft contact lens)
  (1978): Pedersen NB, *Contact Dermatitis* 4(3), 165 (soft contact lens)
Hypersensitivity (local)
  (2001): Ball LK+, *Pediatrics* 107(5):1147
  (2001): van't Veen AJ, *Drugs* 61(5), 565
  (1994): van't Veen AJ+, *Contact Dermatitis* 31(5), 293
  (1991): Aberer W, *Contact Dermatitis* 24(1), 6
  (1991): Noel I+, *Lancet* 338(8768), 705 (in hepatitis B vaccine)
  (1991): Osawa J+, *Contact Dermatitis* 24(3), 178
  (1990): Rietschel RL+, *Dermatol Clin* 8(1), 161
  (1989): Tosti A+, *Contact Dermatitis* 20(3), 173
  (1980): Forstrom L+, *Contact Dermatitis* 6(4), 241
  (1975): Maibach H, *Contact Dermatitis* 1(4), 221
Injection-site pain
  (1984): Lindemayr H+, *Hautarzt* 35, 192
  (1978): Wienert V+, *Z Haut* 53(13), 459
Injection-site urticaria
  (1988): Bork K, *Cutaneous Side Effects Of Drugs* WB Saunders, 114
Systemic reactions (sic)
  (1986): Tosti A+, *Contact Dermatitis* 15(3), 187

THIOGUANINE

Synonyms: TG; 6-TG; 6-thioguanine; tioguanine
Trade name: Thioguanine (GSK)
Other common trade name: *Lanvis*
Indications: Leukemias
Category: Antimetabolite; Antineoplastic
Half-life: 11 hours
Clinically important, potentially hazardous interactions with: aldesleukin, **vaccines**

Reactions

Skin
Exanthems
 (1988): Zimm S+, *J Clin Oncol* 6, 696
Malignancies (sic)
 (1997): Zackheim HS+, *J Am Acad Dermatol* 30, 452 (nonmelanoma)
Painful red hands
 (1988): Shall L+, *Br J Dermatol* 119, 249
Petechiae
Photosensitivity (<1%)
 (1988): Zimm S+, *J Clin Oncol* 6, 696
Pruritus
 (1999): Silvis NG+, *Arch Dermatol* 135, 433
Psoriasis
 (1999): Silvis NG+, *Arch Dermatol* 135, 433
Purpura
Rash (sic) (1–10%)

Hair
Hair – alopecia
 (1999): Murphy FP+, *Arch Dermatol* 135, 1495
 (1988): Zimm S+, *J Clin Oncol* 6, 696

Other
Oral mucosal lesions
Stomatitis (1–10%)
Xerostomia
 (1999): Silvis NG+, *Arch Dermatol* 135, 433

THIOPENTAL

Trade name: Thiopental (Baxter)
Other common trade names: *Anesthal; Hypnostan; Intraval; Nesdonal; Sodipental; Trapanal*
Indications: Induction of anesthesia
Category: Anticonvulsant; Barbiturate anesthetic; Sedative
Half-life: 3–12 hours
Clinically important, potentially hazardous interactions with: ethanol, ethanolamine

Reactions

Skin
Angioedema
 (1975): Brown TP, *Anaesth Intensive Care* 3, 257
 (1972): Almeyda J+, *Br J Dermatol* 86, 313
 (1971): Fox GS+, *Anesthesiology* 35, 655
 (1957): Hayward JR+, *J Oral Surg* 15, 61
Bullous eruption
 (1987): Saiag P+, *Ann Dermatol Venereol* (French) 114, 1440
 (1977): Evans JM+, *BMJ* 2, 735

Erythema (<1%)
Erythema multiforme
 (1947): Hunter AR, *Lancet* 1, 47
 (1946): Peterkin GAG, *BMJ* 2, 52
Exanthems
 (1987): Boittiaux P+, *Ann Fr Anesth Reanim* (French) 6, 324 (3.3%)
 (1971): Fox GS+, *Anesthesiology* 35, 655
 (1946): Peterkin GAG, *BMJ* 2, 52
Exfoliative dermatitis
Fixed eruption
 (1995): Bremang JA+, *Can J Anaesth* 42, 628
 (1990): Desmeules H, *Anesth Analg* 70, 216 (non-pigmenting)
 (1987): Saiag P+, *Ann Dermatol Venereol* (French) 114, 1440
Hypopigmentation
 (1979): Coote N+, *Anaesthesia* 34, 336
Pruritus (<1%)
Purpura
 (1972): Almeyda J+, *Br J Dermatol* 86, 313
 (1946): Peterkin GAG, *BMJ* 2, 52
Rash (sic)
Shivering
 (1987): Boittiaux P+, *Ann Fr Anesth Reanim* (French) 6, 324 (27%)
Stevens–Johnson syndrome
 (1946): Peterkin GAG, *BMJ* 2, 52
Toxic epidermal necrolysis
 (1987): Saiag P+, *Ann Dermatol Venereol* (French) 114, 1440
Urticaria
 (1972): Almeyda J+, *Br J Dermatol* 86, 313
 (1972): Barjenbruch KP+, *Anesth Analg* 51, 113
 (1957): Hayward JR+, *J Oral Surg* 15, 61
 (1946): Peterkin GAG, *BMJ* 2, 52

Other
Anaphylactoid reactions (<1%)
 (2001): Garvey LH+, *Acta Anaesthesiol Scand* 45(10), 1204
 (1993): Seymour DG, *JAMA* 270, 2503 (letter)
 (1992): Breathnach SM+, *Adverse Drug Reactions and the Skin* Blackwell, Oxford, 193 (passim)
 (1988): Cheema AL+, *J Allergy Clin Immunol* 81, 220
 (1975): Brown TP, *Anaesth Intensive Care* 3, 257
 (1973): Kelly AJ+, *Anaesth Intensive Care* 1, 332
 (1972): Barjenbruch KP+, *Anesth Analg* 51, 113
 (1971): Davis J, *Br J Anaesth* 43, 1191
 (1971): Sargent NW, *Br J Anaesth* 43, 591
Headache
Injection-site necrosis
Injection-site pain (>10%)
Injection-site phlebitis
 (1981): Clark RSJ, *Drugs* 22,26 (6%)
Porphyria
 (1993): Harrison GG+, *Anaesthesia* 48, 1008–1010
 (1976): Panica D+, *Folia Med Plovdiv* 18, 161
 (1975): Mees DE+, *South Med J* 68, 29
 (1966): Eales L, *Anesthesiology* 27, 703
Rhabdomyolysis
 (1990): Larpin R+, *Presse Med* 19(30), 1403
Thrombophlebitis (<1%)
Twitching (<1%)

THIORIDAZINE

Trade name: Mellaril (Novartis)
Other common trade names: *Aldazine; Apo-Thioridazine; Calmaril; Dazine; Melleril; Ridazin; Thinin; Thioril*
Indications: Psychotic disorders
Category: Phenothiazine antipsychotic
Half-life: 21–25 hours
Clinically important, potentially hazardous interactions with: antihistamines, arsenic, chlorpheniramine, dofetilide, epinephrine, piperazine, quinolones, sparfloxacin

Reactions

Skin
Acanthosis nigricans
  (1979): Arnold HL+, *J Am Acad Dermatol* 1, 93
Angioedema (<1%)
  (1964): Welsh AL, *Med Clin North Am* 48, 459
Dermatitis (sic)
  (1968): Wolpert A+, *Clin Pharmacol Ther* 9, 456
Erythema multiforme
  (1985): Rees TD, *J Periodontol* 56, 480
Exanthems
  (1974): Rothstein E, *N Engl J Med* 290, 521
Exfoliative dermatitis
Hypohidrosis (>10%)
Lupus erythematosus
  (1971): Fabius AJM+, *Acta Rheumatol Scand* 17, 137
Peripheral edema
Photosensitivity (1–10%)
  (1987): Röhrborn W+, *Contact Dermatitis* 17, 241
  (1976): Suhonen R, *Contact Dermatitis* 2, 179
Phototoxicity
  (1967): Satanove A+, *JAMA* 200, 209
  (1960): Barsa JA+, *Am J Psychiatry* 116, 1028
Pigmentation (<1%) (blue-gray)
  (1970): Ayd FJ, *Int Drug Ther Newsletter* 5, 24
  (1969): Berger H, *Arch Dermatol* 100, 487
Purpura
Rash (sic) (1–10%)
  (1981): Georgotas A+, *Psychopharmacology* 73, 292
  (1969): Doyle JA+, *Curr Ther Res* 11, 429
  (1960): May RH+, *J Nerv Mental Dis* 130, 230
Seborrhea
Toxic epidermal necrolysis
  (1987): Harnar TJ+, *J Burn Care Rehabil* 8, 554
Urticaria
Vasculitis
  (2002): Greenfield JR+, *Br J Dermatol* 147(6), 1265 (confirmed on re-challenge)
Xerosis

Hair
Hair – alopecia
Hair – hypertrichosis
  (1979): Phillips P+, *JAMA* 241, 920

Other
Anaphylactoid reactions
Death
  (2001): Glassman AH+, *Am J Psychiatry* 158(11), 1774
  (2000): Timell AM, *Ann Clin Psychiatry* 12(3), 147 (4 cases)
Galactorrhea (<1%)
Gynecomastia
Headache
Hypersensitivity
Lymphoproliferative disease
  (1992): Aguilar JL+, *Arch Dermatol* 128, 121
Mastodynia (1–10%)
Oral mucosal eruption
  (1985): Rees TD, *J Periodontol* 56, 480
Paresthesias
Parkinsonism (>10%)
Parotitis
  (1974): Rothstein E, *N Engl J Med* 290, 521
Porphyria
  (1985): Kamal S+, *Union Med Can* (French) 114, 330
Priapism (<1%)
  (2001): Compton MT+, *Clin Psychiatry* 62(5), 363 (passim)
Pseudolymphoma
  (1988): Kardaun SH+, *Br J Dermatol* 118, 545
Tardive dyskinesia
  (1990): Miller LG+, *South Med J* 83(5), 525 (27%)
Tremor
Xerostomia
  (1981): Georgotas A+, *Psychopharmacology* 73, 292

THIOTEPA

Synonym: TSPA
Trade name: Thioplex (Immunex)
Indications: Breast, ovarian and bladder carcinomas
Category: Antineoplastic
Half-life: 109 minutes
Clinically important, potentially hazardous interactions with: aldesleukin

Reactions

Skin
Allergic reactions (sic) (1–10%)
Angioedema
  (1992): Breathnach SM+, *Adverse Drug Reactions and the Skin* Blackwell, Oxford, 292 (passim)
  (1987): Lee M+, *J Urol* 138, 143
  (1985): Levine N+, *Cancer Treat Rev* 5, 67
  (1981): Weiss RB+, *Ann Intern Med* 94, 66
  (1969): Veenema RJ+, *J Urol* 101, 711
Bruising
Ecchymoses
Eccrine squamous syringometaplasia
  (1997): Valks R+, *Arch Dermatol* 133, 873
Leucoderma
  (1979): Harben DJ+, *Arch Dermatol* 115, 973 (passim)
  (1976): Rosai J+, *Hum Pathol* 7, 83
  (1969): Berkow JW+, *Arch Ophthalmol* 82, 415 (periorbital)
  (1966): Reed RJ+, *Arch Dermatol* 94, 396
Pigmentation (1–10%)
  (1992): Breathnach SM+, *Adverse Drug Reactions and the Skin* Blackwell, Oxford, 292 (passim)
  (1989): Horn TD+, *Arch Dermatol* 125, 524
  (1974): Hornblass A+, *Ann Ophthalmol* 6, 1155
  (1969): Howitt D+, *Am J Ophthalmol* 68, 473
Pruritus (1–10%)
  (1992): Breathnach SM+, *Adverse Drug Reactions and the Skin* Blackwell, Oxford, 292 (passim)
  (1987): Lee M+, *J Urol* 138, 143
  (1985): Levine N+, *Cancer Treat Rev* 5, 67
  (1981): Weiss RB+, *Ann Intern Med* 94, 66
  (1969): Veenema RJ+, *J Urol* 101, 711

Rash (sic) (1–10%)
Urticaria
  (1992): Breathnach SM+, *Adverse Drug Reactions and the Skin*
      Blackwell, Oxford, 292 (passim)
  (1987): Lee M+, *J Urol* 138, 143
  (1985): Levine N+, *Cancer Treat Rev* 5, 67
  (1981): Weiss RB+, *Ann Intern Med* 94, 66
  (1977): Greenspan E+, *JAMA* 237, 2288 (3.8%)
  (1969): Veenema RJ+, *J Urol* 101, 711

Hair

Hair – alopecia (1–10%)
  (2002): de Jonge ME+, *Bone Marrow Transplantation* 30(9), 593
      (permanent) (with carboplatin and cyclophosphamide)
  (1966): Clavert W, *BMJ* 2, 831

Other

Anaphylactoid reactions (<1%)
Injection-site pain (>10%)
Stomatitis (<1%)

THIOTHIXENE

Synonym: tiotixene
Trade name: Navane (Pfizer)
Other common trade name: *Orbinamon*
Indications: Psychotic disorders
Category: Antipsychotic
Half-life: >24 hours

Reactions

Skin

Diaphoresis
  (1968): Wolpert A+, *Clin Pharmacol Ther* 9, 456 (14%)
Exanthems
  (1994): Shelley WB+, *Cutis* 54, 71 (observation)
  (1968): Wolpert A+, *Clin Pharmacol Ther* 9, 456 (14%)
Hypohidrosis (>10%)
Palmar erythema
  (1982): Matsuoka LY, *J Am Acad Dermatol* 7, 405
Peripheral edema
Photosensitivity (1–10%)
  (1970): *Med Lett* 12, 104
  (1966): Gallant DM+, *Am J Psychiatry* 123, 345
Pigmentation (blue-gray) (<1%)
Pruritus
Rash (sic) (1–10%)
Raynaud's phenomenon
  (1991): McCance-Katz EF, *J Clin Psychiatry* 52, 89
Seborrheic dermatitis
  (1984): Binder RL+, *J Clin Psychiatry* 45, 125
  (1983): Binder RL+, *Arch Dermatol* 119, 473
Sensitivity (sic)
  (1982): Matsuoka LY, *J Am Acad Dermatol* 7, 405
Telangiectasia
  (1982): Matsuoka LY, *J Am Acad Dermatol* 7, 405
Urticaria

Hair

Hair – alopecia

Other

Anaphylactoid reactions
Black tongue
  (2000): Heymann WR, *Cutis* 66, 25
Dysgeusia

(2000): Heymann WR, *Cutis* 66, 25
Galactorrhea (<1%)
Gynecomastia
Mastodynia (1–10%)
Paresthesias
Parkinsonism (>10%)
Priapism (<1%)
Sialorrhea
Xerostomia
  (2000): Heymann WR, *Cutis* 66, 25
  (1987): Sarai K+, *Pharmacopsychiatry* 20, 38

TIAGABINE

Trade name: Gabitril (Cephalon)
Indications: Partial seizures
Category: Anticonvulsant
Half-life: 7–9 hours

Reactions

Skin

Acne (>1%)
Allergic reactions (sic) (<1%)
Carcinoma (sic) (<1%)
Dermatitis (<1%)
Diaphoresis (<1%)
Ecchymoses (>1%)
Eczema (sic) (<1%)
Edema (<1%)
Exanthems (<1%)
Exfoliative dermatitis (<1%)
Facial edema (<1%)
Furunculosis (<1%)
Herpes simplex (<1%)
Herpes zoster (<1%)
Neoplasms (benign) (<1%)
Nodules (sic) (<1%)
Peripheral edema (<1%)
Petechiae (<1%)
Photosensitivity (<1%)
Pigmentation (<1%)
Pruritus (2%)
Psoriasis (<1%)
Rash (sic) (5%)
Stevens–Johnson syndrome
Ulcerations (<1%)
Urticaria (<1%)
Vesiculobullous eruption (<1%)
Xerosis (<1%)

Hair

Hair – alopecia (<1%)
Hair – hirsutism (<1%)

Other

Ageusia (<1%)
Depression
  (2001): Kalvianen R, *Epilepsia* 42(Suppl 3), 46
Dysgeusia (<1%)
Foetor ex ore (halitosis) (<1%)
Gingival hyperplasia (<1%)
Gingivitis (<1%)
Glossitis (<1%)

Gynecomastia (<1%)
Mastodynia (<1%)
Myalgia (>1%)
Oral ulceration (2%)
Paresthesias (4%)
Parosmia (<1%)
Sialorrhea (<1%)
Stomatitis (<1%)
Thrombophlebitis (<1%)
Tremor (>1%)
  (2001): Kalvianen R, *Epilepsia* 42(Suppl 3), 43
  (2000): Fakhoury T+, *Seizure* 9, 431 (31%)
Ulcerative stomatitis (<1%)
Vaginitis (<1%)
Xerostomia (>1%)

TICARCILLIN

Trade names: Ticar (GSK); Timentin
Indications: Various infections caused by susceptible organisms
Category: Penicillinase-sensitive penicillin
Half-life: 1.0–1.2 hours
**Clinically important, potentially hazardous interactions
with:** anticoagulants, cyclosporine, demeclocycline, doxycycline,
methotrexate, minocycline, oxytetracycline, tetracycline

Reactions

Skin

Allergic reactions (sic)
  (1994): Pleasants RA+, *Chest* 106, 1124 (in patients with cystic
  fibrosis)
Angioedema
Bullous eruption
Ecchymoses
Erythema multiforme
Erythema nodosum
Exanthems
  (1980): Brogden RN+, *Drugs* 20, 325 (1%)
Exfoliative dermatitis
Hematomas
Jarisch–Herxheimer reaction (<1%)
Pruritus
Purpura
Rash (sic) (<1%)
Stevens–Johnson syndrome
Toxic epidermal necrolysis
Urticaria
Vasculitis

Other

Anaphylactoid reactions (<1%)
Black tongue
Dysgeusia
Glossitis
Glossodynia
Hypersensitivity (<1%)
Injection-site pain
  (1980): Brogden RN+, *Drugs* 20, 325
Injection-site phlebitis
  (1980): Brogden RN+, *Drugs* 20, 325
Oral candidiasis
Serum sickness
Stomatitis

Stomatodynia
Thrombophlebitis (<1%)
Vaginitis
Xerostomia

TICLOPIDINE

Trade name: Ticlid (Roche)
Other common trade names: *Anagregal; Panaldine; Ticlidil;
Ticlodix; Ticlodone; Tiklid; Tiklyd*
Indications: To reduce risk of thrombotic stroke
Category: Antithrombotic; Platelet aggregation inhibitor
Half-life: 24 hours
**Clinically important, potentially hazardous interactions
with:** alteplase, **dong quai**, fondaparinux, **garlic**, **ginger**,
ginseng, horse chestnut (bark, flower, leaf, seed), **red clover**

Reactions

Skin

Acute generalized exanthematous pustulosis (AGEP)
  (2000): Cannavò SP+, *Br J Dermatol* 142, 577
Angioedema (<1%)
  (1999): Chassany O+, *Presse Med* (French) 28, 18
Bleeding (sic)
  (1990): McTavish D+, *Drugs* 40, 238 (1–5%)
  (1984): Stiegler H+, *Dtsch Med Wochenschr* (German) 109, 1240
  (4.4%)
Dermatitis (sic)
  (1998): Ceylan C+, *Am J Hematol* 59, 260
Diaphoresis
  (1984): Stiegler H+, *Dtsch Med Wochenschr* (German) 109, 1240
  (1.7%)
Ecchymoses (<1%)
Erythema
  (1990): McTavish D+, *Drugs* 40, 238
Erythema multiforme (<1%)
  (1999): Yosipovitch G+, *J Am Acad Dermatol* 41, 473
Erythema nodosum (<1%)
Exanthems (1–11.9%)
  (2000): Prost C+, *Presse Med* (French) 29, 303
  (1999): Yosipovitch G+, *J Am Acad Dermatol* 41, 473
  (1997): Litt JZ, Beachwood, OH (personal case) (observation)
  (1990): McTavish D+, *Drugs* 40, 238 (7%)
  (1989): Hass WK+, *N Engl J Med* 321, 501 (11.9%)
  (1987): Saltiel E+, *Drugs* 34, 222 (1–5%)
Exfoliative dermatitis (<1%)
Facial erythema
  (1999): Yosipovitch G+, *J Am Acad Dermatol* 41, 473
Fixed eruption
  (2001): Garcia CM+, *Contact Dermatitis* 44, 40
  (1999): Yosipovitch G+, *J Am Acad Dermatol* 41, 473
Hematomas
  (1984): Stiegler H+, *Dtsch Med Wochenschr* (German) 109, 1240
  (2.7%)
Lupus erythematosus (positive ANA) (<1%)
  (2002): Spiera RF+, *Arch Intern Med* 162(19), 2240 (4 cases)
Petechiae
  (1984): Stiegler H+, *Dtsch Med Wochenschr* (German) 109, 1240
  (1.7%)
Phenytoin toxicity (sic)
  (1998): Klaasen SL, *Ann Pharmacother* 32, 1295
Pruritus (1.3%)
  (1999): Yosipovitch G+, *J Am Acad Dermatol* 41, 473
  (1990): McTavish D+, *Drugs* 40, 238

(1987): Saltiel E+, *Drugs* 34, 222

Purpura (2.2%)
  (2000): Chemnitz JM+, *Med Klin* (German) 95, 96
  (2000): Tsai HM+, *Ann Intern Med* 132, 794

Rash (sic) (5.1%)
  (1999): Quinn MJ+, *Circulation* 100, 1667
  (1999): Whetsel TR+, *Pharmacotherapy* 19, 228

Side effects (sic)
  (1984): Stiegler H+, *Dtsch Med Wochenschr* (German) 109, 1240
    (8%)

Stevens–Johnson syndrome (<1%)

Thrombocytopenic purpura (2.2%)
  (2001): Medina PJ+, *Curr Opin Hematol* 8(5), 286
  (2001): Naseer N+, *Heart Dis* 3(4), 221
  (2001): Yang CW+, *Ren Fail* 23(6), 851 (2 cases)
  (2000): Tsai H-M+, *Ann Intern Med* 132, 794
  (1999): Bennett CL+, *Ann Intern Med* 159, 2524
  (1999): Chen DK+, *Arch Intern Med* 159, 311
  (1999): Elangovan L, *Arch Int Med* 159, 1624
  (1999): Mauro M+, *Blood* 94, 1–646a
  (1999): Steinhubl SR+, *JAMA* 281, 806
  (1998): Bennett CL+, *Ann Intern Med* 128, 541
  (1998): Bennett CL+, *Lancet* 352, 1036
  (1998): Jamar S+, *Acta Cardiol* 53, 285
  (1998): Mukamal KJ+, *Ann Intern Med* 129, 837
  (1998): Muszkat M+, *Pharmacotherapy* 18, 1352
  (1997): Kupfer Y+, *N Engl J Med* 337, 1245
  (1996): Wysowski DK+, *JAMA* 276, 952
  (1991): Page Y+, *Lancet* 337, 774
  (1990): McTavish D+, *Drugs* 40, 238 (1–5%)
  (1990): Takishita S+, *N Engl J Med* 323, 1487
  (1989): Hass WK+, *N Engl J Med* 321, 501 (4%)
  (1984): Stiegler H+, *Dtsch Med Wochenschr* (German) 109, 1240
    (1–5%)
  (1982): de Fraiture WH+, *Ned Tijdschr Geneeskd* (Dutch)
    126, 1051

Toxic erythroderma (sic)
  (1999): Hsi DH+, *N Engl J Med* 340, 1212

Urticaria (<1%)
  (1999): Yosipovitch G+, *J Am Acad Dermatol* 41, 473
  (1990): McTavish D+, *Drugs* 40, 238
  (1989): Hass WK+, *N Engl J Med* 321, 501 (2%)
  (1987): Saltiel E+, *Drugs* 34, 222 (1–5%)

Vasculitis (<1%)
  (2001): Pintor E+, *Rev Esp Cardiol* 54(1), 114

Other

Erythromelalgia
  (1999): Yosipovitch G+, *J Am Acad Dermatol* 41, 473
Headache
Serum sickness
Tinnitus

TIMOLOL

Trade names: Betimol; Blocadren (Merck); CoSopt (Merck);
Timolide (Merck); Timoptic (ophthalmic) (Merck)
Other common trade names: Apo-Timol; Aquanil; Dispatim;
Nu-Timolol; Tenopt; Tiloptic; Timacor; Timoptol
Indications: Hypertension
Category: Antihypertensive; Beta-adrenoceptor blocker
Half-life: 2–2.7 hours
**Clinically important, potentially hazardous interactions
with:** clonidine, epinephrine, ergot, verapamil

CoSopt is timolol and dorzolamide; Timolide is timolol and
hydrochlorothiazide. Dorzolamide and hydrochlorothiazide are
sulfonamides and can be absorbed systemically. Sulfonamides can
produce severe, possibly fatal, reactions such as toxic epidermal
necrolysis and Stevens–Johnson syndrome

Reactions

Skin

Angioedema
Burning (from ophthalmic)
Dermatitis (sic) (eyedrops)
  (2001): Holdiness MR, *Am J Contact Dermat* 12(4), 217
  (2000): Quiralte J+, *Contact Dermatitis* 42, 245
  (1998): Lewis B, Colorado Springs, CO (from Internet)
    (observation) (glans penis)
  (1995): Koch P, *Contact Dermatitis* 33, 140
  (1993): Corazza M+, *Contact Dermatitis* 28, 188
  (1993): O'Donnell BF+, *Contact Dermatitis* 28, 121
  (1991): Cameli N+, *Contact Dermatitis* 25, 129
  (1991): Kubota K+, *Br J Clin Pharmacol* 31, 471
  (1988): Kanzaki T+, *Contact Dermatitis* 19, 388
  (1986): Fernandez-Vozmediano JM+, *Contact Dermatitis* 14, 252
  (1986): Romaguera C+, *Contact Dermatitis* 14, 248
Diaphoresis
Eczema (sic)
  (1991): Cameli N+, *Contact Dermatitis* 25, 129
  (1979): van Joost T, *Br J Dermatol* 101, 171
Edema (0.6%)
Erythema multiforme
Erythroderma
  (1997): Shelley WB+, *J Am Acad Dermatol* 37, 799
  (1993): Shelley WB+, *Cutis* 51, 330 (observation)
Exanthems
Exfoliative dermatitis
Hyperkeratosis (palms and soles)
Lichenoid eruption
  (1978): Savage RL+, *BMJ* 1, 987
Lupus erythematosus
  (1994): Cohen MG, *J Rheumatol* 21, 578
  (1992): Zamber RW+, *J Rheumatol* 19, 977
Pemphigus
  (1987): Fiore PM+, *Arch Ophthalmol* 105, 1660
Photosensitivity
Pigmentation
Pityriasis rubra pilaris
  (1978): Finlay AY+, *BMJ* 1, 987
Pruritus (1–5%)
  (1996): Lazarov A+, *Cutis* 58, 363 (from eye drops)
Psoriasis
  (1992): Germain ML+, *Therapie* (French) 47, 447
  (1989): Puig L+, *Am J Ophthalmol* 108, 455
  (1987): Savola J+, *BMJ* 295, 637 (also aggravation of psoriasis)
  (1986): Czernielewski J+, *Lancet* 1, 808
  (1984): Arntzen N+, *Acta Derm Venereol* (Stockh) 64, 346
Purpura
Rash (sic) (1–10%)
Raynaud's phenomenon
  (1984): Eliasson K+, *Acta Med Scand* 215, 333
  (1976): Marshall AJ+, *BMJ* 1, 1498
Stinging (from ophthalmic)
Toxic epidermal necrolysis
Urticaria
Xerosis

Hair

Hair – alopecia (also from Timoptic eye drops) (1–10%)
  (1990): Fraunfelder FT+, *JAMA* 263, 1493

Nails

Nails – dystrophy
Nails – onycholysis
Nails – pigmentation
   (1981): Feiler-Ofry V, *Ophthalmologica* (Basel) 182, 153

Other

Anaphylactoid reactions
Digital necrosis
   (1989): Dompmartin A+, *Ann Dermatol Venereol* (French)
      115, 593
Dysgeusia
Headache
Myalgia
Ocular allergy
   (1998): LeBlanc RP, *Ophthalmology* 105, 1960
   (1996): Schuman JS, *Surv Ophthalmol* 41, S27
Ocular burning
   (1998): LeBlanc RP, *Ophthalmology* 105, 1960
   (1997): Schuman JS+, *Arch Ophthalmol* 115, 847 (41.9%)
   (1996): Schuman JS, *Surv Ophthalmol* 41, S27
Ocular pemphigoid
   (1992): Shelley WB+, *Advanced Dermatologic Diagnosis* WB
      Saunders, 554 (passim)
Ocular stinging
   (1998): LeBlanc RP, *Ophthalmology* 105, 1960
   (1997): Schuman JS+, *Arch Ophthalmol* 115, 847 (41.9%)
   (1996): Schuman JS, *Surv Ophthalmol* 41, S27
Oculo-mucocutaneous syndrome
   (1982): Cocco G+, *Curr Ther Res* 31, 362
Oral lichenoid eruption
Paresthesias (<1%)
Peyronie's disease
   (1979): Pryor JP+, *Lancet* 1, 331
Tinnitus
Xerostomia
   (1998): LeBlanc RP, *Ophthalmology* 105, 1960
   (1997): Schuman JS+, *Arch Ophthalmol* 115, 847 (19.4%)
   (1996): Schuman JS, *Surv Ophthalmol* 41, S27

Note: Cutaneous side-effects of beta-receptor blockaders are clinically polymorphous. They apparently appear after several months of continuous therapy. Atypical psoriasiform, lichen planus-like, and eczematous chronic rashes are mainly observed. (1983): Hödl St, *Z Hautkr* (German) 1:58, 17

TINZAPARIN

Trade name: Innohep (Pharmion)
Indications: Acute symptomatic deep vein thrombosis
Category: Anticoagulant; Low-molecular weight heparin;
Thrombolytic
Half-life: 3–4 hours
**Clinically important, potentially hazardous interactions
with:** butabarbital

Reactions

Skin

Abscess (<1%)
Allergic reactions (sic)
Angioedema (<1%)
Bullous eruption (1–10%)
Cellulitis (<1%)
Ecchymoses

Exanthems (<1%)
Infections (sic)
Necrosis (sic) (1%)
Neoplasms (sic)
Pruritus (1–10%)
Purpura (<1%)
   (1996): Simpson HK+, *Haemostasis* 26, 90
Rash (sic) (1%)
Urticaria (<1%)

Hair

Hair – alopecia
   (2003): Sarris W+, *Am J Kidney Dis* 41(5)

Other

Anaphylactoid reactions (In sulfite-sensitive people)
Headache
Hypersensitivity
Injection-site bleeding
   (2002): Wong NN, *Heart Dis* 4, 331
Injection-site hematoma (16%)
Injection-site pain
Phlebitis
Priapism (<1%)
   (2002): Wong NN, *Heart Dis* 4, 331
Thrombophlebitis

TIOPRONIN

Trade name: Thiola (Mission)
Other common trade names: *Acadione; Captimer*
Indications: Cystinuria
Category: Antiurolithic
Half-life: N/A

Reactions

Skin

Angioedema
   (1988): Sigaud M+, *Rev Rhum Mal Osteoartic* (French) 55, 467
      (14.5%)
Bullous pemphigoid
   (1988): Nakajima H+, *Nippon Hifuka Gakkai Zasshi* (Japanese)
      98, 803
Dermatitis
   (1995): Romano A+, *Contact Dermatitis* 33, 269
Ecchymoses
Edema
Elastosis perforans serpiginosa
Erythema
   (1990): Sany J+, *Rev Rhum Mal Osteoartic* (French) 57, 105
Erythema multiforme
   (1988): Nakajima H+, *Nippon Hifuka Gakkai Zasshi* (Japanese)
      98, 803
Exanthems
   (1988): Sigaud M+, *Rev Rhum Mal Osteoartic* (French) 55, 467
      (14.5%)
   (1984): Shichiri M+, *Arch Intern Med* 144, 89
Lichenoid eruption
   (1994): Pierard E+, *J Am Acad Dermatol* 31, 665
   (1990): Kurumaji Y+, *J Dermatol* (Tokio) 17, 176
   (1988): Kawabe Y+, *J Dermatol* (Tokio) 15, 434 (bullous)
Lupus erythematosus
   (1986): Katayama I+, *J Dermatol* (Tokio) 13, 151
Pemphigus

(1994): Verdier-Sevrain S+, *Br J Dermatol* 130, 238
(1990): Meuhier L+, *Ann Dermatol Venereol* (French) 117, 959
(1990): Sany J+, *Rev Rhum Mal Osteoartic* (French) 57, 105
(1988): Sigaud M+, *Rev Rhum Mal Osteoartic* (French) 55, 467
(5.8%)
(1987): Enjolras O+, *Ann Dermatol Venereol* (French) 114, 25
Pemphigus erythematosus
(1982): Alinovi A+, *Acta Derm Venereol* (Stockh) 62, 452
Pemphigus foliaceus
(1983): Lucky PA+, *J Am Acad Dermatol* 8, 667
Photosensitivity
(1988): Sigaud M+, *Rev Rhum Mal Osteoartic* (French) 55, 467
(1.5%)
Pityriasis rosea
(1990): Sany J+, *Rev Rhum Mal Osteoartic* (French) 57, 105
(1988): Sigaud M+, *Rev Rhum Mal Osteoartic* (French) 55, 467
(5.8%)
Pruritus
Rash (sic)
Side effects (sic)
(1988): Sigaud M+, *Rev Rhum Mal Osteoartic* (French) 55, 467
(27.5%)
Toxic epidermal necrolysis
Urticaria
Wrinkling (sic)

Hair
Hair – alopecia
(1990): Sany J+, *Rev Rhum Mal Osteoartic* (French) 57, 105
Hair – hypertrichosis
(1993): Arnaud M+, *Joint Bone Spine Dis* 60, 548

Other
Ageusia
(1989): Mordini M+, *Minerva Med* 80(9), 1019
Hypogeusia
Mucocutaneous reactions (sic)
(1990): Sany J+, *Rev Rhum Mal Osteoartic* (French) 57, 105
(32.8%)
Myopathy
(1988): Menkes CJ+, *Presse Med* (French) 17, 1156
Oral mucosal lesions
(1988): Sigaud M+, *Rev Rhum Mal Osteoartic* (French) 55, 467
(4.4%)
(1984): Shichiri M+, *Arch Intern Med* 144, 89
Oral ulceration
(2000): Madinier I+, *Ann Med Interne (Paris)* (French) 151, 248
Parageusia
Parosmia
Polymyositis
(1999): Cacoub B+, *Presse Med* (French) 28, 911
Stomatitis
(1990): Sany J+, *Rev Rhum Mal Osteoartic* (French) 57, 105
(1988): Sigaud M+, *Rev Rhum Mal Osteoartic* (French) 55, 467
Xerostomia

TIROFIBAN

Trade name: Aggrastat (Merck)
Indications: Acute coronary syndrome
Category: Platelet aggregation inhibitor
Half-life: 2 hours
**Clinically important, potentially hazardous interactions
with:** aspirin, fondaparinux, heparin, NSAIDs

Reactions

Skin
Bleeding (sic)
Diaphoresis (2%)
Edema (2%)
Rash (sic) (<1%)
Urticaria (<1%)

Other
Limb pain (3%)

TIZANIDINE

Trade name: Zanaflex (Elan)
Other common trade names: *Sirdalud; Ternalax; Ternelin*
Indications: Muscle spasticity, multiple sclerosis
Category: Alpha-2-adrenoceptor blocker
Half-life: 2.5 hours

Reactions

Skin
Acne (<1%)
Allergic reactions (sic) (<1%)
Candidiasis (<1%)
Cellulitis (<1%)
Diaphoresis (>1%)
Ecchymoses (<1%)
Edema (<1%)
Exanthems (<1%)
Exfoliative dermatitis (<1%)
Herpes simplex (<1%)
Herpes zoster (<1%)
Petechiae (<1%)
Pruritus (1–10%)
Purpura (<1%)
Rash (sic) (1–10%)
Ulcerations (>1%)
Urticaria (<1%)
Xerosis (<1%)

Hair
Hair – alopecia (<1%)

Other
Paresthesias (>1%)
Tremor (1–10%)
Vaginal candidiasis (<1%)
Xerostomia (49%)

TOBRAMYCIN

Trade names: Nebcin (Lilly); TOBI (Chiron); TobraDex (Alcon);
Tobrex
Other common trade names: *AKTob Ophthalmic; Oftalmotrisol-T; Tobra*
Indications: Various serious infections caused by susceptible
organisms, superficial ocular infections
Category: Aminoglycoside antibiotic
Half-life: 2–3 hours
**Clinically important, potentially hazardous interactions
with:** adefovir, aldesleukin, aminoglycosides, atracurium,
bumetanide, doxacurium, ethacrynic acid, furosemide,
neuromuscular blockers, pancuronium, polypeptide antibiotics,
rocuronium, succinylcholine, torsemide, vecuronium

TobraDex is tobramycin and dexamethasone

Reactions

Skin
Dermatitis (from ophthalmic preparations) (<1%)
    (2002): Litt JZ, Beachwood, OH (personal observation) (eyelids)
    (1998): Litt JZ, Beachwood, OH (personal case) (observation)
    (1995): Caraffini S+, *Contact Dermatitis* 32, 186
    (1990): Menendez-Ramos F+, *Contact Dermatitis* 22, 305
Eczema (sic)
Erythema multiforme
    (1983): Ansel J+, *Arch Dermatol* 119, 1006
Exanthems
    (2002): Spigarelli MG+, *Pediatr Pulmonol* 33(4), 311
    (1991): Karp S+, *Cutis* 47, 331
    (1976): Brogden RN+, *Drugs* 12, 166
Exfoliative dermatitis
    (1991): Karp S+, *Cutis* 47, 331
Eyelid edema (from ophthalmic preparations) (<1%)
Pruritus (<1%)
    (1976): Brogden RN+, *Drugs* 12, 166
Purpura
Radiation recall
    (2001): Krishnan RS+, *J Am Acad Dermatol* 44, 1045 (ultraviolet)
        (with piperacillin & ciprofloxacin)
Rash (sic) (<1%)
    (2002): Spigarelli MG+, *Pediatr Pulmonol* 33(4), 311
Side effects (sic)
    (1976): Brogden RN+, *Drugs* 12, 166 (<1%)
Urticaria

Other
Headache
Hypersensitivity
    (2002): Spigarelli MG+, *Pediatr Pulmonol* 33(4), 311
    (1995): Schretlen-Doherty JS+, *Ann Pharmacother* 29, 704
Injection-site pain
Paresthesias (<1%)
Sialorrhea
Tinnitus
    (2002): *Prescrire Int* 11(62), 177
Tremor (<1%)

TOCAINIDE

Trade name: Tonocard (AstraZeneca)
Indications: Ventricular arrhythmias
Category: Antiarrhythmic class I B
Half-life: 11–14 hours

Reactions

Skin
Allergic reactions (sic)
    (1987): Arrowsmith JB+, *Ann Intern Med* 107, 693
    (1985): Coulter DM+, *N Z Med J* 98, 553
Clammy skin
Diaphoresis (<1%)
Erythema multiforme (<1%)
Exanthems
    (1988): Dunn JM+, *Drug Intell Clin Pharm* 22, 142
Exfoliative dermatitis (<1%)
Lupus erythematosus (<1%)
    (1994): Gelfand MS+, *South Med J* 87, 839
    (1988): Oliphant LD+, *Chest* 94, 427
Pallor (<1%)
Pruritus (<1%)
Rash (sic) (0.5–8.4%)
Stevens–Johnson syndrome (<1%)
Vasculitis (<1%)

Hair
Hair – alopecia (<1%)

Other
Dysgeusia (8.4%)
Gingivitis
    (1988): Dunn JM+, *Drug Intell Clin Pharm* 22, 142
Headache
Hypersensitivity (<1%)
Myalgia (<1%)
Paresthesias (3.5–9%)
Parosmia (<1%)
Stomatitis (<1%)
Tinnitus
Xerostomia (<1%)

TOLAZAMIDE

Trade name: Tolinase (Pharmacia)
Other common trade names: *Diabewas; Diadutos; Norglycin;
Tolanase; Tolisan*
Indications: Non-insulin dependent diabetes type II
Category: First generation sulfonylurea hypoglycemic
Half-life: 7 hours
**Clinically important, potentially hazardous interactions
with:** phenylbutazones

Reactions

Skin
Dermatitis (sic)
    (1966): Beidleman P+, *J Fla Med Assoc* 53, 191
Diaphoresis
Eczema (sic)
    (1985): Frosch PJ+, *Contact Dermatitis* 13, 272
Erythema (0.4%)

Exanthems (0.4%)
Lichenoid eruption
  (1990): Franz CB+, *J Am Acad Dermatol* 22, 128
  (1984): Barnett JH+, *Cutis* 34, 542
Lupus erythematosus
Photosensitivity (1–10%)
Pruritus (0.4%)
Purpura
Rash (sic) (1–10%)
Urticaria (1–10%)

Other
Acute intermittent porphyria
Dysgeusia
Paresthesias
Porphyria cutanea tarda
Tongue ulceration
  (1984): Barnett JH+, *Cutis* 34, 542

*Note: Tolazamide is a sulfonamide and can be absorbed systemically. Sulfonamides can produce severe, possibly fatal, reactions such as toxic epidermal necrolysis and Stevens–Johnson syndrome

TOLAZOLINE

Trade name: Priscoline (Novartis)
Indications: Pulmonary hypertension in the newborn
Category: Alpha-adrenoceptor blocker; Antihypertensive (of the newborn); Peripheral vasodilator
Half-life: 3–10 hours (neonates)

Reactions

Skin
Dermatitis
  (1985): Frosch PJ+, *Contact Dermatitis* 13, 272
Edema
Exanthems
  (1989): Cambazard F+, *Ann Dermatol Venereol* (French) 116, 499
Flushing
  (1972): Coffman JD+, *Ann Intern Med* 76, 35 (66%)
Rash (sic)
Urticaria

Other
Injection-site burning (>10%)

TOLBUTAMIDE

Trade name: Orinase (Pharmacia)
Other common trade names: *Abemin; Aglycid; Diaben; Diatol; Dolipol; Mobenol; Novo-Butamid; Orabet; Rastinon*
Indications: Non-insulin dependent diabetes type II
Category: First generation sulfonylurea hypoglycemic
Half-life: 4–25 hours
Clinically important, potentially hazardous interactions with: aprepitant, phenylbutazones

Reactions

Skin
Allergic reactions (sic)
  (1965): Bernhard H, *Diabetes* 14, 59 (0.8%)

Bullous eruption (<1%)
Bullous pemphigoid
  (1975): Glander HJ+, *Derm Monatsschr* (German) 161, 455
Dermatitis
  (1982): Fisher AA, *Cutis* 29, 551 (systemic)
Erythema (1.1%)
Erythema multiforme (<1%)
Exanthems (1–5%)
  (1972): Kuokkanen K, *Acta Allergol* 27, 407
  (1971): Harris EL, *BMJ* 3, 29 (1–5%)
  (1969): *Postgrad Med* 45, 211
Fixed eruption (<1%)
Flushing
  (1981): Capretti L+, *BMJ* 283, 1361
  (1966): Cohen P+, *JAMA* 197, 817
  (1966): Muller SA, *Proc Staff Meet Mayo Clin* 41, 689
Lichenoid eruption
  (1963): Hurlbut WB, *Arch Dermatol* 88, 105
Photosensitivity (1–10%)
  (1984): Kar PK+, *J Indian Med Assoc* 82, 289
  (1978): Meneghini CL+, *Z Haut* (German) 53, 329
Poikiloderma
  (1965): Esteves J+, *Hautarzt* (German) 16, 281
Pruritus (1.1%)
Purpura
  (1965): Horowitz HI+, *Semin Hematol* 2, 287
  (1959): Bradley RF, *Ann N Y Acad Sci* 82, 513
Rash (sic) (1–10%)
Side effects (sic)
  (1967): McKiddie MT+, *Scott Med J* 12, 6 (1.65%)
  (1965): Ferguson BD, *Med Clin North Am* 49, 929 (0.35%)
  (1959): O'Donovan CJ, *Curr Ther Res* 1, 69 (1.1%)
Toxic epidermal necrolysis (<1%)
Urticaria (1–10%)
  (1960): Boshell BR, *N Engl J Med* 262, 80

Other
Acute intermittent porphyria
Disulfiram-like reaction
Dysgeusia
Headache
Hypersensitivity (<1%)
Injection-site thrombophlebitis (<1%)
Oral lichenoid eruption
Paresthesias
Porphyria
  (1968): De Matteis F, *Semin Hematol* 5, 409
Porphyria cutanea tarda
  (1960): Rook A+, *BMJ* 1, 860
Thrombophlebitis (<1%)

*Note: Tolbutamide is a sulfonamide and can be absorbed systemically. Sulfonamides can produce severe, possibly fatal, reactions such as toxic epidermal necrolysis and Stevens–Johnson syndrome

TOLCAPONE

Trade name: Tasmar (Roche)
Indications: Parkinsonism
Category: Antiparkinsonian
Half-life: 2–3 hours

Reactions

Skin

Allergic reactions (sic) (<1%)
Burning (sic) (2%)
Cellulitis (<1%)
Diaphoresis (7%)
Eczema (sic) (<1%)
Edema (<1%)
Erythema multiforme (<1%)
Facial edema (<1%)
Fungal infections (sic) (<1%)
Furunculosis (<1%)
Herpes simplex (<1%)
Herpes zoster (<1%)
Pigmentation (<1%)
Pruritus (<1%)
Rash (sic) (<1%)
Seborrhea (<1%)
Urticaria (<1%)
Vitiligo
   (1999): Sabate M+, *Ann Pharmacother* 33, 1228 (with levodopa)

Hair

Hair – alopecia (1%)

Other

Headache
Hyperesthesia (<1%)
Myalgia (<1%)
Oral ulceration (<1%)
Paresthesias (3%)
Parosmia (<1%)
Sialorrhea (<1%)
Tongue disorder (<1%)
Tooth disorder (<1%)
Tumors (sic) (1%)
Twitching (<1%)
Vaginitis (<1%)
Xerostomia (5%)

TOLMETIN

Trade name: Tolectin (Ortho-McNeil)
Other common trade names: *Donison; Midocil; Novo-Tolmetin; Reutol; Safitex*
Indications: Arthritis
Category: Nonsteroidal anti-inflammatory (NSAID) analgesic
Half-life: 1–2 hours
Clinically important, potentially hazardous interactions with: methotrexate

Reactions

Skin

Angioedema (<1%)

   (1994): Shapiro N, *J Oral Maxillofac Surg* 52, 626
   (1985): Ponte CD+, *Drug Intell Clin Pharm* 19, 479
Bullous eruption
Diaphoresis
Edema (3–9%)
Erythema multiforme (<1%)
Exanthems
   (1985): Bigby M+, *J Am Acad Dermatol* 12, 866
   (1984): Stern RS+, *JAMA* 252, 1433
   (1981): Reimer GW, *S Afr Med J* 60, 843
   (1977): Aylward M+, *Curr Res Med Opin* 4, 695 (9%)
Hot flashes (<1%)
Photodermatitis
   (1993): Shelley WB+, *Cutis* 52, 201 (observation)
Pruritus (1–10%)
   (1985): Bigby M+, *J Am Acad Dermatol* 12, 866
   (1981): Reimer GW, *S Afr Med J* 60, 843
   (1978): Restivo C+, *JAMA* 240, 246
Purpura
   (1984): Stern RS+, *JAMA* 252, 1433
Rash (sic) (>10%)
Stevens–Johnson syndrome (<1%)
Toxic epidermal necrolysis (<1%)
   (1992): Breathnach SM+, *Adverse Drug Reactions and the Skin*
      Blackwell, Oxford, 191 (passim)
   (1985): Bigby M+, *J Am Acad Dermatol* 12, 866
   (1984): Stern RS+, *JAMA* 252, 1433
Urticaria (1–5%)
   (1985): Bigby M+, *J Am Acad Dermatol* 12, 866
   (1985): Ponte CD+, *Drug Intell Clin Pharm* 19, 479
   (1984): Stern RS+, *JAMA* 252, 1433
   (1980): Ahmad S, *N Engl J Med* 303, 1417
   (1978): Restivo C+, *JAMA* 240, 246

Other

Anaphylactoid reactions
   (1985): Bretza JA+, *Western J Med* 143, 55
   (1985): O'Brien WM, *J Rheumatol* 12, 13
   (1983): Paulus HE, *Arthritis Rheum* 26, 1397
   (1982): Rossi AC+, *N Engl J Med* 307, 499
   (1980): Ahmad S, *N Engl J Med* 303, 1417
   (1980): McCall CY+, *JAMA* 243, 1263
   (1978): Restivo C+, *JAMA* 240, 246
Aphthous stomatitis
Dysgeusia
Gingival ulceration
Glossitis (<1%)
Gynecomastia
Headache
Myalgia
Oral ulceration
Serum sickness (<1%)
Stomatitis (<1%)
Tinnitus
Xerostomia

TOLTERODINE

Trade name: Detrol (Pharmacia)
Indications: Urinary incontinence
Category: Anticholinergic; Muscarinic antagonist (overactive bladder)
Half-life: 2–4 hours

Reactions

Skin
Erythema (1.9%)
Flu-like syndrome (sic) (4.4%)
Fungal infections (sic) (1.1%)
Pruritus (1.3%)
Rash (sic) (1.9%)
Upper respiratory infection (sic) (5.9%)
Xerosis (1.7%)

Other
Headache
Paresthesias (1.1%)
Xerostomia (40%)
  (2002): Zinner NR+, *J Am Geriatr Soc* 50(5), 799
  (2001): Crandall C, *J Womens Health Gend Based Med* 10(8), 735
  (2001): Harvey MA+, *Am J Obstet Gynecol* 185(1), 56
  (2001): Malone-Lee J+, *J Urol* 165(5), 1452 (37%)
  (2001): Olsson B+, *Clin Pharmacokinet* 40(3), 227
  (2001): Van Kerrebroeck+, *Urology* 57(3), 414
  (1999): Drutz HP+, *Int Urogynecol J Pelvic Floor Dysfunct* 10, 283
  (1999): Millard R+, *J Urol* 161, 1551
  (1999): Ruscin JM+, *Ann Pharmacother* 33, 1073
  (1997): Appell RA, *Urology* 50, 90
  (1997): Jonas U+, *World J Urol* 15, 144 (9%)

TOPIRAMATE

Trade name: Topamax (Ortho-McNeil)
Indications: Partial onset seizures
Category: Anticonvulsant
Half-life: 21 hours

Reactions

Skin
Acne (>1%)
Basal cell carcinoma (<1%)
Dermatitis (sic) (<1%)
Diaphoresis (1.8%)
Eczema (sic) (<1%)
Edema (1.8%)
Exanthems (<1%)
Facial edema (<1%)
  (2002): Nieto-Barrera M+, *Rev Neurol* 34(2), 114
Flu-like syndrome (sic) (1–10%)
Flushing (<1%)
Folliculitis (<1%)
Hot flashes (1–10%)
Hypohidrosis (<1%)
  (2002): Nieto-Barrera M+, *Rev Neurol* 34(2), 114
  (2001): Arcas J+, *Epilepsia* 42(10), 1363
Photosensitivity (<1%)
Pigmentation (<1%)
Pruritus (1.8%)

Purpura (<1%)
Rash (sic) (4.4%)
Seborrhea (<1%)
Urticaria (<1%)
Xerosis (<1%)

Hair
Hair – abnormal texture (<1%)
Hair – alopecia (>1%)
  (2002): Chuang Y-C+, *Dermatology Psychosomatics* 3, 183

Nails
Nails – changes (sic) (<1%)

Other
Ageusia (<1%)
Bromhidrosis (1.8%)
Depression
  (2001): Klufas A+, *Am J Psychiatry* 158(10), 1736
Dysgeusia (>1%)
  (2001): Storey JR+, *Headache* 41(10), 968
Foetor ex ore (halitosis)
Gingival hyperplasia (<1%)
Gingivitis (1.8%)
Gynecomastia (8.3%)
Hyperesthesia (<1%)
Mastodynia (3–9%)
Myalgia (1.8%)
Paresthesias (15%)
  (2002): Appolinario JC+, *Can J Psychiatry* 47(3), 271
  (2002): Mathew NT+, *Headache* 42(8), 796 (12%)
  (2002): Silberstein SD, *Headache* 42(1), 85
  (2001): Chengappa KN+, *Bipolar Disord* 3(5), 215
  (2001): Ghaemi SN+, *Ann Clin Psychiatry* 13(4), 185
  (2001): Storey JR+, *Headache* 41(10), 968
  (1999): Glauser TA, *Epilepsia* 40, S71
Parosmia (<1%)
Sialorrhea
  (2001): Buck ML, *Pediatr Pharmacol* 7 (4–5%)
Stomatitis (<1%)
Tongue edema (<1%)
Tremor (>10%)
Vaginitis
Xerostomia (2.7%)

TOPOTECAN

Synonyms: hycamptamine; SKF 104864; TOPO; TPT
Trade name: Hycamtin (GSK)
Indications: Metastatic ovarian carcinoma
Category: Antineoplastic antibiotic
Half-life: 3 hours

Reactions

Skin
Erythema (<1%)
Fixed eruption (cellulitis-like)
  (2002): Senturk N+, *J Eur Acad Dermatol Venereol* 16(4), 414
Neutrophilic eccrine hidradenitis
  (2002): Marini M+, *J Dermatolog Treat* 13(1), 35
Purpura (<1%)
Scleroderma
  (2002): Ene-Stroescu D+, *Arthritis Rheum* 46(3), 844

Hair

Hair – alopecia (59%)
  (2001): Clarke-Pearson DL+, *J Clin Oncol* 19(19), 3967
  (2001): Gore M+, *Br J Cancer* 84(8), 1043
  (2001): Mobus V+, *Anticancer Res* 21(5), 3551
  (1999): Ormrod D+, *Drugs* 58, 533

Other

Death
  (2002): Miller DS+, *Gynecol Oncol* 87(3), 247
  (2001): Seiter K+, *Leuk Lymphoma* 42(5), 963
Headache
Mucositis
  (2001): Seiter K+, *Leuk Lymphoma* 42(5), 963
Paresthesias (9%)
Stomatitis (24%)

TOREMIFENE

Trade name: Fareston (Shire)
Indications: Metastatic breast cancer
Category: Antiestrogen; Antineoplastic
Half-life: ~5 days

Reactions

Skin

Dermatitis (sic)
Diaphoresis (20%)
  (1997): Wiseman LR+, *Drugs* 54, 141
  (1990): Valavaara R+, *J Steroid Biochem* 36, 229
Edema (5%)
  (1997): Wiseman LR+, *Drugs* 54, 141
Hot flashes (35%)
  (1997): Wiseman LR+, *Drugs* 54, 141
Pigmentation
Pruritus

Other

Galactorrhea (1–10%)
Headache
Priapism (1–10%)
Thrombophlebitis (1%)
Vaginal discharge (13%)
  (1997): Wiseman LR+, *Drugs* 54, 141

TORSEMIDE

Trade name: Demadex (Roche)
Other common trade name: *Unat*
Indications: Edema
Category: Antihypertensive; Sulfonylurea loop diuretic
Half-life: 2–4 hours
**Clinically important, potentially hazardous interactions
with:** amikacin, aminoglycosides, gentamicin, kanamycin,
neomycin, streptomycin, tobramycin

Reactions

Skin

Angioedema
Edema (1.1%)
Exanthems

Lichenoid eruption
  (1997): Byrd DR+, *Mayo Clin Proc* 72, 930 (photosensitive)
Photosensitivity (1–10%)
Pruritus
Purpura
  (1998): Sanfelix Genoves J+, *Aten Primaria* (Spanish) 21, 252
Rash (sic) (<1%)
Stevens–Johnson syndrome
  (1997): Billon S, *The Schoch Letter* 47, 32 (observation)
Urticaria (1–10%)
Vasculitis
  (1998): Palop-Larrea V+, *Lancet* 352, 1909
  (1998): Sanfelix Genoves J+, *Aten Primaria* (Spanish) 21, 252

Other

Headache
Injection-site erythema (<1%)
Myalgia (1.6%)
Tinnitus
Xerostomia

*Note: Torsemide is a sulfonamide and can be absorbed
systemically. Sulfonamides can produce severe, possibly fatal,
reactions such as toxic epidermal necrolysis and Stevens–Johnson
syndrome

TRAMADOL

Trade names: Ultracet (Ortho-McNeil); Ultram (Ortho-McNeil)
Other common trade names: *Contramal; Tadol; Tradol; Tramal;
Tramed; Tramol; Tridol; Zipan*
Indications: Pain
Category: Centrally-acting synthetic analgesic
Half-life: 6–7 hours
**Clinically important, potentially hazardous interactions
with:** citalopram, desflurane, fluoxetine, fluvoxamine, MAO
inhibitors, nefazodone, phenelzine, tranylcypromine, venlafaxine

Reactions

Skin

Allergic reactions (sic) (<1%)
Angioedema
  (1996): Kind B+, *Schweiz Med Wochenschr* (German) 85, 567
Diaphoresis (9%)
Exanthems
  (1999): Ghislain PD+, *Ann Dermatol Venereol* (French) 126, 38
Pruritus (10%)
  (2002): Finkel JC+, *Anesth Analg* 94(6), 1469 (7%)
  (1999): Ghislain PD+, *Ann Dermatol Venereol* (French) 126, 38
Rash (sic) (1–5%)
  (2002): Finkel JC+, *Anesth Analg* 94(6), 1469
Toxic dermatitis (sic)
  (1999): Ghislain PD+, *Ann Dermatol Venereol* (French) 126, 38
Urticaria (<1%)
  (2003): Asero R, *J Investig Allergol Clin Immunol* 13(1), 56 (18%)

Other

Anaphylactoid reactions
  (1999): Moore PA, *J Am Dent Assoc* 130, 1075
Death
  (2001): Musshoff F+, *Forensic Sci Int* 116(2), 197
Dysgeusia (<1%)
Headache
Paresthesias (<1%)
Serotonin syndrome

(2002): Lange-Asschenfeldt C+, *J Clin Psychopharmacol* 22(4), 440 (with fluoxetine)
Stomatitis
Tremor (5–10%)
Xerostomia (10%)
(2003): Jarernsiripornkul N+, *Eur J Pain* 7(3), 219

TRANDOLAPRIL

Trade names: Mavik (Abbott); Tarka (Abbott)
Other common trade names: *Gopten; Odrik; Udrik*
Indications: Hypertension
Category: Angiotensin-converting enzyme (ACE) inhibitor; Antihypertensive; Calcium channel blocker (with verapamil)
Half-life: 24 hours
Clinically important, potentially hazardous interactions with: amiloride, spironolactone, triamterene

Tarka is trandolapril and verapamil

Reactions

Skin
Angioedema (0.15%)
(2001): Cohen EG+, *Ann Otol Rhinol Laryngol* 110(8), 701 (64 cases)
(1996): *Med Lett Drugs Ther* 38, 104
Edema (>3%)
Flushing (>3%)
Pemphigus (<1%)
Pemphigus foliaceus
(2000): Ong CS+, *Australas J Dermatol* 41(4), 242
Pruritus (>3%)
Rash (sic) (>10%)

Other
Cough
(2001): Adigun AQ+, *West Afr J Med* 20(1), 46–7
(2001): Lee SC+, *Hypertension* 38(2), 166
Headache
Hyperesthesia (>3%)
Myalgia (>3%)
Paresthesias (>3%)
Rhabdomyolysis
(2000): Gokel Y+, *Am J Emerg Med* 18(6), 738 (with verapamil)
Xerostomia (>3%)

TRANYLCYPROMINE

Trade name: Parnate (GSK)
Other common trade name: *Siciton*
Indications: Depression
Category: Antidepressant; Monoamine oxidase (MAO) inhibitor
Half-life: 2.5 hours
Clinically important, potentially hazardous interactions with: amitriptyline, amoxapine, amphetamines, bupropion, citalopram, clomipramine, cyproheptadine, desipramine, dextroamphetamine, dextromethorphan, diethylpropion, dopamine, doxepin, entacapone, ephedrine, epinephrine, fluoxetine, fluvoxamine, imipramine, levodopa, mazindol, meperidine, methamphetamine, nefazodone, nortriptyline, paroxetine, phendimetrazine, phentermine, phenylephrine, phenylpropanolamine, protriptyline, pseudoephedrine, rizatriptan, sertraline, sibutramine, sumatriptan, sympathomimetics, tramadol, tricyclic antidepressants, trimipramine, **tryptophan**, **tyramine-containing foods***, venlafaxine, zolmitriptan

Reactions

Skin
Diaphoresis
(1963): Adams PH+, *Lancet* 2, 692
Edema (<1%)
Exanthems
Flushing
(1963): Adams PH+, *Lancet* 2, 692
Neuroleptic malignant syndrome
(2002): Lappa A+, *Intensive Care Med* 28(7), 976 (with trifluoperazine)
Peripheral edema
Photosensitivity (<1%)
Pruritus
Rash (sic) (<1%)
Urticaria

Other
Acute intermittent porphyria
(1963): Adams PH+, *Lancet* 2, 692
Black tongue
Headache
Paresthesias
Priapism
Tinnitus
Tremor
Twitching
Xerostomia (<1%)

***Note:** Tyramine-containing foods include the following: aged cheeses, avocados, banana skins, bologna and other processed luncheon meats, chicken livers, chocolate, figs, canned pickled herring, meat extracts, pepperoni, raisins, raspberries, soy sauce, vermouth, sherry and red wines

TRASTUZUMAB

Trade name: Herceptin (Genentech)
Indications: Metastatic breast cancer
Category: Monoclonal antibody
Half-life: 5.8 days

Reactions

Skin

Acne (2%)
Acral erythrodysesthesia syndrome (hand–foot syndrome*)
  (2000): Merimsky O+, *Isr Med Assoc* 2(10), 786
Allergic reactions (sic) (3%)
Angioedema (<1%)
Cellulitis (<1%)
Chills (32%)
  (2002): McKeage K+, *Drugs* 62(1), 209
  (2002): Vogel CL+, *J Clin Oncol* 20(3), 719
  (2001): Cook-Bruns N, *Oncology* 61, 58
  (2001): Vogel CL+, *Oncology* 61, 37
  (2000): Treish I+, *Am J Health Syst Pharm* 57(22), 2063
  (1999): Goldenberg MM, *Clin Ther* 21(2), 309
Diaphoresis
  (1999): Dillman RO, *Cancer Metastasis Rev* 18(4), 465
Edema (8%)
Flu-like syndrome (10%)
  (2001): *Prescrire Int* 10(54), 102 (40%)
  (1999): Dillman RO, *Cancer Metastasis Rev* 18(4), 465
Herpes simplex (2%)
Herpes zoster (~1%)
Infections (sic) (20%)
  (1999): Goldenberg MM, *Clin Ther* 21(2), 309
Peripheral edema (10%)
Rash (sic) (18%)
  (2001): Vogel CL+, *Oncology* 61, 37
  (1999): Dillman RO, *Cancer Metastasis Rev* 18(4), 465
Ulcerations (~1%)

Other

Anaphylactoid reactions (<1%)
  (2002): McKeage K+, *Drugs* 62(1), 209
Arthralgia (6%)
Back pain (22%)
Bone or joint pain (7%)
Cough (26%)
  (1999): Goldenberg MM, *Clin Ther* 21(2), 309
Death
  (2002): McKeage K+, *Drugs* 62(1), 209
Depression (6%)
Headache
Injection-site reactions (<1%)
  (2002): Tokuda Y+, *Gan To Kagaku Ryoho* 29(4), 645
  (2001): Cook-Bruns N, *Oncology* 61, 58
  (2001): Smith IE, *Anticancer Drugs* 12, S3
  (2001): Vogel CL+, *Oncology* 61, 37
  (2000): Treish I+, *Am J Health Syst Pharm* 57(22), 2063
Myopathy (~1%)
Pain (47%)
  (2002): Vogel CL+, *J Clin Oncol* 20(3), 719 (18%)
  (1999): Goldenberg MM, *Clin Ther* 21(2), 309
Paresthesias (9%)
Stomatitis (<1%)

*Note: Hand–foot syndrome is also known as Acral dysesthesia syndrome

TRAVOPROST

Trade name: Travatan (Alcon)
Indications: Open-angle glaucoma, ocular hypertension
Category: Ophthalmic prostaglandin
Half-life: N/A

Reactions

Skin

Blepharitis (1–4%)
Eyelid crusting (1–4%)
Infections (sic)
Ocular hyperemia (35–50%)
Ocular pruritus (5–10%)
  (2001): Goldberg I+, *J Glaucoma* 10(5), 414
Pruritus
  (2001): Goldberg I+, *J Glaucoma* 10(5), 414

Hair

Eyelashes – growth
  (2002): Eisenberg DL+, *Surv Ophthalmol* 47(Suppl 1), S105

Other

Arthritis (1–5%)
Depression (1–5%)
Headache
Ocular irritation (5–10%)
  (2001): Goldberg I+, *J Glaucoma* 10(5), 414
Ocular pigmentation (1–4%)
  (2002): Novack GD+, *J Am Geriatr Soc* 50(5), 956
  (2002): Stjernschantz JW+, *Surv Ophthalmol* 47(Suppl 1), S162
  (2001): Goldberg I+, *J Glaucoma* 10(5), 414
  (2001): Netland PA+, *Am J Ophthalmol* 132(4), 472 (5%)
Pain
  (2001): Goldberg I+, *J Glaucoma* 10(5), 414
Tearing

TRAZODONE

Trade name: Desyrel (Apothecon)
Other common trade names: *Alti-Trazodone; Bimaran; Deprax; Desirel; Molipaxin; Sideril; Taxagon; Trazalon*
Indications: Depression
Category: Heterocyclic antidepressant
Half-life: 3–6 hours
Clinically important, potentially hazardous interactions with: citalopram, fluoxetine, fluvoxamine, linezolid, nefazodone, paroxetine, sertraline, venlafaxine

Reactions

Skin

Angioedema
  (2001): Adson DE+, *Ann Pharmacother* 35(11), 1375
Diaphoresis (>1%)
Edema (1–10%)
Erythema multiforme
  (1985): Ford HE+, *J Clin Psychiatry* 46, 294
Exanthems
  (1988): Warnock JK+, *Am J Psychiatry* 145, 425
  (1986): Rongioletti F+, *J Am Acad Dermatol* 14, 274
  (1984): Cohen LE, *J Am Acad Dermatol* 10, 303
  (1984): Cohen LE, *J Am Acad Dermatol* 11, 526

(1980): Al-Yassiri MM+, *Neuropharmacology* 19, 1191
(1979): Trapp GA+, *Psychopharmacol Bull* 15, 25
Exfoliative dermatitis
(1983): Chu AG+, *Ann Intern Med* 99, 128
Formication
(1987): Peabody CA, *J Clin Psychiatry* 48, 385
Photosensitivity
(1994): Berger TG+, *Arch Dermatol* 130, 609 (in HIV-infected)
(1986): Rongioletti F+, *J Am Acad Dermatol* 14, 274
Pruritus (<1%)
Psoriasis (exacerbation)
(1992): Breathnach SM+, *Adverse Drug Reactions and the Skin*
Blackwell, Oxford, 197 (passim)
(1986): Barth JH+, *Br J Dermatol* 115, 629 (generalized and
pustular)
Purpura
Rash (sic) (<1%)
(1985): Longstreth GF+, *J Am Acad Dermatol* 13, 149
Urticaria
(1988): Warnock JK+, *Am J Psychiatry* 145, 425
(1984): Cohen LE, *J Am Acad Dermatol* 10, 303
(1983): Fabre LF+, *J Clin Psychiatry* 44, 17
Vasculitis
(1984): Mann SC+, *J Am Acad Dermatol* 10, 669

Hair

Hair – alopecia
(2000): Mercke Y+, *Ann Clin Psychiatry* 12, 35
(1988): Warnock JK+, *Am J Psychiatry* 145, 425

Nails

Nails – leukonychia
(1985): Longstreth GF+, *J Am Acad Dermatol* 13, 149

Other

Dysgeusia (>10%)
Galactorrhea
Gynecomastia
Headache
Hypersensitivity
Myalgia (1–10%)
Paresthesias (>1%)
Parkinsonism
(2002): Fukunishi I+, *Nephron* 90(2), 222
Priapism
(2001): Warner MD+, *Pharmacopsychiatry* 34(4), 128 (12%)
(2000): Correas Gomez MA+, *Actas Urol Esp* (Spanish)
24(10), 840
(1998): Myrick H+, *Ann Clin Psychiatry* 10, 81
(1994): Thavundayil JX+, *Neuropsychobiology* 30, 4
(1993): Pescatori ES+, *J Urol* 149, 1557
Priapism (clitoral)
(2002): Kem DL+, *J Am Acad Child Adolesc Psychiatry* 41(7), 758
(2002): Medina CA, *Obstet Gynecol* 100(5 Pt 2), 1089 (clitoral)
Serotonin syndrome
(2001): Adson DE+, *Ann Pharmacother* 35(11), 1375
(2001): McCue RE+, *Am J Psychiatry* 158(12), 2088
Sialorrhea
Tremor (1–10%)
Xerostomia (>10%)
(1982): Rawls WN, *Drug Intell Clin Pharm* 16, 7

TREPROSTINIL

Trade name: Remodulin (United Therapeutics)
Indications: Pulmonary hypertension
Category: Prostacyclin analog; Vasodilator
Half-life: 2–4 hours
**Clinically important, potentially hazardous interactions
with:** anticoagulants

Reactions

Skin

Diaphoresis
Edema (9%)
Erythema
Flushing
Peripheral edema
Pruritus (8%)
Rash (sic) (14%)

Other

Dizziness (9%)
Injection-site bleeding (33%)
Injection-site induration
Injection-site pain (85%)
(2002): Simonneau G+, *Am J Respir Crit Care Md* 165(6), 800
(2002): Vachiery JL+, *Chest* 121(5), 1561
Injection-site reactions (83%)
Pain (13%)
Pharyngitis (12%)

TRETINOIN

Synonym: All-trans-retinoic acid
Trade names: Aberela; Acnavit; Aknemycin Plus (Hermal);
ATRA; Atragen; Avita (Bertek); Avitoin; Dermojuventus; Relief;
Renova (Ortho); Retin-A Micro (Ortho); Retinoic Acid; Retinova;
SolagJJ (Bristol-Myers Squibb); SteiVAA; Tri-Luma (Galderma);
Vesanoid (Roche)
Other common trade names: *A-Acido; Aberal; Acid A Vit; Acta;
Airol; Alquingel; Alten; Avitcid; Cordes VAS; Derm A; Dermairol; Epi-
Aberel; Eudyna; Stieva-A; Vitamin A Acid*
Indications: Acne vulgaris, skin aging, facial roughness, fine
wrinkles, hyperpigmentation [T], acute promyelocytic leukemia
(APL) [O]
Category: Retinoid
Half-life: 0.5–2 hours
**Clinically important, potentially hazardous interactions
with:** aldesleukin, bexarotene

Note: [T] = Topical, [O] = Oral

Reactions

Skin

Acne (1%)
(1996): Shalita A+, *J Am Acad Dermatol* 34, 482
Acute febrile neutrophilic dermatosis (Sweet's syndrome)
(1999): Takada S+, *Int J Hematol* 70(1), 26
(1997): Hatake K+, *Int J Hematol* 66(1), 13
(1996): Christ E+, *Leukemia* 10(4), 731
Bullous eruption
(1998): Webster GF, *J Am Acad Dermatol* 39, S38–44
(1997): Cunliffe WJ+, *J Am Acad Dermatol* 36, S126–34

Burning (10–40%) ([O][T])
(2001): Vandana B+, *AAPS PharmSciTech* 2(3), Technical Note 4
(1998): Ellis CN+, *Br J Dermatol* 139 Suppl 52, 41
(1998): Webster GF, *J Am Acad Dermatol* 39, S38–44
(1997): Cunliffe WJ+, *J Am Acad Dermatol* 36, S126–34
(1997): Gilchrest B, *J Am Acad Dermatol* 36, S27–36
(1997): *Drug Information Handbook* Fifth Ed., American
    Pharmaceutical Association, Hudson, OH
(1996): Shalita A+, *J Am Acad Dermatol* 34, 482
(1996): Shroot B, *Presented at Dermatology Update '95* (Montreal,
    Canada)
(1995): Hall R, *Inpharma* December, 13
(1995): *Package Insert* Hoffman-LaRoche, Inc. (Nutley, NJ)
(1992): Olsen EA+, *J Am Acad Dermatol* 26, 215
(1991): Weinstein GD+, *Arch Dermatol* 127, 659
(1989): Goldfarb MT+, *J Am Acad Dermatol* 21, 645
(1989): Leyden JJ+, *J Am Acad Dermatol* 21, 638
(1988): Cohen BA+, *Pediatric Dermatology* 1, New York:
    Churchill Livingstone, 663
(1977): Muller SA+, *Arch Dermatol* 113(8), 1052
Carcinoma ([O])
Cellulitis (1–10%) ([O])
(1997): *Drug Information Handbook* Fifth Ed., American
    Pharmaceutical Association (Hudson, OH)
(1995): Gillis JC+, *Drugs* 50(5), 897
(1995): *Package insert* Hoffman-LaRoche, Inc. (Nutley, NJ)
Cheilitis (10%) ([O])
(1997): *Drug Information Handbook* Fifth Ed. (American
    Pharmaceutical Association, Hudson, OH)
(1995): *Package insert* (Hoffman-LaRoche, Inc., Nutley, NJ)
Crusting
(1998): Webster GF, *J Am Acad Dermatol* 39, S38–44
(1997): Cunliffe WJ+, *J Am Acad Dermatol* 36, S126–34
Dermatitis (sic)
(1997): Gilchrest B, *J Am Acad Dermatol* 36, S27–36
(1992): Olsen EA+, *J Am Acad Dermatol* 26, 215
(1991): Weinstein GD+, *Arch Dermatol* 127, 659
(1989): Goldfarb MT+, *J Am Acad Dermatol* 21, 645
(1989): Leyden JJ+, *J Am Acad Dermatol* 21, 638
Desquamation (14%)
Diaphoresis (20%)
Dry skin (49–100%) ([O])
(1998): Soignet SL+, *Leukema* 12(10), 1518
(1995): Dockx P+, *Br J Dermatol* 133(3), 426
(1995): Gillis JC+, *Drugs* 50(5), 897
(1992): Fenaux P+, *Blood* 80(9), 2176
(1991): Chen ZX+, *Blood* 78(6), 1413
(1988): Huang ME+, *Blood* 72(2), 567
Edema (29%) ([O])
(1997): *Drug Information Handbook* Fifth Ed. (American
    Pharmaceutical Association, Hudson, OH)
(1995): *Package insert* (Hoffman-LaRoche, Inc., Nutley, NJ)
Erythema (1–49%) ([O][T])
(2001): Vandana B+, *AAPS PharmSciTech* 2(3), Technical Note 4
(2000): Kreusch+, *Curr Med Res & Opinion* 16(1), 1
(1998): Ellis CN+, *Br J Dermatol* 139 Suppl 52, 41
(1998): Webster GF, *J Am Acad Dermatol* 39(2), S38–44
(1997): Cunliffe WJ+, *J Am Acad Dermatol* 36(6), S126–34
(1997): Gilchrest BA, *J Am Acad Dermatol* 36(3), S27–36
(1997): *Drug Information Handbook* Fifth Ed (American
    Pharaceutical Association, Hudson, OH)
(1996): Shalita A+, *J Am Acad Dermatol* 34(3), 482
(1996): Shroot B, *Presented at Dermatology Update '95*,
    Montreal, Canada
(1995): Hall R, *Inpharma* December, 13
(1995): *Package insert* Hoffman-LaRoche, Inc., Nutley, NJ
(1992): Olsen EA+, *J Am Acad Dermatol* 26(2), 215
(1991): Weinstein GD+, *Arch Dermatol* 127, 659
(1989): Goldfarb MT+, *J Am Acad Dermatol* 21, 645

(1989): Leyden JJ+, *J Am Acad Dermatol* 21, 638
(1988): Cohen BA+, *Pediatric Dermatology* 1. New York:
    Churchill Livingstone, 663
(1977): Muller SA+, *Arch Dermatol* 113(8), 1052
Erythema nodosum
Exfoliation (8.3%) ([O])
(1998): Webster GF, *J Am Acad Dermatol* 39, S38–44
(1997): Cunliffe WJ+, *J Am Acad Dermatol* 36, S126–34
(1988): Huang ME+, *Blood* 72(2), 567
Facial edema (1–10%) ([O])
(1997): *Drug Information Handbook* Fifth Ed. American
    Pharmaceutical Association, Hudson, OH
(1995): *Package insert* Hoffman-LaRoche, Inc., Nutley NJ
Flaking (23%) ([O])
Flushing
(1997): *Drug Information Handbook* Fifth Ed. American
    Pharmaceutical Association, Hudson, OH
(1996): Miller VA+, *Clin Cancer Res* 2(3), 471
(1995): *Package insert* Hoffman-LaRoche, Inc., Nutley, NJ
Hyperkeratosis (78%) ([O])
(1991): Chen ZX+, *Blood* 78, 1413
Hypopigmentation (5%)
(1998): Webster GF, *J Am Acad Dermatol* 39, S38–44
(1997): Cunliffe WJ+, *J Am Acad Dermatol* 36, S126–34
Infections (sic) (58%) ([O])
(1997): *Drug Information Handbook* Fifth Ed. American
    Pharaceutical Association, Hudson, OH
(1995): *Package insert* Hoffman-LaRoche, Inc,. Nutley, NJ
(1991): Chen ZX+, *Blood* 78(6), 1413
Irritation (sic) (5%)
(2001): Vandana B+, *AAPS PharmSciTech* 2(3), Technical Note 4
(1998): Cohen BA+, *Pediatric Dermatology* 1, New York:
    Churchill Livingstone, 663
(1997): Clucas A+, *J Am Acad Dermatol* 36, S116–8
(1996): Shalita A+, *J Am Acad Dermatol* 34(3), 482
Localized edema
(1998): Webster GF, *J Am Acad Dermatol* 39, S38–44
(1997): Cunliffe WJ+, *J Am Acad Dermatol* 36, S126–34
(1997): Gilchrest BA, *J Am Acad Dermatol* 36, S27–36
(1992): Olsen EA+, *J Am Acad Dermatol* 26, 215
(1991): Weinstein GD+, *Arch Dermatol* 127, 659
(1989): Goldfarb MT+, *J Am Acad Dermatol* 21, 645
(1989): Leyden JJ+, *J Am Acad Dermatol* 21, 638
Ocular pruritus (10%) ([O])
(1997): *Drug Information Handbook* Fifth Ed. American
    Pharmaceutical Association, Hudson, OH
(1995): *Package insert* Hoffman-LaRoche, Inc., Natley, NJ
Pallor (1–10%) ([O])
(1997): *Drug Information Handbook* Fifth Ed. American
    Pharmaceutical Association, Hudson, OH
(1995): *Package insert* Hoffman-LaRoche, Inc., Nutley, NJ
Palmar–plantar peeling (1–10%) ([O])
(1997): *Drug Information Handbook* Fifth Ed. American
    Pharmaceutical Association, Hudson, OH
(1995): *Package insert* Hoffman-LaRoche, Inc., Nutley, NJ
Photosensitivity (10%) ([O][T])
(1998): Webster GF, *J Am Acad Dermatol* 39, S38–44
(1997): Cunliffe WJ+, *J Am Acad Dermatol* 36, S126–34
(1997): *Drug Information Handbook* Fifth Ed. American
    Pharmaceutical Association, Hudson, OH
(1995): *Package insert* Hoffman-LaRoche, Inc., Nutley, NJ
Pigmentation (5%)
(1998): Webster GF, *J Am Acad Dermatol* 39, S38–44
(1997): Cunliffe WJ+, *J Am Acad Dermatol* 36, S126–34
Pruritus (10–40%) ([O][T])
(2001): Vandana B+, *AAPS PharmSciTech* 2(3), Technical Note 4
(2000): Kreusch+, *Curr Med Res & Opinion* 16(1), 1
(1998): Ellis CN+, *Br J Dermatol* 139 Suppl 52, 41
(1998): Webster GF, *J Am Acad Dermatol* 39, S38–44

(1997): Cunliffe WJ+, *J Am Acad Dermatol* 36, S126–34
(1997): *Drug Information Handbook* Fifth Ed. American
  Pharmaceutical Association, Hudson, OH
(1996): Shalita A+, *J Am Acad Dermatol* 34, 482
(1995): Gillis JC+, *Drugs* 50(5), 897
(1995): *Package insert* Hoffman-LaRoche, Inc., Nutley, NJ
(1988): Cohen BA+, *Pediatric Dermatology* 1, New
  York:Churchill Livingstone, 663
(1977): Muller SA+, *Arch Dermatol* 113(8), 1052
Rash (sic) (54%) ([O][T])
(1998): Webster GF, *J Am Acad Dermatol* 39, S38–44
(1997): Cunliffe WJ+, *J Am Acad Dermatol* 36, S126–34
(1997): *Drug Information Handbook* Fifth Ed American
  Pharmaceutical Association, Hudson, OH
(1995): *Package insert* Hoffman-LaRoche, Inc.,Nutley, NJ
(1991): Warrell RP+, *N Engl J Med* 324, 1385
Scaling (10–40%)
(2001): Vandana B+, *AAPS PharmSciTech* 2(3), Technical Note 4
(2000): Kreusch+, *Curr Med Res & Opinion* 16(1), 1
(1998): Ellis CN+, *Br J Dermatol* 139 Suppl 52, 41
(1997): Gilchrest BA, *J Am Acad Dermatol* 36, S27–36
(1996): Shalita A+, *J Am Acad Dermatol* 34, 482
(1996): Shroot B, *Presented ar Dermatology Update '95* Montreal,
  Canada
(1995): Hall R, *Inpharma* December, 13
(1992): Olsen EA+, *J Am Acad Dermatol* 26, 215
(1991): Weinstein GD+, *Arch Dermatol* 127, 659
(1989): Goldfarb MT+, *J Am Acad Dermatol* 21, 645
(1988): Cohen BA+, *Pediatric Dermatology* 1 New York:
  Chrurchill Livingstone, 663
Shivering (63%) ([O])
(1997): *Drug Information Handbook* Fifth Ed. American
  Pharmaceutical Association, Hudson, OH
(1995): *Package insert* Hoffman-LaRoche, Inc., Nutley, NJ
Stinging (1–26%)
(1997): Gilchrest BA, *J Am Acad Dermatol* 36, S27–36
(1996): Shalita A+, *J Am Acad Dermatol* 34, 482
(1992): Olsen EA+, *J Am Acad Dermatol* 26, 215
(1991): Weinstein GD+, *Arch Dermatol* 127, 659
(1989): Goldfarb MT+, *J Am Acad Dermatol* 21, 645
(1989): Leyden JJ+, *J Am Acad Dermatol* 21, 638
Sunburn (1%)
(1996): Shalita A+, *J Am Acad Dermatol* 34, 482
Ulcerations (penile)
(2000): Esser AC+, *J Am Acad Dermatol* 43(2 Pt 1), 316
(1995): Gillis JC+, *Drugs* 50, 897
Vesiculobullous eruption
Xerosis (77%)
(2000): Kreusch+, *Curr Med Res & Opinion* 16(1), 1
(1997): Gilchrest BA, *J Am Acad Dermatol* 36, S27
(1996): Shalita A+, *J Am Acad Dermatol* 34, 482
(1992): Olsen EA+, *J Am Acad Dermatol* 26, 215
(1991): Weinstein GD+, *Arch Dermatol* 127, 659
(1989): Leyden JJ+, *J Am Acad Dermatol* 21, 638

Hair

Hair – alopecia areata (14%) ([O])
(1997): *Drug Information Handbook* Fifth Ed American
  Pharmaceutical Association, Hudson, OH
(1995): *Package insert* Hoffman-LaRoche, Inc., Nutley, NJ

Other

Arthralgia (10%) ([O])
(1997): *Drug Information Handbook* American Pharmaceutical
  Association, Hudson, OH
(1995): Gillis JC+, *Drugs* 50, 897
(1995): *Package insert* Hoffman-LaRoche, Inc., Nutley, NJ
Bone or joint pain (77%) ([O])
(1995): Gillis JC+, *Drugs* 50, 897
(1992): Fenaux P+, *Blood* 80, 2176

(1988): Huang ME+, *Blood* 72, 567
Conjunctivitis (<1%) ([O])
(1997): *Drug Information Handbook* Fifth Ed. American
  Pharmaceutical Association, Hudson, OH
(1995): *Package insert* Hoffman-LaRoche, Inc., Nutley, NJ
Death ([O])
(1997): Fenaux P+, *N Engl J* 337, 1076
(1997): Larson RA+ In: Hall JB+, *Principles of Critical Care*
  Second Ed. New York, McGraw-Hill
(1995): *Package insert* Hoffman-LaRoche, Inc., Nutley, NJ
Depression (14%) ([O])
(1997): *Drug Information Handbook* Fifth Ed, American
  Pharmaceutical Association, Hudson, OH
(1995): *Package insert* Hoffman-LaRoche, Inc., Nutley, NJ
Dry eyes (1–10%) ([O])
(1997): *Drug Information Handbook* Fifth Ed. American
  Pharmaceutical Association, Hudson, OH
(1995): *Package insert* Hoffman-LaRoche, Inc., Nutley, NJ
Fever ([O])
(1997): Fenaux P+, *N Engl J Med* 337, 1076
(1997): Larson RA+ In: Halll JB+, *Principles of Critical Care*
  Second Ed., New York, McGraw
(1995): *Package insert* Hoffman-LaRoche, Inc., Nutley, NJ
Gingivitis (<1%) ([O])
(1997): *Drug Information Handbook* Fifth Ed. American
  Pharmaceutical Association, Hudson, OH
(1995): *Package insert* Hoffman-LaRoche, Inc., Nutley, NJ
Headache
Injection-site reactions (17%)
Myalgia (14%) ([O])
(1997): *Drug Information Handbook* Fifth Ed. American
  Pharmaceutical Association, Hudson, OH
(1995): *Package insert* Hoffman-LaRoche, Inc., Nutley, NJ
Myositis
Ocular pigmentation (1–10%) ([O])
(1997): *Drug Information Handbook* Fifth Ed. American
  Pharmaceutical Association, Hudson, OH
(1995): *Package insert* Hoffman-LaRoche, Inc., Nutley, NJ
Pain (37%) ([O])
(1997): *Drug Information Handbook* Fifth Ed. American
  Pharmaceutical Association, Hudson, OH
(1995): *Package insert* Hoffman-LaRoche, Inc., Nutley, NJ
Paresthesias (17%) ([O])
(1997): *Drug Information Handbook* Fifth Ed. American
  Pharmaceutical Association, Hudson, OH
(1995): *Package insert* Hoffman-LaRoche, Inc., Nutley, NJ
Phlebitis (11%)
Pseudotumor cerebri (<1%) ([O])
(2003): Colucciello M, *Arch Ophthalmol* 121(7), 1064
(1997): Tallman MS+, *N Engl J Med* 337, 1021
(1996): Visani G+, *Leuk Lymphoma* 23(5–6), 437
(1995): *Package insert* Hoffman-LaRoche, Inc., Nutley, NJ
(1994): *Drug Information Handbook* Fifth Ed. American
  Pharmaceutical Association, Hudson, OH
(1993): Mahmoud HH+, *Lancet* 342(8884), 1394
(1991): Warrell RP+, *N Engl J Med* 324, 1385
Retinoic Acid–APL (RA-APL) syndrome * (25%) ([O])
(1997): Fenaux P+, *N Engl J Med* 337, 1076
(1997): Sacchi S+, *Haematologica* 82(1), 106
(1997): Tallman MS+, *N Engl J Med* 337, 1021
(1995): Gillis JC+, *Drugs* 50, 897
(1995): *Package insert* Hoffman-LaRoche, Inc., Nutley, NJ
(1992): Fenaux P+, *Blood* 80, 2176
Tingling (26%)
Tremor (1–10%) ([O])
(1997): *Drug Information Handbook* Fifth Ed. American
  Pharmaceutical Association, Hudson, OH
(1995): *Package insert* Hoffman-LaRoche, Inc., Nutley, NJ

Xerostomia (10%) ([O])
(1997): *Drug Information Handbook* Fifth Ed American
Pharmaceutical Association, Hudson, OH
(1995): *Package insert* Hoffman-LaRoche, Inc., Nutley, NJ

Note: Oral tretinoin can cause birth defects, and women should
avoid Tretinoin when pregnant or trying to conceive. Avoid
prolonged exposure to sunlight

*Note: The RA-APL syndrome is characterized by fever, dyspnea,
weight gain, pulmonary infiltrates and pleural effusions. Some patients
have expired due to multiorgan failure

TRIAMTERENE

Trade names: Dyazide (GSK); Dyrenium (Wellspring); Maxzide
(Bertek)
Other common trade names: *Amterene; Diarrol; Diuteren;
Dytac; Reviten; Suloton; Trian*
Indications: Edema
Category: Antihypertensive; Potassium-sparing antihypertensive
diuretic
Half-life: 1–2 hours
**Clinically important, potentially hazardous interactions
with:** ACE inhibitors, benazepril, captopril, cyclosporine,
enalapril, fosinopril, indomethacin, **juniper**, lisinopril, moexipril,
potassium iodide, potassium salts, quinapril, ramipril,
spironolactone, trandolapril

Dyazide is triamterene and hydrochlorothiazide*; Maxzide is
triamterene and hydrochlorothiazide*

Reactions

Skin
Chills
Diaphoresis
(1979): Fan WJ+, *Pediatrics* 64, 698
Edema (1–10%)
Exanthems
Flushing (<1%)
Lupus erythematosus (with hydrochlorothiazide)
(1991): Wollenberg A+, *Hautarzt* (German) 42, 709
(1988): Darken M+, *J Am Acad Dermatol* 18, 38
Perleche
Photosensitivity
(1989): Rosen C, *Semin Dermatol* 8, 149
(1987): Fernandez de Corres L+, *Contact Dermatitis* 17, 114
Pruritus
Purpura
Rash (sic) (1–10%)
Urticaria
Vasculitis

Other
Anaphylactoid reactions
Dysgeusia
(1999): Sorkin M, Denver, CO (from Internet) (observation)
Glossitis
Gynecomastia (<1%)
Headache
Paresthesias
Pseudoporphyria
(1990): Motley RJ, *BMJ* 300, 1468
Stomatodynia
(1999): Sorkin M, Denver, CO (from Internet) (observation)

Xerostomia
(1987): Fernandez de Corres L+, *Contact Dermatitis* 17, 114

*Note: Hydrochlorothiazide is a sulfonamide and can be absorbed
systemically. Sulfonamides can produce severe, possibly fatal,
reactions such as toxic epidermal necrolysis and Stevens–Johnson
syndrome

TRIAZOLAM

Trade name: Halcion (Pharmacia)
Other common trade names: *Dumozolam; Novo-Triolam; Nu-
Triazo; Nuctane; Somese; Somniton; Songar; Trialam*
Indications: Insomnia
Category: Benzodiazepine sedative-hypnotic
Half-life: 1.5–5.5 hours
**Clinically important, potentially hazardous interactions
with:** atazanavir, clarithromycin, delavirdine, efavirenz,
erythromycin, indinavir, itraconazole, ketoconazole, rifampin,
ritonavir

Reactions

Skin
Dermatitis (sic) (1–10%)
(1984): Greenblatt DJ+, *J Clin Psychiatry* 45, 192
Diaphoresis (>10%)
(1983): Kroboth PD+, *Drug Intell Clin Pharm* 17, 495
(1979): van der Kroef C, *Lancet* 2, 526
Exanthems
Photosensitivity
(1984): Hussar DA, *Am Drug* 190, 109
Pruritus
(1983): Poeldinger W+, *Neuropsychobiology* 9, 135
(1981): Cobden I+, *Postgrad Med J* 57, 730
Purpura
Rash (sic) (>10%)
(1985): Jerram TC, *Side Effects Drugs Annu* 9, 39
Urticaria

Hair
Hair – alopecia
Hair – hirsutism

Other
Dysesthesia (<1%)
Dysgeusia (<1%)
(1979): van der Kroef C, *Lancet* 2, 526
(1978): Fabre LF Jr+, *J Clin Psychiatry* 39, 679
Gingivitis
Glossitis (<1%)
Glossodynia (<1%)
Headache
Paresthesias (<1%)
(1979): van der Kroef C, *Lancet* 2, 526
Sialopenia (>10%)
(1995): Loesche WJ+, *J Am Geriatr Soc* 43, 401
Sialorrhea (1–10%)
Stomatitis (<1%)
Tinnitus
Tremor (1–10%)
Xerostomia (>10%)
(1995): Loesche WJ+, *J Am Geriatr Soc* 43, 401
(1986): Hughes RRL+, *Br J Clin Pract* 40, 279
(1984): Greenblatt DJ+, *J Clin Psychiatry* 45, 192
(1983): Cohn JB, *J Clin Psychiatry* 44, 401

TRICHLORMETHIAZIDE

Trade names: Metahydrin (Aventis); Naqua (Schering)
Other common trade names: *Anatran; Aquacot; Carvacron; Diurese; Doqua; Esmarin; Flute; Iopran; Niazide; Trichlon; Trichlorex*
Indications: Edema, hypertension
Category: Antihypertensive; Thiazide diuretic
Half-life: N/A
Clinically important, potentially hazardous interactions with: digoxin, lithium

Reactions

Skin
Exanthems
Lichenoid eruption (<1%)
Lupus erythematosus
  (1978): Pereyo-Torellas N, *Arch Dermatol* 114, 1097
Photosensitivity (<1%)
Purpura
  (1962): Loftus LR+, *JAMA* 180, 410
Rash (sic)
Urticaria
Vasculitis
  (1962): Loftus LR+, *JAMA* 180, 410

Other
Anaphylactoid reactions
Paresthesias
Xerostomia

*Note: Trichlormethiazide is a sulfonamide and can be absorbed systemically. Sulfonamides can produce severe, possibly fatal, reactions such as toxic epidermal necrolysis and Stevens–Johnson syndrome

TRIENTINE

Trade name: Syprine (Merck)
Indications: Wilson's disease
Category: Antidote (copper toxicity); Chelating agent
Half-life: N/A

Reactions

Skin
Dermatitis (sic)
  (1980): Rudzki E, *Contact Dermatitis* 6, 235
Desquamation
Lupus erythematosus (<1%)
Thickening (sic) (<1%)

Other
Aphthous stomatitis
Oral mucosal lesions

TRIFLUOPERAZINE

Trade name: Stelazine (GSK)
Other common trade names: *Calmazine; Domilium; Flupazine; Fluzine; Nerolet; Psyrazine; Sedizine; Tfp*
Indications: Psychoses, anxiety
Category: Antipsychotic; Anxiolytic; Phenothiazine tranquilizer
Half-life: 10–20 hours
Clinically important, potentially hazardous interactions with: antihistamines, arsenic, chlorpheniramine, dofetilide, piperazine, quinolones, sparfloxacin

Reactions

Skin
Angioedema
  (1974): Panikarskii VG, *Vrach Delo* (Russian) February, 118
Dermatitis
Diaphoresis
Eczema (sic)
Erythema
Exanthems
Exfoliative dermatitis
Fixed eruption
  (1987): Kanwar AJ+, *Br J Dermatol* 117, 798
Hypohidrosis
Lupus erythematosus
Neuroleptic malignant syndrome
  (2002): Lappa A+, *Intensive Care Med* 28(7), 976 (with tranylcypromine)
Peripheral edema
Photosensitivity (1–10%)
  (1970): *Med Lett* 12, 104
Pigmentation (blue-gray) (<1%)
  (1994): Buckley C+, *Clin Exp Dermatol* 19, 149
Pruritus
Purpura
Rash (sic) (1–10%)
Seborrhea
Urticaria
Xerosis

Other
Anaphylactoid reactions
Galactorrhea (<1%)
Gynecomastia
Headache
Mastodynia (1–10%)
Oral mucosal eruption
  (1988): Ward DF+, *Postgrad Med* 84, 99
Parkinsonism (>10%)
Priapism (<1%)
Tongue edema
  (1988): Ward DF+, *Postgrad Med* 84, 99
Tremor
Xerostomia

TRIHEXYPHENIDYL

Trade name: Artane (Wyeth)
Other common trade names: *Acamed; Aparkane; Bentex; Hexinal; Hipokinon; Parkines; Partane; Tridyl; Trihexy; Trihexyphen*
Indications: Parkinsonism
Category: Anticholinergic; Antidyskinetic; Antiparkinsonian
Half-life: 3–4 hours
Clinically important, potentially hazardous interactions with: anticholinergics, arbutamine

Reactions

Skin
Chills
Diaphoresis
Flushing
Hypohidrosis (>10%)
Photosensitivity (1–10%)
Rash (sic) (<1%)
Spider angiomas
　(1953): Holt CL, *N Engl J Med* 249, 318
Urticaria
Xerosis (>10%)

Other
Glossitis
Glossodynia
Paresthesias
Xerostomia (30–50%)

TRIMEPRAZINE

Trade name: Temaril (Allergan)
Other common trade names: *Nedeltran; Panectyl; Theralene; Vallergan; Variargil*
Indications: Pruritus, urticaria
Category: Antihistamine; Phenothiazine tranquilizer
Duration of action: 3–6 hours

Reactions

Skin
Angioedema (<1%)
　(1959): Wright W, *JAMA* 171, 1642
Dermatitis (sic)
Diaphoresis
Edema (<1%)
Exanthems
　(1959): Wright W, *JAMA* 171, 1642
Lupus erythematosus
Peripheral edema
Photosensitivity (<1%)
Pruritus
　(1959): Wright W, *JAMA* 171, 1642
Purpura
Rash (sic) (<1%)
Urticaria

Other
Anaphylactoid reactions
Gynecomastia
Myalgia (<1%)

Paresthesias (<1%)
Stomatitis
Tinnitus
Xerostomia (1–10%)
　(1992): Chambers FA+, *Anaesthesia* 47, 585

TRIMETHADIONE

Trade name: Tridione (Abbott)
Other common trade name: *Mino Aleviatin*
Category: Anticonvulsant
Half-life: N/A

Reactions

Skin
Acne
Bullous eruption
Erythema multiforme
　(1992): Breathnach SM+, *Adverse Drug Reactions and the Skin*
　　Blackwell, Oxford, 210 (passim)
　(1972): Levantine A+, *Br J Dermatol* 87, 646
　(1961): Rallison ML+, *Am J Dis Child* 101, 725
　(1948): Kevin JC, *Lancet* 1, 267
Exanthems
　(1972): Levantine A+, *Br J Dermatol* 87, 646
　(1962): LeVan P+, *Arch Dermatol* 86, 254
　(1948): Kevin JC, *Lancet* 1, 267
Exfoliative dermatitis
　(1992): Breathnach SM+, *Adverse Drug Reactions and the Skin*
　　Blackwell, Oxford, 210 (passim)
　(1948): Kevin JC, *Lancet* 1, 267
Fixed eruption
Infections (sic)
　(2002): Sarris AH+, *J Clin Oncol* 20(12), 2876 (3%)
Lupus erythematosus
　(1993): Drory VE+, *Clin Neuropharmacol* 16, 19
　(1980): Condemi JJ, *Geriatrics* 35(3), 81
　(1976): Singsen BH+, *Pediatrics* 57, 529
　(1973): Beernink DH+, *J Pediatr* 82, 113
　(1962): LeVan P+, *Arch Dermatol* 86, 254
　(1961): Rallison ML+, *Am J Dis Child* 101, 725
Petechiae
Photosensitivity
　(1962): LeVan P+, *Arch Dermatol* 86, 254
Pruritus
　(1961): Weingartner L, *Monatsschr Kinderheilkd* (German)
　　109, 517
Purpura
　(1956): Wintrobe MM+, *Arch Intern Med* 98, 559
Stevens–Johnson syndrome
　(1961): Rallison ML+, *Am J Dis Child* 101, 725
Urticaria
　(1992): Breathnach SM+, *Adverse Drug Reactions and the Skin*
　　Blackwell, Oxford, 210 (passim)
　(1964): Beall GN, *Medicine* (Baltimore) 43, 131
　(1948): Kevin JC, *Lancet* 1, 267
Vasculitis
　(1993): Drory VE+, *Clin Neuropharmacol* 16, 19
　(1986): Hannedouche T+, *Ann Med Interne Paris* (French)
　　137, 57

Hair
Hair – alopecia
　(1960): Holowach J+, *N Engl J Med* 263, 1187

Other
Acute intermittent porphyria
Gingivitis
Mucositis
   (2002): Sarris AH+, *J Clin Oncol* 20(12), 2876 (4%)
Paresthesias

TRIMETHOBENZAMIDE

Trade names: Arrestin; Benzacot; Bio-Gan; Navogan; Stemetic; T-Gene; Tebamide; Tegamide; Ticon; Tigan (Monarch); Triban; Tribenzagen; Trimazide
Other common trade names: *Anaus; Elen; Ibikin*
Indications: Prevention and treatment of nausea and vomiting
Category: Antiemetic
Half-life: N/A

Reactions

Skin
Allergic reactions (sic) (<1%)

Other
Headache
Hypersensitivity (<1%)
Injection-site reactions (sic)
Parkinsonism

TRIMETHOPRIM*

Trade names: Bactrim (Women First); Polytrim; Septra (Monarch)
Other common trade names: *Abaprim; Alprim; Bactin; Idotrim; Ipral; Lidaprim; Methoprim; Monotrim; Primosept; Syraprim; Tiempe; Triprim; Unitrim; Wellcprim*
Indications: Various urinary tract infections caused by susceptible organisms
Category: Sulfonamide antibiotic
Half-life: 8–10 hours
Clinically important, potentially hazardous interactions with: dofetilide, methotrexate

Reactions

Skin
Erythema multiforme
Erythema nodosum
   (1983): *Ugeskr Laeger* (Danish) 145, 1070
Exanthems
Exfoliative dermatitis (<1%)
Photosensitivity
Pruritus (1–10%)
Rash (sic) (2.9–6.7%)
Stevens–Johnson syndrome
Toxic epidermal necrolysis

Other
Anaphylactoid reactions
Dysgeusia
Glossitis
Headache

*Note: Although trimethoprim has been known to elicit occasional adverse reactions by itself, it is most commonly used in conjunction with sulfamethoxazole (co-trimoxazole). The trade names for this combination are: Bactrim; Cotrim; Septra. Please see co-trimoxazole for the specific reaction patterns and references

TRIMETREXATE

Trade name: Neutrexin (US Bioscience)
Indications: *Pneumocystis carinii* pneumonia
Category: Antineoplastic; Antiprotozoal; Folate antagonist
Half-life: 15–17 hours

Reactions

Skin
Angioedema
   (1990): Grem JL+, *Drugs* 8, 211
Exanthems
   (1987): Leiby J+, *Invest New Drugs* 5, 136
Fixed eruption
Flu-like syndrome (sic) (1–10%)
Flushing
   (1990): Grem JL+, *Drugs* 8, 211
Photosensitivity
Pruritus (5.5%)
   (1990): Grem JL+, *Drugs* 8, 211
Rash (sic) (1–10%)

Other
Hypersensitivity (1–10%)
Oral mucosal lesions
   (1987): Leiby J+, *Invest New Drugs* 5, 136
Stomatitis (1–10%)

TRIMIPRAMINE

Trade name: Surmontil (Odyssey)
Other common trade names: *Apo-Trimip; Rhotrimine; Stangyl; Sumontil*
Indications: Major depression
Category: Antineuralgic; Tricyclic antidepressant
Half-life: 20–26 hours
Clinically important, potentially hazardous interactions with: amprenavir, arbutamine, bupropion, clonidine, epinephrine, formoterol, guanethidine, isocarboxazid, linezolid, MAO inhibitors, phenelzine, quinolones, sparfloxacin, tranylcypromine

Reactions

Skin
Allergic reactions (sic) (<1%)
Diaphoresis (1–10%)
Exanthems
Petechiae
Photosensitivity (<1%)
Pruritus
Purpura
Rash (sic)
Urticaria

Hair
Hair – alopecia (<1%)

Other
Dysgeusia (>10%)
Galactorrhea (<1%)
Glossitis
Gynecomastia (<1%)
Paresthesias
Parkinsonism (1–10%)
Seizures
(2001): Enns MW, *J Clin Psychiatry* 62(6), 476 (with bupropion)
Stomatitis
Tinnitus
Tremor
Xerostomia (>10%)

TRIOXSALEN

Trade name: Trisoralen (ICN)
Other common trade names: *Neosoralen; Puvadin*
Indications: Vitiligo, hypopigmentation
Category: Psoralen; Repigmenting agent
Half-life: ~2 hours

Reactions

Skin
Acne
(1978): Nielsen EB+, *Acta Derm Venereol* (Stockh) 58, 374
Bullous eruption (with UVA)
(1999): Chuan MT+, *J Formos Med Assoc* 98, 335
(1979): Abel EA+, *Arch Dermatol* 115, 988
(1977): Melski JW+, *J Invest Dermatol* 68, 328
(1976): Thomsen K+, *Br J Dermatol* 95, 568
Eczema (sic)
(1979): Saihan EM, *BMJ* 2, 20
Freckles
(1984): Kietzmann E+, *Dermatologica* 168, 306
(1983): Kanerva L+, *Dermatologica* 166, 281
Granuloma annulare
(1979): Dorval JC+, *Ann Dermatol Venereol* (French) 106, 79
Herpes simplex
(1982): Stüttgen G, *Int J Dermatol* 21, 198
Herpes zoster
(1982): Stüttgen G, *Int J Dermatol* 21, 198
(1977): Roenigk HH+, *Arch Dermatol* 113, 1667
Lupus erythematosus
(1985): Bruze M+, *Acta Derm Venereol* (Stockh) 65, 31
Melanoma
(1980): Forrest JB+, *J Surg Oncol* 13, 337
Pemphigus
(1978): Robinson JK, *Br J Dermatol* 99, 709
Photosensitivity
(1978): Plewig G+, *Arch Derm Res* 261, 201
(1977): Ljunggren B, *Contact Dermatitis* 3, 85
(1976): Jonelis FJ+, *Arch Dermatol* 112, 1036
Phototoxicity
(2001): Snellman E+, *Acta Derm Venereol* 81(3), 171
(1992): George SA+, *Br J Dermatol* 127, 444
(1979): Fischer T+, *Acta Derm Venereol* (Stockh) 59, 171
Pigmentation
(1989): Weiss E+, *Int J Dermatol* 28, 188
(1987): Bruce DR+, *J Am Acad Dermatol* 16, 1087
(1986): MacDonald KJS+, *Br J Dermatol* 114, 395
Porokeratosis (actinic)
(1988): Beiteke U+, *Photodermatology* 5, 274
(1985): Hazen PG+, *J Am Acad Dermatol* 12, 1077

(1980): Reymond JL, *Acta Derm Venereol* (Stockh) 60, 539
Pruritus (>10%)
(1999): Chuan MT+, *J Formos Med Assoc* 98, 335
Scleroderma
(1976): Duperrat B+, *Bull Soc Franc Dermatol Syphiligr* (French) 83, 79
Seborrheic dermatitis
(1983): Tegner E, *Acta Derm Venereol* (Stockh) Suppl 107, 5
Skin pain (sic)
(1987): Norris PG+, *Clin Exp Dermatol* 12, 403
(1983): Tegner E, *Acta Derm Venereol* (Stockh) Suppl 107, 5
Vasculitis
(1981): Barriere H+, *Presse Med* (French) 10, 37
Vitiligo
(1983): Tegner E, *Acta Derm Venereol* (Stockh) Suppl 107, 5
(1976): Duperrat B+, *Bull Soc Franc Dermatol Syphiligr* (French) 83, 79
Xerosis
(1999): Chuan MT+, *J Formos Med Assoc* 98, 335

Hair
Hair – hypertrichosis
(1983): Rampen FHJ, *Br J Dermatol* 109, 657
(1967): Singh G+, *Br J Dermatol* 79, 501

Nails
Nails – photo-onycholysis
(1987): Baran R+, *J Am Acad Dermatol* 17, 1012
Nails – pigmentation
(1990): Trattner A+, *Int J Dermatol* 29, 310
(1989): Weiss E+, *Int J Dermatol* 28, 188
(1986): MacDonald KJS+, *Br J Dermatol* 114, 395
(1982): Naik RPC+, *Int J Dermatol* 21, 275

Other
Lymphoproliferative disease
(1989): Aschinoff R+, *J Am Acad Dermatol* 21, 1134
Tumors (sic)
(1995): Halder RM+, *Arch Dermatol* 131, 734
(1989): Hannuksela M+, *J Am Acad Dermatol* 21, 813
(1988): Gupta AK+, *J Am Acad Dermatol* 19, 67
(1987): Henseler T+, *J Am Acad Dermatol* 16, 108
(1986): Kahn JR+, *Clin Exp Dermatol* 11, 398

TRIPELENNAMINE

Trade name: PBZ (Novartis)
Other common trade names: *Azaron; Pyribenzamine; Triplen*
Indications: Allergic rhinitis, urticaria
Category: Antihistamine H$_1$-blocker
Half-life: N/A
Clinically important, potentially hazardous interactions with: alcohol, barbiturates, chloral hydrate, ethchlorvynol, paraldehyde, phenothiazines

Reactions

Skin
Angioedema (<1%)
(1951): Guiducci A+, *Arch Dermatol* 63, 263
Diaphoresis
Edema (<1%)
Fixed eruption
(1961): Welsh AL+, *Arch Dermatol* 84, 1004
Flushing
Lichenoid eruption
(1947): Epstein E, *JAMA* 134, 782

Lupus erythematosus
Peripheral edema
Photosensitivity (<1%)
Pityriasis rosea
(1947): Epstein E, *JAMA* 134, 782
Purpura
(1956): Wintrobe MM+, *Arch Intern Med* 98, 559
(1951): Uvitsky IH, *J Allergy* 22, 544
Rash (sic) (<1%)
Systemic eczematous contact dermatitis
Urticaria
(1949): London ID, *J Invest Dermatol* 13, 317

Other
Anaphylactoid reactions
Myalgia (<1%)
Paresthesias (<1%)
Stomatitis
Tremor (<1%)
Xerostomia (1–10%)

TRIPROLIDINE

Trade names: Actagen; Actidil; Actifed; Allerphed; Cenafed;
Genac; Myidil; Trifed; Triofed; Triposed*
Other common trade name: *Actidilon*
Indications: Allergic rhinitis
Category: Antihistamine H₁-blocker; Sympathomimetic
Half-life: N/A

Reactions

Skin
Angioedema (<1%)
Diaphoresis (1–10%)
Edema (<1%)
Exanthems
Fixed eruption
(1968): Brownstein MH, *Arch Dermatol* 97, 115
Flushing
Lichenoid eruption
(1964): Alexander S, *BMJ* 2, 512
Photosensitivity (<1%)
Purpura
Rash (sic) (<1%)
Urticaria

Other
Myalgia (<1%)
Paresthesias (<1%)
Xerostomia (1–10%)

*Note: Most of the trade name drugs contain pseudoephedrine as well

TRIPTORELIN

Synonym: Decapeptyl
Trade name: Trelstar (Debio Recherche)
Indications: Palliative treatment of advanced prostate carcinoma
Category: Antineoplastic; Luteinizing hormone-releasing hormone analog
Half-life: 2.8–1.2 hours

Reactions

Skin
Angioedema (<1%)
Hot flashes (59%)
(1996): Choktanasiri W+, *Int J Gynaecol Obstet* 54, 237
(1994): Neskovic-Konstantinovic ZB+, *Oncology* 51, 95
(1994): Vercellini P+, *Fertil Steril* 62, 938
Pruritus (1%)
Vasculitis
(1993): Amichai B+, *Eur J Obstet Gynecol Reprod Biol* 52, 217

Hair
Hair – alopecia
(1997): Kauschansky A+, *Acta Derm Venereol* 77, 333

Other
Anaphylactoid reactions (<1%)
Headache
Hypersensitivity (<1%)
Injection-site pain (4%)
Limb pain (2%)

TROLEANDOMYCIN

Trade name: TAO (Pfizer)
Indications: Various infections caused by susceptible organisms
Category: Macrolide antibiotic
Half-life: N/A
Clinically important, potentially hazardous interactions with: aprepitant, carbamazepine, colchicine, cyclosporine, dihydroergotamine, ergot alkaloids, fluoxetine, fluvoxamine, methysergide, oral contraceptives, paroxetine, pimozide, sertraline, warfarin

Reactions

Skin
Angioedema
(1971): *Med Lett* 13, 55
Erythema multiforme
Exanthems
(1961): Saslaw S, *Med Clin North Am* 45, 839
(1960): Welsh AL+, *Antibiotic Med Clin Ther* 7, 179
Pruritus
(1971): *Med Lett* 13, 55
Rash (sic) (1–10%)
Urticaria (1–10%)
(1971): *Med Lett* 13, 55

Other
Anaphylactoid reactions
Oral mucosal lesions
(1971): *Med Lett* 13, 55

TROVAFLOXACIN*

Trade name: Trovan (Pfizer)
Indications: Various infections caused by susceptible organisms
Category: Fourth generation fluoroquinolone antibiotic
Half-life: 9.5 hours

Reactions

Skin
Acne
Allergic reactions (sic) (<1%)
Angioedema (<1%)
Balanoposthitis (<1%)
Candidiasis (<1%)
Cheilitis (<1%)
Dermatitis (sic) (<1%)
Diaphoresis (<1%)
Edema (<1%)
Erythema multiforme
Exanthems
   (1999): Litt JZ, Beachwood, OH (personal case) (observation)
Exfoliation (<1%)
Facial edema (<1%)
Flushing (<1%)
Lichen planus
   (1999): Smith KC, Niagara Falls, NY (from Internet)
      (observation)
Periorbital edema (<1%)
Peripheral edema (<1%)
Photosensitivity (0.03%)
   (2000): Ferguson J+, J Antimicrob Chemother 45, 503
Phototoxicity
   (2000): Traynor NJ+, Toxicol Vitr 14, 275
Pruritus (2%)
   (1999): Litt JZ, Beachwood, OH (personal case) (observation)
   (1998): Mayne JT+, J Antimicrob Chemother 39, 67
Pruritus ani (<1%)
Rash (sic) (2%)
Seborrhea (<1%)
Stevens–Johnson syndrome (<1%)
Toxic epidermal necrolysis
   (1999): Matthews MR+, Arch Intern Med 159, 2225
Ulcerations (<1%)
Urticaria (<1%)
Vasculitis

Other
Anaphylactoid reactions (<1%)
Dysgeusia (<1%)
Foetor ex ore (halitosis) (<1%)
Gingivitis (<1%)
Headache
Hypersensitivity
Injection-site edema (<1%)
Injection-site inflammation (<1%)
Injection-site pain (<1%)
Myalgia (<1%)
Paresthesias (<1%)
Serum sickness
Sialorrhea (<1%)
Stomatitis (<1%)
Tendon rupture
Thrombophlebitis (<1%)

Tongue disorder (<1%)
Tongue edema (<1%)
Vaginitis (<10%)
Xerostomia (<1%)

*__Note:__ Trovafloxacin has been withdrawn in the USA except for intravenous hospital use

TRYPTOPHAN

Scientific name: *L-2-amino-3-(indole-3yl) propionic acid*
Family: None
Trade and other common names: 5-HT; 5-HTP; 5-hydroxytryptophan; 5-OHTrp; L-trypt; L-tryptophan
Category: Sedative; Serotonin modulator
Purported indications and other uses: Insomnia, depression, myofascial pain, premenstrual syndrome, smoking cessation, bruxism
Half-life: N/A
Clinically important, potentially hazardous interactions with: fluoxetine, fluvoxamine, isocarboxazid, phenelzine, sibutramine, tranylcypromine

Reactions

Skin
Diaphoresis (with phenelzine)
Scleroderma
   (2000): Egermayer P, J Intern Med 247(1), 11
   (2000): Nietert PJ+, Curr Opin Rheumatol 12(6), 520
   (1998): Haustein UF+, Clin Dermatol 16(3), 353
   (1990): Silver RM+, N Engl J Med 322(13), 874

Other
Death
   (2002): Avarello TP+, Neurol Sci 23, S55 (from contaminants)
Eosinophilia–myalgia syndrome
   (2003): Klarskov K+, J Rheumatol 30(1), 89
   (2000): Fernstrom JD, Am J Clin Nutr 71(6), 1669
   (1999): Barth H+, Adv Exp Med Biol 467, 487
   (1999): Hess EV, Environ Health Perspect 107, 709
   (1999): Klarskov K+, Adv Exp Med Biol 467, 461
   (1999): Muller B+, Adv Exp Med Biol 467, 481
   (1999): Terao T+, Ryoikibetsu Shokogun Shirizu 27 Pt 2, 650
   (1998): Bohme A+, Ann Hematol 77(5), 235
   (1998): Haustein UF+, Clin Dermatol 16(3), 353
   (1998): Williamson BL+, Biomed Chromatogr 12(5), 255
   (1998): Williamson BL+, Toxicol Lett 99, 13
   (1997): Blackburn WD Jr, Semin Arthritis Rheum 26, 788
   (1996): Clauw DJ+, J Rheumatol Suppl 46, 2
   (1990): Edison M+, Lancet 335, 645
   (1990): Hertzman PA+, N Engl J Med 322(13), 869
   (1990): Martin RW+, Ann Intern Med 113, 124
   (1990): Medsger TA, N Engl J Med 322, 926
Fever
   (2002): Avarello TP+, Neurol Sci 23, S55
Parkinsonism
Serotonin syndrome
   (2002): Avarello TP+, Neurol Sci 23, S55
Shivering (with phenelzine)

__Note:__ Tryptophan is an essential amino acid. It is a precursor of serotonin and is also converted to nicotinic acid and nicotinamide

TURMERIC

Scientific names: *Curcuma aromatica; Curcuma domestica; Curcuma longa; Curcuma xanthorrhiza*
Family: Zingiberaceae
Trade and other common names: Calebin-A; Chiang Huang; Curcumin; E100; Haridra; Indian Saffron; Jiang Huang; Yellow Root; Yu Jin; Zedoary
Category: Anti-inflammatory
Purported indications and other uses: Arthritis, anticarcinogen, stimulant, carminative, amenorrhea, angina, asthma, colorectal cancer, delirium, diarrhea, dyspepsia, flatulence, hemorrhage, hepatitis, hypercholesterolemia, hypertension, jaundice, mania, menstrual disorders, ophthalmia, tendonitis. Topical: conjuctivitis, skin cancer, smallpox, chickenpox, leg ulcers. Food coloring in cheese, margarine, sweets, snack foods, cosmetics, essential oil in perfumes, culinary spice
Half-life: N/A

Reactions

Skin

Allergic reactions (sic) (rare)
Dermatitis
(1997): Hata M+, *Contact Dermatitis* 36(2), 107
(1993): Futrell JM+, *Cutis* 52(5), 288
(1987): Goh CL+, *Contact Dermatitis* 17(3), 186

Note: Persons with symptoms of gallstones or obstruction of bile passages should avoid turmeric

UNOPROSTONE

Synonym: UF-021
Trade name: Rescula (Novartis)
Indications: Open-angle glaucoma
Category: Antiglaucoma
Half-life: 14 minutes

Reactions

Skin
Allergic reactions (sic) (1–10%)
Diaphoresis
Eyelid edema
Flu-like syndrome (6%)
Local irritation
    (1999): Hejkal TW+, *Semin Ophthalmol* 14, 114
Ocular burning (10–25%)
Ocular erythema
    (2001): Aung T+, *Am J Ophthalmol* 131(5), 636
Ocular pruritus (10–25%)
Shivering

Hair
Eyelashes – growth
    (1999): Hejkal TW+, *Semin Ophthalmol* 14, 114
Eyelashes – hypertrichosis (10–14%)
Eyelashes – length decreased (7%)

Other
Headache
Myalgia
Ocular pigmentation
    (2002): Novack GD+, *J Am Geriatr Soc* 50(5), 956
    (2002): Stjernschantz JW+, *Surv Ophthalmol* 47, S162
    (1999): Hejkal TW+, *Semin Ophthalmol* 14, 114
Ocular stinging (10–25%)
Paresthesias (tongue)
    (1998): Stewart WC+, *J Glaucoma* 7, 388
    (1996): Haria M+, *Drugs Aging* 9, 213
    (1993): Azuma I+, *Jpn J Ophthalmol* 37, 514
Xerostomia
    (1998): Stewart WC+, *J Glaucoma* 7, 388
    (1996): Haria M+, *Drugs Aging* 9, 213
    (1993): Azuma I+, *Jpn J Ophthalmol* 37, 514

UROFOLLITROPIN

Trade names: Bravelle; Fertinex; Metrodin
Other common trade names: *Fertinorm; Follegon; Follimon; Gonotrop F; Medtrodine HP; Metrodin HP*
Indications: Infertility, Polycystic ovary syndrome, Follicle stimulation
Category: Hormone; Hormone modifier; Ovarian stimulant
Half-life: N/A

Reactions

Skin
Chills
Exanthems
Hot flashes
Urticaria
Xerosis

Hair
Hair – alopecia

Other
Abdominal pain
Fatigue
Fever
Injection-site edema
Injection-site irritation
Injection-site pain
Injection-site rash
Mastodynia
Myalgia
Thrombophlebitis

UROKINASE

Trade name: Abbokinase (Abbott)
Other common trade name: *Ukidan*
Indications: Acute myocardial infarction, coronary artery thrombosis, pulmonary embolism
Category: Thrombolytic enzyme
Half-life: 10–20 minutes
Clinically important, potentially hazardous interactions with: aspirin, bivalirudin, ibuprofen, indomethacin

Reactions

Skin
Angioedema (>10%)
    (2001): Pechlaner C+, *Blood Coagul Fibrinolysis* 12(6), 491
Bleeding (44%)
Bullous eruption (hemorrhagic)
    (1995): Ejaz AA+, *Am J Nephrol* 15, 178
Chills
Diaphoresis (<1%)
Ecchymoses
Exanthems
Flushing
Periorbital edema (>10%)
Pruritus
Purpura
Rash (sic) (<1%)
Urticaria

Other
Anaphylactoid reactions (>10%)
    (2001): Pechlaner C+, *Blood Coagul Fibrinolysis* 12(6), 491
Hypersensitivity
    (2001): Pechlaner C+, *Blood Coagul Fibrinolysis* 12(6), 491
Injection-site phlebitis

URSODIOL

Synonym: Ursodeoxycholic Acid
Trade names: Actigall (Watson); Urso (Axcan Scandipharm)
Other common trade names: *Adursall; Arsacol; Biliepar; Cholacid; Cholit-Ursan; Cholofalk; Coledos; Delursan; Desocol; Desoxil; Destolit; Deurcil; Dexo; Estazor; Fraurs; Galmax; Lentorsil; Litanin; Litocure; Litoff; Litursol; Lyeton; Peptaron; Solutrat; UDC; UDC Hexal; Urdafalk; Urdes; Urosofalk; Urso Heumann; Urso Vinas; Ursochol; Ursofal; Ursoflor; Ursolac; Ursolism; Ursolvan; Ursolvan; Urson; Ursoproge; Ursosan; Ursotan; USCA*
Indications: Cholelithiasis
Category: Gallstone dissolution agent
Half-life: 100 hours

Reactions

Skin

Allergic reactions (sic) (5%)
Dermatitis herpetiformis
   (2001): Stroubou E+, *J Am Acad Dermatol* 45(2), 319
Diaphoresis
Lichen planus
   (1992): Ellul JP+, *Dig Dis Sci* 37, 628
Lichenoid eruption
   (2002): Matsuzaki Y+, *Gastroenterology* 122(5), 1547
   (2001): Horiuchi Y, *Gastroenterology* 121(2), 501
Pruritus (<1%)
Psoriasis
Rash (sic) (1–3%)
Urticaria
Xerosis

Hair

Hair – alopecia (<1% to 5%)

Other

Arthralgia
Depression
Dizziness (~17%)
Dysgeusia (<1%) (metallic taste)
Fatigue (<1%)
Myalgia
Stomatitis

VALACYCLOVIR

Trade name: Valtrex (GSK)
Indications: Genital herpes, herpes simplex, herpes zoster
Category: Antiviral
Half-life: 3 hours
**Clinically important, potentially hazardous interactions
with:** immunosuppressants, meperidine

Reactions

Skin

Facial edema (3–5%)
  (2000): Colin J+, *Ophthalmology* (107) 1507 (3–5%)
Periorbital edema (3–5%)
  (2000): Colin J+, *Ophthalmology* 107, 1507 (3–5%)
Pruritus (generalized)
  (2001): Vaughan TK, Tacoma, WA (from Internet) (observation)
Purpura
  (2000): Rivaud E+, *Arch Intern Med* 160, 1705
Systemic contact dermatitis
  (2001): Lammintausta K+, *Contact Dermatitis* 45(3), 181

Other

Headache
Paresthesias
  (2003): Baker D+, *Cutis* 71(3), 239

VALDECOXIB

Trade name: Bextra (Pfizer)
Indications: Osteoarthritis, adult rheumatoid arthritis,
dysmenorrhea
Category: Nonsteroidal anti-inflammatory (NSAID) COX-2
inhibitor
Half-life: 8–11 hours
**Clinically important, potentially hazardous interactions
with:** aspirin, dextromethorphan, lithium, warfarin

Reactions

Skin

Acne (<2%)
Allergic reactions (sic) (<2%)
Basal cell carcinoma
Candidiasis
Cellulitis (<2%)
Chills (<2%)
Dermatitis (sic) (<2%)
Diaphoresis (<2%)
Ecchymoses (<2%)
Eczema (sic) (<2%)
Edema (<2%)
Erythema multiforme
  (2003): Sharma R, Aligarh, India (from Internet) (observation)
Exanthems (<2%)
  (2002): Litt JZ, Beachwood, OH (personal case)
  (2002): Smith JG, Mobile, AL (from Internet) (observation)
Facial edema (<2%)
Flu-like syndrome (2%)
Hemangioma (<2%)
Hematomas (<2%)
Herpes simplex

Herpes zoster
Hot flashes (<2%)
Malignant melanoma
Periorbital edema (<2%)
Peripheral edema (2–3%)
Photosensitivity (<2%)
Pruritus (<2%)
Psoriasis (<2%)
Rash (sic) (1–2)
Toxic epidermal necrolysis
  (2003): Glasser DL+, *Pharmacotherapy* 23(4), 551
Ulcerations (<2%)
Upper respiratory infection (6–7%)
Urticaria (<2%)
Xerosis (<2%)

Hair

Hair – alopecia (<2%)

Other

Arthralgia (<2%)
Back pain (2–3%)
Cough (<2%)
Depression (<2%)
Dysgeusia (<2%)
Foetor ex ore (halitosis) (<2%)
Headache
Hyperesthesia (<2%)
Lipoma (<2%)
Myalgia (2%)
Paresthesias (<2%)
Stomatitis (<2%)
Tendinitis (<2%)
Thrombophlebitis (<2%)
Tinnitus (2–10%)
Tooth disorder (sic)
Tremor (<2%)
Twitching (<2%)
Vaginal candidiasis
Xerostomia (<2%)

Note: Valdecoxib is a sulfonamide and can be absorbed systemically.
Sulfonamides can produce severe, possibly fatal, reactions such as
toxic epidermal necrolysis and Stevens–Johnson syndrome

VALERIAN

Scientific names: *Valeriana edulis; Valeriana jatamansii; Valeriana officinalis; Valeriana sitchensis; Valeriana wallichii*
Family: Valerianaceae
Trade and other common names: All-Heal; Amantilla; Baldrian; Garden Heliotrope
Category: Anxiolytic; Sedative-hypnotic
Purported indications and other uses: Depression, tremors, epilepsy, attention deficit hyperactivity disorder, rheumatism, nervous asthma, gastric spasms, colic, menstrual cramps, hot flashes. Flavoring in foods and beverages
Half-life: N/A
Clinically important, potentially hazardous interactions with: escitalopram

Reactions

Skin
Adverse effects (sic)
  (2002): Haller CA+, *Adverse Drug React Toxicol Rev* 21(3), 143

Other
Toxicity
  (2001): Boniel T+, *Harefuah* 140(8), 780
Tremor
  (2001): Boniel T+, *Harefuah* 140(8), 780

VALGANCICLOVIR*

Trade name: Valcyte (Roche)
Indications: Cytomegalovirus retinitis (in patients with AIDS)
Category: Antiviral
Half-life: 4 hours (In severe renal impairment up to 68%)

*****Note:** Valganciclovir is rapidly converted to ganciclovir in the body

Reactions

Skin
Allergic reactions (sic) (<5%)
Infections (sic) (<5%)
Rash (sic)

Other
Headache
Paresthesias (8%)
  (2001): Curran M+, *Drugs* 61(8), 1145

VALPROIC ACID

Trade names: Depakene (Abbott); Depacon (Abbott)
Indications: Seizures, migraine
Category: Anticonvulsant
Half-life: 6–16 hours
Clinically important, potentially hazardous interactions with: aspirin, cholestyramine, ivermectin

Reactions

Skin
Acne

Allergic reactions (sic) (<5%)
Bullous eruption
  (2001): Christ EA+ (poster at meeting of the American Federation for Medical Research)
Dermatitis
Diaphoresis
  (2001): Hebert AA+, *J Clin Psychiatry* 62(suppl 14), 22
Ecchymoses (<5%)
  (2001): Christ EA+ (poster at meeting of the American Federation for Medical Research)
  (2000): Picart N+, *Presse Med* (French) 29, 648
  (1983): Bruni J+, *Arch Neurol* 40, 135
  (1978): Lewis JR, *JAMA* 240, 2190
Edema
  (2002): Witters I+, *Prenat Diagn* 22(9), 834
Erythema multiforme (<1%)
  (2001): Hebert AA+, *J Clin Psychiatry* 62(suppl 14), 22
  (1990): Chan HL+, *Arch Dermatol* 126, 43
Exanthems (5%)
Facial edema (>5%)
Fixed eruption
  (1997): Chan HL+, *J Am Acad Dermatol* 36, 259
Furunculosis (<5%)
Lupus erythematosus
  (1996): Gigli GL+, *Epilepsia* 37(6), 587
  (1996): Park-Matsumoto YC+, *J Neurol Sci* 143, 185
  (1994): Fritzler MJ, *Lupus* 3, 455
  (1993): Drory VE+, *Clin Neuropharmacol* 16, 19 (passim)
  (1990): Bleck TP+, *Epilepsia* 31, 343
Morphea
  (1980): Goihman-Yahr M+, *Arch Dermatol* 116, 621
Peripheral edema (<5%)
Petechiae (<5%)
  (2001): Hebert AA+, *J Clin Psychiatry* 62(suppl 14), 22
Photosensitivity
  (2001): Hebert AA+, *J Clin Psychiatry* 62(suppl a4), 22
Pruritus (>5%)
  (2001): Hebert AA+, *J Clin Psychiatry* 62(suppl 14), 22
Psoriasis
Purpura
  (1984): *Drugs Ther Bull* 22, 23
  (1976): Winfield DA+, *BMJ* 2, 98
Rash (sic) (>5%)
  (2002): Gallagher RM+, *J Am Osteopath Assoc* 102(2), 92
  (1978): Lewis JR, *JAMA* 240, 2190
Scleroderma
  (1980): Goihman-Yahr M+, *Arch Dermatol* 116, 621
Seborrhea
Stevens–Johnson syndrome
  (1999): Rzany B+, *Lancet* 353, 2190
  (1998): Tsai SJ+, *J Clin Psychopharmacol* 18, 420
Toxic epidermal necrolysis
  (1999): Rzany B+, *Lancet* 353, 2190
  (1991): Porteous DM+, *Arch Dermatol* 127, 740
Urticaria
Vasculitis
  (2003): Bonnet F+, *J Rheumatol* 30(1), 208
  (1991): Kamper AM+, *Lancet* 1, 497

Hair
Hair – alopecia (7%)
  (2002): Gallagher RM+, *J Am Osteopath Assoc* 102(2), 92
  (2001): Hebert AA+, *J Clin Psychiatry* 62(suppl 14), 22
  (1998): Fetterman M (Miami FL) (from Internet) (observation)
  (1996): McKinney PA+, *Ann Clin Psychiatry* 8, 183
  (1996): Wallace SJ, *Drug Saf* 15, 378
  (1995): Fatemi SH+, *Ann Pharmacother* 29, 1302
  (1981): Herranz JL, *Dev Med Child Neurol* 23, 386

(1978): *Drug Ther Bull* 16, 77 (up to 10%)
(1978): Lewis JR, *JAMA* 240, 2190
(1977): Pinder RM+, *Drugs* 13, 81 (.5%)
(1976): Winfield DA+, *BMJ* 2, 981
(1975): Barnes SE+, *Dev Med Child Neurol* 17, 175
(1974): Jeavons PM+, *BMJ* 2, 584
Hair – curly
(2001): Caneppele S+, *Ann Dermatol Venereol* 128(2), 134
(1988): Gupta AK, *Br J Clin Pract* 42, 75
(1977): Jeavons PM+, *Lancet* 1, 359
Hair – depigmentation
(1981): Herranz JL+, *Dev Med Child Neurol* 23, 386

Other
Acute intermittent porphyria
(1989): Herrick AL+, *Br J Clin Pharmacol* 27, 491
(1980): Garcia-Merino JA+, *Lancet* 2, 856
Anticonvulsant hypersensitivity syndrome
(2003): Bin-Nakhi HA+, *Med Princ Pract* 12(3), 197
Aplasia cutis congenita
Death
(2002): Yazdani K+, *Medicine* (Baltimore) 81(4), 305
Dysgeusia (<5%)
Galactorrhea
(1983): Kollipara S+, *J Pediatr* 103, 501
Gingival hyperplasia
(1997): Anderson HH+, *ASDC J Dent Child* 64, 294
(1991): Behari M, *J Neurol Neurosurg Psychiatry* 54, 279
Glossitis (<5%)
Gynecomastia
(1983): Kollipara S+, *J Pediatr* 103, 501
Headache
Hyperesthesia
Hypersensitivity
(2000): Moore SJ+, *J Med Genet* 37, 489
(1994): Garcia-Bravo B+, *Contact Dermatitis* 30, 40
Myalgia (<5%)
Paresthesias (<5%)
Parkinsonism
(2002): Barroso B, *Therapie* 57(4), 410
(2002): Iijima M, *J Clin Psychiatry* 63(1), 75
Porphyria
(1991): Jalil P+, *Rev Med Chil* 119, 920
(1981): Doss M+, *Lancet* 2, 91
Pseudolymphoma
(2001): Cogrel O+, *Br J Dermatology* 144, 1235
Rhabdomyolysis
(2001): Kottlors M+, *Neuromuscul Disord* 11(8), 757
Seizures
(2001): Lerman-Sagie T+, *Epilepsia* 42(7), 941
Sialorrhea
Stomatitis (<5%)
Tinnitus
(2000): Reeves RR+, *South Med J* 93(10), 1030
Tremor
(2002): Gallagher RM+, *J Am Osteopath Assoc* 102(2), 92
(2002): Thibault M+, *Epilepsy Res* 50(3), 243
(2002): Tohen M+, *Arch Gen Psychiatry* 59(1), 62 (with lithium)
Vaginitis (<5%)
Xerostomia (<5%)
(2002): Tohen M+, *Arch Gen Psychiatry* 59(1), 62 (with olanzapine)

VALRUBICIN

Trade name: Valstar (Celltech)
Indications: Bladder carcinoma
Category: Antineoplastic (Analog of doxorubicin)
Half-life: N/A

Reactions

Skin
Irritation (sic) (<1%)
Peripheral edema (1%)
Pruritus (<1%)
Rash (sic) (3%)

Other
Abdominal pain (5%)
Ageusia (<1%)
Back pain (3%)
Dizziness (3%)
Fever (2%)
Myalgia (1%)
Pneumonia (1%)

VALSARTAN

Trade name: Diovan (Novartis)
Indications: Hypertension
Category: Angiotensin II receptor antagonist; Antihypertensive
Half-life: 9 hours

Reactions

Skin
Allergic reactions (sic) (>2%)
Angioedema (>2%)
(2000): de la Serna Higuera C, *Med Clin (Barc)* (Spanish) 114, 599
(1998): Frye Cb+, *Pharmacotherapy* 18, 866
Edema (>1%)
(2000): Prat H, *Rev Med Chil* (Spanish) 128, 475
(1996): Corea L+, *Clin Pharmacol Ther* 60, 341
Flushing
(2000): Prat H, *Rev Med Chil* (Spanish) 128, 475
Photosensitivity
(1998): Frye Cb+, *Pharmacotherapy* (18) 866
Pruritus (>2%)
Rash (sic) (>2%)
Urticaria
(2000): de la Serna Higuera C, *Med Clin (Barc)* (Spanish) 114, 599

Nails
Nails – bed changes (sic)
Nails – pigmentation

Other
Aphthous stomatitis (1–10%)
Arthralgia (1–10%)
Cough
(2000): Prat H, *Rev Med Chil* 128, 475
Death
(2001): Briggs GG+, *Ann Pharmacother* 35(7), 859
Dysgeusia (>10%)
Headache
Injection-site extravasation (<1%)

Injection-site pain
Injection-site phlebitis
Injection-site reactions (sic)
Myalgia (10–29%)
Paresthesias (>2%)
Xerostomia (>10%)

VANCOMYCIN

Trade name: Vancocin (Lilly)
Other common trade names: *Balcoran; Diatracin; Vanmicina*
Indications: Various infections caused by susceptible organisms
Category: Narrow-spectrum antibiotic
Half-life: 5–11 hours
Clinically important, potentially hazardous interactions with: succinylcholine

Reactions

Skin

Acute generalized exanthematous pustulosis (AGEP)
  (1996): Sawhney RA+, *Int J Dermatol* 35, 826
  (1995): Moreau A+, *Int J Dermatol* 34, 263 (passim)
  (1991): Roujeau J-C+, *Arch Dermatol* 127, 1333
Allergic reactions (sic) (<5%)
  (2001): Bernedo N+, *Contact Dermatitis* 45(1), 43
  (1997): Kahata S+, *Bone Marrow Transplant* 20, 1001
  (1997): Korman TM+, *J Antimicrob Chemother* 39(3), 371
  (1992): Breathnach SM+, *Adverse Drug Reactions and the Skin*
    Blackwell, Oxford, 158 (passim)
Angioedema
  (1989): Koestner B+, *Schweiz Med Wochenschr* (German)
    119, 28
  (1959): Rothenberg HJ, *JAMA* 171, 1102
Bullous eruption
  (1996): Heald PW, *Skin and Allergy News* 27, 18
  (1992): Carpenter S+, *J Am Acad Dermatol* 26, 45
  (1990): Forrence EA+, *Drug Intell Clin Pharm* 24, 369
  (1988): Baden LA+, *Arch Dermatol* 124, 1186
Chills (>10%)
Erythema multiforme
  (2001): Hsu SI, *Pharmacotherapy* 21(10), 1233
  (2000): Padial MA+, *Allergy* 55, 1201
  (1992): Laurencin CT, *Ann Pharmacotherapy* 26, 1520
  (1988): Gutfeld MB+, *Drug Intell Clin Pharm* 22, 881
Exanthems
  (1991): McCullough JM+, *Drug Intell Clin Pharm* 25, 1326
  (1991): Valero R+, *J Cardiothorac Vasc Anesth* 5, 574
  (1988): Neal D+, *BMJ* 296, 137
  (1988): Schlemmer B+, *N Engl J Med* 318, 1127
  (1987): Lacouture PG+, *J Pediatr* 111, 615 (35%)
  (1987): Longon P+, *Presse Med* (French) 16, 682
  (1986): Davis RL+, *Ann Intern Med* 104, 285
  (1986): Markman M+, *South Med J* 79, 382 (passim)
  (1986): McElrath MJ+, *Lancet* 1, 47
  (1985): Schifter S+, *Lancet* 2, 499 (8%)
  (1984): Odio C+, *Am J Dis Child* 138, 17
  (1984): Rimailho A+, *Presse Med* (French) 13, 567
  (1960): Kirby WMM+, *N Engl J Med* 262, 49 (1–5%)
Exfoliative dermatitis
  (1990): Forrence EA+, *Drug Intell Clin Pharm* 24, 369
  (1988): Gutfeld MB+, *Drug Intell Clin Pharm* 22, 881
  (1988): Neal D+, *BMJ* 296, 137
Flushing (1–10%)
Linear IgA bullous dermatosis
  (2003): Dellavalle RP+, *J Am Acad Dermatol* 48(5), S56

  (2002): Cohen LM+, *J Am Acad Dermatol* 46(2), S32
  (2002): Neughebauer BI+, *Am J Med Sci* 323(5), 273
  (2001): Ahkami R+, *Cutis* 67, 423
  (2001): Chang A+, *Arch Dermatol* 137, 815
  (2001): Palmer RA+, *Br J Dermatol* 145(5), 816 (2 cases)
  (2001): Wiadrowski TP+, *Austral J Dermatol* 42, 196 (with
    ciprofloxacin)
  (2000): Klein PA+, *J Am Acad Dermatol* 42, 316
  (1999): Nousari HC+, *Medicine* 78, 1
  (1998): Bernstein EF+, *Ann Intern Med* 129, 508
  (1998): Nousari HC+, *Ann Intern Med* 129, 507
  (1997): Norland A, Minneapolis, American Academy of
    Dermatology Meeting (SF) (Gross and Microscopic)
  (1996): Bitman LM+, *Arch Dermatol* 1289
  (1996): Primka E+, *J Cutan Pathol* 58
  (1996): Tranvan A+, *J Am Acad Dermatol* 865
  (1996): Whitworth JM+, *J Am Acad Dermatol* 890
  (1995): Geissmann C+, *J Am Acad Dermatol* 296
  (1995): Richards S+, *Arch Dermatol* 1447
  (1994): Kuechle MK+, *J Am Acad Dermatol* 187
  (1994): Piketty C+, *Br J Dermatol* 130
  (1992): Carpenter S+, *J Am Acad Dermatol* 45
  (1988): Baden LA+, *Arch Dermatol* 1186
Lupus erythematosus
  (1993): Ena J+, *JAMA* 269, 598
  (1986): Markman M+, *South Med J* 79, 382
Photoallergic reaction
  (2001): Zabawski E, Longview, TX (from Internet) (observation)
Pruritus
  (1991): Killian AD+, *Ann Intern Med* 115, 410
  (1991): McCullough JM+, *Drug Intell Clin Pharm* 25, 1326
  (1989): Koestner B+, *Schweiz Med Wochenschr* (German)
    119, 28
  (1986): Davis RL+, *Ann Intern Med* 104, 285
  (1959): Rothenberg HJ, *JAMA* 171, 1102
Purpura
  (1998): Michael S+, *Scand J Rheumatol* 27, 233
Rash (sic)
  (2001): Hsu SI, *Pharmacotherapy* 21(10), 1233
  (1997): Reis AG+, *Rev Paul Med* 115, 1452
  (1993): Ena J+, *JAMA* 269, 598
  (1983): Farber BF+, *Antimicrob Agents Chemother* 23, 138
  (1978): Hook EW+, *Am J Med* 65, 411
  (1976): Arndt KA+, *JAMA* 235, 918 (10%)
Red man syndrome* (1–10%)
  (2002): Cohen E+, *J Antimicrob Chemother* 49(1), 155 (10–14%)
  (2002): Hui YL+, *Acta Anaesthesiol Sin* 40(3), 149
  (2001): Wazny LD+, *Ann Pharmacother* 35(11), 1458
  (2000): Wood MJ, *J Chemother* 12, 21
  (1999): Khurana C+, *Postgrad Med J* 75, 41
  (1998): Polk RE, *Ann Pharmacother* 32, 840
  (1996): Szymusiak-Mutnick BA+, *Am J Health Syst Pharm*
    53, 2098
  (1995): Lilley LL+, *Am J Nurs* 95, 14
  (1994): Bergeron L+, *Ann Pharmacother* 28, 581
  (1993): Ena J+, *JAMA* 269, 598
  (1993): O'Sullivan TL+, *J Infect Dis* 168, 773
  (1993): Polk RE+, *Antimicrob Agents Chemother* 37, 2139
  (1992): Levy M+, *Harefuah* (Hebrew) 122, 36
  (1992): Rengo C+, *Recenti Prog Med* (Italian) 83, 726
  (1991): Killian AD+, *Ann Intern Med* 115, 410
  (1991): Maccabruni A+, *Recenti Prog Med* (Italian) 82, 17
  (1991): Valero R+, *J Cardiothorac Vasc Anesth* 5, 574
  (1991): Wallace MR+, *J Infect Dis* 164, 1180
  (1990): Bailie GR+, *Clin Pharm* 9, 671
  (1990): Healey DP+, *Antimicrob Agents Chemother* 34, 550
  (1990): Levy M+, *Pediatrics* 86, 572
  (1990): No Author, *Lancet* 335, 1006
  (1990): Sahai J+, *Antimicrob Agents Chemother* 34, 765
  (1989): Pearson DA, *J Am Dent Assoc* 118, 59

(1989): Sahai J+, *J Infect Dis* 160, 876
(1988): Polk RE+, *J Infect Dis* 157, 502
(1988): Rubin M+, *Ann Intern Med* 108, 30 (3%)
(1987): Duro JC+, *Med Clin (Barc)* (Spanish) 89, 218
(1986): Daly BM+, *Drug Intell Clin Pharm* 20, 986
(1986): Davis RL+, *Ann Intern Med* 104, 285
(1986): Rolston KV+, *JAMA* 255, 2445
(1986): Wade TP+, *Arch Surg* 121, 859
(1985): Cole DR+, *Lancet* 2, 280
(1985): Garrelts JC+, *N Engl J Med* 312, 245
(1985): Holliman R, *Lancet* 1, 1399
Red neck syndrome (sic)
(1985): Ackerman BH+, *Ann Intern Med* 102, 723
(1985): Pau AK+, *N Engl J Med* 313, 756
Stevens–Johnson syndrome (<1%)
(1996): Alexander II+, *Allergy Asthma Proc* 17, 75
(1995): Patterson R+, *Allergy Proc* 16, 115
(1992): Laurencin CT+, *Ann Pharmacother* 26, 1520
(1990): Forrence EA+, *Drug Intell Clin Pharm* 24, 369
Toxic epidermal necrolysis
(2001): Hsu SI, *Pharmacotherapy* 21(10), 1233
(2000): Chan-Tack K, *Mo Med* 97, 131
(1992): Vidal C+, *Ann Allergy* 68, 345
(1990): Hannah BA+, *South Med J* 83, 720
(1985): Heng MCY, *Br J Dermatol* 113, 597
Urticaria
(1989): Koestner B+, *Schweiz Med Wochenschr* (German) 119, 28
(1988): Neal D+, *BMJ* 296, 137
(1987): Longon P+, *Presse Med* (French) 16, 682
(1986): Davis RL+, *Ann Intern Med* 104, 285
(1986): Markman M+, *South Med J* 79, 382 (passim)
(1960): Kirby WMM+, *N Engl J Med* 262, 49 (1–5%)
(1959): Rothenberg HJ, *JAMA* 171, 1102 (1–5%)
Vasculitis (<1%)
(1987): Rawlinson WD+, *Med J Australia* 147, 470
(1986): Markman M+, *South Med J* 79, 382

Other

Anaphylactoid reactions
(2001): Wazny LD+, *Ann Pharmacother* 35(11), 1458
(2000): Chopra N+, *Ann Allergy Asthma Immunol* 84, 633
(1992): Breathnach SM+, *Adverse Drug Reactions and the Skin*
    Blackwell, Oxford, 158 (passim)
(1988): Rubin M+, *Ann Intern Med* 108, 30 (1 in 63 patients)
(1987): Longon P+, *Presse Med* (French) 16, 682
(1986): Markman M+, *Southern Med J* 79, 382 (passim)
Death
(2001): Hsu SI, *Pharmacotherapy* 21(10), 1233
Dysgeusia (>10%)
Hypersensitivity
(2001): Hsu SI, *Pharmacotherapy* 21(10), 1233
(1997): Marik PE+, *Pharmacotherapy* 17, 1341
Injection-site thrombophlebitis
Paresthesias
Phlebitis
(2002): Cohen E+, *J Antimicrob Chemother* 49(1), 155 (14–23%)
(1983): Farber BF+, *Antimicrob Agents Chemother* 23, 138
(1978): Hook EW+, *Am J Med* 65, 411
Priapism
(1998): Czachor JS+, *N Engl J Med* 338, 1701
Tinnitus

*Note: The vancomycin-induced red man syndrome is characterized by pruritus, erythema and, in severe cases, angioedema, hypotension, and cardiovascular collapse

VASOPRESSIN

Synonyms: ADH; antidiuretic hormone
Trade name: Pitressin (Monarch)
Other common trade name: *Pressyn*
Indications: Diabetes insipidus
Category: Antidiuretic pituitary hormone; Vasoconstrictor
Half-life: 10–20 minutes

Reactions

Skin

Allergic reactions (sic) (<1%)
Angioedema
Bullous eruption
(2002): Kahn JM+, *Crit Care Med* 30(8), 1899
(1997): Lin RY+, *Dermatology* 195, 271
(1991): Colemont LJ+, *J Clin Gastroenterol* 13, 91
(1986): Korenberg RJ+, *J Am Acad Dermatol* 15, 393
Diaphoresis (1–10%)
Ecchymoses
(1997): Lin RY+, *Dermatology* 195, 271
(1985): Thomas TK, *Am J Gastroenterol* 80, 704
Exanthems
Pallor (1–10%)
Purpura
(1996): Lemlich G+, *Cutis* 57, 330
(1985): Thomas TK, *Am J Gastroenterol* 80, 704
Rash (sic)
Urticaria (1–10%)

Hair

Hair – alopecia
(1994): Maceyko RD+, *J Am Acad Dermatol* 31, 111

Other

Anaphylactoid reactions
Death
(2001): Rizzo V+, *J Pediatr Endocrinol Metab* 14(7), 861
Gangrene
(1997): Lin RY+, *Dermatology* 195, 271
Headache
Injection-site inflammation
(2002): Kahn JM+, *Crit Care Med* 30(8), 1899
(1997): Lin RY+, *Dermatology* 195, 271 (amber-like)
(1996): Lemlich G+, *Cutis* 57, 330
(1991): Colemont LJ+, *J Clin Gastroenterol* 13, 91
(1990): Stump DL+, *Drugs* 39, 38
(1986): Korenberg RJ+, *J Am Acad Dermatol* 15, 393
(1985): Thomas TK, *Am J Gastroenterol* 80, 704
Injection-site necrosis
(2002): Kahn JM+, *Crit Care Med* 30(8), 1899
Rhabdomyolysis
(1995): Hino A+, *Rinsho Shinkeigaku* 35(8), 911
(1993): de Cuenca Moron B+, *Rev Clin Esp* 192(2), 79
(1993): Pierce ST+, *Am J Gastroenterol* 88(3), 424
(1991): Moreno-Sanchez D+, *Gastroenterology* 101(2), 529
(1991): Moreno-Sanchez D+, *Rev Esp Enferm Dig* 79(2), 160
Trembling
Tremor (1–10%)

VECURONIUM

Trade name: Norcuron
Other common trade name: *Vecuron*
Indications: Adjunct to general anesthesia
Category: Anesthetic; Non-depolarizing neuromuscular blocker; Skeletal muscle relaxant
Half-life: 65–75 minutes
Clinically important, potentially hazardous interactions
with: aminoglycosides, gentamicin, halothane, kanamycin, neomycin, streptomycin, tobramycin, inhalational anesthetics, magnesium salts, quinidine, succinylcholine

Reactions

Other
Anaphylactoid reactions
Injection-site pain
(2003): Blunk JA+, *Eur J Anaesthesiol* 20(3), 245

VENLAFAXINE

Trade name: Effexor (Wyeth)
Indications: Depression
Category: Heterocyclic antidepressant; Selective serotonin reuptake inhibitor (SSRI)
Half-life: 3–7 hours
Clinically important, potentially hazardous interactions
with: isocarboxazid, linezolid, MAO inhibitors, metoclopramide, phenelzine, selegiline, sibutramine, sumatriptan, tramadol, tranylcypromine, trazodone

Reactions

Skin
Acne (<1%)
Allergic reactions (sic) (<1%)
Candidiasis
Dermatitis
Ecchymoses (<1%)
Eczema (sic) (<1%)
Edema (<1%)
Exanthems (<1%)
Exfoliative dermatitis (<1%)
Facial edema (<1%)
Furunculosis (<1%)
Herpes simplex (<1%)
Herpes zoster (<1%)
Lichenoid eruption (<1%)
Peripheral edema
Photosensitivity (<1%)
Pruritus (1–10%)
Psoriasis (<1%)
Pustules (<1%)
Rash (sic) (3%)
Urticaria (<1%)
Vesiculobullous eruption (<1%)
Xerosis (<1%)

Hair
Hair – alopecia (<1%)
(2001): Pitchot W+, *Am J Psych* 158, 1159

Hair – hirsutism (<1%)
Hair – pigmentation (<1%)

Other
Ageusia (<1%)
Bromhidrosis (<1%)
Bruxism
(2000): Jaffee MS+, *Psychosomatics* 41(6), 535
Dysgeusia (2%)
Galactorrhea
(2003): Sternbach H, *J Clin Psychopharmacol* 23(1), 109
Gingivitis (<1%)
Glossitis (<1%)
Gynecomastia (<1%)
Headache
Hyperesthesia (<1%)
Mastodynia
(2000): Bhatia SC+, *J Clin Psychopharmacol* 20(5), 590
(1996): Bhatia SC+, *J Clin Psychiatry* 57, 423
Myalgia (>1%)
Oral ulceration (<1%)
Paresthesias (3%)
Parosmia (<1%)
Serotonin syndrome
(2003): Pan JJ+, *Ann Pharmacother* 37(2), 209
(2002): Fisher AA+, *Ann Pharmacother* 36(1), 67
(2001): McCue RE+, *Am J Psychiatry* 158(12), 2088
Sialorrhea (<1%)
Stomatitis (<1%)
Thrombophlebitis (<1%)
Tinnitus
Tongue edema (<1%)
Tongue pigmentation (<1%)
Tremor (1–10%)
Vaginal candidiasis (<1%)
Vaginitis
Xerostomia (22%)
(2000): Gelenberg AJ+, *JAMA* 283, 3082

VERAPAMIL

Trade names: Calan (Pharmacia); Covera-HS (Pharmacia); Isoptin (Abbott); Tarka (Abbott); Verelan (Schwartz)
Other common trade names: *APO-Verap; Arpamyl LP; Azupamil; Berkatens; Chronovera; Cordilox; Geangin; Isoptine; Nu-Verap; Veraken*
Indications: Angina, hypertension
Category: Antianginal; Antihypertensive; Calcium channel blocker
Half-life: 2–8 hours
Clinically important, potentially hazardous interactions
with: acebutolol, amiodarone, aspirin, atenolol, atorvastatin, betaxolol, carbamazepine, carteolol, clonidine, dantrolene, digoxin, dofetilide, epirubicin, eplerenone, esmolol, lovastatin, metoprolol, **mistletoe**, nadolol, penbutolol, pindolol, propranolol, quinidine, sibutramine, simvastatin, timolol

Tarka is trandolapril and verapamil

Reactions

Skin
Acne
(1989): Stern R+, *Arch Intern Med* 149, 829

Acute febrile neutrophilic dermatosis (Sweet's syndrome)
(1998): Knowles S+, *J Am Acad Dermatol* 38, 201 (passim)
Angioedema
(1998): Knowles S+, *J Am Acad Dermatol* 38, 201 (passim)
(1989): Sadick NS+, *J Am Acad Dermatol* 21, 132
(1989): Stern R+, *Arch Intern Med* 149, 829
Ankle edema
Dermatitis (sic)
Diaphoresis (<1%)
(1989): Stern R+, *Arch Intern Med* 149, 829
(1983): Lewis JG, *Drugs* 25, 196
Ecchymoses (<1%)
(1989): Sadick NS+, *J Am Acad Dermatol* 21, 132
Edema (1.9%)
Erythema multiforme (<1%)
(1991): Kürkçüoglu N+, *J Am Acad Dermatol* 24, 511
(1989): Lin AYF+, *Drug Intell Clin Pharm* 23, 987
(1989): Stern R+, *Arch Intern Med* 149, 829
(1987): Naito S+, *Skin Res* (Japanese) 29, 602
Erythema nodosum
(1998): Knowles S+, *J Am Acad Dermatol* 38, 201 (passim)
Exanthems
(1998): Knowles S+, *J Am Acad Dermatol* 38, 201 (passim)
(1989): McTavish D+, *Drugs* 38, 19
(1989): Sadick NS+, *J Am Acad Dermatol* 21, 132
(1989): Stern R+, *Arch Intern Med* 149, 829
(1983): Lewis JG, *Drugs* 25, 196 (3.2%)
(1982): Anon, *Lakartidningen* (Swedish) 79, 3822
(1980): Midtbo K+, *Curr Ther Res* 27, 830
Exfoliative dermatitis
(1998): Knowles S+, *J Am Acad Dermatol* 38, 201 (passim)
(1989): Stern R+, *Arch Intern Med* 149, 829
Flushing (1–7%)
(1992): Shelley WB+, *Advanced Dermatologic Diagnosis* WB
Saunders, 583 (passim)
(1989): McTavish D+, *Drugs* 38, 19 (1–5.4%)
(1983): Lewis JG, *Drugs* 25, 196 (4–7%)
(1980): Raftos J, *Med J Aust* 2, 78
Hyperkeratosis (palms) (<1%)
(1989): Sadick NS+, *J Am Acad Dermatol* 21, 132
(1983): Major P, *Tidsskr Nor Laegeforen* (Norwegian), 103, 2061
Lichenoid eruption
Lupus erythematosus
(1998): Callen JP, Academy '98 Meeting (4 patients)
(1997): Crowson AN+, *Hum Pathol* 28, 67 (subacute cutaneous)
Peripheral edema (1–10%)
(2002): No author, *Medscape Primary Care* 4
Photosensitivity
(1994): Berger TG+, *Arch Dermatol* 130, 609 (in HIV-infected)
(1989): McTavish D+, *Drugs* 38, 19
(1983): Lewis JG, *Drugs* 25, 196
(1979): Anon, *Med J Aust* 2, 204
Prurigo (sic)
(1983): Lewis JG, *Drugs* 25, 196
Pruritus
(1998): Knowles S+, *J Am Acad Dermatol* 38, 201 (passim)
(1989): McTavish D+, *Drugs* 38, 19
(1989): Stern R+, *Arch Intern Med* 149, 829
(1988): Burgunder JM+, *Hepatogastroenterology* 35, 169
(1983): Lewis JG, *Drugs* 25, 196
(1982): Fischer Hansen J+, *Clin Exp Pharmacol Physiol* 6, 31
Purpura (<1%)
(1982): *Lakartidningen* (Swedish) 79, 3822
Rash (sic) (1.2%)
(1989): Stern R+, *Arch Intern Med* 149, 829
(1987): Johnson BF+, *Clin Pharmacol Ther* 42, 66
Side effects (sic)
(1993): Kitamura K+, *J Dermatol* 20, 279 (psoriasiform)

(1989): McTavish D+, *Drugs* 38, 19. (0.6%)
Stevens–Johnson syndrome (<1%)
(1998): Knowles S+, *J Am Acad Dermatol* 38, 201 (passim)
(1992): Gonski PN, *Med J Aust* 156, 672
(1989): Lin AYF+, *Drug Intell Clin Pharm* 23, 987
(1989): Stern R+, *Arch Intern Med* 149, 829
Urticaria (<1%)
(1998): Knowles S+, *J Am Acad Dermatol* 38, 201 (passim)
(1989): McTavish D+, *Drugs* 38, 19
(1989): Sadick NS+, *J Am Acad Dermatol* 21, 132
(1989): Stern R+, *Arch Intern Med* 149, 829
(1983): Lewis JG, *Drugs* 25, 196
Vasculitis (<1%)
(1989): Sadick NS+, *J Am Acad Dermatol* 21, 132
(1983): Lewis JG, *Drugs* 25, 196

Hair
Hair – alopecia (<1%)
(1994): Litt JZ, Beachwood, OH (personal case) (observation)
(1991): Shelley WB+, *Cutis* 48, 364 (observation)
(1989): Sadick NS+, *J Am Acad Dermatol* 21, 132
(1989): Stern R+, *Arch Intern Med* 149, 829
(1981): Rosing DR+, *Am J Cardiol* 48, 545
(1980): Rosing DR+, *Chest* 78 (Suppl), 239
Hair – hypertrichosis
(1991): Sever PS, *Lancet* 338, 1215
Hair – pigmentation
(1991): Read GM, *Lancet* 338, 1520

Nails
Nails – dystrophy
(1989): Stern R+, *Arch Intern Med* 149, 829

Other
Erythromelalgia
(1992): Drenth JP+, *Br J Dermatol* 127, 292
Galactorrhea (<1%)
Gingival hyperplasia (19%)
(1995): Moghadam BKH+, *Cutis* 56, 46 (passim)
(1993): Steele RM+, *Arch Intern Med* 120, 663
(1989): Pernu HE+, *J Oral Pathol Med* 18, 422
(1987): Giustiniani S+, *Int J Cardiol* 15, 247
Gynecomastia (<1%)
(2000): Hugues FC+, *Ann Med Interne (Paris)* (French) 151, 10
(passim)
(1994): Deniel-Rosanas J, *Med Clin* (Barc) (Spanish) 102, 399
(1994): *BMJ* 308, 503
(1988): Tanner LA+, *Arch Intern Med* 148, 379
Headache
Paresthesias (<1%)
Parkinsonism
(2003): *Prescrire Int* 12(64), 62
Rhabdomyolysis
(2000): Gokel Y+, *Am J Emerg Med* 18, 738 (with trandolapril)
Serum sickness
(1989): Pascual-Velasco F, *Med Clin* (Barc) (Spanish) 92, 719
Xerostomia (<1%)

VERTEPORFIN

Trade name: Visudyne (Novartis)
Indications: Wet form of age-related macular degeneration
Category: Macular degeneration adjunct; Photosensitizer
Half-life: 5–6 hours

Reactions

Skin
Cheilitis
  (1998): Mitchell D, Thomasville, GA (from Internet)
    (observation)
Chills
Diaphoresis
Eczema (sic) (1–10%)
Erythema
Flu-like syndrome (1–10%)
Ocular pruritus
Pallor
Photosensitivity (<3%)
  (2002): Houle JM+, *Retina* 22(6), 691
  (2000): Scott LJ+, *Drugs Aging* 16, 139
Pigmentation
Pruritus
Purpura
Rash (sic)
Shivering
Ulcerations
Urticaria
  (1998): Mitchell D, Thomasville, GA (generalized) (from
    Internet) (observation)
Vesicular eruptions
  (1998): Mitchell D, Thomasville, GA (from Internet)
    (observation)

Other
Arthralgia (1–10%)
Burning mouth syndrome (1–10%)
  (1998): Mitchell D, Thomasville, GA (from Internet)
    (observation)
Chest pain
  (2003): *Prescrire Int* 12(63), 17
  (2002): Cahill MT+, *Am J Ophthalmol* 134(2), 281
Hyperesthesia (1–10%)
Injection-site pain
  (2000): Scott LJ+, *Drugs Aging* 16, 139
Injection-site reactions (sic)
Pain (chest and neck)
  (2002): Cahill MT+, *Am J Ophthalmol* 134(2), 281
Paresthesias

VIDARABINE

Synonyms: adenine arabinoside; ara-A
Trade name: Vira-A Ophthalmic (Parke-Davis)
Other common trade names: *Adena a Ungena; Arasena*
Indications: Herpetic keratoconjunctivitis
Category: Ophthalmic antiviral
Half-life: 3.3 hours
Clinically important, potentially hazardous interactions with: insulin

Reactions

Skin
Ocular burning
Ocular erythema
Ocular pruritus
Pruritus
Rash (sic)

VINBLASTINE

Trade name: Velban (Lilly)
Indications: Lymphomas, melanoma, carcinomas
Category: Antineoplastic
Half-life: initial phase: 3.7 minutes; terminal phase: 24.8 hours
Clinically important, potentially hazardous interactions with: aldesleukin, aprepitant, erythromycin, fluconazole, itraconazole, ketoconazole, miconazole

Reactions

Skin
Acne
  (1962): Falkson G+, *Br J Dermatol* 74, 229
Acral gangrene
  (1998): Reiser M+, *Eur J Clin Microbiol Infect Dis* 17, 58
  (1997): Hladunewich M+, *J Rheumatol* 24, 2371
Bullous eruption (<1%)
Cellulitis
  (1983): Bronner AK+, *J Am Acad Dermatol* 9, 645
Dermatitis (sic) (1–10%)
Erythema
  (1969): Lampkin BC, *Lancet* 1, 891
Erythema multiforme
  (1991): Arias D+, *J Cutan Pathol* 18, 344
Exanthems
Photosensitivity (1–10%)
  (1992): Breathnach SM+, *Adverse Drug Reactions and the Skin*
    Blackwell, Oxford, 302 (passim)
  (1975): Breza TS+, *Arch Dermatol* 111, 1168
Phototoxicity
Pigmentation
  (2001): Mutafoglu-Uysal K+, *Turk J Pediatr* 43(2), 172
  (1997): Smith KJ+, *J Am Acad Dermatol* 36, 329
  (1994): Cecchi R+, *Dermatology* 188, 244
Purpura
Radiation recall
  (1992): Nemechek PM+, *Cancer* 70, 1605
Radiodermatitis (reactivation)
  (1969): Lampkin BC, *Lancet* 1, 891
Rash (sic) (1–10%)
Raynaud's phenomenon (1–10%)

(1998): Reiser M+, *Eur J Clin Microbiol Infect Dis* 17, 58
(1997): Hladunewich M+, *J Rheumatol* 24, 2371
(1993): von Gunten CF+, *Cancer* 72, 2004
(1992): Doll DC+, *Semin Oncol* 19(5), 580
(1981): Harvey HA+, *Ann Intern Med* 94, 542
(1981): Vogelzang NJ+, *Ann Intern Med* 95, 288
(1978): Rothberg H, *Cancer Treat Rep* 62, 569
(1977): Teutsch C+, *Cancer Treat Rep* 61, 925
Urticaria

Hair

Hair – alopecia (>10%)
(1992): Breathnach SM+, *Adverse Drug Reactions and the Skin*
Blackwell, Oxford, 302 (passim)
Hair – changes (sic)
(1971): Kostanecki W+, *Z Haut Geschlechtskr* (German) 46, 704

Other

Dysgeusia (>10%) (metallic taste)
Headache
Hypersensitivity
(2001): Mutafoglu-Uysal K+, *Turk J Pediatr* 43(2), 172
Injection-site extravasation
(2000): Kassner E, *J Pediatr Oncon Nurs* 17, 135
Injection-site necrosis
(1992): Misery L+, *Presse Med* (French) 21, 2153
(1991): Arias D+, *J Cutan Pathol* 18, 344
Injection-site pain
Myalgia (1–10%)
Oral mucosal lesions
(1978): Levine N+, *Cancer Treat Rev* 5, 67 (1–5%)
Paresthesias (1–10%)
Phlebitis
(1989): Kerker BJ+, *Semin Dermatol* 8, 173
Rhabdomyolysis
(1995): Anderlini P+, *Cancer* 76(4), 678
Stomatitis (>10%)
Ulceration due to extravasation
Vesiculation of mouth (sic)

VINCRISTINE

Trade names: Oncovin (Lilly); Vincasar (Pharmacia)
Indications: Leukemias, lymphomas, neuroblastoma, Wilm's
tumor
Category: Antineoplastic
Half-life: 24 hours
**Clinically important, potentially hazardous interactions
with:** aldesleukin, aprepitant, fluconazole, itraconazole,
ketoconazole, miconazole

Reactions

Skin

Acral erythema
(1995): Komamura H+, *J Dermatol* 22(2), 116 (with
cyclophosphamide, doxorubicin and GCSF)
Actinic keratoses
(1987): Johnson TM+, *J Am Dermatol* 17(2 Pt 1), 192
Angioedema
(1984): Gassel WD+, *Oncology* 41, 403
Dermatitis herpetiformis
(1986): Gottlieb D+, *Med J Aust* 145, 241 (flare)
Edema

Erythroderma
(1989): Matsumoto N+, *Gan To Kagaku Ryoho* (Japanese)
16, 2297
(1984): Gassel WD+, *Oncology* 41, 403
Exanthems
(1984): Gassel WD+, *Oncology* 41, 403
(1978): Levine N+, *Cancer Treat Rev* 5, 67
(1972): Zanoni G+, *Blut* (German) 25, 20
Palmar–plantar dysesthesia
(2002): Hussein MA+, *Cancer* 95(10), 2160 (with
dexamethasone)
Palmar–plantar erythema
(1990): Pagliuca A+, *Postgrad Med J* 66, 242
Pruritus
(1978): Levine N+, *CancerTreat Rev* 5, 67
Rash (sic) (1–10%)
Raynaud's phenomenon
(1998): Reiser M+, *Eur J Clin Microbiol Infect Dis* 17, 58
Serpentine supravenous hyperpigmentation (sic)
(2000): Marcoux D+, *J Am Acad Dermatol* 43, 540 (with
dactinomycin)
Sjøgren's syndrome
(1989): Monno S+, *Jpn J Med* 28, 399
Urticaria

Hair

Hair – alopecia (20–70%)
(2002): Klasa RJ+, *J Clin Oncol* 20(24), 4649 (with
cyclophosphamide and prednisone)
(1987): David J+, *Nurs Times* 83, 36
(1973): Levantine A+, *Br J Dermatol* 89, 549 (>5%)
(1971): Helson L+, *N Engl J Med* 284, 336
(1970): O'Brien R+, *N Engl J Med* 283, 1469
(1966): Simister JM, *BMJ* 2, 1138
(1964): Knock FE, *Med Clin North Am* 48, 501 (>5%)
(1963): Martin J+, *Lancet* 2, 1080 (47%)

Nails

Nails – Beau's lines (transverse nail bands)
(1994): Ben-Dayan D+, *Acta Haematol* 91, 89
Nails – leukonychia
(1990): Bader-Meunier B+, *Ann Pediatr Paris* (French) 37, 337
(transverse)
Nails – Mees' lines
(1983): James WD+, *Arch Dermatol* 119, 334
(1982): Jeanmougin M+, *Ann Dermatol Venereol* (French)
109, 169
Nails – onychodermal band
(1993): Kowal-Vern A+, *Cutis* 52, 43 (plus erythema of proximal
nail fold)

Other

Anaphylactoid reactions
Dysgeusia (1–10%) (metallic taste)
Headache
Injection-site cellulitis (>10%)
(1983): BronnerAK+, *J Am Acad Dermatol* 9, 645
Injection-site extravasation
(2000): Kassner E, *J Pediatr Oncon Nurs* 17, 135
Injection-site necrosis (>10%)
Myalgia (1–10%)
Oral mucosal lesions (1–10%)
(1989): KerkerBJ+, *Semin Dermatol* 8, 173 (1–5%)
(1964): Knock FE, *Med Clin North Am* 48, 501
Oral ulceration (1–10%)
Paresthesias (1–10%)
Phlebitis (1–10%)
Stomatitis (<1%)

VINORELBINE

Trade name: Navelbine (GSK)
Indications: Non-small cell lung cancer
Category: Antineoplastic
Half-life: 28–44 hours
Clinically important, potentially hazardous interactions with: aldesleukin

Reactions

Skin

Acral erythrodysesthesia syndrome (hand–foot syndrome)
(1998): Hoff PM+, *Cancer* 82, 965
Angioedema
Erythema
Flushing
Infections
(2002): Bonneterre J+, *Br J Cancer* 87(11), 1210 (with fluorouracil)
Pigmentation
(1994): Cecchi R+, *Dermatology* 188, 244
Pruritus
Rash (sic) (<5%)
Toxic epidermal necrolysis
(1992): Misery L+, *Presse Med* (French) 21, 2153

Hair

Hair – alopecia (12%)
(1994): Gasparini G+, *J Clin Oncol* 12, 2094
(1989): Marty M+, *Nouv Rev Fr Hematol* (French) 31, 77

Other

Anaphylactoid reactions
Dysgeusia (>10%) (metallic taste)
Extravasation
(2001): Bertelli G+, *Tumori* 87(2), 112
Hyperesthesia (1–10%)
Injection-site irritation (1–10%)
Injection-site necrosis (1–10%)
Injection-site pain
(2001): Long TD+, *Am J Clin Oncol* 24(4), 414
Injection-site phlebitis
(1998): Sauter C+, *Schweiz Med Wochenschr* (German) 128, 343
(1989): Marty M+, *Nouv Rev Fr Hematol* (French) 31, 77 (12%)
Myalgia (<5%)
Paresthesias (1–10%)
Phlebitis (7%)
Stomatitis (>10%)
(2002): Bonneterre J+, *Br J Cancer* 87(11), 1210 (40%) (with fluorouracil)
(1989): Marty M+, *Nouv Rev Fr Hematol* (French) 31, 77 (12%)

VITAMIN A

Trade names: Aquasol A (AstraZeneca); Del-Vi-A (Del-Ray); Palmitate A
Other common trade names: *Acaren; Acon; Afaxin; Arovit; Avipur; Avitin; Axerol; Dolce; Vogan*
Indications: Vitamin A deficiency
Category: Fat-soluble vitamin
Half-life: N/A
Clinically important, potentially hazardous interactions with: acitretin, bexarotene, **fish oil supplements**, isotretinoin, minocycline, tetracycline, warfarin

Reactions

Skin

Cheilitis
Dermatitis
(1996): Bazzano C+, *Contact Dermatitis* 35, 261
(1995): Heidenheim M+, *Contact Dermatitis* 33, 439
(1994): Manzano A+, *Contact Dermatitis* 31, 324
(1994): Sanz de Galdeano C+, *Contact Dermatitis* 30, 50
(1984): Blondeel A, *Contact Dermatitis* 11, 191
Dermatitis (sic) (dry, scaly and keratotic – mainly palms and soles)
(1971): Muenter MD+, *Am J Med* 50, 129
(1958): Oliver TK, *Am J Dis Child* 95, 57
Eczema (pellagra-like)
(1982): Hamann K+, *Hautarzt* (German) 33, 559
Erythema
(1992): Breathnach SM+, *Adverse Drug Reactions and the Skin* Blackwell, Oxford, 254 (passim)
Erythema multiforme (<1%)
(1971): Muenter MD+, *Am J Med* 50, 129
Exanthems
(1971): Muenter MD+, *Am J Med* 50, 129
Exfoliation (sic)
(1970): Nater P+, *Acta Derm Venereol* (Stockh) 50, 109
Exfoliative dermatitis
Fissures
(1992): Breathnach SM+, *Adverse Drug Reactions and the Skin* Blackwell, Oxford, 254 (passim)
Hyperkeratosis
(1992): Breathnach SM+, *Adverse Drug Reactions and the Skin* Blackwell, Oxford, 254 (passim)
Perleche
(1971): Muenter MD+, *Am J Med* 50, 129
Photosensitivity
Pigmentation (yellow-orange)
(1971): Muenter MD+, *Am J Med* 50, 129
Pruritus (<1%)
(1992): Breathnach SM+, *Adverse Drug Reactions and the Skin* Blackwell, Oxford, 254 (passim)
(1971): Muenter MD+, *Am J Med* 50, 129
Stevens–Johnson syndrome
(1971): Muenter MD+, *Am J Med* 50, 129
Xerosis (1–10%)
(1975): Stüttgen G, *Acta Derm Venereol* (Stockh) 55 (Suppl 74), 174

Hair

Hair – alopecia
(1992): Breathnach SM+, *Adverse Drug Reactions and the Skin* Blackwell, Oxford, 254 (passim)
(1979): Schmunes E, *Arch Dermatol* 115, 882
(1975): Stüttgen G, *Acta Derm Venereol* (Stockh) 55 (Suppl 74), 174

(1973): Levantine A+, *Br J Dermatol* 89, 549
(1972): Mausle R+, *Fortschr Med* (German) 90, 687
(1971): Muenter MD+, *Am J Med* 50, 129
(1970): Ippen H, *Dtsch Med Wochenschr* (German) 95, 1411
(1967): di Benedetto RJ, *JAMA* 201, 700
(1965): Rook A, *Br J Dermatol* 77, 115
(1960): Morrice G+, *JAMA* 173, 1802

Other

Anaphylactoid reactions
Gingivitis
Hypersensitivity
    (1995): Shelley WB+, *BMJ* 311, 232
Oral mucosal eruption
    (1971): Muenter MD+, *Am J Med* 50, 129
    (1964): Smith JH, *Oral Surg* 17 (Suppl 3), 305
Pseudotumor cerebri
Stomatodynia
Xerostomia
    (1992): Breathnach SM+, *Adverse Drug Reactions and the Skin*
        Blackwell, Oxford, 254 (passim)

VITAMIN B₁

(See THIAMINE)

VITAMIN B₁₂

(See CYANOCOBALAMIN)

VITAMIN B₂

(See RIBOFLAVIN)

VITAMIN B₃

(See NIACINAMIDE)

VITAMIN B₅

(See PANTOTHENIC ACID)

VITAMIN B₆

(See PYRIDOXINE)

VITAMIN B₉

(See FOLIC ACID)

VITAMIN C

(See ASCORBIC ACID)

VITAMIN D

(See ERGOCALCIFEROL)

VITAMIN E

Synonym: alpha tocopherol
Trade names: Aquasol E (AstraZeneca); E-Vitamin Succinate; Eprolin; Pheryl-E; Vita Plus E; Vitec
Other common trade names: *Bio E; Davitamon E; Detulin; E Perle; Ephynal; Optovit-E; Vita-E*
Indications: Vitamin E deficiency
Category: Fat-soluble vitamin
Half-life: N/A
Clinically important, potentially hazardous interactions with: amprenavir, warfarin

Reactions

Skin

Dermatitis (sic) (<1%)
    (1997): Parsad D+, *Contact Dermatitis* 37, 294 (xanthomatous)
    (1994): Manzano D+, *Contact Dermatitis* 31, 324
    (1994): Perrenoud D+, *Dermatology* 189, 225
    (1992): Garcia-Bravo B+, *Contact Dermatitis* 26, 280 (generalized)
    (1991): de Groot AC+, *Contact Dermatitis* 25, 302
    (1991): Fisher AA, *Cutis* 48, 272
    (1991): Hunter D+, *Cutis* 47, 193
    (1986): Goldman MP+, *J Am Acad Dermatol* 14, 133
    (1976): Roed-Petersen J+, *Br J Dermatol* 94, 233
    (1975): Roed-Petersen J+, *Contact Dermatitis* 1, 391
    (1975): Schorr WF, *Am Fam Physician* 12, 90
    (1973): Aeling JL+, *Arch Dermatol* 108, 579
Erythema multiforme
    (1994): Spreux A+, *Therapie* (French) 49, 460
    (1986): Fisher AA, *Cutis* 37, 158 and 262 (topical administration)
    (1984): Saperstein H+, *Arch Dermatol* 120, 906
Exanthems
Lupus erythematosus
    (1995): Whittam J+, *Am J Clin Nutr* 62, 1025
Urticaria

Hair

Hair – depigmentation (at injection sites)
    (1972): Sehgal VN, *Dermatologica* 145, 56

Other

Gingivitis
    (1998): Liede KE+, *Ann Med* 30, 542
Gynecomastia
    (1994): Roberts HJ, *Hosp Pract Off Ed* 29, 12
Sclerosing lipogranuloma
    (1983): Foucar E+, *J Am Acad Dermatol* 9, 103
Thrombophlebitis
    (1979): Roberts HS, *Angiology* 30, 169
Tooth pigmentation

VITAMIN K

(See PHYTONADIONE)

VORICONAZOLE

Synonym: UK109496
Trade name: Vfend (Pfizer)
Indications: Invasive aspergillosis
Category: Triazole antifungal
Half-life: 6–24 hours (dose dependent)
**Clinically important, potentially hazardous interactions
with:** barbiturates, carbamazepine, ergot alkaloids, pimozide,
quinidine, rifabutin, rifampin, sirolimus

Reactions

Skin
Adverse effects (sic)
  (2003): Jeu L+, *Clin Ther* 25(5), 1321 (20%)
Allergic reactions (sic) (<1%)
Angioedema (<1%)
Cellulitis (<1%)
Cheilitis (<1%)
Chills (3.1%)
  (2002): Herbrecht R+, *N Engl J Med* 347(6), 408
Dermatitis (<1%)
Diaphoresis (<1%)
Ecchymoses (<1%)
Eczema (<1%)
Edema (<1%)
Erythema multiforme
Exfoliative dermatitis (<1%)
Facial edema (<1%)
Facial erythema
  (2001): Denning DW+, *Clin Exp Dermatol* 26(8), 648
Fixed eruption (<1%)
Flu-like syndrome (<1%)
Furunculosis (<1%)
Graft-versus-host reaction (<1%)
Granulomas (<1%)
Herpes simplex (<1%)
Infections (sic) (<1%)
Lupus erythematosus (<1%)
Peripheral edema (1%)
Petechiae (<1%)
Photosensitivity (8.2%)
  (2003): Johnson LB+, *Clin Infect Dis* 36(5), 630
  (2002): Herbrecht R+, *N Engl J Med* 347(6), 408 (8.2%)
Pigmentation (<1%)
Pruritus (8.2%)
  (2002): Herbrecht R+, *N Engl J Med* 347(6), 408 (8.2%)
Psoriasis (<1%)
Purpura (<1%)
Rash (sic) (8.2%)
  (2003): Johnson LB+, *Clin Infect Dis* 36(5), 630
  (2002): Herbrecht R+, *N Engl J Med* 347(6), 408 (8.2%)
  (2002): Purkins L+, *Antimicrob Agents Chemother* 46(8), 2546
Scrotal edema (<1%)
Stevens–Johnson syndrome
Toxic epidermal necrolysis
Urticaria (<1%)
Xerosis (<1%)

Hair
Hair – alopecia (<1%)

Other
Ageusia (<1%)
Anaphylactoid reactions (<1%)
Arthralgia (<1%)
Arthritis (<1%)
Back pain (<1%)
Bone or joint pain (<1%)
Depression (<1%)
Dysgeusia (<1%)
Gingival hemorrhage (<1%)
Gingival hyperplasia (<1%)
Gingivitis (<1%)
Glossitis (<1%)
Guillain–Barré syndrome (<1%)
Headache
Hyperesthesia (<1%)
Injection-site infection (sic) (<1%)
Injection-site inflammation (<1%)
Injection-site pain (<1%)
Myalgia (<1%)
Myopathy (<1%)
Oral ulceration (<1%)
Pain (<1%)
Paresthesias (<1%)
Phlebitis (<1%)
Stomatitis (<1%)
Thrombophlebitis (<1%)
Tongue edema (<1%)
Tremor (<1%)
Visual disturbances
  (2002): Herbrecht R+, *N Engl J Med* 347(6), 408 (44.8%)
  (2002): Walsh TJ+, *N Engl J Med* 346(4), 225
  (2001): Ally R+, *Clin Infect Dis* 33(9), 1447 (23%)
Xerostomia (1%)

WARFARIN

Trade name: Coumadin (Bristol-Myers Squibb)
Other common trade names: *Aldocumar; Coumadine; Marevan; Waran; Warfilone*
Indications: Thromboembolic disease, pulmonary embolism
Category: Anticoagulant
Half-life: 1.5–2.5 days (highly variable)
Clinically important, potentially hazardous interactions with: amiodarone, amobarbital, antithyroid agents, aprepitant, aprobarbital, **arnica**, aspirin, azithromycin, barbiturates, bismuth, bivalirudin, bosentan, butabarbital, **capsicum**, **chamomile**, cimetidine, clarithromycin, clofibrate, clopidogrel, clorazepate, co-trimoxazole, **coenzyme Q-10**, cyclosporine, **dan-shen**, danazol, delavirdine, **devil's claw**, dirithromycin, disulfiram, **dong quai**, erythromycin, fenofibrate, **feverfew**, fluconazole, fluoxymesterone, **garlic**, gemfibrozil, **ginger**, **ginkgo biloba**, ginseng, glucagon, **green tea**, **horse chestnut (bark, flower, leaf, seed)**, imatinib, itraconazole, ketoconazole, levothyroxine, liothyronine, **melatonin**, mephobarbital, methimazole, methyltestosterone, metronidazole, miconazole, nalidixic acid, PEG-interferon alfa-2b, penicillins, pentobarbital, phenobarbital, phenylbutazones, phytonadione, piperacillin, primidone, propoxyphene, propylthiouracil, quinidine, quinine, **red clover**, rifampin, rifapentine, rofecoxib, salicylates, **saw palmetto**, secobarbital, **St John's wort**, stanozolol, sulfamethoxazole, sulfinpyrazone, sulfisoxazole, sulfonamides, sulindac, testosterone, thyroid, troleandomycin, valdecoxib, vitamin A, vitamin E, zileuton

Note: Alternative remedies, including herbals, may potentially increase the risk of bleeding or potentiate the effects of warfarin therapy. Some of these include the following: angelica root, arnica flower, anise, asafetida, bogbean, borage seed oil, bromelain, dan shen, devil's claw, fenugreek, feverfew, garlic, ginger, ginkgo biloba, ginseng, horse chestnut, lovage root, meadowsweet, onion, parsley, passionflower herb, poplar, quassia, red clover, rue, turmeric and willow bark

Reactions

Skin

Abscess
  (1997): Clayton BD, *J Geriatr Dermatology* 5, 314
Acral purpura
  (1986): Stone MS+, *J Am Acad Dermatol* 14, 796
Angioedema (<1%)
Bullous eruption
  (1993): Elis A+, *J Intern Med* 234, 615 (hemorrhagic)
  (1986): Stone MS+, *J Am Acad Dermatol* 14, 796 (passim)
Dermatitis (sic)
  (1992): Breathnach SM+, *Adverse Drug Reactions and the Skin* Blackwell, Oxford, 248 (passim)
  (1991): Quintavalla R+, *Int Angiol* 10, 103
Ecchymoses
  (2000): Juaneza MA+, *Am J Med Sci* 320(6), 388
  (1988): Cole MS+, *Surgery* 103, 271 (passim)
Exanthems
  (2003): Spyropoulos AC+, *Pharmacotherapy* 23(4), 533
  (1993): Antony SJ+, *South Med J* 86, 1413
  (1989): Kruis-de Vries MH+, *Dermatologica* 178, 109
  (1988): Cole MS+, *Surgery* 103, 271 (passim)
  (1978): Kwong P+, *JAMA* 239, 1884
  (1968): Schiff BL+, *Arch Dermatol* 98, 136
  (1960): Adams CW+, *Circulation* 22, 947
Exfoliative dermatitis

Hematomas
  (1997): Clayton BD, *J Geriatr Dermatology* 5, 314
Hemorrhage
  (1989): Geoghegan+, *BMJ* 298, 902
  (1988): Cole MS, *Surgery* 103, 271
  (1980): Schleicher SM+, *Arch Dermatol* 116, 444
Lingual hemorrhage
  (2000): Shojania KG, *Am J Med* 109, 77
Livedo reticularis
  (1993): Park S+, *Arch Dermatol* 129, 775
Necrosis (>10%)
  (2003): Parsi K+, *Australas J Dermatol* 44(1), 57
  (2003): Roche-Nagle G+, *Eur J Vasc Endovasc Surg* 25(5), 481
  (2002): Clark JA+, *J Arthroplasty* 17(8), 1070
  (2002): Francesconi Do Valle F+, *World Congress Dermatol* Poster, 0101 (2 cases)
  (2002): Piccoli GB+, *Med Sci Monit* 8(11), CS83
  (2002): Scarff CE+, *Australas J Dermatol* 43(3), 202
  (2002): Sharkey MP+, *Australas J Dermatol* 43(3), 218
  (2000): Ad-El DD+, *Br J Plast Surg* 53(7), 624
  (2000): Chan YC+, *Br J Surgery* 87, 266
  (2000): Zimbelman J+, *J Pediatr* 137, 266
  (1999): Gailine D+, *Am J Hematol* 60, 231
  (1999): Martin FL, *Am J Nursing* 99, 53
  (1999): Stewart AJ+, *Postgrad Med J* 75, 233
  (1999): Yang Y+, *N Engl J Med* 340, 735
  (1998): Essex DW+, *Am J Hematol* 57, 233
  (1998): Gelwix TJ+, *Am J Emerg Med* 16, 541
  (1998): Sallah S+, *Haemostasis* 28, 25
  (1997): English JC+, *J Am Acad Dermatol* 37, 1 (passim)
  (1997): Hermes B+, *Acta Derm Venereol* 77, 35
  (1997): Sallah S+, *Thromb Haemost* 78, 785
  (1997): Wynn SS+, *Haemostasis* 27, 246
  (1996): Jillella AP+, *Am J Hematol* 52, 117
  (1996): Makris M+, *Thromb Haemost* 75, 523
  (1995): DeFranzo AJ+, *Ann Plast Surg* 34, 203
  (1995): Hauben M, *N Engl J Med* 332, 959
  (1995): Sternberg ML+, *Ann Emerg Med* 26, 94
  (1994): Lewandowski K+, *Thromb Haemost* 69, 311
  (1994): Soisson AP+, *Mil Med* 159, 252
  (1993): Bauer KA, *Arch Dermatol* 129, 766
  (1993): Colman RW+, *Am J Hematol* 43, 300
  (1993): Eby CS, *Hematol Oncol Clin North Am* 7, 1291
  (1993): Hiers CL, *J Ark Med Soc* 89, 443
  (1993): LaPrade RF+, *Orthopedics* 16, 703
  (1993): Locht H+, *J Intern Med* 233, 287
  (1993): Schramm W+, *Arch Dermatol* 129, 753
  (1993): Yates P+, *Clin Exp Dermatol* 18, 138
  (1992): Anderson DR+, *Haemostasis* 22, 124
  (1992): McKnight JT+, *Arch Fam Med* 1, 105
  (1992): Sharafuddin MA+, *Arch Dermatol* 128, 105
  (1992): Viegas GV, *J Am Podiatr Med Assoc* 82, 463
  (1991): Berkompas DC, *Indiana Med* 84, 788
  (1991): Brooks LW+, *J Am Osteopath Assoc* 91, 601
  (1991): Humphries JE+, *Am J Hematol* 37, 197
  (1991): Ritchie AJ+, *Ulster Med J* 60, 248
  (1990): Comp PC+, *Semin Thromb Hemost* 16, 293
  (1989): Barkley C+, *J Urology* 141, 946
  (1989): Grimaudo V+, *BMJ* 289, 233
  (1988): Cole MS+, *Surgery* 103, 271
  (1988): Conlan MG+, *Am J Hematol* 29, 226
  (1988): Dominic W+, *Burns Incl Therm Inj* 14, 139
  (1988): Kandrotas RJ+, *Pharmacotherapy* 8, 351
  (1988): Konrad P+, *Vasa*, 17, 208
  (1987): Gladson CL+, *Arch Dermatol* 123, 1701
  (1987): Haimovici H+, *J Vasc Surg* 5, 655
  (1987): Norris PG, *Clin Exp Dermatol* 12, 370
  (1986): Brennan M+, *J Tenn Med Assoc* 79, 210
  (1986): Everett RN+, *Postgrad Med* 79, 97
  (1986): Rowbotham B+, *Aust N Z J Med* 16, 513

(1986): Sjoberg A+, *Lakartidningen* (Swedish) 83, 4089
(1986): Zauber NP+, *Ann Intern Med* 104, 659
(1984): Franson TR+, *Arch Dermatol* 120, 927
(1984): McGehee WG+, *Ann Intern Med* 101, 59
(1984): Schwartz RA+, *Dermatologica* 168, 31 (linear localized)
(1984): Slutzki S+, *Int J Dermatol* 23, 117
(1983): Caldwell EH+, *Plast Reconstr Surg* 72, 231
(1983): Leath MC, *Tex Med* 79, 62
(1983): Papa MA+, *Harefuah* (Hebrew) 104, 504
(1982): Faraci PA, *Int J Dermatol* 21, 329
(1982): Torngren S+, *Acta Chir Scand* 148, 471
(1981): Horn JR+, *Am J Hosp Pharm* 38, 1763
(1980): Hislop IG+, *Aust N Z J Med* 10, 51
(1980): Schleicher SM+, *Arch Dermatol* 116, 444
(1979): Boss JM+, *Br J Dermatol* 100, 617
(1979): Jones RR+, *Br J Dermatol* 101, 561
(1978): Faraci PA+, *Surg Gynecol Obstet* 146, 695
(1978): Kirby JD+, *Br J Dermatol* 98, 707
(1976): Kirby JD+, *Br J Dermatol* 94, 97
(1976): Renick AM, *South Med J* 69, 775
(1975): Lacy JP+, *Ann Intern Med* 82, 381
(1971): Nalbandian RM+, *Obstet Gynecol* 38, 395
(1970): Martin CM+, *Calif Med* 113, 78
(1969): Korbitz BD+, *Am J Cardiol* 24, 420
(1969): Lipp H+, *Med J Aust* 2, 351
(1969): Vaughan ED+, *JAMA* 210, 2282 (genitalia)
(1954): Verhagen H, *Acta Med Scand* 148, 453

Pruritus (<1%)
(2003): Spyropoulos AC+, *Pharmacotherapy* 23(4), 533
(1978): Kwong P+, *JAMA* 239, 1884

Purple toe syndrome
(2003): Talmadge DB+, *Pharmacotherapy* 23(5), 674

Purplish erythema (sic) (feet and toes) (<1%)
(1998): Krahn MJ+, *Can J Cardiol* 14, 90 ('purple toes')
(1997): Sallah S+, *Thromb Haemost* 78, 785 ('purple toes')
(1994): Soisson AP+, *Mil Med* 159, 252
(1993): Park S+, *Arch Dermatol* 129, 775
(1982): Lebsack CS+, *Postgrad Med* 71, 81 ('purple toes')
(1981): Akle CA+, *J R Soc Med* 74, 219 (purple toe syndrome)
(1978): Kwong P+, *JAMA* 239, 1884
(1961): Feder W+, *Ann Intern Med* 55, 911

Purpura
(2002): Scarff CE+, *Australas J Dermatol* 43(3), 202
(1988): Cole MS+, *Surgery* 103, 271 (passim)
(1978): Friedenberg WR+, *Arch Dermatol* 114, 578 (fulminans)

Rash (sic) (<1%)
(2003): Spyropoulos AC+, *Pharmacotherapy* 23(4), 533

Ulcerations
(2002): Scarff CE+, *Australas J Dermatol* 43(3), 202

Urticaria
(1988): Cole MS+, *Surgery* 103, 271 (passim)
(1986): Stone MS+, *J Am Acad Dermatol* 14, 796 (passim)
(1959): Sheps ES+, *Am J Cardiol* 3, 118

Vasculitis
(1998): Krahn MJ+, *Can J Cardiol* 14, 90
(1994): Tamir A+, *Acta Derm Venereol* 74, 138
(1982): Howitt AJ+, *Postgrad Med J* 58, 233
(1982): Tanay A+, *Dermatologica* 165, 178

Vesicular eruptions
(1986): Stone MS+, *J Am Acad Dermatol* 14, 796 (passim)

Hair

Hair – alopecia (>10%)
(1995): Nagao T+, *Lancet* 346, 1004
(1989): Kruis-de Vries MH+, *Dermatologica* 178, 109 (passim)
(1988): Umlas J+, *Cutis* 42, 63
(1986): Stone MS+, *J Am Acad Dermatol* 14, 796 (passim)
(1969): Baker H+, *Br J Dermatol* 81, 236
(1957): Cornbleet T+, *Arch Dermatol* 75, 440

Other

Death
(2002): Clark JA+, *J Arthroplasty* 17(8), 1070
Gangrene
(1978): Hardisty CA, *Postgrad Med J* 54, 123
(1976): Shnider M+, *Can J Surg* 19, 64
(1973): Chua FS+, *J Thorac Cardiovasc Surg* 65, 238
Hypersensitivity
(2002): Kristensen SR, *Blood* 100(7), 2676
(1968): Schiff BL+, *Arch Dermatol* 98, 136
Oral ulceration (<1%)
Priapism
(2000): Zimbelman J+, *J Pediatr* 137, 266
(1997): Daryanani S+, *Clin Lab Haematol* 19, 213

WILLOW BARK

Scientific names: *Salix alba; Salix fragilis; Salix purpurea*
Family: Salicaceae
Trade and other common names: Basket Willow; Brittle Willow; Crack Willow; White Willow; Willowbark
Category: Anti-inflammatory; Antinociceptive; Antipyretic
Purported indications and other uses: Colds, infections, headaches, pain, muscle and joint aches, influenza, gouty arthritis, ankylosing spondylitis, rheumatoid arthritis, osteoarthritis
Half-life: N/A
Clinically important, potentially hazardous interactions with: NSAIDs, salicylates

Reactions

Skin

Rash (sic)

Other

Anaphylactoid reactions
(2003): Boullata JI+, *Ann Pharmacother* 37(6), 832

YARROW

Scientific name: *Achillea millefolium*
Family: Compositae
Trade and other common names: Angel flower; Bad Man's Plaything; Bloodwort; Carpenter's Weed; Devil's Nettle; Devil's Plaything; Herbe Militaris; Knight's Milfoil; Milfoil; Millefoil; Nose Bleed; Nosebleed; Old Man's Pepper; Sanguinary; Soldier's Woundwort; Staunchgrass; Staunchweed; Thousand Weed; Thousand-leaf; Yarroway
Category: Anti-inflammatory; Antipyretic; Astringent; Diaphoretic; Diuretic; Haemostatic
Purported indications and other uses: Fevers, common cold, essential hypertension, digestive complaints, loss of appetite, amenorrhoea, dysentery, diarrhoea, cerebral and coronary thromboses, menstrual pain, bleeding piles, toothache, muscle spasms, gastrointestinal disorders. Topical: slow-healing wounds, skin inflammations, cosmetics
Half-life: N/A
Clinically important, potentially hazardous interactions with: anticoagulants hypotensives, antiepileptics, hypertensives

Reactions

Skin
Allergic reactions (sic)
  (1996): Hausen BM, *Am J Contact Dermat* 7(2), 94
Dermatitis
  (2002): Schempp CM+, *Hautarzt* 53(2), 93
  (1991): Hausen BM+, *Contact Dermatitis* 24(4), 274
  (1991): Rucker G+, *Arch Pharm* (Weinheim) 324(12), 979
  (1983): Hausen BM+, *Acta Derm Venereol* 63(4), 308
Photosensitivity
  (2002): Schempp CM+, *Hautarzt* 53(2), 93
Rash (sic)
  (2002): Schempp CM+, *Hautarzt* 53(2), 93
Rhinoconjunctivitis
  (2001): Uter W+, *Am J Contact Dermat* 12(3), 182
Urticaria
  (2001): Uter W+, *Am J Contact Dermat* 12(3), 182

YOHIMBINE

Scientific name: *Pausinystalia yohimbe*
Family: Rubiaceae
Trade and other common names: Actibane (Consolidated Midland); Aphrodyne (Star); Yocon (Palisades); Yohimex (Kramer); Yomax
Category: Anesthetic; Aphrodisiac (purported)
Purported indications and other uses: Impotence, alpha2-adrenergic blocker, orthostatic hypertension
Half-life: 36 minutes
Clinically important, potentially hazardous interactions with: tricyclic antidepressants

Reactions

Skin
Adverse effects (sic)
  (2002): Haller CA+, *Adverse Drug React Toxicol Rev* 21(3), 143
Diaphoresis
Exfoliative dermatitis
  (1993): Sandler B+, *Urology* 41, 343
Flushing
Lupus erythematosus
  (1993): Sandler B+, *Urology* 41, 343

Other
Death

ZAFIRLUKAST

Trade name: Accolate (AstraZeneca)
Indications: Asthma
Category: Antiasthmatic; Leukotriene receptor antagonist
Half-life: 10 hours
Clinically important, potentially hazardous interactions with: CYP3A4 substrates, **high protein foods**

Reactions

Skin
Granulomatous dermatitis (Churg–Strauss syndrome)
  (1999): Green RL+, *Lancet* 353, 725 (2 cases)
  (1999): Wechsler ME+, *Chest* 116, 266
  (1999): Wechsler ME+, *Lancet* 353, 1970
  (1998): Churg J+, *JAMA* 279, 1949
  (1998): Holloway J+, *J Am Osteopath Assoc* 98, 275
  (1998): Honsinger RW, *JAMA* 279, 1949
  (1998): Katz RS+, *JAMA* 279, 1949
  (1998): Knoell DL+, *Chest* 114, 332
  (1998): Wechsler ME+, *JAMA* 279, 457
Lupus erythematosus
  (1999): Finkel TH+, *J Allergy Clin Immunol* 103, 533
Vasculitis
  (2002): Soy M+, *Clin Rheumatol* 21(4), 328

Other
Cough
  (2001): Spector SL, *Ann Allergy Asthma Immunol* 86(6 Suppl 1), 18
Fatigue
  (1999): Finkel TH+, *J Allergy Clin Immunol* 103(3), 533
Headache
Myalgia (1.6%)
  (1999): Finkel TH+, *J Allergy Clin Immunol* 103(3), 533
Oral ulceration
  (1999): Finkel TH+, *J Allergy Clin Immunol* 103(3), 533

ZALCITABINE

Synonyms: ddC; dideoxycytidine
Trade name: Hivid (Roche)
Indications: Advanced HIV disease
Category: Antiretroviral; Nucleoside reverse transcriptase inhibitor (NRTI)
Half-life: 2.9 hours

Reactions

Skin
Acne (<1%)
Angioedema
  (1988): Yarchoan R+, *Lancet* 1, 76 (5%)
Ankle edema
  (1989): Jeffries DJ, *J Antimicrob Chemother* 23, 29
Bullous eruption (<1%)
Dermatitis (sic) (<1%)
Diaphoresis (<1%)
Edema (<1%)
  (1991): Pluda JM+, *Hematol Oncol Clin North Am* 5, 229
  (1991): Yarchoan R+, *Blood* 78, 859
  (1989): McNeely MC+, *J Am Acad Dermatol* 21, 1213 (70%)
    (dose-related)
Erythema multiforme

  (1995): Wardropper AG+, *Int J STD AIDS* 6, 450
Erythroderma
  (1989): McNeely MC+, *J Am Acad Dermatol* 21, 1213 (10%)
Exanthems (1–66%)
  (1991): Fischl MA, *Recent Advances in Antiretroviral Therapy* New York, Triclinica Communications
  (1991): Merigan TC, *Am J Med* 90, 8S
  (1991): Pluda JM+, *Hematol Oncol Clin North Am* 5, 229
  (1990): Pizzo PA+, *J Pediatr* 117, 799
  (1989): McNeely MC+, *J Am Acad Dermatol* 21, 1213 (40%)
  (1989): Merigan TC+, *Ann Intern Med* 110, 189 (66%)
  (1989): Yarchoan R+, *N Engl J Med* 321, 726 (1–5%)
  (1988): Yarchoan R+, *Lancet* 1, 76 (65%)
  (1987): Richman DD+, *N Engl J Med* 317, 192 (1–5%)
Exfoliative dermatitis (<1%)
Flushing (<1%)
Folliculitis
Granuloma annulare
  (2001): Peñas PF+, *Arch Dermatol* 137, 964
Penile edema (<1%)
Photosensitivity (<1%)
Pruritus (3–5%)
Rash (sic) (2–11%)
  (1990): Bozzette SA+, *Am J Med* 88, 24S
  (1989): Jeffries DJ, *J Antimicrob Chemother* 23, 29
Side effects (sic)
  (1991): Yarchoan R+, *Blood* 78, 859
  (1990): Broder S+, *Am J Med* 88, 31S
Urticaria (3.4%)
  (1992): Roche Laboratories Monograph
Xerosis (<1%)

Hair
Hair – alopecia

Nails
Nails – changes (sic)
  (1989): Jeffries DJ, *J Antimicrob Chemother* 23, 29

Other
Ageusia (<1%)
Anaphylactoid reactions
  (1992): Roche Laboratories Monograph
Aphthous stomatitis
  (1991): Fischl MA, *Recent Advances in Antiretroviral Therapy* . New York, Triclinica Communications
  (1991): Merigan TC, *Am J Med* 90, 8S
  (1991): Pluda JM+, *Hematol Oncol Clin North Am* 5, 229
  (1989): Jeffries DJ, *J Antimicrob Chemother* 23, 29
  (1989): Yarchoan R+, *N Engl J Med* 321, 726
  (1988): Yarchoan R+, *Lancet* 1, 76
Dysgeusia (<1%)
Gingivitis (<1%)
Glossitis (<1%)
Glossodynia (<1%)
Headache
Myalgia (1–6%)
Myopathy (<1%)
Oral mucosal lesions (40–73%)
  (1991): Fischl MA, *Recent Advances in Antiretroviral Therapy* . New York, Triclinica Communications
  (1989): Merigan TC+, *Ann Intern Med* 110, 189 (73%)
  (1988): Yarchoan R+, *Lancet* 1, 76 (40%)
Oral ulceration (3–64%)
  (1990): Bozzette SA+, *Am J Med* 88, 24S
  (1990): Pizzo PA+, *J Pediatr* 117, 799 (painful)
  (1989): McNeely MC+, *J Am Acad Dermatol* 21, 1213 (64%)
Paresthesias
Parosmia (<1%)

Stomatitis (3%)
  (1991): Yarchoan R+, *Blood* 78, 859
Tinnitus
Tongue disorder (sic) (<1%)
Xerostomia (<1%)

ZALEPLON

Trade name: Sonata (Wyeth)
Indications: Insomnia
Category: Nonbenzodiazepine sedative-hypnotic
Half-life: 1 hour

Reactions

Skin
Acne (<1%)
Cheilitis (<1%)
Chills (<1%)
Dermatitis (<1%)
Diaphoresis (<1%)
Ecchymoses (<1%)
Eczema (<1%)
Edema (<1%)
Exanthems (<1%)
Facial edema (<1%)
Peripheral edema (1–10%)
Photosensitivity (1–10%)
Pigmentation (<1%)
Pruritus (<1%)
Psoriasis (<1%)
Purpura (<1%)
Pustules (<1%)
Rash (sic) (<1%)
Vesiculobullous eruption (<1%)
Xerosis (<1%)

Hair
Hair – alopecia (<1%)

Other
Ageusia (<1%)
Aphthous stomatitis (<1%)
Gingival hemorrhage (<1%)
Gingivitis (<1%)
Glossitis (<1%)
Headache
Hyperesthesia (<1%)
Mastodynia (<1%)
Myalgia (5%)
Oral ulceration (<1%)
Paresthesias (3%)
Parosmia (2%)
Sialorrhea (<1%)
Stomatitis (<1%)
Thrombophlebitis (<1%)
Tongue discoloration (<1%)
Tremor (1–10%)
Vaginitis (<1%)
Xerostomia (1–10%)

ZANAMIVIR

Trade name: Relenza (GSK)
Indications: Influenza A and B
Category: Viral neuranimidase inhibitor (by oral inhalation)
Half-life: 2.5–5.1 hours

Reactions

Skin
Infections (sic) (2%)
Upper respiratory infection
  (2001): McNicholl IR+, *Ann Pharmacother* 35(1), 57
Urticaria (<1.5%)

Other
Myalgia (<1.5%)
  (2001): McNicholl IR+, *Ann Pharmacother* 35(1), 57

ZIDOVUDINE

Synonyms: azidothymidine; AZT; compound S
Trade names: Combivir (GSK); Retrovir (GSK); Trizivir
Other common trade names: *Novo-AZT; Retrovis*
Indications: HIV infection
Category: Antiretroviral; Nucleoside reverse transcriptase inhibitor (NRTI)
Half-life: 1 hour
Clinically important, potentially hazardous interactions with: clarithromycin, ganciclovir, PEG-interferon alfa-2b, ribavirin

Reactions

Skin
Acne (<5%)
  (1988): McEvoy GK, *Am Hosp Formulary Service: Drug Info* 392
Allergic reactions (sic)
  (1988): Diven DG+, *Arch Intern Med* 148, 2296
Blue vitiligo (sic)
  (1994): Ivker R+, *J Am Acad Dermatol* 30, 829
Bullous eruption
  (1989): Caumes E+, *Presse Med* (French) 18, 1708 (fatal in AIDS)
Diaphoresis (5–19%)
  (1988): McEvoy GK, *Am Hosp Formulary Service: Drug Info* 392
Ecchymoses
  (1992): Breathnach SM+, *Adverse Drug Reactions and the Skin*
    Blackwell, Oxford, 172 (passim)
Edema of lip (<5%)
  (1988): McEvoy GK, *Am Hosp Formulary Service: Drug Info* 392
Erythema multiforme
  (1989): Langtry HD+, *Drugs* 37, 408
  (1989): Yarchoan R+, *N Engl J Med* 321, 726
Erythroderma
  (1996): Duque S+, *J Allergy Clin Immunol* 98, 234
Exanthems
  (1990): Petty BG+, *Lancet* 335, 1044 (1–5%) (in AIDS patients)
  (1989): Gelman K+, *AIDS* 3, 555 (>5%)
  (1989): Langtry HD+, *Drugs* 37, 408
  (1987): Richman DD+, *N Engl J Med* 317, 192
Neutrophilic eccrine hidradenitis
  (1990): Smith KJ+, *J Am Acad Dermatol* 23, 945
Pigmentation
  (1993): Hermanns-Le T+, *Ann Pathol* (French) 13, 328
  (1992): Baudo F+, *Eur J Dermatol* 2, 448
  (1992): Hill DA+, *Hosp Pract Off Ed* 27, 29

(1991): Poizot-Martin I+, *Presse Med* (French) 20, 632
(1991): Tal A+, *Cutis* 48, 153
(1990): Greenberg RG+, *J Am Acad Dermatol* 22, 327
(1989): Bendick C+, *Arch Dermatol* 125, 1285 (palms and soles)
(1989): Merenich JA+, *Am J Med* 86, 469
(1989): Valencia ME+, *Med Clin (Barc)* (Spanish) 92, 357
Pruritus
(1989): Gelman K+, *AIDS* 3, 555 (>5%)
(1988): McEvoy GK, *Am Hosp Formulary Service: Drug Info* 392
Purpura
Rash (sic) (17%)
(1996): Henry K+, *Ann Intern Med* 124, 855
(1987): Richman DD+, *N Engl J Med* 317, 192
Stevens–Johnson syndrome
(1989): Langtry HD+, *Drugs* 37, 408
(1989): Yarchoan R+, *N Engl J Med* 321, 726
Toxic epidermal necrolysis
(1996): Murri R+, *Clin Infect Dis* 23, 640
Urticaria (<5%)
(1990): McKinley GF+, *Lancet* 336, 384
(1988): McEvoy GK, *Am Hosp Formulary Service: Drug Info* 392
Vasculitis
(1992): Torres RA+, *Arch Intern Med* 152, 850
(1990): Lee MH+, *Int Conf AIDS* 6, 360 (leukocytoclastic)

Hair

Hair – alopecia
(1996): Geletko SM+, *Pharmacotherapy* 16, 69
Hair – hypertrichosis (eyelashes)
(1991): Klutman NE+, *N Engl J Med* 324, 1896
(1991): Sahai J+, *AIDS* 5, 1395

Nails

Nails – paronychia
(1999): Russo F+, *J Am Acad Dermatol* 40, 322
Nails – pigmentation (42%)
(1992): Rahav G+, *Scand J Infect Dis* 24, 557
(1991): Sahai J+, *AIDS* 5, 1395
(1990): Don PC+, *Ann Intern Med* 112, 145 (42%) (bluish)
(1990): Greenberg RG+, *J Am Acad Dermatol* 22, 327
(1990): Poizot-Martin I+, *Int Conf AIDS* 6, 357
(1990): Ramos C+, *Rev Clin Esp* (Spanish) 187, 94
(1989): Anders KH+, *J Am Acad Dermatol* 21, 792
(1989): Bendick C+, *Arch Dermatol* 125, 1285
(1989): Depaoli MA+, *G Ital Dermatol Venereol* (Italian) 124, 71
(1989): Dupon M+, *Scand J Infect Dis* 21, 237
(1989): Fisher CA+, *Cutis* 43, 552
(1989): Groark SP+, *J Am Acad Dermatol* 21, 1032
(1989): Langtry HD+, *Drugs* 37, 408
(1989): Merenich JA+, *Am J Med* 86, 469
(1989): Yarchoan R+, *N Engl J Med* 321, 726
(1988): Azon-Masoliver A+, *Arch Dermatol* 124, 1570
(1988): Gonzalez-Lahoz JM+, *Rev Clin Esp* (Spanish) 183, 278 (bluish)
(1988): Vaiopoulos G+, *Ann Intern Med* 108, 777
(1987): Furth PA+, *Ann Intern Med* 107, 350
Nails – pigmentation
(1991): Tadini G+, *Arch Dermatol* 127, 267
(1990): Grau-Massanes M+, *J Am Acad Dermatol* 22, 687
(1990): Tosti A+, *Dermatologica* 180, 217 (longitudinal)
(1989): Bendick C+, *Z Hautkr* (German) 64, 91
(1989): Valencia ME+, *Rev Clin Esp* (Spanish) 185, 167 (blue striae)

Other

Bromhidrosis (<5%)
(1988): McEvoy GK, *Am Hosp Formulary Service: Drug Info* 392
Death
Dysgeusia (5–19%)
(1988): McEvoy GK, *Am Hosp Formulary Service: Drug Info* 392

(1987): Richman DD+, *N Engl J Med* 317, 192
Foetor ex ore (halitosis)
Gingivitis
Headache
Hypersensitivity
Lipodystrophy
(2001): Bogner JR+, *J Acquir Immune Defic Syndr* 27(3), 237
Myopathy (<1%)
(1993): Simpson DM+, *Neurology* 43, 971
(1989): Gertner E+, *Am J Medicine* 86, 814
(1988): Helbert M+, *Lancet* 2, 689
Oral lichenoid eruption
(2001): Scully C+, *Oral Dis* 7(4), 205 (passim)
(1993): Ficarra G+, *Oral Surg Oral Med Oral Pathol* 76, 460
Oral mucosal eruption
(1989): Gelman K+, *AIDS* 3, 555 (>5%)
Oral mucosal pigmentation
(1991): Poizot-Martin I+, *Presse Med* (French) 20, 632
(1991): Tadini G+, *Arch Dermatol* 127, 267
(1990): Ficarra G+, *Oral Surg Oral Med Oral Pathol* 70, 748
(1990): Grau-Massanes M+, *J Am Acad Dermatol* 22, 687
(1990): Greenberg RG+, *J Am Acad Dermatol* 22, 327
(1990): Poizot-Martin I+, *Int Conf AIDS* 6, 357
(1989): Merenich JA+, *Am J Med* 86, 469
Oral ulceration (<5%)
(1988): McEvoy GK, *Am Hosp Formulary Service: Drug Info* 392
Paresthesias (<8%)
(1988): McEvoy GK, *Am Hosp Formulary Service: Drug Info* 392
Polymyositis
(1988): Bessen LJ+, *N Engl J Med* 318, 708 (4 patients)
Porphyria cutanea tarda
(1988): Ong EL+, *Postgrad Med J* 64, 956
Tongue edema (<5%)
(1988): McEvoy GK, *Am Hosp Formulary Service: Drug Info* 392
Tongue pigmentation
(1991): Tadini G+, *Arch Dermatol* 127, 267
(1991): Tal A+, *Cutis* 48, 153
(1990): Grau-Massanes M+, *J Am Acad Dermatol* 22, 687
(1990): Greenberg RG+, *J Am Acad Dermatol* 22, 327
Tongue ulceration
(1993): Schwander S+, *Med Klin* (German) 88, 60

ZILEUTON

Trade name: Zyflo (Abbott)
Indications: Asthma
Category: Antiasthmatic bronchodilator; Leukotriene receptor antagonist
Half-life: 2.5 hours
Clinically important, potentially hazardous interactions with: anisindione, anticoagulants, dicumarol, pimozide, warfarin

Reactions

Skin

Eosinophilic fasciitis
(2000): Dellaripa PF+, *Mayo Clin Proc* 75(6), 643
Erythema nodosum
(2000): Dellaripa PF+, *Mayo Clin Proc* 75, 643
Granulomatous dermatitis (Churg–Strauss syndrome)
(2000): Dellaripa PF+, *Mayo Clin Proc* 75(6), 643
Morphea
(2000): Dellaripa PF+, *Mayo Clin Proc* 75(6), 643
Pruritus (>1%)
Scleroderma
(2000): Dellaripa PF+, *Mayo Clin Proc* 75(6), 643

Other
Cough
(2001): Spector SL, *Ann Allergy Asthma Immunol* 86(6 Suppl 1), 18
Myalgia (3.2%)
Paresthesias (1%)
Vaginitis (>1%)

ZIPRASIDONE

Synonym: Zeldox
Trade name: Geodon (Pfizer)
Indications: Schizophrenia
Category: Antipsychotic (benzothiazolylpiperazine); Serotonin & dopamine antagonist
Half-life: 4–5 hours

Reactions

Skin
Chills (<1%)
Dermatitis
Ecchymoses (<1%)
Eczema (<1%)
Exanthems (<1%)
Exfoliative dermatitis (<1%)
Facial edema (<1%)
Fungal dermatitis (sic) (2%)
Peripheral edema (<1%)
Photosensitivity (<1%)
Rash (sic) (4%)
Upper respiratory infection (8%)
Urticaria (5%)
Vesiculobullous eruption (<1%)

Hair
Hair – alopecia (<1%)

Other
Gingival hemorrhage (<1%)
Gynecomastia (<1%)
Headache
Hyperesthesia (<1%)
Myalgia (1%)
Myopathy (<1%)
Paresthesias (<1%)
Priapism
(2002): Reeves RR+, *Pharmacotherapy* 22(8), 1070
Rhabdomyolysis
(2002): Yang SH+, *Am J Psychiatry* 159(8), 1435
Sialorrhea
Thrombophlebitis (<1%)
Tinnitus (<1%)
Tongue edema (<1%)
Tremor (<1%)
Xerostomia (4%)

ZOLEDRONIC ACID

Trade name: Zometa (Novartis)
Indications: Hypercalcemia of malignancy, Paget's disease
Category: Biphosphonate (bone resorption inhibitor)
Half-life: 7 days

Reactions

Skin
Candidiasis
Flu-like syndrome (1–10%)
(2001): Berenson JR+, *Clin Cancer Res* 7(3), 478
Upper respiratory infection
(2001): Berenson JR+, *Clin Cancer Res* (10%)

Other
Arthralgia
Bone or joint pain (1–10%)
(2001): Berenson JR+, *Cancer* 91(1), 144
(2001): Berenson JR+, *Cancer* 91(7), 1191
(2001): Berenson JR+, *Clin Cancer Res* 7(3), 478
(2001): Rosen LS+, *Cancer J* 7(5), 377
Headache
Myalgia

ZOLMITRIPTAN

Trade name: Zomig (AstraZeneca)
Indications: Migraine attacks
Category: Antimigraine; Serotonin agonist
Half-life: 3 hours
Clinically important, potentially hazardous interactions with: dihydroergotamine, ergot, isocarboxazid, MAO inhibitors, methysergide, naratriptan, phenelzine, rizatriptan, sibutramine, sumatriptan, tranylcypromine

Reactions

Skin
Allergic reactions (sic) (<1%)
Diaphoresis (2%)
Ecchymoses (<1%)
Edema (<1%)
Facial edema (<1%)
Flushing
Hot flashes (>10%)
Photosensitivity (<1%)
Pruritus (<1%)
Rash (sic) (<1%)
Urticaria (<1%)

Other
Headache
Hyperesthesia (<1%)
Myalgia (2%)
Paresthesias (11%)
(1998): Multiple Authors, *Headache* 38, 173 (11%)
Parosmia (<1%)
Serotonin syndrome
(2001): Lucas C+, *Cephalalgia* 21, 421
Thrombophlebitis (<1%)
Tongue edema (<1%)

Twitching (<1%)
Xerostomia (3%)
  (1997): Edmeads JG+, *Cephalalgia* 17, 41

ZOLPIDEM

Trade name: Ambien (Sanofi-Synthelabo)
Other common trade names: *Niotal; Stilnoct; Stilnox*
Indications: Insomnia
Category: Nonbenzodiazepine sedative-hypnotic
Half-life: 2.6 hours
**Clinically important, potentially hazardous interactions
with:** antihistamines, azatadine, azelastine, brompheniramine,
buclizine, chlorpheniramine, clemastine, dexchlorpheniramine,
meclizine, ritonavir

Reactions

Skin
Acne (<1%)
Allergic reactions (sic) (4%)
Bullous eruption (<1%)
Dermatitis (sic) (<1%)
Diaphoresis (<1%)
Edema (<1%)
Facial edema (<1%)
Flushing (<1%)
Furunculosis (<1%)
Herpes simplex (<1%)
Herpes zoster (<1%)
Hot flashes (<1%)
Periorbital edema (<1%)
Photosensitivity (<1%)
Pruritus
  (1994): Litt JZ, Beachwood, OH (personal case) (observation)
Purpura (<1%)
Rash (sic) (2%)
Urticaria (<1%)

Other
Anaphylactoid reactions (<1%)
Dysgeusia (<1%)
Hallucinations
  (2002): Andrade C, *Aust N Z J Psychiatry* 36(3), 425
  (2002): *Prescrire Int* 11(60), 117
Headache
Hyperesthesia (<1%)
Injection-site inflammation (<1%)
Mastodynia (<1%)
Myalgia (7%)
Paresthesias (<1%)
Tinnitus
Tremor (<1%)
Vaginitis (<1%)
Xerostomia (3%)

ZONISAMIDE*

Trade name: Zonegran (Elan)
Indications: Epilepsy
Category: Anticonvulsant sulfonamide
Half-life: 63 hours

**Clinically important, potentially hazardous interactions
with: caffeine**

Reactions

Skin
Acne (<1%)
Allergic reactions (sic) (<1%)
Diaphoresis (<1%)
Ecchymoses (2%)
Eczema (<1%)
Edema (<1%)
Exanthems (<1%)
Facial edema (<1%)
Lupus erythematosus (<1%)
Peripheral edema (<1%)
Petechiae (<1%)
Pruritus (<1%)
Purpura (2%)
Pustules (<1%)
Rash (sic) (3%)
Stevens–Johnson syndrome
  (1985): Wilensky AJ+, *Epilepsia* 26, 212
Toxic epidermal necrolysis
Urticaria (<1%)
Vesiculobullous eruption (<1%)
Xerosis (<1%)

Hair
Hair – alopecia (<1%)
Hair – hirsutism (<1%)

Other
Dysgeusia (2%)
Gingival hyperplasia (<1%)
Gingivitis (<1%)
Glossitis (<1%)
Gynecomastia (<1%)
  (1998): Ikeda A+, *J Neurol Neurosurg Psychiatry* 65, 803
Headache
Hyperesthesia (<1%)
Hyperpyrexia
  (1997): Shimizu T+, *Brain Dev* 19, 366
Hypersensitivity
Myalgia (<1%)
Oligohydrosis
  (2003): Knudsen JF+, *Pediatr Neurol* 28(3), 184 (6 cases)
  (1999): Isumi H+, *No To Hattatsu* (Japanese) 31, 468
  (1997): Shimizu T+, *Brain Dev* 19, 366
  (1996): Okumura A+, *No To Hattatsu* (Japanese) 28, 44
Oral ulceration (<1%)
Paresthesias (4%)
Parosmia (<1%)
Restless legs syndrome
  (2003): Chen JT+, *Neurology* 60(1), 147
Stomatitis (<1%)
Thrombophlebitis (<1%)
Tremor (<1%)
  (1992): Taira T, *No To Shinkei* (Japanese) 44, 61
Ulcerative stomatitis (<1%)
Xerostomia (2%)

*Note: Zonisamide is a sulfonamide and can be absorbed
systemically. Sulfonamides can produce severe, possibly fatal,
reactions such as toxic epidermal necrolysis and Stevens–Johnson
syndrome

Drugs responsible for 101 common reaction patterns

Acanthosis Nigricans
Azathioprine
Corticosteroids
Diethylstilbestrol
Estrogens
Gemfibrozil
Heroin
Lithium
Mechlorethamine
Methsuximide
Methyltestosterone
Niacin
Niacinamide
Oral contraceptives
Protease inhibitors
Thioridazine

Acneform Lesions
Acyclovir
Adapalene
Alosetron
Alprazolam
Amitriptyline
Amobarbital
Amoxapine
Androstenedione
Aripiprazole
Atorvastatin
Azathioprine
Basiliximab
Betaxolol
Bexarotene
Bisoprolol
Botulinum toxin (A & B)
Bupropion
Buspirone
Butabarbital
Cabergoline
Carbamazepine
Carteolol
Cefamandole
Cefpodoxime
Ceftazidime
Cetirizine
Chasteberry
Chloral hydrate
Chlorotrianisene
Cidofovir
Cimetidine
Ciprofloxacin
Clofazimine
Clomiphene
Clomipramine
Corticosteroids
Creatine
Cyanocobalamin
Cyclosporine
Dactinomycin
Danazol
Dantrolene
Deferoxamine
Demeclocycline
Desipramine
Diazepam
Diethylstilbestrol

Diltiazem
Disulfiram
Eflornithine
Epoetin alfa
Erythromycin
Escitalopram
Esmolol
Esomeprazole
Estazolam
Estrogens
Ethambutol
Ethionamide
Famotidine
Felbamate
Fenoprofen
Fexofenadine
Floxuridine
Fluconazole
Fluoxetine
Fluoxymesterone
Fluvoxamine
Folic acid
Foscarnet
Fosphenytoin
Gabapentin
Ganciclovir
Gefitinib
Glatiramer
Gold and gold compounds
Granulocyte colony-
    stimulating factor (GCSF)
Grepafloxacin
Haloperidol
Halothane
Heroin
Imipramine
Interferons, alfa-2
Isoniazid
Isotretinoin
Lamotrigine
Lansoprazole
Leflunomide
Leuprolide
Levothyroxine
Lithium
Maprotiline
MDMA
Medroxyprogesterone
Mephenytoin
Mesalamine
Methotrexate
Methoxsalen
Methyltestosterone
Minoxidil
Mirtazapine
Mycophenolate
Nabumetone
Nafarelin
Naltrexone
Naratriptan
Nefazodone
Nimodipine
Nisoldipine
Nizatidine

Nortriptyline
Olsalazine
Oral contraceptives
Oxcarbazepine
Pantoprazole
Paramethadione
Paroxetine
Pentobarbital
Pentostatin
Pergolide
Phenobarbital
Phenytoin
Potassium iodide
Primidone
Progestins
Propafenone
Propranolol
Propylthiouracil
Protriptyline
Psoralens
Pyrazinamide
Pyridoxine
Quinidine
Quinine
Ramipril
Riboflavin
Rifampin
Rifapentine
Risperidone
Ritonavir
Saquinavir
Sertraline
Sibutramine
Sirolimus
Sparfloxacin
Stanozolol
Tacrine
Testosterone
Tetracycline
Tiagabine
Tizanidine
Topiramate
Trastuzumab
Tretinoin
Trimethadione
Trioxsalen
Trovafloxacin
Valdecoxib
Valproic acid
Venlafaxine
Verapamil
Vinblastine
Zalcitabine
Zaleplon
Zidovudine
Zolpidem
Zonisamide

Acral Erythema
Bleomycin
Capecitabine
Cisplatin
Cyclophosphamide
Cytarabine
Didanosine

Doxorubicin
Fluorouracil
Granulocyte colony-
    stimulating factor (GCSF)
Hydroxyurea
Idarubicin
Lomustine
Mercaptopurine
Methotrexate
Mitotane
Paclitaxel
Quinine
Vincristine

**Acute Febrile Neutrophilic
Dermatosis
(Sweet's syndrome)**
Arnica
Capsicum
Celecoxib
Clofazimine
Clozapine
Co-trimoxazole
Cytarabine
Furosemide
Gabapentin
Glucagon
Granulocyte colony-
    stimulating factor (GCSF)
Hydralazine
Hydroxyurea
Infliximab
Isotretinoin
Minocycline
Nitrofurantoin
Oral contraceptives
Sulfamethoxazole
Tretinoin
Verapamil

**Acute Generalized
Exanthematous Pustulosis
(AGEP)**
Acetaminophen
Acetazolamide
Allopurinol
Amoxapine
Amoxicillin
Ampicillin
Aspirin
Bacampicillin
Carbamazepine
Cefaclor
Cefazolin
Ceftazidime
Cefuroxime
Cephalexin
Cephradine
Chloramphenicol
Chloroquine
Clindamycin
Clozapine
Co-trimoxazole
Codeine
Corticosteroids
Diltiazem

527

Doxycycline
Erythromycin
Famotidine
Fluconazole
Furosemide
Galantamine
Hydrochlorothiazide
Hydroxychloroquine
Imatinib
Imipenem/cilastatin
Isoniazid
Itraconazole
Lamotrigine
Lansoprazole
Methoxsalen
Metronidazole
Mexiletine
Minocycline
Nifedipine
Nimodipine
Nystatin
Penicillins
Phenobarbital
Phenytoin
Piperacillin
Progestins
Protease inhibitors
Pyrimethamine
Quinidine
Ranitidine
Streptomycin
Sulfamethoxazole
Sulfasalazine
Terbinafine
Ticlopidine
Vancomycin

Ageusia
Acarbose
Acetazolamide
Amitriptyline
Aspirin
Atorvastatin
Azelastine
Benazepril
Betaxolol
Captopril
Cetirizine
Cisplatin
Clidinium
Clomipramine
Clopidogrel
Cocaine
Cyclobenzaprine
Diazoxide
Dicyclomine
Enalapril
Etidronate
Feverfew
Fluoxetine
Fluvoxamine
Fosinopril
Glatiramer
Grepafloxacin
Hyoscyamine
Indomethacin
Interferon beta-1b
Interferons, alfa-2
Isotretinoin
Levodopa
Losartan

Methantheline
Methimazole
Mirtazapine
Nefazodone
Paroxetine
Penicillamine
Pentamidine
Phenytoin
Propantheline
Propylthiouracil
Ramipril
Rifabutin
Rimantadine
Ritonavir
Rivastigmine
Spironolactone
Sulfadoxine
Sulindac
Terbinafine
Tiagabine
Tiopronin
Topiramate
Valrubicin
Venlafaxine
Voriconazole
Zalcitabine
Zaleplon

Anaphylactoid Reactions
Abacavir
Abciximab
Acetaminophen
Acetazolamide
Acetylcysteine
Acyclovir
Alemtuzumab
Aloe vera (gel, juice, leaf)
Alteplase
Amiloride
Aminocaproic acid
Aminoglutethimide
Amitriptyline
Amoxicillin
Amphotericin B
Ampicillin
Anistreplase
Anthrax vaccine
Aprotinin
Asparaginase
Aspartame
Aspirin
Atenolol
Atropine sulfate
Azathioprine
Azithromycin
Aztreonam
Bacampicillin
Basiliximab
Benactyzine
Bendroflumethiazide
Betaxolol
Bisoprolol
Bleomycin
Bortezomib
Botulinum toxin (A & B)
Bromocriptine
Bupropion
Butalbital
Caffeine
Calcitonin
Captopril

Caraway
Carbenicillin
Carboplatin
Carisoprodol
Carteolol
Carvedilol
Caspofungin
Cefaclor
Cefadroxil
Cefamandole
Cefazolin
Cefdinir
Cefditoren
Cefepime
Cefixime
Cefmetazole
Cefonicid
Cefotaxime
Cefotetan
Cefoxitin
Cefpodoxime
Cefprozil
Ceftazidime
Ceftizoxime
Ceftriaxone
Cefuroxime
Celecoxib
Cephalexin
Cephalothin
Cephapirin
Cephradine
Cetirizine
Cetrorelix
Chamomile
Chloramphenicol
Chlorhexidine
Chlorothiazide
Chlorpromazine
Chlorzoxazone
Cimetidine
Cinoxacin
Ciprofloxacin
Cisatracurium
Cisplatin
Clarithromycin
Clemastine
Clidinium
Clindamycin
Cloxacillin
Co-trimoxazole
Codeine
Colchicine
Corticosteroids
Creatine
Cromolyn
Cyanocobalamin
Cyclobenzaprine
Cyclophosphamide
Cyclosporine
Cyproheptadine
Cytarabine
Dacarbazine
Dactinomycin
Dalteparin
Dantrolene
Daunorubicin
Deferoxamine
Demeclocycline
Denileukin
Desloratadine

Dexchlorpheniramine
Dextromethorphan
Diazepam
Diclofenac
Dicloxacillin
Dicyclomine
Didanosine
Diflunisal
Dimenhydrinate
Diphenhydramine
Diphenoxylate
Dipyridamole
Dirithromycin
Dolasetron
Domperidone
Doxorubicin
Doxycycline
Echinacea
Edrophonium
Enalapril
Enoxaparin
Epirubicin
Epoetin alfa
Eptifibatide
Ertapenem
Erythromycin
Escitalopram
Ethambutol
Ethanolamine
Etoposide
Felbamate
Fenoprofen
Fentanyl
Floxuridine
Fluconazole
Flucytosine
Fluorouracil
Fluoxetine
Fluoxymesterone
Fluphenazine
Flurbiprofen
Fluvastatin
Fluvoxamine
Folic acid
Formoterol
Fosfomycin
Fosinopril
Furosemide
Ganciclovir
Garlic
Gatifloxacin
Gemcitabine
Gemfibrozil
Gemifloxacin
Gentamicin
Glatiramer
Gold and gold compounds
Goserelin
Granisetron
Granulocyte colony-
    stimulating factor (GCSF)
Griseofulvin
Heparin
Hepatitis B vaccine
Horse chestnut (bark, flower,
    leaf, seed)
Hyoscyamine
Ibritumomab
Ibuprofen
Ifosfamide

Indapamide
Indomethacin
Infliximab
Insulin
Interferon beta 1-a
Interferon beta-1b
Ipodate
Ipratropium
Isoetharine
Isoniazid
Itraconazole
Ketoconazole
Ketoprofen
Ketorolac
Labetalol
Lamivudine
Lamotrigine
Lansoprazole
Leflunomide
Leucovorin
Levamisole
Levobupivacaine
Levofloxacin
Lidocaine
Lincomycin
Linseed
Lisinopril
Loratadine
Losartan
Mafenide
Marihuana
Mechlorethamine
Medroxyprogesterone
Mefenamic acid
Meloxicam
Melphalan
Meprobamate
Mesoridazine
Metaxalone
Methantheline
Methicillin
Methocarbamol
Methohexital
Methotrexate
Methoxsalen
Methyclothiazide
Methyltestosterone
Metolazone
Mezlocillin
Miconazole
Midazolam
Minocycline
Minoxidil
Misoprostol
Mistletoe
Moexipril
Moxifloxacin
Nabumetone
Nafcillin
Nalidixic acid
Naproxen
Neomycin
Niacin
Nitrofurantoin
Nitroglycerin
Norfloxacin
Octreotide
Ofloxacin
Omeprazole
Ondansetron

Orphenadrine
Oxacillin
Oxaliplatin
Oxaprozin
Oxytetracycline
Paclitaxel
Palivizumab
Pancuronium
Pantoprazole
PEG-interferon alfa-2b
Pegfilgrastim
Pegvisomant
Penicillins
Pentostatin
Perindopril
Perphenazine
Phenazopyridine
Phytonadione
Piperacillin
Piroxicam
Pravastatin
Prazosin
Probenecid
Prochlorperazine
Progestins
Promethazine
Propantheline
Propofol
Propranolol
Protamine
Protamine sulfate
Psoralens
Pyrilamine
Pyrimethamine
Quinupristin/dalfopristin
Ramipril
Ranitidine
Rasburicase
Repaglinide
Reteplase
Riboflavin
Rifampin
Risperidone
Ritodrine
Ritonavir
Salsalate
Scopolamine
Simvastatin
Sparfloxacin
Spectinomycin
Spironolactone
Streptokinase
Streptomycin
Succinylcholine
Sulfadiazine
Sulfadoxine
Sulfamethoxazole
Sulfasalazine
Sulfisoxazole
Sulindac
Sumatriptan
Tacrolimus
Tartrazine
Temazepam
Tenecteplase
Terazosin
Terbinafine
Terfenadine
Testosterone
Tetracycline

Thiabendazole
Thiamine
Thiopental
Thioridazine
Thiotepa
Thiothixene
Ticarcillin
Timolol
Tinzaparin
Tolmetin
Tramadol
Trastuzumab
Triamterene
Trichlormethiazide
Trifluoperazine
Trimeprazine
Trimethoprim
Tripelennamine
Triptorelin
Troleandomycin
Trovafloxacin
Urokinase
Vancomycin
Vasopressin
Vecuronium
Vincristine
Vinorelbine
Vitamin A
Voriconazole
Willow bark
Zalcitabine
Zolpidem

Angioedema
Acetaminophen
Acetylcysteine
Albuterol
Aldesleukin
Alefacept
Alemtuzumab
Allopurinol
Alteplase
Aminoglutethimide
Aminosalicylate sodium
Amiodarone
Amitriptyline
Amobarbital
Amoxicillin
Amphotericin B
Ampicillin
Anistreplase
Anthrax vaccine
Aprepitant
Aprobarbital
Aprotinin
Ascorbic acid
Asparaginase
Aspartame
Aspirin
Atomoxetine
Azatadine
Azathioprine
Azithromycin
Aztreonam
Bacampicillin
Benactyzine
Benazepril
Betaxolol
Bismuth
Bisoprolol
Bleomycin

Brompheniramine
Bupropion
Butabarbital
Caffeine
Candesartan
Captopril
Carbamazepine
Carbenicillin
Carisoprodol
Carteolol
Carvedilol
Cefaclor
Cefadroxil
Cefepime
Cefoxitin
Cefprozil
Ceftazidime
Ceftriaxone
Cefuroxime
Celecoxib
Cephalexin
Cetirizine
Chloral hydrate
Chlorambucil
Chloramphenicol
Chlordiazepoxide
Chloroquine
Chlorpheniramine
Chlorpromazine
Chlorpropamide
Chlorzoxazone
Cimetidine
Cinoxacin
Ciprofloxacin
Cisplatin
Clemastine
Clonazepam
Clonidine
Clopidogrel
Cloxacillin
Co-trimoxazole
Cocaine
Codeine
Colchicine
Corticosteroids
Cromolyn
Cyanocobalamin
Cyclamate
Cyclobenzaprine
Cyclophosphamide
Cyclosporine
Cyproheptadine
Dacarbazine
Danazol
Daunorubicin
Deferoxamine
Delavirdine
Demeclocycline
Desipramine
Dexchlorpheniramine
Diazepam
Diclofenac
Dicloxacillin
Dicumarol
Diethylstilbestrol
Diflunisal
Digoxin
Diltiazem
Dimenhydrinate
Diphenhydramine

Diphenoxylate
Dipyridamole
Disopyramide
Docetaxel
Dofetilide
Doxorubicin
Doxycycline
Echinacea
Enalapril
Enoxaparin
Epoetin alfa
Eprosartan
Esomeprazole
Estrogens
Ethambutol
Etidronate
Etodolac
Famotidine
Fenoprofen
Feverfew
Fluconazole
Fluorouracil
Fluoxetine
Fluphenazine
Flurbiprofen
Fluvastatin
Fluvoxamine
Formoterol
Fosfomycin
Fosinopril
Gatifloxacin
Gemfibrozil
Gemifloxacin
Glatiramer
Glucagon
Glyburide
Gold and gold compounds
Griseofulvin
Halothane
Heparin
Hepatitis B vaccine
Heroin
Hydralazine
Hydroxychloroquine
Hydroxyzine
Ibritumomab
Ibuprofen
Imipenem/cilastatin
Imipramine
Indapamide
Indomethacin
Insulin
Interferons, alfa-2
Irbesartan
Isoniazid
Itraconazole
Ketoconazole
Ketoprofen
Ketorolac
Labetalol
Lamivudine
Lamotrigine
Levamisole
Levobupivacaine
Levothyroxine
Lidocaine
Lincomycin
Lisinopril
Lithium
Loratadine

Losartan
Mebendazole
Mecamylamine
Mechlorethamine
Meclizine
Meclofenamate
Medroxyprogesterone
Mefenamic acid
Meloxicam
Melphalan
Meperidine
Mephenytoin
Mephobarbital
Meprobamate
Mesna
Mesoridazine
Methadone
Methicillin
Methohexital
Methylphenidate
Metoclopramide
Metoprolol
Metronidazole
Mezlocillin
Miconazole
Midazolam
Minocycline
Mitomycin
Mitotane
Moexipril
Montelukast
Nabumetone
Nafcillin
Nalidixic acid
Naloxone
Naproxen
Neomycin
Nifedipine
Nisoldipine
Nitrofurantoin
Nitroglycerin
Norfloxacin
Ofloxacin
Olanzapine
Olmesartan
Omeprazole
Ondansetron
Oral contraceptives
Oxacillin
Oxaliplatin
Oxaprozin
Oxcarbazepine
Oxytetracycline
Paclitaxel
Pamidronate
Pantoprazole
Paroxetine
PEG-interferon alfa-2b
Penicillins
Pentagastrin
Pentobarbital
Pentoxifylline
Perindopril
Perphenazine
Phenelzine
Phenindamine
Phenobarbital
Phenolphthalein
Phenytoin
Pioglitazone

Piperacillin
Piroxicam
Potassium iodide
Pravastatin
Prazosin
Primaquine
Procainamide
Procarbazine
Progestins
Promethazine
Propranolol
Propylthiouracil
Protamine
Protamine sulfate
Protriptyline
Pseudoephedrine
Pyrilamine
Pyrimethamine
Quetiapine
Quinapril
Quinestrol
Quinidine
Quinine
Ramipril
Ranitidine
Riboflavin
Rifampin
Risperidone
Ritonavir
Rituximab
Rofecoxib
Salmeterol
Salsalate
Secobarbital
Sertraline
Simvastatin
Sparfloxacin
Streptokinase
Streptomycin
Sucralfate
Sulfamethoxazole
Sulfasalazine
Sulfisoxazole
Sulindac
Sumatriptan
Tamsulosin
Tartrazine
Telmisartan
Tenecteplase
Terbinafine
Terfenadine
Tetracycline
Thiabendazole
Thiamine
Thiopental
Thioridazine
Thiotepa
Ticarcillin
Ticlopidine
Timolol
Tinzaparin
Tiopronin
Tolmetin
Torsemide
Tramadol
Trandolapril
Trastuzumab
Trazodone
Trifluoperazine
Trimeprazine

Trimetrexate
Tripelennamine
Triprolidine
Triptorelin
Troleandomycin
Trovafloxacin
Urokinase
Valsartan
Vancomycin
Vasopressin
Verapamil
Vincristine
Vinorelbine
Voriconazole
Warfarin
Zalcitabine

Anosmia
Acetazolamide
Ciprofloxacin
Cocaine
Cromolyn
Doxycycline
Enalapril
Ganciclovir
Interferons, alfa-2
Methazolamide
Minoxidil
Paroxetine
Pentamidine
Sparfloxacin
Terbinafine

Aphthous Stomatitis
Aldesleukin
Anagrelide
Asparaginase
Aspirin
Atazanavir
Azathioprine
Azelastine
Aztreonam
Captopril
Cidofovir
Co-trimoxazole
Cyclosporine
Delavirdine
Diclofenac
Diflunisal
Doxepin
Fenoprofen
Fluoxetine
Flurbiprofen
Gold and gold compounds
Hepatitis B vaccine
Ibuprofen
Imiquimod
Indinavir
Indomethacin
Interferon beta-1b
Interferons, alfa-2
Ketoprofen
Ketorolac
Losartan
Meclofenamate
Midodrine
Mirtazapine
Naproxen
Olanzapine
Pantoprazole
Paroxetine
Penicillamine

Piroxicam
Rofecoxib
Sertraline
Sirolimus
Sulfamethoxazole
Sulfasalazine
Sulfisoxazole
Sulindac
Terbinafine
Tolmetin
Trientine
Valsartan
Zalcitabine
Zaleplon

Black Hairy Tongue (Lingua Villosa Nigra)
Amitriptyline
Amoxapine
Amoxicillin
Ampicillin
Bacampicillin
Benztropine
Carbenicillin
Chloramphenicol
Clarithromycin
Clomipramine
Clonazepam
Cloxacillin
Co-trimoxazole
Cocaine
Corticosteroids
Desipramine
Dicloxacillin
Fluoxetine
Griseofulvin
Imipramine
Isocarboxazid
Lansoprazole
Maprotiline
Methicillin
Methyldopa
Mezlocillin
Minocycline
Nafcillin
Nortriptyline
Oxacillin
Oxytetracycline
Penicillins
Phenelzine
Protriptyline
Streptomycin
Sulfamethoxazole
Tetracycline
Thiothixene
Ticarcillin
Tranylcypromine

Bullous Eruptions
Acetazolamide
Acitretin
Aldesleukin
Alemtuzumab
Alitretinoin
Aminocaproic acid
Aminosalicylate sodium
Amitriptyline
Amobarbital
Ampicillin
Argatroban
Arsenic
Aspirin

Atropine sulfate
Benactyzine
Bergamot
Bleomycin
Bumetanide
Buspirone
Busulfan
Butabarbital
Butalbital
Caffeine
Capsicum
Captopril
Carbamazepine
Carbenicillin
Cetirizine
Cevimeline
Chloral hydrate
Chloramphenicol
Chlorothiazide
Chlorpromazine
Chlorpropamide
Ciprofloxacin
Clopidogrel
Co-trimoxazole
Cocaine
Codeine
Colchicine
Corticosteroids
Cyanocobalamin
Cyclamate
Cyclosporine
Cytarabine
Dalteparin
Dapsone
Demeclocycline
Denileukin
Dextromethorphan
Diazepam
Diclofenac
Dicloxacillin
Dicumarol
Diethylstilbestrol
Diflunisal
Digoxin
Dirithromycin
Disulfiram
Ephedrine
Estrogens
Ethambutol
Ethchlorvynol
Ethotoin
Etodolac
Felbamate
Fenoprofen
Floxuridine
Fluconazole
Fluorouracil
Fluoxetine
Flutamide
Fluvoxamine
Fondaparinux
Fosphenytoin
Frovatriptan
Furosemide
Ganciclovir
Garlic
Glyburide
Gold and gold compounds
Granulocyte colony-
    stimulating factor (GCSF)

Griseofulvin
Henna
Hydralazine
Hydrochlorothiazide
Hydroxychloroquine
Ibuprofen
Ibutilide
Idarubicin
Imipramine
Imiquimod
Indapamide
Indomethacin
Infliximab
Insulin
Interferons, alfa-2
Isoniazid
Ivermectin
Ketoprofen
Lamotrigine
Leflunomide
Lidocaine
Lindane
Lisinopril
Lithium
Mafenide
Mechlorethamine
Meclofenamate
Meloxicam
Mephenytoin
Meprobamate
Methicillin
Methotrexate
Methoxsalen
Mezlocillin
Miconazole
Minoxidil
Mitomycin
Mycophenolate
Nabumetone
Nafcillin
Nalidixic acid
Naproxen
Neomycin
Nifedipine
Nitrofurantoin
Norfloxacin
Ofloxacin
Omeprazole
Oral contraceptives
Oxacillin
Penicillamine
Pentamidine
Pentobarbital
Pentostatin
Phenobarbital
Phenolphthalein
Phenytoin
Piperacillin
Piroxicam
Promethazine
Propranolol
Pyridoxine
Pyrimethamine
Quinapril
Quinethazone
Quinidine
Quinine
Reserpine
Rifampin
Risperidone

Ritonavir
Rivastigmine
Rofecoxib
Saquinavir
Senna
Sertraline
Smallpox vaccine
Sparfloxacin
Streptomycin
Sulfadoxine
Sulfamethoxazole
Sulfasalazine
Sulfisoxazole
Tacrine
Temazepam
Testosterone
Tetracycline
Thalidomide
Thiopental
Ticarcillin
Tinzaparin
Tolbutamide
Tolmetin
Tretinoin
Trimethadione
Trioxsalen
Urokinase
Valproic acid
Vancomycin
Vasopressin
Vinblastine
Warfarin
Zalcitabine
Zidovudine
Zolpidem

Bullous Pemphigoid
Aldesleukin
Amoxicillin
Ampicillin
Bumetanide
Captopril
Cephalexin
Chloroquine
Ciprofloxacin
Dactinomycin
Enalapril
Fosinopril
Furosemide
Gold and gold compounds
Hepatitis B vaccine
Ibuprofen
Ivermectin
Mefenamic acid
Methoxsalen
Nadolol
Omeprazole
Penicillamine
Penicillins
Potassium iodide
Psoralens
Risperidone
Spironolactone
Sulfasalazine
Tiopronin
Tolbutamide

Candidiasis
Ampicillin
Aripiprazole
Basiliximab
Cefaclor

Cefadroxil
Cefdinir
Cefepime
Cefixime
Cefmetazole
Cefonicid
Cefoperazone
Cefotaxime
Cefotetan
Cefoxitin
Cefpodoxime
Cefprozil
Ceftazidime
Ceftibuten
Ceftizoxime
Ceftriaxone
Cefuroxime
Celecoxib
Cephalothin
Cephapirin
Chlorotrianisene
Ciprofloxacin
Corticosteroids
Danazol
Demeclocycline
Diazoxide
Doxycycline
Eletriptan
Ertapenem
Esomeprazole
Famotidine
Fluoxetine
Gatifloxacin
Gemifloxacin
Griseofulvin
Heroin
Imipenem/cilastatin
Infliximab
Interferons, alfa-2
Lansoprazole
Levofloxacin
Linezolid
Loracarbef
Methotrexate
Metronidazole
Minocycline
Moxifloxacin
Ofloxacin
Olanzapine
Oral contraceptives
Pamidronate
Paroxetine
Pentostatin
Piperacillin
Quetiapine
Quinupristin/dalfopristin
Riluzole
Saquinavir
Tetracycline
Tizanidine
Trovafloxacin
Valdecoxib
Venlafaxine
Zoledronic acid

Cheilitis
Acitretin
Aripiprazole
Atorvastatin
Bexarotene
Busulfan

Clofazimine
Clomipramine
Cyanocobalamin
Dactinomycin
Eflornithine
Frovatriptan
Gatifloxacin
Gold and gold compounds
Grepafloxacin
Indinavir
Interferon beta-1b
Isotretinoin
Lithium
Methoxsalen
Methyldopa
Peppermint
Propolis
Propranolol
Psoralens
Ritonavir
Saquinavir
Simvastatin
Streptomycin
Sulfasalazine
Tetracycline
Thimerosal
Tretinoin
Trovafloxacin
Verteporfin
Vitamin A
Voriconazole
Zaleplon

Chills
Abacavir
Acetylcysteine
Acitretin
Albuterol
Alefacept
Alemtuzumab
Allopurinol
Almotriptan
Amifostine
Amphotericin B
Anagrelide
Anastrozole
Anisindione
Anistreplase
Anthrax vaccine
Aripiprazole
Asparaginase
Azathioprine
Benzonatate
Bexarotene
Bleomycin
Caffeine
Caspofungin
Ceftriaxone
Cidofovir
Cilostazol
Dantrolene
Daunorubicin
Denileukin
Dexchlorpheniramine
Dextroamphetamine
Didanosine
Dolasetron
Droperidol
Eletriptan
Enfuvirtide
Enoxacin

Ertapenem
Escitalopram
Estazolam
Ethacrynic acid
Ethambutol
Floxuridine
Fludarabine
Fosphenytoin
Ganciclovir
Gatifloxacin
Gemtuzumab
Glatiramer
Goserelin
Heparin
Hepatitis B vaccine
Hydralazine
Ibritumomab
Infliximab
Interferon beta 1-a
Interferon beta-1b
Interferons, alfa-2
Irbesartan
Irinotecan
Ketoconazole
Lamivudine
Levalbuterol
Levobupivacaine
Lomefloxacin
MDMA
Metolazone
Miconazole
Midodrine
Mifepristone
Mirtazapine
Mistletoe
Mitoxantrone
Modafinil
Moxifloxacin
Naltrexone
Nifedipine
Nisoldipine
Nitrofurantoin
Ofloxacin
Ondansetron
Paricalcitol
Pergolide
Perindopril
Pilocarpine
Procainamide
Promethazine
Rabeprazole
Riluzole
Ritodrine
Rituximab
Rizatriptan
Sirolimus
Smallpox vaccine
Spectinomycin
Spironolactone
Stanozolol
Stavudine
Sufentanil
Sulfadiazine
Tenofovir
Terconazole
Trastuzumab
Triamterene
Trihexyphenidyl
Urofollitropin
Urokinase

Valdecoxib
Vancomycin
Verteporfin
Voriconazole
Zaleplon
Ziprasidone

Dermatitis
Acebutolol
Acetaminophen
Acetylcysteine
Acitretin
Acyclovir
Adapalene
Albendazole
Albuterol
Aldesleukin
Almotriptan
Aloe vera (gel, juice, leaf)
Alprazolam
Altretamine
Amantadine
Amikacin
Aminocaproic acid
Aminolevulinic acid
Aminophylline
Amitriptyline
Amlodipine
Amoxapine
Amoxicillin
Amphotericin B
Ampicillin
Amyl nitrite
Anisindione
Apraclonidine
Arnica
Arsenic
Aspartame
Atenolol
Atorvastatin
Atropine sulfate
Azathioprine
Azelastine
Azithromycin
Bacampicillin
Baclofen
Benazepril
Bendroflumethiazide
Bergamot
Beta-carotene
Betaxolol
Biperiden
Bismuth
Bleomycin
Bloodroot
Brinzolamide
Bumetanide
Capecitabine
Capsicum
Captopril
Caraway
Carbamazepine
Carmustine
Carteolol
Cefaclor
Cefazolin
Ceftriaxone
Celecoxib
Cephalexin
Cetirizine
Cevimeline

Chamomile
Chicory
Chloral hydrate
Chloramphenicol
Chlordiazepoxide
Chlorhexidine
Chloroquine
Chlorotrianisene
Chlorpheniramine
Chlorpromazine
Chlorpropamide
Cimetidine
Cisplatin
Citalopram
Clindamycin
Clofibrate
Clomiphene
Clomipramine
Clonazepam
Clonidine
Clorazepate
Clotrimazole
Cloxacillin
Clozapine
Co-trimoxazole
Codeine
Colchicine
Colestipol
Corticosteroids
Cromolyn
Cyanocobalamin
Cyclobenzaprine
Cyclophosphamide
Cycloserine
Cyproheptadine
Dacarbazine
Dactinomycin
Dantrolene
Daunorubicin
Deferoxamine
Delavirdine
Dexchlorpheniramine
Diazepam
Diclofenac
Dicloxacillin
Dicumarol
Diltiazem
Diphenhydramine
Disopyramide
Disulfiram
Docetaxel
Docusate
Donepezil
Dong quai
Dorzolamide
Doxepin
Doxorubicin
Eflornithine
Enalapril
Ephedrine
Epinephrine
Epoetin alfa
Ertapenem
Erythromycin
Escitalopram
Esomeprazole
Estazolam
Estrogens
Ethambutol
Ethanolamine

Etodolac
Famciclovir
Famotidine
Feverfew
Floxuridine
Fluorouracil
Fluoxetine
Fluoxymesterone
Fluphenazine
Flurazepam
Flurbiprofen
Fluvoxamine
Folic acid
Foscarnet
Furazolidone
Garlic
Gemcitabine
Gemfibrozil
Gemifloxacin
Gentamicin
Ginger
Ginkgo biloba
Glatiramer
Gold and gold compounds
Grepafloxacin
Guanethidine
Guanfacine
Haloperidol
Henna
Heparin
Heroin
Horse chestnut (bark, flower,
    leaf, seed)
Hydrochlorothiazide
Hydroxychloroquine
Hydroxyurea
Hydroxyzine
Ibuprofen
Ibutilide
Ifosfamide
Indinavir
Indomethacin
Insulin
Interferon beta 1-a
Interferon beta-1b
Interferons, alfa-2
Ipratropium
Irbesartan
Irinotecan
Isoniazid
Isoxsuprine
Itraconazole
Ivermectin
Juniper
Ketoconazole
Ketoprofen
Ketorolac
Labetalol
Lamivudine
Lansoprazole
Lavender
Leflunomide
Leuprolide
Levamisole
Levobetaxolol
Levobunolol
Licorice
Lidocaine
Lincomycin
Lindane

Lithium
Loratadine
Lorazepam
Losartan
Loxapine
Mafenide
Mechlorethamine
Mefloquine
Meprobamate
Mercaptopurine
Mesoridazine
Metaxalone
Methotrexate
Methoxsalen
Methyltestosterone
Metronidazole
Mezlocillin
Miconazole
Minoxidil
Misoprostol
Mistletoe
Mitomycin
Mupirocin
Nadolol
Naproxen
Naratriptan
Nelfinavir
Neomycin
Niacin
Nicotine
Nifedipine
Nitrofurantoin
Nitroglycerin
Nizatidine
Norfloxacin
Nystatin
Ofloxacin
Olanzapine
Omeprazole
Oral contraceptives
Orlistat
Oxazepam
Oxcarbazepine
Oxytetracycline
Palivizumab
Pantoprazole
Paroxetine
PEG-interferon alfa-2b
Penicillamine
Penicillins
Pentazocine
Pentostatin
Peppermint
Perphenazine
Phenindamine
Phenoxybenzamine
Phenylephrine
Phenytoin
Phytonadione
Pilocarpine
Piroxicam
Prazepam
Probenecid
Procainamide
Procarbazine
Progestins
Promazine
Promethazine
Propantheline
Propolis

Propranolol
Propylthiouracil
Protriptyline
Pseudoephedrine
Psoralens
Pyrazinamide
Pyridoxine
Pyrilamine
Pyrimethamine
Quazepam
Quinacrine
Quinidine
Quinine
Ramipril
Ranitidine
Rifampin
Risperidone
Ritonavir
Rivastigmine
Rofecoxib
Ropinirole
Rue
Saccharin
Salsalate
Saquinavir
Scopolamine
Selenium
Senna
Sertraline
Sildenafil
Simvastatin
Sirolimus
Sparfloxacin
Spectinomycin
Spironolactone
Streptomycin
Succinylcholine
Sulfamethoxazole
Sulfasalazine
Sulfinpyrazone
Sulindac
Tacrine
Tartrazine
Tea tree
Telmisartan
Temazepam
Terbinafine
Terbutaline
Terfenadine
Testosterone
Tetracycline
Thalidomide
Thiabendazole
Thiamine
Thimerosal
Thioridazine
Tiagabine
Ticlopidine
Timolol
Tiopronin
Tobramycin
Tolazamide
Tolazoline
Tolbutamide
Tolmetin
Topiramate
Toremifene
Tramadol
Tretinoin
Triazolam

Trientine
Trifluoperazine
Trimeprazine
Trovafloxacin
Turmeric
Valacyclovir
Valdecoxib
Valproic acid
Venlafaxine
Verapamil
Vinblastine
Vitamin A
Vitamin E
Voriconazole
Warfarin
Yarrow
Zalcitabine
Zaleplon
Ziprasidone
Zolpidem

Dermatitis Herpetiformis (DH)

Amitriptyline
Aspirin
Cyclophosphamide
Diclofenac
Doxorubicin
Flurbiprofen
Ibuprofen
Indomethacin
Interferons, alfa-2
Levothyroxine
Lithium
Mycophenolate
Oral contraceptives
Potassium iodide
Sirolimus
Ursodiol
Vincristine

Diaphoresis

Acebutolol
Acetaminophen
Acetohexamide
Acitretin
Acyclovir
Adenosine
Albuterol
Allopurinol
Almotriptan
Alprazolam
Alprostadil
Amiloride
Aminophylline
Amiodarone
Amitriptyline
Amlodipine
Amoxapine
Amphotericin B
Amyl nitrite
Anastrozole
Anistreplase
Anthrax vaccine
Aprepitant
Arbutamine
Aripiprazole
Asparaginase
Aspirin
Atazanavir
Atenolol
Atorvastatin

Atovaquone
Azatadine
Aztreonam
Baclofen
Benazepril
Bendroflumethiazide
Benzphetamine
Bepridil
Betaxolol
Bethanechol
Bicalutamide
Biperiden
Bisacodyl
Bisoprolol
Black cohosh
Blue cohosh
Bretylium
Bumetanide
Bupropion
Buspirone
Butorphanol
Candesartan
Capecitabine
Capsicum
Carbamazepine
Carisoprodol
Carteolol
Carvedilol
Caspofungin
Cefamandole
Cefditoren
Cefpodoxime
Ceftazidime
Ceftriaxone
Celecoxib
Cetirizine
Cevimeline
Chlordiazepoxide
Chlorpheniramine
Cidofovir
Ciprofloxacin
Cisplatin
Citalopram
Cladribine
Clemastine
Clofibrate
Clomiphene
Clomipramine
Clonazepam
Clonidine
Clorazepate
Clozapine
Cocaine
Codeine
Corticosteroids
Cyclobenzaprine
Cyclophosphamide
Cyproheptadine
Danazol
Dantrolene
Delavirdine
Denileukin
Desipramine
Desmopressin
Dexchlorpheniramine
Dexmedetomidine
Dextroamphetamine
Diazepam
Diazoxide
Diclofenac

Didanosine
Diethylpropion
Diflunisal
Digoxin
Diltiazem
Dimenhydrinate
Diphenhydramine
Diphenoxylate
Dipyridamole
Dirithromycin
Disulfiram
Docusate
Dofetilide
Dolasetron
Domperidone
Donepezil
Doxapram
Doxazosin
Doxepin
Dronabinol
Droperidol
Edrophonium
Eletriptan
Enalapril
Enoxacin
Entacapone
Ephedrine
Epinephrine
Eprosartan
Ertapenem
Escitalopram
Esmolol
Esomeprazole
Estazolam
Ethambutol
Ethchlorvynol
Etodolac
Etoposide
Exemestane
Felbamate
Felodipine
Fenoprofen
Fentanyl
Flecainide
Flumazenil
Fluoxetine
Fluphenazine
Flurazepam
Flurbiprofen
Flutamide
Fluvoxamine
Foscarnet
Fosinopril
Frovatriptan
Fulvestrant
Furosemide
Ganciclovir
Gatifloxacin
Gemcitabine
Glatiramer
Glimepiride
Goserelin
Granulocyte colony-
  stimulating factor (GCSF)
Grepafloxacin
Guanfacine
Haloperidol
Hawthorn (fruit, leaf, flower
  extract)
Hepatitis B vaccine

Hydralazine
Hydrochlorothiazide
Hydrocodone
Hydromorphone
Hydroxyzine
Ibritumomab
Ibuprofen
Imipenem/cilastatin
Imipramine
Indapamide
Indinavir
Indomethacin
Insulin
Interferon beta 1-a
Interferon beta-1b
Interferons, alfa-2
Irinotecan
Isocarboxazid
Isoproterenol
Isosorbide dinitrate
Isosorbide mononitrate
Isotretinoin
Isradipine
Ketoprofen
Ketorolac
Labetalol
Lamotrigine
Lansoprazole
Leflunomide
Letrozole
Leuprolide
Levalbuterol
Levobupivacaine
Levodopa
Levofloxacin
Levothyroxine
Liothyronine
Lisinopril
Lomefloxacin
Loratadine
Lorazepam
Losartan
Loxapine
Maprotiline
Mazindol
MDMA
Medroxyprogesterone
Mefenamic acid
Meperidine
Mesalamine
Methadone
Methamphetamine
Methylphenidate
Metoclopramide
Metoprolol
Mexiletine
Milk thistle
Mirtazapine
Misoprostol
Mitoxantrone
Modafinil
Moexipril
Moricizine
Morphine
Moxifloxacin
Mycophenolate
Nabumetone
Nadolol
Nalbuphine
Naloxone

Naltrexone
Naproxen
Naratriptan
Nelfinavir
Nesiritide
Nicotine
Nifedipine
Nimodipine
Nisoldipine
Nitazoxanide
Nitroglycerin
Nizatidine
Norfloxacin
Nortriptyline
Octreotide
Ofloxacin
Olanzapine
Omeprazole
Oxaliplatin
Oxaprozin
Oxazepam
Oxcarbazepine
Oxycodone
Pantoprazole
Papaverine
Paroxetine
PEG-interferon alfa-2b
Penbutolol
Penicillins
Pentagastrin
Pentazocine
Pentostatin
Pentoxifylline
Pergolide
Perindopril
Perphenazine
Phendimetrazine
Phenelzine
Phenindamine
Phenolphthalein
Phentermine
Physostigmine
Phytonadione
Pilocarpine
Pimozide
Pindolol
Piroxicam
Potassium iodide
Pramipexole
Prazepam
Praziquantel
Prazosin
Procarbazine
Prochlorperazine
Progestins
Promethazine
Propafenone
Propantheline
Propoxyphene
Propranolol
Protriptyline
Pseudoephedrine
Pyrilamine
Quazepam
Quetiapine
Quinapril
Quinine
Quinupristin/dalfopristin
Rabeprazole
Raloxifene

Ramipril
Rapacuronium
Rifampin
Risperidone
Ritodrine
Ritonavir
Rituximab
Rivastigmine
Rizatriptan
Rofecoxib
Ropinirole
Saquinavir
Selegiline
Selenium
Sertraline
Sibutramine
Sildenafil
Simvastatin
Sirolimus
Sodium oxybate
Sotalol
Sparfloxacin
Spironolactone
Stavudine
Streptokinase
Sulfasalazine
Sulindac
Sumatriptan
Tacrine
Tacrolimus
Tamoxifen
Tegaserod
Telmisartan
Temazepam
Terazosin
Terbutaline
Terfenadine
Teriparatide
Tetracycline
Thalidomide
Thiamine
Thiothixene
Tiagabine
Ticlopidine
Timolol
Tirofiban
Tizanidine
Tocainide
Tolazamide
Tolcapone
Tolmetin
Topiramate
Toremifene
Tramadol
Tranylcypromine
Trastuzumab
Trazodone
Treprostinil
Tretinoin
Triamterene
Triazolam
Trifluoperazine
Trihexyphenidyl
Trimeprazine
Trimipramine
Tripelennamine
Triprolidine
Trovafloxacin
Tryptophan
Unoprostone

Urokinase
Ursodiol
Valdecoxib
Valproic acid
Vasopressin
Verapamil
Verteporfin
Voriconazole
Yohimbine
Zalcitabine
Zaleplon
Zidovudine
Zolmitriptan
Zolpidem
Zonisamide
Dysgeusia
Acebutolol
Acetaminophen
Acetazolamide
Acyclovir
Adenosine
Albuterol
Aldesleukin
Alemtuzumab
Alendronate
Allopurinol
Almotriptan
Alosetron
Alprazolam
Amifostine
Amiloride
Amiodarone
Amitriptyline
Amlodipine
Amoxapine
Amoxicillin
Amprenavir
Apraclonidine
Aprepitant
Arbutamine
Aripiprazole
Arsenic
Aspirin
Atazanavir
Atorvastatin
Atovaquone
Atropine sulfate
Azelastine
Aztreonam
Bacampicillin
Baclofen
Benazepril
Benzthiazide
Benztropine
Bepridil
Betaxolol
Bismuth
Bisoprolol
Bortezomib
Botulinum toxin (A & B)
Brimonidine
Brinzolamide
Bromocriptine
Bupropion
Buspirone
Busulfan
Butorphanol
Calcitonin
Captopril
Carbamazepine

Carbenicillin
Carteolol
Cefaclor
Cefamandole
Cefditoren
Cefmetazole
Cefpodoxime
Ceftazidime
Ceftibuten
Ceftriaxone
Celecoxib
Cetirizine
Cevimeline
Chloral hydrate
Chlorhexidine
Chlormezanone
Chlorothiazide
Cholestyramine
Cidofovir
Cinoxacin
Ciprofloxacin
Citalopram
Clarithromycin
Clidinium
Clindamycin
Clofazimine
Clofibrate
Clomipramine
Clonazepam
Clonidine
Clotrimazole
Clozapine
Co-trimoxazole
Codeine
Cromolyn
Cyclobenzaprine
Cyproheptadine
Dacarbazine
Dantrolene
Delavirdine
Desipramine
Devil's claw
Dextroamphetamine
Diazoxide
Diclofenac
Dicloxacillin
Dicyclomine
Diethylpropion
Dihydroergotamine
Dihydrotachysterol
Diltiazem
Dipyridamole
Dirithromycin
Disulfiram
Docetaxel
Docusate
Dolasetron
Donepezil
Dorzolamide
Doxazosin
Doxepin
Doxycycline
Efavirenz
Eletriptan
Enalapril
Enfuvirtide
Enoxacin
Entacapone
Eprosartan
Ergocalciferol

Ertapenem
Escitalopram
Esmolol
Esomeprazole
Estazolam
Ethchlorvynol
Ethionamide
Etidronate
Etoposide
Famotidine
Felbamate
Fenoprofen
Fentanyl
Flecainide
Fluconazole
Fludarabine
Fluorouracil
Fluoxetine
Flurazepam
Flurbiprofen
Fluvastatin
Fluvoxamine
Fomepizole
Foscarnet
Fosinopril
Fosphenytoin
Frovatriptan
Ganciclovir
Gatifloxacin
Gemcitabine
Gemfibrozil
Gemifloxacin
Glatiramer
Glyburide
Glycopyrrolate
Gold and gold compounds
Granisetron
Grepafloxacin
Griseofulvin
Guanabenz
Guanfacine
Hydrochlorothiazide
Hydroflumethiazide
Hydromorphone
Hydroxychloroquine
Hyoscyamine
Imipenem/cilastatin
Imipramine
Indinavir
Interferon beta-1b
Interferons, alfa-2
Ipratropium
Irinotecan
Isotretinoin
Ketoprofen
Ketorolac
Labetalol
Lamotrigine
Lansoprazole
Leflunomide
Leuprolide
Levamisole
Levobetaxolol
Levodopa
Levofloxacin
Linezolid
Lisinopril
Lithium
Lomefloxacin
Loratadine

Losartan
Lovastatin
Maprotiline
Mazindol
Mechlorethamine
Meclofenamate
Meloxicam
Mesalamine
Mesna
Metformin
Methamphetamine
Methantheline
Methazolamide
Methicillin
Methimazole
Methocarbamol
Methotrexate
Methyclothiazide
Metolazone
Metoprolol
Metronidazole
Mexiletine
Mezlocillin
Midazolam
Minoxidil
Mirtazapine
Modafinil
Moexipril
Moricizine
Moxifloxacin
Mupirocin
Nadolol
Nafcillin
Nalbuphine
Naratriptan
Nedocromil
Nefazodone
Nicotine
Nifedipine
Nisoldipine
Norfloxacin
Nortriptyline
Ofloxacin
Olanzapine
Olopatadine
Omeprazole
Ondansetron
Oxacillin
Oxaliplatin
Oxaprozin
Oxcarbazepine
Pamidronate
Pantoprazole
Paroxetine
PEG-interferon alfa-2b
Pegfilgrastim
Penbutolol
Penicillamine
Penicillins
Pentamidine
Pentazocine
Pentostatin
Pentoxifylline
Pergolide
Perindopril
Phendimetrazine
Phentermine
Phytonadione
Pilocarpine
Pimozide

Pindolol
Pirbuterol
Plicamycin
Potassium iodide
Pramipexole
Pravastatin
Procainamide
Propafenone
Propantheline
Propofol
Propranolol
Propylthiouracil
Protriptyline
Pyrimethamine
Quazepam
Quinapril
Quinidine
Ramipril
Ranitidine
Ribavirin
Rifabutin
Riluzole
Rimantadine
Risperidone
Ritonavir
Rivastigmine
Saccharin
Saquinavir
Selegiline
Selenium
Sermorelin
Sertraline
Sibutramine
Simvastatin
Sirolimus
Sotalol
Sparfloxacin
Sulfamethoxazole
Sulfasalazine
Sulfisoxazole
Sulindac
Sumatriptan
Tacrine
Tamoxifen
Temazepam
Terbinafine
Terbutaline
Teriparatide
Thiothixene
Tiagabine
Ticarcillin
Timolol
Tocainide
Tolazamide
Tolbutamide
Tolmetin
Topiramate
Tramadol
Trazodone
Triamterene
Triazolam
Trimethoprim
Trimipramine
Trovafloxacin
Ursodiol
Valdecoxib
Valproic acid
Valsartan
Vancomycin
Venlafaxine

Vinblastine
Vincristine
Vinorelbine
Voriconazole
Zalcitabine
Zidovudine
Zolpidem
Zonisamide

Ecchymoses
Allopurinol
Alprostadil
Alteplase
Amiodarone
Amoxicillin
Anagrelide
Anakinra
Anisindione
Anistreplase
Atazanavir
Atorvastatin
Bacampicillin
Benactyzine
Beta-carotene
Botulinum toxin (A & B)
Bupropion
Buspirone
Caffeine
Carbenicillin
Celecoxib
Chlorzoxazone
Cholestyramine
Cilostazol
Cloxacillin
Corticosteroids
Delavirdine
Denileukin
Desipramine
Dicloxacillin
Dicumarol
Diethylpropion
Diltiazem
Donepezil
Enfuvirtide
Enoxaparin
Etodolac
Etoposide
Fluvoxamine
Fosphenytoin
Gatifloxacin
Gemtuzumab
Glatiramer
Heparin
Hepatitis B vaccine
Ibritumomab
Indomethacin
Interferon beta 1-a
Interferons, alfa-2
Irbesartan
Lamotrigine
Latanoprost
Leuprolide
Levetiracetam
Lindane
Losartan
Meprobamate
Mesalamine
Methicillin
Methotrexate
Mezlocillin
Mitoxantrone

Modafinil
Nafcillin
Naproxen
Nefazodone
Nisoldipine
Ofloxacin
Olanzapine
Oxacillin
Oxaprozin
Pantoprazole
Paroxetine
Penicillamine
Pentosan
Pentostatin
Perindopril
Piperacillin
Piroxicam
Plicamycin
Rabeprazole
Reteplase
Risedronate
Ritonavir
Sibutramine
Sirolimus
Sparfloxacin
Streptokinase
Sulindac
Tacrolimus
Tenecteplase
Thiotepa
Tiagabine
Ticarcillin
Ticlopidine
Tinzaparin
Tiopronin
Tizanidine
Urokinase
Valdecoxib
Valproic acid
Vasopressin
Venlafaxine
Verapamil
Voriconazole
Warfarin
Zaleplon
Zidovudine
Ziprasidone
Zolmitriptan
Zonisamide

Eczema
Acetohexamide
Adapalene
Aldesleukin
Amantadine
Aminocaproic acid
Aminosalicylate sodium
Aripiprazole
Ascorbic acid
Atazanavir
Atorvastatin
Azelastine
Bisoprolol
Carbamazepine
Cevimeline
Chloral hydrate
Chloramphenicol
Citalopram
Clindamycin
Clonidine
Clopidogrel

Clozapine
Corticosteroids
Cromolyn
Cyanocobalamin
Diazepam
Diclofenac
Dimenhydrinate
Diphenhydramine
Disulfiram
Doxazosin
Efavirenz
Eprosartan
Erythromycin
Escitalopram
Esmolol
Estrogens
Ethionamide
Fluorouracil
Fluoxetine
Fluphenazine
Flurbiprofen
Gemfibrozil
Gemifloxacin
Gentamicin
Glatiramer
Glipizide
Glucosamine
Glyburide
Gold and gold compounds
Henna
Heparin
Hepatitis B vaccine
Hydralazine
Hydrochlorothiazide
Ibuprofen
Indomethacin
Interferons, alfa-2
Irbesartan
Isoniazid
Isotretinoin
Kanamycin
Ketoconazole
Ketoprofen
Labetalol
Lamotrigine
Latanoprost
Leflunomide
Lidocaine
Lindane
Lithium
Lomefloxacin
Meprobamate
Mesalamine
Mesoridazine
Metformin
Methenamine
Methoxsalen
Methyldopa
Metoprolol
Minoxidil
Nadolol
Nefazodone
Neomycin
Nitrofurantoin
Nitroglycerin
Nystatin
Olanzapine
Omeprazole
Oral contraceptives
Oxcarbazepine

Palivizumab
Pantoprazole
Paroxetine
Penicillins
Pentostatin
Perphenazine
Phytonadione
Pindolol
Potassium iodide
Pravastatin
Procainamide
Prochlorperazine
Promethazine
Propranolol
Pseudoephedrine
Psoralens
Quinidine
Quinine
Ranitidine
Ribavirin
Riluzole
Ritonavir
Ropinirole
Salmeterol
Saquinavir
Simvastatin
Spironolactone
Streptomycin
Sulfasalazine
Sulfisoxazole
Tacrine
Tamsulosin
Tea tree
Telmisartan
Terbinafine
Tetracycline
Thiamine
Thimerosal
Tiagabine
Timolol
Tobramycin
Tolazamide
Tolcapone
Topiramate
Trifluoperazine
Trioxsalen
Tripelennamine
Valdecoxib
Venlafaxine
Verteporfin
Vitamin A
Voriconazole
Zaleplon
Ziprasidone
Zonisamide

Edema
Abacavir
Abciximab
Acebutolol
Acetaminophen
Acitretin
Acyclovir
Adalimumab
Adapalene
Aldesleukin
Alefacept
Alemtuzumab
Alitretinoin
Allopurinol
Alprazolam

Alprostadil
Amantadine
Aminocaproic acid
Aminolevulinic acid
Amiodarone
Amitriptyline
Amlodipine
Amoxapine
Amoxicillin
Amyl nitrite
Anagrelide
Anthrax vaccine
Apraclonidine
Aprepitant
Aripiprazole
Arsenic
Asparaginase
Atazanavir
Atenolol
Atorvastatin
Atracurium
Atropine sulfate
Azatadine
Azithromycin
Bacampicillin
Baclofen
Basiliximab
Benactyzine
Benazepril
Bendroflumethiazide
Bepridil
Betaxolol
Bexarotene
Bicalutamide
Bisoprolol
Bortezomib
Bosentan
Botulinum toxin (A & B)
Brimonidine
Bumetanide
Bupropion
Buspirone
Butorphanol
Butterbur
Cabergoline
Caffeine
Calcitonin
Candesartan
Capecitabine
Carbamazepine
Carbenicillin
Carboplatin
Carisoprodol
Carteolol
Carvedilol
Caspofungin
Cefaclor
Cefamandole
Cefdinir
Cefmetazole
Cefonicid
Cefpodoxime
Ceftazidime
Ceftizoxime
Celecoxib
Cetirizine
Cetrorelix
Cevimeline
Chlorambucil
Chlordiazepoxide

Chlorhexidine	Epoetin alfa	Isosorbide mononitrate	Nimodipine
Chlormezanone	Eprosartan	Isotretinoin	Nisoldipine
Chlorotrianisene	Ertapenem	Isradipine	Nitroglycerin
Chlorpropamide	Escitalopram	Itraconazole	Nizatidine
Chlortetracycline	Esmolol	Ivermectin	Norfloxacin
Cholestyramine	Esomeprazole	Juniper	Nortriptyline
Chondroitin	Estazolam	Kanamycin	Nystatin
Cidofovir	Estramustine	Ketoprofen	Octreotide
Cilostazol	Estrogens	Ketorolac	Ofloxacin
Cinoxacin	Ethosuximide	Labetalol	Olanzapine
Ciprofloxacin	Etodolac	Lamotrigine	Olmesartan
Cisplatin	Etoposide	Lansoprazole	Olopatadine
Citalopram	Exemestane	Latanoprost	Omeprazole
Cladribine	Famotidine	Leuprolide	Oral contraceptives
Clemastine	Felbamate	Levamisole	Oxaliplatin
Clindamycin	Felodipine	Levobupivacaine	Oxaprozin
Clofazimine	Fentanyl	Levofloxacin	Oxazepam
Clomiphene	Finasteride	Licorice	Oxcarbazepine
Clomipramine	Flecainide	Lidocaine	Paclitaxel
Clonazepam	Floxuridine	Linseed	Palivizumab
Clonidine	Fludarabine	Lisinopril	Pamidronate
Clopidogrel	Fluorouracil	Lithium	Pancuronium
Clotrimazole	Fluoxetine	Lomefloxacin	Pantoprazole
Clozapine	Fluoxymesterone	Losartan	Paroxetine
Codeine	Fluphenazine	Loxapine	Pegvisomant
Colestipol	Flurbiprofen	Mafenide	Penbutolol
Collagen	Flutamide	Maprotiline	Penicillamine
Corticosteroids	Fluvoxamine	Mazindol	Pentamidine
Cromolyn	Fondaparinux	Meclofenamate	Pentazocine
Cyclobenzaprine	Foscarnet	Medroxyprogesterone	Pentostatin
Cyclosporine	Fosinopril	Mefenamic acid	Pentoxifylline
Cyproheptadine	Fosphenytoin	Meloxicam	Pergolide
Cytarabine	Fulvestrant	Melphalan	Perindopril
Dalteparin	Gabapentin	Mephenytoin	Phellodendron
Danaparoid	Galantamine	Mercaptopurine	Phenazopyridine
Danazol	Ganciclovir	Mesalamine	Phenelzine
Darbepoetin alfa	Gatifloxacin	Mesoridazine	Phenobarbital
Deferoxamine	Gemcitabine	Methadone	Phenytoin
Delavirdine	Gentamicin	Methenamine	Pilocarpine
Denileukin	Ginseng	Methimazole	Pimozide
Desipramine	Glatiramer	Methohexital	Pindolol
Desmopressin	Glimepiride	Methoxsalen	Pioglitazone
Dexchlorpheniramine	Glipizide	Methyldopa	Piperacillin
Diazoxide	Glyburide	Methylphenidate	Pirbuterol
Diclofenac	Goserelin	Methyltestosterone	Piroxicam
Diethylstilbestrol	Grepafloxacin	Metolazone	Pramipexole
Diflunisal	Guanabenz	Metoprolol	Prazepam
Dihydroergotamine	Guanfacine	Mexiletine	Praziquantel
Diltiazem	Henna	Minoxidil	Prazosin
Dimenhydrinate	Hepatitis B vaccine	Mirtazapine	Procarbazine
Diphenhydramine	Heroin	Mistletoe	Progestins
Dipyridamole	Hydralazine	Mitomycin	Promazine
Dirithromycin	Hydrocodone	Mitoxantrone	Propafenone
Disopyramide	Hydroxyzine	Modafinil	Propofol
Docetaxel	Ibuprofen	Molindone	Propoxyphene
Dofetilide	Imatinib	Moricizine	Propranolol
Dolasetron	Imipramine	Morphine	Propylthiouracil
Domperidone	Imiquimod	Moxifloxacin	Protriptyline
Donepezil	Indinavir	Mupirocin	Psoralens
Dorzolamide	Indomethacin	Mycophenolate	Quetiapine
Doxazosin	Infliximab	Nabumetone	Quinapril
Doxepin	Insulin	Nadolol	Quinestrol
Doxercalciferol	Insulin glargine	Nafarelin	Quinine
Eflornithine	Interferon beta 1-a	Naltrexone	Quinupristin/dalfopristin
Eletriptan	Interferon beta-1b	Naproxen	Rabeprazole
Enalapril	Interferons, alfa-2	Naratriptan	Raloxifene
Enfuvirtide	Irbesartan	Nefazodone	Ramipril
Enoxacin	Irinotecan	Nicardipine	Rapacuronium
Enoxaparin	Isoproterenol	Nicotine	Rasburicase
Ephedrine	Isosorbide dinitrate	Nifedipine	Reserpine

Rifampin
Riluzole
Rimantadine
Risedronate
Risperidone
Ritonavir
Rivastigmine
Rizatriptan
Rofecoxib
Ropinirole
Rosiglitazone
Rue
Scopolamine
Senna
Sermorelin
Sertraline
Sibutramine
Sildenafil
Simvastatin
Sirolimus
Sotalol
Sparfloxacin
Spironolactone
Stanozolol
Streptokinase
Streptomycin
Streptozocin
Sucralfate
Sulfacetamide
Sulfinpyrazone
Sulindac
Tacrine
Tacrolimus
Tamoxifen
Tartrazine
Tegaserod
Telmisartan
Temozolomide
Terazosin
Teriparatide
Testosterone
Thalidomide
Tiagabine
Timolol
Tiopronin
Tirofiban
Tizanidine
Tobramycin
Tolazoline
Tolcapone
Tolmetin
Topiramate
Toremifene
Torsemide
Trandolapril
Tranylcypromine
Trastuzumab
Trazodone
Treprostinil
Tretinoin
Triamterene
Trifluoperazine
Trimeprazine
Tripelennamine
Triprolidine
Trovafloxacin
Unoprostone
Urofollitropin
Valacyclovir
Valdecoxib

Valproic acid
Valsartan
Venlafaxine
Verapamil
Vincristine
Voriconazole
Zalcitabine
Zaleplon
Zidovudine
Ziprasidone
Zolmitriptan
Zolpidem
Zonisamide

Erythema
Acarbose
Acetaminophen
Acetohexamide
Acitretin
Acyclovir
Adalimumab
Adapalene
Albuterol
Aldesleukin
Alendronate
Allopurinol
Almotriptan
Aminocaproic acid
Aminoglutethimide
Aminolevulinic acid
Amiodarone
Amitriptyline
Amobarbital
Amphotericin B
Anakinra
Anisindione
Anthrax vaccine
Aprotinin
Arsenic
Ascorbic acid
Asparaginase
Atracurium
Atropine sulfate
Azithromycin
Benzphetamine
Bergamot
Betaxolol
Bexarotene
Bimatoprost
Bismuth
Bleomycin
Brimonidine
Busulfan
Butterbur
Capecitabine
Capsicum
Carbamazepine
Carboplatin
Carmustine
Caspofungin
Cefadroxil
Cefamandole
Cefonicid
Ceftazidime
Celecoxib
Cetrorelix
Chloral hydrate
Chlorambucil
Chloramphenicol
Chlorotrianisene
Chlortetracycline

Cisplatin
Cladribine
Clomiphene
Clomipramine
Clonidine
Clotrimazole
Clozapine
Collagen
Corticosteroids
Cromolyn
Cyclophosphamide
Cyclosporine
Cyproheptadine
Cytarabine
Dacarbazine
Dactinomycin
Dantrolene
Dapsone
Daunorubicin
Deferoxamine
Delavirdine
Desipramine
Desmopressin
Diclofenac
Dicumarol
Diethylpropion
Diltiazem
Dobutamine
Docetaxel
Domperidone
Donepezil
Doxapram
Doxepin
Doxorubicin
Efavirenz
Eflornithine
Enalapril
Enfuvirtide
Enoxaparin
Epirubicin
Ertapenem
Esmolol
Etanercept
Etoposide
Felodipine
Fentanyl
Floxuridine
Fluorouracil
Fluphenazine
Flutamide
Folic acid
Formoterol
Furosemide
Gatifloxacin
Gentamicin
Ginkgo biloba
Glatiramer
Glimepiride
Glipizide
Glyburide
Granulocyte colony-
    stimulating factor (GCSF)
Henna
Heparin
Hepatitis B vaccine
Hydroxyurea
Idarubicin
Imipenem/cilastatin
Imipramine
Imiquimod

Interferon beta 1-a
Interferon beta-1b
Interferons, alfa-2
Irbesartan
Juniper
Kanamycin
Ketamine
Lamotrigine
Latanoprost
Leucovorin
Levobunolol
Levobupivacaine
Levofloxacin
Lidocaine
Lincomycin
Lindane
Linseed
Lisinopril
Lithium
Losartan
Lovastatin
Mafenide
Maprotiline
Mefloquine
Meperidine
Meprobamate
Mercaptopurine
Mesalamine
Mesna
Mesoridazine
Metformin
Methohexital
Methotrexate
Methoxsalen
Metronidazole
Miconazole
Minoxidil
Mistletoe
Mitomycin
Mitoxantrone
Modafinil
Mupirocin
Nabumetone
Naratriptan
Nedocromil
Nelfinavir
Niacin
Nicotine
Nifedipine
Nitroglycerin
Norfloxacin
Nortriptyline
Octreotide
Omeprazole
Ondansetron
Oral contraceptives
Oxaliplatin
Oxaprozin
Paclitaxel
Palivizumab
Pancuronium
Penicillins
Pentamidine
Pentostatin
Perindopril
Perphenazine
Phenindamine
Physostigmine
Phytonadione
Piroxicam

Plicamycin
Prochlorperazine
Propofol
Propranolol
Protamine sulfate
Protriptyline
Pseudoephedrine
Psoralens
Quinacrine
Quinestrol
Quinine
Ramipril
Rapacuronium
Rifampin
Ritodrine
Rofecoxib
Rue
Saquinavir
Scopolamine
Sermorelin
Sertraline
Simvastatin
Spironolactone
Streptomycin
Streptozocin
Succinylcholine
Sufentanil
Sulfacetamide
Sulindac
Sumatriptan
Tacrolimus
Teriparatide
Testosterone
Thalidomide
Thiopental
Thiothixene
Ticlopidine
Tiopronin
Tolazamide
Tolbutamide
Tolterodine
Topotecan
Torsemide
Treprostinil
Tretinoin
Trifluoperazine
Unoprostone
Verteporfin
Vidarabine
Vinblastine
Vincristine
Vinorelbine
Vitamin A
Voriconazole
Warfarin

Erythema Annulare Centrifugum (EAC)
Amitriptyline
Ampicillin
Chloroquine
Cimetidine
Gold and gold compounds
Hydrochlorothiazide
Hydroxychloroquine
Levamisole
Penicillins
Phenolphthalein
Piroxicam
Spironolactone

Erythema Multiforme
Acarbose
Acebutolol
Acetaminophen
Acetazolamide
Alendronate
Allopurinol
Amantadine
Aminosalicylate sodium
Amiodarone
Amlodipine
Amoxapine
Amoxicillin
Amphotericin B
Ampicillin
Anisindione
Arsenic
Aspirin
Atenolol
Atovaquone
Atropine sulfate
Azathioprine
Aztreonam
Bacampicillin
Benactyzine
Bleomycin
Botulinum toxin (A & B)
Bumetanide
Bupropion
Busulfan
Butabarbital
Butalbital
Capsicum
Carbamazepine
Carbenicillin
Carisoprodol
Cefaclor
Cefadroxil
Cefamandole
Cefazolin
Cefdinir
Cefditoren
Cefepime
Cefixime
Cefonicid
Cefoperazone
Cefotaxime
Cefotetan
Cefpodoxime
Cefprozil
Ceftazidime
Ceftriaxone
Cefuroxime
Celecoxib
Cephalexin
Cephalothin
Cephapirin
Cephradine
Chloral hydrate
Chlorambucil
Chloramphenicol
Chlordiazepoxide
Chlormezanone
Chloroquine
Chlorothiazide
Chlorotrianisene
Chlorpromazine
Chlorpropamide
Chlorthalidone
Chlorzoxazone

Cimetidine
Cinoxacin
Ciprofloxacin
Clindamycin
Clofibrate
Clomiphene
Clonazepam
Cloxacillin
Clozapine
Co-trimoxazole
Codeine
Corticosteroids
Cyclophosphamide
Dactinomycin
Danazol
Dapsone
Deferoxamine
Delavirdine
Diclofenac
Dicloxacillin
Didanosine
Diethylpropion
Diethylstilbestrol
Diflunisal
Diltiazem
Dipyridamole
Doxycycline
Enalapril
Enoxacin
Erythromycin
Estrogens
Ethambutol
Ethosuximide
Etodolac
Etoposide
Famotidine
Fenoprofen
Fluconazole
Fluorouracil
Fluoxetine
Flurbiprofen
Fluvastatin
Fosphenytoin
Furazolidone
Furosemide
Gemfibrozil
Glucagon
Gold and gold compounds
Griseofulvin
Henna
Hepatitis B vaccine
Hydrochlorothiazide
Hydrocodone
Hydroxychloroquine
Hydroxyurea
Hydroxyzine
Ibuprofen
Imipenem/cilastatin
Indapamide
Indinavir
Indomethacin
Isoniazid
Isotretinoin
Itraconazole
Ketoprofen
Lamotrigine
Levamisole
Levofloxacin
Lidocaine
Lincomycin

Lithium
Loracarbef
Loratadine
Lorazepam
Lovastatin
Maprotiline
Mechlorethamine
Meclofenamate
Mefenamic acid
Mefloquine
Meloxicam
Mephenytoin
Meprobamate
Methenamine
Methicillin
Methotrexate
Methsuximide
Methyclothiazide
Methyldopa
Methylphenidate
Metoprolol
Mezlocillin
Midodrine
Minocycline
Minoxidil
Mitomycin
Mitotane
Nabumetone
Nadolol
Nafcillin
Nalidixic acid
Naproxen
Neomycin
Nifedipine
Nitrofurantoin
Nitroglycerin
Norfloxacin
Nystatin
Ofloxacin
Omeprazole
Oral contraceptives
Oxacillin
Oxaprozin
Oxazepam
Oxcarbazepine
Oxybutynin
Pantoprazole
Paramethadione
Paroxetine
Penicillamine
Penicillins
Pentobarbital
Phenobarbital
Phenolphthalein
Phensuximide
Phenytoin
Pindolol
Piroxicam
Pravastatin
Primidone
Probenecid
Progestins
Promethazine
Propranolol
Pseudoephedrine
Pyrazinamide
Pyrimethamine
Quinidine
Quinine
Ramipril

Ranitidine
Ribavirin
Rifampin
Ritodrine
Saquinavir
Scopolamine
Sertraline
Simvastatin
Smallpox vaccine
Spironolactone
Streptomycin
Sulfacetamide
Sulfadiazine
Sulfadoxine
Sulfamethoxazole
Sulfasalazine
Sulfisoxazole
Sulindac
Tamsulosin
Tea tree
Terbinafine
Tetracycline
Thiabendazole
Thiopental
Thioridazine
Ticarcillin
Ticlopidine
Timolol
Tiopronin
Tobramycin
Tocainide
Tolbutamide
Tolcapone
Tolmetin
Trazodone
Trimethadione
Trimethoprim
Troleandomycin
Trovafloxacin
Valdecoxib
Valproic acid
Vancomycin
Verapamil
Vinblastine
Vitamin A
Vitamin E
Voriconazole
Zalcitabine
Zidovudine

Erythema Nodosum
Acetaminophen
Acyclovir
Aldesleukin
Amiodarone
Arsenic
Aspirin
Azathioprine
Busulfan
Carbamazepine
Carbenicillin
Cefdinir
Chlordiazepoxide
Chlorotrianisene
Chlorpropamide
Ciprofloxacin
Clomiphene
Co-trimoxazole
Codeine
Colchicine
Dapsone

Diclofenac
Dicloxacillin
Diethylstilbestrol
Disopyramide
Echinacea
Enoxacin
Estrogens
Fluoxetine
Furosemide
Glatiramer
Glucagon
Gold and gold compounds
Granulocyte colony-
  stimulating factor (GCSF)
Hepatitis B vaccine
Hydralazine
Hydroxychloroquine
Ibuprofen
Indomethacin
Interferon beta-1b
Interferons, alfa-2
Isotretinoin
Levofloxacin
Loperamide
Meclofenamate
Medroxyprogesterone
Meprobamate
Mesalamine
Methicillin
Methimazole
Methyldopa
Mezlocillin
Minocycline
Montelukast
Naproxen
Nifedipine
Nitrofurantoin
Ofloxacin
Omeprazole
Oral contraceptives
Oxacillin
Paroxetine
Penicillamine
Penicillins
Piperacillin
Progestins
Propylthiouracil
Smallpox vaccine
Sparfloxacin
Streptomycin
Sulfamethoxazole
Sulfasalazine
Sulfisoxazole
Thalidomide
Ticarcillin
Ticlopidine
Tretinoin
Trimethoprim
Verapamil
Zileuton

Erythroderma
Abacavir
Acitretin
Aldesleukin
Amitriptyline
Aspirin
Captopril
Carbamazepine
Chloroquine
Cimetidine

Ciprofloxacin
Clindamycin
Clofazimine
Co-trimoxazole
Colchicine
Cytarabine
Dapsone
Dicloxacillin
Diflunisal
Doxepin
Doxycycline
Epirubicin
Hydroxychloroquine
Lansoprazole
Meclofenamate
Methotrexate
Minocycline
Minoxidil
Nitroglycerin
Nystatin
Omeprazole
Pentostatin
Phenobarbital
Phenytoin
Piroxicam
Propolis
St John's wort
Sulfamethoxazole
Sulfasalazine
Terbinafine
Thalidomide
Timolol
Vincristine
Zalcitabine
Zidovudine

Exanthems
Abacavir
Acebutolol
Acetaminophen
Acetazolamide
Acetohexamide
Acitretin
Acyclovir
Albuterol
Aldesleukin
Alendronate
Allopurinol
Alprazolam
Altretamine
Amantadine
Amikacin
Amiloride
Aminocaproic acid
Aminoglutethimide
Aminophylline
Aminosalicylate sodium
Amiodarone
Amitriptyline
Amlodipine
Amobarbital
Amoxapine
Amoxicillin
Amphotericin B
Ampicillin
Amprenavir
Anisindione
Anistreplase
Aprobarbital
Aprotinin
Aripiprazole

Arsenic
Asparaginase
Aspartame
Aspirin
Atenolol
Atorvastatin
Atovaquone
Atropine sulfate
Azatadine
Azathioprine
Azelastine
Azithromycin
Aztreonam
Bacampicillin
Baclofen
Benactyzine
Benazepril
Bendroflumethiazide
Benztropine
Betaxolol
Bexarotene
Bicalutamide
Biperiden
Bisacodyl
Bismuth
Bisoprolol
Bleomycin
Bromocriptine
Brompheniramine
Bumetanide
Bupropion
Buspirone
Busulfan
Butabarbital
Butalbital
Butorphanol
Calcitonin
Candesartan
Captopril
Carbamazepine
Carbenicillin
Carboplatin
Carisoprodol
Carmustine
Carteolol
Carvedilol
Cefaclor
Cefadroxil
Cefamandole
Cefazolin
Cefdinir
Cefepime
Cefoperazone
Cefotaxime
Cefotetan
Cefoxitin
Cefprozil
Ceftazidime
Ceftriaxone
Cefuroxime
Celecoxib
Cephalexin
Cephalothin
Cephradine
Cetirizine
Cevimeline
Chloral hydrate
Chlorambucil
Chloramphenicol
Chlordiazepoxide

Chlormezanone	Docetaxel	Granulocyte colony-	Mefenamic acid
Chloroquine	Docusate	stimulating factor (GCSF)	Mefloquine
Chlorothiazide	Dopamine	Grepafloxacin	Meloxicam
Chlorpromazine	Doxazosin	Griseofulvin	Melphalan
Chlorpropamide	Doxepin	Guanethidine	Mephenytoin
Chlorthalidone	Doxorubicin	Guanfacine	Mephobarbital
Chlorzoxazone	Doxycycline	Haloperidol	Meprobamate
Cholestyramine	Efavirenz	Halothane	Mercaptopurine
Cimetidine	Eletriptan	Heparin	Mesalamine
Ciprofloxacin	Enalapril	Heroin	Mesna
Cisplatin	Enfuvirtide	Hydralazine	Metformin
Citalopram	Enoxacin	Hydrochlorothiazide	Methadone
Cladribine	Enoxaparin	Hydrocodone	Methantheline
Clarithromycin	Ephedrine	Hydromorphone	Methazolamide
Clemastine	Epinephrine	Hydroxychloroquine	Methenamine
Clindamycin	Epoetin alfa	Hydroxyurea	Methicillin
Clofazimine	Eprosartan	Hydroxyzine	Methimazole
Clofibrate	Erythromycin	Ibuprofen	Methocarbamol
Clomiphene	Esomeprazole	Idarubicin	Methohexital
Clomipramine	Estramustine	Imipenem/cilastatin	Methotrexate
Clonazepam	Estrogens	Imipramine	Methoxsalen
Clonidine	Etanercept	Indapamide	Methsuximide
Clopidogrel	Ethacrynic acid	Indinavir	Methyclothiazide
Clorazepate	Ethambutol	Indomethacin	Methyldopa
Cloxacillin	Ethionamide	Insulin	Methylphenidate
Clozapine	Ethosuximide	Interferon beta 1-a	Methyltestosterone
Co-trimoxazole	Etidronate	Interferon beta-1b	Methysergide
Codeine	Etodolac	Interferons, alfa-2	Metoclopramide
Colchicine	Etoposide	Ipodate	Metolazone
Colestipol	Famotidine	Ipratropium	Metoprolol
Corticosteroids	Felodipine	Irinotecan	Metronidazole
Cromolyn	Fenofibrate	Isocarboxazid	Mexiletine
Cyanocobalamin	Fenoprofen	Isoniazid	Mezlocillin
Cyclamate	Fentanyl	Isotretinoin	Miconazole
Cyclophosphamide	Flavoxate	Isradipine	Midazolam
Cycloserine	Flecainide	Itraconazole	Minocycline
Cyclosporine	Floxuridine	Ivermectin	Minoxidil
Cyclothiazide	Fluconazole	Kanamycin	Misoprostol
Cyproheptadine	Flucytosine	Ketamine	Mitomycin
Cytarabine	Fludarabine	Ketoconazole	Mitotane
Dacarbazine	Fluorouracil	Ketoprofen	Moexipril
Dactinomycin	Fluoxetine	Ketorolac	Moricizine
Dalteparin	Fluoxymesterone	Labetalol	Morphine
Danazol	Fluphenazine	Lamivudine	Moxifloxacin
Dantrolene	Flurazepam	Lamotrigine	Nabumetone
Dapsone	Flurbiprofen	Lansoprazole	Nadolol
Daunorubicin	Flutamide	Letrozole	Nafarelin
Deferoxamine	Fluvoxamine	Leuprolide	Nafcillin
Delavirdine	Folic acid	Levamisole	Nalidixic acid
Demeclocycline	Foscarnet	Levodopa	Naloxone
Denileukin	Fosfomycin	Levofloxacin	Naltrexone
Desipramine	Fosphenytoin	Lidocaine	Naproxen
Diazepam	Furazolidone	Lincomycin	Naratriptan
Diazoxide	Furosemide	Lisinopril	Nateglinide
Diclofenac	Gabapentin	Lithium	Nefazodone
Dicloxacillin	Ganciclovir	Lomefloxacin	Nelfinavir
Dicumarol	Gatifloxacin	Loperamide	Neomycin
Dicyclomine	Gemcitabine	Loratadine	Nevirapine
Didanosine	Gemfibrozil	Lorazepam	Niacin
Diethylpropion	Gemifloxacin	Losartan	Nicardipine
Diethylstilbestrol	Gentamicin	Lovastatin	Nifedipine
Diflunisal	Ginkgo biloba	Loxapine	Nimodipine
Digoxin	Glatiramer	Maprotiline	Nisoldipine
Dihydrotachysterol	Glimepiride	Marihuana	Nitisinone
Diltiazem	Glipizide	Mazindol	Nitrofurantoin
Dimenhydrinate	Glucagon	Mebendazole	Nitroglycerin
Diphenhydramine	Glyburide	Mechlorethamine	Nizatidine
Dipyridamole	Gold and gold compounds	Meclizine	Norfloxacin
Disopyramide	Granisetron	Meclofenamate	Nortriptyline
Disulfiram		Medroxyprogesterone	Nystatin

Octreotide
Ofloxacin
Olanzapine
Olsalazine
Omeprazole
Ondansetron
Oral contraceptives
Orphenadrine
Oxacillin
Oxaliplatin
Oxaprozin
Oxazepam
Oxcarbazepine
Oxytetracycline
Paclitaxel
Pamidronate
Pantoprazole
Pantothenic acid
Papaverine
Paramethadione
Paromomycin
Paroxetine
Pemoline
Penbutolol
Penicillamine
Penicillins
Pentagastrin
Pentamidine
Pentazocine
Pentobarbital
Pentostatin
Pentoxifylline
Pergolide
Perindopril
Perphenazine
Phenazopyridine
Phenelzine
Phenobarbital
Phenolphthalein
Phenytoin
Phytonadione
Pimozide
Pindolol
Piperacillin
Piroxicam
Plicamycin
Polythiazide
Potassium iodide
Pravastatin
Prazepam
Prazosin
Primaquine
Primidone
Probenecid
Procainamide
Procarbazine
Prochlorperazine
Progestins
Promazine
Promethazine
Propafenone
Propantheline
Propofol
Propoxyphene
Propranolol
Propylthiouracil
Protamine
Protriptyline
Pseudoephedrine
Pyrazinamide

Pyrimethamine
Quinacrine
Quinapril
Quinethazone
Quinidine
Quinine
Quinupristin/dalfopristin
Ramipril
Ranitidine
Rapacuronium
Reserpine
Ribavirin
Rifampin
Ritodrine
Ritonavir
Rituximab
Rivastigmine
Rofecoxib
Ropinirole
Rosiglitazone
Saccharin
Salmeterol
Salsalate
Saquinavir
Scopolamine
Secobarbital
Sertraline
Simvastatin
Smallpox vaccine
Sotalol
Sparfloxacin
Spectinomycin
Spironolactone
Stanozolol
Streptokinase
Streptomycin
Streptozocin
Succinylcholine
Sucralfate
Sulfadiazine
Sulfadoxine
Sulfamethoxazole
Sulfasalazine
Sulfinpyrazone
Sulfisoxazole
Sulindac
Sumatriptan
Tacrine
Tacrolimus
Tamoxifen
Temazepam
Terazosin
Terbinafine
Terbutaline
Terfenadine
Testosterone
Tetracycline
Thalidomide
Thiabendazole
Thiamine
Thioguanine
Thiopental
Thioridazine
Thiothixene
Tiagabine
Ticarcillin
Ticlopidine
Timolol
Tinzaparin
Tiopronin

Tizanidine
Tobramycin
Tocainide
Tolazamide
Tolazoline
Tolbutamide
Tolmetin
Topiramate
Torsemide
Tramadol
Tranylcypromine
Trazodone
Triamterene
Triazolam
Trichlormethiazide
Trifluoperazine
Trimeprazine
Trimethadione
Trimethoprim
Trimetrexate
Trimipramine
Triprolidine
Troleandomycin
Trovafloxacin
Urofollitropin
Urokinase
Valdecoxib
Valproic acid
Vancomycin
Vasopressin
Venlafaxine
Verapamil
Vinblastine
Vincristine
Vitamin A
Vitamin E
Warfarin
Zalcitabine
Zaleplon
Zidovudine
Ziprasidone
Zonisamide

Exfoliative Dermatitis
Acebutolol
Acetaminophen
Acitretin
Aldesleukin
Alitretinoin
Allopurinol
Aminoglutethimide
Aminophylline
Aminosalicylate sodium
Amiodarone
Amitriptyline
Amobarbital
Amoxicillin
Amphotericin B
Ampicillin
Anisindione
Aprobarbital
Aripiprazole
Arsenic
Aspirin
Atropine sulfate
Aztreonam
Bacampicillin
Benactyzine
Bendroflumethiazide
Betaxolol
Bexarotene

Bismuth
Bisoprolol
Bumetanide
Bupropion
Butabarbital
Butalbital
Capecitabine
Captopril
Carbamazepine
Carbenicillin
Carteolol
Carvedilol
Cefdinir
Cefoxitin
Celecoxib
Chlorambucil
Chloroquine
Chlorothiazide
Chlorpromazine
Chlorpropamide
Chlorthalidone
Cimetidine
Ciprofloxacin
Cisplatin
Clofazimine
Clofibrate
Cloxacillin
Co-trimoxazole
Codeine
Cromolyn
Cytarabine
Dapsone
Demeclocycline
Desipramine
Diazepam
Diclofenac
Dicloxacillin
Diethylstilbestrol
Diflunisal
Diltiazem
Doxorubicin
Doxycycline
Eletriptan
Enalapril
Enoxacin
Ephedrine
Epirubicin
Esmolol
Estrogens
Ethambutol
Ethosuximide
Etodolac
Fenoprofen
Fentanyl
Flecainide
Fluconazole
Fluoxetine
Fluphenazine
Flurbiprofen
Fluvoxamine
Fosinopril
Fosphenytoin
Furosemide
Ganciclovir
Gemfibrozil
Gentamicin
Gold and gold compounds
Granulocyte colony-
    stimulating factor (GCSF)
Grepafloxacin

Griseofulvin
Guanfacine
Haloperidol
Hydrochlorothiazide
Hydroxychloroquine
Imipramine
Indomethacin
Interferon beta-1b
Isoniazid
Ketoconazole
Ketoprofen
Ketorolac
Labetalol
Levamisole
Levofloxacin
Lidocaine
Lincomycin
Lithium
Meclofenamate
Mefenamic acid
Mefloquine
Mephenytoin
Mephobarbital
Meprobamate
Mesoridazine
Methantheline
Methicillin
Methimazole
Methoxsalen
Methsuximide
Methylphenidate
Metolazone
Metoprolol
Mexiletine
Mezlocillin
Minocycline
Mirtazapine
Mitomycin
Nadolol
Nafcillin
Nalidixic acid
Naproxen
Nifedipine
Nisoldipine
Nitisinone
Nitrofurantoin
Nitroglycerin
Nizatidine
Norfloxacin
Ofloxacin
Omeprazole
Oxacillin
Oxaprozin
Oxytetracycline
Paramethadione
Penicillamine
Penicillins
Pentobarbital
Pentostatin
Perphenazine
Phenobarbital
Phenolphthalein
Phenytoin
Pindolol
Piperacillin
Piroxicam
Primidone
Procarbazine
Prochlorperazine
Propranolol

Propylthiouracil
Pseudoephedrine
Pyrimethamine
Quinacrine
Quinapril
Quinidine
Quinine
Rifampin
Riluzole
Risperidone
Rivastigmine
Rosiglitazone
Secobarbital
Sildenafil
Smallpox vaccine
Sparfloxacin
Streptomycin
Sulfacetamide
Sulfadiazine
Sulfadoxine
Sulfamethoxazole
Sulfasalazine
Sulfisoxazole
Sulindac
Tetracycline
Thalidomide
Thiopental
Thioridazine
Tiagabine
Ticarcillin
Ticlopidine
Timolol
Tizanidine
Tobramycin
Tocainide
Trazodone
Trifluoperazine
Trimethadione
Trimethoprim
Vancomycin
Venlafaxine
Verapamil
Vitamin A
Voriconazole
Warfarin
Yohimbine
Zalcitabine
Ziprasidone

Fixed Eruptions

Acetaminophen
Acyclovir
Albendazole
Alendronate
Allopurinol
Aminosalicylate sodium
Amitriptyline
Amoxicillin
Amphotericin B
Ampicillin
Arsenic
Aspirin
Atenolol
Atropine sulfate
Azathioprine
Azithromycin
Bacampicillin
Benactyzine
Bisacodyl
Bismuth
Bleomycin

Butabarbital
Butalbital
Cabergoline
Carbamazepine
Carisoprodol
Cefazolin
Cephalexin
Cetirizine
Chloral hydrate
Chloramphenicol
Chlordiazepoxide
Chlorhexidine
Chlormezanone
Chloroquine
Chlorothiazide
Chlorpromazine
Chlorpropamide
Cimetidine
Ciprofloxacin
Clarithromycin
Clindamycin
Co-trimoxazole
Codeine
Colchicine
Corticosteroids
Cyclosporine
Dacarbazine
Dapsone
Demeclocycline
Dextromethorphan
Diazepam
Diclofenac
Diflunisal
Dimenhydrinate
Diphenhydramine
Disulfiram
Docetaxel
Doxycycline
Ephedrine
Epinephrine
Erythromycin
Estrogens
Ethchlorvynol
Ethotoin
Etodolac
Fentanyl
Fluconazole
Flurbiprofen
Foscarnet
Ganciclovir
Gatifloxacin
Gold and gold compounds
Griseofulvin
Guanethidine
Heparin
Heroin
Hydralazine
Hydrochlorothiazide
Hydroxychloroquine
Hydroxyurea
Hydroxyzine
Ibuprofen
Imipramine
Indapamide
Indomethacin
Isotretinoin
Itraconazole
Ketoconazole
Lamotrigine
Levamisole

Lidocaine
Loratadine
Lorazepam
Meclofenamate
Mefenamic acid
Melatonin
Meprobamate
Mesna
Metaxalone
Methenamine
Methimazole
Methyldopa
Methylphenidate
Metronidazole
Minocycline
Moxifloxacin
Naproxen
Neomycin
Niacin
Nifedipine
Nitrofurantoin
Norfloxacin
Nystatin
Ofloxacin
Omeprazole
Ondansetron
Oral contraceptives
Orphenadrine
Oxaprozin
Oxazepam
Oxytetracycline
Paclitaxel
Papaverine
Penicillins
Pentobarbital
Phenobarbital
Phenolphthalein
Phenylpropanolamine
Phenytoin
Piroxicam
Procarbazine
Prochlorperazine
Promethazine
Propofol
Pseudoephedrine
Pyrazinamide
Pyridoxine
Pyrimethamine
Quinacrine
Quinidine
Quinine
Ranitidine
Rifampin
Rofecoxib
Saccharin
Saquinavir
Scopolamine
Sertraline
Sildenafil
Sparfloxacin
Streptomycin
Sulfadiazine
Sulfamethoxazole
Sulfasalazine
Sulfisoxazole
Sulindac
Tartrazine
Temazepam
Terbinafine
Terfenadine

Tetracycline
Thiabendazole
Thiopental
Ticlopidine
Tolbutamide
Topotecan
Trifluoperazine
Trimethadione
Trimetrexate
Tripelennamine
Triprolidine
Valproic acid
Voriconazole

Flushing
Acetaminophen
Acetylcysteine
Adenosine
Albuterol
Alemtuzumab
Alitretinoin
Alprostadil
Amifostine
Amiloride
Aminophylline
Amiodarone
Amitriptyline
Amlodipine
Amoxapine
Amphotericin B
Amyl nitrite
Anastrozole
Anistreplase
Aprepitant
Arbutamine
Ascorbic acid
Asparaginase
Aspirin
Atracurium
Atropine sulfate
Azatadine
Azelastine
Baclofen
Benazepril
Benzphetamine
Betaxolol
Bethanechol
Biperiden
Bisoprolol
Bleomycin
Bosentan
Bretylium
Bromocriptine
Bupropion
Buspirone
Butorphanol
Calcitonin
Capsicum
Captopril
Carboplatin
Carisoprodol
Carmustine
Carteolol
Caspofungin
Cefaclor
Cefamandole
Cefoxitin
Cefpodoxime
Ceftazidime
Ceftriaxone
Cetirizine

Chloral hydrate
Chlormezanone
Chlorpropamide
Chlorzoxazone
Ciprofloxacin
Cisatracurium
Cisplatin
Clemastine
Clidinium
Clomiphene
Clomipramine
Co-trimoxazole
Codeine
Colchicine
Corticosteroids
Cromolyn
Cyclobenzaprine
Cyclophosphamide
Cyclosporine
Cyproheptadine
Dacarbazine
Danazol
Daunorubicin
Deferoxamine
Denileukin
Desipramine
Desmopressin
Diazepam
Diazoxide
Diclofenac
Dicyclomine
Diethylpropion
Diethylstilbestrol
Diflunisal
Diltiazem
Dimenhydrinate
Diphenoxylate
Dipyridamole
Disulfiram
Docetaxel
Dolasetron
Donepezil
Doxapram
Doxazosin
Doxepin
Doxorubicin
Dronabinol
Edrophonium
Efavirenz
Enalapril
Ephedra
Epinephrine
Epirubicin
Ertapenem
Escitalopram
Esmolol
Esomeprazole
Estazolam
Estramustine
Estrogens
Etodolac
Etoposide
Famotidine
Felbamate
Felodipine
Fentanyl
Flecainide
Flumazenil
Fluoxetine
Fluoxymesterone

Flurazepam
Flurbiprofen
Fluvastatin
Folic acid
Fomepizole
Foscarnet
Fosinopril
Frovatriptan
Furazolidone
Furosemide
Gemifloxacin
Glatiramer
Glipizide
Glyburide
Glycopyrrolate
Granulocyte colony-
    stimulating factor (GCSF)
Griseofulvin
Haloperidol
Hepatitis B vaccine
Hydralazine
Hydrocodone
Hydromorphone
Hydroxyzine
Hyoscyamine
Ibritumomab
Ibuprofen
Imipenem/cilastatin
Imipramine
Indapamide
Indinavir
Indomethacin
Insulin
Ipratropium
Irbesartan
Irinotecan
Isoniazid
Isoproterenol
Isosorbide dinitrate
Isosorbide mononitrate
Isotretinoin
Isradipine
Ketorolac
Labetalol
Lamotrigine
Leuprolide
Levodopa
Levothyroxine
Lisinopril
Lomefloxacin
Lomustine
Loratadine
Losartan
Lovastatin
Maprotiline
MDMA
Medroxyprogesterone
Meperidine
Mesna
Mesoridazine
Methadone
Methantheline
Methocarbamol
Methyltestosterone
Methysergide
Metoclopramide
Metronidazole
Miconazole
Midodrine
Minoxidil

Mitotane
Moexipril
Morphine
Nafarelin
Nalbuphine
Nefazodone
Niacin
Nicardipine
Nicotine
Nifedipine
Nimodipine
Nisoldipine
Nitrofurantoin
Nitroglycerin
Nortriptyline
Octreotide
Ondansetron
Orphenadrine
Oxaliplatin
Oxybutynin
Paclitaxel
Pancuronium
Papaverine
Paroxetine
PEG-interferon alfa-2b
Penbutolol
Penicillamine
Pentagastrin
Pentazocine
Pentostatin
Pentoxifylline
Phendimetrazine
Phenindamine
Phentolamine
Phytonadione
Pilocarpine
Plicamycin
Pravastatin
Probenecid
Procainamide
Procarbazine
Progestins
Promethazine
Propafenone
Propofol
Propoxyphene
Propranolol
Protamine
Protamine sulfate
Protriptyline
Pyrazinamide
Pyrilamine
Quinapril
Quinidine
Quinine
Ramipril
Rapacuronium
Reserpine
Rifampin
Risperidone
Rituximab
Rivastigmine
Rizatriptan
Rofecoxib
Ropinirole
Scopolamine
Selenium
Sermorelin
Sertraline
Sildenafil

Simvastatin
Spironolactone
Streptokinase
Succinylcholine
Sulfamethoxazole
Sulfasalazine
Sulfinpyrazone
Sulfisoxazole
Sumatriptan
Tacrine
Tacrolimus
Tamoxifen
Tegaserod
Telmisartan
Terbutaline
Terfenadine
Testosterone
Thiabendazole
Tolazoline
Tolbutamide
Topiramate
Trandolapril
Tranylcypromine
Treprostinil
Tretinoin
Triamterene
Trihexyphenidyl
Trimetrexate
Tripelennamine
Triprolidine
Trovafloxacin
Urokinase
Valsartan
Vancomycin
Verapamil
Vinorelbine
Yohimbine
Zalcitabine
Zolmitriptan
Zolpidem

Galactorrhea
Alprazolam
Amitriptyline
Amoxapine
Buspirone
Chlordiazepoxide
Chlorpromazine
Cimetidine
Citalopram
Clomipramine
Cyclobenzaprine
Desipramine
Domperidone
Doxepin
Estrogens
Fluoxetine
Fluphenazine
Haloperidol
Imipramine
Isotretinoin
Loxapine
Maprotiline
Medroxyprogesterone
Mesoridazine
Methyldopa
Metoclopramide
Minocycline
Molindone
Nitrofurantoin
Nortriptyline

Octreotide
Olanzapine
Oral contraceptives
Paroxetine
Perphenazine
Pimozide
Prochlorperazine
Progestins
Promazine
Promethazine
Protease inhibitors
Protriptyline
Risperidone
Sertraline
Tamoxifen
Terfenadine
Thalidomide
Thioridazine
Thiothixene
Toremifene
Trazodone
Trifluoperazine
Trimipramine
Valproic acid
Venlafaxine
Verapamil

Gingival Hyperplasia
Amlodipine
Basiliximab
Cevimeline
Co-trimoxazole
Cyclosporine
Diltiazem
Erythromycin
Estrogens
Ethosuximide
Ethotoin
Felodipine
Fosphenytoin
Ganciclovir
Isradipine
Ketoconazole
Lamotrigine
Lithium
Mephenytoin
Methsuximide
Mycophenolate
Nicardipine
Nifedipine
Nisoldipine
Oral contraceptives
Oxcarbazepine
Phensuximide
Phenytoin
Primidone
Sertraline
Sirolimus
Tacrolimus
Tartrazine
Tiagabine
Topiramate
Valproic acid
Verapamil
Voriconazole
Zonisamide

Glossitis
Aldesleukin
Amitriptyline
Amoxapine
Amoxicillin

Ampicillin
Aripiprazole
Atorvastatin
Azelastine
Bacampicillin
Betaxolol
Bleomycin
Bupropion
Captopril
Carbamazepine
Carbenicillin
Cefaclor
Cefadroxil
Cefamandole
Cefpodoxime
Cefprozil
Ceftazidime
Ceftriaxone
Chloramphenicol
Chlorhexidine
Clarithromycin
Clomipramine
Cloxacillin
Co-trimoxazole
Cyclosporine
Demeclocycline
Dicloxacillin
Doxepin
Doxycycline
Enalapril
Estazolam
Etidronate
Etodolac
Felbamate
Floxuridine
Fluoxetine
Fluvoxamine
Gabapentin
Gatifloxacin
Gold and gold compounds
Grepafloxacin
Guanadrel
Guanethidine
Hydroxyurea
Imipenem/cilastatin
Imipramine
Interferon beta-1b
Lansoprazole
Lincomycin
Mecamylamine
Mefenamic acid
Mercaptopurine
Methicillin
Methotrexate
Metronidazole
Mezlocillin
Minocycline
Mirtazapine
Moxifloxacin
Nabumetone
Nafcillin
Nefazodone
Nisoldipine
Olanzapine
Oxacillin
Pantoprazole
Paroxetine
Penicillamine
Penicillins
Peppermint

Phenelzine
Pirbuterol
Protriptyline
Pyrimethamine
Quetiapine
Rabeprazole
Riluzole
Risedronate
Rivastigmine
Ropinirole
Saquinavir
Sertraline
Sildenafil
Streptomycin
Sulfadoxine
Sulfamethoxazole
Sulfasalazine
Sulfisoxazole
Sulindac
Tacrine
Tetracycline
Tiagabine
Ticarcillin
Tolmetin
Triamterene
Triazolam
Trihexyphenidyl
Trimethoprim
Trimipramine
Valproic acid
Venlafaxine
Voriconazole
Zalcitabine
Zaleplon
Zonisamide

Gynecomastia
Alprazolam
Amiloride
Amitriptyline
Amlodipine
Amoxapine
Amprenavir
Androstenedione
Aripiprazole
Arsenic
Atazanavir
Atorvastatin
Bendroflumethiazide
Benzphetamine
Bicalutamide
Bupropion
Busulfan
Captopril
Carmustine
Chlordiazepoxide
Chlorotrianisene
Chlorpromazine
Cimetidine
Ciprofloxacin
Citalopram
Cladribine
Clofibrate
Clomiphene
Clomipramine
Clonidine
Cyclobenzaprine
Cyclosporine
Delavirdine
Desipramine
Diazepam

Didanosine
Diethylpropion
Diethylstilbestrol
Digoxin
Diltiazem
Disopyramide
Domperidone
Dong quai
Doxepin
Dutasteride
Efavirenz
Enalapril
Eplerenone
Estazolam
Estramustine
Estrogens
Ethionamide
Etodolac
Famotidine
Felodipine
Finasteride
Fluoxetine
Fluoxymesterone
Fluphenazine
Flutamide
Fluvastatin
Foscarnet
Fosinopril
Gabapentin
Ginseng
Glatiramer
Goserelin
Griseofulvin
Guanabenz
Haloperidol
Ibuprofen
Imatinib
Imipramine
Indinavir
Indomethacin
Isoniazid
Isotretinoin
Itraconazole
Ketoconazole
Ketoprofen
Lamivudine
Lansoprazole
Latanoprost
Leuprolide
Loratadine
Lovastatin
Loxapine
Maprotiline
Medroxyprogesterone
Melphalan
Meprobamate
Mesoridazine
Methotrexate
Methyldopa
Methyltestosterone
Metoclopramide
Metronidazole
Minocycline
Minoxidil
Mirtazapine
Misoprostol
Molindone
Morphine
Nafarelin
Nefazodone

Nelfinavir
Nifedipine
Nisoldipine
Nizatidine
Nortriptyline
Octreotide
Omeprazole
Penicillamine
Pentostatin
Perphenazine
Phenytoin
Pimozide
Pravastatin
Procarbazine
Prochlorperazine
Progestins
Promazine
Promethazine
Protriptyline
Pyrilamine
Quinestrol
Rabeprazole
Ranitidine
Reserpine
Risperidone
Ritonavir
Ropinirole
Saquinavir
Sertraline
Sildenafil
Simvastatin
Spironolactone
Stanozolol
Stavudine
Sulindac
Terfenadine
Testosterone
Thalidomide
Thioridazine
Thiothixene
Tiagabine
Tolmetin
Topiramate
Trazodone
Triamterene
Trifluoperazine
Trimeprazine
Trimipramine
Valproic acid
Venlafaxine
Verapamil
Vitamin E
Ziprasidone
Zonisamide

Hair – Alopecia
Acebutolol
Acetaminophen
Acetohexamide
Acitretin
Acyclovir
Albendazole
Aldesleukin
Alitretinoin
Allopurinol
Altretamine
Amantadine
Amiloride
Aminophylline
Aminosalicylate sodium
Amiodarone

Amitriptyline
Amlodipine
Amoxapine
Amphotericin B
Anagrelide
Anastrozole
Androstenedione
Anisindione
Anthrax vaccine
Aprepitant
Aripiprazole
Arsenic
Asparaginase
Aspirin
Atazanavir
Atenolol
Atorvastatin
Azathioprine
Balsalazide
Bendroflumethiazide
Benzphetamine
Betaxolol
Bexarotene
Bicalutamide
Bismuth
Bisoprolol
Bleomycin
Brinzolamide
Bromocriptine
Bupropion
Buspirone
Busulfan
Capecitabine
Captopril
Carbamazepine
Carboplatin
Carmustine
Carteolol
Carvedilol
Celecoxib
Cetirizine
Cevimeline
Chlorambucil
Chloramphenicol
Chlordiazepoxide
Chloroquine
Chlorothiazide
Chlorotrianisene
Chlorpropamide
Chlorthalidone
Chondroitin
Cidofovir
Cimetidine
Cisplatin
Citalopram
Clofibrate
Clomiphene
Clomipramine
Clonazepam
Clonidine
Colchicine
Corticosteroids
Cyclobenzaprine
Cyclophosphamide
Cyclosporine
Cytarabine
Dacarbazine
Dactinomycin
Dalteparin
Danazol

Daunorubicin
Delavirdine
Desipramine
Diazoxide
Diclofenac
Dicumarol
Didanosine
Diethylpropion
Diethylstilbestrol
Diflunisal
Digoxin
Diltiazem
Disopyramide
Docetaxel
Donepezil
Dopamine
Doxazosin
Doxepin
Doxorubicin
Efavirenz
Eflornithine
Eletriptan
Enalapril
Epinephrine
Epirubicin
Epoetin alfa
Escitalopram
Esmolol
Estramustine
Estrogens
Ethambutol
Ethionamide
Ethosuximide
Etidronate
Etodolac
Etoposide
Exemestane
Famotidine
Felbamate
Fenofibrate
Fenoprofen
Finasteride
Flecainide
Floxuridine
Fluconazole
Fludarabine
Fluorouracil
Fluoxetine
Fluoxymesterone
Flurbiprofen
Fluvastatin
Fluvoxamine
Foscarnet
Gabapentin
Ganciclovir
Gemcitabine
Gemfibrozil
Gentamicin
Glatiramer
Gold and gold compounds
Goserelin
Granisetron
Granulocyte colony-
    stimulating factor (GCSF)
Grepafloxacin
Guanethidine
Guanfacine
Haloperidol
Halothane
Heparin

Hepatitis B vaccine
Hydromorphone
Hydroxychloroquine
Hydroxyurea
Ibuprofen
Idarubicin
Ifosfamide
Imipramine
Indinavir
Indomethacin
Interferon beta 1-a
Interferon beta-1b
Interferons, alfa-2
Ipratropium
Irinotecan
Isoniazid
Isotretinoin
Itraconazole
Ketoconazole
Ketoprofen
Labetalol
Lamivudine
Lamotrigine
Lansoprazole
Leflunomide
Letrozole
Leucovorin
Leuprolide
Levamisole
Levobetaxolol
Levobunolol
Levodopa
Levothyroxine
Liothyronine
Lisinopril
Lithium
Lomustine
Loperamide
Loratadine
Lorazepam
Losartan
Lovastatin
Loxapine
Maprotiline
Mebendazole
Mechlorethamine
Meclofenamate
Medroxyprogesterone
Mefloquine
Melphalan
Mephenytoin
Mercaptopurine
Mesalamine
Mesoridazine
Metformin
Methimazole
Methotrexate
Methsuximide
Methyldopa
Methylphenidate
Methyltestosterone
Methysergide
Metoprolol
Mexiletine
Minocycline
Minoxidil
Misoprostol
Mitomycin
Mitotane
Mitoxantrone

Moexipril
Mycophenolate
Nabumetone
Nadolol
Nalidixic acid
Naltrexone
Naproxen
Naratriptan
Nefazodone
Neomycin
Nifedipine
Nimodipine
Nisoldipine
Nitisinone
Nitrofurantoin
Nortriptyline
Octreotide
Olanzapine
Omeprazole
Ondansetron
Oral contraceptives
Oxaliplatin
Oxaprozin
Oxcarbazepine
Paclitaxel
Pantoprazole
Paramethadione
Paroxetine
PEG-interferon alfa-2b
Pegfilgrastim
Penbutolol
Penicillamine
Penicillins
Pentosan
Pentostatin
Pergolide
Phensuximide
Phentermine
Phenytoin
Pindolol
Pirbuterol
Piroxicam
Pravastatin
Prazepam
Prazosin
Probenecid
Procarbazine
Progestins
Propafenone
Propranolol
Propylthiouracil
Protriptyline
Pyrimethamine
Quazepam
Quinacrine
Quinapril
Quinidine
Rabeprazole
Ramipril
Ranitidine
Ribavirin
Riluzole
Risperidone
Ritonavir
Rivastigmine
Rofecoxib
Ropinirole
Saquinavir
Selegiline
Selenium

Sertraline
Simvastatin
Sotalol
Sparfloxacin
Spironolactone
St John's wort
Stanozolol
Sulfasalazine
Sulfisoxazole
Sulindac
Tacrine
Tacrolimus
Tamoxifen
Terbinafine
Terfenadine
Testosterone
Thalidomide
Thioguanine
Thioridazine
Thiotepa
Thiothixene
Tiagabine
Timolol
Tinzaparin
Tiopronin
Tizanidine
Tocainide
Tolcapone
Topiramate
Topotecan
Trazodone
Triazolam
Trimethadione
Trimipramine
Triptorelin
Urofollitropin
Ursodiol
Valdecoxib
Valproic acid
Vasopressin
Venlafaxine
Verapamil
Vinblastine
Vincristine
Vinorelbine
Vitamin A
Voriconazole
Warfarin
Zalcitabine
Zaleplon
Zidovudine
Ziprasidone
Zonisamide

Hair – Alopecia Areata
Carboplatin
Clomipramine
Cyclosporine
Fluvoxamine
Haloperidol
Imipramine
Interferons, alfa-2
Leflunomide
Lithium
Oral contraceptives
Paclitaxel
Propranolol
Rifampin
Terbinafine
Tretinoin

Hair – Hirsutism
Acetazolamide
Aminoglutethimide
Androstenedione
Bupropion
Chlorotrianisene
Clonazepam
Corticosteroids
Danazol
Diethylstilbestrol
Diltiazem
Donepezil
Estrogens
Ethosuximide
Fluoxetine
Fluoxymesterone
Gemfibrozil
Interferon beta-1b
Isotretinoin
Lamotrigine
Lorazepam
Medroxyprogesterone
Methsuximide
Methyltestosterone
Minoxidil
Nafarelin
Olanzapine
Oral contraceptives
Penicillamine
Pergolide
Phensuximide
Phenytoin
Prazepam
Progestins
Quazepam
Sertraline
Sirolimus
Spironolactone
Stanozolol
Tacrolimus
Tamoxifen
Testosterone
Tiagabine
Triazolam
Venlafaxine
Zonisamide

Hair – Hypertrichosis
Amantadine
Amiodarone
Basiliximab
Betaxolol
Cetirizine
Citalopram
Clomiphene
Clomipramine
Corticosteroids
Cyclosporine
Diazoxide
Epoetin alfa
Interferons, alfa-2
Latanoprost
Methoxsalen
Minoxidil
Phenytoin
Psoralens
Risperidone
Selegiline
Streptomycin
Tamoxifen
Thioridazine

Tiopronin
Trioxsalen
Unoprostone
Verapamil
Zidovudine

Herpes Simplex
Alefacept
Aspirin
Azathioprine
Azelastine
Basiliximab
Butabarbital
Butalbital
Celecoxib
Chlorambucil
Cidofovir
Cladribine
Clonidine
Collagen
Corticosteroids
Cyclosporine
Diazoxide
Eflornithine
Enfuvirtide
Eprosartan
Fluoxetine
Flurbiprofen
Foscarnet
Gemtuzumab
Glatiramer
Grepafloxacin
Indinavir
Infliximab
Interferon beta 1-a
Interferons, alfa-2
Isotretinoin
Latanoprost
Leflunomide
Meperidine
Methotrexate
Methoxsalen
Mirtazapine
Modafinil
Mycophenolate
Naltrexone
Nisoldipine
Oral contraceptives
Pantoprazole
Pentobarbital
Pentostatin
Perindopril
Phenobarbital
Pimecrolimus
Psoralens
Ribavirin
Rivastigmine
Rofecoxib
Ropinirole
Saquinavir
Sibutramine
Sildenafil
Smallpox vaccine
Sparfloxacin
Tacrine
Tacrolimus
Tiagabine
Tizanidine
Tolcapone
Trastuzumab
Trioxsalen

Valdecoxib
Venlafaxine
Voriconazole
Zolpidem

Herpes Zoster
Acyclovir
Adalimumab
Azathioprine
Basiliximab
Bortezomib
Celecoxib
Chlorambucil
Corticosteroids
Cyclosporine
Cytarabine
Enalapril
Etanercept
Fluoxetine
Flurbiprofen
Glatiramer
Gold and gold compounds
Griseofulvin
Hepatitis B vaccine
Indinavir
Infliximab
Interferon beta 1-a
Isoniazid
Mechlorethamine
Mercaptopurine
Methoxsalen
Naltrexone
Nisoldipine
Pantoprazole
Pentostatin
Procarbazine
Psoralens
Rabeprazole
Rofecoxib
Ropinirole
Saquinavir
Smallpox vaccine
Tacrine
Tiagabine
Tizanidine
Tolcapone
Trastuzumab
Trioxsalen
Valdecoxib
Venlafaxine
Zolpidem

Hot Flashes
Adefovir
Anastrozole
Anthrax vaccine
Arbutamine
Bicalutamide
Bupropion
Cabergoline
Cefmetazole
Celecoxib
Cevimeline
Citalopram
Clomiphene
Cyclosporine
Doxazosin
Efavirenz
Epirubicin
Eprosartan
Escitalopram
Estramustine

Estrogens
Exemestane
Fenoprofen
Flumazenil
Fluoxetine
Flurbiprofen
Flutamide
Frovatriptan
Fulvestrant
Ganirelix
Gemifloxacin
Goserelin
Granisetron
Hydrocodone
Ibuprofen
Indomethacin
Interferons, alfa-2
Ketoprofen
Lamotrigine
Letrozole
Leuprolide
Levodopa
Meclofenamate
Medroxyprogesterone
Mefenamic acid
Meloxicam
Mexiletine
Modafinil
Nabumetone
Nafarelin
Naltrexone
Naproxen
Oxaliplatin
Oxcarbazepine
Oxybutynin
Piroxicam
Raloxifene
Rasburicase
Rivastigmine
Rizatriptan
Sirolimus
Sulindac
Sumatriptan
Tamoxifen
Tolmetin
Topiramate
Toremifene
Triptorelin
Urofollitropin
Valdecoxib
Zolmitriptan
Zolpidem

Hypersensitivity
Abacavir
Acetaminophen
Acetylcysteine
Acyclovir
Alefacept
Alendronate
Allopurinol
Aloe vera (gel, juice, leaf)
Alteplase
Aminophylline
Aminosalicylate sodium
Amitriptyline
Amobarbital
Amoxicillin
Ampicillin
Anakinra
Anisindione

Anistreplase
Anthrax vaccine
Aprotinin
Asparaginase
Aspirin
Azathioprine
Azithromycin
Aztreonam
Bacampicillin
Balsalazide
Basiliximab
Benazepril
Benzonatate
Benzphetamine
Bismuth
Bleomycin
Bortezomib
Bupropion
Butterbur
Caffeine
Calcitonin
Capecitabine
Capsicum
Caraway
Carbamazepine
Carbenicillin
Carboplatin
Cefaclor
Cefadroxil
Cefamandole
Cefazolin
Cefepime
Cefixime
Cefmetazole
Cefonicid
Cefoperazone
Cefotaxime
Cefotetan
Cefpodoxime
Cefprozil
Ceftazidime
Ceftibuten
Ceftriaxone
Cefuroxime
Cephalexin
Cephapirin
Cephradine
Chamomile
Chloral hydrate
Chlorambucil
Chloramphenicol
Chlorhexidine
Chlorpheniramine
Chlorzoxazone
Cimetidine
Cinoxacin
Ciprofloxacin
Cisatracurium
Cisplatin
Clarithromycin
Clemastine
Clindamycin
Clopidogrel
Cloxacillin
Co-trimoxazole
Colchicine
Collagen
Corticosteroids
Cromolyn
Cyanocobalamin

Cyclamate
Cyclophosphamide
Cyclosporine
Cytarabine
Dacarbazine
Dapsone
Denileukin
Desipramine
Desloratadine
Diazepam
Diazoxide
Diclofenac
Dicloxacillin
Dicumarol
Didanosine
Diflunisal
Diltiazem
Diphenhydramine
Dobutamine
Docetaxel
Domperidone
Doxycycline
Echinacea
Edrophonium
Efavirenz
Enfuvirtide
Enoxacin
Enoxaparin
Ephedra
Epirubicin
Epoetin alfa
Ertapenem
Erythromycin
Ethambutol
Ethchlorvynol
Etidronate
Etoposide
Famciclovir
Flavoxate
Fluconazole
Fluoxetine
Fluoxymesterone
Flurbiprofen
Garlic
Gatifloxacin
Gemifloxacin
Gentamicin
Glatiramer
Glucosamine
Glyburide
Gold and gold compounds
Goserelin
Granisetron
Grepafloxacin
Haloperidol
Hawthorn (fruit, leaf, flower extract)
Henna
Heparin
Hepatitis B vaccine
Heroin
Hydralazine
Hydroxyzine
Ibritumomab
Ibuprofen
Imipenem/cilastatin
Inamrinone
Indomethacin
Infliximab
Insulin

Interferon beta 1-a
Interferons, alfa-2
Ipodate
Isoniazid
Kanamycin
Kava
Ketoconazole
Ketorolac
Labetalol
Lamivudine
Lamotrigine
Lansoprazole
Leucovorin
Levalbuterol
Levobunolol
Levothyroxine
Lidocaine
Liothyronine
Lomefloxacin
Loperamide
Lovastatin
Mafenide
Meadowsweet
Mechlorethamine
Meclofenamate
Meloxicam
Melphalan
Meprobamate
Mesalamine
Methazolamide
Methicillin
Methyldopa
Methylphenidate
Methyltestosterone
Metronidazole
Mezlocillin
Minocycline
Nafarelin
Nafcillin
Naproxen
Nelfinavir
Neomycin
Nevirapine
Nicotine
Nisoldipine
Nitrofurantoin
Nystatin
Ofloxacin
Olanzapine
Ondansetron
Orphenadrine
Oxacillin
Oxaliplatin
Oxcarbazepine
Oxytetracycline
Paclitaxel
Pamidronate
Pancuronium
PEG-interferon alfa-2b
Pegvisomant
Penicillamine
Penicillins
Pentagastrin
Pentobarbital
Peppermint
Phenobarbital
Phenylephrine
Phenytoin
Phytonadione
Pilocarpine

Piperacillin
Pravastatin
Primidone
Probenecid
Procarbazine
Promethazine
Propolis
Propylthiouracil
Protamine
Protamine sulfate
Protease inhibitors
Pyrazinamide
Pyridoxine
Pyrimethamine
Quinapril
Quinethazone
Quinidine
Quinine
Ramipril
Ranitidine
Rasburicase
Salmeterol
Secobarbital
Simvastatin
Sparfloxacin
Spectinomycin
St John's wort
Succinylcholine
Sulfacetamide
Sulfadiazine
Sulfadoxine
Sulfamethoxazole
Sulfasalazine
Sulfisoxazole
Sulindac
Tartrazine
Tea tree
Terbinafine
Testosterone
Tetracycline
Thalidomide
Thiabendazole
Thimerosal
Thioridazine
Ticarcillin
Tinzaparin
Tobramycin
Tocainide
Tolbutamide
Trazodone
Trimethobenzamide
Trimetrexate
Triptorelin
Trovafloxacin
Urokinase
Valproic acid
Vancomycin
Vinblastine
Vitamin A
Warfarin
Zidovudine
Zonisamide

Jarisch-Herxheimer Reaction
Amoxicillin
Bacampicillin
Carbenicillin
Ceftriaxone
Cefuroxime
Cloxacillin
Co-trimoxazole

Dicloxacillin
Griseofulvin
Ketoconazole
Methicillin
Mezlocillin
Nafcillin
Oxacillin
Penicillins
Pentamidine
Piperacillin
Thiabendazole
Ticarcillin

Kaposi's Sarcoma
Aldesleukin
Aminocaproic acid
Azathioprine
Busulfan
Captopril
Chlorambucil
Corticosteroids
Cyclosporine
Heroin
Interferons, alfa-2

Lichen Planus (LP)
Allopurinol
Amitriptyline
Amlodipine
Arsenic
Aspirin
Captopril
Carbamazepine
Diflunisal
Doxazosin
Felbamate
Gemfibrozil
Glipizide
Gold and gold compounds
Hepatitis B vaccine
Hydroxyurea
Imipramine
Indomethacin
Interferons, alfa-2
Labetalol
Levamisole
Levobunolol
Lithium
Mesalamine
Methyldopa
Naproxen
Omeprazole
Penicillamine
Phenytoin
Prazosin
Procainamide
Psoralens
Quinidine
Quinine
Simvastatin
Spironolactone
Sulfasalazine
Sulindac
Thimerosal
Trovafloxacin
Ursodiol

Lichenoid (Lichen Planus-like) Eruptions
Acebutolol
Acetohexamide
Acyclovir
Aminosalicylate sodium

Amlodipine
Aspirin
Atenolol
Atorvastatin
Azathioprine
Captopril
Carbamazepine
Chloral hydrate
Chloroquine
Chlorothiazide
Chlorpromazine
Chlorpropamide
Clopidogrel
Co-trimoxazole
Colchicine
Cycloserine
Cyclosporine
Cyproheptadine
Dapsone
Demeclocycline
Diazoxide
Diclofenac
Diflunisal
Diltiazem
Doxazosin
Enalapril
Epoetin alfa
Ethambutol
Fluoxetine
Fluoxymesterone
Flurbiprofen
Furosemide
Glipizide
Glyburide
Gold and gold compounds
Granulocyte colony-
   stimulating factor (GCSF)
Griseofulvin
Henna
Hepatitis B vaccine
Hydrochlorothiazide
Hydroxychloroquine
Hydroxyurea
Ibuprofen
Indomethacin
Interferons, alfa-2
Isoniazid
Isotretinoin
Ketoconazole
Labetalol
Lansoprazole
Levamisole
Lisinopril
Lorazepam
Mercaptopurine
Mesalamine
Metformin
Methamphetamine
Methyldopa
Methyltestosterone
Metoprolol
Minocycline
Nadolol
Naproxen
Nelfinavir
Nifedipine
Omeprazole
Oral contraceptives
Pantoprazole
Penicillamine

Peppermint
Phenytoin
Pindolol
Piroxicam
Pravastatin
Prazosin
Propranolol
Propylthiouracil
Pyrimethamine
Quinacrine
Quinidine
Quinine
Ramipril
Ranitidine
Risperidone
Salsalate
Sildenafil
Simvastatin
Sotalol
Sparfloxacin
Spironolactone
Streptomycin
Sulfadoxine
Sulfamethoxazole
Sulindac
Temazepam
Terazosin
Terbinafine
Testosterone
Tetracycline
Thimerosal
Timolol
Tiopronin
Tolazamide
Tolbutamide
Torsemide
Trichlormethiazide
Tripelennamine
Triprolidine
Ursodiol
Venlafaxine
Verapamil
Zidovudine

Linear IgA Bullous
Dermatosis (LABD)
Acetaminophen
Aldesleukin
Amiodarone
Ampicillin
Atorvastatin
Candesartan
Captopril
Carbamazepine
Cefamandole
Ceftriaxone
Ciprofloxacin
Co-trimoxazole
Cyclosporine
Diclofenac
Furosemide
Glyburide
Granulocyte colony-
   stimulating factor (GCSF)
Ibuprofen
Interferons, alfa-2
Lithium
Metronidazole
Naproxen
Penicillins
Phenytoin

Piroxicam
Rifampin
Sulfamethoxazole
Sulfisoxazole
Vancomycin
Livedo Reticularis
Amantadine
Anistreplase
Arsenic
Bromocriptine
Ciprofloxacin
Dihydrotachysterol
Diphenhydramine
Estrogens
Felbamate
Heparin
Ibuprofen
Minocycline
Quinidine
Tenecteplase
Warfarin
Lupus Erythematosus
Acebutolol
Acetazolamide
Adalimumab
Albuterol
Allopurinol
Aminoglutethimide
Aminosalicylate sodium
Amiodarone
Amitriptyline
Amlodipine
Anthrax vaccine
Atenolol
Benazepril
Betaxolol
Bisoprolol
Butabarbital
Butalbital
Captopril
Carbamazepine
Carteolol
Chlorambucil
Chlordiazepoxide
Chlorothiazide
Chlorpromazine
Chlorpropamide
Chlorthalidone
Cimetidine
Clofibrate
Clonidine
Clozapine
Co-trimoxazole
Corticosteroids
Cyclophosphamide
Cyclosporine
Cyproheptadine
Danazol
Dapsone
Demeclocycline
Diclofenac
Diethylstilbestrol
Diltiazem
Disopyramide
Domperidone
Doxazosin
Doxycycline
Enalapril
Estrogens
Etanercept

Ethambutol
Ethionamide
Ethosuximide
Ethotoin
Felbamate
Fluoxetine
Fluoxymesterone
Fluphenazine
Flutamide
Fluvastatin
Fosphenytoin
Furosemide
Gemfibrozil
Glatiramer
Gold and gold compounds
Griseofulvin
Guanethidine
Hepatitis B vaccine
Hydralazine
Hydrochlorothiazide
Hydroxyurea
Ibuprofen
Imipramine
Infliximab
Interferon beta 1-a
Interferons, alfa-2
Isoniazid
Labetalol
Lamotrigine
Leuprolide
Levodopa
Lidocaine
Lisinopril
Lithium
Lovastatin
Meclofenamate
Mephenytoin
Meprobamate
Mercaptopurine
Mesalamine
Mesoridazine
Methimazole
Methoxsalen
Methsuximide
Methyldopa
Methyltestosterone
Methysergide
Metoprolol
Mexiletine
Minocycline
Minoxidil
Nadolol
Nalidixic acid
Naproxen
Nifedipine
Nitrofurantoin
Olsalazine
Omeprazole
Oral contraceptives
Oxcarbazepine
Oxytetracycline
Pantoprazole
Paramethadione
Penicillamine
Penicillins
Pentobarbital
Perphenazine
Phenelzine
Phenindamine
Phenobarbital

Phenolphthalein
Phensuximide
Phenytoin
Pindolol
Piroxicam
Potassium iodide
Pravastatin
Prazosin
Primidone
Procainamide
Prochlorperazine
Promethazine
Propafenone
Propranolol
Propylthiouracil
Psoralens
Pyrilamine
Quinidine
Quinine
Ranitidine
Reserpine
Rifabutin
Rifampin
Selenium
Sertraline
Simvastatin
Smallpox vaccine
Spironolactone
Streptomycin
Sulfadiazine
Sulfadoxine
Sulfamethoxazole
Sulfasalazine
Sulfisoxazole
Terbinafine
Terfenadine
Testosterone
Tetracycline
Thioridazine
Ticlopidine
Timolol
Tiopronin
Tocainide
Tolazamide
Triamterene
Trichlormethiazide
Trientine
Trifluoperazine
Trimeprazine
Trimethadione
Trioxsalen
Tripelennamine
Valproic acid
Vancomycin
Verapamil
Vitamin E
Voriconazole
Yohimbine
Zafirlukast
Zonisamide
Mastodynia
Anastrozole
Aripiprazole
Azelastine
Aztreonam
Betaxolol
Bexarotene
Bicalutamide
Black cohosh
Cabergoline

Celecoxib
Cetirizine
Chlorotrianisene
Chlorpromazine
Citalopram
Clomiphene
Clomipramine
Clozapine
Diethylstilbestrol
Dipyridamole
Doxazosin
Dutasteride
Eletriptan
Eplerenone
Estramustine
Estrogens
Fenoprofen
Finasteride
Fluoxetine
Fluoxymesterone
Fluphenazine
Fluvoxamine
Ganciclovir
Gatifloxacin
Ginseng
Glatiramer
Goserelin
Haloperidol
Interferon beta 1-a
Interferon beta-1b
Lansoprazole
Leuprolide
Levobupivacaine
Lisinopril
Loratadine
Medroxyprogesterone
Mesoridazine
Methyltestosterone
Metoclopramide
Minoxidil
Mirtazapine
Nafarelin
Nefazodone
Nitrofurantoin
Pantoprazole
Pergolide
Perphenazine
Prochlorperazine
Promazine
Promethazine
Quinestrol
Raloxifene
Riluzole
Risperidone
Rivastigmine
Sparfloxacin
Spironolactone
Temozolomide
Testosterone
Thioridazine
Thiothixene
Tiagabine
Topiramate
Trifluoperazine
Urofollitropin
Venlafaxine
Zaleplon
Zolpidem
Melanoma
Adalimumab

Aminolevulinic acid
Arsenic
Clomiphene
Cyclosporine
Diazepam
Gemfibrozil
Interferons, alfa-2
Levodopa
Methotrexate
Oral contraceptives
Paroxetine
Psoralens
Selenium
Smallpox vaccine
Tacrine
Trioxsalen
Myalgia
Abacavir
Abciximab
Acebutolol
Albendazole
Aldesleukin
Alefacept
Alemtuzumab
Alitretinoin
Allopurinol
Almotriptan
Aminocaproic acid
Aminoglutethimide
Amphotericin B
Anagrelide
Anastrozole
Anistreplase
Anthrax vaccine
Apraclonidine
Aprepitant
Aripiprazole
Aspirin
Atorvastatin
Azatadine
Azathioprine
Azelastine
Aztreonam
Balsalazide
Basiliximab
Benazepril
Benzphetamine
Bepridil
Betaxolol
Bexarotene
Bicalutamide
Bisoprolol
Blue cohosh
Bortezomib
Brompheniramine
Bupropion
Buspirone
Candesartan
Capecitabine
Captopril
Carteolol
Carvedilol
Caspofungin
Cefditoren
Cefonicid
Celecoxib
Cetirizine
Cevimeline
Chloroquine
Chlorpheniramine

Cidofovir
Cilostazol
Cimetidine
Cisplatin
Citalopram
Cladribine
Clemastine
Clofibrate
Clomiphene
Clomipramine
Co-trimoxazole
Colchicine
Colesevelam
Creatine
Cromolyn
Cyclophosphamide
Cyclosporine
Cyproheptadine
Cytarabine
Dacarbazine
Dactinomycin
Dantrolene
Darbepoetin alfa
Delavirdine
Denileukin
Desflurane
Desloratadine
Dexchlorpheniramine
Dicloxacillin
Didanosine
Diethylpropion
Dihydroergotamine
Dihydrotachysterol
Dimenhydrinate
Diphenhydramine
Dipyridamole
Dirithromycin
Docetaxel
Dolasetron
Doxazosin
Doxorubicin
Dronabinol
Efavirenz
Eletriptan
Enalapril
Enfuvirtide
Enoxacin
Ephedra
Ephedrine
Epirubicin
Epoetin alfa
Eprosartan
Ergocalciferol
Escitalopram
Estazolam
Ezetimibe
Famotidine
Felbamate
Felodipine
Fenofibrate
Flecainide
Fludarabine
Fluoxetine
Fluvastatin
Fluvoxamine
Formoterol
Foscarnet
Fosfomycin
Fosinopril
Frovatriptan

Fulvestrant
Gabapentin
Ganciclovir
Gatifloxacin
Gemcitabine
Gemfibrozil
Gemifloxacin
Glatiramer
Glipizide
Glyburide
Granulocyte colony-
    stimulating factor (GCSF)
Grepafloxacin
Guanethidine
Hepatitis B vaccine
Hydralazine
Hydroxyzine
Ibritumomab
Imatinib
Imiquimod
Indinavir
Infliximab
Interferon beta 1-a
Interferon beta-1b
Interferons, alfa-2
Isotretinoin
Itraconazole
Ivermectin
Ketoprofen
Ketorolac
Lamivudine
Lamotrigine
Lansoprazole
Latanoprost
Leflunomide
Leuprolide
Levalbuterol
Levamisole
Levofloxacin
Levothyroxine
Liothyronine
Lisinopril
Lomefloxacin
Loratadine
Losartan
Lovastatin
MDMA
Meclizine
Mefloquine
Mesalamine
Methimazole
Methotrexate
Methyldopa
Methysergide
Minocycline
Mirtazapine
Mitotane
Modafinil
Moexipril
Moxifloxacin
Mycophenolate
Nabumetone
Nafarelin
Naltrexone
Naproxen
Nebivolol
Nefazodone
Nelfinavir
Nevirapine
Nicardipine

Nicotine
Nifedipine
Nitrofurantoin
Nizatidine
Norfloxacin
Ofloxacin
Olanzapine
Olmesartan
Omeprazole
Orlistat
Oseltamivir
Oxaliplatin
Paclitaxel
Pamidronate
Pancuronium
Pantoprazole
Paroxetine
PEG-interferon alfa-2b
Pegfilgrastim
Pentamidine
Pentostatin
Pergolide
Perindopril
Phentermine
Pilocarpine
Pimozide
Pindolol
Pioglitazone
Pramipexole
Pravastatin
Procainamide
Procarbazine
Promethazine
Propofol
Propranolol
Propylthiouracil
Pyrazinamide
Quetiapine
Quinapril
Quinidine
Quinupristin/dalfopristin
Rabeprazole
Raloxifene
Ranitidine
Rapacuronium
Rasburicase
Ribavirin
Rifabutin
Rifampin
Risedronate
Risperidone
Ritonavir
Rituximab
Rivastigmine
Rizatriptan
Rofecoxib
Salmeterol
Selenium
Sibutramine
Sildenafil
Simvastatin
Sirolimus
Smallpox vaccine
Sotalol
Sparfloxacin
Stavudine
Succinylcholine
Sulfasalazine
Sulfisoxazole
Sumatriptan

Tacrine
Tacrolimus
Telmisartan
Temozolomide
Terazosin
Terfenadine
Tiagabine
Timolol
Tocainide
Tolcapone
Tolmetin
Topiramate
Torsemide
Trandolapril
Trazodone
Tretinoin
Trimeprazine
Tripelennamine
Triprolidine
Trovafloxacin
Unoprostone
Urofollitropin
Ursodiol
Valdecoxib
Valproic acid
Valrubicin
Valsartan
Venlafaxine
Vinblastine
Vincristine
Vinorelbine
Voriconazole
Zafirlukast
Zalcitabine
Zaleplon
Zanamivir
Zileuton
Ziprasidone
Zoledronic acid
Zolmitriptan
Zolpidem
Zonisamide

Nails – Onycholysis
Acebutolol
Allopurinol
Atenolol
Bleomycin
Capecitabine
Captopril
Chloramphenicol
Chlorpromazine
Clofazimine
Clorazepate
Cloxacillin
Demeclocycline
Diflunisal
Docetaxel
Doxorubicin
Doxycycline
Estrogens
Etoposide
Fluorouracil
Gold and gold compounds
Hydroxyurea
Ibuprofen
Indomethacin
Irinotecan
Isoniazid
Isotretinoin
Ketoprofen

Methotrexate
Methoxsalen
Metoprolol
Minocycline
Mycophenolate
Nadolol
Nitrofurantoin
Norfloxacin
Ofloxacin
Oral contraceptives
Paclitaxel
Pindolol
Piroxicam
Propranolol
Psoralens
Quinine
Tetracycline
Timolol
Trioxsalen

Nails – Pigmented
Arsenic
Betaxolol
Bleomycin
Busulfan
Chloroquine
Chlorpromazine
Cyclophosphamide
Dacarbazine
Daunorubicin
Demeclocycline
Docetaxel
Doxorubicin
Epirubicin
Fluorouracil
Flurbiprofen
Gold and gold compounds
Hydroxychloroquine
Hydroxyurea
Idarubicin
Kava
Ketoconazole
Methotrexate
Methoxsalen
Minocycline
Mitomycin
Oxytetracycline
Paclitaxel
Phenytoin
Psoralens
Quinacrine
Timolol
Trioxsalen
Valsartan
Zidovudine

Neuroleptic Malignant Syndrome
Aripiprazole
Citalopram
Clozapine
Domperidone
Donepezil
Haloperidol
Levodopa
Loxapine
Olanzapine
Pravastatin
Quetiapine
Risperidone
Tranylcypromine
Trifluoperazine

Oral Candidiasis
Amoxicillin
Ampicillin
Aripiprazole
Atovaquone
Bacampicillin
Botulinum toxin (A & B)
Capecitabine
Carbenicillin
Cefaclor
Cefadroxil
Cefamandole
Cefazolin
Cefditoren
Cefepime
Cefpodoxime
Cefprozil
Ceftazidime
Ceftibuten
Ceftizoxime
Cefuroxime
Cephalexin
Cidofovir
Ciprofloxacin
Clarithromycin
Cloxacillin
Corticosteroids
Dicloxacillin
Ertapenem
Erythromycin
Gatifloxacin
Glatiramer
Grepafloxacin
Griseofulvin
Interferon beta-1b
Leflunomide
Linezolid
Mesalamine
Methicillin
Mezlocillin
Mirtazapine
Mycophenolate
Nafcillin
Nefazodone
Olanzapine
Omeprazole
Oxacillin
Palivizumab
Pantoprazole
Penicillins
Piperacillin
Quinupristin/dalfopristin
Riluzole
Ritonavir
Salmeterol
Sirolimus
Sparfloxacin
Tacrolimus
Ticarcillin

Oral Ulceration
Abacavir
Aldesleukin
Alendronate
Allopurinol
Alprazolam
Aminoglutethimide
Anisindione
Aripiprazole
Aspirin
Atorvastatin

Azathioprine
Aztreonam
Betaxolol
Bleomycin
Butabarbital
Butalbital
Capecitabine
Captopril
Carbamazepine
Cefadroxil
Cefditoren
Chloral hydrate
Chlorambucil
Chloramphenicol
Chloroquine
Chlorpromazine
Cidofovir
Cisplatin
Clofibrate
Clonazepam
Clorazepate
Co-trimoxazole
Codeine
Colesevelam
Cyclophosphamide
Cyclosporine
Cytarabine
Delavirdine
Diclofenac
Dicumarol
Diflunisal
Dirithromycin
Doxorubicin
Enalapril
Epirubicin
Ertapenem
Erythromycin
Estazolam
Ethionamide
Ethosuximide
Fenoprofen
Feverfew
Flavoxate
Floxuridine
Fluconazole
Fluorouracil
Fluoxetine
Foscarnet
Ganciclovir
Gatifloxacin
Glatiramer
Gold and gold compounds
Grepafloxacin
Heroin
Hydralazine
Hydroxychloroquine
Hydroxyurea
Ibuprofen
Imipramine
Indomethacin
Ipratropium
Irinotecan
Isoniazid
Lamotrigine
Leflunomide
Leucovorin
Levamisole
Lithium
Losartan
Meclofenamate

Mefenamic acid
Melphalan
Meprobamate
Mesalamine
Mesna
Methimazole
Methotrexate
Methsuximide
Methyldopa
Metronidazole
Minocycline
Mitomycin
Modafinil
Mycophenolate
Nabumetone
Naproxen
Nefazodone
Nelfinavir
Nisoldipine
Olanzapine
Paroxetine
Penicillamine
Penicillins
Pentobarbital
Pentosan
Peppermint
Phenobarbital
Phenolphthalein
Phensuximide
Phenytoin
Promethazine
Propolis
Propranolol
Propylthiouracil
Quazepam
Quetiapine
Quinidine
Quinine
Rabeprazole
Ritonavir
Rofecoxib
Saquinavir
Sirolimus
Sparfloxacin
Streptomycin
Sulfadoxine
Sulfamethoxazole
Sulfasalazine
Sulfisoxazole
Sulindac
Tacrolimus
Terbutaline
Tetracycline
Tiagabine
Tiopronin
Tolcapone
Tolmetin
Venlafaxine
Vincristine
Voriconazole
Warfarin
Zafirlukast
Zalcitabine
Zaleplon
Zidovudine
Zonisamide

Paresthesias
Abacavir
Acetazolamide
Acetohexamide

Acitretin
Acyclovir
Adalimumab
Adenosine
Alitretinoin
Allopurinol
Almotriptan
Alprazolam
Altretamine
Amikacin
Amiloride
Amiodarone
Amitriptyline
Amlodipine
Amoxapine
Amphotericin B
Amprenavir
Anagrelide
Anastrozole
Anthrax vaccine
Apraclonidine
Arbutamine
Aspirin
Atorvastatin
Azatadine
Aztreonam
Baclofen
Basiliximab
Benactyzine
Benazepril
Bendroflumethiazide
Benzthiazide
Benztropine
Bepridil
Betaxolol
Bicalutamide
Biperiden
Bisoprolol
Bleomycin
Bortezomib
Bromocriptine
Brompheniramine
Bupropion
Buspirone
Butorphanol
Cabergoline
Caffeine
Calcitonin
Candesartan
Capecitabine
Captopril
Carisoprodol
Carteolol
Carvedilol
Caspofungin
Cefaclor
Cefamandole
Cefotaxime
Cefpodoxime
Cefprozil
Ceftazidime
Ceftibuten
Ceftizoxime
Celecoxib
Cephapirin
Cetirizine
Cevimeline
Chloramphenicol
Chlordiazepoxide
Chlorothiazide

Chlorpheniramine	Ethchlorvynol	Ketorolac	Nitrofurantoin
Chlorpropamide	Etidronate	Labetalol	Nizatidine
Chlorthalidone	Etodolac	Lamivudine	Norfloxacin
Cholestyramine	Etoposide	Lamotrigine	Nortriptyline
Cidofovir	Exemestane	Lansoprazole	Ofloxacin
Cilostazol	Famciclovir	Leflunomide	Omeprazole
Cinoxacin	Famotidine	Leuprolide	Ondansetron
Ciprofloxacin	Felbamate	Levalbuterol	Orphenadrine
Citalopram	Felodipine	Levamisole	Oxaliplatin
Clemastine	Fenofibrate	Levetiracetam	Oxazepam
Clomipramine	Fentanyl	Levobupivacaine	Oxytetracycline
Clonazepam	Flecainide	Levodopa	Paclitaxel
Clopidogrel	Floxuridine	Levofloxacin	Pantoprazole
Clorazepate	Fluconazole	Lidocaine	Paramethadione
Codeine	Flucytosine	Lindane	Paroxetine
Cromolyn	Fludarabine	Lisinopril	Pegvisomant
Cyanocobalamin	Flumazenil	Lomefloxacin	Penbutolol
Cyclamate	Fluorouracil	Loratadine	Pentagastrin
Cyclobenzaprine	Fluoxetine	Lorazepam	Pentazocine
Cycloserine	Fluoxymesterone	Losartan	Pentostatin
Cyclosporine	Flurazepam	Lovastatin	Pentoxifylline
Cyclothiazide	Flurbiprofen	Loxapine	Pergolide
Cyproheptadine	Flutamide	Mazindol	Perindopril
Dacarbazine	Fluvastatin	MDMA	Phenylephrine
Danaparoid	Fluvoxamine	Mecamylamine	Phenytoin
Danazol	Foscarnet	Meclizine	Pindolol
Delavirdine	Fosfomycin	Meclofenamate	Pirbuterol
Demeclocycline	Fosinopril	Medroxyprogesterone	Piroxicam
Denileukin	Fosphenytoin	Meloxicam	Polythiazide
Desipramine	Frovatriptan	Meprobamate	Potassium iodide
Dexchlorpheniramine	Fulvestrant	Mesalamine	Pramipexole
Diazepam	Furosemide	Mesoridazine	Pravastatin
Diazoxide	Gabapentin	Methazolamide	Prazepam
Diclofenac	Galantamine	Methimazole	Prazosin
Didanosine	Ganciclovir	Methyclothiazide	Procarbazine
Diflunisal	Gatifloxacin	Methyldopa	Promethazine
Dihydroergotamine	Gemcitabine	Methyltestosterone	Propafenone
Diltiazem	Gemfibrozil	Methysergide	Propranolol
Dimenhydrinate	Gentamicin	Metoclopramide	Propylthiouracil
Diphenhydramine	Glatiramer	Metolazone	Protriptyline
Diphenoxylate	Glipizide	Metoprolol	Pyridoxine
Dipyridamole	Glyburide	Metronidazole	Pyrilamine
Dirithromycin	Grepafloxacin	Mexiletine	Quazepam
Disopyramide	Griseofulvin	Midazolam	Quetiapine
Disulfiram	Guanadrel	Midodrine	Quinapril
Dobutamine	Guanethidine	Minocycline	Quinethazone
Docetaxel	Guanfacine	Minoxidil	Quinupristin/dalfopristin
Dofetilide	Hepatitis B vaccine	Mirtazapine	Rabeprazole
Dolasetron	Hydralazine	Mitomycin	Ramipril
Donepezil	Hydrochlorothiazide	Modafinil	Rasburicase
Doxapram	Hydroflumethiazide	Moricizine	Repaglinide
Doxazosin	Hydromorphone	Moxifloxacin	Rifabutin
Doxepin	Ibuprofen	Mycophenolate	Riluzole
Doxycycline	Imipenem/cilastatin	Nabumetone	Risedronate
Dronabinol	Imipramine	Nadolol	Risperidone
Echinacea	Indapamide	Nafarelin	Ritonavir
Efavirenz	Indinavir	Nalbuphine	Rivastigmine
Eflornithine	Indomethacin	Nalidixic acid	Rizatriptan
Eletriptan	Infliximab	Naratriptan	Rofecoxib
Enalapril	Insulin	Nebivolol	Ropinirole
Enfuvirtide	Interferon beta 1-a	Nefazodone	Salmeterol
Enoxacin	Interferon beta-1b	Nelfinavir	Saquinavir
Epoetin alfa	Interferons, alfa-2	Nesiritide	Selegiline
Eprosartan	Ipratropium	Nevirapine	Selenium
Ertapenem	Irbesartan	Niacin	Sertraline
Escitalopram	Isoniazid	Niacinamide	Sibutramine
Esmolol	Isradipine	Nicardipine	Sildenafil
Esomeprazole	Kanamycin	Nicotine	Simvastatin
Estazolam	Ketoconazole	Nifedipine	Sirolimus
Ethambutol	Ketoprofen	Nisoldipine	Sotalol

Sparfloxacin
Spironolactone
St John's wort
Stavudine
Streptomycin
Sulindac
Sumatriptan
Tacrine
Tacrolimus
Tartrazine
Telmisartan
Temazepam
Temozolomide
Tenofovir
Terazosin
Terfenadine
Teriparatide
Testosterone
Tetracycline
Thalidomide
Thiabendazole
Thiamine
Thioridazine
Thiothixene
Tiagabine
Timolol
Tizanidine
Tobramycin
Tocainide
Tolazamide
Tolbutamide
Tolcapone
Tolterodine
Topiramate
Topotecan
Tramadol
Trandolapril
Tranylcypromine
Trastuzumab
Trazodone
Tretinoin
Triamterene
Triazolam
Trichlormethiazide
Trihexyphenidyl
Trimeprazine
Trimethadione
Trimipramine
Tripelennamine
Triprolidine
Trovafloxacin
Unoprostone
Valacyclovir
Valdecoxib
Valganciclovir
Valproic acid
Valsartan
Vancomycin
Venlafaxine
Verapamil
Verteporfin
Vinblastine
Vincristine
Vinorelbine
Voriconazole
Zalcitabine
Zaleplon
Zidovudine
Zileuton
Ziprasidone

Zolmitriptan
Zolpidem
Zonisamide
Parkinsonism
Amitriptyline
Amlodipine
Bupropion
Buspirone
Busulfan
Carboplatin
Citalopram
Cyclosporine
Diltiazem
Domperidone
Doxepin
Entacapone
Flucytosine
Fluphenazine
Haloperidol
Imipramine
Infliximab
Interferons, alfa-2
Kava
Lithium
Loxapine
Maprotiline
MDMA
Methyldopa
Metoclopramide
Nabumetone
Nortriptyline
Olanzapine
Pemoline
Perphenazine
Phenelzine
Prochlorperazine
Promazine
Promethazine
Protriptyline
Reserpine
Risperidone
Ritonavir
Tacrine
Thioridazine
Thiothixene
Trazodone
Trifluoperazine
Trimethobenzamide
Trimipramine
Tryptophan
Valproic acid
Verapamil
Parosmia
Almotriptan
Alosetron
Aminophylline
Amiodarone
Amlodipine
Apraclonidine
Atorvastatin
Buspirone
Cetirizine
Cevimeline
Clarithromycin
Doxazosin
Efavirenz
Eletriptan
Esomeprazole
Fluoxetine
Flurbiprofen

Fluvoxamine
Fomepizole
Gatifloxacin
Grepafloxacin
Interferon beta-1b
Isotretinoin
Levamisole
Mirtazapine
Nifedipine
Ofloxacin
Propafenone
Rimantadine
Ritonavir
Sumatriptan
Terbinafine
Tiagabine
Tiopronin
Tocainide
Tolcapone
Topiramate
Venlafaxine
Zalcitabine
Zaleplon
Zolmitriptan
Zonisamide
Periorbital Edema
Acyclovir
Aspirin
Cabergoline
Carbamazepine
Cefmetazole
Chlorambucil
Clozapine
Creatine
Diltiazem
Donepezil
Ethosuximide
Famotidine
Foscarnet
Furosemide
Ibuprofen
Imatinib
Indomethacin
Methsuximide
Moricizine
Nifedipine
Omeprazole
Phensuximide
Phenylephrine
Pimozide
Rivastigmine
Sertraline
Streptokinase
Sulfadiazine
Sulfadoxine
Sulfasalazine
Sulfisoxazole
Trovafloxacin
Urokinase
Valacyclovir
Valdecoxib
Zolpidem
Peripheral Edema
Abciximab
Acyclovir
Adalimumab
Aldesleukin
Alemtuzumab
Alendronate
Amantadine

Amlodipine
Anagrelide
Anastrozole
Aripiprazole
Atazanavir
Basiliximab
Benazepril
Bepridil
Bexarotene
Bicalutamide
Bosentan
Botulinum toxin (A & B)
Bupropion
Cabergoline
Candesartan
Carteolol
Carvedilol
Cefditoren
Celecoxib
Cetrorelix
Cevimeline
Chlorotrianisene
Chlorpromazine
Chondroitin
Cilostazol
Clonidine
Cyproheptadine
Danaparoid
Darbepoetin alfa
Delavirdine
Diclofenac
Diethylstilbestrol
Diflunisal
Diltiazem
Dirithromycin
Docetaxel
Dofetilide
Dolasetron
Doxazosin
Efavirenz
Eletriptan
Enoxaparin
Eprosartan
Esomeprazole
Estrogens
Etodolac
Exemestane
Felodipine
Fenoprofen
Fluoxetine
Fluphenazine
Flurbiprofen
Foscarnet
Fulvestrant
Gabapentin
Galantamine
Gatifloxacin
Gemcitabine
Gemtuzumab
Glatiramer
Granulocyte colony-
    stimulating factor (GCSF)
Grepafloxacin
Guanadrel
Guanethidine
Guanfacine
Heparin
Hydroxyurea
Ibritumomab
Imatinib

Indapamide
Indomethacin
Isocarboxazid
Isosorbide dinitrate
Isradipine
Itraconazole
Ivermectin
Ketoprofen
Labetalol
Lansoprazole
Leflunomide
Leuprolide
Lisinopril
Loratadine
Meclofenamate
Meprobamate
Mesalamine
Mesoridazine
Methyldopa
Methysergide
Metoprolol
Midazolam
Minoxidil
Mirtazapine
Moexipril
Molindone
Montelukast
Morphine
Moxifloxacin
Mycophenolate
Naproxen
Nefazodone
Nicardipine
Nifedipine
Nimodipine
Nisoldipine
Nitroglycerin
Olanzapine
Olmesartan
Omeprazole
Oxaliplatin
Pantoprazole
Paricalcitol
Paroxetine
Pegfilgrastim
Pegvisomant
Penbutolol
Penicillamine
Pentostatin
Pergolide
Perphenazine
Phenelzine
Phentermine
Pindolol
Piroxicam
Pramipexole
Prochlorperazine
Propranolol
Quinapril
Quinestrol
Quinupristin/dalfopristin
Rabeprazole
Raloxifene
Rapacuronium
Reserpine
Rifapentine
Riluzole
Risedronate
Risperidone
Ritonavir

Rituximab
Rivastigmine
Rofecoxib
Ropinirole
Selegiline
Sibutramine
Sildenafil
Sirolimus
Sotalol
Sparfloxacin
Tacrine
Tacrolimus
Tamoxifen
Telmisartan
Temozolomide
Terazosin
Terbinafine
Testosterone
Thalidomide
Thioridazine
Thiothixene
Tiagabine
Tranylcypromine
Trastuzumab
Treprostinil
Trifluoperazine
Trimeprazine
Tripelennamine
Trovafloxacin
Valdecoxib
Valproic acid
Valrubicin
Venlafaxine
Verapamil
Voriconazole
Zaleplon
Ziprasidone
Zonisamide

Petechiae
Abciximab
Aldesleukin
Alendronate
Allopurinol
Amitriptyline
Amlodipine
Amoxapine
Amoxicillin
Anisindione
Aspirin
Atorvastatin
Aztreonam
Benactyzine
Black cohosh
Carbamazepine
Chlorzoxazone
Cladribine
Clozapine
Cytarabine
Danazol
Delavirdine
Denileukin
Desipramine
Diltiazem
Floxuridine
Fluconazole
Fludarabine
Fluoxetine
Gemcitabine
Gemfibrozil
Gemtuzumab

Griseofulvin
Heparin
Hepatitis B vaccine
Ibritumomab
Imatinib
Imipramine
Indomethacin
Interferon beta 1-a
Lamotrigine
Maprotiline
Melphalan
Meprobamate
Mercaptopurine
Methyldopa
Minocycline
Mirtazapine
Mitoxantrone
Nisoldipine
Nortriptyline
Octreotide
Ofloxacin
Pentostatin
Piroxicam
Plicamycin
Procarbazine
Protriptyline
Riluzole
Simvastatin
Sparfloxacin
Tacrine
Thioguanine
Tiagabine
Ticlopidine
Tizanidine
Trimethadione
Trimipramine
Valproic acid
Voriconazole
Zonisamide

Peyronie's Disease
Acebutolol
Atenolol
Betaxolol
Bisoprolol
Carteolol
Interferon beta 1-a
Labetalol
Methotrexate
Metoprolol
Nadolol
Penbutolol
Phenytoin
Pindolol
Propranolol
Ropinirole
Timolol

Photosensitivity
Acetaminophen
Acetazolamide
Acetohexamide
Acitretin
Acyclovir
Aldesleukin
Alitretinoin
Allopurinol
Almotriptan
Alprazolam
Amantadine
Amiloride
Aminolevulinic acid

Aminosalicylate sodium
Amiodarone
Amitriptyline
Amobarbital
Amoxapine
Anagrelide
Anthrax vaccine
Arsenic
Atazanavir
Atenolol
Atorvastatin
Atropine sulfate
Azatadine
Azathioprine
Azithromycin
Benazepril
Bendroflumethiazide
Benzthiazide
Benztropine
Bergamot
Betaxolol
Bexarotene
Bisoprolol
Brompheniramine
Bumetanide
Bupropion
Butabarbital
Butalbital
Capecitabine
Captopril
Carbamazepine
Carisoprodol
Carteolol
Carvedilol
Cefazolin
Ceftazidime
Celecoxib
Cetirizine
Cevimeline
Chlorambucil
Chlordiazepoxide
Chlorhexidine
Chloroquine
Chlorothiazide
Chlorotrianisene
Chlorpheniramine
Chlorpromazine
Chlorpropamide
Chlortetracycline
Chlorthalidone
Cinoxacin
Ciprofloxacin
Citalopram
Clemastine
Clofazimine
Clofibrate
Clomipramine
Clopidogrel
Clorazepate
Clozapine
Co-trimoxazole
Cromolyn
Cyclamate
Cyclobenzaprine
Cyclothiazide
Cyproheptadine
Dacarbazine
Danazol
Dantrolene
Dapsone

Demeclocycline
Desipramine
Dexchlorpheniramine
Diazoxide
Diclofenac
Diflunisal
Diltiazem
Dimenhydrinate
Diphenhydramine
Disopyramide
Docetaxel
Doxepin
Doxycycline
Efavirenz
Enalapril
Enoxacin
Epirubicin
Epoetin alfa
Esomeprazole
Estazolam
Estrogens
Ethacrynic acid
Ethambutol
Ethionamide
Etodolac
Felbamate
Fenofibrate
Floxuridine
Flucytosine
Fluorouracil
Fluoxetine
Fluphenazine
Flurbiprofen
Flutamide
Fluvastatin
Fluvoxamine
Fosinopril
Furazolidone
Furosemide
Ganciclovir
Gatifloxacin
Gemifloxacin
Gentamicin
Glatiramer
Glimepiride
Glipizide
Glyburide
Glycopyrrolate
Gold and gold compounds
Grepafloxacin
Griseofulvin
Haloperidol
Henna
Heroin
Hydralazine
Hydrochlorothiazide
Hydroflumethiazide
Hydroxychloroquine
Hydroxyurea
Hydroxyzine
Hyoscyamine
Ibuprofen
Imatinib
Imipramine
Indapamide
Indomethacin
Infliximab
Interferon beta 1-a
Interferon beta-1b
Interferons, alfa-2

Isocarboxazid
Isoniazid
Isotretinoin
Itraconazole
Kanamycin
Kava
Ketoconazole
Ketoprofen
Ketotifen
Lamotrigine
Leuprolide
Levofloxacin
Lincomycin
Lisinopril
Lomefloxacin
Loratadine
Losartan
Loxapine
Maprotiline
Meclizine
Meclofenamate
Medroxyprogesterone
Mefenamic acid
Melatonin
Meloxicam
Meprobamate
Mercaptopurine
Mesalamine
Mesoridazine
Metformin
Methazolamide
Methenamine
Methotrexate
Methoxsalen
Methyclothiazide
Methyldopa
Methylphenidate
Metolazone
Minocycline
Minoxidil
Mirtazapine
Mitomycin
Moexipril
Molindone
Moxifloxacin
Nabumetone
Nalidixic acid
Naproxen
Naratriptan
Nefazodone
Nifedipine
Nisoldipine
Nitrofurantoin
Norfloxacin
Nortriptyline
Ofloxacin
Olanzapine
Oral contraceptives
Oxaprozin
Oxcarbazepine
Oxytetracycline
Paclitaxel
Pantoprazole
Paroxetine
Pentobarbital
Pentosan
Pentostatin
Perphenazine
Phenelzine
Phenindamine

Phenobarbital
Pimozide
Piroxicam
Polythiazide
Pravastatin
Procarbazine
Prochlorperazine
Procyclidine
Promazine
Promethazine
Propranolol
Propylthiouracil
Protriptyline
Psoralens
Pyridoxine
Pyrilamine
Pyrimethamine
Quetiapine
Quinacrine
Quinapril
Quinestrol
Quinethazone
Quinidine
Quinine
Rabeprazole
Ramipril
Ranitidine
Ribavirin
Riluzole
Risperidone
Ritonavir
Rofecoxib
Ropinirole
Saccharin
Saquinavir
Scopolamine
Selegiline
Sertraline
Sildenafil
Simvastatin
Smallpox vaccine
Sotalol
Sparfloxacin
Spironolactone
St John's wort
Streptomycin
Sulfacetamide
Sulfadiazine
Sulfadoxine
Sulfamethoxazole
Sulfasalazine
Sulfisoxazole
Sulindac
Sumatriptan
Tacrolimus
Tartrazine
Terbinafine
Terfenadine
Tetracycline
Thioguanine
Thioridazine
Thiothixene
Tiagabine
Timolol
Tiopronin
Tolazamide
Tolbutamide
Topiramate
Torsemide
Tranylcypromine

Trazodone
Tretinoin
Triamterene
Triazolam
Trichlormethiazide
Trifluoperazine
Trihexyphenidyl
Trimeprazine
Trimethadione
Trimethoprim
Trimetrexate
Trimipramine
Trioxsalen
Tripelennamine
Triprolidine
Trovafloxacin
Valdecoxib
Valproic acid
Valsartan
Venlafaxine
Verapamil
Verteporfin
Vinblastine
Vitamin A
Voriconazole
Yarrow
Zalcitabine
Zaleplon
Ziprasidone
Zolmitriptan
Zolpidem

Phototoxic Reactions
Acitretin
Alprazolam
Aspirin
Bendroflumethiazide
Bergamot
Captopril
Cefazolin
Cetirizine
Chlorpromazine
Ciprofloxacin
Clarithromycin
Demeclocycline
Docetaxel
Dong quai
Doxycycline
Enoxacin
Fenofibrate
Fluorouracil
Fluoxetine
Furosemide
Glipizide
Grepafloxacin
Haloperidol
Hydrochlorothiazide
Hydroxychloroquine
Itraconazole
Levofloxacin
Lomefloxacin
Methotrexate
Methoxsalen
Minocycline
Nabumetone
Nalidixic acid
Naproxen
Norfloxacin
Nortriptyline
Ofloxacin
Oxaprozin

Pantoprazole
Prochlorperazine
Promazine
Propranolol
Protriptyline
Psoralens
Rofecoxib
Sparfloxacin
Sulfisoxazole
Sulindac
Terazosin
Tetracycline
Thioridazine
Trioxsalen
Trovafloxacin
Vinblastine

Pigmentation
Acebutolol
Alitretinoin
Aminolevulinic acid
Amiodarone
Amitriptyline
Amphotericin B
Arsenic
Azathioprine
Bergamot
Betaxolol
Bimatoprost
Bismuth
Bisoprolol
Bleomycin
Busulfan
Capecitabine
Captopril
Carbamazepine
Carboplatin
Carmustine
Carteolol
Chlorhexidine
Chloroquine
Chlorotrianisene
Chlorpromazine
Cidofovir
Ciprofloxacin
Cisplatin
Citalopram
Clofazimine
Clomipramine
Clonazepam
Clonidine
Corticosteroids
Cyclobenzaprine
Cyclophosphamide
Cyclosporine
Dactinomycin
Dapsone
Daunorubicin
Deferoxamine
Demeclocycline
Desipramine
Diazepam
Dicumarol
Diethylstilbestrol
Diltiazem
Donepezil
Doxorubicin
Doxycycline
Eletriptan
Enoxacin
Epirubicin

Esmolol
Estramustine
Estrogens
Etodolac
Etoposide
Floxuridine
Fluorouracil
Fluoxetine
Fluphenazine
Fluvoxamine
Foscarnet
Ganciclovir
Glatiramer
Gold and gold compounds
Grepafloxacin
Griseofulvin
Haloperidol
Henna
Heroin
Hydroxychloroquine
Hydroxyurea
Ifosfamide
Imipramine
Imiquimod
Indapamide
Indinavir
Insulin
Interferon beta 1-a
Interferons, alfa-2
Irinotecan
Isotretinoin
Kava
Ketoconazole
Ketoprofen
Labetalol
Latanoprost
Leflunomide
Leuprolide
Levobupivacaine
Lidocaine
Linezolid
Lomefloxacin
Loxapine
Mechlorethamine
Medroxyprogesterone
Mephenytoin
Mercaptopurine
Mesoridazine
Methamphetamine
Methimazole
Methotrexate
Methoxsalen
Methyldopa
Methysergide
Metoprolol
Minocycline
Minoxidil
Mitomycin
Mitotane
Mitoxantrone
Molindone
Niacin
Nisoldipine
Ofloxacin
Olanzapine
Oral contraceptives
Orphenadrine
Oxytetracycline
Paclitaxel
Pantoprazole

Paroxetine
Pentazocine
Pentostatin
Perphenazine
Phenazopyridine
Phenolphthalein
Phenytoin
Pimozide
Procarbazine
Prochlorperazine
Progestins
Promazine
Promethazine
Propranolol
Propylthiouracil
Psoralens
Pyrimethamine
Quinacrine
Quinestrol
Quinidine
Quinine
Rabeprazole
Rifabutin
Rifapentine
Risperidone
Ropinirole
Saquinavir
Smallpox vaccine
Sparfloxacin
Spironolactone
Stanozolol
Sulfadiazine
Sulfasalazine
Tacrolimus
Terbinafine
Tetracycline
Thioridazine
Thiotepa
Thiothixene
Tiagabine
Timolol
Tolcapone
Topiramate
Toremifene
Tretinoin
Trifluoperazine
Trioxsalen
Venlafaxine
Verteporfin
Vinblastine
Vincristine
Vinorelbine
Vitamin A
Voriconazole
Zaleplon
Zidovudine

Pityriasis Rosea
Acetaminophen
Ampicillin
Arsenic
Aspirin
Captopril
Clonidine
Codeine
Corticosteroids
Gold and gold compounds
Griseofulvin
Isotretinoin
Ketotifen
Meprobamate

Metronidazole
Mitomycin
Naproxen
Omeprazole
Penicillins
Terbinafine
Tiopronin
Tripelennamine

Porphyria
Amlodipine
Butabarbital
Butalbital
Carbamazepine
Chloral hydrate
Chlorambucil
Chloramphenicol
Chlordiazepoxide
Chlormezanone
Chloroquine
Chlorotrianisene
Chlorpropamide
Cimetidine
Cisplatin
Clonidine
Clorazepate
Cocaine
Cyclophosphamide
Danazol
Dapsone
Demeclocycline
Diazepam
Diclofenac
Dimenhydrinate
Estrogens
Ethchlorvynol
Ethosuximide
Flurazepam
Furosemide
Glipizide
Gold and gold compounds
Griseofulvin
Hydroxychloroquine
Indinavir
Isoniazid
Ketoprofen
Lamotrigine
Lidocaine
Mafenide
Meclofenamate
Meprobamate
Methyldopa
Metoclopramide
Metronidazole
Nalidixic acid
Nitisinone
Nortriptyline
Ondansetron
Oral contraceptives
Pentobarbital
Phenobarbital
Phensuximide
Phenytoin
Primidone
Pyrazinamide
Quinestrol
Quinidine
Quinine
Ranitidine
Rifampin
Sodium oxybate

Spironolactone
Thiopental
Thioridazine
Tolazamide
Tolbutamide
Tranylcypromine
Trimethadione
Valproic acid
Priapism
Alprostadil
Androstenedione
Anisindione
Aripiprazole
Bromocriptine
Bupropion
Chlorpromazine
Citalopram
Clozapine
Cocaine
Codeine
Dicumarol
Fluoxetine
Fluoxymesterone
Fluphenazine
Fluvoxamine
Gabapentin
Glatiramer
Guanethidine
Haloperidol
Heparin
Hydroxyzine
Labetalol
Levodopa
Loxapine
MDMA
Mesoridazine
Methyltestosterone
Nefazodone
Olanzapine
Oxcarbazepine
Papaverine
Paroxetine
Pergolide
Perphenazine
Phenelzine
Phenoxybenzamine
Phentolamine
Prazosin
Prochlorperazine
Promazine
Promethazine
Quetiapine
Risperidone
Sertraline
Sildenafil
Stanozolol
Terazosin
Testosterone
Thioridazine
Thiothixene
Tinzaparin
Toremifene
Tranylcypromine
Trazodone
Trifluoperazine
Vancomycin
Warfarin
Ziprasidone
Pruritus
Abacavir

Abciximab
Acebutolol
Acetaminophen
Acetazolamide
Acetohexamide
Acetylcysteine
Acitretin
Acyclovir
Adapalene
Albendazole
Albuterol
Aldesleukin
Alefacept
Alemtuzumab
Alendronate
Alfentanil
Alitretinoin
Allopurinol
Almotriptan
Alprazolam
Alprostadil
Altretamine
Amantadine
Amikacin
Amiloride
Aminocaproic acid
Aminoglutethimide
Aminolevulinic acid
Aminophylline
Aminosalicylate sodium
Amiodarone
Amitriptyline
Amlodipine
Amoxapine
Amoxicillin
Amphotericin B
Ampicillin
Amprenavir
Anagrelide
Anastrozole
Anthrax vaccine
Apraclonidine
Aprotinin
Aripiprazole
Arsenic
Asparaginase
Aspartame
Aspirin
Atazanavir
Atenolol
Atomoxetine
Atorvastatin
Atovaquone
Atracurium
Atropine sulfate
Azithromycin
Aztreonam
Bacampicillin
Baclofen
Balsalazide
Basiliximab
Benactyzine
Benazepril
Bendroflumethiazide
Benzonatate
Benztropine
Betaxolol
Bexarotene
Bicalutamide
Bimatoprost

Bismuth
Bisoprolol
Black cohosh
Bleomycin
Bortezomib
Bosentan
Botulinum toxin (A & B)
Brimonidine
Brinzolamide
Bumetanide
Bupropion
Buspirone
Butabarbital
Butalbital
Butorphanol
Butterbur
Cabergoline
Caffeine
Calcitonin
Capecitabine
Captopril
Carbamazepine
Carbenicillin
Carboplatin
Carisoprodol
Carteolol
Carvedilol
Caspofungin
Cefaclor
Cefadroxil
Cefamandole
Cefazolin
Cefdinir
Cefditoren
Cefepime
Cefixime
Cefmetazole
Cefonicid
Cefoperazone
Cefotaxime
Cefotetan
Cefoxitin
Cefpodoxime
Cefprozil
Ceftazidime
Ceftibuten
Ceftizoxime
Ceftriaxone
Cefuroxime
Celecoxib
Cephalexin
Cephalothin
Cephapirin
Cephradine
Cetirizine
Cetrorelix
Cevimeline
Chloral hydrate
Chlorambucil
Chloramphenicol
Chlordiazepoxide
Chlormezanone
Chloroquine
Chlorothiazide
Chlorpromazine
Chlorpropamide
Chlortetracycline
Chlorzoxazone
Cidofovir
Cilostazol

Cimetidine
Cinoxacin
Ciprofloxacin
Cisplatin
Citalopram
Cladribine
Clarithromycin
Clindamycin
Clofazimine
Clofibrate
Clomiphene
Clomipramine
Clonazepam
Clonidine
Clopidogrel
Clorazepate
Clotrimazole
Cloxacillin
Clozapine
Co-trimoxazole
Codeine
Colchicine
Corticosteroids
Cromolyn
Cyanocobalamin
Cyclamate
Cyclobenzaprine
Cyclophosphamide
Cycloserine
Cyclosporine
Cytarabine
Dactinomycin
Dalteparin
Dan-shen
Danaparoid
Danazol
Dantrolene
Dapsone
Darbepoetin alfa
Daunorubicin
Deferoxamine
Delavirdine
Demeclocycline
Denileukin
Desflurane
Desipramine
Diazepam
Diazoxide
Diclofenac
Dicloxacillin
Dicumarol
Dicyclomine
Didanosine
Diethylpropion
Diethylstilbestrol
Diflunisal
Digoxin
Dihydroergotamine
Dihydrotachysterol
Diltiazem
Diphenhydramine
Diphenoxylate
Dipyridamole
Dirithromycin
Disopyramide
Dobutamine
Docetaxel
Dolasetron
Domperidone
Donepezil

Dopamine	Gentamicin	Levobupivacaine	Mupirocin
Doxapram	Ginkgo biloba	Levofloxacin	Mycophenolate
Doxazosin	Ginseng	Levothyroxine	Nabumetone
Doxepin	Glatiramer	Lidocaine	Nadolol
Doxercalciferol	Glimepiride	Lincomycin	Nafarelin
Doxorubicin	Glipizide	Lindane	Nafcillin
Doxycycline	Glyburide	Linezolid	Nalbuphine
Droperidol	Gold and gold compounds	Lisinopril	Nalidixic acid
Efavirenz	Granulocyte colony-	Lithium	Naloxone
Eflornithine	stimulating factor (GCSF)	Lomefloxacin	Naltrexone
Eletriptan	Grepafloxacin	Loperamide	Naproxen
Enalapril	Griseofulvin	Loracarbef	Nefazodone
Enfuvirtide	Guanabenz	Loratadine	Nelfinavir
Enoxacin	Guanfacine	Lorazepam	Neomycin
Enoxaparin	Haloperidol	Losartan	Nesiritide
Epirubicin	Henna	Lovastatin	Nevirapine
Epoetin alfa	Heparin	Loxapine	Niacin
Eprosartan	Hepatitis B vaccine	Mafenide	Niacinamide
Ergocalciferol	Heroin	Maprotiline	Nicotine
Ertapenem	Hydralazine	Marihuana	Nifedipine
Erythromycin	Hydrochlorothiazide	Mebendazole	Nimodipine
Escitalopram	Hydrocodone	Mechlorethamine	Nisoldipine
Esomeprazole	Hydromorphone	Meclofenamate	Nitazoxanide
Estazolam	Hydroxychloroquine	Medroxyprogesterone	Nitisinone
Estramustine	Hydroxyurea	Mefenamic acid	Nitrofurantoin
Estrogens	Ibritumomab	Mefloquine	Nizatidine
Etanercept	Ibuprofen	Meloxicam	Norfloxacin
Ethambutol	Imatinib	Melphalan	Nortriptyline
Ethchlorvynol	Imipenem/cilastatin	Meperidine	Nystatin
Ethosuximide	Imipramine	Mephenytoin	Octreotide
Etidronate	Imiquimod	Meprobamate	Ofloxacin
Etodolac	Indapamide	Mercaptopurine	Olanzapine
Etoposide	Indinavir	Mesalamine	Olopatadine
Exemestane	Indomethacin	Mesna	Olsalazine
Famciclovir	Infliximab	Mesoridazine	Omeprazole
Famotidine	Insulin	Metaxalone	Ondansetron
Felbamate	Insulin glargine	Metformin	Oral contraceptives
Felodipine	Interferon beta 1-a	Methadone	Orphenadrine
Fenofibrate	Interferons, alfa-2	Methazolamide	Oxacillin
Fenoprofen	Ipodate	Methenamine	Oxaliplatin
Fentanyl	Ipratropium	Methicillin	Oxaprozin
Flecainide	Irbesartan	Methimazole	Oxazepam
Floxuridine	Irinotecan	Methocarbamol	Oxcarbazepine
Fluconazole	Isocarboxazid	Methotrexate	Oxybutynin
Flucytosine	Isoniazid	Methoxsalen	Oxycodone
Fluorouracil	Isoproterenol	Methsuximide	Oxytetracycline
Fluoxetine	Isosorbide mononitrate	Methyldopa	Paclitaxel
Fluoxymesterone	Isotretinoin	Methylphenidate	Pancuronium
Fluphenazine	Isradipine	Methyltestosterone	Pantoprazole
Flurazepam	Itraconazole	Methysergide	Pantothenic acid
Flurbiprofen	Ivermectin	Metolazone	Papaverine
Fluvastatin	Kanamycin	Metoprolol	Paramethadione
Fluvoxamine	Kava	Metronidazole	Paromomycin
Folic acid	Ketamine	Mexiletine	Paroxetine
Fondaparinux	Ketoconazole	Mezlocillin	PEG-interferon alfa-2b
Formoterol	Ketoprofen	Miconazole	Pegvisomant
Foscarnet	Ketorolac	Midazolam	Penbutolol
Fosfomycin	Ketotifen	Midodrine	Penicillamine
Fosinopril	Labetalol	Minocycline	Penicillins
Fosphenytoin	Lamivudine	Minoxidil	Pentagastrin
Frovatriptan	Lamotrigine	Mirtazapine	Pentamidine
Furazolidone	Lansoprazole	Mistletoe	Pentazocine
Furosemide	Latanoprost	Mitomycin	Pentobarbital
Gabapentin	Leflunomide	Mitotane	Pentosan
Ganciclovir	Letrozole	Modafinil	Pentostatin
Ganirelix	Leucovorin	Moexipril	Pentoxifylline
Gatifloxacin	Leuprolide	Molindone	Pergolide
Gefitinib	Levalbuterol	Moricizine	Perindopril
Gemcitabine	Levamisole	Morphine	Perphenazine
Gemfibrozil	Levobunolol	Moxifloxacin	Phenazopyridine

Phenelzine
Phenobarbital
Phenolphthalein
Phensuximide
Phenytoin
Pilocarpine
Pimecrolimus
Pimozide
Pindolol
Piperacillin
Pirbuterol
Piroxicam
Pramipexole
Pravastatin
Prazepam
Praziquantel
Prazosin
Primaquine
Probenecid
Procainamide
Procarbazine
Prochlorperazine
Progestins
Propafenone
Propofol
Propoxyphene
Propranolol
Propylthiouracil
Protriptyline
Psoralens
Pyrazinamide
Pyrimethamine
Quazepam
Quinacrine
Quinapril
Quinethazone
Quinidine
Quinine
Quinupristin/dalfopristin
Rabeprazole
Ramipril
Ranitidine
Rapacuronium
Reserpine
Ribavirin
Rifampin
Rifapentine
Riluzole
Risedronate
Risperidone
Ritonavir
Rituximab
Rizatriptan
Rofecoxib
Ropinirole
Saccharin
Salmeterol
Salsalate
Saquinavir
Selenium
Senna
Sermorelin
Sertraline
Sibutramine
Sildenafil
Simvastatin
Sirolimus
Sotalol
Sparfloxacin
Spectinomycin

Spironolactone
St John's wort
Streptokinase
Streptomycin
Streptozocin
Succinylcholine
Sucralfate
Sufentanil
Sulfacetamide
Sulfadiazine
Sulfadoxine
Sulfamethoxazole
Sulfasalazine
Sulfisoxazole
Sulindac
Sumatriptan
Tacrine
Tacrolimus
Tamoxifen
Tamsulosin
Tartrazine
Tea tree
Tegaserod
Telmisartan
Temazepam
Temozolomide
Terazosin
Terbinafine
Terbutaline
Terconazole
Terfenadine
Testosterone
Tetracycline
Thalidomide
Thiabendazole
Thiamine
Thioguanine
Thiopental
Thiotepa
Thiothixene
Tiagabine
Ticarcillin
Ticlopidine
Timolol
Tinzaparin
Tiopronin
Tizanidine
Tobramycin
Tocainide
Tolazamide
Tolbutamide
Tolcapone
Tolmetin
Tolterodine
Topiramate
Toremifene
Torsemide
Tramadol
Trandolapril
Tranylcypromine
Travoprost
Trazodone
Treprostinil
Tretinoin
Triamterene
Triazolam
Trifluoperazine
Trimeprazine
Trimethadione
Trimethoprim

Trimetrexate
Trimipramine
Trioxsalen
Triptorelin
Troleandomycin
Trovafloxacin
Unoprostone
Urokinase
Ursodiol
Valacyclovir
Valdecoxib
Valproic acid
Valrubicin
Valsartan
Vancomycin
Venlafaxine
Verapamil
Verteporfin
Vidarabine
Vincristine
Vinorelbine
Vitamin A
Voriconazole
Warfarin
Zalcitabine
Zaleplon
Zidovudine
Zileuton
Zolmitriptan
Zolpidem
Zonisamide

Pseudolymphoma
Allopurinol
Alprazolam
Amitriptyline
Aspirin
Atenolol
Captopril
Carbamazepine
Cefixime
Chlorpromazine
Cimetidine
Clarithromycin
Clonazepam
Clonidine
Co-trimoxazole
Cyclosporine
Dapsone
Desipramine
Diclofenac
Diflunisal
Diltiazem
Doxepin
Estrogens
Ethotoin
Fluoxetine
Furosemide
Gemcitabine
Gemfibrozil
Gold and gold compounds
Ibuprofen
Indomethacin
Ketoprofen
Lamotrigine
Lithium
Lorazepam
Losartan
Lovastatin
Methotrexate
Mexiletine

Nabumetone
Naproxen
Nitrofurantoin
Nizatidine
Oxaprozin
Penicillins
Perphenazine
Phenytoin
Procainamide
Ranitidine
Sulfamethoxazole
Sulfasalazine
Sulindac
Terfenadine
Thioridazine
Valproic acid

Psoriasis
Acebutolol
Acitretin
Aldesleukin
Amiodarone
Amoxicillin
Ampicillin
Aripiprazole
Arsenic
Aspirin
Atenolol
Betaxolol
Bisoprolol
Botulinum toxin (A & B)
Captopril
Carbamazepine
Carteolol
Carvedilol
Celecoxib
Chlorambucil
Chloroquine
Chlorthalidone
Cimetidine
Citalopram
Clarithromycin
Clomipramine
Clonidine
Co-trimoxazole
Cyclosporine
Diclofenac
Digoxin
Diltiazem
Dipyridamole
Doxycycline
Eletriptan
Enalapril
Esmolol
Flecainide
Fluorouracil
Fluoxetine
Fluoxymesterone
Foscarnet
Ganciclovir
Gemfibrozil
Glatiramer
Glimepiride
Glipizide
Glyburide
Gold and gold compounds
Granulocyte colony-
    stimulating factor (GCSF)
Henna
Hydroxychloroquine
Hydroxyurea

Ibuprofen
Indomethacin
Infliximab
Interferon beta-1b
Interferons, alfa-2
Ketoprofen
Labetalol
Letrozole
Levamisole
Levobetaxolol
Lithium
Meclofenamate
Mefloquine
Mesalamine
Methotrexate
Methyltestosterone
Metoprolol
Modafinil
Nadolol
Omeprazole
Oral contraceptives
PEG-interferon alfa-2b
Penbutolol
Penicillamine
Pentostatin
Perindopril
Pindolol
Primaquine
Propranolol
Psoralens
Quinidine
Quinine
Rabeprazole
Ranitidine
Risperidone
Ritonavir
Rivastigmine
Rofecoxib
Ropinirole
Saquinavir
Sotalol
Sulfamethoxazole
Sulfasalazine
Sulfisoxazole
Tacrine
Terbinafine
Terfenadine
Testosterone
Tetracycline
Thalidomide
Thiabendazole
Thioguanine
Tiagabine
Timolol
Trazodone
Ursodiol
Valdecoxib
Valproic acid
Venlafaxine
Voriconazole
Zaleplon
Purpura
Acetaminophen
Acetazolamide
Acitretin
Aldesleukin
Alemtuzumab
Allopurinol
Alprazolam
Alteplase

Amiloride
Aminocaproic acid
Aminoglutethimide
Aminosalicylate sodium
Amiodarone
Amitriptyline
Amlodipine
Amobarbital
Amoxapine
Amoxicillin
Amphotericin B
Ampicillin
Anistreplase
Aprobarbital
Arsenic
Aspartame
Aspirin
Atazanavir
Atenolol
Azatadine
Azathioprine
Aztreonam
Bendroflumethiazide
Benzthiazide
Beta-carotene
Betaxolol
Bisoprolol
Botulinum toxin (A & B)
Bromocriptine
Bumetanide
Buspirone
Busulfan
Butabarbital
Butalbital
Caffeine
Capecitabine
Captopril
Carbamazepine
Carbenicillin
Carteolol
Carvedilol
Cefaclor
Cefamandole
Cefdinir
Cefmetazole
Cefonicid
Cefoxitin
Ceftriaxone
Cefuroxime
Cephalexin
Cephalothin
Cephradine
Cetirizine
Chloral hydrate
Chlorambucil
Chloramphenicol
Chlordiazepoxide
Chlorothiazide
Chlorpromazine
Chlorpropamide
Chlorthalidone
Cilostazol
Cimetidine
Ciprofloxacin
Citalopram
Cladribine
Clarithromycin
Clemastine
Clidinium
Clindamycin

Clofibrate
Clomiphene
Clomipramine
Clonazepam
Clopidogrel
Clorazepate
Clozapine
Co-trimoxazole
Colchicine
Corticosteroids
Cyclobenzaprine
Cyclophosphamide
Cyclosporine
Cyclothiazide
Cyproheptadine
Danaparoid
Danazol
Dapsone
Deferoxamine
Delavirdine
Demeclocycline
Denileukin
Desipramine
Diazepam
Diazoxide
Diclofenac
Dicloxacillin
Dicumarol
Didanosine
Diethylpropion
Diethylstilbestrol
Diflunisal
Digoxin
Diltiazem
Diphenhydramine
Dipyridamole
Disopyramide
Disulfiram
Dolasetron
Donepezil
Doxazosin
Doxepin
Doxorubicin
Doxycycline
Drotrecogin alfa
Enalapril
Enoxacin
Enoxaparin
Entacapone
Ephedrine
Eprosartan
Escitalopram
Esmolol
Estazolam
Estramustine
Estrogens
Etanercept
Ethacrynic acid
Ethambutol
Ethchlorvynol
Ethionamide
Ethosuximide
Ethotoin
Etodolac
Etoposide
Famotidine
Felbamate
Felodipine
Fenoprofen
Fentanyl

Floxuridine
Fluconazole
Flucytosine
Fluoxetine
Fluoxymesterone
Fluphenazine
Flurazepam
Flurbiprofen
Fluvastatin
Fluvoxamine
Fondaparinux
Frovatriptan
Furosemide
Gabapentin
Galantamine
Ganciclovir
Gentamicin
Glatiramer
Glipizide
Glyburide
Gold and gold compounds
Griseofulvin
Guanethidine
Guanfacine
Haloperidol
Heparin
Hepatitis B vaccine
Heroin
Horse chestnut (bark, flower,
  leaf, seed)
Hydralazine
Hydrochlorothiazide
Hydroflumethiazide
Hydroxychloroquine
Hydroxyurea
Hydroxyzine
Ibritumomab
Ibuprofen
Imipramine
Indapamide
Indomethacin
Insulin
Interferons, alfa-2
Ipodate
Isoniazid
Itraconazole
Ketoconazole
Ketoprofen
Ketorolac
Labetalol
Leflunomide
Leuprolide
Levamisole
Levobupivacaine
Levodopa
Levofloxacin
Lidocaine
Lincomycin
Lindane
Lisinopril
Lithium
Lomefloxacin
Loratadine
Lorazepam
Losartan
Lovastatin
Loxapine
Maprotiline
Mechlorethamine
Meclofenamate

Medroxyprogesterone
Mefenamic acid
Meloxicam
Melphalan
Mephenytoin
Mephobarbital
Meprobamate
Mercaptopurine
Metformin
Methadone
Methazolamide
Methicillin
Methimazole
Methotrexate
Methoxsalen
Methsuximide
Methyclothiazide
Methyldopa
Methylphenidate
Methyltestosterone
Metolazone
Metoprolol
Mexiletine
Miconazole
Minocycline
Mitomycin
Mitoxantrone
Nalidixic acid
Naltrexone
Naproxen
Naratriptan
Nifedipine
Nimodipine
Nitrofurantoin
Nitroglycerin
Nortriptyline
Octreotide
Ofloxacin
Omeprazole
Oral contraceptives
Oxaliplatin
Oxaprozin
Oxazepam
Oxcarbazepine
Oxytetracycline
Paclitaxel
Paroxetine
PEG-interferon alfa-2b
Penbutolol
Penicillamine
Penicillins
Pentagastrin
Pentamidine
Pentobarbital
Pentosan
Pentostatin
Pentoxifylline
Perindopril
Perphenazine
Phenindamine
Phenobarbital
Phensuximide
Phentermine
Phenytoin
Pindolol
Piperacillin
Pirbuterol
Piroxicam
Plicamycin
Polythiazide

Potassium iodide
Pravastatin
Prazepam
Procainamide
Procarbazine
Prochlorperazine
Promazine
Promethazine
Propafenone
Propranolol
Propylthiouracil
Protriptyline
Pyrazinamide
Pyridoxine
Pyrilamine
Pyrimethamine
Quazepam
Quinethazone
Quinidine
Quinine
Rabeprazole
Ramipril
Ranitidine
Rapacuronium
Reserpine
Reteplase
Rifampin
Rifapentine
Riluzole
Risperidone
Rivastigmine
Rofecoxib
Ropinirole
Salsalate
Secobarbital
Sertraline
Simvastatin
Sirolimus
Smallpox vaccine
Sparfloxacin
Spironolactone
Streptokinase
Streptomycin
Streptozocin
Sulfadiazine
Sulfadoxine
Sulfamethoxazole
Sulfasalazine
Sulfinpyrazone
Sulfisoxazole
Sulindac
Tacrine
Tacrolimus
Tamoxifen
Tartrazine
Temazepam
Tenecteplase
Tenofovir
Terfenadine
Tetracycline
Thalidomide
Thiamine
Thioguanine
Thiopental
Thioridazine
Ticarcillin
Ticlopidine
Timolol
Tinzaparin
Tizanidine

Tobramycin
Tolazamide
Tolbutamide
Tolmetin
Topiramate
Topotecan
Torsemide
Trazodone
Triamterene
Triazolam
Trichlormethiazide
Trifluoperazine
Trimeprazine
Trimethadione
Trimipramine
Tripelennamine
Triprolidine
Urokinase
Valacyclovir
Valproic acid
Vancomycin
Vasopressin
Verapamil
Verteporfin
Vinblastine
Voriconazole
Warfarin
Zaleplon
Zidovudine
Zolpidem
Zonisamide

Pustular Eruption
Acetazolamide
Allopurinol
Aminolevulinic acid
Amoxicillin
Ampicillin
Azithromycin
Bacampicillin
Bexarotene
Capsicum
Captopril
Carbamazepine
Cefaclor
Cefazolin
Cefoxitin
Cefuroxime
Cephalexin
Cephradine
Chloramphenicol
Chloroquine
Chlorpromazine
Clarithromycin
Clomipramine
Co-trimoxazole
Dactinomycin
Diltiazem
Disulfiram
Erythromycin
Felbamate
Fentanyl
Fluoxetine
Furosemide
Glatiramer
Heroin
Hydroxychloroquine
Imipenem/cilastatin
Infliximab
Isoniazid
Ivermectin

Lithium
Lomefloxacin
Minocycline
Nadolol
Naproxen
Nisoldipine
Norfloxacin
Olanzapine
Oxytetracycline
Paclitaxel
Perindopril
Phenobarbital
Phenytoin
Pyrimethamine
Quinidine
Ranitidine
Ritodrine
Simvastatin
Sparfloxacin
Streptomycin
Sulfadoxine
Sulfamethoxazole
Sulfasalazine
Sulfisoxazole
Tacrolimus
Terbinafine
Tetracycline
Venlafaxine
Zaleplon
Zonisamide

Pustular Psoriasis
Acetazolamide
Aminoglutethimide
Amiodarone
Amoxicillin
Ampicillin
Aspirin
Atenolol
Chloroquine
Cimetidine
Corticosteroids
Cyclosporine
Diclofenac
Diltiazem
Doxorubicin
Hydroxychloroquine
Indomethacin
Interferon beta-1b
Lithium
Methicillin
Morphine
Penicillins
Potassium iodide
Propranolol
Terbinafine

Radiation Recall
Acyclovir
Bleomycin
Buspirone
Capecitabine
Ciprofloxacin
Co-trimoxazole
Codeine
Dactinomycin
Docetaxel
Doxorubicin
Epirubicin
Etoposide
Fluorouracil
Gemcitabine

Hydroxyurea
Idarubicin
Interferons, alfa-2
Mercaptopurine
Methotrexate
Oxaliplatin
Paclitaxel
Piperacillin
Simvastatin
Sulfamethoxazole
Tamoxifen
Tobramycin
Vinblastine

Rash

Abacavir
Acarbose
Acebutolol
Acetaminophen
Acetazolamide
Acetohexamide
Acetylcysteine
Acitretin
Acyclovir
Adalimumab
Adapalene
Adenosine
Albendazole
Aldesleukin
Alemtuzumab
Alendronate
Alfentanil
Alitretinoin
Allopurinol
Almotriptan
Alprazolam
Alprostadil
Alteplase
Altretamine
Amantadine
Amifostine
Amikacin
Amiloride
Aminocaproic acid
Aminoglutethimide
Aminophylline
Amiodarone
Amitriptyline
Amlodipine
Amobarbital
Amoxapine
Amoxicillin
Amphotericin B
Ampicillin
Amprenavir
Amyl nitrite
Anagrelide
Anastrozole
Anistreplase
Anthrax vaccine
Aprepitant
Aprobarbital
Aprotinin
Arbutamine
Argatroban
Aripiprazole
Asparaginase
Aspartame
Aspirin
Atazanavir
Atenolol

Atomoxetine
Atorvastatin
Atovaquone
Atropine sulfate
Azatadine
Azathioprine
Azithromycin
Aztreonam
Bacampicillin
Baclofen
Balsalazide
Basiliximab
Benazepril
Bendroflumethiazide
Benzonatate
Benzphetamine
Benzthiazide
Benztropine
Bepridil
Betaxolol
Bexarotene
Bicalutamide
Biperiden
Bismuth
Bisoprolol
Black cohosh
Bortezomib
Botulinum toxin (A & B)
Bretylium
Bromocriptine
Brompheniramine
Bumetanide
Bupropion
Buspirone
Butabarbital
Butalbital
Butorphanol
Butterbur
Caffeine
Calcitonin
Candesartan
Captopril
Carbamazepine
Carbenicillin
Carboplatin
Carisoprodol
Carteolol
Carvedilol
Caspofungin
Cefaclor
Cefadroxil
Cefamandole
Cefazolin
Cefdinir
Cefditoren
Cefepime
Cefixime
Cefmetazole
Cefonicid
Cefoperazone
Cefotaxime
Cefotetan
Cefoxitin
Cefpodoxime
Cefprozil
Ceftazidime
Ceftibuten
Ceftizoxime
Ceftriaxone
Cefuroxime

Celecoxib
Cephalexin
Cephalothin
Cephapirin
Cephradine
Cetirizine
Cevimeline
Chasteberry
Chloral hydrate
Chlorambucil
Chloramphenicol
Chlordiazepoxide
Chlorhexidine
Chlormezanone
Chlorothiazide
Chlorotrianisene
Chlorpromazine
Chlorpropamide
Chlortetracycline
Chlorthalidone
Chlorzoxazone
Cholestyramine
Cidofovir
Cilostazol
Cimetidine
Cinoxacin
Ciprofloxacin
Cisatracurium
Cisplatin
Citalopram
Cladribine
Clarithromycin
Clemastine
Clindamycin
Clofazimine
Clofibrate
Clomiphene
Clomipramine
Clonazepam
Clonidine
Clopidogrel
Clorazepate
Cloxacillin
Clozapine
Co-trimoxazole
Codeine
Colchicine
Collagen
Corticosteroids
Creatine
Cromolyn
Cyclobenzaprine
Cyclophosphamide
Cycloserine
Cyclosporine
Cyclothiazide
Cyproheptadine
Cytarabine
Dacarbazine
Dalteparin
Danaparoid
Danazol
Dantrolene
Dapsone
Darbepoetin alfa
Daunorubicin
Deferoxamine
Delavirdine
Denileukin
Desipramine

Desmopressin
Dexchlorpheniramine
Dextroamphetamine
Diazepam
Diazoxide
Diclofenac
Dicloxacillin
Dicumarol
Dicyclomine
Didanosine
Diethylpropion
Diethylstilbestrol
Diflunisal
Digoxin
Diltiazem
Dimenhydrinate
Diphenhydramine
Dipyridamole
Dirithromycin
Disopyramide
Disulfiram
Docetaxel
Docusate
Dofetilide
Dolasetron
Domperidone
Dorzolamide
Doxacurium
Doxazosin
Doxepin
Doxorubicin
Doxycycline
Echinacea
Edrophonium
Efavirenz
Eflornithine
Eletriptan
Enalapril
Enfuvirtide
Enoxacin
Epirubicin
Epoetin alfa
Eprosartan
Ertapenem
Erythromycin
Escitalopram
Esmolol
Estazolam
Estramustine
Estrogens
Etanercept
Ethacrynic acid
Ethambutol
Ethchlorvynol
Ethionamide
Ethosuximide
Ethotoin
Etidronate
Etodolac
Etoposide
Exemestane
Famotidine
Felbamate
Felodipine
Fenofibrate
Fenoprofen
Fentanyl
Finasteride
Flavoxate
Flecainide

Floxuridine
Fluconazole
Flucytosine
Fludarabine
Flumazenil
Fluoxetine
Fluphenazine
Flurazepam
Flurbiprofen
Flutamide
Fluvastatin
Fluvoxamine
Folic acid
Fomepizole
Fondaparinux
Formoterol
Foscarnet
Fosfomycin
Fosinopril
Fosphenytoin
Frovatriptan
Fulvestrant
Furazolidone
Furosemide
Gabapentin
Ganciclovir
Gatifloxacin
Gefitinib
Gemcitabine
Gemfibrozil
Gemtuzumab
Gentamicin
Ginkgo biloba
Glatiramer
Glimepiride
Glipizide
Glucagon
Glyburide
Glycopyrrolate
Gold and gold compounds
Goserelin
Granisetron
Granulocyte colony-
    stimulating factor (GCSF)
Grepafloxacin
Griseofulvin
Guanabenz
Guanfacine
Haloperidol
Hawthorn (fruit, leaf, flower
    extract)
Henna
Heparin
Hepatitis B vaccine
Hydralazine
Hydrochlorothiazide
Hydrocodone
Hydroflumethiazide
Hydromorphone
Hydroxychloroquine
Hydroxyurea
Hydroxyzine
Hyoscyamine
Ibritumomab
Ibuprofen
Idarubicin
Imatinib
Imipenem/cilastatin
Imipramine
Indapamide

Indinavir
Indomethacin
Infliximab
Insulin glargine
Interferons, alfa-2
Ipodate
Ipratropium
Irbesartan
Irinotecan
Isocarboxazid
Isoniazid
Isoproterenol
Isosorbide
Isosorbide mononitrate
Isotretinoin
Isradipine
Itraconazole
Ivermectin
Kanamycin
Kava
Ketamine
Ketoconazole
Ketoprofen
Ketorolac
Ketotifen
Labetalol
Lamivudine
Lamotrigine
Lansoprazole
Latanoprost
Leflunomide
Letrozole
Leucovorin
Leuprolide
Levamisole
Levetiracetam
Levobetaxolol
Levobunolol
Levobupivacaine
Levodopa
Levofloxacin
Levothyroxine
Lidocaine
Lincomycin
Linezolid
Liothyronine
Lisinopril
Lithium
Lomefloxacin
Lomustine
Loperamide
Loracarbef
Loratadine
Lorazepam
Losartan
Lovastatin
Loxapine
Mafenide
Maprotiline
Mazindol
MDMA
Meadowsweet
Mebendazole
Mechlorethamine
Meclizine
Meclofenamate
Medroxyprogesterone
Mefenamic acid
Mefloquine
Meloxicam

Melphalan
Meperidine
Mephobarbital
Meprobamate
Mercaptopurine
Mesalamine
Mesna
Mesoridazine
Metaxalone
Metformin
Methadone
Methamphetamine
Methazolamide
Methenamine
Methicillin
Methimazole
Methocarbamol
Methohexital
Methotrexate
Methoxsalen
Methsuximide
Methyclothiazide
Methyldopa
Methylphenidate
Methysergide
Metoclopramide
Metolazone
Metoprolol
Metronidazole
Mexiletine
Mezlocillin
Miconazole
Midazolam
Midodrine
Miglitol
Milk thistle
Minocycline
Minoxidil
Mirtazapine
Misoprostol
Mitomycin
Mitotane
Mitoxantrone
Modafinil
Moexipril
Molindone
Montelukast
Moricizine
Morphine
Moxifloxacin
Mupirocin
Mycophenolate
Nabumetone
Nadolol
Nafarelin
Nafcillin
Nalidixic acid
Naloxone
Naltrexone
Naproxen
Naratriptan
Nateglinide
Nedocromil
Nefazodone
Nelfinavir
Neomycin
Nesiritide
Nevirapine
Niacin
Niacinamide

Nicardipine
Nicotine
Nifedipine
Nimodipine
Nisoldipine
Nitisinone
Nitrofurantoin
Nitroglycerin
Nizatidine
Norfloxacin
Nortriptyline
Nystatin
Octreotide
Ofloxacin
Olanzapine
Olmesartan
Olsalazine
Omeprazole
Ondansetron
Orlistat
Orphenadrine
Oxacillin
Oxaliplatin
Oxaprozin
Oxazepam
Oxcarbazepine
Oxybutynin
Oxycodone
Paclitaxel
Palivizumab
Pamidronate
Pancuronium
Pantoprazole
Papaverine
Paroxetine
PEG-interferon alfa-2b
Pegfilgrastim
Pemoline
Penbutolol
Penicillamine
Penicillins
Pentagastrin
Pentamidine
Pentazocine
Pentobarbital
Pentosan
Pentostatin
Pentoxifylline
Peppermint
Pergolide
Perindopril
Perphenazine
Phenazopyridine
Phenelzine
Phenindamine
Phenobarbital
Phensuximide
Phentermine
Phenytoin
Phytonadione
Pilocarpine
Pimozide
Pindolol
Pipecuronium
Piperacillin
Pirbuterol
Piroxicam
Polythiazide
Potassium iodide
Pramipexole

Pravastatin
Prazepam
Praziquantel
Prazosin
Primidone
Probenecid
Procainamide
Procarbazine
Prochlorperazine
Procyclidine
Progestins
Promazine
Promethazine
Propafenone
Propantheline
Propofol
Propoxyphene
Propranolol
Propylthiouracil
Protamine sulfate
Protriptyline
Psoralens
Pyrazinamide
Pyrilamine
Pyrimethamine
Quazepam
Quetiapine
Quinapril
Quinestrol
Quinethazone
Quinidine
Quinine
Quinupristin/dalfopristin
Rabeprazole
Raloxifene
Ramipril
Ranitidine
Rapacuronium
Rasburicase
Reserpine
Ribavirin
Rifabutin
Rifampin
Rifapentine
Rimantadine
Risedronate
Risperidone
Ritodrine
Ritonavir
Rituximab
Rivastigmine
Rofecoxib
Ropinirole
Salmeterol
Salsalate
Saquinavir
Scopolamine
Secobarbital
Selegiline
Selenium
Senna
Sertraline
Sibutramine
Sildenafil
Simvastatin
Sirolimus
Smallpox vaccine
Sotalol
Sparfloxacin
Spectinomycin

Spironolactone
Stavudine
Streptokinase
Streptomycin
Succinylcholine
Sucralfate
Sufentanil
Sulfadiazine
Sulfadoxine
Sulfamethoxazole
Sulfasalazine
Sulfinpyrazone
Sulfisoxazole
Sulindac
Sumatriptan
Tacrine
Tacrolimus
Tamoxifen
Tamsulosin
Tartrazine
Tea tree
Telmisartan
Temazepam
Temozolomide
Tenecteplase
Tenofovir
Terazosin
Terbinafine
Terfenadine
Teriparatide
Testosterone
Tetracycline
Thalidomide
Thiabendazole
Thiamine
Thioguanine
Thiopental
Thioridazine
Thiotepa
Thiothixene
Tiagabine
Ticarcillin
Ticlopidine
Timolol
Tinzaparin
Tiopronin
Tirofiban
Tizanidine
Tobramycin
Tocainide
Tolazamide
Tolazoline
Tolbutamide
Tolcapone
Tolmetin
Tolterodine
Topiramate
Torsemide
Tramadol
Trandolapril
Tranylcypromine
Trastuzumab
Trazodone
Treprostinil
Tretinoin
Triamterene
Triazolam
Trichlormethiazide
Trifluoperazine
Trihexyphenidyl

Trimeprazine
Trimethoprim
Trimetrexate
Trimipramine
Tripelennamine
Triprolidine
Troleandomycin
Trovafloxacin
Urofollitropin
Urokinase
Ursodiol
Valdecoxib
Valganciclovir
Valproic acid
Valrubicin
Valsartan
Vancomycin
Vasopressin
Venlafaxine
Verapamil
Verteporfin
Vidarabine
Vinblastine
Vincristine
Vinorelbine
Voriconazole
Warfarin
Willow bark
Yarrow
Zalcitabine
Zaleplon
Zidovudine
Ziprasidone
Zolmitriptan
Zolpidem
Zonisamide

Raynaud's Phenomenon
Acebutolol
Amphotericin B
Arsenic
Atenolol
Azathioprine
Betaxolol
Bisoprolol
Bleomycin
Bromocriptine
Carteolol
Cisplatin
Clonidine
Cyclosporine
Dopamine
Doxorubicin
Estrogens
Ethosuximide
Fluoxetine
Gemfibrozil
Hepatitis B vaccine
Interferon beta 1-a
Interferons, alfa-2
Labetalol
Methysergide
Metoprolol
Minocycline
Nadolol
Octreotide
Phentermine
Pindolol
Propofol
Propranolol
Sotalol

Spironolactone
Sulfasalazine
Sulindac
Sumatriptan
Thiothixene
Timolol
Vinblastine
Vincristine
Rhabdomyolysis
Acetaminophen
Aldesleukin
Aminocaproic acid
Aminophylline
Amitriptyline
Amobarbital
Amphotericin B
Aprobarbital
Aripiprazole
Atorvastatin
Azathioprine
Bupropion
Butabarbital
Butalbital
Caffeine
Carbamazepine
Cisplatin
Clarithromycin
Clofibrate
Clopidogrel
Clozapine
Co-trimoxazole
Cocaine
Colchicine
Creatine
Cyclophosphamide
Cyclosporine
Cytarabine
Dacarbazine
Danazol
Delavirdine
Dextroamphetamine
Diazepam
Diclofenac
Diltiazem
Diphenhydramine
Domperidone
Doxepin
Enflurane
Erythromycin
Esomeprazole
Fenofibrate
Fluoxetine
Fluphenazine
Fluvastatin
Gemfibrozil
Haloperidol
Halothane
Heroin
Ibuprofen
Interferon beta 1-a
Interferons, alfa-2
Isoniazid
Isotretinoin
Itraconazole
Lamivudine
Licorice
Lindane
Lithium
Lorazepam
Lovastatin

Loxapine
MDMA
Mephobarbital
Meprobamate
Methadone
Methamphetamine
Methohexital
Minocycline
Mirtazapine
Morphine
Naltrexone
Nefazodone
Nelfinavir
Norfloxacin
Olanzapine
Pancuronium
Pemoline
Pentamidine
Pentobarbital
Perphenazine
Phenelzine
Phenobarbital
Phenylpropanolamine
Phenytoin
Pravastatin
Primidone
Propofol
Protamine sulfate
Protriptyline
Rabeprazole
Risperidone
Ritonavir
Secobarbital
Simvastatin
Sodium oxybate
Succinylcholine
Tenecteplase
Terbutaline
Theophylline
Thiopental
Trandolapril
Valproic acid
Vasopressin
Verapamil
Vinblastine
Ziprasidone

Scleroderma
Aldesleukin
Arsenic
Azathioprine
Bleomycin
Bromocriptine
Cocaine
Dapsone
Diethylpropion
Docetaxel
Estrogens
Fosinopril
Heparin
Hepatitis B vaccine
Interferon beta-1b
Lithium
Medroxyprogesterone
Melphalan
Mephenytoin
Methoxsalen
Methysergide
Metoprolol
Paclitaxel
Penicillamine

Pentazocine
Phenytoin
Phytonadione
Psoralens
Selenium
Sotalol
Topotecan
Trioxsalen
Tryptophan
Valproic acid
Zileuton

Seborrhea
Acitretin
Aripiprazole
Atazanavir
Atorvastatin
Cetirizine
Clomipramine
Danazol
Delavirdine
Doxycycline
Fluoxetine
Fluoxymesterone
Fluphenazine
Flurbiprofen
Fluvoxamine
Foscarnet
Gemfibrozil
Indinavir
Interferon beta 1-a
Interferon beta-1b
Loxapine
Mesoridazine
Methyltestosterone
Minoxidil
Mirtazapine
Nafarelin
Naltrexone
Olanzapine
Oral contraceptives
Palivizumab
Pentostatin
Pergolide
Perphenazine
Prochlorperazine
Risperidone
Ritonavir
Tacrine
Testosterone
Thioridazine
Tolcapone
Topiramate
Trifluoperazine
Trovafloxacin
Valproic acid

Seborrheic Dermatitis
Buspirone
Chlorpromazine
Cimetidine
Ethionamide
Fluorouracil
Fluoxymesterone
Gold and gold compounds
Griseofulvin
Haloperidol
Interferons, alfa-2
Kava
Lithium
Methoxsalen
Methyldopa

Methyltestosterone
Psoralens
Saquinavir
Stanozolol
Testosterone
Thiothixene
Trioxsalen

Serum Sickness
Amobarbital
Amoxicillin
Ampicillin
Anistreplase
Aprobarbital
Asparaginase
Azathioprine
Bacampicillin
Bupropion
Carbamazepine
Carbenicillin
Cefaclor
Cefadroxil
Cefamandole
Cefazolin
Cefdinir
Cefditoren
Cefixime
Cefmetazole
Cefonicid
Cefoperazone
Cefotaxime
Cefotetan
Cefoxitin
Cefpodoxime
Cefprozil
Ceftazidime
Ceftibuten
Ceftizoxime
Ceftriaxone
Cefuroxime
Cephalexin
Cephalothin
Cephapirin
Cephradine
Ciprofloxacin
Cloxacillin
Co-trimoxazole
Cromolyn
Diclofenac
Dicloxacillin
Doxycycline
Fluoxetine
Furazolidone
Gatifloxacin
Glatiramer
Griseofulvin
Hepatitis B vaccine
Heroin
Ibuprofen
Indomethacin
Ipodate
Isoniazid
Itraconazole
Lincomycin
Loracarbef
Meclofenamate
Mephobarbital
Mercaptopurine
Methicillin
Methimazole
Metronidazole

Mezlocillin
Minocycline
Nafcillin
Nizatidine
Ofloxacin
Oxacillin
Oxaprozin
Penicillamine
Penicillins
Pentoxifylline
Phenytoin
Piperacillin
Piroxicam
Potassium iodide
Propranolol
Rifampin
Rituximab
Secobarbital
Sparfloxacin
Streptokinase
Sulfadiazine
Sulfamethoxazole
Sulfasalazine
Sulfisoxazole
Sulindac
Tartrazine
Terbinafine
Tetracycline
Ticarcillin
Ticlopidine
Tolmetin
Trovafloxacin
Verapamil

Sialorrhea
Acitretin
Almotriptan
Alprazolam
Amiodarone
Amitriptyline
Amoxapine
Aprepitant
Aripiprazole
Betaxolol
Bethanechol
Bupropion
Buspirone
Cetirizine
Cevimeline
Chlordiazepoxide
Citalopram
Clomipramine
Clonazepam
Clorazepate
Clozapine
Delavirdine
Diazepam
Diazoxide
Echinacea
Edrophonium
Eletriptan
Estazolam
Ethionamide
Etodolac
Fluoxetine
Fluphenazine
Flurazepam
Fluvoxamine
Frovatriptan
Gabapentin
Galantamine

Gentamicin	**Stevens–Johnson Syndrome**	Co-trimoxazole	Methazolamide
Guanabenz	Abacavir	Cyclophosphamide	Methicillin
Guanethidine	Acetaminophen	Cycloserine	Methotrexate
Guanfacine	Acetazolamide	Danazol	Methsuximide
Haloperidol	Acyclovir	Dapsone	Methyclothiazide
Ifosfamide	Albendazole	Delavirdine	Methyldopa
Imipenem/cilastatin	Allopurinol	Demeclocycline	Metolazone
Interferon beta-1b	Aminophylline	Diclofenac	Mexiletine
Irinotecan	Amiodarone	Dicloxacillin	Mezlocillin
Kanamycin	Amobarbital	Didanosine	Minocycline
Ketamine	Amoxicillin	Diflunisal	Minoxidil
Ketoprofen	Ampicillin	Diltiazem	Nabumetone
Lamotrigine	Amprenavir	Dipyridamole	Nafcillin
Levodopa	Aprepitant	Doxycycline	Naproxen
Lithium	Aprobarbital	Enalapril	Nevirapine
Loratadine	Arsenic	Enoxacin	Nifedipine
Lorazepam	Aspirin	Erythromycin	Nitrofurantoin
Maprotiline	Atropine sulfate	Ethambutol	Norfloxacin
Mefenamic acid	Azithromycin	Ethosuximide	Nystatin
Mesoridazine	Bacampicillin	Etidronate	Ofloxacin
Methohexital	Bleomycin	Etodolac	Omeprazole
Midazolam	Bupropion	Etoposide	Oral contraceptives
Mirtazapine	Butabarbital	Felbamate	Oxacillin
Modafinil	Butalbital	Fenoprofen	Oxaprozin
Molindone	Captopril	Fluconazole	Oxcarbazepine
Nabumetone	Carbamazepine	Fluoxetine	Pantoprazole
Nefazodone	Carbenicillin	Flurbiprofen	Penicillamine
Nicotine	Carvedilol	Fluvastatin	Penicillins
Olanzapine	Cefaclor	Fluvoxamine	Pentamidine
Oxazepam	Cefadroxil	Fosphenytoin	Pentobarbital
Pancuronium	Cefamandole	Furosemide	Phenobarbital
Pantoprazole	Cefazolin	Gabapentin	Phenolphthalein
Paroxetine	Cefdinir	Ganciclovir	Phensuximide
Pentoxifylline	Cefditoren	Gatifloxacin	Phenytoin
Perphenazine	Cefepime	Ginseng	Piperacillin
Physostigmine	Cefixime	Griseofulvin	Piroxicam
Pilocarpine	Cefmetazole	Hepatitis B vaccine	Pravastatin
Pimozide	Cefonicid	Hydrochlorothiazide	Promethazine
Potassium iodide	Cefoperazone	Hydrocodone	Propranolol
Pramipexole	Cefotaxime	Hydroxychloroquine	Pyrimethamine
Prazepam	Cefotetan	Ibuprofen	Quinine
Prochlorperazine	Cefoxitin	Imatinib	Ranitidine
Propofol	Cefpodoxime	Indapamide	Rifampin
Quazepam	Cefprozil	Indinavir	Ritonavir
Quetiapine	Ceftazidime	Indomethacin	Rituximab
Ramipril	Ceftibuten	Isoniazid	Saquinavir
Rapacuronium	Ceftizoxime	Itraconazole	Secobarbital
Reserpine	Ceftriaxone	Ketoprofen	Sertraline
Risperidone	Cefuroxime	Ketorolac	Simvastatin
Rivastigmine	Celecoxib	Lamotrigine	Smallpox vaccine
Ropinirole	Cephalexin	Leflunomide	Sparfloxacin
Selenium	Cephalothin	Levamisole	Streptomycin
Sertraline	Cephapirin	Levofloxacin	Sulfacetamide
Sodium oxybate	Cephradine	Lidocaine	Sulfadiazine
Succinylcholine	Chlorambucil	Lincomycin	Sulfadoxine
Tacrine	Chloramphenicol	Lisinopril	Sulfamethoxazole
Temazepam	Chlormezanone	Lomefloxacin	Sulfasalazine
Thiothixene	Chloroquine	Loracarbef	Sulfisoxazole
Tiagabine	Chlorothiazide	Lorazepam	Sulindac
Tobramycin	Chlorpropamide	Lovastatin	Terbinafine
Tolcapone	Chlorthalidone	Maprotiline	Tetracycline
Topiramate	Cimetidine	Mebendazole	Thalidomide
Trazodone	Cinoxacin	Mechlorethamine	Thiabendazole
Triazolam	Ciprofloxacin	Meclofenamate	Thiopental
Trovafloxacin	Cisplatin	Mefenamic acid	Tiagabine
Valproic acid	Clarithromycin	Mefloquine	Ticarcillin
Venlafaxine	Clindamycin	Meloxicam	Ticlopidine
Zaleplon	Clofibrate	Mephenytoin	Tocainide
Ziprasidone	Cloxacillin	Mephobarbital	Tolmetin
	Clozapine	Meprobamate	Torsemide

Trimethadione
Trimethoprim
Trovafloxacin
Valproic acid
Vancomycin
Verapamil
Vitamin A
Voriconazole
Zidovudine
Zonisamide

Stomatitis

Acetylcysteine
Acitretin
Aldesleukin
Alemtuzumab
Allopurinol
Amitriptyline
Amoxapine
Amoxicillin
Amphotericin B
Ampicillin
Anisindione
Aripiprazole
Arsenic
Atorvastatin
Azathioprine
Azelastine
Bacampicillin
Basiliximab
Benactyzine
Bismuth
Bleomycin
Bortezomib
Botulinum toxin (A & B)
Bupropion
Busulfan
Capecitabine
Carbamazepine
Carbenicillin
Carboplatin
Carmustine
Cefaclor
Cefdinir
Cefditoren
Celecoxib
Cetirizine
Cevimeline
Chloral hydrate
Chlorambucil
Chloramphenicol
Chlorhexidine
Chloroquine
Cidofovir
Ciprofloxacin
Citalopram
Clarithromycin
Clofibrate
Clomipramine
Cloxacillin
Co-trimoxazole
Corticosteroids
Cyclobenzaprine
Cyclophosphamide
Cyclosporine
Cytarabine
Dacarbazine
Dactinomycin
Daunorubicin
Delavirdine
Desipramine

Diclofenac
Dicloxacillin
Diflunisal
Docetaxel
Doxepin
Doxorubicin
Eletriptan
Enalapril
Enoxacin
Epirubicin
Ertapenem
Esomeprazole
Ethionamide
Etidronate
Etodolac
Etoposide
Fenoprofen
Floxuridine
Fludarabine
Fluorouracil
Fluoxetine
Fluoxymesterone
Flurbiprofen
Fluvoxamine
Foscarnet
Frovatriptan
Furosemide
Gabapentin
Gatifloxacin
Gemcitabine
Gemtuzumab
Gentamicin
Ginkgo biloba
Glatiramer
Gold and gold compounds
Granulocyte colony-
    stimulating factor (GCSF)
Grepafloxacin
Griseofulvin
Hydroxychloroquine
Hydroxyurea
Ibuprofen
Idarubicin
Ifosfamide
Imipramine
Indomethacin
Interferons, alfa-2
Ipratropium
Irinotecan
Ketoprofen
Ketorolac
Lamotrigine
Lansoprazole
Leflunomide
Levamisole
Lidocaine
Lincomycin
Lithium
Lomustine
Loratadine
Lovastatin
Maprotiline
Meclofenamate
Meloxicam
Melphalan
Mephenytoin
Meprobamate
Mercaptopurine
Methenamine
Methicillin

Methotrexate
Methyltestosterone
Metronidazole
Mezlocillin
Mirtazapine
Mitomycin
Moxifloxacin
Mupirocin
Nabumetone
Nafcillin
Naproxen
Nefazodone
Nevirapine
Nicotine
Norfloxacin
Nortriptyline
Olanzapine
Olsalazine
Oxacillin
Oxaliplatin
Oxaprozin
Oxcarbazepine
Paclitaxel
Pamidronate
Pantoprazole
Paroxetine
Pegfilgrastim
Penicillamine
Penicillins
Pentostatin
Peppermint
Piroxicam
Plicamycin
Pravastatin
Procarbazine
Propolis
Protriptyline
Pyrilamine
Quetiapine
Quinupristin/dalfopristin
Rabeprazole
Rifampin
Riluzole
Rimantadine
Risperidone
Rivastigmine
Ropinirole
Saquinavir
Sertraline
Sildenafil
Sirolimus
Sparfloxacin
Streptokinase
Streptomycin
Sulfadiazine
Sulfadoxine
Sulfamethoxazole
Sulfasalazine
Sulfisoxazole
Sulindac
Tacrine
Terbinafine
Terfenadine
Testosterone
Thioguanine
Thiotepa
Tiagabine
Ticarcillin
Tiopronin
Tocainide

Tolmetin
Topiramate
Topotecan
Tramadol
Trastuzumab
Triazolam
Trimeprazine
Trimetrexate
Trimipramine
Tripelennamine
Trovafloxacin
Ursodiol
Valdecoxib
Valproic acid
Venlafaxine
Vinblastine
Vincristine
Vinorelbine
Voriconazole
Zalcitabine
Zaleplon
Zonisamide

Stomatodynia

Alemtuzumab
Amoxicillin
Anisindione
Bacampicillin
Benztropine
Biperiden
Carbenicillin
Dicloxacillin
Erythromycin
Ethionamide
Floxuridine
Garlic
Griseofulvin
Lithium
Methicillin
Mezlocillin
Nafcillin
Oxacillin
Piperacillin
Potassium iodide
Ticarcillin
Triamterene
Vitamin A

Telangiectasia

Amlodipine
Carmustine
Corticosteroids
Estrogens
Felodipine
Hydroxychloroquine
Hydroxyurea
Interferon beta 1-a
Interferons, alfa-2
Isocarboxazid
Isotretinoin
Lisinopril
Lithium
Methotrexate
Methysergide
Nifedipine
Oral contraceptives
Phenelzine
Progestins
Thiothixene

Tendinitis

Adalimumab
Adenosine

Amlodipine
Aripiprazole
Celecoxib
Cevimeline
Ciprofloxacin
Eprosartan
Gatifloxacin
Grepafloxacin
Indinavir
Levobetaxolol
Levofloxacin
Methotrexate
Minoxidil
Moxifloxacin
Norfloxacin
Orlistat
Risedronate
Rofecoxib
Valdecoxib

Tendon Rupture
Ciprofloxacin
Enoxacin
Gatifloxacin
Grepafloxacin
Leflunomide
Levofloxacin
Lomefloxacin
Mirtazapine
Moxifloxacin
Norfloxacin
Ofloxacin
Sparfloxacin
Trovafloxacin

Toxic Epidermal Necrolysis (TEN)
Acebutolol
Acetaminophen
Acetazolamide
Aldesleukin
Allopurinol
Alprostadil
Amifostine
Aminosalicylate sodium
Amiodarone
Amobarbital
Amoxapine
Amoxicillin
Ampicillin
Asparaginase
Aspirin
Atenolol
Atorvastatin
Azathioprine
Aztreonam
Betaxolol
Butabarbital
Butalbital
Captopril
Carbamazepine
Carbenicillin
Cefaclor
Cefadroxil
Cefamandole
Cefazolin
Cefdinir
Cefditoren
Cefepime
Cefmetazole
Cefonicid
Cefoperazone

Cefotaxime
Cefotetan
Cefoxitin
Cefpodoxime
Cefprozil
Ceftazidime
Ceftibuten
Ceftizoxime
Ceftriaxone
Cefuroxime
Celecoxib
Cephalexin
Cephalothin
Cephapirin
Cephradine
Chlorambucil
Chloramphenicol
Chlormezanone
Chloroquine
Chlorothiazide
Chlorpromazine
Chlorpropamide
Chlorthalidone
Cimetidine
Cinoxacin
Ciprofloxacin
Cladribine
Clarithromycin
Clindamycin
Clofibrate
Co-trimoxazole
Codeine
Colchicine
Cyclophosphamide
Cyclosporine
Cytarabine
Dactinomycin
Dapsone
Deferoxamine
Demeclocycline
Dextroamphetamine
Diclofenac
Dicloxacillin
Diflunisal
Diltiazem
Diphenhydramine
Dipyridamole
Disulfiram
Docetaxel
Doxycycline
Enalapril
Enoxacin
Ephedrine
Erythromycin
Ethambutol
Etidronate
Etodolac
Famotidine
Felbamate
Fenofibrate
Fenoprofen
Fluconazole
Fluoxetine
Fluphenazine
Flurbiprofen
Flutamide
Fluvastatin
Fluvoxamine
Foscarnet
Fosphenytoin

Furosemide
Gatifloxacin
Gentamicin
Gold and gold compounds
Grepafloxacin
Griseofulvin
Heparin
Heroin
Hydrochlorothiazide
Hydrocodone
Hydroxychloroquine
Ibuprofen
Imipenem/cilastatin
Indapamide
Indomethacin
Isoniazid
Isotretinoin
Ketoprofen
Ketorolac
Lamotrigine
Leflunomide
Levofloxacin
Lisinopril
Lovastatin
Meclofenamate
Mefenamic acid
Mefloquine
Meloxicam
Meperidine
Mephenytoin
Meprobamate
Mercaptopurine
Methamphetamine
Methazolamide
Methicillin
Methotrexate
Methyldopa
Metolazone
Metoprolol
Metronidazole
Mezlocillin
Nabumetone
Nadolol
Nafcillin
Nalidixic acid
Naproxen
Neomycin
Nevirapine
Nifedipine
Nitrofurantoin
Norfloxacin
Ofloxacin
Omeprazole
Oxacillin
Oxaprozin
Oxazepam
Oxcarbazepine
Pantoprazole
Papaverine
Paroxetine
Penicillamine
Penicillins
Pentamidine
Pentazocine
Pentobarbital
Phenobarbital
Phenolphthalein
Phenytoin
Pindolol
Piperacillin

Piroxicam
Plicamycin
Pravastatin
Primidone
Procarbazine
Prochlorperazine
Promethazine
Propranolol
Pyridoxine
Pyrimethamine
Quinidine
Quinine
Ranitidine
Reserpine
Rifampin
Simvastatin
Smallpox vaccine
Sparfloxacin
Streptomycin
Streptozocin
Sulfacetamide
Sulfadiazine
Sulfadoxine
Sulfamethoxazole
Sulfasalazine
Sulfisoxazole
Sulindac
Terbinafine
Terconazole
Tetracycline
Thalidomide
Thiabendazole
Thiopental
Thioridazine
Ticarcillin
Timolol
Tiopronin
Tolbutamide
Tolmetin
Trimethoprim
Trovafloxacin
Valdecoxib
Valproic acid
Vancomycin
Vinorelbine
Voriconazole
Zidovudine
Zonisamide

Urticaria
Acarbose
Acebutolol
Acetaminophen
Acetazolamide
Acetohexamide
Acetylcysteine
Acitretin
Acyclovir
Albendazole
Albuterol
Aldesleukin
Alefacept
Alemtuzumab
Alfentanil
Allopurinol
Alprazolam
Alprostadil
Alteplase
Amantadine
Amikacin
Amiloride

Aminocaproic acid
Aminoglutethimide
Aminophylline
Aminosalicylate sodium
Amiodarone
Amitriptyline
Amlodipine
Amobarbital
Amoxapine
Amoxicillin
Amphotericin B
Ampicillin
Anagrelide
Anisindione
Anistreplase
Anthrax vaccine
Aprepitant
Aprobarbital
Aprotinin
Aripiprazole
Arsenic
Asparaginase
Aspartame
Aspirin
Atazanavir
Atenolol
Atomoxetine
Atorvastatin
Atracurium
Atropine sulfate
Azatadine
Azathioprine
Azithromycin
Aztreonam
Bacampicillin
Baclofen
Benactyzine
Benazepril
Bendroflumethiazide
Benzphetamine
Benzthiazide
Benztropine
Betaxolol
Biperiden
Bisacodyl
Bisoprolol
Bleomycin
Botulinum toxin (A & B)
Brinzolamide
Bromocriptine
Bumetanide
Bupropion
Buspirone
Busulfan
Butabarbital
Butalbital
Butorphanol
Caffeine
Calcitonin
Capsicum
Captopril
Caraway
Carbamazepine
Carbenicillin
Carboplatin
Carisoprodol
Cefaclor
Cefadroxil
Cefamandole
Cefazolin

Cefdinir
Cefditoren
Cefepime
Cefixime
Cefmetazole
Cefonicid
Cefoperazone
Cefotaxime
Cefotetan
Cefoxitin
Cefpodoxime
Cefprozil
Ceftazidime
Ceftibuten
Ceftizoxime
Ceftriaxone
Cefuroxime
Celecoxib
Cephalexin
Cephalothin
Cephapirin
Cephradine
Cetirizine
Chasteberry
Chloral hydrate
Chlorambucil
Chloramphenicol
Chlordiazepoxide
Chlorhexidine
Chlormezanone
Chloroquine
Chlorothiazide
Chlorotrianisene
Chlorpromazine
Chlorpropamide
Chlorthalidone
Chlorzoxazone
Cholestyramine
Cidofovir
Cilostazol
Cimetidine
Cinoxacin
Ciprofloxacin
Cisplatin
Citalopram
Clarithromycin
Clemastine
Clidinium
Clindamycin
Clofazimine
Clofibrate
Clomiphene
Clomipramine
Clonazepam
Clonidine
Clopidogrel
Clorazepate
Clotrimazole
Cloxacillin
Clozapine
Co-trimoxazole
Cocaine
Codeine
Colchicine
Colestipol
Collagen
Corticosteroids
Cromolyn
Cyanocobalamin
Cyclamate

Cyclobenzaprine
Cyclophosphamide
Cycloserine
Cyclosporine
Cyclothiazide
Cyproheptadine
Cytarabine
Dacarbazine
Dactinomycin
Danazol
Dantrolene
Dapsone
Darbepoetin alfa
Daunorubicin
Deferoxamine
Delavirdine
Demeclocycline
Denileukin
Desipramine
Dexchlorpheniramine
Dextroamphetamine
Diazepam
Diazoxide
Diclofenac
Dicloxacillin
Dicumarol
Dicyclomine
Didanosine
Diethylpropion
Diethylstilbestrol
Diflunisal
Digoxin
Diltiazem
Dimenhydrinate
Diphenhydramine
Diphenoxylate
Dipyridamole
Dirithromycin
Disopyramide
Disulfiram
Docetaxel
Dolasetron
Domperidone
Donepezil
Dopamine
Doxacurium
Doxazosin
Doxepin
Doxorubicin
Doxycycline
Echinacea
Edrophonium
Efavirenz
Eletriptan
Enalapril
Enoxacin
Enoxaparin
Ephedrine
Epinephrine
Epirubicin
Epoetin alfa
Ertapenem
Erythromycin
Esmolol
Esomeprazole
Estazolam
Estramustine
Estrogens
Etanercept
Ethacrynic acid

Ethambutol
Ethchlorvynol
Ethionamide
Ethosuximide
Etidronate
Etodolac
Etoposide
Famotidine
Felbamate
Felodipine
Fenofibrate
Fenoprofen
Fentanyl
Finasteride
Flavoxate
Flecainide
Fluconazole
Flucytosine
Flumazenil
Fluorouracil
Fluoxetine
Fluoxymesterone
Fluphenazine
Flurazepam
Flurbiprofen
Flutamide
Fluvastatin
Fluvoxamine
Folic acid
Formoterol
Foscarnet
Fosinopril
Furazolidone
Furosemide
Gabapentin
Ganciclovir
Garlic
Gatifloxacin
Gemfibrozil
Gemifloxacin
Gentamicin
Glatiramer
Glimepiride
Glipizide
Glucagon
Glyburide
Glycopyrrolate
Gold and gold compounds
Goserelin
Granisetron
Granulocyte colony-
    stimulating factor (GCSF)
Grepafloxacin
Griseofulvin
Guanethidine
Guanfacine
Haloperidol
Halothane
Henna
Heparin
Hepatitis B vaccine
Heroin
Hydralazine
Hydrochlorothiazide
Hydrocodone
Hydroflumethiazide
Hydromorphone
Hydroxychloroquine
Hydroxyurea
Hydroxyzine

Hyoscyamine	Mercaptopurine	Oral contraceptives	Pyrimethamine
Ibritumomab	Mesalamine	Orphenadrine	Quazepam
Ibuprofen	Mesna	Oxacillin	Quinacrine
Idarubicin	Mesoridazine	Oxaliplatin	Quinapril
Imipenem/cilastatin	Metaxalone	Oxaprozin	Quinestrol
Imipramine	Metformin	Oxazepam	Quinethazone
Indapamide	Methadone	Oxybutynin	Quinidine
Indinavir	Methamphetamine	Oxycodone	Quinine
Indomethacin	Methantheline	Oxytetracycline	Quinupristin/dalfopristin
Infliximab	Methazolamide	Paclitaxel	Rabeprazole
Insulin	Methenamine	Pantoprazole	Ramipril
Interferon beta 1-a	Methicillin	Pantothenic acid	Ranitidine
Interferon beta-1b	Methimazole	Papaverine	Rapacuronium
Interferons, alfa-2	Methocarbamol	Paroxetine	Reserpine
Ipodate	Methohexital	PEG-interferon alfa-2b	Ribavirin
Ipratropium	Methotrexate	Pegfilgrastim	Riboflavin
Irbesartan	Methoxsalen	Penicillamine	Rifabutin
Isoniazid	Methsuximide	Penicillins	Rifampin
Isoproterenol	Methyclothiazide	Pentagastrin	Rifapentine
Isotretinoin	Methyldopa	Pentamidine	Risperidone
Isradipine	Methylphenidate	Pentazocine	Ritodrine
Itraconazole	Methyltestosterone	Pentobarbital	Ritonavir
Ivermectin	Methysergide	Pentosan	Rituximab
Kanamycin	Metoclopramide	Pentostatin	Rivastigmine
Ketoconazole	Metolazone	Pentoxifylline	Rofecoxib
Ketoprofen	Metoprolol	Pergolide	Ropinirole
Ketorolac	Metronidazole	Perphenazine	Saccharin
Labetalol	Mexiletine	Phendimetrazine	Salmeterol
Lamivudine	Mezlocillin	Phenelzine	Salsalate
Lamotrigine	Miconazole	Phenindamine	Saquinavir
Lansoprazole	Midazolam	Phenobarbital	Scopolamine
Leflunomide	Milk thistle	Phenolphthalein	Secobarbital
Leucovorin	Minocycline	Phentermine	Secretin
Leuprolide	Minoxidil	Phenytoin	Sermorelin
Levamisole	Mitomycin	Phytonadione	Sertraline
Levobunolol	Mitotane	Pilocarpine	Sildenafil
Levobupivacaine	Mitoxantrone	Pimozide	Simvastatin
Levodopa	Moexipril	Pindolol	Smallpox vaccine
Levofloxacin	Montelukast	Pipecuronium	Sotalol
Levothyroxine	Moricizine	Piperacillin	Sparfloxacin
Lidocaine	Moxifloxacin	Piroxicam	Spectinomycin
Lincomycin	Nabumetone	Polythiazide	Spironolactone
Lindane	Nadolol	Potassium iodide	Stanozolol
Liothyronine	Nafarelin	Pravastatin	Streptokinase
Lisinopril	Nafcillin	Prazepam	Streptomycin
Lithium	Nalbuphine	Praziquantel	Succinylcholine
Lomefloxacin	Nalidixic acid	Prazosin	Sucralfate
Loperamide	Naloxone	Primaquine	Sufentanil
Loracarbef	Naproxen	Primidone	Sulfadiazine
Loratadine	Naratriptan	Probenecid	Sulfadoxine
Lorazepam	Nefazodone	Procainamide	Sulfamethoxazole
Losartan	Nelfinavir	Procarbazine	Sulfasalazine
Lovastatin	Neomycin	Prochlorperazine	Sulfisoxazole
Loxapine	Niacin	Procyclidine	Sulindac
Maprotiline	Nicardipine	Progestins	Sumatriptan
Marihuana	Nicotine	Promazine	Tacrine
Mazindol	Nifedipine	Promethazine	Tacrolimus
Mebendazole	Nisoldipine	Propafenone	Tamoxifen
Mechlorethamine	Nitrofurantoin	Propantheline	Tartrazine
Meclizine	Nitroglycerin	Propofol	Temazepam
Meclofenamate	Nizatidine	Propoxyphene	Tenecteplase
Medroxyprogesterone	Norfloxacin	Propranolol	Terbinafine
Mefenamic acid	Nortriptyline	Propylthiouracil	Terbutaline
Mefloquine	Nystatin	Protamine	Terfenadine
Meloxicam	Octreotide	Protamine sulfate	Testosterone
Melphalan	Ofloxacin	Protriptyline	Tetracycline
Meperidine	Olanzapine	Pseudoephedrine	Thalidomide
Mephenytoin	Olsalazine	Psoralens	Thiabendazole
Mephobarbital	Omeprazole	Pyrazinamide	Thiamine
Meprobamate	Ondansetron	Pyrilamine	Thimerosal

Thiopental
Thioridazine
Thiotepa
Thiothixene
Tiagabine
Ticarcillin
Ticlopidine
Timolol
Tinzaparin
Tiopronin
Tirofiban
Tizanidine
Tobramycin
Tolazamide
Tolazoline
Tolbutamide
Tolcapone
Tolmetin
Topiramate
Torsemide
Tramadol
Tranylcypromine
Trazodone
Triamterene
Triazolam
Trichlormethiazide
Trifluoperazine
Trihexyphenidyl
Trimeprazine
Trimethadione
Trimipramine
Tripelennamine
Triprolidine
Troleandomycin
Trovafloxacin
Urofollitropin
Urokinase
Ursodiol
Valdecoxib
Valproic acid
Valsartan
Vancomycin
Vasopressin
Venlafaxine
Verapamil
Verteporfin
Vinblastine
Vincristine
Vitamin E
Voriconazole
Warfarin
Yarrow
Zalcitabine
Zanamivir
Zidovudine
Ziprasidone
Zolmitriptan
Zolpidem
Zonisamide

Vaginal Candidiasis
Acitretin
Ampicillin
Aripiprazole
Aztreonam
Botulinum toxin (A & B)
Cefamandole
Cefdinir
Cefditoren
Cefixime
Cefpodoxime

Ceftazidime
Celecoxib
Chlorotrianisene
Delavirdine
Diethylstilbestrol
Dirithromycin
Enoxacin
Ertapenem
Estrogens
Lamotrigine
Leflunomide
Lomefloxacin
Metronidazole
Norfloxacin
Paroxetine
Riluzole
Ropinirole
Sibutramine
Sparfloxacin
Tizanidine
Valdecoxib
Venlafaxine

Vaginitis
Acyclovir
Amitriptyline
Amoxapine
Amoxicillin
Azithromycin
Aztreonam
Bacampicillin
Bupropion
Carbenicillin
Cefaclor
Cefadroxil
Cefamandole
Cefazolin
Cefdinir
Cefditoren
Cefepime
Cefixime
Cefmetazole
Cefonicid
Cefotaxime
Cefpodoxime
Cefprozil
Ceftazidime
Ceftibuten
Ceftizoxime
Ceftriaxone
Cefuroxime
Celecoxib
Cephalexin
Cephapirin
Cephradine
Cetirizine
Cevimeline
Chlorotrianisene
Cilostazol
Ciprofloxacin
Clomipramine
Cloxacillin
Dicloxacillin
Dirithromycin
Donepezil
Doxycycline
Eletriptan
Enoxacin
Ertapenem
Esomeprazole
Fenofibrate

Fluvoxamine
Fosfomycin
Fulvestrant
Gatifloxacin
Gemifloxacin
Glatiramer
Gold and gold compounds
Grepafloxacin
Imipramine
Interferon beta 1-a
Lamotrigine
Leuprolide
Levofloxacin
Lincomycin
Lomefloxacin
Loratadine
Medroxyprogesterone
Methicillin
Mezlocillin
Mifepristone
Mirtazapine
Moxifloxacin
Nafarelin
Nafcillin
Nefazodone
Nisoldipine
Nortriptyline
Nystatin
Octreotide
Ofloxacin
Olanzapine
Orlistat
Oxacillin
Oxcarbazepine
Pantoprazole
Paroxetine
Pentostatin
Perindopril
Piperacillin
Quinupristin/dalfopristin
Raloxifene
Rivastigmine
Sertraline
Sparfloxacin
Tetracycline
Tiagabine
Ticarcillin
Tolcapone
Topiramate
Trovafloxacin
Valproic acid
Venlafaxine
Zaleplon
Zileuton
Zolpidem

Vasculitis
Acebutolol
Acetaminophen
Acyclovir
Allopurinol
Amiloride
Aminosalicylate sodium
Amiodarone
Amitriptyline
Amlodipine
Amoxapine
Amoxicillin
Ampicillin
Anistreplase
Aspartame

Aspirin
Atenolol
Azathioprine
Bendroflumethiazide
Benzthiazide
Bexarotene
Bismuth
Bromocriptine
Bumetanide
Busulfan
Butabarbital
Butalbital
Captopril
Carbamazepine
Carbenicillin
Caspofungin
Cefdinir
Celecoxib
Cevimeline
Chloramphenicol
Chlordiazepoxide
Chloroquine
Chlorothiazide
Chlorpromazine
Chlorpropamide
Chlorthalidone
Cimetidine
Ciprofloxacin
Citalopram
Cladribine
Clarithromycin
Clindamycin
Clomipramine
Clorazepate
Clozapine
Co-trimoxazole
Cocaine
Colchicine
Corticosteroids
Cromolyn
Cyclophosphamide
Cyclosporine
Cyclothiazide
Cyproheptadine
Cytarabine
Dacarbazine
Delavirdine
Desipramine
Diazepam
Diclofenac
Dicloxacillin
Didanosine
Diflunisal
Digoxin
Diltiazem
Diphenhydramine
Disulfiram
Doxepin
Doxycycline
Efavirenz
Enalapril
Ephedrine
Erythromycin
Estrogens
Etanercept
Ethacrynic acid
Etodolac
Famotidine
Fluoxetine
Flurbiprofen

Fluvastatin
Fosinopril
Furosemide
Gatifloxacin
Gemcitabine
Gemfibrozil
Gentamicin
Ginkgo biloba
Glucagon
Glyburide
Gold and gold compounds
Granulocyte colony-
    stimulating factor (GCSF)
Griseofulvin
Guanethidine
Heparin
Hepatitis B vaccine
Heroin
Hydralazine
Hydrochlorothiazide
Hydroflumethiazide
Hydroxychloroquine
Hydroxyurea
Ibuprofen
Imipenem/cilastatin
Imipramine
Indapamide
Indinavir
Indomethacin
Infliximab
Insulin
Interferon beta-1b
Interferons, alfa-2
Isoniazid
Isotretinoin
Itraconazole
Ketoconazole
Leflunomide
Levamisole
Levofloxacin
Lisinopril
Lithium
Lomefloxacin
Lovastatin
Maprotiline
Meclofenamate
Mefenamic acid
Mefloquine
Meloxicam
Melphalan
Meprobamate
Mercaptopurine
Mesalamine
Metformin
Methazolamide
Methicillin
Methimazole
Methotrexate
Methoxsalen
Methyldopa
Methylphenidate
Metolazone
Metronidazole
Mezlocillin
Minocycline
Mitotane
Nabumetone
Nafcillin
Naproxen
Nelfinavir

Nicotine
Nifedipine
Nizatidine
Norfloxacin
Nortriptyline
Ofloxacin
Omeprazole
Oxacillin
Oxaprozin
Oxytetracycline
Paroxetine
Penicillamine
Penicillins
Pentamidine
Pentobarbital
Pergolide
Phenobarbital
Phenytoin
Phytonadione
Piperacillin
Piroxicam
Polythiazide
Potassium iodide
Pravastatin
Procainamide
Propylthiouracil
Protriptyline
Psoralens
Pyridoxine
Pyrimethamine
Quinapril
Quinethazone
Quinidine
Quinine
Ramipril
Ranitidine
Rifampin
Ritodrine
Rofecoxib
Simvastatin
Sotalol
Sparfloxacin
Spironolactone
Streptokinase
Streptomycin
Sulfamethoxazole
Sulfasalazine
Sulfisoxazole
Sulindac
Tamoxifen
Tartrazine
Terbutaline
Tetracycline
Thalidomide
Thiamine
Thioridazine
Ticarcillin
Ticlopidine
Tocainide
Torsemide
Trazodone
Triamterene
Trichlormethiazide
Trimethadione
Trioxsalen
Triptorelin
Trovafloxacin
Valproic acid
Vancomycin
Verapamil

Warfarin
Zafirlukast
Zidovudine
Vesicular Eruption
Acyclovir
Aminolevulinic acid
Amoxicillin
Amphotericin B
Aripiprazole
Atazanavir
Bexarotene
Carbenicillin
Carteolol
Clofibrate
Clonidine
Clotrimazole
Colchicine
Delavirdine
Denileukin
Dicloxacillin
Dicumarol
Enoxaparin
Estrogens
Etodolac
Fenoprofen
Gatifloxacin
Ginkgo biloba
Glatiramer
Glyburide
Grepafloxacin
Ibuprofen
Imiquimod
Interferon beta-1b
Juniper
Letrozole
Lincomycin
Meclofenamate
Melphalan
Naproxen
Nefazodone
Olanzapine
Penicillamine
Penicillins
Piperacillin
Piroxicam
Propylthiouracil
Pyridoxine
Tiagabine
Tretinoin
Venlafaxine
Verteporfin
Vinblastine
Warfarin
Zaleplon
Ziprasidone
Zonisamide
Xerosis
Acebutolol
Acitretin
Adapalene
Aldesleukin
Alitretinoin
Alprazolam
Amiloride
Amlodipine
Amoxapine
Amphotericin B
Apraclonidine
Aripiprazole
Atazanavir

Atenolol
Atorvastatin
Atropine sulfate
Benztropine
Betaxolol
Bexarotene
Bicalutamide
Bisoprolol
Bleomycin
Bupropion
Buspirone
Busulfan
Capecitabine
Captopril
Carteolol
Celecoxib
Cetirizine
Cevimeline
Chlorpromazine
Chlortetracycline
Cidofovir
Cilostazol
Cimetidine
Citalopram
Clindamycin
Clofazimine
Clofibrate
Clomipramine
Delavirdine
Desipramine
Dexmedetomidine
Diazoxide
Dicyclomine
Disopyramide
Docetaxel
Doxazosin
Eflornithine
Eletriptan
Escitalopram
Estazolam
Estramustine
Famotidine
Floxuridine
Fluorouracil
Fluoxetine
Fluphenazine
Flurbiprofen
Fluvastatin
Fluvoxamine
Foscarnet
Gemfibrozil
Glatiramer
Glycopyrrolate
Gold and gold compounds
Grepafloxacin
Hydroxyurea
Hyoscyamine
Imipramine
Indinavir
Interferons, alfa-2
Isotretinoin
Kava
Ketoconazole
Labetalol
Lamotrigine
Leflunomide
Leuprolide
Levamisole
Levobetaxolol
Levothyroxine

Liothyronine
Lithium
Loratadine
Losartan
Mechlorethamine
Medroxyprogesterone
Mesalamine
Mesoridazine
Methantheline
Methoxsalen
Metolazone
Metoprolol
Mexiletine
Midodrine
Minoxidil
Mirtazapine
Modafinil
Moricizine
Moxifloxacin
Mupirocin
Nabumetone
Nadolol
Naratriptan
Nefazodone
Niacin
Nisoldipine
Nitisinone
Nizatidine
Nortriptyline
Olanzapine
Omeprazole
Orlistat
Oxaliplatin
Oxybutynin
Pantoprazole
Paroxetine
PEG-interferon alfa-2b
Penicillamine
Pentamidine
Pentostatin
Pergolide
Perindopril
Perphenazine
Pindolol
Prochlorperazine
Procyclidine
Promazine
Propantheline
Propranolol
Protriptyline
Quetiapine
Rabeprazole
Ranitidine
Risperidone
Ritonavir
Rofecoxib
Saquinavir
Scopolamine
Sertraline
Sparfloxacin
Spironolactone
Sulfasalazine
Tacrine
Tamoxifen
Thalidomide
Thioridazine
Tiagabine
Timolol
Tizanidine
Tolterodine

Topiramate
Tretinoin
Trifluoperazine
Trihexyphenidyl
Trioxsalen
Urofollitropin
Ursodiol
Valdecoxib
Venlafaxine
Vitamin A
Voriconazole
Zalcitabine
Zaleplon
Zonisamide

Xerostomia
Acebutolol
Acetazolamide
Acitretin
Albendazole
Albuterol
Aldesleukin
Almotriptan
Alprazolam
Alprostadil
Amantadine
Amifostine
Amiloride
Amitriptyline
Amlodipine
Amoxapine
Amoxicillin
Amphotericin B
Anastrozole
Apraclonidine
Arbutamine
Aripiprazole
Atomoxetine
Atropine sulfate
Azatadine
Azathioprine
Azelastine
Bacampicillin
Baclofen
Balsalazide
Benactyzine
Bendroflumethiazide
Benzphetamine
Benztropine
Bepridil
Betaxolol
Bexarotene
Bicalutamide
Biperiden
Bismuth
Bisoprolol
Botulinum toxin (A & B)
Brimonidine
Brinzolamide
Bromocriptine
Brompheniramine
Buclizine
Bumetanide
Bupropion
Buspirone
Butorphanol
Cabergoline
Caffeine
Captopril
Carbamazepine
Carbenicillin

Carisoprodol
Carteolol
Carvedilol
Cefditoren
Cefixime
Ceftibuten
Celecoxib
Cetirizine
Cevimeline
Chloramphenicol
Chlordiazepoxide
Chlormezanone
Chlorpheniramine
Chlorpromazine
Chlortetracycline
Cidofovir
Cimetidine
Ciprofloxacin
Citalopram
Clarithromycin
Clemastine
Clidinium
Clomipramine
Clonazepam
Clonidine
Clorazepate
Clozapine
Codeine
Cromolyn
Cyclobenzaprine
Cyproheptadine
Delavirdine
Desipramine
Desloratadine
Dexchlorpheniramine
Dextroamphetamine
Diazepam
Diazoxide
Diclofenac
Dicloxacillin
Dicyclomine
Didanosine
Diethylpropion
Diflunisal
Dihydroergotamine
Dihydrotachysterol
Diltiazem
Dimenhydrinate
Diphenhydramine
Diphenoxylate
Dirithromycin
Disopyramide
Donepezil
Doxazosin
Doxepin
Dronabinol
Efavirenz
Enalapril
Enoxacin
Entacapone
Ephedra
Ephedrine
Epinephrine
Eprosartan
Ergocalciferol
Escitalopram
Esmolol
Esomeprazole
Estazolam
Ethacrynic acid

Ethionamide
Etodolac
Famotidine
Felbamate
Felodipine
Fenoprofen
Fentanyl
Flavoxate
Flecainide
Fluconazole
Flucytosine
Flumazenil
Fluoxetine
Fluphenazine
Flurazepam
Flurbiprofen
Fluvoxamine
Formoterol
Foscarnet
Fosfomycin
Fosinopril
Fosphenytoin
Frovatriptan
Furosemide
Gabapentin
Galantamine
Ganciclovir
Gemifloxacin
Glatiramer
Glycopyrrolate
Grepafloxacin
Griseofulvin
Guanabenz
Guanadrel
Guanethidine
Guanfacine
Haloperidol
Hydrochlorothiazide
Hydrocodone
Hydromorphone
Hydroxyzine
Hyoscyamine
Ibuprofen
Imipramine
Indapamide
Indinavir
Indomethacin
Interferon beta 1-a
Interferon beta-1b
Interferons, alfa-2
Ipratropium
Isocarboxazid
Isoetharine
Isoniazid
Isoproterenol
Isosorbide dinitrate
Isotretinoin
Isradipine
Itraconazole
Ketoprofen
Ketorolac
Labetalol
Lamotrigine
Lansoprazole
Leflunomide
Levodopa
Levofloxacin
Lisinopril
Lithium
Lomefloxacin

Loperamide	Niacin	Prochlorperazine	Terbutaline
Loratadine	Nicardipine	Procyclidine	Terfenadine
Lorazepam	Nicotine	Promazine	Thalidomide
Losartan	Nifedipine	Promethazine	Thiabendazole
Lovastatin	Nisoldipine	Propafenone	Thioguanine
Loxapine	Nitrofurantoin	Propantheline	Thioridazine
Maprotiline	Nitroglycerin	Propofol	Thiothixene
Mazindol	Nizatidine	Propoxyphene	Tiagabine
MDMA	Norfloxacin	Propranolol	Ticarcillin
Mebendazole	Nortriptyline	Protriptyline	Timolol
Mecamylamine	Octreotide	Pseudoephedrine	Tiopronin
Meclizine	Ofloxacin	Pyrilamine	Tizanidine
Meclofenamate	Olanzapine	Pyrimethamine	Tocainide
Mefenamic acid	Omeprazole	Quazepam	Tolcapone
Meloxicam	Ondansetron	Quetiapine	Tolmetin
Meperidine	Orphenadrine	Quinapril	Tolterodine
Meprobamate	Oxacillin	Quinethazone	Topiramate
Mesoridazine	Oxaliplatin	Rabeprazole	Torsemide
Methadone	Oxazepam	Ramipril	Tramadol
Methamphetamine	Oxcarbazepine	Reserpine	Trandolapril
Methantheline	Oxybutynin	Riluzole	Tranylcypromine
Methazolamide	Oxycodone	Rimantadine	Trazodone
Methicillin	Pantoprazole	Risperidone	Tretinoin
Methyldopa	Papaverine	Ritonavir	Triamterene
Methylphenidate	Paricalcitol	Rivastigmine	Triazolam
Metoclopramide	Paroxetine	Rizatriptan	Trichlormethiazide
Metolazone	Penicillins	Rofecoxib	Trifluoperazine
Metronidazole	Pentamidine	Ropinirole	Trihexyphenidyl
Mexiletine	Pentazocine	Saquinavir	Trimeprazine
Mezlocillin	Pentoxifylline	Scopolamine	Trimipramine
Midodrine	Pergolide	Selegiline	Tripelennamine
Mirtazapine	Perindopril	Sertraline	Triprolidine
Modafinil	Perphenazine	Sibutramine	Trovafloxacin
Moexipril	Phendimetrazine	Sildenafil	Unoprostone
Molindone	Phenelzine	Sotalol	Valdecoxib
Moricizine	Phenindamine	Sparfloxacin	Valproic acid
Morphine	Phenobarbital	Spironolactone	Valsartan
Moxifloxacin	Phenoxybenzamine	St John's wort	Venlafaxine
Mupirocin	Phentermine	Sucralfate	Verapamil
Nabumetone	Phenylpropanolamine	Sulfasalazine	Vitamin A
Nadolol	Pimozide	Sulindac	Voriconazole
Nafcillin	Pirbuterol	Sumatriptan	Zalcitabine
Nalbuphine	Piroxicam	Tacrine	Zaleplon
Naltrexone	Pramipexole	Tamoxifen	Ziprasidone
Naproxen	Prazepam	Telmisartan	Zolmitriptan
Nedocromil	Prazosin	Temazepam	Zolpidem
Nefazodone	Procarbazine	Terazosin	Zonisamide

DESCRIPTION OF THE 31 MOST COMMON REACTION PATTERNS

Acanthosis nigricans

Acanthosis nigricans (AN) is a process characterized by a soft, velvety, brown or grayish-black thickening of the skin that is symmetrically distributed over the axillae, neck, inguinal areas and other body folds.

While most cases of AN are seen in obese and prepubertal children, it can occur as a marker for various endocrinopathies as well as in female patients with elevated testosterone levels, irregular menses, and hirsutism.

It is frequently a concomitant of an underlying malignant condition, principally an adenocarcinoma of the intestinal tract.

Acneform lesions

Acneform eruptions are inflammatory follicular reactions that resemble acne vulgaris and that are manifested clinically as papules or pustules. They are monomorphic reactions, have a monomorphic appearance, and are found primarily on the upper parts of the body. Unlike acne vulgaris, there are rarely comedones present. Consider a drug-induced acneform eruption if:

- The onset is sudden

- There is a worsening of existing acne lesions

- The extent is considerable from the outset

- The appearance is monomorphic

- The localization is unusual for acne as, for example, when the distal extremities are involved

- The patient's age is unusual for regular acne

- There is an exposure to a potentially responsible drug.

The most common drugs responsible for acneform eruptions are: ACTH, androgenic hormones, anticonvulsants (hydantoin derivatives, phenobarbital, trimethadione), corticosteroids, danazol, disulfiram, halogens (bromides, chlorides, iodides), lithium, oral contraceptives, tuberculostatics (ethionamide, isoniazid, rifampin), vitamins B_2, B_6, and B_{12}.

Acute generalized exanthematous pustulosis

Arising on the face or intertriginous areas, acute generalized exanthematous pustulosis (AGEP) is characterized by a rapidly evolving, widespread, scarlatiniform eruption covered with hundreds of small superficial pustules.

Often accompanied by a high fever, AGEP is most frequently associated with penicillin and macrolide antibiotics, and usually occurs within 24 hours of the drug exposure.

Alopecia

Many drugs have been reported to occasion hair loss. Commonly appearing as a diffuse alopecia, it affects women more frequently than men and is limited in most instances to the scalp. Axillary and pubic hairs are rarely affected except with anticoagulants.

The hair loss from cytostatic agents, which is dose-dependent and begins about 2 weeks after the onset of therapy, is a result of the interruption of the anagen (growing) cycle of hair. With other drugs the hair loss does not begin until 2–5 months after the medication has been begun. With cholesterol-lowering drugs, diffuse alopecia is a result of interference with normal keratinization.

The scalp is normal and the drug-induced alopecia is almost always reversible within 1–3 months after the therapy has been discontinued. The regrown hair is frequently depigmented and occasionally more curly.

The most frequent offenders are cytostatic agents and anticoagulants, but hair loss can occur with a variety of common drugs, including hormones, anticonvulsants, amantadine, amiodarone, captopril, cholesterol-lowering drugs, cimetidine, colchicine, etretinate, isotretinoin, ketoconazole, heavy metals, lithium, penicillamine, valproic acid, and propranolol.

Angioedema

Angioedema is a term applied to a variant of urticaria in which the subcutaneous tissues, rather than the dermis, are mainly involved.

Also known as Quincke's edema, giant urticaria, and angioneurotic edema, this acute, evanescent, skin-colored, circumscribed edema usually affects the most distensible tissues: the lips, eyelids, earlobes, and genitalia. It can also affect the mucous membranes of the tongue, mouth, and larynx.

Symptoms of angioedema, frequently unilateral, asymmetrical and non-pruritic, last for an hour or two but can persist for 2–5 days.

The etiological factors associated with angioedema are as varied as that of urticaria (which see).

Aphthous stomatitis

Aphthous stomatitis – also known as canker sores – is a common disease of the oral mucous membranes.

Arising as tiny, discrete or grouped, papules or vesicles, these painful lesions develop into small (2–5 mm in diameter), round, shallow ulcerations having a grayish, yellow base surrounded by a thin red border.

Located predominantly over the labial and buccal mucosae, these aphthae heal without scarring in 10–14 days. Recurrences are common.

Black hairy tongue (lingua villosa nigra)

Black hairy tongue (BHT) represents a benign hyperplasia of the filiform papillae of the anterior two-thirds of the tongue.

These papillary elongations, usually associated with black, brown, or yellow pigmentation attributed to the overgrowth of pigment-producing bacteria, may be as long as 2 cm.

Occurring only in adults, BHT has been associated with the administration of oral antibiotics, poor dental hygiene, and excessive smoking.

Bullous eruptions

Bullous and vesicular drug eruptions are diseases in which blisters and vesicles occur as a complication of the administration of drugs. Blisters are a well-known manifestation of cutaneous reactions to drugs.

In many types of drug reactions, bullae and vesicles may be found in addition to other manifestations. Bullae are usually noted in erythema multiforme, Stevens–Johnson syndrome, toxic epidermal necrolysis, fixed eruptions when very intense, urticaria, vasculitis, porphyria cutanea tarda, and phototoxic reactions (from furosemide and nalidixic acid). Tense, thick-walled bullae can be seen in bromoderma and iododerma as well as in barbiturate overdosage.

Common drugs that cause bullous eruptions and bullous pemphigoid are: nadalol, penicillamine, piroxicam, psoralens, rifampin, clonidine, furosemide, diclofenac, mefenamic acid, bleomycin, and others.

Erythema multiforme and Stevens–Johnson syndrome

Erythema multiforme is a relatively common, acute, self-limited, inflammatory reaction pattern that is often associated with a preceding herpes simplex or mycoplasma infection. Other causes are associated with connective tissue disease, physical agents, X-ray therapy, pregnancy and internal malignancies, to mention a few. In 50% of the cases, no cause can be found. In a recent prospective study of erythema multiforme, only 10% were drug related.

The eruption rapidly occurs over a period of 12 to 24 hours. In about half the cases there are prodromal symptoms of an upper respiratory infection accompanied by fever, malaise, and varying degrees of muscular and joint pains.

Clinically, bluish-red, well-demarcated, macular, papular, or urticarial lesions, as well as the classical 'iris' or 'target lesions', sometimes with central vesicles, bullae, or purpura, are distributed preferentially over the distal extremities, especially over the dorsa of the hands and extensor aspects of the forearms. Lesions tend to spread peripherally and may involve the palms and trunk as well as the mucous membranes of the mouth and genitalia. Central healing and overlapping lesions often lead to arciform, annular and gyrate patterns. Lesions appear over the course of a week or 10 days and resolve over the next 2 weeks.

The Stevens–Johnson syndrome (erythema multiforme major), a severe and occasionally fatal variety of erythema multiforme, has an abrupt onset and is accompanied by any or all of the following: fever, myalgia, malaise, headache, arthralgia, ocular involvement, with occasional bullae and erosions covering less than 10% of the body surface. Painful stomatitis is an early and conspicuous symptom. Hemorrhagic bullae may appear over the lips, mouth and genital mucous membranes. Patients are often acutely ill with high fever. The course from eruption to the healing of the lesions may extend up to 6 weeks.

The following drugs have been most often associated with erythema multiforme and Stevens–Johnson syndrome: allopurinol, lamotrigine phenytoin, barbiturates, carbamazepine, estrogens/progestins, gold, NSAIDs, penicillamine, sulfonamides, tetracycline, and tolbutamide.

Erythema nodosum

Erythema nodosum is a cutaneous reaction pattern characterized by erythematous, tender or painful subcutaneous nodules commonly distributed over the anterior aspect of the lower legs, and occasionally elsewhere.

More common in young women, erythema nodosum is often associated with increased estrogen levels as occurs during pregnancy and with the ingestion of oral contraceptives. It is also an occasional manifestation of streptococcal infection, sarcoidosis, secondary syphilis, tuberculosis, certain deep fungal infections, Hodgkin's disease, leukemia, ulcerative colitis, and radiation therapy and is often preceded by fever, fatigue, arthralgia, vomiting, and diarrhea.

The incidence of erythema nodosum due to drugs is low and it is impossible to distinguish clinically between erythema nodosum due to drugs and that caused by other factors.

Some of the drugs that are known to occasion erythema nodosum are: antibiotics, estrogens, amiodarone, gold, NSAIDs, oral contraceptives, sulfonamides, and opiates.

Exanthems

Exanthems, commonly resembling viral rashes, represent the most common type of cutaneous drug eruption. Described as maculopapular or morbilliform eruptions, these flat, barely raised, erythematous patches, from one to several millimeters in diameter, are usually bilateral and symmetrical. They commonly begin on the head and neck or upper torso and progress downward to the limbs. They may present or develop into confluent areas and may be accompanied by pruritus and a mild fever.

The exanthems caused by drugs can be classified as either:

- Morbilliform eruptions: fingernail-sized erythematous patches

- Scarlatiniform eruptions: punctate, pinpoint, or pinhead-sized lesions in erythematous areas that have a tendency to coalesce. Circumoral pallor and the subsequent appearance of scaling may also be noted.

Maculopapular drug eruptions usually fade with desquamation and, occasionally, postinflammatory hyperpigmentation, in about 2 weeks. They invariably recur on rechallenge.

Exanthems often have a sudden onset during the first 2 weeks of administration, except for semisynthetic penicillins that frequently develop after the first 2 weeks following the initial dose.

The drugs most commonly associated with exanthems are: amoxicillin, ampicillin, bleomycin, captopril, carbamazepine, chlorpromazine, co-trimoxazole, gold, nalidixic acid, naproxen, phenytoin, penicillamine, and piroxicam.

Exfoliative dermatitis

Exfoliative dermatitis is a rare but serious reaction pattern that is characterized by erythema, pruritus and scaling over the entire body (erythroderma).

Drug-induced exfoliative dermatitis usually begins a few weeks or longer following the administration of a culpable drug. Beginning as erythematous, edematous patches, often on the face, it spreads to involve the entire integument. The skin becomes swollen and scarlet and may ooze a straw-colored fluid; this is followed in a few days by desquamation.

High fever, severe malaise and chills, along with enlargement of lymph nodes, often coexist with the cutaneous changes.

One of the most dangerous of all reaction patterns, exfoliative dermatitis can be accompanied by any or all of the following: hypothermia, fluid and electrolyte loss, cardiac failure, and gastrointestinal hemorrhage. Death may supervene if the drug is continued after the onset of the eruption. Secondary infection often complicates the course of the disease. Once the active dermatitis has receded, hyperpigmentation as well as loss of hair and nails may ensue. The following drugs, among others, can bring about exfoliative dermatitis: barbiturates, captopril, carbamazepine, cimetidine, furosemide, gold, isoniazid, lithium, nitrofurantoin, NSAIDs, penicillamine, phenytoin, pyrazolons, quinidine, streptomycin, sulfonamides, and thiazides.

Fixed eruptions

A fixed eruption is an unusual hypersensitivity reaction characterized by one or more well demarcated erythematous plaques that recur at the same cutaneous (or mucosal) site or sites each time exposure to the offending agent occurs. The sizes of the lesions vary from a few millimeters to as much as 20 centimeters in diameter. Almost any drug that is ingested, injected, inhaled, or inserted into the body can trigger this skin reaction.

The eruption typically begins as a sharply marginated, solitary edematous papule or plaque – occasionally surmounted by a large bulla – which usually develops 30 minutes to 8 hours following the administration of a drug. If the offending agent is not promptly eliminated, the inflammation intensifies, producing a dusky red, violaceous or brown patch that may crust, desquamate, or blister within 7 to 10 days. The lesions are rarely pruritic. Favored sites are the hands, feet, face, and genitalia – especially the glans penis.

The reason for the specific localization of the skin lesions in a fixed drug eruption is unknown. The offending drug cannot be detected at the skin site. Certain drugs cause a fixed eruption at specific sites, for example, tetracycline and ampicillin often elicit a fixed eruption on the penis, whereas aspirin usually causes skin lesions on the face, limbs and trunk.

Common causes of fixed eruptions are: ampicillin, aspirin, barbiturates, dapsone, metronidazole, NSAIDs, oral contraceptives, phenolphthalein, phenytoin, quinine, sulfonamides, and tetracyclines.

Gingival hyperplasia

Gingival hyperplasia, a common, undesirable, non-allergic drug reaction begins as a diffuse swelling of the interdental papillae.

Particularly prevalent with phenytoin therapy, gingival hyperplasia begins about 3 months after the onset of therapy, and occurs in 30 to 70% of patients receiving it. The severity of the reaction is dose-dependent and children and young adults are more frequently affected. The most severe cases are noted in young women.

In many cases, gingival hyperplasia is accompanied by painful and bleeding gums. There is often superimposed secondary bacterial gingivitis. This can be so extensive that the teeth of the maxilla and mandible are completely overgrown.

While it is characteristically a side effect of hydantoin derivatives, it may occur during the administration of phenobarbital, nifedipine, diltiazem and other medications.

Lichenoid (lichen planus-like) eruptions

Lichenoid eruptions are so called because of their resemblance to lichen planus, a papulosquamous disorder that characteristically presents as multiple, discrete, violaceous, flat-topped papules, often polygonal in shape and which are extremely pruritic.

Not infrequently, lichenoid lesions appear weeks or months following exposure to the responsible drug. As a rule, the symptoms begin to recede a few weeks following the discontinuation of the drug.

Common drug causes of lichenoid eruptions are: anti-malarials, beta-blockers, chlorpropamide, furosemide, gold, methyldopa, phenothiazines, quinidine, thiazides, and tolazamide.

Lupus erythematosus

A reaction, clinically and pathologically resembling idiopathic systemic lupus erythematosus (SLE), has been reported in association with a large variety of drugs. There is some evidence that drug-induced SLE, invariably accompanied by a positive ANA reaction with 90% having antihistone antibodies, may have a genetically determined basis. These symptoms of SLE, a relatively benign form of lupus, recede within days or weeks following the discontinuation of the responsible drug. Skin lesions occur in about 20% of cases. Drugs cause fewer than 8% of all cases of systemic LE.

The following drugs have been commonly associated with inducing, aggravating or unmasking SLE: beta-blockers, carbamazepine, chlorpromazine, estrogens, griseofulvin, hydralazine, isoniazid (INH), lithium, methyldopa, minoxidil, oral contraceptives, penicillamine, phenytoin (diphenyl-hydantoin), procainamide, propylthiouracil, quinidine, and testosterone.

Neuroleptic Malignant Syndrome (NMS)

NMS is a rare, potentially life-threatening neuroleptic-induced movement disorder characterized by fever, muscular rigidity, altered mental status, and autonomic dysfunction.

NMS is a result of complex neurochemical changes induced by neuroleptics, particularly haloperidol and trifluoperazine – during the initial stages of treatment.

Diagnostic criteria for NMS include administration of neuroleptics; hyperthermia (>38°C) (in 100% of patients); extreme muscle rigidity (90%), described as 'lead-pipe', is a core feature of NMS; and diaphoresis (60%). Other signs and symptoms include mental status change, tremor, tachycardia, incontinence, labile blood pressure, metabolic acidosis, CPK elevation, sialorrhea, and leukocytosis.

Almost all classes of drugs, primarily antipsychotics that induce dopamine-2 receptor blockade – dopamine agonists and levodopa – have been associated with NMS.

Onycholysis

Onycholysis, the painless separation of the nail plate from the nail bed, is one of the most common nail disorders.

The unattached portion, which is white and opaque, usually begins at the free margin and proceeds proximally, causing part or most of the nail plate to become separated. The attached, healthy portion of the nail, by contrast, is pink and translucent.

Pemphigus vulgaris

Pemphigus vulgaris (PV) is a rare, serious, acute or chronic, blistering disease involving the skin and mucous membranes.

Characterized by thin-walled, easily ruptured, flaccid bullae that are seen to arise on normal or erythematous skin and over mucous membranes, the lesions of PV appear initially in the mouth (in about 60% of the cases) and then spread, after weeks or months, to involve the axillae and groin, the scalp, face and neck. The lesions may become generalized.

Because of their fragile roofs, the bullae rupture leaving painful erosions and crusts may develop principally over the scalp.

Photosensitivity

A photosensitive reaction is a chemically induced change in the skin that makes an individual unusually sensitive to electromagnetic radiation (light). On absorbing light of a specific wavelength, an oral, injected or topical drug may be chemically altered to produce a reaction ranging from macules and papules, vesicles and bullae, edema, urticaria, or an acute eczematous reaction.

Any eruption that is prominent on the face, the dorsa of the hands, the 'V' of the neck, and the presternal area should suggest an adverse reaction to light. The distribution is the key to the diagnosis.

Initially the eruption, which consists of erythema, edema, blisters, weeping and desquamation, involves the forehead, rims of the ears, the nose, the malar eminences and cheeks, the sides and back of the neck, the extensor surfaces of the forearms and the dorsa of the hands. These reactions commonly spare the shaded areas: those under the chin, under the nose, behind the ears and inside the fold of the upper eyelids. There is usually a sharp cut-off at the site of jewelry and at clothing margins. All light-exposed areas need not be affected equally.

There are two main types of photosensitive reactions: the phototoxic and the photoallergic reaction.

Phototoxic reactions, the most common type of drug-induced photosensitivity, resemble an exaggerated sunburn and occur within 5 to 20 hours after the skin has been exposed to a photosensitizing substance and light of the proper wavelength and intensity. It is not a form of allergy – prior sensitization is not required – and, theoretically, could occur in anyone given enough drug and light. Phototoxic reactions are dose-dependent both for drug and sunlight. Patients with phototoxicity reactions are commonly sensitive to ultraviolet A (UVA radiation), the so-called 'tanning rays' at 320–400 nm. Phototoxic reactions may cause onycholysis, as the nailbed is particularly susceptible because of its lack of melanin protection.

Patients with a true photoallergy (the interaction of drug, light and the immune system), a less common form of drug-induced photosensitivity, are often sensitive to UVB radiation, the so-called 'burning rays' at 290–320 nm. Photoallergic reactions, unlike phototoxic responses, represent an immunologic change and require a latent period of from 24 to 48 hours during which sensitization occurs. They are not dose-related.

If the photosensitizer acts internally, it is a photodrug reaction; if it acts externally, it is photocontact dermatitis.

Drugs that are likely to cause phototoxic reactions are: amiodarone, nalidixic acid, various NSAIDs, phenothiazines (especially chlorpromazine), and tetracyclines (particularly demeclocycline).

Photoallergic reactions may occur as a result of exposure to systemically-administered drugs such as griseofulvin, NSAIDs, phenothiazines, quinidine, sulfonamides, sulfonylureas, and thiazide diuretics as well as to external agents such as para-aminobenzoic acid (found in sunscreens), bithionol (used in soaps and cosmetics), paraphenylenediamine, and others.

Pigmentation

Drug-induced pigmentation on the skin, hair, nails, and mucous membranes is a result of either melanin synthesis, increased lipofuscin synthesis, or post-inflammatory pigmentation.

Color changes, which can be localized or widespread, can also be a result of a deposition of bile pigments (jaundice), exogenous metal compounds, and direct deposition of elements such as carotene or quinacrine.

Post-inflammatory pigmentation can follow a variety of drug-induced inflammatory cutaneous reactions; fixed eruptions are known to leave a residual pigmentation that can persist for months.

The following is a partial list of those drugs that can cause various pigmentary changes: anticonvulsants, antimalarials, cytostatics, hormones, metals, tetracyclines, phenothiazine tranquilizers, psoralens, amiodarone, etc.

Pityriasis rosea-like eruptions

Pityriasis rosea, commonly mistaken for ringworm, is a unique disorder that usually begins as a single, large, round or oval pinkish patch known as the 'mother' or 'herald' patch. The most common sites for this solitary lesion are the chest, the back, or the abdomen. This is followed in about 2 weeks by a blossoming of small, flat, round or oval, scaly patches of similar color, each with a central collarette scale, usually distributed in a Christmas tree pattern over the trunk and, to a lesser degree, the extremities. This eruption seldom itches and usually limits itself to areas from the neck to the knees.

While the etiology of idiopathic pityriasis rosea is unknown, we do know that various medications have been reported to give rise to this friendly disorder. These are: barbiturates, beta-blockers, bismuth, captopril, clonidine, gold, griseofulvin, isotretinoin, labetalol, meprobamate, metronidazole, penicillin, and tripelennamine.

In drug-induced pityriasis rosea, the 'herald patch' is usually absent, and the eruption will often not follow the classic pattern.

Pruritus

Generalized itching, without any visible signs, is one of the least common adverse reactions to drugs. More frequently than not, drug-induced itching – moderate or severe – is fairly generalized.

For most drugs it is not known in what way they elicit pruritus; some drugs can cause itching directly or indirectly through cholestasis. Pruritus may develop by different pathogenetic mechanisms: allergic, pseudoallergic (histamine release), neurogenic, by vasodilatation, cholestatic effect, and others.

A partial list of those drugs that can cause pruritus are as follows: aspirin, NSAIDs, penicillins, sulfonamides, chloroquine, ACE inhibitors, amiodarone, nicotinic acid derivatives, lithium, bleomycin, tamoxifen, interferons, gold, penicillamine, methoxsalen, isotretinoin, etc.

Psoriasis

Many drugs, as a result of their pharmacological action, have been implicated in the precipitation or exacerbation of psoriasis or psoriasiform eruptions.

Psoriasis is a common, chronic, papulosquamous disorder of unknown etiology with characteristic histopathological features and many biochemical, physiological, and immunological abnormalities.

Drugs that can precipitate psoriasis are, among others, beta-blockers and lithium. Drugs that are reported to aggravate psoriasis are antimalarials, beta-blockers, lithium, NSAIDs, quinidine, and photosensitizing drugs. The effect and extent of these drug-induced psoriatic eruptions are dose-dependent.

Purpura

Purpura, a result of hemorrhage into the skin, can be divided into thrombocytopenic purpura and non-thrombocytopenic purpura (vascular purpura). Both thrombocytopenic and vascular purpura may be due to drugs, and most of the drugs producing purpura may do so by giving rise to vascular damage and thrombocytopenia. In both types of purpura, allergic or toxic (nonallergic) mechanisms may be involved.

Some drugs combine with platelets to form an antigen, stimulating formation of antibody to the platelet–drug combination. Thus, the drug appears to act as a hapten; subsequent antigen–antibody reaction causes platelet destruction leading to thrombocytopenia.

The purpuric lesions are usually more marked over the lower portions of the body, notably the legs and dorsal aspects of the feet in ambulatory patients.

Other drug-induced cutaneous reactions – erythema multiforme, erythema nodosum, fixed eruption, necrotizing vasculitis, and others – can have a prominent purpuric component.

A whole host of drugs can give rise to purpura, the most common being: NSAIDs, thiazide diuretics, phenothiazines, cytostatics, gold, penicillamine, hydantoins, thiouracils, and sulfonamides.

Raynaud's phenomenon

Raynaud's phenomenon is the paroxysmal, cold-induced constriction of small arteries and arterioles of the fingers and, less often, the toes.

Occurring more frequently in women, Raynaud's phenomenon is characterized by blanching, pallor, and cyanosis. In severe cases, secondary changes may occur: thinning and ridging of the nails, telangiectases of the nail folds, and, in the later stages, sclerosis and atrophy of the digits.

Rhabdomyolysis

Rhabdomyolysis is the breakdown of muscle fibers, the result of skeletal muscle injury, that leads to the release of potentially toxic intracellular contents into the plasma. The causes are diverse: muscle trauma from vigorous exercise, electrolyte imbalance, extensive thermal burns, crush injuries, infections, various toxins and drugs, and a host of other factors.

Rhabdomyolysis can result from direct muscle injury by myotoxic drugs such as cocaine, heroin and alcohol. About 10 to 40 percent of patients with rhabdomyolysis develop acute renal failure.

The classic triad of symptoms of rhabdomyolysis is muscle pain, weakness and dark urine. Most frequently, the involved muscle groups are those of the back and lower calves. The primary diagnostic indicator of this syndrome is significantly elevated serum creatine phosphokinase.

Some of the drugs that have been reported to cause rhabdomyolysis are salicylates, amphotericin, quinine, statin drugs, SSRIs, theophylline, amphetamines, and others.

Toxic epidermal necrolysis (TEN)

Also known as Lyell's syndrome, toxic epidermal necrolysis is a rare, serious, acute exfoliative, bullous eruption of the skin and mucous membranes that usually develops as a reaction to diverse drugs. TEN can also be a result of a bacterial or viral infection and can develop after radiation therapy or vaccinations.

In the drug-induced form of TEN, a morbilliform eruption accompanied by large red, tender areas of the skin will develop shortly after the drug has been administered. This progresses rapidly to blistering, and a widespread exfoliation of the epidermis develops dramatically over a very short period accompanied by high fever. The hairy parts of the body are usually spared. The mucous membranes and eyes are often involved.

The clinical picture resembles an extensive second-degree burn; the patient is acutely ill. Fatigue, vomiting, diarrhea and angina are prodromal symptoms. In a few hours the condition becomes grave.

TEN is a medical emergency and unless the offending agent is discontinued immediately, the outcome may be fatal in the course of a few days.

Drugs that are the most common cause of TEN are: allopurinol, ampicillin, amoxicillin, carbamazepine, NSAIDs, phenobarbital, pentamidine, phenytoin (diphenylhydantoin), pyrazolones, and sulfonamides.

Urticaria

Urticaria induced by drugs is, after exanthems, the second most common type of drug reaction. Urticaria, or hives, is a vascular reaction of the skin characterized by pruritic, erythematous wheals. These welts – or wheals – caused by localized edema, can vary in size from one millimeter in diameter to large palm-sized swellings, favor the covered areas (trunk, buttocks, chest), and are, more often than not, generalized. Urticaria usually develops within 36 hours following the administration of the responsible drug. Individual lesions rarely persist for more than 24 hours.

Urticaria may be the only symptom of drug sensitivity, or it may be a concomitant or followed by the manifestations of serum sickness. Urticaria may be accompanied by angioedema of the lips or eyelids. It may, on rare occasions, progress to anaphylactoid reactions or to anaphylaxis.

The following are the most common causes of drug-induced urticaria: antibiotics, notably penicillin (more commonly following parenteral administration than by ingestion), barbiturates, captopril, levamisole, NSAIDs, quinine, rifampin, sulfonamides, thiopental, and vancomycin.

Vasculitis

Drug-induced cutaneous necrotizing vasculitis, a clinicopathologic process characterized by inflammation and necrosis of blood vessels, often presents with a variety of small, palpable purpuric lesions most frequently distributed over the lower extremities: urticaria-like lesions, small ulcerations, and occasional hemorrhagic vesicles and pustules. The basic process involves an immunologically mediated response to antigens that result in vessel wall damage.

Beginning as small macules and papules, they ultimately eventuate into purpuric lesions and, in the more severe cases, into hemorrhagic blisters and frank ulcerations. A polymorphonuclear infiltrate and fibrinoid changes in the small dermal vessels characterize the vasculitic reaction.

Drugs that are commonly associated with vasculitis are: ACE inhibitors, amiodarone, ampicillin, cimetidine, coumadin, furosemide, hydantoins, hydralazine, NSAIDs, pyrazolons, quinidine, sulfonamides, thiazides, and thiouracils.

Xerostomia

Xerostomia is a dryness of the oral cavity that makes speaking, chewing and swallowing difficult.

Resulting from a partial or complete absence of saliva production, xerostomia can be caused by a variety of medications.

DRUG ERUPTIONS ILLUSTRATED

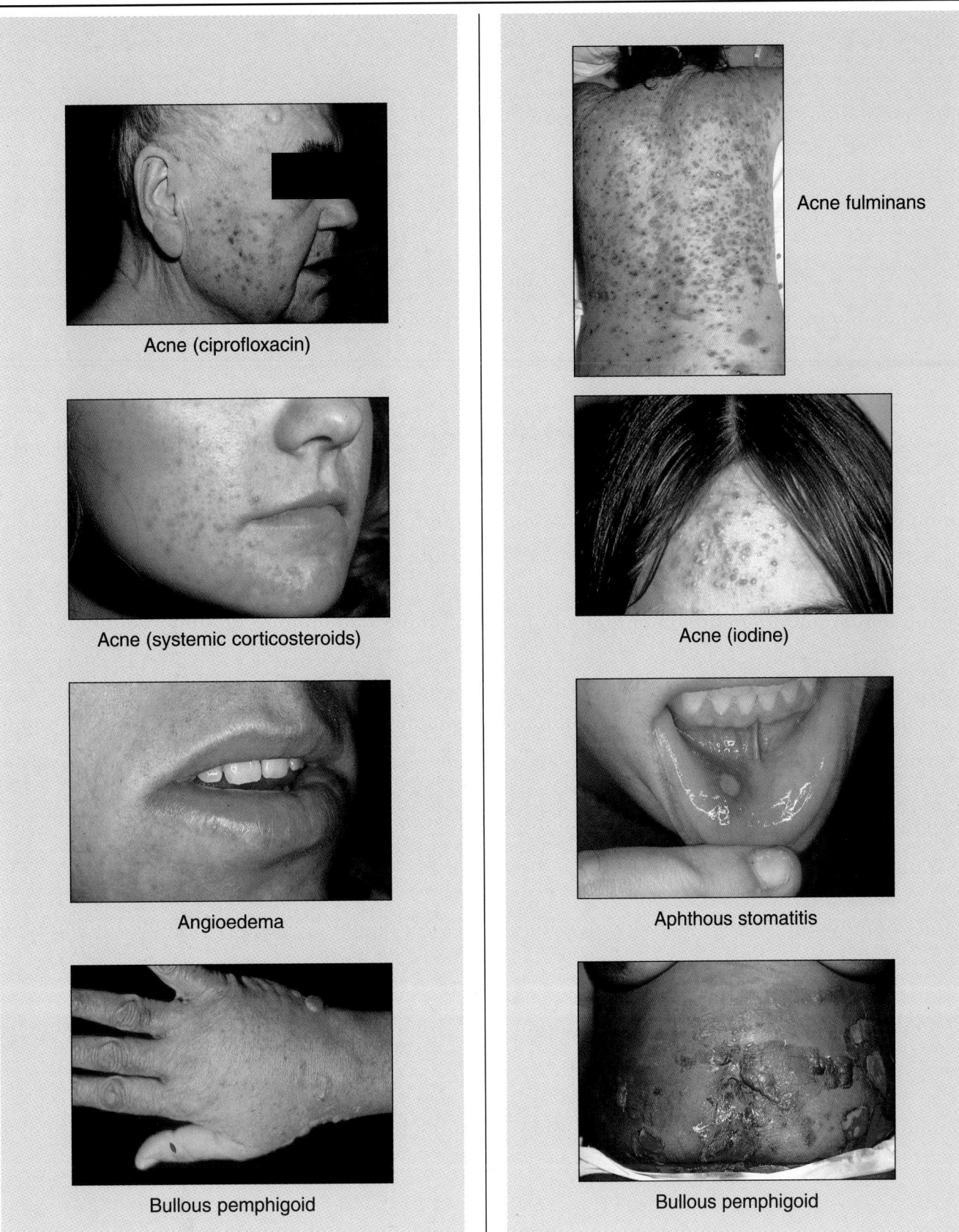

Acne (ciprofloxacin)

Acne (systemic corticosteroids)

Angioedema

Bullous pemphigoid

Acne fulminans

Acne (iodine)

Aphthous stomatitis

Bullous pemphigoid

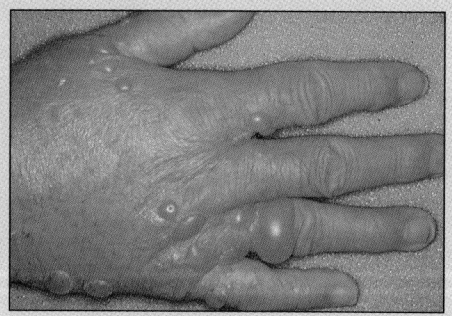

Bullous pemphigoid

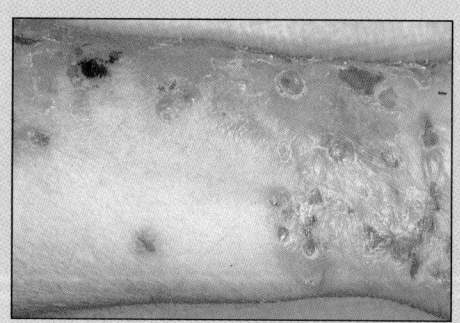

Bullous pemphigoid

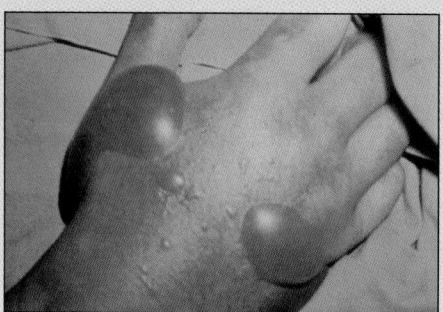

Bullous drug eruption

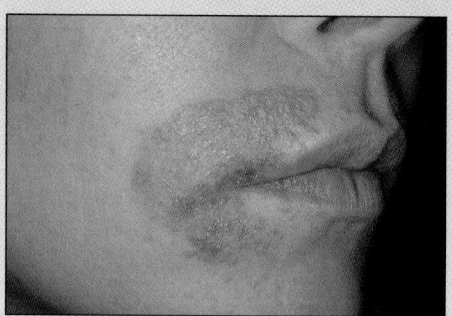

Contact (mycolog cream)

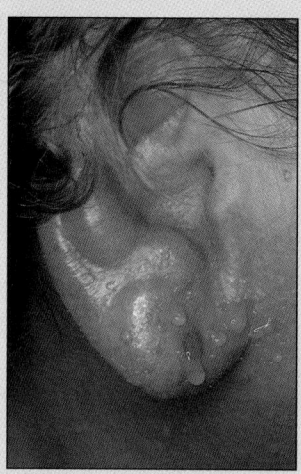

Contact (neomycin)

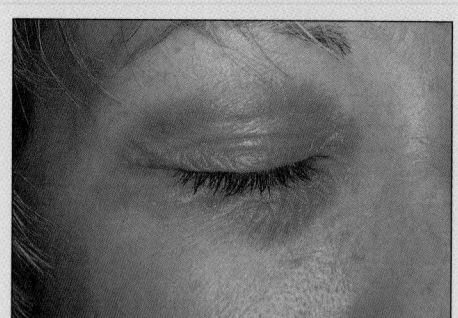

Contact (vitamin E cream)

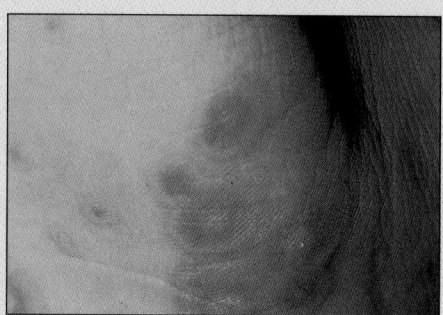

Erythema multiforme

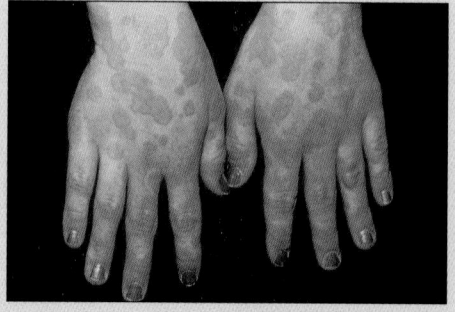

Erythema multiforme

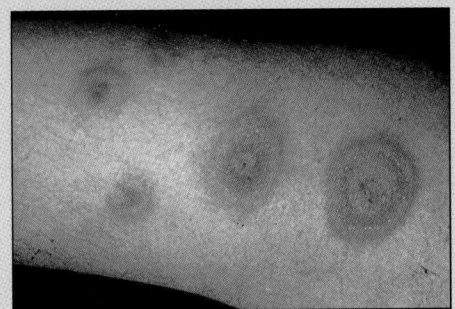

Erythema multiforme

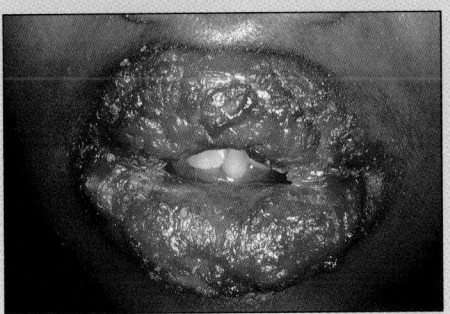

Erythema multiforme

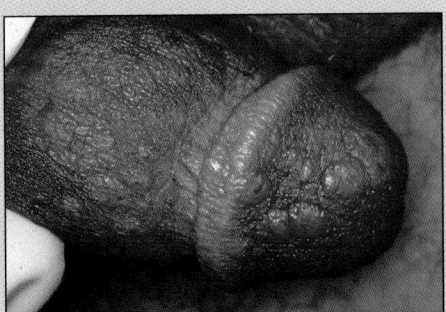

Erythema multiforme

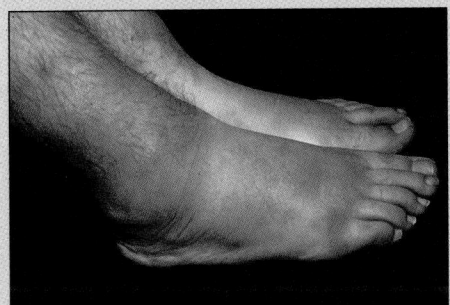

Erythema nodosum

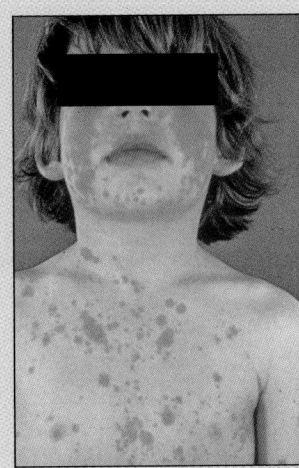

Erythema
multiforme

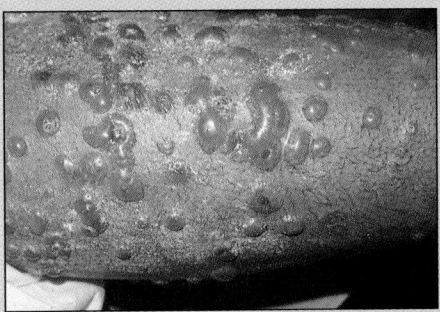

Erythema multiforme

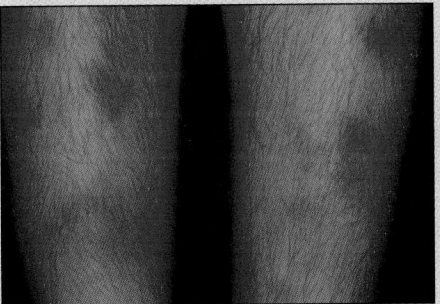

Erythema nodosum

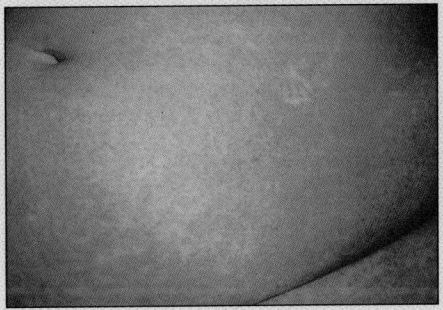

Erythroderma

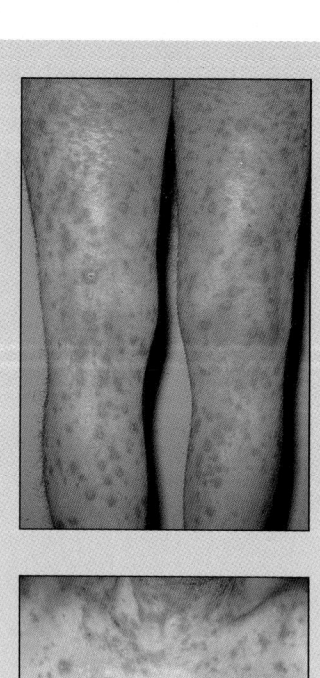

Exanthem
(phenobarbital)

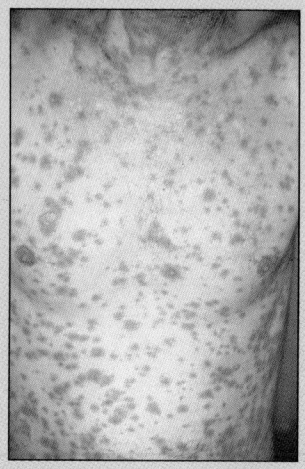

Exanthem
(griseofulvin)

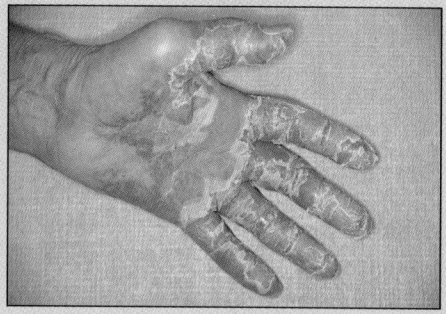

Exfoliative dermatitis

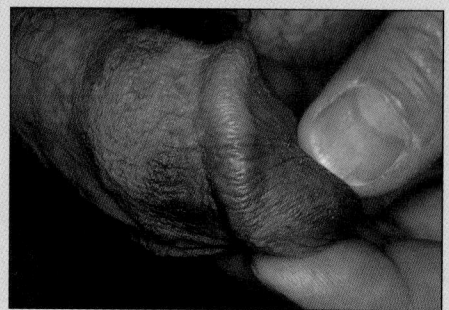

Fixed eruption

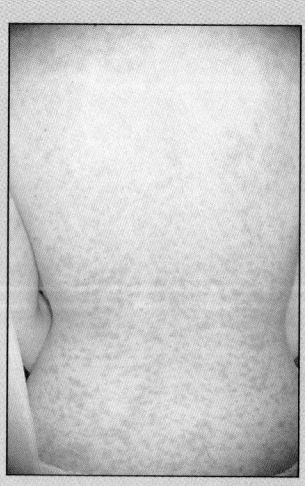

Exanthem
(ampicillin)

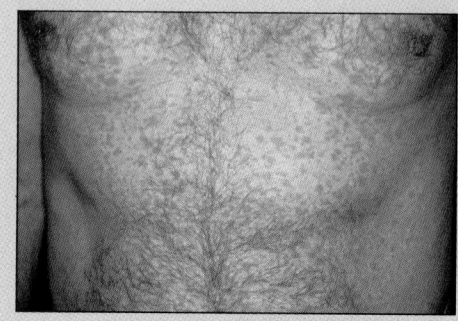

Exanthem (cotrimoxazole)

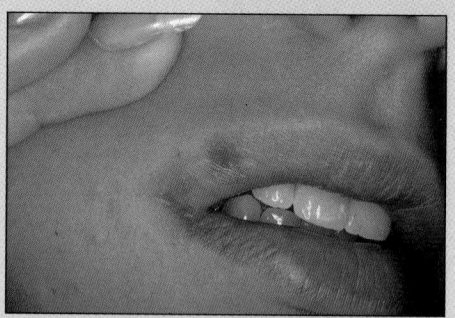

Fixed eruption

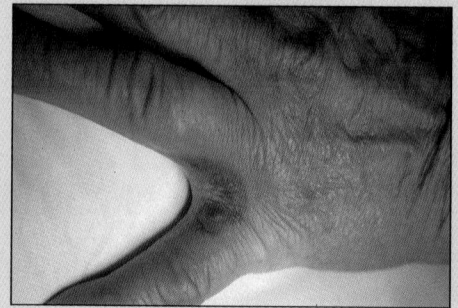

Fixed eruption

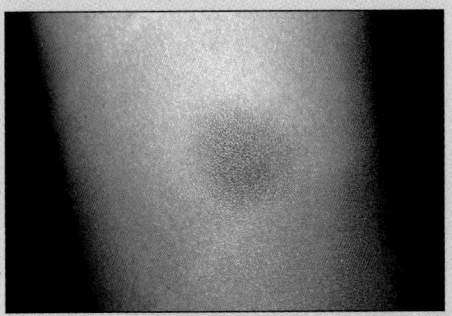

Fixed eruption (cyclophosphamide)

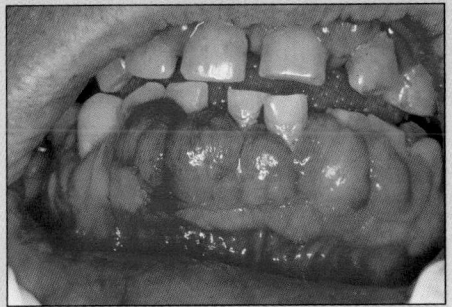

Gingival hyperplasia (verapamil)

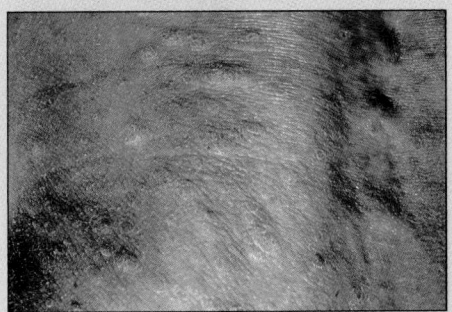

Lichenoid eruption

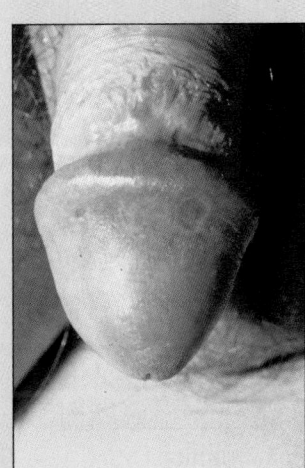

Lichen planus

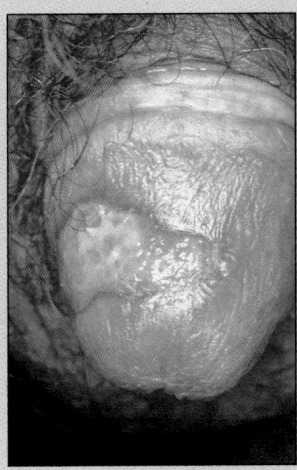

Fixed eruption

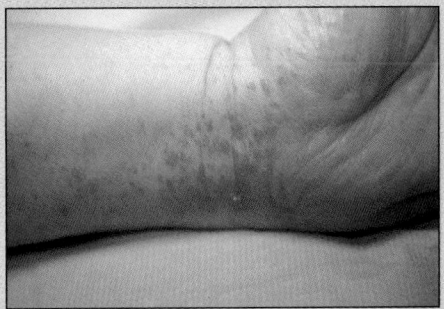

Lichenoid eruption

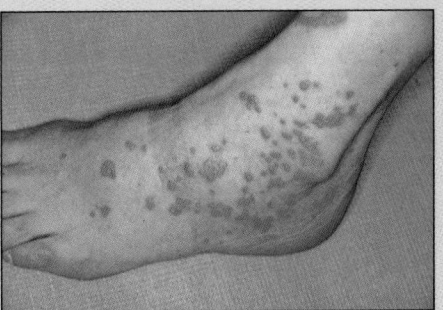

Lichen planus

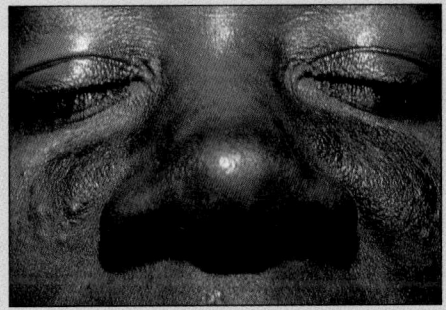

Lupus erythematosus

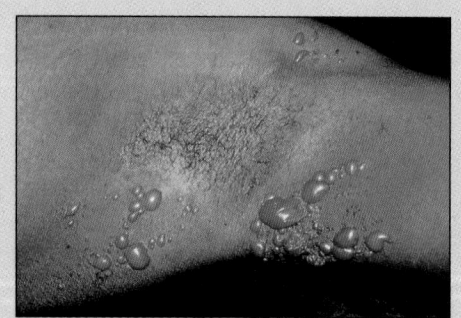

Bullous lupus erythematosus

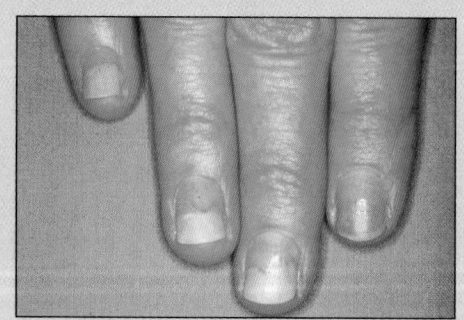

Photo-onycholysis (tetracycline)

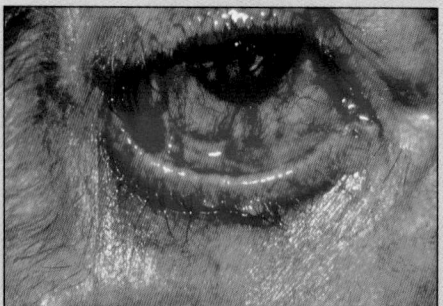

Cicatricial pemphigoid

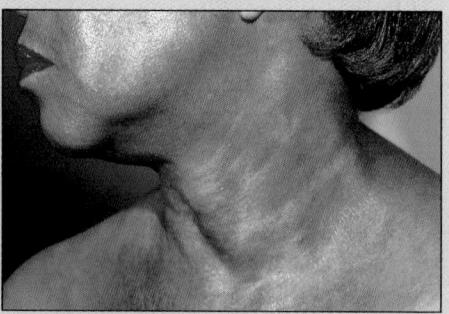

Photocontact dermatitis

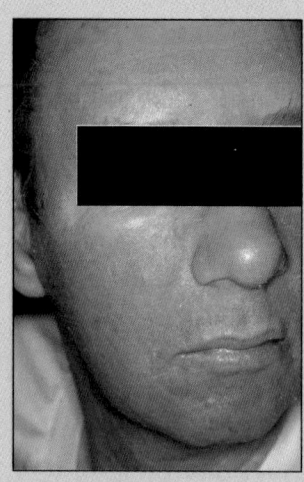

Photosensitivity

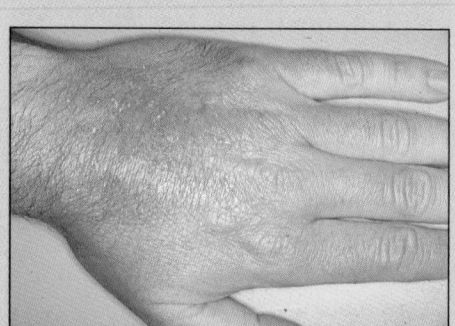

Photosensitivity

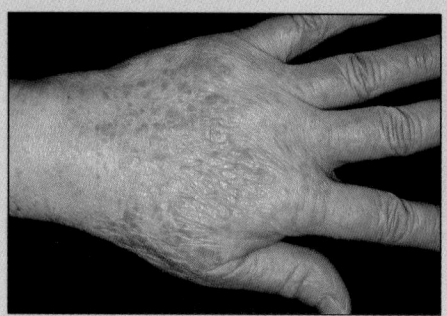

Photosensitivity (lichenoid)

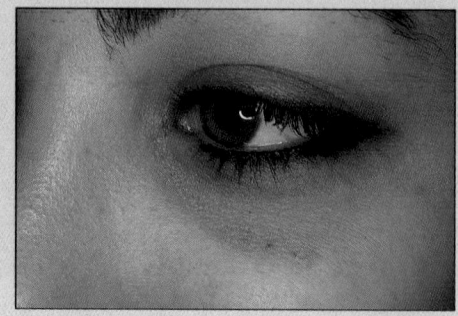

Pigmentation

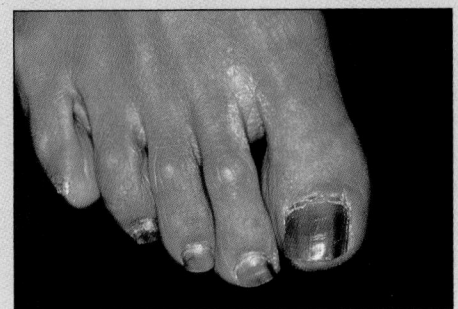

Pigmentation (zidovudine)

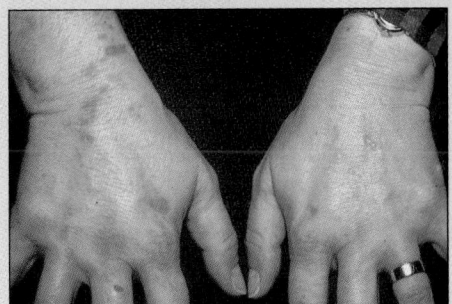

Porphyria (estrogens)

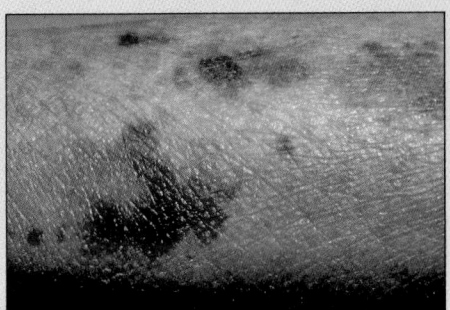

Purpura (aspirin)

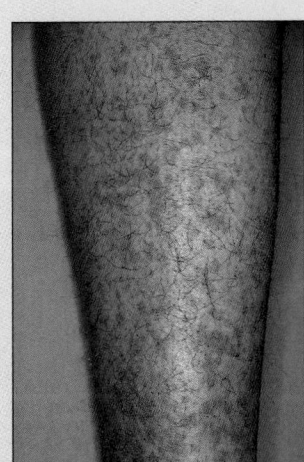

Purpura (naproxen)

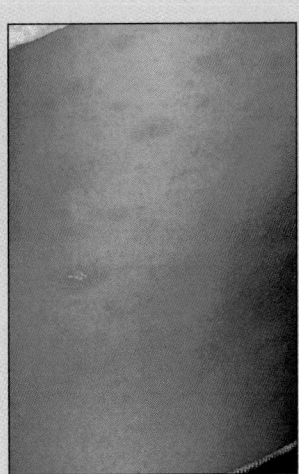

Pityriasis rosea

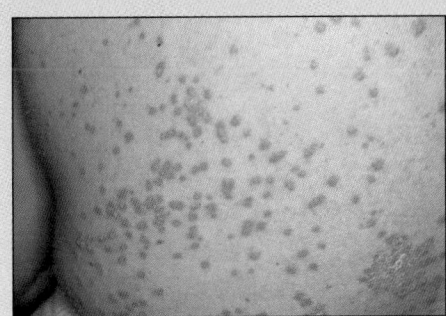

Psoriasis

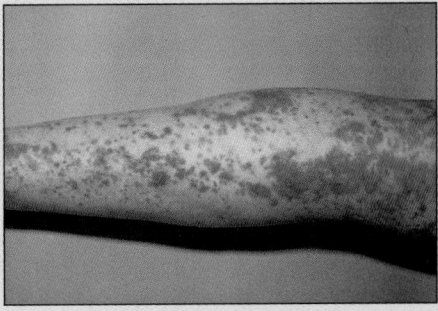

Purpura

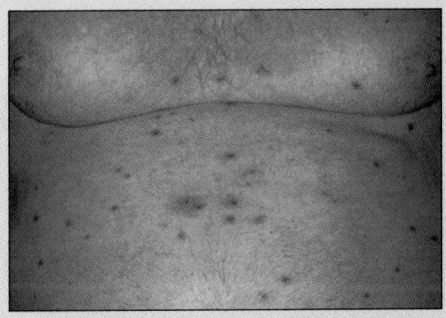

Pustular eruption (lithium)

593

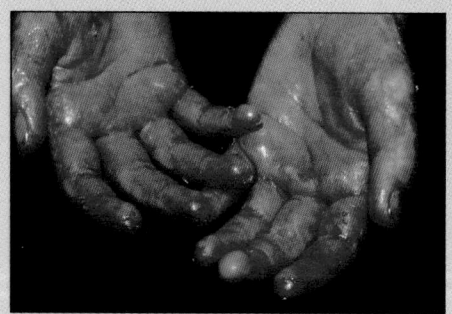

Stevens–Johnson syndrome (dilantin)

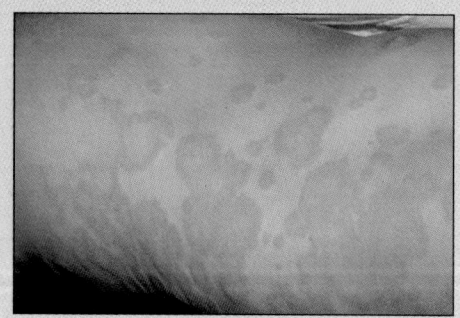

Urticaria

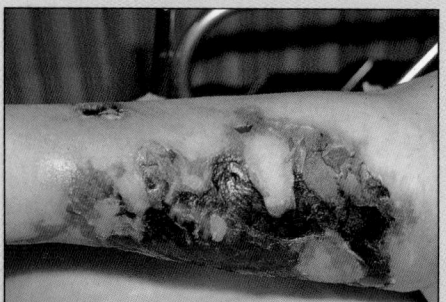

Necrosis

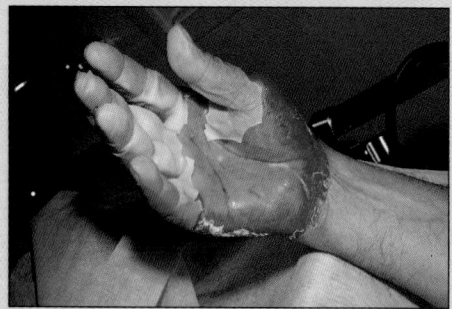

Toxic epidermal necrolysis

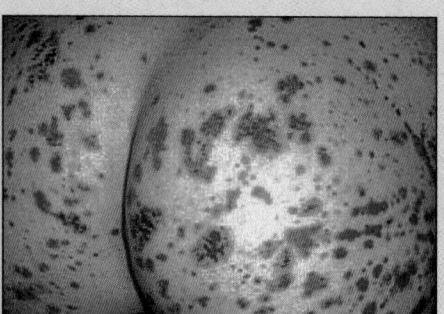

Vasculitis

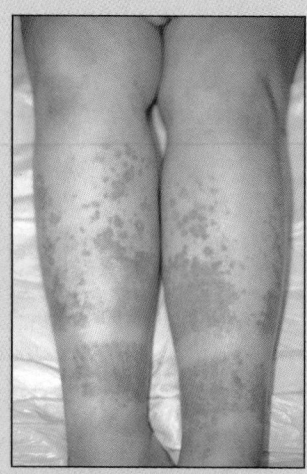

Vasculitis

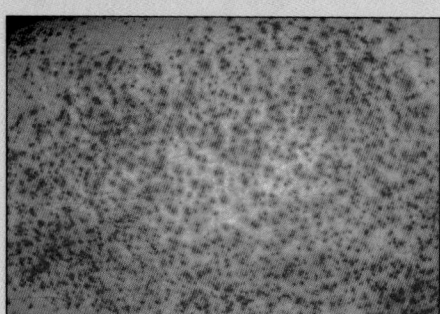

Leukocytoclastic vasculitis

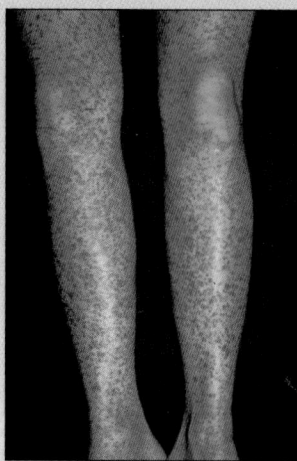

Vasculitis

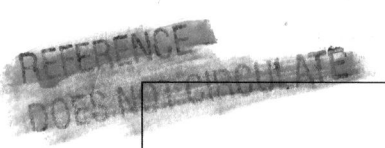

Litt's
DRUG ERUPTION REFERENCE MANUAL
on CD-ROM

This CD-ROM allows users to search the whole database in a highly sophisticated and flexible way. Drugs can be searched by generic name or trade name – or searches can be made on the basis of reaction patterns. The CD-ROM also has the added capacity for multiple drug searching – the user may enter, for example, the names of all the drugs taken by a patient and it will identify if any of these are responsible for an adverse reaction. Results of all searches can be printed out.

Instructions for installing

To install Litt's DRUG ERUPTION REFERENCE MANUAL, double click on the file 'Setup'.

Minimum System Requirements for CD Users

Windows

- Intel-compatible computer
- Microsoft® Windows® 95, Windows 98, Windows 2000, or Windows NT® Pack 3.51 or later
- 8 MB of available RAM (16 MB recommended)
- 10 MB of available hard disk space
- CD-ROM drive

Macintosh

- MacOS-based computer
- MacOS software version 7.1 or later
- 8 MB of available RAM (16 MB recommended)
- 10 MB of available hard disk space
- CD-ROM drive
- 800 x 600 (SVGA) with 16 bit high color display (recommended)

Technical support

Technical support enquiries can be emailed from the Litt Drug Eruption Database website Help section support@drugeruptiondata.com.

Litt's
DRUG ERUPTION REFERENCE DATABASE is
continuously updated and is available to paid subscribers on
the Internet. For further information, please refer to
http://www.drugeruptiondata.com